RECONSTRUCTIVE PREPROSTHETIC ORAL AND MAXILLOFACIAL SURGERY

RAYMOND J. FONSECA, DMD

Chairman, Department of Oral and Maxillofacial Surgery,
School of Dentistry, University of Michigan,
Ann Arbor, Michigan

W. HOWARD DAVIS, DDS, FACD

Clinical Professor, School of Dentistry,
University of Southern California, Los Angeles, California;
Private Practice, Bellflower, California

W. B. SAUNDERS COMPANY

Philadelphia
London
Toronto
Mexico City
Rio de Janeiro
Sydney
Tokyo
Hong Kong

W. B. Saunders Company: West Washington Square
Philadelphia, PA 19105

Library of Congress Cataloging in Publication Data

Fonseca, Raymond J.
  Reconstructive preprosthetic oral and maxillofacial surgery.

  1. Mouth—Surgery. 2. Maxilla—Surgery. 3. Face—
Surgery. 4. Surgery, Plastic. 5. Prosthodontics.
I. Davis, W. Howard. II. Title. III. Title: Prepros-
thetic oral and maxillofacial surgery. {DNLM:
1. Maxillofacial Injuries—surgery. 2. Surgery, Oral,
Preprosthetic. WU 600 F676r]
RK529.F66   1986   617'.522   85-8295
ISBN 0-7216-3797-3

Acquisition Editor: Darlene Pedersen

Manuscript Editor: Donna Walker

Production Manager: Frank Polizzano

Reconstructive Preprosthetic Oral and Maxillofacial Surgery   ISBN 0-7216-3797-3

©1986 by W. B. Saunders Company. Copyright under the Uniform Copyright Convention. Simultaneously published in Canada. All rights reserved. This book is protected by copyright. No part of it may be reproduced, stored in a retrieval system, or transmitted in any form or by any means, electronic, mechanical, photocopying, recording, or otherwise, without written permission from the publisher. Made in the United States of America. Press of W. B. Saunders Company. Library of Congress catalog card number 85-8295.

Last digit is the print number: 9   8   7   6   5   4   3   2

To our wives,
Marilyn and Jane,
who have sacrificed so much for so many years.

CONTRIBUTORS

TOMAS ALBREKTSSON, M.D., Ph.D.

Associate Professor of Anatomy, and Professor in Handicap Research, University of Gothenburg. Assistant Surgeon, Sahlgren University Clinic, Gothenburg, Sweden.

CHARLES A. BABBUSH, D.D.S., M.Sc.D.

Associate Clinical Professor, Oral and Maxillofacial Surgery, Case Western Reserve University, Cleveland, Ohio; Associate Visiting Professor, Department of Oral Surgery, University of Miami School of Medicine, Miami, Florida. Senior Visiting Oral and Maxillofacial Surgeon, Mount Sinai Medical Center, Cleveland, Ohio.

ROBERT A. BAYS, D.D.S.

Associate Clinical Professor of Anatomy and Oral and Maxillofacial Surgery, Medical Surgery of Georgia; Active Staff, University Hospital and Medical College of Georgia Hospital and Clinics, Augusta, Georgia.

JOHN BEUMER, III, D.D.S., M.S.

Director and Professor, Maxillofacial Prosthodontic Hospital Dentistry Group, UCLA School of Dentistry, Los Angeles, California.

CRAIG BLOOM, D.M.D.

Private Practitioner, Berkeley, California. Attending Dentist, Alta Bates and Herrick Hospitals, Berkeley; Children's Hospital Medical Center of Northern California, Oakland; and Pacific Medical Center, San Francisco, California.

HANS BOSKER, D.M.D.

Senior Associate, University of Utrecht, Netherlands. Private Practice, Groningen, Netherlands.

PER-INGVAR BRÅNEMARK, M.D., Ph.D.

Professor of Anatomy, University of Gothenburg. Surgeon, Sahlgren University Clinic, Gothenburg, Sweden.

GEORGE J. COLLINGS, D.M.D.

Oral and Maxillofacial Surgeon, Private Practice, Portland, Oregon.

CHRISTOPHER DAVIS, D.D.S., M.D.

Clinical Instructor, Department of Oral and Maxillofacial Surgery, University of Southern California, Los Angeles; Associate Professor, Department of Oral and Maxillofacial Surgery, Loma Linda University, Loma Linda. Attending Physician, Memorial Hospital Medical Center of Long Beach, Downey Community Hospital, and Doctors Hospital of Lakewood, California.

W. HOWARD DAVIS, D.D.S., FACD

Clinical Professor, School of Dentistry, University of Southern California, Los Angeles. Private Practitioner, Bellflower, California.

RICHARD DELO, D.D.S., M.S.

Associate Clinical Professor, Department of Oral and Maxillofacial Surgery, University of Colorado School of Dentistry, Denver. Attending Dentist, Swedish Medical Center, Englewood; Porter Memorial Hospital, Denver; and Presbyterian Aurora and Humana Hospitals, Aurora. Consultant, Veterans Administration Hospital of Denver; Poudre Valley Hospital, Fort Collins; and Longmont United Hospital, Longmont, Colorado.

STEPHEN E. FEINBERG, D.D.S., M.S., Ph.D.

Assistant Professor of Oral and Maxillofacial Surgery, Ohio State University; Attending Oral and Maxillofacial Surgeon, Ohio State University Hospital, Children's Hospital, and St. Anthony's Hospital, Columbus, Ohio.

RAYMOND J. FONSECA, D.M.D.

Chairman, Department of Oral Surgery, School of Dentistry, University of Michigan, Ann Arbor, Michigan.

DAVID E. FROST, D.D.S., M.S.

Teaching Staff, Department of Oral and Maxillofacial Surgery, and Director, Dentofacial Deformities Board, Wilford Hall Medical Center, Lackland Air Force Base, San Antonio, Texas.

JOHN F. HELFRICK, D.D.S., M.S.

Professor and Chairman, Department of Oral and Maxillofacial Surgery, University of Texas, Dental Branch, Houston. Attending Physician, The Methodist Hospital, M.D. Anderson Hospital, Hermann Hospital, Ben Taub General Hospital, Texas Children's Hospital, and Veterans Administration Hospital, Houston, Texas.

FRANCIS V. HOWELL, D.D.S., M.S.

Chairman, Department of Oral Surgery and Stomatology, Scripps Clinic and Research Foundation, La Jolla; Professor of Oral Pathology, Loma Linda University, Loma Linda; Professor of Pathology, University of California at San Diego School of Medicine, La Jolla. Attending Dentist, Green Hospital of Scripps Clinic and Scripps Memorial Hospital, La Jolla; and University Hospital, San Diego, California.

MICHAEL JARCHO, Ph.D.

President, Calcitek, Inc., San Diego, California.

RONALD KAMINISHI, D.D.S.

Assistant Professor, Department of Oral and Maxillofacial Surgery, University of Southern California, Los Angeles; Assistant Professor, Department of Oral and Maxillofacial Surgery, Loma Linda University, Loma Linda. Attending Dentist, Memorial Hospital Medical Center of Long Beach, Downey Community Hospital, and Doctors Hospital of Lakewood, California.

JOHN N. KENT, D.D.S., FACD, FICD

Boyd Professor and Head, Department of Oral and Maxillofacial Surgery, Louisiana State University Medical Center School of Dentistry, New Orleans. Chief, Oral and Maxillofacial Surgery, Charity Hospital of New Orleans; Active Staff, Hotel Dieu Hospital, New Orleans; Academic Staff, Ochsner Hospital, New Orleans; Consultant, Veterans Administration Hospital of New Orleans, Louisiana.

HOWARD LANDESMAN, D.D.S. M. Ed.

Professor, Department of Restorative Dentistry, and Associate Dean for Academic and Faculty Affairs, School of Dentistry, University of Southern California, Los Angeles. Consultant in Fixed and Removable Prosthodontics, Los Angeles County USC Medical Center and Veterans Administration Hospitals of Wadsworth, Sepulveda, and Long Beach, California.

WILLIAM LaVELLE, D.D.S., M.S.

Maxillofacial Prosthodontist and Professor, Department of Otolaryngology, University of Iowa Hospitals and Clinics, Iowa City, Iowa.

ROBERT E. MARX, D.D.S.

Associate Professor of Surgery and Director of Graduate Training and Research, Division of Oral and Maxillofacial Surgery, University of Miami School of Medicine. Director of Head and Neck Cancer Reconstruction Center, Jackson Memorial Medical Center, Miami; Consultant, Veterans Administration Medical Center, Miami, and USAF Hospital, Homestead Air Force Base, Homestead, Florida.

GLENN MINSLEY, D.M.D.

Assistant Professor, Department of Removable Prosthodontics; Director, Maxillofacial Prosthetics Division, University of North Carolina School of Dentistry, Chapel Hill. Assistant Attending Dentist, North Carolina Memorial Hospital, Chapel Hill, North Carolina.

GERALD A. NIZNICK, D.M.D., M.S.D.

President of Core-Vent Corporation, Los Angeles. Private Practice, Encino, California.

ROBERT OLSON, D.M.D.

Associate Professor and Director, Undergraduate Oral and Maxillofacial Surgery Program, University of Iowa College of Dentistry. Staff Dentist, University of Iowa Hospitals and Clinics; Consultant, Veterans Administration Hospital, Iowa City, Iowa.

DONALD B. OSBON, D.D.S.

Professor and Head, Department of Oral and Maxillofacial Surgery, College of Dentistry, University of Iowa. Head, Department of Hospital Dentistry, University of Iowa Hospitals and Clinics; Attending Oral and Maxillofacial Surgeon, Mercy Hospital; Consultant, Veterans Administration Hospital, Iowa City, Iowa.

TIMOTHY R. SAUNDERS, D.D.S.

Assistant Chairman, Department of Prosthodontics, Wilford Hall Medical Center, Lackland Air Force Base, San Antonio, Texas.

RICHARD F. SCOTT, D.D.S., M.S.

Assistant Professor, Department of Oral and Maxillofacial Surgery, University of Michigan School of Dentistry; Assistant Professor, Department of Surgery, University of Michigan School of Medicine, Ann Arbor. Attending Oral and Maxillofacial Surgeon, University Hospitals, University of Michigan, Ann Arbor, and Westland Medical Center, Westland, Michigan.

PAUL V. W. STOELINGA, D.D.S., M.D., Ph.D.

Affiliate Professor, Department of Oral and Maxillofacial Surgery, University of Washington, Seattle. Consultant, Department of Oral and Maxillofacial Surgery, Municipal Hospital, Arnhem, The Netherlands.

BILL C. TERRY, D.D.S.

Professor and Director of Graduate Training, Department of Oral and Maxillofacial Surgery, University of North Carolina, Chapel Hill. Attending Staff, North Carolina Memorial Hospital, Chapel Hill; Dorothea Dix Hospital, Raleigh; and Veterans Administration Hospital, Fayetteville, North Carolina.

JAMES B. TROXELL, D.D.S., M.S.

Private Practice, Fort Collins, Colorado.

TIMOTHY A. TURVEY, D.D.S.

Associate Professor, Department of Oral and Maxillofacial Surgery, University of North Carolina; Co-director, University of North Carolina Dentofacial Deformity Program. Attending Dentist, University of North Carolina Memorial Hospital, Chapel Hill, North Carolina.

LUCAS VANDIJK, D.M.D.

Private Practice, Groningen, Netherlands.

JAY R. WEINER, D.D.S.

Lecturer, UCLA School of Dentistry, Los Angeles. Attending Dentist, Northridge Medical Center, Northridge, and Kaiser Foundation Hospital, Panorama City, California.

DEBORAH ZEITLER, D.D.S., M.S.

Assistant Professor, Hospital Dentistry, Division of Oral and Maxillofacial Surgery, University of Iowa, Iowa City. Staff, University of Iowa Hospitals and Clinics and Veterans Administration Hospital, Iowa City, Iowa.

FOREWORD

It is a great privilege for me to be able to write the foreword to an excellent textbook, especially one dealing with a subject that is part of my own field of study. It was, therefore, with great pleasure that I responded positively to the request of the two editors, Drs. Fonseca and Davis, to write the foreword to this book.

Today the field of preprosthetic surgery, together with its wide-ranging aspects, has gained such importance that it has become indispensible. Drs. Fonseca and Davis have done a great service in compiling the extensive information on the subject into a single book. The complexity of the subject matter, however, has made it necessary to call upon the contributions of specialists, thus turning the textbook into a multiauthor text. The depth of knowledge possessed by each contributing author and their comprehensive coverage of pathophysiology and the biological and biochemical aspects of the materials used have greatly enhanced the quality of the book. The editors have minimized repetition and diversity of opinion.

The many aspects of preprosthetic surgery are dealt with in twelve chapters, including both the theoretical bases and the practical applications of the different methods discussed.

Preprosthetic surgery, in the traditional sense, is described exhaustively; the field of implantology is also included, dealing especially with currently promising modalities. The book deals extensively with the technical particulars of instrumentation and materials that are needed to perform most of the procedures. The possibilities for using hydroxylapatite for augmentation purposes is presented for the first time ever in one concise chapter.

The complicated problems regarding reconstruction of defects of the maxilla and mandible are dealt with, including cases of maxillary defects resulting from cancer surgery, accidental trauma, cleft palate, and other congenital and developmental dentofacial and dentoalveolar deformities.

The abundant illustrations and clearly arranged tabular lists of indications and contraindications and treatment alternatives make the book highly readable and useful. Furthermore, the work distinguishes itself by the list of references at the end of each chapter, including a considerable number from the European literature.

This textbook is the most comprehensive and instructive work at present dealing with the important field of preprosthetic surgery. To all concerned, be they surgeons or prosthodontists, this work will prove itself a great source of information on the literature of reconstructive surgery and a precise guide to operative techniques, indications, and contraindications.

I wish the book great success and I am sure my wish shall be fulfilled.

PROF. H. L. OBWEGESER
University of Zurich

PREFACE

During the last decade, the evolution of knowledge in the area of reconstructive preprosthetic oral and maxillofacial surgery has been significant. A large amount of information based on the experiences of a number of researchers and clinicians has been accumulated. New concepts of inflammation, wound healing, and immunobiology and new techniques in soft and osseous tissue grafting, cleft rehabilitation, orthognathic and tumor surgery, and dental implantology have changed the scope of oral surgery practice and have broadened the horizon of prosthodontic rehabilitation of edentulous patients.

Rehabilitation of the preprosthetic patient involves a complex interaction between the patient and a variety of health professionals, the objective being to restore bodily function to the optimum potential and to prevent additional dysfunction and inconvenience. It has been challenging, exciting, and engrossing for those of us deeply involved in this area of patient care.

Our present reconstructive preprosthetic surgical techniques are the result of previous research. Many questions concerning the future of research and treatment of preprosthetic patients remain unanswered. We hope that this book not only will provide answers to clinical questions but, equally important, will stimulate further research and progress in treatment methods.

Considering the many and recent advances in dental science and practice, we believe that a new book on reconstructive preprosthetic surgery is needed. Our objective has been to write a comprehensive clinical reference on the interdisciplinary art and science of reconstructive preprosthetic surgery. This book was written to provide a concise description of principles and procedures in each important aspect of oral and maxillofacial reconstructive preprosthetic surgery.

Rehabilitation of patients requiring oral and/or maxillofacial prostheses secondary to congenital or acquired problems is a difficult task and requires close interaction among a number of health professionals. Since the oral and maxillofacial surgeon and prosthodontist are the primary professionals involved in the multifaceted care of these patients, much of the text is directed toward these two specialty areas. However, because of the multidisciplinary nature of the topic, we believe the material will also have relevance for other surgical specialists, general practitioners of dentistry, and other health science professionals.

No attempt is made to describe the minor preprosthetic procedures such as traumatic removal of teeth and alveoloplasty techniques. A discussion of these procedures is not within the scope of this book and can be found in other texts.

The purpose of this book is to present a comprehensive review of available information on reconstructive preprosthetic surgery. We have been fortunate to have the assistance of prosthodontists and surgeons experienced in special areas of interest, emphasizing a practical and effective approach to diagnosis and therapy.

The text can be divided into four sections. The first, covering basic principles of reconstructive preprosthetic surgery, is a discussion of the applied gross anatomical and physiological principles as they relate to the edentulous patient. The inflammatory response, repair, and immunobiological response of the related tissues are discussed. Finally, prosthetic and surgical principles as they apply to reconstructive preprosthetic surgery are described.

The second section deals with management of the patients with edentulous bone loss. There is a description of outpatient surgical procedures designed to prepare the ridges for prosthetic function. Comprehensive presentations of the various soft and hard tissue surgical procedures currently available are included. Maxillary and mandibular vestibuloplasty and ridge augmentation procedures are described, with data on stability, complications, and postoperative follow-up. The discussion of dental implants is not all-inclusive, but rather covers those modalities that are rather well-accepted and those which have been recently introduced that appear to hold promise.

Management of the post-traumatic and post–tumor resection patient is the subject of the third section. These two problems are grouped together because the surgical considerations for reconstructing the residual ridges are very similar. Descriptions of the management of continuity defects and of immediate fracture management in the edentulous atrophic mandible are included. Tumor resection rehabilitation is described, including both surgical reconstruction and prosthetic rehabilitation of the tumor patient.

The fourth section deals with the management of patients with congenital or developmental deformities. Cleft rehabilitation and principles of treatment are discussed. The surgical techniques of alveolar cleft grafting and orthognathic procedures in the cleft patient are also presented. Finally, maxillomandibular malrelationships and the diagnosis, treatment planning, and surgical procedures available for the patient requiring preprosthetic orthognathic surgery are considered. Throughout the text, every attempt is made to document the stability of the procedures presented with significant clinical follow-up.

RAYMOND J. FONSECA
W. HOWARD DAVIS

ACKNOWLEDGMENTS

We recognize that there are many in the field of reconstructive preprosthetic surgery and prosthodontics who deserve to be contributors to *Reconstructive Preprosthetic Oral and Maxillofacial Surgery* but for various reasons could not be included. To those who have contributed, may we express our thanks for their outstanding efforts.

RAYMOND J. FONSECA
W. HOWARD DAVIS

I would especially like to extend my gratitude to all of my past and present teaching associates and residents, who have provided the intellectual stimulation, inspiration, and friendship without which this book would not have been written.

I would also like to thank Arlene Dietz and Bonnie Andrews for their assistance in the preparation of this manuscript.

Lastly, a man becomes what he is through the love and strength provided to him by his parents. For this, I acknowledge my father and mother for their support, sacrifice, and love.

RAYMOND J. FONSECA

I wish to thank my partners, Drs. Ronald Maninishi, David Hochwald, Richard Berger, and Christopher Davis, for their constructive criticism and the time they devoted to this effort; a special thanks also to Janice Frembling, Christina Fontecchio, Kathay Woolsey, Robin Dunlap, and the artist, Dr. Randi Landis. I also gratefully acknowledge the sacrifice of my parents and family and the inspiration of my teachers, particularly Professor Hugo Obwegeser and Dr. Adrian Hubbel.

W. HOWARD DAVIS

CONTENTS

1
THE PATHOPHYSIOLOGY AND ANATOMY OF EDENTULOUS BONE LOSS   1
Robert A. Bays, D.D.S.

Physiology of Edentulous Bone Loss	1
Factors Influencing Edentulous Bone Loss	3
Anatomic Considerations	9
Patient Evaluation	11
Bibliography	16

2
BIOLOGIC ASPECTS OF TRANSPLANTATION OF GRAFTS   19
*Stephen E. Feinberg, D.D.S., M.S., Ph.D.,
and Raymond J. Fonseca, D.M.D.*

General Principles of Transplantation	19
Types of Grafts	20
Histocompatibility Antigens	20
Major Histocompatibility Complex	20
Donor-Recipient Matching	22
Immunobiology of Graft Rejection	23
Diagnosis and Prevention of Graft Rejection	24
Problems Unique to the Oral Cavity	25
Bone Grafts	25
Skin Grafts	33
Bibliography	36

3

PROSTHODONTIC AND SURGICAL ASPECTS OF TREATMENT PLANNING FOR RECONSTRUCTIVE SURGERY 41

John Beumer, III, D.D.S., M.S., Howard Landesman, D.D.S., M.Ed., Bill C. Terry, D.D.S., W. Howard Davis, D.D.S., and Christopher L. Davis, D.D.S., M.D.

Prosthodontic Aspects of Reconstructive Preprosthetic Surgery 41
Surgical Aspects of Reconstructive Preprosthetic Surgery 47
Bibliography 58

4

MINOR PREPROSTHETIC PROCEDURES 61

Richard F. Scott, D.D.S., M.S., and Robert A.J. Olson, D.M.D.

Alveoloplasty Along with Tooth Removal 61
Secondary Alveolar Recontouring 62
Redundant Crestal Tissue Removal 62
Maxillary Tuberosity Reduction 62
Hamular Notch Deepening (Tuberoplasty) 64
Abnormal Labial or Buccal Frenum Correction 65
Abnormal Lingual Frenum (Tongue Tie, Ankyloglossia) Correction 66
Mylohyoid Ridge Reduction 66
Mandibular (Lingual) Torus Removal 66
Palatal Torus Removal 67
Palatal Papillary Hyperplasia Removal 68
Bibliography 68

5

SURGICAL MANAGEMENT OF SOFT TISSUE PROBLEMS 69

W. Howard Davis, D.D.S., and Christopher L. Davis, D.D.S., M.D., with contributions by Richard Delo, D.D.S., Jay R. Weiner, D.D.S., Ronald Kaminishi, D.D.S., Craig Bloom, D.M.D., Paul V. W. Stoelinga, D.D.S., M.D., Ph.D., Raymond J. Fonseca, D.M.D., Bill C. Terry, D.D.S., and Glenn Minsley, D.M.D.

Mandibular Procedures 69
Maxillary Procedures 98
Bibliography 115

6

OSSEOUS RECONSTRUCTION OF EDENTULOUS BONE LOSS 117

Raymond J. Fonseca, D.M.D., David Frost, D.D.S., Deborah Zeitler, D.D.S., M.S., and Paul J. W. Stoelinga, D.D.S., M.D., Ph.D.

Maxillary Procedures 117
Mandibular Procedures 142
Bibliography 164

7
IMPLANTS USED IN PREPROSTHETIC RECONSTRUCTIVE SURGERY 167

John Helfrick, D.D.S., M.S., P.-I. Brånemark, M.D., Ph.D., T. Albrektsson, M.D., Ph.D., Hans Bosker, D.M.D., and Lucas VanDijk, D.M.D., Charles A. Babbush, M.Sc.D., D.D.S., George J. Collings, D.M.D., Gerald A. Niznick, D.M.D., M.S.D., and Francis V. Howell, D.D.S.

Implants Used in Reconstructive Surgery 167
Transosteal Implants 175
Endosteal Dental Implants in the Treatment of the Edentulous Jaw 211
Bibliography 299

8
RECONSTRUCTION OF THE ALVEOLAR RIDGE WITH HYDROXYLAPATITE 305

John N. Kent, D.D.S., and Michael Jarcho, Ph.D.

The Edentulous Alveolar Ridge 305
History of Atrophic Ridge Management 305
Preparation and Properties of Calcium Phosphate Biomaterials 307
Basic Biologic Profile of Calcium Phosphate Implant Materials 308
Alveolar Ridge Reconstruction 312
Alveolar Ridge Preservation 340
Summary 344
Bibliography 345

9
RECONSTRUCTION AND REHABILITATION OF CANCER PATIENTS 347

Robert E. Marx, D.D.S., and Timothy R. Saunders, D.D.S.

Patient Assessment 347
Reconstruction of Mandibular Continuity Defects 355
Reconstruction of the Maxilla 412
Rehabilitation Programs 423
Rehabilitation (Versus) Reconstruction 424
Perspective 426
Bibliography 426

10
RECONSTRUCTIVE SURGERY FOR MAXILLOFACIAL INJURIES 429

Donald Osbon, D.D.S.

Early Care 430
Intermediate Care 433

Reconstructive Care 433
Summary 445
Bibliography 446

11
RECONSTRUCTIVE SURGERY FOR THE PATIENT WITH FACIAL CLEFTS 447
*Deborah Zeitler, D.D.S., M.S., Raymond J. Fonseca, D.M.D.,
James B. Troxell, D.D.S., M.S., and William LaVelle, D.D.S., M.S.*

Literature Review 447
Diagnosis and Treatment Planning 448
Presurgical Work-up 452
Surgical Considerations 452
Bibliography 474

12
RECONSTRUCTIVE ORAL AND MAXILLOFACIAL SURGERY FOR THE TOTALLY AND PARTIALLY EDENTULOUS PATIENT WITH DENTOFACIAL AND DENTOALVEOLAR DEFORMITIES 475
*David E. Frost, D.D.S., M.S., Raymond J. Fonseca, D.M.D.,
and Timothy Turvey, D.D.S.*

Totally Edentulous Patient 476
Partially Dentate Patients 482
Summary 483
Case Presentations 483
Bibliography 507

INDEX 509

1

THE PATHOPHYSIOLOGY AND ANATOMY OF EDENTULOUS BONE LOSS

Robert A. Bays, D.D.S.

The restoration of oral functions following loss of the natural dentition is a complex, multidisciplinary problem. Obstacles to satisfactory restoration include both soft and hard tissue aberrations; however, edentulous bone loss (EBL) is by far the greatest etiologic factor in the progressive difficulties encountered in such restoration.[1]

Since bone loss, especially alveolar, always occurs following the removal of teeth, one might assume that EBL is a normal phenomenon. Although some EBL is inevitable, we need to examine the amount that is normal, the factors that influence that amount, and how these factors also affect subsequent reconstructive efforts.

Practically every investigation of EBL has shown wide variation among those individuals studied.[1-3] Interestingly, the *mean* amounts and rates of alveolar ridge loss in groups of people are amazingly consistent throughout the western world. This observation suggests that EBL in many patients is minimal and very slow. One or more factors stimulate resorption at a faster rate in some individuals than in others. In some cases, the initial rapid resorption rate that occurs during the first two years simply never slows down.

Edentulous bone loss is more common in white women than in any other group. Hormonal implications of this finding will be discussed later in the chapter. An important factor is that white women have a normal bone density (in grams of mineral per millimeter of bone) that is less than that of any other racial or sex group. In general, men have higher bone density than women, and blacks and Asians have higher bone density than whites; therefore, white women begin with a lower bone density than any other group.[4]

It is important to note that most edentulous white women do not become atrophic but that some members of other groups do. This indicates that there are other factors that play significant roles in development of excessive EBL; these factors will be discussed later in the chapter.

PHYSIOLOGY OF EDENTULOUS BONE LOSS

Modeling is the appropriate term to characterize the macroscopic changes in bone morphology. *Ridge resorption* and *atrophy* are misnomers because resorption is a part of a process that leads to EBL, whereas atrophy implies a passive process. This loss of bone is actually a detrimental aspect of the physiologic remodeling process.[5] Therefore the term *remodeling* should be used to describe the physiologic process of bone loss. Remodeling of bone involves three steps: (1) activation, (2) resorption, and (3) formation. These three phases are constantly occurring throughout the skeleton at varying rates depending upon the specific location, age, metabolic activity, and local stress on the area. However, the process is essentially the same everywhere with a few minor but important variations.

Activation

Activation is the first phase of the remodeling process and begins as a result of specific local (i.e., stress) and systemic (i.e., hormonal) stimuli. It occurs at the microscopic level on the surface of lamellar bone, whether it be trabecular or cortical. Activation stimulates the rest of the process.

Resorption

The resorption phase begins as osteoclasts adhere to the bone surface; these osteoclasts are probably derived from special circulating monocytes. Resorption may occur on the inside surface of a Haversian system in compact bone or on the outside surface of trabecular bone. Often, this resorption occurs parallel to the stress placed upon the bone, and it influences the formation pattern that follows. This process is followed by the deposition of organic matrix (see *Formation*), which is responsible for the stress resistance of bone after calcification has occurred. Resorption also occurs in the absence of stress, but it does so in a less organized manner. For example, resorption continues until a certain amount of bone has been removed and then it ceases. The specific factors that determine the amount of resorption have not been identified, but there is usually an 8- to 10-day delay period, after which formation begins.

Formation

The formation phase is signaled by the differentiation of local mesenchymal cells into osteoblasts, which concentrate on the same surface and begin to lay down organic matrix. After about eight days, the osteoid begins mineralization. The site at which resorption ceases and formation begins is termed a *cement line*. Formation continues until the approximate amount of bone resorbed has been restored.

The time involved is about three months in compact bone and two months in trabecular bone, indicating that trabecular bone turns over at a higher rate than cortical bone. These units may survive as long as 20 years before replacement is needed, or as short as 3 years, depending upon the variables of age, location, stress, and metabolic activity. Perhaps the most important characteristic of the process is that after cessation of growth, remodeling continues throughout life under a variety of influences. The influences believed to affect the alveolar ridge are discussed in detail below.

There are four skeletal envelopes: periosteum, Haversian system, endosteum, and trabecular system (Table 1–1). Each of these skeletal envelopes has a characteristic bone balance, which is generally not zero (Fig. 1–1). Remodeling under periosteum tends to result in a slight net gain in bone; i.e., the formation somewhat exceeds resorption. The Haversian system has a net bone balance of zero, and the endosteal and trabecular envelopes usually have a net loss of bone due to remodeling. After 25 years of age, it is normal for the total bone mass of the alveolar process to decrease because alveolar bone is mostly trabecular.

Another important factor in understanding remodeling and its influence on alveolar bone loss is the rate at which these cycles of activation, resorption, and formation occur (Fig. 1–2A). If the rate of activation is slowed, the net gain in bone under the periosteum and net loss in the trabecular enve-

TABLE 1–1. THE FOUR SKELETAL ENVELOPES

I. Periosteum
II. Haversian System
III. Endosteum
IV. Trabecular System

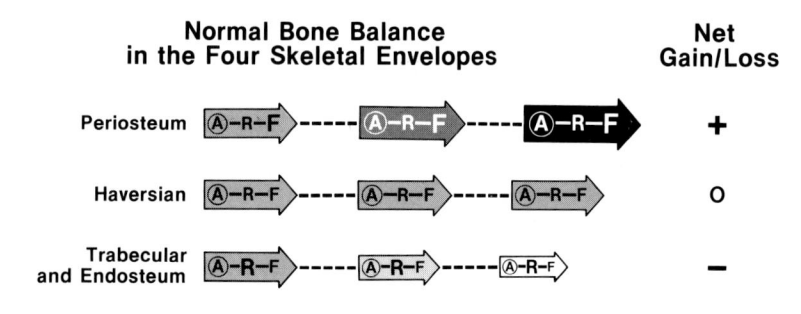

Figure 1–1. The normal progress of bone turnover in the skeletal envelopes. Note that the net change in the periosteal envelope is a gain, and the net change in the endosteal and trabecular envelopes is a loss.

A = Activation   R = Resorption   F = Formation

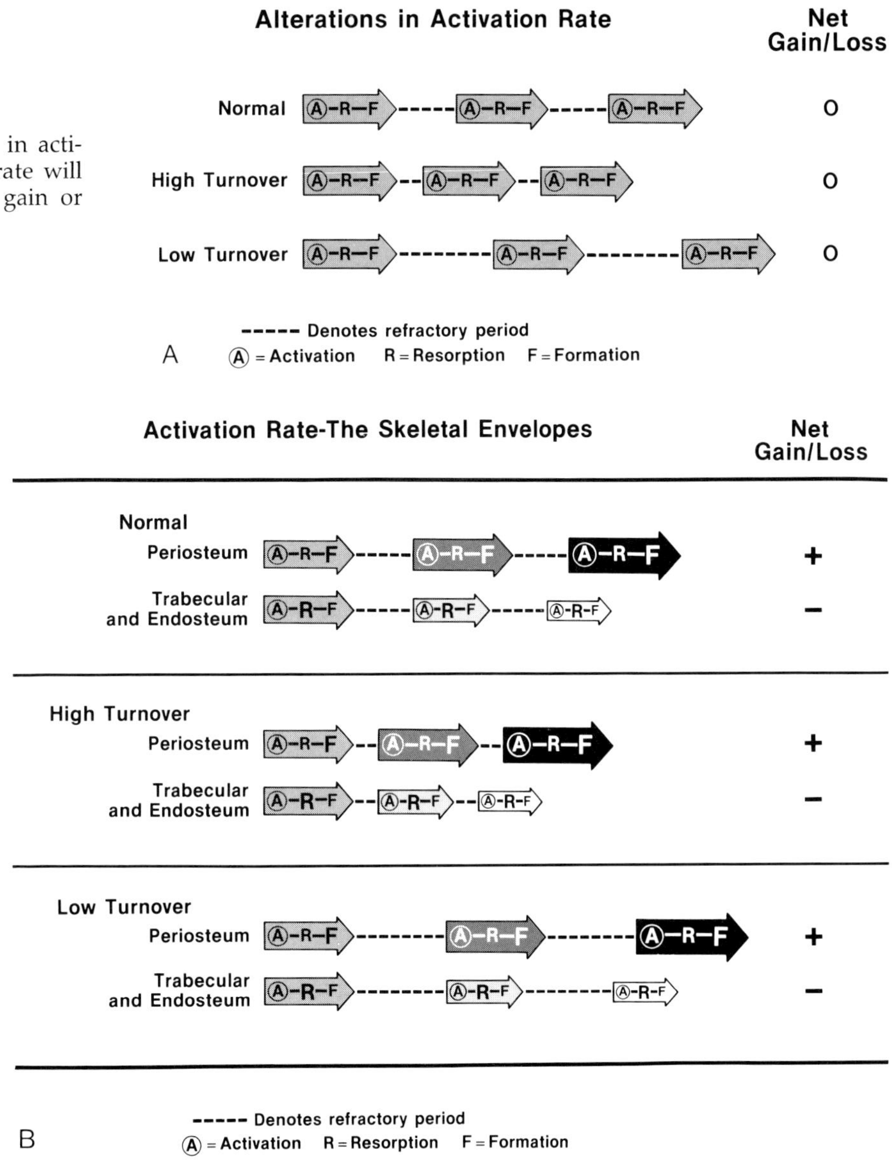

THE PATHOPHYSIOLOGY AND ANATOMY OF EDENTULOUS BONE LOSS / 3

Figure 1–2. The influence of alterations in activation *rate* is illustrated. An increase in rate will hasten whichever process is underway, gain or loss.

lope decrease (Fig. 1–2B). Conversely, if the activation rate is increased, the opposite is true.[5]

Even in osteoporosis it is rare for bones to actually change shape and decrease in volume; however, density may decrease, leaving the bone less resistant to fracture. Interestingly, the maxilla and mandible are unusual in this regard because the size and shape *do* change after the teeth are lost. Because of the widespread use of the term *alveolar ridge atrophy* or *resorption*, it should be understood that the process may include loss not only of the alveolar ridge but sometimes of the body of the maxilla or mandible as well.

Remodeling is a natural phenomenon that is useful to the body in the replenishment of the skeletal system and in the repair of microtrauma. Bone activation, resorption, and formation occur constantly and are influenced by many factors. It is normal for trabecular bone to show a net loss of bone throughout life, but the rate of loss is a function of two factors: (1) the ratio of resorption to formation in each cycle, and (2) the rate at which the activation-resorption-formation cycle is occurring.

FACTORS INFLUENCING EDENTULOUS BONE LOSS

The specific factors that may influence EBL can be categorized as generalized and local.

Generalized Factors

Systemic bone disease (SBD) is any process that influences the normal remodeling process of bones in general. Some common systemic bone diseases are listed in Table 1–2. Many animal studies have shown that alveolar ridge bone may be among the most sensitive to systemic alterations in bone metabolism and remodeling. This is not because alveolar bone resorbs faster under systemic influences than other bone, but because a given amount of bone loss will have a greater net effect on alveolar bone than it will on compact bone. The vertebral bodies are similar to alveolar bone in this respect.[6] Albright and Reifenstein[7] were among the first to recognize that a systemic disease causes a loss of lamina dura around the teeth, which is an early sign of generalized bone loss. The edentulous alveolar ridge must be equally or more sensitive to such influences. Therefore, whatever local factors contribute to excessive alveolar bone loss, systemic abnormalities probably greatly influence the response of the bone to these local factors.

Osteopenia is a clinical term for any loss in bone density. Although most bones do not substantially change in size or shape as bone density decreases, the vertebral body becomes weakened by loss of density and collapses from the stress of the weight placed upon it.[8] This vertebral compression fracture is a type of pathologic fracture. The alveolar process, however, *does* change in size and shape after the teeth are lost. Although the alveolar process does not bear weight, it may bear compression and shear stresses. Therefore, a loss of density due to systemic bone disease that is practically undetectable, and not of any particular clinical significance in most parts of the skeleton, may be just one more factor contributing to the advance of edentulous bone loss.

Osteoporosis

Osteoporosis is a diverse group of diseases characterized by a reduction in the mass of bone per unit volume, resulting in mechanical failure and pain. The ratio of mineral to organic matrix is usually normal, as are the structures of the mineral and matrix. Osteoporosis is a diagnosis that must be made histologically,[8] because many other types of SBD cause a decrease in bone density as detected by radiography or densitometry. Histologically, a decrease in the number and size of trabeculae is seen, with normal width to the osteoid seams. For example, osteomalacia is another form of SBD that can cause a decrease in bone density,[8-12] but is quite different histologically from osteoporosis.

Osteoporosis is the most common form of SBD, and the two most common types of osteoporosis are postmenopausal and senile. Considerable controversy exists, however, regarding the influence of menopause on bone loss. *In vitro* studies have shown that the action of parathyroid hormone (PTH) on bones is inhibited by estrogens and that oophorectomy in rats increases the sensitivity of bone to PTH. This work cannot be directly extrapolated to humans because not all postmenopausal women become osteoporotic and black women rarely do.[8-15]

Women become osteoporotic more often than men and whites more often than blacks. There is an increase in bone loss during menopause and for several years after, which probably contributes to the development of osteoporosis. In addition, women normally have less dense bones than men and over the years an equal loss of bone by men and women usually leaves the woman with a lesser bone mass.

Senile osteoporosis is not easily understood but can be divided into two types (Fig. 1–3). One type exhibits a slow turnover in the remodeling cycle and the other type exhibits an accelerated turnover. It has been suggested that the slow turnover type is due to osteoblastic dysfunction, as there is a scarcity of osteoblasts, osteoclasts, and osteoid seen histologically.[8]

The high turnover type, which may be the same as the postmenopausal type, is characterized by normal rates of bone formation with increased numbers of osteoblasts and osteoclasts. An increase in circulating PTH has also been noted in this type and is probably secondary to poor intestinal absorption of calcium and impaired renal function.[5]

It is difficult to prove that osteoporosis is a factor in EBL because of other factors involved, but several correlations have been made between decrease in generalized bone density (osteopenia) and the presence of alveolar ridge loss.[9] In addition, more trabecu-

TABLE 1–2. COMMON SYSTEMIC BONE DISEASES

Osteoporosis
1. Senile osteoporosis
2. Postmenopausal osteoporosis
3. Hyperparathyroidism
4. Cushing's syndrome

Osteomalacia
1. Vitamin D deficiency
2. Renal osteodystrophy
3. Secondary hyperparathyroidism
4. Malnutrition

Figure 1–3. In osteoporosis bone mineral is lost, but the activation rate influences the speed of loss. *A*, Low turnover osteoporosis. *B*, High turnover osteoporosis.

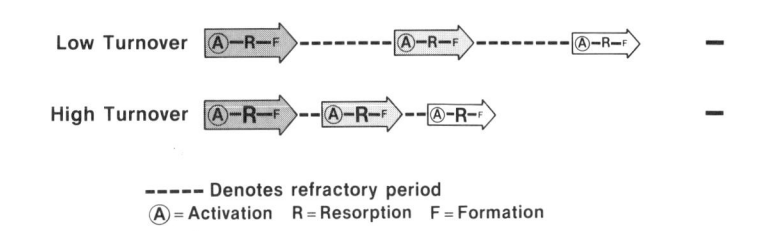

lar bone is lost due to osteoporosis because the trabecular surface area of bone is so much greater than the cortical surface area. Therefore, bones that are primarily trabecular, such as the vertebral bodies, proximal femur, and distal radius, are most affected. Although well-controlled studies are difficult to conduct because biopsies of the alveolar ridge would sacrifice valuable bone, the evidence suggests that the trabecular portion of the alveolar ridge is as sensitive to osteoporosis as are other trabecular bones.

Clinical signs and symptoms of advanced osteoporosis include pain in the spine (especially in the lumbar area), loss of height and/or thoracic kyphosis due to vertebral compression fractures, fractures of other bones secondary to inappropriate trauma, and fractures of the distal radius and ulna (Colles' fracture).

The lumbar region of the spinal column is most often the site of fracture and pain, not because bone loss is more active in this area, but because certain characteristics of this region render it more susceptible to fracture. A large amount of weight is born by a small volume of bone and the surface-to-volume ratio of bone is greatest here. Therefore, a given rate of bone loss will decrease the already small volume of bone to a greater extent than in compact bone.[16]

In most cases of osteoporosis, serum and urine biochemical examinations are normal.[17] Chest radiographs may show vertebral compression fractures, localized vertebral wedging, and thoracic kyphosis (Fig. 1–4). These

Figure 1–4. Radiographic changes seen after 30 to 50 per cent loss in density.

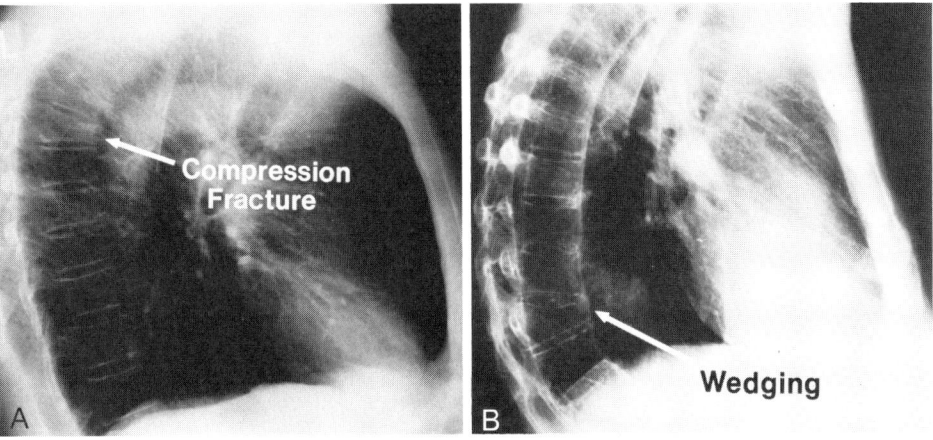

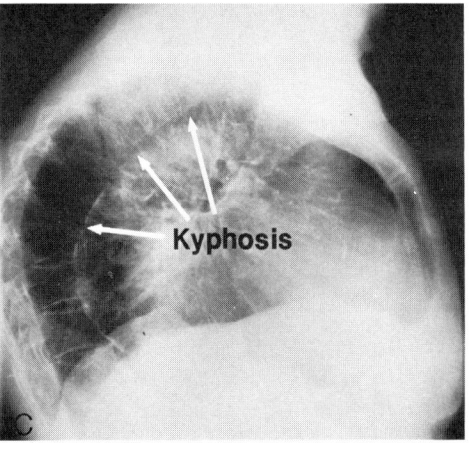

films cannot be used to assess bone density because a 30 to 50 per cent loss in density is necessary before changes are visible radiographically.[18-20] Edelstyn et al.[20] showed that spherical lesions must destroy 50 to 75 per cent of the vertebral spongiosa to be visualized as radiolucencies. Overall, it appears that up to 50 per cent demineralization of bone must occur before consistent radiographic detection of density changes is possible on routine films.[18, 19, 21, 22] Photon absorption densitometry is a much more sensitive determination of bone mineral content and can detect changes in density as small as 2 to 3 per cent.[23] It has been standardized for the distal and midshaft of the radius according to age-, sex-, and race-matched controls.[11] Abnormal results with this test indicate the need for a bone biopsy to diagnose the process causing the loss in density. Decreased bone density of the radius has been loosely associated with alveolar ridge loss, but much more work needs to be done to establish a direct relationship.[24]

Transiliac bone biopsy has been the most successful method for the diagnosis of most systemic bone diseases[11, 15, 25] (Fig. 1–5). Undecalcified specimens should be examined (as well as decalcified ones) so that osteoid can be evaluated.[8, 11] Double tetracycline labeling is also helpful in determining the rate of bone turnover.[11, 26]

Unfortunately, treatment of the two most common types of osteoporosis, senile and postmenopausal, has been relatively unsuccessful in reversing the progress of the disease. Any attempt at a thorough discussion of treatment of osteoporosis is well beyond the scope of this chapter. Estrogen therapy may decrease bone loss after oophorectomy and may be helpful in postmenopausal bone loss[11, 27-29] but also has been associated with increased rates of endometrial carcinoma.[14, 16, 22, 30-34] There is some scientific support for calcium supplementation in perimenopausal and postmenopausal women.[11, 27, 28] Fluoride and vitamin D treatments are controversial.[11, 16] The presence of the signs and symptoms listed previously merit a consultation with a metabolic bone specialist or endocrinologist.

Osteomalacia

Osteomalacia is a term used to describe the diseases in which excess osteoid is not mineralized, or is abnormally mineralized, and impaired bone healing is present. Causes may include vitamin D deficiency, hypophosphatemia, malnutrition, renal osteodystrophy (discussed below), secondary hyperparathyroidism, and metabolic acidosis.[8, 11] In the orthopedic literature, osteomalacia is a contraindication to bone grafting due to impaired healing. Histologic evaluation of undecalcified biopsy specimens is necessary to diagnose osteomalacia.[8, 11] Treatment requires identification of the underlying etiology so that appropriate measures can be taken to correct the specific abnormality.

Endocrine Disorders

A number of endocrine disturbances often associated with drug therapy have been directly or circumstantially associated with a decrease in generalized bone mineral con-

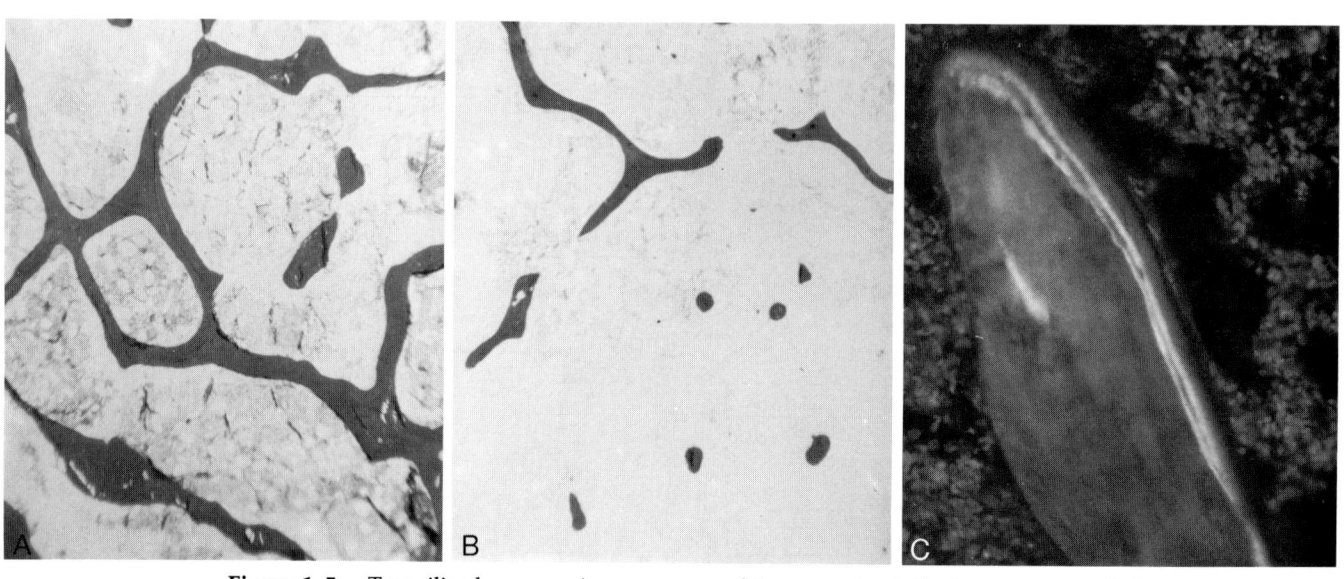

Figure 1–5. Transiliac bone specimens prepared in an undecalcified manner reveal the difference between *(A)* normal bone and *(B)* osteoporosis. *C,* Double tetracycline labeling permits estimation of the rate of bone turnover.

TABLE 1–3. DRUGS ASSOCIATED WITH DECREASED BONE DENSITY

1. Chronic corticosteroid therapy
2. Chronic heparin therapy
3. Anticonvulsant therapy
4. Alcohol

tent. Although the mechanism of bone loss is not always clear, a generalized decrease in bone mass seems to be associated with diabetes mellitus, primary and secondary hyperparathyroidism, alcoholism, renal failure requiring dialysis,[8, 11, 16, 35] and certain types of drug therapy such as chronic corticosteroid therapy, chronic heparin therapy, and anticonvulsant therapy (Table 1–3). Of these, the clearest association has been with renal failure. Given sufficient time, *renal osteodystrophy* occurs in all uremic patients, and dialysis does not seem to prevent or improve the bone disease.[8] Over 90 per cent of all patients on dialysis for over two years have radiographic evidence of renal osteodystrophy.[36] The disease is a combination of osteitis fibrosa, osteosclerosis, and osteomalacia.[37] The quality of the bone is more affected than the quantity, so that fractures may be more prevalent than would be expected from densitometric values.[38]

Renal osteodystrophy has been shown to produce foci of osteitis fibrosa cystica in areas of periodontal trauma. This is usually due to malocclusion and tooth-related infections. These pronounced effects are apparent only in more severe cases, but it seems likely that less obvious cases have some influence on alveolar bone mineral content.

Renal transplantation does reverse the uremic state.[39] However, because it takes years for recovery of parathyroid function, improvement of renal osteodystrophy occurs very slowly. Chronic immunosuppression, which is used to prevent transplant rejection, may also adversely affect the bones.[40]

Diagnosis of renal failure has been described in detail in numerous nephrology texts. Suffice it to say that polyuria, nocturia, or anemia on complete blood count may indicate the need for a more extensive renal evaluation.

Although not related to renal failure, a history of kidney stones is significant because it may reveal a calcium-wasting process that has resulted in stone formation. Obviously, additional investigation is needed to further elucidate a metabolic cause for the stone formation.

Nutritional Disorders

Several studies have shown that *nutritionally induced metabolic disturbances* may contribute to alveolar bone loss in animals.[41–44] The elderly tend to have a low intake of calcium and vitamin D, especially milk,[45] and the western diet is relatively high in phosphates rather than calcium. Red meat, colas, and other items in the diet contribute to this imbalance. It has been shown that high phosphate intake may stimulate a generalized decrease in bone mineral content due to a fall in serum calcium.[4,46–48] Alveolar bone loss has been directly associated with low dietary calcium intake and a poor calcium:phosphorus ratio in both edentulous and dentulous patients.[49–51] One study revealed that EBL in a group of patients was reduced, when compared to controls, by the daily administration of calcium and vitamin D.[52] The "shotgun" use of these agents should be avoided, as examination of the data reveals that those patients whose diet was not deficient in calcium and vitamin D had EBL similar to that of controls. It is appropriate to establish a need for therapy before it is initiated because elevated serum calcium levels may induce kidney stone formation in susceptible individuals.

If a cause and treatment cannot be found for SBD, invasive osseous grafting procedures to augment the alveolar ridge may have a less than ideal prognosis. We have noted poor results with the use of the modified visor and allogeneic bone in a small number of patients with SBD[53] and have avoided grafting procedures in subsequent patients with SBD. Retrospective studies to evaluate large numbers of patients who have been grafted or implanted would be helpful to determine if these procedures are contraindicated in patients with unusually low bone mineral content.

LOCAL FACTORS

Facial Morphology

Facial morphology may influence alveolar ridge loss in at least two ways. First, people with long faces tend to have longer anterior alveolar ridges in the vertical plane[54] (Fig. 1–6A). Although no three-dimensional studies are available, it is presumed that the alveolar ridges in these patients are also more voluminous. Thus, long faces have more anterior alveolar bone than short faces (Fig. 1–6B). Second, it has been shown that faces with low mandibular plane angles and low gonial angles (short faces) are capable of higher biting forces in both the molar and anterior regions.[55] This has implications in the early edentulous stages and later as resorption progresses. Immediately after loss of the teeth, higher biting forces mean that

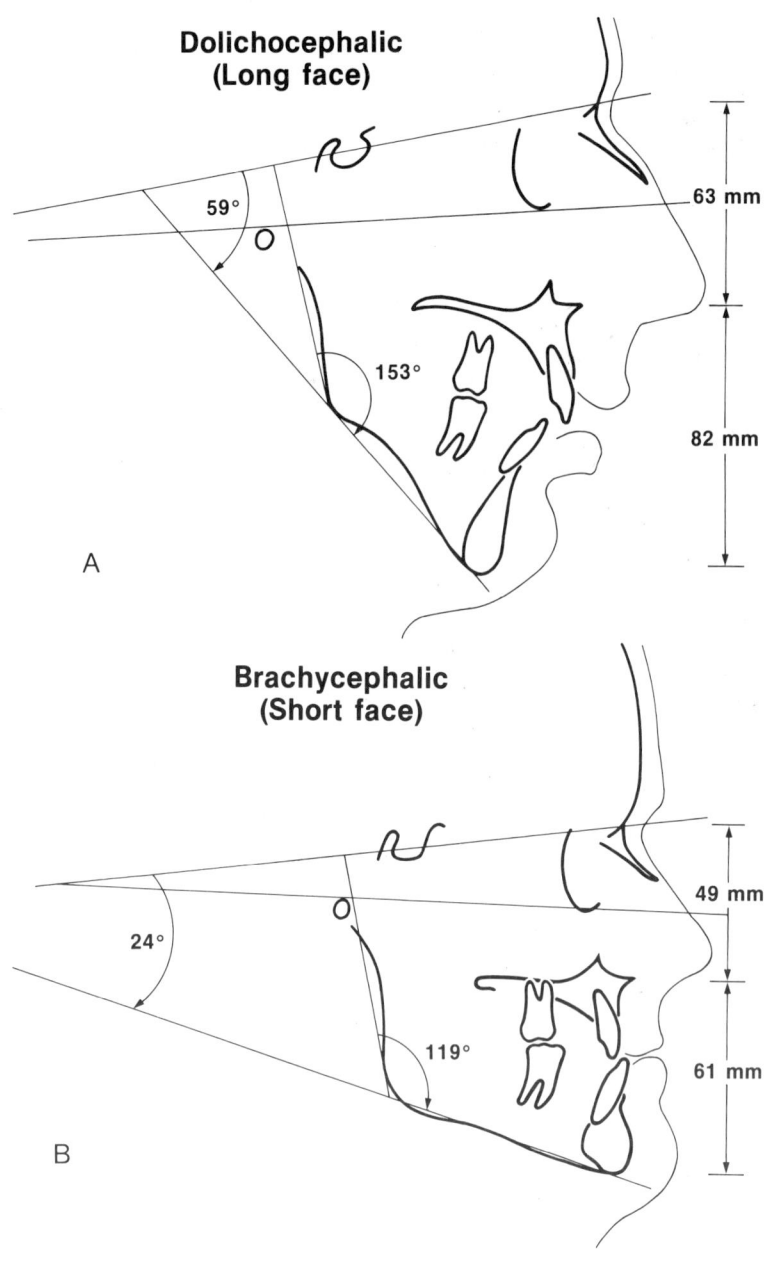

8 / THE PATHOPHYSIOLOGY AND ANATOMY OF EDENTULOUS BONE LOSS

Figure 1–6. Facial morphology influences bone loss. A, Dolichocephalic face. B, Brachycephalic face.

greater compressive forces are delivered to the alveolar ridges under complete dentures. Most observers feel that undue compression forces enhance EBL.[1] This rationale is supported by studies that have compared both low mandibular plane angles and low gonial angles with the amount of remaining alveolar bone. Direct correlations have been found between short faces and alveolar ridge atrophy.[56, 57] In addition, the mandible-to-maxilla relationship becomes worse due to a loss of vertical dimension as atrophy progresses. As vertical dimension decreases, the face becomes even shorter. If people with short faces can abrade their natural teeth, as many of them do, it is reasonable that they can promote EBL. This also correlates with the fact that mandibular alveolar ridges generally resorb four times faster than maxillary ones.[1,58,59] Bone size in women, including the jaws, is smaller and not only do those bones have a lower density, but the absolute dimension is also smaller.[8]

Trauma and Alveolectomy Technique

These two factors determine the amount of bone that remains on the alveolar ridge after loss of teeth. Traumatic loss of alveolar bone through accidental or iatrogenic causes may equal years of resorption. For this reason, maximum conservation of bone should be practiced during extraction and management of the trauma patient. In dentoalveolar fractures that require removal of the teeth, effort should be made to save bone. Occasionally, this may include fixation of nonrestorable teeth while the alveolar bone heals and then extraction of the teeth.

Several studies have evaluated EBL following the removal of all remaining teeth to determine the influence of various extraction techniques.[60] If the buccal and/or lingual plate is removed, the patient begins the postextraction period with less bone. More importantly, EBL progresses more rapidly in these patients than in those with simple extractions. It has also been shown that a modified alveolectomy technique, in which interseptal bone is removed and the buccal and lingual plates are collapsed together, stimulates an increased resorption rate when compared with simple extraction.[61] It is recommended, therefore, that only the least amount of recontouring necessary should be done to the remaining alveolar ridge following extraction.

Prosthetics

Prosthodontic care has been implicated as a factor in alveolar bone loss. Much has been written about the influence of prosthodontic loading of the edentulous alveolar ridge.[59,62,63] While teeth are present, alveolar bone responds to physiologic stresses by aligning the trabeculae appropriately. There are several interpretations that explain EBL after the teeth have been removed. First, disuse atrophy undoubtedly plays a role in a low turnover type remodeling. Secondly, excessive loading may contribute to a higher turnover type of remodeling.[1] There is no reason to assume that these processes are not occurring simultaneously in different parts of the same alveolar ridge. If normal loading of the alveolar ridge by the natural dentition is missing, then disuse atrophy occurs in those areas where load-resisting struts have developed. In the same alveolar ridge, abnormal, unidirectional compressive forces exerted by the denture may also induce an increased remodeling rate.

In bone loss secondary to the influence of dentures, it has been noted that the denture-bearing area of the maxilla is 1.8 times greater than that of the mandible.[59] Therefore, compressive forces (in pounds per square inch) will be greater on the mandible. This may be partly responsible for the increased rate of bone loss in the mandible, which is four times that of the maxilla.[1]

Certain occlusal arrangements of denture teeth are thought to decrease alveolar ridge resorption by improving the efficiency of mastication through decreasing occlusal contact area and balancing the occlusion.[64, 65] It has been suggested that if the occlusion of a denture is initially improper or if EBL has already begun, the shear and tension forces are responsible for increased rates of resorption.[1] However, various studies have not been able to confirm these suspicions.

Atwood[1] theorizes that the overloading of alveolar bone could result in increased vascularity and/or stasis due to compression, piezoelectric effects, and stimulation of bone-resorbing cells by physical force.

An additional factor that must be included in a discussion of prosthetic loading of the alveolar ridge is parafunctional activity (i.e., clenching, bruxing). Tooth contact during mastication occupies less than 15 minutes per day, while the teeth may be forcibly held together several hours per day.[66] The effects of such activities are not clearly understood.

No direct correlation between *bruxism* in complete denture wearers and EBL has been shown. It has been shown, however, that denture wearers may brux as much as 2.5 hours per 8 hours of sleep.[66] If increased compressive forces applied through a denture base contribute to EBL, then bruxism could add to these forces. Instability of the denture has been commonly implicated as one of the factors contributing to EBL.

In summary, it is known that ill-fitting dentures increase alveolar bone loss. Factors that cause high compressive forces on the alveolar ridge are suspected to enhance alveolar bone loss.

ANATOMIC CONSIDERATIONS

Several anatomic considerations that result from EBL deserve mention. As noted in Figure 1–7A and B, the mental foramen becomes closer to the denture-bearing area as the alveolar process decreases in size. The chances of denture impingement upon the mental nerve increases with bone loss, and the nerve is more vulnerable to injury during surgical grafting or implantation procedures. Progressive bone loss leaves the nerve near or at the superior surface of the mandible.

There are a number of possible patterns of EBL in the mandible, as noted in Figure 1–7B. The shape of the mandible is determined by the timing and sequence of tooth loss in the mandible as well as the opposing arch, partial or complete denture wear, and the local factors mentioned above. For example, the presence of mandibular anterior teeth opposing a complete upper denture can lead to excessive alveolar ridge resorption of the anterior maxilla.

The decrease in height and width of the edentulous mandible occurs so that the crest of the ridge moves slightly to the anterior as EBL continues. Also, autorotation of the mandible moves the entire mandible anteriorly and superiorly as vertical dimension is lost. As bone loss progresses, the ridge may become like a knife edge. Generally, the ultimate result of complete alveolar bone loss is a concave superior surface to the mandible. This concave surface represents the upper side of the cortical plate of the mandibular inferior border. In severe cases, the genial tubercles may be superior to the crest of the mandible. Pressure on the mucosa over this area usually causes sharp pain.

Muscle attachments such as the buccinator, mentalis, mylohyoid, and genioglossus do not migrate significantly. EBL leaves the muscle attachments close to the crest of the ridge. Muscle function will often lift the muscles and overlying mucosa above the level of the alveolar ridge, thus reducing the amount of alveolar ridge exposed in the mouth.

As bone loss progresses in the maxilla, the palatal vault becomes relatively more shallow, and redundant soft tissue forms labial to the alveolar crest (Fig.1–7C). The nasopalatine neurovascular bundle may end up on the crest of the ridge or anterior to it. Impingement on this nerve by a denture may occur. However, this is less often a problem than with the mental nerve. The shape of the maxilla after EBL is dictated by many of the same factors as in the mandible. In cases where lower anterior teeth occlude with an upper complete denture, EBL causes loss of anterior ridge height (Fig. 1–7D), which may progress to the point of dehiscence of the bone between the mouth and nose. This usually occurs at or just posterior to the

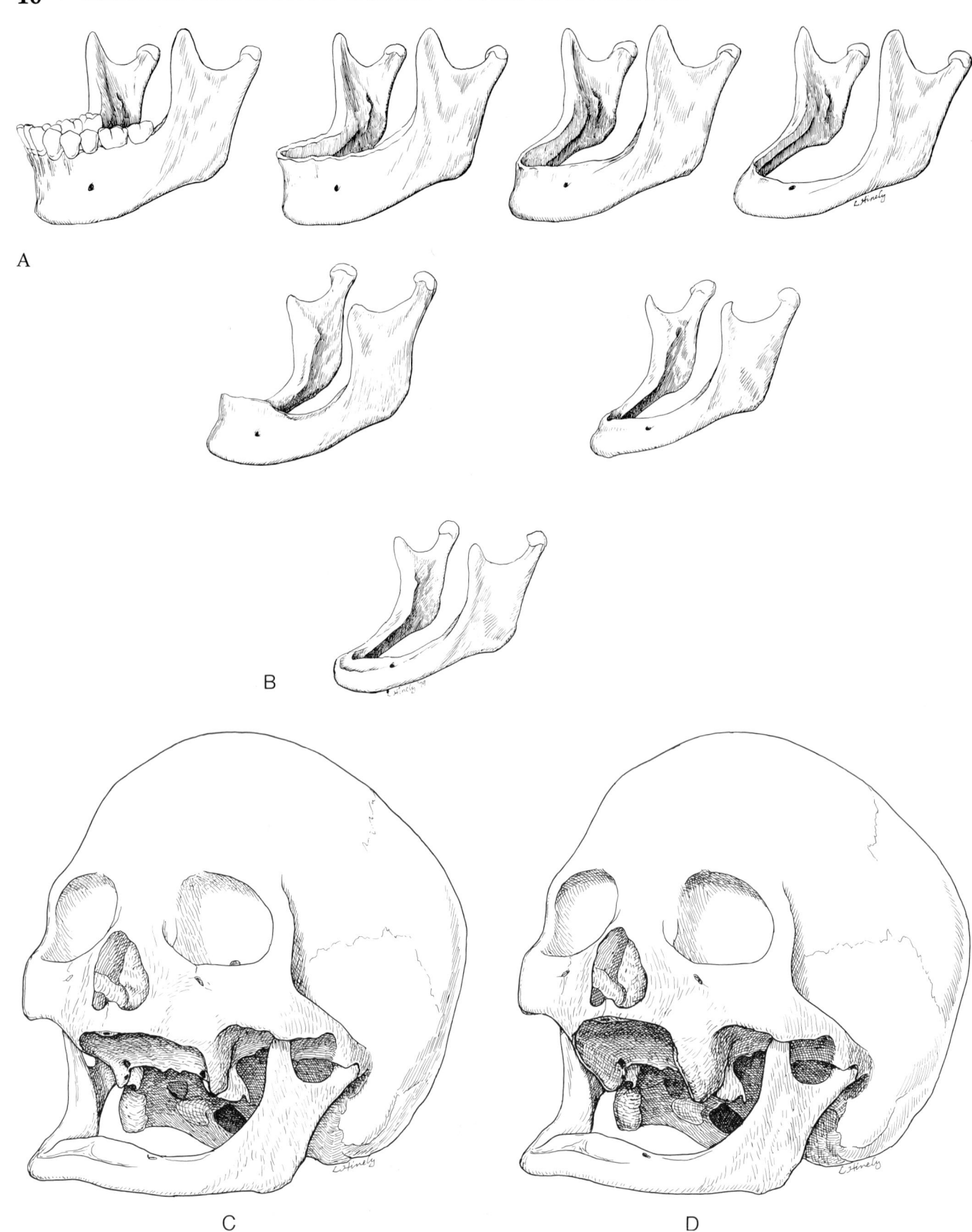

Figure 1–7. Edentulous bone loss (EBL) alters the anatomy and physiology of the mandible and maxilla. *A*, Following loss of teeth, the mandible undergoes remarkable alterations in form. *B*, Several common patterns of bone loss are illustrated. *C*, Total maxillary bone loss. *D*, Anterior maxillary bone loss.

bony piriform rim of the nose. The anterior nasal spine may be almost level with the alveolar crest. EBL in the anterior maxilla occurs mostly on the labial and inferior aspects of the alveolar ridge so that the crest moves posteriorly. Upper lip support is progressively lost as the anterior maxilla decreases in size. This, combined with the relative anterior movement of the mandibular ridge, results in an increasingly Class III facial form and ridge relationship.

Posteriorly, as the maxillary tuberosity decreases in height, it approaches the level of the mucosa that is draped from the mucogingival junction on the posterior aspect of the maxillary tuberosity to the hamulus. This change obliterates the posterior slope of the tuberosity.

As the mandible becomes smaller after the teeth are removed, resistance to fracture is reduced. Fractures in extremely small, edentulous mandibles are especially ominous because of the lack of bone mass for fixation[67] and the changes in the blood supply.[68] As EBL occurs the major source of blood supply to the mandible changes from centrifugal to centripetal (periosteal).[68] The inferior alveolar vessels become smaller and less significant in the nourishment of the mandible. Therefore, surgical procedures that elevate mandibular periosteum compromise the blood supply more as the mandible becomes smaller. The stability of internal fixation must be weighed against the potential complications resulting from a compromised blood supply.

PATIENT EVALUATION

The following recommendations are reasonably comprehensive for the evaluation of patients with edentulous bone loss. Although many of the factors included do not apply to all patients, an attempt has been made to discuss most of the considerations necessary for the screening of patients prior to nonsurgical or surgical intervention. Because many of the historic items are extremely general and many of the laboratory values are normal even in the disease state, considerable judgment must be exercised by the examiner in identifying those patients who require further evaluation and/or referral. Table 1–4 is a sample of a patient information form to be used for patients who present with moderate to severe EBL.

HISTORY OF PRESENT ILLNESS

1. At what age were the teeth extracted? What is the present age of the patient? This information will help the clinician determine the rate of resorption.
2. Why were the teeth extracted? If excessive periodontal bone loss preceded loss of the teeth, this may have caused much of the atrophy rather than actual resorption. However, if periodontal disease bone loss occurred at a relatively young age, it is likely that a host factor(s) played a significant role and might be operative in EBL.
3. Were the extractions especially traumatic, i.e., excessive bone loss?
4. How many relines or new dentures has the patient had since that time? This gives an overall view of dental care and patient motivation.
5. Did the patient grind or brux his or her natural teeth and has the patient persisted with that habit while wearing dentures? (See bruxism in *Local Factors*.)

PAST MEDICAL HISTORY

1. Is there a history of kidney disease? If so, has the patient ever had dialysis or is the patient having dialysis now? (See renal osteodystrophy in *Generalized Factors*.)
2. Is there a history of kidney stones? (See *Generalized Factors*.)
3. In women, has menopause been reached? If so, when? (See osteoporosis in *Generalized Factors*.)
4. Is there a history of alcohol abuse? If so, for how long? (See systemic bone disease in *Generalized Factors*.)
5. Is there a personal history or family history of collagen disorders, rickets, or osteogenesis imperfecta?
6. Operations
    a. Hysterectomy
    b. Oophorectomy
    c. Gastrectomy
    d. Hypophysectomy
    e. Renal transplantation
7. Medication
    a. Chronic corticosteroid therapy
    b. Chronic heparin therapy (>20,000 units/day)
    c. Chronic anticonvulsant therapy
8. History of diabetes mellitus
9. History of bone fractures, especially femoral and hip fractures. The possibility of fractures caused by inappropriate trauma should be explored. Patients may not relate to the examiner that the trauma which caused the fracture was relatively minor unless asked.
10. Nutritional abnormalities should be recorded, especially the absence of dairy products, exposure to sunshine, and exces-

TABLE 1–4. EVALUATION FOR SYSTEMIC BONE DISEASE

Age teeth were extracted _____

History	YES	NO

1. Reason teeth were pulled?
   Decay?
   Gum Disease (pyorrhea)?
   Broken teeth due to accident?
   Other?		

2. Did you ever or do you now grind your teeth (dentures)?		
3. Have you ever had kidney stones?		
4. Have you ever had kidney disease?		
5. Have you ever had dialysis?		
6. Women: Have you reached menopause?		
7. Do you have diabetes?		

8. Have you ever had any of these operations?
   Hysterectomy?
   Ovaries removed?
   Stomach surgery?
   Pituitary gland surgery?
   Kidney (transplant)?		

9. Are you taking any of these medicines?
   Cortisone (or other steroids)?
   Seizure drugs?		

10. Have you ever had a fractured bone when the cause did not seem strong enough to break a bone?		
11. Do you have any unusual dietary restrictions or habits (i.e., do not drink milk, stomach problems)?		
12. Night blindness or dry eyes?		
Review of Systems		
1. Do you have low back pain?		
2. Have you gotten shorter with age?		
3. Do you have to urinate frequently?		
4. Do you urinate several times at night?		

Present Age _____

	YES	NO
5. Are you always thirsty?		
6. Have you lost body hair with age?		
7. Have you lost energy or sexual potence?		
8. Do you have diarrhea or loose stools?		
Physical Examination *Do not write below this line*		

1. GENERAL: —Short torso
   —Obesity or extreme thinness
   —Lack of body/facial hair		

2. HEAD: —Brachycephalic
   —Bossing
   —Moon face
   —Chvostek sign (+ = path)		

3. HAIR: —Sparseness or depigmentation		

4. EYES: —Exophthalmus
   —Papilledema
   —Retinal hemorrhage		

5. MOUTH: —Cheilosis
   —Glossitis
   —Dysphagia		

6. NECK: —Thyroid enlargement		

7. SKIN: —Pallor
   —Abdominal striae
   —Pigmentation
   —Petechiae
   —Dermatitides		

8. C-V: —Tachycardia —Cardiac enlargement		
9. G-I: —Hepatomegaly —Ascites		

10. MUSCULO-SKEL: —Lumbar pain
   —Scoliosis
   —Thoracic kyphosis
   —Proximal muscle weakness		

11. NEURO: —Tetany, Chvostek, or Trousseau
   —Nervousness or irritability
   —Hyperreflexia
   —Hyporeflexia		

sive amounts of phosphate-containing foods such as colas and other carbonated beverages, red meats, etc. Such evaluations are time-consuming and may not be productive unless performed by professionals in nutrition or a well-informed clinician.

The interested practitioner should note the description by DePaola and Alfano[69] of a triphasic nutritional analysis that incorporates a computer-assisted dietary analysis service (Nutran™, Atlanta, Georgia). Table 1–5 is a checklist from DePaola and Alfano and is recommended to identify the high-risk patient.

Review of Systems

1. The musculoskeletal system
   a. Low back pain. It is important to determine if the pain is localized or generalized. It is also significant to determine the degree of pain, e.g., does it keep the patient awake at night? One would also like to know the duration of the pain, what relieves the pain, and if the patient has ever sought professional help for low back pain.
   b. Loss of height. Normally a patient will be able to tell if there has been a significant decrease in his or her height. This may indicate vertebral compression fractures. Women especially will note the change in the waistline of their clothing.
2. The endocrine system
   a. Polydipsia, polyuria, nocturia, fatigue, or any of the other classic signs and symptoms of diabetes

TABLE 1–5. CHECKLIST FOR ASSESSMENT OF NUTRITIONAL STATUS*

	YES	NO
Usual body weight 20 per cent above or below desirable?		
Recent loss or gain of 10 per cent of usual body weight?		
Any evidence that income and meals are not adequate for needs?		
More than half of meals eaten away from home?		
Does patient live alone and prepare own meals?		
Ill fitting dentures?		
Excessive use of alcohol?		
Frequent use of fad diets or monotonous diets?		
Any chronic disease of gastrointestinal tract? (describe)		
Has there been any surgical procedure on gastrointestinal tract other than appendectomy? (describe)		
Recent major surgery, illness, or injury?		
Recent use of large doses of:		
catabolic steroids?		
immunosuppressants?		
antitumor agents?		
anticonvulsants?		
antibiotics?		
oral contraceptives?		
vitamins?		
other?		
Has patient been maintained more than 10 days on intravenous fluids?		
Any reason to anticipate that patient will be unable to eat for 10 days or longer?		
Is patient known to have:		
diabetes?		
hypertension?		
hyperlipidemia?		
coronary artery disease?		
malabsorption?		
chronic lung disease?		
chronic renal disease?		
chronic liver disease?		
circulatory problem or heart failure?		
neurological disorder or paralysis?		
mental retardation?		

(Note: If all answers to the above items are "No," the patient may be regarded as a "low-risk" or "acceptable risk." The risk increases in direct proportion to the number of "Yes" answers. Patients with more than 3 "Yes" answers should be considered at an increased risk of developing medical complications, unless special attention is given to providing their nutritional requirements.)

*Reproduced with permission from DePaola DP, and Alfano MC: Triphasic nutritional analysis and dietary counseling. Dent Clin North Am 20:613–633, 1976.

    b. Loss of secondary sexual characteristics in males such as absence of facial and/or body hair, loss of sex drive, impotence, muscle weakness, or any other signs of hypogonadism in the male
3. The gastrointestinal system
    a. Steatorrhea indicates fat in the feces and a possible malabsorption syndrome.
4. The urinary system
    a. Polyuria
    b. Nocturia
    c. Weakness and/or easy fatigability, possibly indicating anemia

Physical Examination

The following items may indicate systemic disorders that would require additional examination and/or laboratory tests. Many of the findings listed below signal endocrine dysfunction or nutritional deficiencies, many of which are associated with malabsorption problems.

General

1. Body proportions—An unusually short torso may indicate a loss of vertical height. The arm span should be within 1.5 inches of the height for Caucasians and slightly more in blacks.
2. Extreme obesity or thinness—Obesity may indicate hormonal disturbances such as Cushing's syndrome. In elderly women, osteoporosis and obesity may be the first signs of a corticosteroid imbalance. Extreme thinness may indicate hyperthyroidism or nutritional insufficiency.
3. Lack of facial and/or body hair—Loss

of body hair is seen with hypogonadism in men, hyperthyroidism, or vitamin C deficiency.

Face and Skull

1. Facial morphology—Brachycephalic facial types with low mandibular plane angle and low gonial angle exert greater biting forces on the alveolar ridges.
2. Bossing—This is seen in acromegaly and Paget's disease.
3. Moon face—The collection of adipose tissue in the upper face gives it a round appearance.
4. Positive Chvostek sign—Elicited by a gentle tapping with the fingers over the facial nerve directly in front of the ear. A positive test is observed when the facial muscles contract as the nerve is tapped and is an indication of hypocalcemia.

Eyes

1. Exophthalmos—Hyperthyroidism produces exophthalmos, especially when it is long-standing. Urinary calcium should be elevated.
2. Papilledema—Prolonged corticosteroid therapy may cause increased intraocular pressure leading to papilledema.
3. Retinal hemorrhage—Diabetic retinal hemorrhages may be seen along with osteoporosis.
4. Band keratopathy—A band of calcium may develop across the cornea and conjunctiva in hyperparathyroidism, hypercalcemia, and renal failure.

Mouth

1. Cheilosis and
2. Glossitis—Both of these are associated with diabetes and vitamin C deficiency.

Neck

1. Thyroid enlargement—This is seen in hyperthyroidism.

Skin

1. Pallor—Poor skin color may be associated with hyperthyroidism, malnutrition, and renal failure.
2. Abdominal striae—Water retention and fat deposition in the abdomen in Cushing's syndrome produce striae.
3. Pigmentation — Hyperpigmentation may be due to malnutrition and chronic liver disease (cirrhosis).
4. Petechiae—Petechiae are seen in vitamin C deficiency.

Cardiovascular

1. Tachycardia—Thyrotoxicosis increases heart rate.
2. Hypertrophy—Hypertension, diabetes, Cushing's syndrome, and chronic steroid therapy are all associated with cardiac hypertrophy.

Gastrointestinal

1. Hepatomegaly—Associated with cirrhosis.
2. Ascites—This is seen with cirrhosis and renal failure.

Musculoskeletal

1. Pain in lumbar spine—Pain in this area may indicate a compression fracture.
2. Scoliosis—This may be exaggerated by osteoporosis.
3. Thoracic kyphosis—Compression fractures of the vertebral bodies usually occur on the anterior aspect of the vertebrae, which produces kyphosis.
4. Proximal muscle weakness—The waddling gait of osteomalacia is due to muscle weakness, which may be due to calcium and/or vitamin D deficiency.

Neurologic

1. Tetany (see Chvostek sign)—Also Trousseau sign may be elicited by applying a sphygmomanometer to the upper arm and inflating it until the pulse is obliterated. It is left in that position not more than 3 minutes. The test is positive if carpal spasm occurs with apposition of the thumb. The forearm remains painful and tingling for a few minutes as the carpal spasm slowly subsides.
2. Nervousness or irritability—These are seen in hyperthyroidism.
3. Hyperreflexia—Severe calcium deficiency stimulates hyperreflexia or tetany.
4. Hyporeflexia—This is seen in renal diseases.

LABORATORY EXAMINATIONS

1. Chest radiograph—One should look for evidence of vertebral compression fractures, localized vertebral wedging, and asymmetric biconcavity of the vertebral bodies. Assessment of bone density from the chest film is extremely inaccurate.
2. Complete blood count with special attention to the presence of anemia.
3. Photon absorption densitometry—This particular examination may be unavailable to those not located near teaching centers, but over a hundred instruments are in use in the United States. This measurement is attractive because it is relatively inexpensive, is noninvasive, involves a minimum of radiation exposure to the patient, and is extremely sensitive. It is a nonspecific test that

determines the amount of bone mineral per millimeter of bone. The distal or midshaft radius is used most frequently for the examination. The values obtained are compared with control values determined from large numbers of patients and matched to the patient in question as to age, sex, and race. Values more than two standard deviations below the age-, sex-, race-matched controls are considered abnormal enough to require the following:

a. Serum levels of calcium—Calcium determination should be performed on fasting patients. The values are often normal in osteoporosis, which includes the greatest number of patients with systemic bone disease. However, the values for calcium may be high in primary hyperparathyroidism, vitamin D overdose, and thyrotoxicosis. Calcium values may be low in osteomalacia, especially if there is an absence of secondary hyperparathyroidism. Calcium values are also normal in vitamin D–resistant rickets and other forms of renal tubular rickets. Serum calcium is low in hypoparathyroidism and pseudohypoparathyroidism.
b. Serum levels of phosphate—Inorganic phosphate values are generally low in primary hyperparathyroidism and in hyperparathyroidism secondary to malabsorption. Inorganic phosphate is usually normal in osteoporosis. There is a tendency toward high serum phosphate levels in patients with active SBD.
c. Alkaline phosphatase activity—Alkaline phosphatase activity is generally normal in adult osteoporosis. It may be increased in osteomalacia due to vitamin D deficiency or malabsorption but is usually normal in osteomalacia due to renal tubular disorders. It is also normal in primary hyperparathyroidism.
d. Serum levels of parathyroid hormone (PTH)
e. Serum levels of vitamin D
f. Serum levels of calcitonin—Evaluation of items d, e, and f would not normally be within the purview of those not specializing in systemic bone disease. Values are generally normal in osteoporosis. Values for these substances generally must be obtained from special laboratories located throughout the country.
g. 24-hour urine calcium—24-hour specimens of urine are required. Urine calcium in these examinations may be low in certain forms of osteomalacia and renal glomerular failure. Urine calcium may be abnormally high in primary hyperparathyroidism and in certain cases of excessive bone resorption.
h. 24-hour urine creatinine—Creatinine values are used as a standard by which the excretion of other substances is measured. The ratio of creatinine to other substances, therefore, is generally the most important factor to be noted.
i. 24-hour urine hydroxyproline—Hydroxyproline is derived almost exclusively from collagen, and most of the hydroxyproline found in the urine comes from bone. In general, hydroxyproline excretion reflects a turnover in bone collagen, i.e., the organic matrix of bone, and is often increased in SBD. However, hydroxyproline values are usually normal in osteoporosis and moderately increased in osteomalacia, depending upon the degree of secondary hyperparathyroidism.
j. 24-hour urine phosphate—The value of this measurement is generally low because of the variability associated with phosphate intake.
k. Bone biopsy—Standardized methods for transileal bone biopsies have been developed. These can be performed under local anesthesia with or without intravenous sedation. This examination should be conducted by the systemic bone specialist or endocrinologist who will be analyzing the bone specimen so that it can be done by a standard method. Decalcified and undecalcified specimens should be prepared. The examination of specimens permits the assessment of the amount of osteoid. Two doses of tetracycline are given at approximately a three-week interval in order that a double tetracycline label can be found in the bone at the mineralization front. The distance separating the two tetracycline labels permits the estimation of the rate of bone formation.

The diagnosis of SBD, or of other generalized factors that may influence the overall remodeling rate of bone in the body, is made by a comprehensive evaluation of many of the above historic, physical, and laboratory findings. Unfortunately, even in the face of such an extensive work-up, the SBD expert may not be able to identify an etiologic factor in many cases of osteoporosis. Treatment may therefore be difficult to prescribe and the prognosis of treatment may be uncertain. In such instances, it is up to the surgeon in consultation with the systemic bone specialist and the patient to determine the relative risks and values of bone grafting and/or implantation. No clear guidelines have been established at this time.

Acknowledgments

The author extends a special thank you to Karin Paulin and June Shafer for their assistance in the preparation of this chapter.

BIBLIOGRAPHY

1. Atwood DA. Bone loss of edentulous alveolar ridges. Eighth James A. English Symposium on Oral Perspectives on Bone Biology, 1979, Buffalo, New York. J Periodontol 50 (4):11–21, 1979.
2. Atwood DA: Reduction of residual ridges: A major oral disease entity. J Prosthet Dent 26:266–279, 1971.
3. Tallgren A: The continuing reduction of the residual alveolar ridges in complete denture wearers: A mixed longitudinal study covering 25 years. J Prosthet Dent 27:120–132, 1972.
4. Laflamme GH, and Jowsey J: Bone and soft tissue changes with oral phosphate supplements. J Clin Invest 51:2834–2840, 1972.
5. Frost HM: Skeletal physiology and bone remodeling: An overview. In Urist MR (ed.): Fundamental and Clinical Bone Physiology. Philadelphia, JP Lippincott Co, 1980, pp 208–241.
6. Messer HH, Goebel NK, and Wilcox L: A comparison of bone loss from different skeletal sites during acute calcium deficiency in mice. Arch Oral Biol 26:1001–1004, 1981.
7. Albright F, and Reifenstein EC: The Parathyroid Glands and Metabolic Bone Disease. Selected Studies. Baltimore, The Williams and Wilkins Co, 1948.
8. Teitelbaum S: Metabolic and other nontumorous disorders of the bone. In Anderson WAD: Pathology. St Louis, The CV Mosby Co, 1980.
9. Baxter JC: Relationship of osteoporosis to excessive residual ridge resorption. J Prosthet Dent 46:123–125, 1981.
10. Paterson CR: Metabolic Disorders of Bone. Oxford, Blackwell Scientific Publications, 1974, pp 165–191.
11. Smith R: Biochemical Disorders of the Skeleton. London, Butterworths, 1979, pp 95–132.
12. Thomson DL, and Frame B: Involutional osteopenia: Current concepts. Ann Intern Med 85:789–803, 1976.
13. Jowsey J, and Gilbert G: Bone turnover and osteoporosis. In Bourne G (ed.): The Biochemistry and Physiology of Bone. New York, Academic Press, 1971, pp 202–235.
14. Krane SM, and Holick MF: Metabolic bone disease. In Petersdorf RG, Adams RD, Braunwald E, Isselbacher KJ, Martin JB, and Wilson JD (eds.): Harrison's Principles of Internal Medicine. New York, McGraw-Hill Book Co, 1983, pp 1949–1960.
15. Lichtenstein L: Osteoporosis in Diseases of Bone and Joints. St. Louis, The CV Mosby Co, 1975.
16. Bourne GH (ed.): The Biochemistry and Physiology of Bone. Vol III (Development and Growth). 2nd ed. New York, Academic Press, 1971.
17. Kelly PJ, Jowsey J, Riggs BL, and Elveback LR: Relationship between serum phosphate concentration and bone resorption in osteoporosis. J Lab Clin Med 69:110–115, 1967.
18. Ardan GM: Bone destruction not demonstrable by radiography. Br J Radiol 24:107–109, 1951.
19. Borak J: Relationship between the clinical and roentgenological findings in bone metastases. Surg Gynecol Obstet 75:599–604, 1942.
20. Edelstyn GA, Gillespie PJ, and Grebbell FS: The radiological demonstration of osseous metastasis. Experimental observations. Clin Radiol 18:158–162, 1967.
21. Gates GF: Radionuclide diagnosis. In Laskin DM (ed.): Oral and Maxillofacial Surgery. Vol I, The Biomedical and Clinical Basis for Surgical Practice. St. Louis, The CV Mosby Co, 1980, pp 463–545.
22. Weiss NS, Szekely DR, and Austin DF: Increasing incidence of endometrial cancer in the United States. N Engl J Med 294:1259–1262, 1976.
23. Cameron JR, and Sorenson JA: Measurement of bone mineral in vitro: An improved method. Science 142:230–232, 1963.
24. Rosenquist JB, Baylink DJ, and Berger JS: Alveolar atrophy and decreased skeletal mass of the radius. Int J Oral Surg 7:479–481, 1978.
25. Nordin BEC: Metabolic Bone and Stone Disease. Baltimore, The Williams and Wilkins Co, 1973, pp 1–53.
26. Jowsey J.: Metabolic diseases of bone. Saunders Monographs in Clinical Orthopaedics, Vol I. Philadelphia, WB Saunders Co, 1977, pp 124–126.
27. Recker RR: Continuous treatment of osteoporosis: Current status. Orthop Clin North Am 12:611–627, 1981.
28. Recker RR, Saville PD, and Heaney RP: Effect of estrogens and calcium carbonate on bone loss in postmenopausal women. Ann Intern Med 87:649–655, 1977.
29. Weiss NS, Ure CL, Barrard JH, Williams AR, and Daling JR: Decreased risk of fractures of the hip and lower forearm with postmenopausal use of estrogen. N Engl J Med 303:1195–1198, 1980.
30. Gordan GS, and Greenberg BG: Exogenous estrogens and endometrial cancer. Postgrad Med 59:66–77, 1976.
31. Mack TM, Pike MC, Henderson BE, et al.: Estrogens and endometrial cancer in a retirement community. N Engl J Med 294:1262–1267, 1976.
32. Smith DC, Prentice R, Thompson DJ, and Herrmann WL: Association of exogenous estrogen and endometrial carcinoma. N Engl J Med 293:1164–1167, 1975.
33. Weiss NS: Risks and benefits of estrogen use. N Engl J Med 293:1200–1202, 1975.
34. Ziel HK, and Finkle WD: Increased risk of endometrial carcinoma among users of conjugated estrogens. N Engl J Med 293:1167–1170, 1975.
35. Walter JB, and Israel MS: Calcium metabolism and heterotopic calcification. In General Pathology, 5th ed. Edinburgh, Churchill Livingstone, 1979, pp 457–466.
36. Massry S, Coburn JW, Popvtzer MM, Shinaberger JH, Maxwell MH, and Kleeman CR: Secondary hyperparathyroidism in chronic renal failure. The clinical spectrum in uremia, during hemodialysis, and after renal transplantation. Arch Intern Med 124:431–441, 1969.
37. Ellis HA, and Peart KM: Azotaemic renal osteodystrophy: A quantitative study on iliac bone. J Clin Pathol 26:83–101, 1973.

38. Russell JE, Termine JD, and Avioli LV: Abnormal bone maturation in chronic uremic state. J Clin Invest 52:2848–2852, 1973.
39. Katz AI, Hampers CL, and Merrill JP: Secondary hyperparathyroidism and renal osteodystrophy in chronic failure. Analysis of chronic dialysis, kidney transplantation and subtotal parathyroidectomy. Medicine 48:333–474, 1969.
40. Pierides AM, Simpson W, Stainsby D, Alvarez-Ude F, and Uldall PR: Avascular necrosis of bone following renal transplantation. Q J Med 44:459–480, 1975.
41. Kassirer JP: Hyperphosphatemia, hyperparathyroidism and bighead. N Engl J Med 289:1367–1368, 1973.
42. Krook L, Whalen JP, Lesser GV, et al.: Experimental studies on osteoporosis. Methods Achiev Exp Pathol 7:72–108, 1975.
43. Massry SG, Ritz E, and Verberckmoes R: Role of phosphate in the genesis of secondary hyperparathyroidism of renal failure. Nephron 18:77–81, 1977.
44. Reiss E, and Slatapolsky E: Secondary (adaptive) hyperparathyroidism. In DeGroot LJ, Cahill GF, Jr., Odell WD, et al. (eds.): Endocrinology, Vol 2. New York, Grune and Stratton, 1980, pp 745–749.
45. Heaney RP: Calcium intake requirement and bone mass in the elderly. (Editorial) J Lab Clin Med 100:309–312, 1982.
46. Jowsey J, Reiss E, and Canterbury JM: Long-term effects of high phosphate intake on parathyroid hormone levels and bone metabolism. Acta Orthop Scand 45:801–808, 1974.
47. Morrin PAF, Gedney WB, and Reiss E: Phosphate homeostasis: Sensitivity of parathyroid-mediated response of renal excretion. J Lab Clin Med 59:387–395, 1962.
48. Reiss E, Canterbury JM, Bercovitz MA, and Kaplan EL: The role of parathyroid hormone in man. J Clin Invest 49:2146–2149, 1970.
49. Reynolds FC, Oliver DR, and Ramsey R: Clinical evaluation of the merthiolate bone bank and homogenous bone grafts. J Bone Joint Surg [Am] 33:873–883, 1951.
50. Sorenson RL: A study of dietary calcium and phosphorus intakes in relation to residual ridge resorption. Thesis, School of Health, Loma Linda University, 1977.
51. Wical KE, and Swoope CC: Studies of residual ridge resorption. Part II. The relationship of dietary calcium and phosphorus to residual ridge resorption. J Prosthet Dent 32:13–22, 1974.
52. Wical KE, and Brussee P: Effects of calcium and vitamin D supplement on alveolar ridge resorption in immediate denture patients. J Prosthet Dent 41:4–11, 1979.
53. Bays RA: The influence of systemic bone disease on bone resorption following mandibular augmentation. Oral Surg 55:223–231, 1983.
54. Bell WH, and Proffit WR: Maxillary excess. In Bell WH, Proffit WR, and White RP, Jr. (eds.): Surgical Correction of Dentofacial Deformities. Philadelphia, WB Saunders Co, 1980, pp 234–441.
55. Throckmorton GS, Finn RA, and Bell WH: Biomechanics of differences in lower facial height. Am J Orthod 77:410–420, 1980.
56. Mercier P, and Lafontant R: Residual alveolar ridge atrophy: Classification and influence of facial morphology. J Prosthet Dent 41:90–100, 1979.
57. Tallgren A: Alveolar bone loss in denture wearers as related to facial morphology. Acta Odontol Scand 28:251–270, 1970.
58. Jaul DH, McNamara JA, Carlson DS, and Upton LG: A cephalometric evaluation of edentulous Rhesus monkeys (Macaca mulatta): A long-term study. J Prosthet Dent 44:453–460, 1980.
59. Woelfel JB, Winter CM, and Igaraski T: Five-year cephalometric study of mandibular ridge resorption with different posterior occlusal forms. Part I. Denture construction and initial comparison. J Prosthet Dent 36:602–623, 1976.
60. Michael CG, and Barsoum WM: Comparing ridge resorption with various surgical techniques in immediate dentures. J Prosthet Dent 35:142–155, 1976.
61. Gazabatt C, Parra N, and Meissner E: A comparison of bone resorption following intraseptal alveolotomy and labial alveolectomy. J Prosthet Dent 15:435–443, 1965.
62. Cutright DE, Brudvik JS, Gay WD, and Selting WJ: Tissue pressure under complete maxillary dentures. J Prosthet Dent 35:160–170, 1976.
63. Ohashi M, Woelfel JB, and Paffenbarger GC: Pressures exerted on complete dentures during swallowing. J Am Dent Assoc 73:625–630, 1966.
64. Ortman HR: The role of occlusion in preservation and prevention in complete denture prosthodontics. J Prosthet Dent 25:121–138, 1971.
65. Page ME: Systemic and prosthodontic treatment to prevent bone resorption in edentulous patients. J Prosthet Dent 33:483–488, 1975.
66. Brewer AA: Prosthodontic research in progress at the School of Aerospace Medicine. J Prosthet Dent 13:49–69, 1963.
67. Bruce RA, and Strachan DS: Fractures of the edentulous mandible: The Chalmers J. Lyons Academy Study. J Oral Surg 34:973–979, 1976.
68. Cobetto GA, McClary SA, and Zallen RD: Treatment of mandibular fractures with malleable titanium mesh plates: A review of 20 cases. J Oral Maxillofac Surg 41:597–600, 1983.
69. DePaola DP, and Alfano MC: Triphasic nutritional analysis and dietary counseling. Dent Clin North Am 20:613–633, 1976.

2
BIOLOGIC ASPECTS OF TRANSPLANTATION OF GRAFTS

Stephen E. Feinberg, D.D.S., M.S., Ph.D., and Raymond J. Fonseca, D.M.D.

GENERAL PRINCIPLES OF TRANSPLANTATION

For many years, surgeons have attempted to graft normal tissues or organs from one animal to another. In the past, most tissues of higher animals have had a record of repeated failures until strains of mice were bred (by careful brother-sister mating and selection) whose genetic constitution was identical, or isogeneic, in all members. When skin grafts are exchanged between isogeneic individuals, they become vascularized, persistent, and indefinitely functioning. Therefore, the general difficulties experienced in the transplantation of tissues are not due to faulty transplantation techniques but to the fact that in ordinary populations every individual is likely to differ genetically from every other, except in the cases of uniovular (identical) twins. Genetic differences are expressed ultimately by the synthesis of chemically unique materials, whether these be required for the structure or the function of the cells. Individuals with different genetic constitutions, termed heterogeneic, are likely to differ in their chemical makeup.

These chemical materials, or glycoproteins, which are so important in determining the fate of the graft, are associated with the surface membranes of most nucleated cells of the body and are referred to as "transplantation antigens." The investigation of transplantation antigens emerged in the early part of the century from the work of P. Medawar, P. Gorer, G. Snell, and their associates. The analysis of transplantation antigens began with the discovery that some tumors are transplantable, but the successful "take" and subsequent growth of transplantable tumors does not regularly occur. In fact, the success rate was low when outbred or heterogeneic animals were used but could be high when inbred or isogeneic animals were used. Successful transplantation was dependent upon the genetic constitutions of the donor and recipient.

Despite the identification of the genetic control of tumor transplant rejection by different strains, little was known about the mechanism of rejection. In 1936, Gorer and associates conducted a series of serologic studies that led to the demonstration of cell surface alloantigenic differences between inbred strains of mice. When appropriate mating combinations were tested, it was possible to show that some of the genes responsible for susceptibility to transplantable tumors were closely linked or identical to the genes controlling the cell surface antigens. In addition, the serum of the animals that rejected a tumor frequently contained antibodies that were directed against antigens shared by the tumor and normal tissues of the strain in which the tumor originated. This suggested that the rejection process was immunologic in nature and that the rejection was not due to "tumor-specific" antigens. Later, these tumor rejection studies were confirmed using normal tissues, such as spleen and skin.

TYPES OF GRAFTS

There are four basic terms used to describe transplants or grafts between individuals and species (Fig. 2–1):

1. *Autografts* are transplants from one region to another in the same individual.
2. *Isografts* are transplants from one individual to a genetically identical individual. These are possible only between monozygotic twins and between members of certain strains of mice and other rodents that have been so highly inbred (by brother-sister mating) as to be syngeneic or isogeneic, i.e., genetically identical.
3. *Allografts* or *homografts* are transplants from one individual to a genetically nonidentical (i.e., allogeneic) individual of the same species.
4. *Xenografts* or *heterografts* (Gr. *xenos* = foreign) are transplants from one species to another.

In these four types of grafts the donors are designated, respectiveley, autologous, isologous, homologous, and heterologous with respect to recipient.

HISTOCOMPATIBILITY ANTIGENS

The cell surface proteins that give an organ its recognizable antigenicity and evoke the rejection phenomenon are referred to as histocompatibility (transplantation) antigens. In all animal species studied sufficiently, similar antigens have been identified on the surface of the nucleated cells of the transplanted tissue. These glycoprotein molecules are responsible for the induction of rejection and appear to be inherited in a systemic fashion, in all cases, bearing a relationship to parenteral antigens. Nearly 30 such antigens have been detected in the mouse and each of them varies in nonbred populations. This genetic diversity provides biologic uniqueness for each individual in a normal population. Studies of histocompatibility antigens suggest that the number of possible combinations is so large that (with the exception of identical twins) exact matches are very rare.

Histocompatibility antigens differ in their ability to elicit an immunologic response in a graft recipient. In mice, one set of antigens known as the H-2 system provides the strongest barrier to transplantation. If skin grafts are exchanged between mice having different H-2 antigens on their cells, the grafts will invariably be rejected within 14 days. Grafts differing in "weak" histocompatibility antigens outside the H-2 system, however, can take up to 200 days to be rejected. The strong H-2 antigens of the mouse have their counterpart in the HLA (Human Leukocyte Antigens) of man, which were first detected on the surface of white blood cells in the early 1950's (Fig. 2–2).

The H-2 and HLA antigens are protein molecules firmly attached to the surface of nearly all cells. Part of the molecule is embedded in or passes through the cell's outer membrane. Like other protein molecules, the antigens consist of chains of amino acids, but they also contain a small amount of carbohydrate; hence, they are termed glycoproteins. They are detected and classified by their ability to bind to specific antibodies, which are manufactured when cells from one animal are injected into a genetically different animal of the same species. Some of the molecules on the injected cells could be identical to those of the recipient; others, because of the genetic differences, are not. The recipient typically makes antibodies against the molecules that are different, and those antibodies define the antigenic specificities of the injected cells. A given antigenic specificity may reflect the presence of an antigen molecule on the donor's cells that is not present on the recipient's cells, or it may reflect structural differences between variants of a histocompatibility antigen that is present on both the donor's and the recipient's cells.

MAJOR HISTOCOMPATIBILITY COMPLEX

The strip of chromosome that codes for the histocompatibility antigens of man is

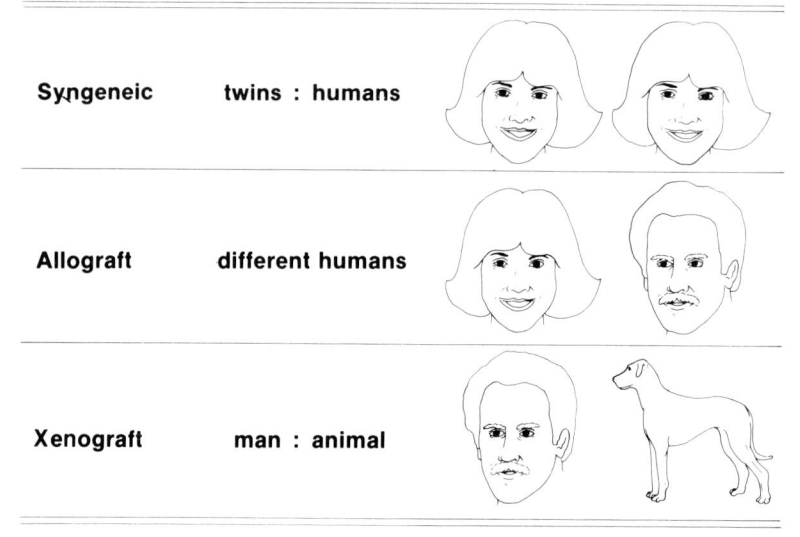

Syngeneic	twins : humans	
Allograft	different humans	
Xenograft	man : animal	

Figure 2–1. Types of grafts.

known as the histocompatibility, or HLA, complex. Mice and rats have analogous systems known as H-2 and AGB, respectively, that have been studied to provide an understanding of the HLA complex of man. In these systems, there are genes capable of coding for the production of cell surface antigens, which can be recognized by the recipient as self or foreign. On each of two chromosomes there are at least four known loci, each containing a series of codominant allelic forms. At present, in man, 51 antigens have been recognized in the HLA system; 2 on locus A, 2 on locus B, 5 on locus C, and 6 on locus D. Each individual inherits one chromosome from each parent and thus one allele from each of these four loci from each parent. A parent will share exactly half of the antigens with an offspring, and siblings may share all, some, or none of these antigens.

One of the very important distinctions among the antigens of the various loci within the histocompatibility complex is that the gene product antigens of the various loci are capable of stimulating recognition by different limbs of the immune response. The human A and B loci antigens stimulate recognition by the humoral immune system, i.e., the serologically determined (SD) antigens, whereas the human D locus appears to stimulate recognition by the thymus-derived (T) lymphocytes, i.e., the lymphocytically determined (LD) antigens. Thus, sensitization against SD antigens of the A or B locus induces circulating antibodies against the specific antigens of these loci. In contrast, individuals sensitized against the LD antigens of the D locus will have enhanced mixed lymphocyte reactivity, or sensitized cells of the lymphocyte lineage (Fig. 2–2).

The HLA or major histocompatibility complex (MHC) of humans, which is homologous to the H-2 region in the mouse, has other biologic roles besides the placement of determinants on cellular membranes to thwart the success of clinical tissue transplantation. The HLA-A and HLA-B loci, corresponding to the K and D regions of the H-2 in the mouse (serologically defined, SD), are the regions recognized during allograft rejection by cytotoxic T lymphocytes. It has also been shown that when cells are treated with viruses or chemical haptens, they seem to be specifically associated with the SD regions; and cytotoxic T lymphocytes are lytic only if the target cells that are modified with virus or chemical carry the same modifying antigen and the same K and D (or A and B) region molecules as the originating stimulating cells (Figs. 2–3 and 2–4).

The I region in the mouse (or HLA-D re-

MHC MAN (HLA)

6th Chromosome

MHC MOUSE (H-2)

17th Chromosome

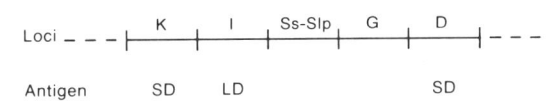

Figure 2–2. Comparison of major histocompatibility complex (MHC) of man and mouse.

gion in man) is a region of the MHC that controls many major immunologic phenomena. Most importantly, it controls the genetics of immune response to certain defined antigens, e.g., myeloma proteins and synthetic polypeptides. The antigens coded for by this region are termed Ia (I region–associated) antigens. The Ia antigens have a molecular weight between 28,000 and 32,000 daltons as compared to 48,000 daltons for H-2 antigens, i.e., K and D (HLA-A and HLA-B). While products of the K and D regions (H-2 antigens) of the MHC are located on all tissues except sperm, Ia antigens are located on lymphocytes, macrophages, sperm, and possibly epidermal cells. It has been shown, by the use of specific antisera directed against antigens coded for by the I region, that it controls such immune functions as genetic control of specific immune responses, graft-versus-host reactions, regulation of immune suppression, and the surface membrane structures that regulate interactions between T and B lymphocytes and macrophages (helper and suppressor T lymphocytes) (Fig. 2–4).

Another region of the MHC in the mouse is the Ss-Slp region, which maps to the left of the H-2 region (in man to the left of HLA-B) and controls the synthesis of component C4 in the complement cascade.

Also, the MHC immune response genes code for a portion of the T lymphocyte recognition structure. The H regions encode for the synthesis of heavy chains of immunoglobulins that function, in part, as the antigen-combining sites of the molecule on the T lymphocyte.

Finally, certain HLA phenotypes have been found in association with some human

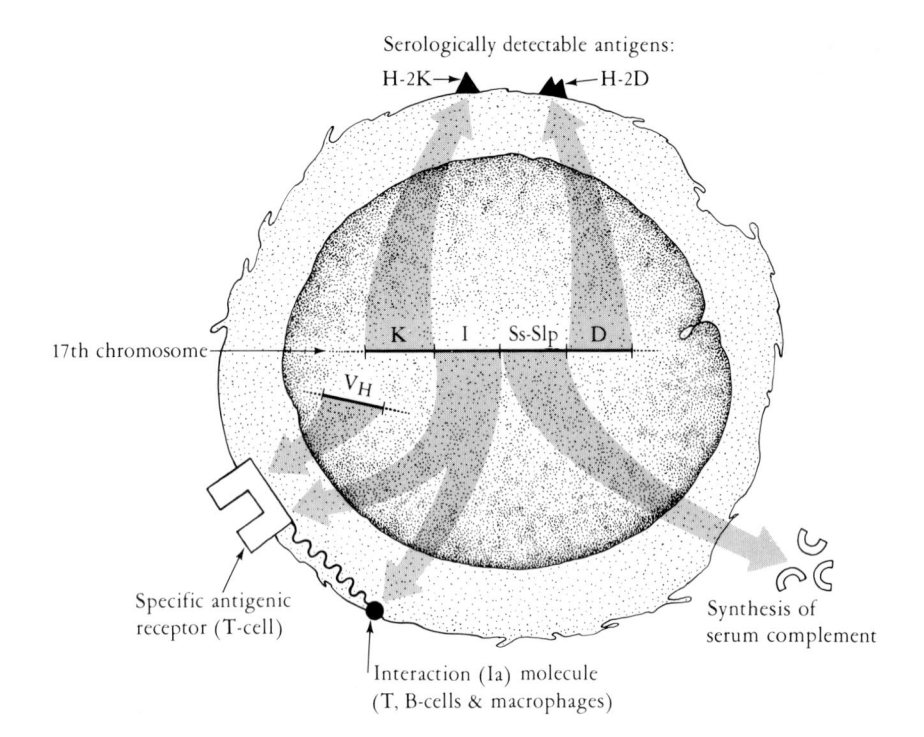

22 / BIOLOGIC ASPECTS OF TRANSPLANTATION OF GRAFTS

Figure 2–3. Functions of regions of MHC. (From Bellanti JA: Immunology II. Philadelphia, W.B. Saunders Co., p 82, 1978.)

diseases. The relationship of HLA phenotypes with human diseases, i.e., immunopathologic diseases, suggests that similar Ir-type (immune response) genes are linked to the HLA system—for instance, HLA-B27 is associated with ankylosing spondylitis and Reiter's syndrome, HLA-B8 with myasthenia gravis, and HLA-A3 with multiple sclerosis.

DONOR-RECIPIENT MATCHING

The closer the match of histocompatability antigens between the donor and the recipient, the more likely it is that the transplant will be successful. This is clearly apparent with graft survival in identical twin donor-recipient pairs as compared to that in unrelated pairs.

There are two basic principles in donor-recipient matching that are inviolable, whereas the remainder are relative requisites. First, transplantation will not be successful in the presence of ABO incompatibility. It can, however, be performed in the presence of minor blood group disparities, including Rh factors. Secondly, a positive cross-match, i.e., demonstrable circulating antibodies in the recipient against the tissue antigens of the donor, is also a contra-

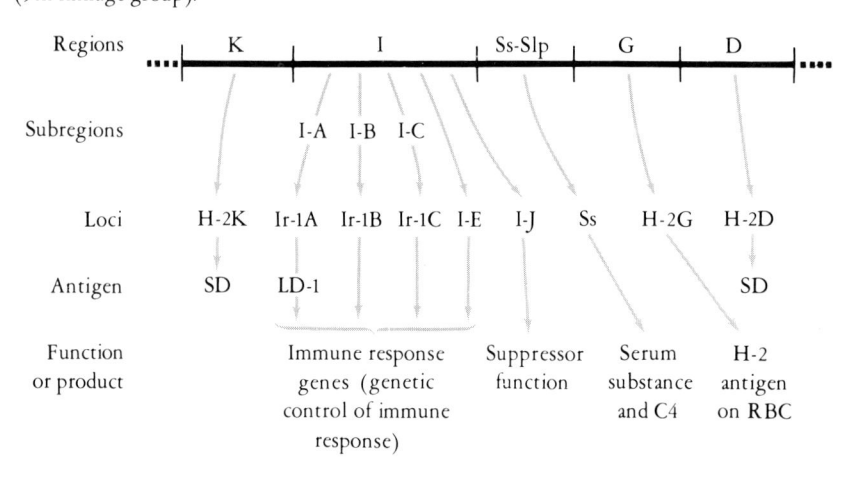

Figure 2–4. Functions of regions of MHC. (From Bellanti JA: Immunology II. Philadelphia, W.B. Saunders Co., 1978, p 83.)

indication to transplantation. Such circulating cytotoxic antibodies are routinely tested for by incubating donor lymphoid cells in recipient serum in the presence of a source of complement. After a period of incubation, a marker of cell death (such as trypan blue) is added to the cell suspension and the proportion of dead cells is counted. The presence of significant numbers of dead cells indicates a positive cross-match.

The lack of histocompatibility between recipient and donor is not a contraindication to transplantation; however, in most cases every effort is made to obtain the closest possible antigenic match for the recipient. This is done by tissue typing, i.e., identifying the antigens of loci HLA-A, HLA-B, and HLA-C on the cells of the recipient by means of monospecific antisera obtained from sensitized individuals and performing a series of individual cross-match tests with the recipient's lymphoid cells. The same is done with the cells of all potential donors, and in the absence of other critical factors, the closest match is selected to be the donor. Critical factors that might eliminate a potential donor include ABO incompatibility, antibodies in the recipient against the donor's cells, medical disability of the donor, and unwillingness to donate an organ.

Living related donors may be further matched to recipients by evaluating HLA-D locus compatibility. Compatibility for this locus is evaluated by mixed lymphocyte culture (MLC) reactivity, i.e., the degree to which recipient lymphocytes undergo blast transformation on exposure to donor lymphocytes.

IMMUNOBIOLOGY OF GRAFT REJECTION

Rejection may be defined as the process by which the immune system of the host recognizes, becomes sensitized against, and attempts to eliminate the antigenic differences of the donor organ. With the exception of autografts and isografts, some degree of rejection occurs with every transplant.

The prototype of the immunobiology of rejection is primary (first-set) rejection. In this form of rejection, the host encounters the histocompatibility antigens (mouse H-2 K and D; human HLA-A and B) on the surface of the cells of the transplant for the first time. In some as yet poorly defined manner, locally or within regional lymph nodes, macrophages process antigenic material and present it to B and T lymphocytes for sensitization. Sensitized lymphocytes may then en-

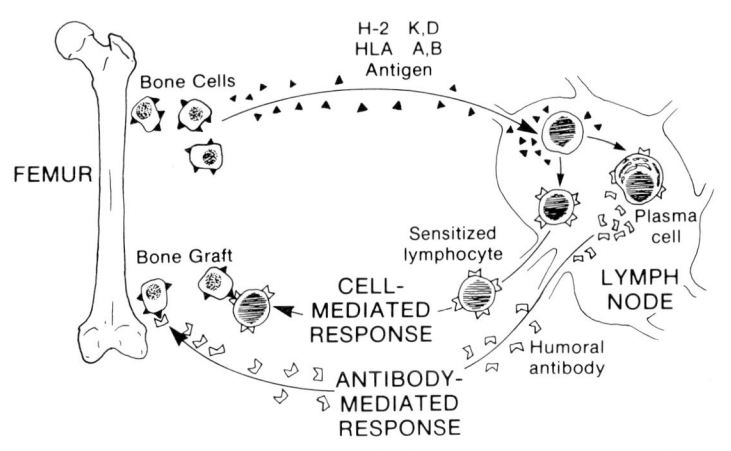

Figure 2–5. Host sensitization and effector response to a graft.

ter the peripheral circulation. Upon arriving in the grafted organ and encountering the specific antigens of the graft, sensitized lymphoid cells initiate immune injury. The immune injury may be mediated by either the humoral or the cellular path of the immune response in a variety of ways: (1) directly, by cytotoxic T cells; (2) indirectly, by soluble T cell mediators of immune injury (lymphokines); (3) by B cell–mediated (humoral) antibody; or (4) by antibody-dependent cellular cytotoxicity (ADCC) attack on the target organ. This process of primary rejection is the classic model and can become clinically evident after the first week posttransplantation (Fig. 2–5).

In contrast to primary rejection is hyperacute (secondary) rejection in which the recipient has been sensitized to the histocompatibility antigens of the graft by previous transfusions, pregnancy, or transplantation. Circulating cytotoxic antibodies to the HLA antigens of the graft may be found in the serum of recipients hyperacutely rejecting their grafts. Upon completion of the vascular anastomosis of the graft, there is prompt deposition of antibody along the vascular endothelium with activation of the complement and the coagulation systems, resulting in fibrin deposition, polymorphonuclear leukocyte infiltration, platelet thrombosis, and prompt coagulation necrosis with invariable loss of the graft (Fig. 2–6).

Acute rejection describes the clinical situation associated with abrupt onset of signs and symptoms of rejection. The graft is tender, and it is heavily infiltrated with mononuclear and inflammatory cells. Chronic rejection occurs after an extended period of time and is characterized by gradual loss of functions of the graft. On histopathologic examination, the chronically rejected graft appears infiltrated with large numbers of

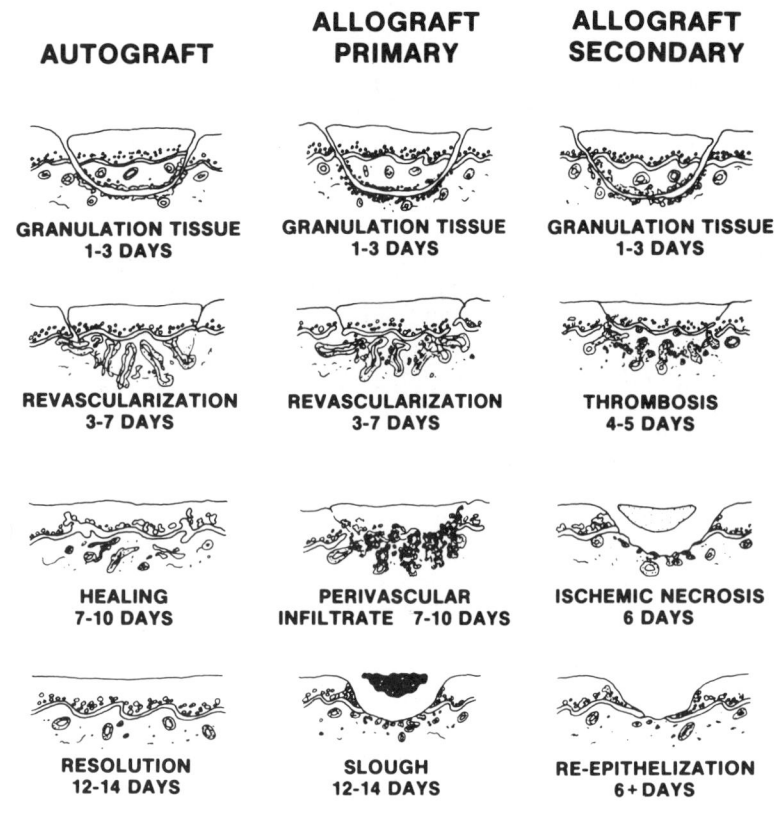

Figure 2–6. Stages of skin graft rejection: Comparison of primary and secondary (hyperacute) rejection of allogeneic grafts to a syngeneic (autologous) graft.

DIAGNOSIS AND PREVENTION OF GRAFT REJECTION

The clinical diagnosis of allograft rejection is dependent in part on the identity of the recipient and donor, since no two could be alike; thus, variations will exist in the immune response. For example, the underlying state of health of one recipient will differ from that of another, or the type of tissue being transplanted might differ. Factors affecting the recipient (host) in graft transplantation are immunologic integrity; previous sensitization; underlying disease that either may affect the immune response (uremia) or metabolism of immunosuppressive drugs (liver disease), or may exacerbate the rejection (diabetes); nutritional status; and patient compliance. The donor can be affected by the type of tissue being transplanted, his relationship to the recipient, the degree of match, and if it is a cadaver, the cause of death.

Symptoms commonly seen in graft rejection include fever, malaise, and graft tenderness. General signs seen in graft rejection are leukocytosis, hypocomplementemia, and an elevated sedimentation rate. There are more specific signs and symptoms depending on the type of tissue being transplanted. For example, in renal transplantation one can see oliguria, lymphocyturia, hematuria, proteinuria, and rising blood urea nitrogen and creatinine.

The treatment of rejection, i.e., immunosuppression, varies considerably depending on the type of transplant. The goal of immunosuppression is to prevent or minimize sensitization, because once sensitization has occurred, the suppression of the immune response becomes considerably more difficult. The recipient will usually receive the largest dose of immunosuppression just prior to or during the first week after transplantation, the period during which primary sensitization occurs. In the unfortunate instance in which the recipient has been presensitized, prompt graft rejection (hyperacute or accelerated) will ensue, defying in most cases the most strenuous attempts at immunosuppression. If no early rejection occurs, the drugs used for immunosuppression are tapered over succeeding days to weeks until a stable maintenance dose is achieved. In the event of an acute rejection, the dose of immunosuppressive agents may be increased or different drugs added to the regimen until rejection is brought under control or the graft is lost. Drugs used in immunosuppression fall into three general categories: acute inflammatory agents, antimetabolites, and cytotoxic agents.

mononuclear cells, predominantly of the T cell lineage, although B cells may also be involved.

Specific antibodies and sensitized lymphocytes interact with an allograft by virtue of the transplantation antigens expressed on living cells within the graft. For solid tissue grafts such as bone and skin, the relevant antigens are expressed fully on parenchymal (epithelial) cells, as well as on stromal and supporting tissues. For example, in skin, HLA antigens are expressed strongly on the epidermal cells that (1) form the stratified squamous surface and (2) comprise the glands and hair roots that dip down into the dermis. In addition, endothelial cells that line vascular channels within the graft also express HLA antigens. A third source of transplantation antigens within a graft is cells of the lymphoid system that populate the extravascular spaces as passenger cells. The susceptibility of a graft to rejection can be attributed to the aggregate contributions of parenchymal cells, vascular endothelial cells, and passenger leukocytes; all can provide antigenic stimulation and can serve as targets.

PROBLEMS UNIQUE TO THE ORAL CAVITY

The same genetic principles and immunologic rules that apply to other tissues and organs are applicable to transplantation in the oral region. There are, however, certain specific features that exist in the oral cavity that demand a different approach. The most obvious is that the oral cavity is densely populated with a wide variety of bacteria. The host cannot combat these microbes because of the difficulty of the host's humoral factors to diffuse through acellular, avascular grafts, i.e., bone; therefore, aseptic conditions for storage and post-transplantation are essential.

The tissue transplanted to the oral cavity can, in most cases, remain functional in a nonviable state. For example, the value of a bone graft is actually the mechanical scaffold that it provides, rather than the potential for persistent viability of its original cell population. The bony matrix will eventually become repopulated by invading cells from the host, i.e., "creeping substitution." This is not true for skin or mucous membrane, for which the persistent viability of the original cell population is essential for the usefulness of the graft.

In most cases, grafting of tissue to the oral cavity, i.e., bone, skin, or mucous membrane, does not involve the alleviation of a life-threatening situation, as with a renal or cardiac transplantation. This being the case, it is not warranted to immunologically suppress a graft recipient too severely in an attempt to salvage the transplant. The approach in oral and maxillofacial surgery has been to decrease the immunogenicity, that is to say, the property of a substance (immunogen) that endows it with the capacity to provoke a specific immune response, rather than suppress the immune system of the recipient. In the following sections, we will elaborate on the inherent immunogenicity of bone and skin (mucous membrane) and the attempts at minimizing or eliminating its immunogenicity.

BONE GRAFTS

IMMUNOBIOLOGY OF BONE

Allograft Immunogenicity

Bone is one of the most frequently transplanted tissues in the body, and it is routinely used for the repair of defects resulting from injury, neoplasms, congenital malformations, or infections. Tissue banks issue far more units of bone than any other tissue. The reason is that bone performs an allostructural function and its incorporation does not depend upon tissue survival.

Present knowledge of bone graft surgery encompasses the field of bone cell differentiation, the mechanism of osteoinduction, and the immunology of allogeneic transplants and implants. The international terminology relating to the principles and practices of bone graft surgery conforms to the general field of transplantation surgery. The terminology is based on the genome of the donor and the recipient's immune surveillance, not only of viable bone grafts but also of biochemical components of nonviable alloimplants. The term *implant* applies to nonviable bone that has been frozen, freeze dried, or sterilized by irradiation. The term also applies to bone exposed to chemical solutions for extraction of antigenic substances or chemosterilization.

A major problem that has plagued surgeons is the availability of appropriate bone transplant material. The acquisition of autogenous bone transplant material is accomplished with certain costs to the patient, which can include (1) additional surgical incision, (2) increased postoperative morbidity, (3) weakened donor bone sites, and (4) potential serious complications from any of the previous conditions. If at all possible, it is desirable to reduce the amount of surgery and surgical morbidity associated with an operative procedure; principally for this reason, allogeneic tissue has been suggested as a substitute for autogenous bone in grafting procedures. To establish the possibility of using allogeneic bone, the question of its biological acceptability for transplantation must be addressed. If allogeneic bone is indeed antigenic, what kind of immunologic response does it stimulate? Bone is composed of living osteogenic cells, some on the surface, others buried in a nonviable matrix, and has a bone marrow contact. If these tissues contain transplantation antigens, they will elicit an immune response on transplantation.

Experimental allogeneic bone grafts have been shown to produce an immune response on transplantation.[1-7] Although allogeneic bone transplantation elicits a host immunologic response, it is not known whether the immunogens responsible for the reaction come entirely from the transplanted bone. The major immunogenic component in allogeneic bone transplants is thought to be the marrow.[1-3, 8] The cells and serum within the transplant are presumed to be antigenic, whereas the matrix of the transplant, which is composed of glycoprotein, collagen, and mucopolysaccharides, may or may not be antigenic. In a study by

Brooks and others,[9] fresh and decalcified bone transplants were used to show that the bony matrix was immunogenic, since transplants were rejected at an accelerated rate if preceded by skin transplants.

Evidence for bone immunogenicity was obtained in experiments that demonstrated either second-set reactions in lymph node tissues by increased inflammation about allografts and visibly prolonged inflammatory reactions, or altered patterns of allograft repair in recipients who were presented to the donor.[3,6,7,10,11]

Some investigators have suggested that the immune response to allogeneic bone transplants is preferentially directed toward the marrow contained in the bone.[8] Thus, grafts devoid of marrow did not elicit a regional lymph node response or a second-set response when skin, syngeneic with the bone, was transplanted to the same recipient prior to the bone.[3,7,8]

The Humoral Component of Allograft Immunogenicity

Histologic studies have shown that allografts of bone become infiltrated with small round cells, plasma cells, and macrophages, suggesting that an immune response is occurring.[1,2,11,12] Elves[13] reviewed the literature on humoral antibodies produced by allografts and observed that marrow-containing cancellous bone elicited a pattern of antibody production similar to that seen following skin grafting. In contrast, the response to allogeneic spleen cells injected intradermally is more rapid. Grafts of marrow-free cancellous or cortical allografted bone gave rise to an antibody response that was delayed in onset. Elves[13] postulated that the delayed humoral response to bone and skin grafts is due to a delay in the antigen leaving the graft until vascular and lymphatic connections are made. He suggested that the antigen that triggers the immune response to these grafts is in the form of viable cells. Elves showed that removal of bone marrow from cancellous bone allografts does result in an alteration of the pattern of antibody production. The interval between grafting and appearance of antibodies in the majority of recipients of such grafts is at least six weeks. In the case of cortical grafts, the interval is longer. With both of these types of marrow-depleted grafts, there was a higher proportion of animals that never developed antibody. In marrow-depleted bone grafts the sensitizing antigens are derived from either endosteal osteoblasts or from osteocytes that are exposed secondary to bone graft matrix resorption.

Langer and others[14] assessed the humoral and cellular immune response to allografted bone using the leukocyte migration test. They observed varying levels of immunity: at two weeks a good response was evident, at four weeks a much weaker response was seen, and at eight weeks the response returned. When a comparison of the leukocyte migration test was performed in serum-free medium and in media containing syngeneic sera, the greater immune response was noted with media containing no serum. Langer and colleagues[14] suggested that substances are present in the sera of bone-graft recipients which can act to abrogate the normally observed transplantation immunity to allografts. They postulated that these substances were blocking antibodies; that is, antibodies are produced to surface antigens on the target cells in the allogeneic bone. The antibodies combine with the surface antigens of the target cells and the histocompatibility antigens are then no longer visibly accessible to the receptors of the aggressor lymphocytes. This phenomenon is called enhancement and results in prolongation of the presence of the allografted bone. The possible role of enhancement (blocking) in bone transplantation was first suggested by Bonfiglio and Jeter[10] when they noted a decreased cellular response around bone allografts in rabbits that had received prior inoculations with bone extract. Chalmers[5] also referred to this possibility to explain the prolonged survival of skin grafts in rats that had received grafts of frozen bone.

Muscolo and others[15] noted, using a cytotoxicity assay to measure the humoral response to allogeneic bone grafts, that a complete first-set and second-set graft response was detectable. They postulated that cellular alloantigens present in marrow-free bone may be responsible for the humoral cytotoxic reactivity. In a later study, Muscolo and associates[16] used *in vitro* studies on isolated bone cells to detect the presence of transplantation (histocompatibility) antigens. Bone cells were cultured with allogeneic lymphocytes and exposed to cytotoxic sera containing antibodies against transplantation antigens to determine their antigenic profile. Their results suggested that bone cells were killed by specifically raised cytotoxic antibodies directed only against serologically defined (SD) transplantation antigens on the cell surface. Additionally, studies with adsorbed sera suggested "sharing" of histocompatibility antigens between bone cells and lymphocytes.

Halloran and others[17,18] studied the alloantibody response of inbred strains of mice receiving orthotopic cortical bone allografts. They found that such grafts were highly immunogenic, resulting in antibody responses at least as strong as those to skin allografts in the same combinations of inbred strains of mice. The duration of the response to a single bone allograft was prolonged (> 10 months). The antibody response was shown to be directed against H-2K, H-2D, Ia, and at least two non–H-2 antigens. Although the great majority of the parenchymal cells of the graft were dead, the immunogenicity of the graft required living cells, since bone that had previously been frozen and thawed was nonimmunogenic. By retransplantation of the bone allografts to a second recipient, they showed it was possible to demonstrate that the grafts remained immunogenic for at least four weeks after transplantation, indicating that the living immunogenic cells survived in the recipient for at least four weeks. Such cells may be of the cortical bone itself (osteocytes) or else residual bone marrow elements, "passenger leukocytes," or vascular endothelium.

The Cell-Mediated Component of Immunogenicity

The cell-mediated response is probably the most important immune mechanism in the rejection of tissue (bone) allografts. In the case of adult bone allografts, a prolonged inflammatory reaction in which small lymphocytes are prominent has been observed.[1,2,5,6,10,11] There have been several attempts to quantify the immune response to bone grafts using various parameters. Burwell and Gowland[1,2] assayed variations in weight and histologic changes in draining regional lymph nodes as an assay of cell-mediated immunity. They found an increase in weight of the regional lymph nodes draining subcutaneously implanted allogeneic cancellous bone in rabbits. A smaller increase in weight of draining nodes was also found following an autograft of bone. In histologic sections, the enlarged nodes draining allografts showed the typical enlargement in areas of the paracortical zone with the appearance of large lymphoid cells in increasing numbers, up to five days after grafting. Increased numbers of plasma cells were also seen in the medullary portion of those nodes, and, in addition, germinal center changes occurred; both of these latter phenomena would suggest that the nodes are also active in antibody production.

Bonfiglio and Jeter[10] observed numerous lymphocytes, macrophages, and scattered eosinophils between an allogeneic graft cortex and surrounding muscle at one week after grafting. This reaction reaches its maximum intensity at three weeks. They failed to detect serum-bound antibodies by any of the "usual" serologic tests and postulated that the reaction was a delayed-type hypersensitivity (cell-mediated) response. To test the effect of a second allograft, a series of rabbits was operated upon in pairs, each receiving a first graft in the right foreleg, followed by right foreleg amputation at intervals of one to twelve weeks. A second graft from the same donor was then placed in the left ulna. A comparison of the inflammatory reactions of the primary and secondary allografts revealed an "increase in persistence of the reaction after three weeks." A secondary fresh autograft at four weeks showed inflammatory cells between the cortex and overlying necrotic periosteal new bone. This observation paralleled the second-set reaction described for other allografted tissues.

Bonfiglio and Jeter[10] suggested that an immune reaction between host and antigenic allogeneic bone existed. The character and timing of the reaction were suggestive of a delayed-type (cell-mediated) hypersensitivity response.

Ray[19] took this one step further. He took fresh allogeneic bone and transplanted it to a host animal and developed a delayed rejection response. If he took the serum of plasma from the sensitized host and injected it into another animal of the same strain, there was no transfer of immunity. In other words, if the second animal was challenged with a similar allogeneic bone graft, it too showed a first-set (primary) delayed rejection. But if lymph or spleen cells are taken from the first animal and transferred to a related animal, the second animal when challenged with an identical bone allograft shows an accelerated rejection or a second-set reaction. This indicates that the immune response involved in rejection of the osseous allograft is cell-bound rather than circulating or humoral antibodies.

A cellular immune response was also confirmed by Langer et al.[14] using a leukocyte migration test and by Muscolo et al.,[16] who studied a mixed lymphocyte culture assay. Muscolo and others[16] concluded that the cellular reaction was immunologically specific in nature, since there was no reaction to a third party. They stated that the reaction time was related to major histocompatibility antigens of grafted bone and that the reaction was stronger with complete bone than with grafted bone free of marrow.

In summary, the accumulated evidence suggests that bone is immunogenic and that marrow contributes significantly to this immunogenicity. The histocompatibility antigens in allogeneic transplants of bone are presumably the protein of glycoproteins on cell surfaces, whereas cytoplasmic and nuclear components or matrix constituents are not known to elicit transplant rejection.[15, 19, 20] At present, it is not known whether the rejection of a bone allograft is antibody-mediated, cell-mediated, or both.[20] If sensitized lymphocytes contact foreign cell surfaces, a series of unknown reactions occurs that results in graft cell destruction. Cytotoxic antibodies can participate in organ graft destruction if complement is present. Other immunologic factors in the immune rejection might include chemotactic and osteoclastic activating factors (OAF),[21, 22] release of anaphylatoxins, and the associated inflammatory hallmarks such as vasoconstriction, vasodilation, sticky platelets, and thrombus formation.

Histopathology of Immune Response to Bone Allografts

The initial histologic reponse of the host to a fresh allograft is similar to that of an autograft. At the end of the first week post-transplantation, an inflammatory response at the periphery of the graft is seen.[1,2,6,8,10,11,13] The inflammatory reaction reaches a peak of activity toward the end of the second week, with lymphocytes as the major cell type present. During the next two months, lymphocytes continue to predominate and a fibrous tissue barrier encapsulating the allograft develops. The inflammatory response either abates at this point or can continue as chronic inflammation, persisting for eight months or more.[10]

The initial regenerating vascular pattern surrounding the allograft is less extensive than that occurring in the autograft, and end-to-end anastomoses occur infrequently.[23-25] At the end of the first week, inflammatory cells are around the vessels, the vessels become occluded, and hyalinization of the vascular walls is apparent.[6, 7, 25] Subsequently, progressive necrosis of the periosteal cells ensues and peripheral osteocyte death occurs.[1, 2, 6, 8, 10, 11]

The rate at which a transplant is incorporated into the host skeleton indicates whether a transplant is accepted or rejected. Successful incorporation includes the formation of callus around the transplant-host junction as well as the internal repair of the transplant. New bone formation has been observed at the periphery of the autograft within the first week, with a maximal osteogenic peak near the end of the first week.[26] A similar process occurs in the allograft, although osteogenesis may be quantitatively inferior.[3]

Once the allograft undergoes necrosis as a result of vascular insufficiency, a second phase of osteogenesis may be initiated by the host tissue approximately four weeks after transplantation.[27-29] This secondary osteogenic phase in allografts is not as successful as osteogenesis in fresh autografts, since remodeling at two months is less complete than that found in comparable autogenous transplants, with resorption and new bone formation absent throughout the allogeneic transplant.[1-3, 8, 10, 11, 30] At eight months post-transplantation, transplant revascularization is not as complete as the autogenous vascularity at one month.[23, 25, 31]

In a six-month study of a fibula allograft in a dog, two basic courses of allograft repair were observed.[32] One repair course reflected strong genetic transplantation differences between the donor and host, as the allograft was rapidly and completely resorbed. Roentgenographic, microradiographic, and tetracycline fluorescence studies suggested that this vigorous rejection of an allograft occurs by continuous resorption at the periphery without any internal creeping substitutional repair.

The second allograft repair course was chronic and suggested less marked genetic transplantation differences between the donor and host. This second repair course was characterized by (1) nonunion or delayed graft-host union; (2) an increased incidence of fatigue fractures concomitant with a loss in the transplant's diameter; (3) considerably less internal repair (i.e., the amount of viable bone formed to replace necrotic bone; creeping substitution) than that seen for autografts; and (4) the formation of a callus that bridged the transplanted segments. Despite the formation of a bridging callus, the allografts were structurally weak, since fatigue fractures and nonunions occurred frequently.

Effect of Immune Response on Healing of Allogeneic Bone Grafts

In a series of papers by Halloran and others,[17, 18, 33, 34] it was postulated that impaired healing of allogeneic bone grafts was immunologically mediated. Halloran and others developed a technique for orthotopic bone transplantation in inbred mice.[17, 18] A section of a recipient mouse's tibia was removed and replaced by a similar section from the donor animal. The graft was held in place by internal fixation. Bone healing was assessed clinically, histologically, radiologically, and by torsion testing. The degree of bone healing in donor-recipient combinations differing at H-2 (major histocompatibility), non–H-2 (minor histocompatibility), or H-Y (sex) antigens was compared to the degree of healing in syngeneic controls. The incidence of nonunion was significantly increased in H-2–disparate groups. In the mouse strain combinations tested, the order of importance of the genetic disparities influencing allogeneic bone grafts was H-2, H-Y, non–H-2. The adverse effect on healing was accompanied by accelerated rejection of subsequent skin grafts, implying that the delayed healing has an immunologic basis.

Previous histologic studies have suggested that the interference with bone healing is attributable to an immunologic response by the host against the graft, which interfered with the revascularization of the grafts.[12,35] With this thought in mind, Halloran's group speculated that immunosuppression may improve the healing of allogeneic bone. In a pilot project, bone graft healing was studied in BALB/c nude mice (mice that lacked circulating T cells; no cell-mediated immunity), receiving either H-2^d identical bone from heterozygous (nu/+) littermates, or fully allogeneic bone from C57BL/b (H-2^b) donors.[36] The results showed that no antibody was produced and no impairment of bone healing could be demonstrated in allogeneic bone transplanted into nu/nu recipients; syngeneic and allogeneic bone healed equally well. In comparison, antibody responses were strong, and healing was always impaired when immunocompetent animals received H-2 disparate bone. This result demonstrated that, in the absence of host immune responses, healing of allogeneic bone may be entirely normal. Their next series of experiments compared the effects on healing of various methods of reducing the induced immune response to allogeneic bone grafts, either by pretreating the graft or by immunosuppressing the recipient.[34] Tibial grafts from an inbred strain of mice, B10.D2 (H-2^d), either untreated or pretreated in various ways, were transplanted into allogeneic B10 recipient mice (H-2^a). The antibody response was followed and the extent of bone healing at four months was assessed. Pretreatment of the graft by x-irradiation, freezing, or incubation in alloantisera (either anti–H-2 or anti-Ia) reduced or abolished the immunogenicity of the graft.

Immunosuppression of the recipient with methotrexate (MTX) or antilymphocyte serum (ALS) also greatly depressed the antibody response. But when graft healing was assessed, this being the most important parameter in determining successful bone grafting, none of these treatments except ALS improved the delayed healing of the bone allografts. It was postulated that x-irradiation, freezing, alloantiserum pretreatment, and MTX all interfered with bone healing directly by removing or devitalizing any remaining living donor cells in the graft. In contrast, treatment with ALS did not remove this critical osteogenic precursor population of Ia-positive cells and therefore did not delay healing of the allogeneic bone graft. It would seem that if one desires to use immunosuppression to improve bone healing, it must be done only with agents that have no direct effect on the healing of the graft itself.

Michejda and others[37] investigated *in utero* allogeneic bone transplantation in primates in the hope of finding a material to repair anomalous skeletal development during prenatal growth and differentiation. They theorized that the fetal-placental allograft and malignant neoplasia are the only naturally occurring biologic conditions in which antigenic tissue is fully tolerated by the immune system. In their present study, they performed allogeneic transplantation within the humeral midshaft of fetal rhesus monkeys *in utero*. Two types of fetus-to-fetus bone transplants were applied: (1) the humerus was severed cross-sectionally and a segment or link of bone was replaced; (2) particles of crushed humerus, mixed in an agar-enriched medium (bone paste), were applied to refill a cavity after extensive surgical ablation in the humeral midshaft without complete severance of the shaft. Incorporation and/or fusion of the allograft tissue with endogenous bone was studied during the remainder of intrauterine development and up to six months postnatally, using radiographic analysis of long bone growth and histologic evaluation of osteoblastic activity within the osteotomized humeral midshaft. Concurrently, they observed neonatal monkeys to assess limb dexterity postoperatively. The findings of Michejda and coworkers[37] indicate that the immune surveillance system of fetal monkeys may be tolerant of these bone allografts; alternatively, healing by substitution may also occur. The radiographic and histologic results demonstrated that both of the transplantation procedures used in this study achieved restoration of the long bone. The use of bone paste allowed the investigators to sculpt the allograft to the desired conformation. The results were encouraging and indicated that fetal allogeneic bone transplantation may be useful for intrauterine repair of skeletal anomalies in man.

Types of Allografts

Numerous techniques have been devised to minimize the antigenic differences between the donor and the recipient of a bone allograft. Blocking the host's immune response and destroying the antigens within the bone allograft have been suggested as means of minimizing antigenic differences. Bone allografts that have been treated to destroy the antigenicity prior to use lack viable cells and therefore should be referred to as implants rather than transplants.

Frozen Allografts. Frozen bone implants were frequently used as substitute materials for autografts because of their lack of antigenicity. However, the following experimental and clinical findings demonstrated that bone immunogenicity was partially retained: (1) a cellular foreign body reaction occurred which was less intense than that of fresh allogeneic transplants but which sometimes persisted for seven months[10, 11]; (2) second-set skin transplant rejections could be experimentally induced[10, 11]; (3) frozen cortico-cancellous,[14, 38-41] allogeneic bone elicited cytotoxic antibodies; this is in contrast to Elves' finding of no antibody production[13]; (4) revascularization of frozen implants was delayed at least one month[42]; (5) freezing destroyed the early osteogenic peak and adversely affected the amount and incidence of new bone and callus formation[43]; and (6) fracture implants usually did not reunite.[43]

Freeze-dried Allografts. The most commonly used bone substitute for autogenous bone transplants is the lyophilized allogeneic bone. Freeze-drying, as the term implies, involves the removal of water from tissues that are frozen. In addition to reduced allograft antigenicity, freeze-drying results in long-term presentation of biologically useful tissues. Although tissue viability is not maintained, freeze-drying preserves three major specimen characteristics: morphology, solubility, and chemistry. Present philosophy states that the preservation technique of freeze-drying is associated with a marked reduction in antigenicity as judged by a variety of parameters.

Chalmers[12] demonstrated an early-onset but less intense inflammatory infiltrate of freeze-dried bone allograft (FDBA) when compared to fresh allografts. Burwell and Gowland[8] and Bonfiglio and others[11] noted a reduction in tissue response to FDBA as compared to fresh allografts. Several studies[35, 44, 45] have shown no accelerated rejection of a fresh skin allograft following a primary FDBA from the same tissue donor. Burwell and Gowland[8] noted that FDBA failed to cause an appreciable response in regional lymph nodes. Elves,[13] using inbred rats, failed to detect cytotoxic antibodies after first-set implants of FDBA. This was confirmed by Langer and others,[14] who also demonstrated the presence of "blocking" antibodies induced by FDBA. Friedlaender, Strong, and Sell[40] studied fresh and preserved bone allografts in a skeletal bed in rabbits. Peripheral lymphocytes from the allograft donors served as target cells, and these were exposed to either serum or lymphocytes from the graft recipients four to five weeks following surgery. Freeze-dried cortical bone failed to sensitize the recipients as judged by this assay, and freeze-dried cancellous bone appeared to be weakly antigenic. In humans, Lundgren, Moller, and Thorsby[46] were unable to demonstrate the presence of cytotoxic lymphocytes in two patients following FDBA.

Autolyzed Antigen-Extracted Allogeneic (AAA) Bone. Autolyzed antigen-extracted allogeneic (AAA) bone is a demineralized cortical bone that can stimulate or induce osteogenesis.[47, 48] This implant material has been advocated over freeze-dried bone because of the maintenance of a diffusible bone morphogenetic protein (BMP) in its preparation.[49, 50] Freeze-drying destroys BMP, and thus the allogeneic bone has no osteogenic induction capability.[50] The test for BMP is the differentiation of somatic mesenchymal cells into bone in response to the matrix residue.[48] Urist claims that transplantation antigens can be extracted by chloroform methanol. Autodigestion of bone in neutral buffer solutions, *in vitro*, removes from the tissue soluble proteins that are capable of producing an alloimmune (delayed hypersensitivity) response.[49, 50] Tissue typing is stated to be unnecessary in recipients of AAA bone.[50]

Xenografts

Numerous xenograft materials have been used clinically as substitutes for autogenous bone grafts. Bovine bone was a relatively popular alternative to autogenous bone during the 1950's and early 1960's. The clinician had two choices: Kiel bone, which was bovine bone treated with hydrogen peroxide that converted protein into protein urates with urea,[51] and Boplant, which was bovine bone treated with beta-propiolactone and freeze-dried.[52] Both types of xenogenic implants became clinically unacceptable because the antigens were not destroyed, and they therefore elicited rejection episodes characterized by fever, inflammation, resorption, or sequestration.[52, 53] Emmings[33] decalcified Boplant specimens and implanted them in mongrel dogs and humans. There were no signs histologically or clinically of any rejection of the decalcified Boplant, and he claimed that the material was immunologically inert.

Deproteinized bone implants were obtained by ethylenediamine extraction.[26, 54] These implants were found to cause accelerated rejections of secondary fresh skin allografts.[44] Other reports have shown that deproteinized implants were not well incorporated into the host skeleton as compared with autografts, although second-set rejection was not observed.[52, 55] Anderson and others[26] determined that the deproteinized implants did not provoke an inflammatory response, although greater numbers of multinucleated giant cells were associated with the implant than were observed with fresh allogeneic transplants.

Healing and Revascularization of Bone Grafts

Grafting systems should be immunologically inert, have an osteogenic effect on the surrounding bone and soft tissues, thus stimulating new bone formation to replace host bone, have a minimal inflammatory response that would precipitate a rejection phenomenon, and, lastly, withstand the forces of function.[56] Both autologous and allogeneic bone grafts have been used experimentally and clinically. Moderate success for various types of ridge augmentation has been shown using these systems.[57-59] Although other metallic and bone substitute systems are also currently utilized, bone grafting techniques are still a viable option in many clinical instances.

A review of the basic stages of healing and revascularization of bone grafts is important in understanding their fate. The vascular response to a bone graft placed either on, or within, the edentulous ridge follows a well-documented sequence of steps.[60-63] When the bone graft is first placed in the area, the cortical portion of bone is avascular and has very few viable cells on its surface. This bone graft subsequently becomes replaced by host bone. During this replacement, a vascular sequence is observed. The area surrounding the bone graft becomes hypervascular. The bone graft elicits a proliferation of angioblasts and small capillaries in the early stages of healing. This proliferation is temporally different between the allogeneic and autologous bone grafts. The autologous bone grafts tend to initiate an earlier angioblastic proliferation within the first week of grafting, whereas the allogeneic bone graft tends to elicit a later (7 to 14 days) proliferative response after the hypervascular response of blood vessels are seen penetrating the bone graft on its superior, inferior, lateral, and medial surfaces. These blood vessels bring with them the elements of osteogenic bone formation and replacement. Osteoclasts are seen resorbing the bone at the periphery of the bone graft. This avascular acellular bone graft is gradually replaced while new bone is laid down at the periphery and within the cortical bone graft. Autologous bone grafts have a far greater amount of intracortical bone replacement than allogeneic grafts.[63, 64] Once the bone graft is replaced, which occurs at approximately three to six months in the autologous graft system and at six months to one year in the allogeneic graft system, the hypervascular response gradually disappears.[63, 64]

The histologic response that corresponds to the vascular response is also sequential in both the allogeneic and the autologous graft system.[60-64] Granulation tissue with fibroblastic and angioblastic proliferation is followed by a proliferation of immature osteoid tissue at the periphery of the graft. The temporal sequence of this response is delayed in the allogeneic graft when compared to the autologous graft. After the osteoid is replaced by mature bone, there is no evidence of the grafted avascular acellular bone graft. Occasionally, small pieces of graft become sequestered in an area of the graft site and are surrounded by a chronic inflammatory response. These little areas of sequestration are gradually resorbed and at six months to one year there is very little evidence of any sequestration in the graft site.

It would be helpful to review the physiology of bone healing and its relationship to bone grafting to understand and evaluate the sequence of graft healing. Graft healing and the subsequent formation of new bone occurs in one of three ways: osteogenesis (survival theory),[65] osteoinduction,[66, 67] or osteoconduction (creeping substitution).[68, 69] Osteogenesis occurs when the graft itself supplies viable osteoblasts as the source of new bone. Osteoinduction occurs when the graft in some way "turns on" the surrounding host tissues to stimulate osteoblastic activity and subsequent new bone formation. Lastly, osteoconduction occurs when undifferentiated mesenchymal cells invade the graft followed by the formation of cartilage that subsequently undergoes ossification. With most autologous bone grafts, few osteoblasts survive the early weeks of transplantation. No viable osteoblasts are observed to survive the transplant with allogeneic bone grafts. Thus, the survival theory does not appear to be valid for the allogeneic grafted bone but may be valid for the autologous grafted bone early in the postgrafting period. At no time during the resorption phase are fibroblastic ingrowths and associated cartilage formation seen within the allografts. There is evidence of fibroblastic ingrowths in autografts. Therefore, osteoconduction does occur in autografts, but there is little evidence to suggest that any osteoconduction occurs in allografts. Immature new bone is seen forming along the resorbing host cortical bone in both allografts and autografts, supporting the theory of osteoinduction.[60-64]

There are many variables in bone grafting, and an understanding of these variables will help to clarify the fate of various bone graft systems. These variables can be divided into donor site and recipient site variables.

The donor site variables are specific to the type of bone (i.e., allogeneic vs. autologous), the quality of bone (i.e., cancellous vs. cortical), and the particle size of the bone. Autologous bone is far more osteoinductive than allogeneic bone. Allogeneic bone has been shown to have a very slow and very minimal osteoinductive potential.[60, 62, 63] Autologous bone, although far more osteoinductive, has two major disadvantages. The donor site surgery is not without associated morbidity, which is one of the major disadvantages of autologous bone grafting. The second drawback is associated with the intense and early osteoinductive response that the autologous graft elicits. Along with this response, there is an increased amount of osteoclastic activity with subsequent bone resorption. The net result of this intense response is not only an increased osteogenic induction but also an increased resorption. Hence, the net augmentation of the edentulous ridge is decreased when compared to the allogeneic bone grafts.[60-64]

Allogeneic bone grafts tend to be retained by the body longer because of slow replacement and tend to have a greater bulk of augmentation as a net result.[60, 62, 64] In general, allogeneic bone grafts, because of their lack of vascularity and cellularity and because of a minimal but present immunologic response, tend to be used sporadically in the clinical situation. Care must be taken in using allogeneic bone to make sure that minimal oral contamination occurs during graft placement, since there seems to be an increased rejection phenomenon with subsequent dehiscence and loss of bone with this rejection. There are significant differences between the host response to cortical vs. cancellous bone. The cortical bone grafts tend to be slowly replaced and to act as a scaffold for new bone proliferation. The host response is very gradual, and very little viability can be expected of grafted cortical bone. Again, autologous cortical bone tends to have more viable cells and has greater survival than allogeneic cortical bone.[61-63] Cancellous bone has very little scaffolding effect and should not be used when one hopes to obtain osseous bulk by replacement or osteoinduction. Cancellous bone tends to be resorbed rather rapidly with very little net osseous bulk.[60, 61] It should be used in combination with cortical grafting to help induce osteogenesis or for a three-walled discontinuity defect such as an alveolar cleft defect in the maxilla.

Particle size has been shown to be critical in cortical cancellous bone augmentation. Two sizes of autologous bone chips were compared to determine the size that revascularizes faster and what effect this has on the resorption of the graft.[60] To accomplish this, autologous chips of iliac corticocancellous bone of either $2 \times 2 \times 2$ mm or $5 \times 5 \times 2$ mm were placed bilaterally in the mandibular cortex of monkeys. In general, the small-particle graft was quicker to revascularize, showed more osteoclastic activity, and resorbed much more quickly and completely than did the large-particle graft. Therefore, the resultant net gain in alveolar ridge contour was less with the small-particle grafts. Additionally, Burwell[1] has demonstrated that very small bone particles are not recognized as bone and are resorbed.

A similar study was performed utilizing allogeneic particles of the same dimensions as in the previous study.[60] Both the large and the small particle grafts showed complete revascularization and a significant increase in the dimensions of the lateral cortical plate. Unlike the findings with autologous particulate onlay bone grafts, the sites of the allogeneic lyophilized grafts were clinically evident as exostoses along the lateral cortical plate, even six months postoperatively. The allogeneic bone is slowly removed by the host and during the interim acts as a scaffold to allow new subperiosteal and endosteal bone formation.

Recipient site variables include the vascular quality of the tissue bed, the presence or absence of oral contamination, and the type of graft system needed, i.e., interpositional, onlay, or discontinuity grafting.

Irradiated or previously scarred tissue beds present serious obstacles to free bone grafting. Tissue that has been previously irradiated should be evaluated for the amount and type of irradiation received and the physical characteristics of the contemplated recipient bed. In many instances, hyperbaric oxygen therapy will be indicated to improve tissue vascularity and increase the probability of graft success.

If scarring is present from trauma or previous surgical intervention, excision of excessive scar should be considered to eliminate poorly vascularized tissue.

Bone grafts to the oral and maxillofacial region have an increased incidence of success if oral contamination is eliminated or reduced. Whenever possible, an extraoral route should be utilized to minimize oral contamination. When this is not achievable, care should be taken to enhance the intraoral closure to minimize oral contamination.

Lastly, the type of graft system used has a marked effect on the success of the graft. Interpositional grafts fare better than onlay grafts. They have an enhanced vascular bed, tend to increase the scaffold effect, and are not directly subjected to the stresses of masticatory function.[62] Discontinuity grafts have special requirements, which will be discussed in Chapter 10.

SKIN GRAFTS

A skin graft is a segment of dermis and epidermis that has been completely separated from its blood supply and donor-site attachment before being transplanted to another area of the body, its recipient site. Skin grafts consist of the epidermis and a portion of the dermis if they are of the partial-thickness type (split-thickness skin graft). The complete-thickness type (full-thickness skin graft) contains the epidermis and all of the dermis. Full-thickness grafts contain varying portions of the sweat glands, sebaceous glands, hair follicles, and capillaries of the skin, depending on their thickness.

Skin grafts can be classified as autografts, allografts, or xenografts; split-thickness or full-thickness. In oral and maxillofacial surgery, the use of autogenous split-thickness skin or mucosal grafts predominates.

Split-thickness skin grafts contain epidermis and a portion of the dermis. The split-thickness graft is further subdivided, depending on the amount of dermis included. Surgeons tend to refer to skin grafts as being either thin, intermediate, or thick grafts (depending on the setting of the dermatome at 10 to 25 thousandths of an inch, the translucency of the graft, and the bleeding pattern of the donor site). The translucency of a skin graft will vary from the thin split-thickness graft, with its translucent tissue-paper appearance, to that of the thick split-thickness graft, which is nearly opaque. The pattern of bleeding at the donor site also varies from a high intensity of fine bleeding points with the thin graft to a lower intensity of bleeding from larger points with the thick split-thickness graft.[70]

The thinner a skin graft, the more the interface of fibrous tissue between the graft and the recipient site contracts during the first few months after transplantation. The thick split-thickness skin graft contracts less than an intermediate-thickness graft, whereas the full-thickness graft contracts hardly at all.

The thin split-thickness skin graft (STSG) is more likely to survive on its recipient site because it can survive well during the phase of plasmatic absorption and can therefore wait longer for vascularization. Also, skin from a more vascular donor site becomes vascularized more rapidly.[71]

The thin STSG taken from a hirsute donor site will not have hair growing following transplantation, whereas the thick STSG and full-thickness graft will usually contain some hair follicles to permit the growth of hair.

The donor site for a thin STSG re-epithelializes more rapidly than that for a thick STSG. The donor site of a full-thickness skin graft does not re-epithelialize because no accessory skin structures remain.

In order for a skin graft to take, it must have a vascular recipient bed, fixed contact to its recipient bed, and proper preparation of any granulation tissue.

The Vascularity of the Recipient Bed. A skin graft requires a sufficiently good blood supply in its recipient site for survival. A quantitative estimate of this need can be judged by observing whether ample support for growth of granulation tissue exists. This does not imply that the skin graft has to be placed on granulation tissue but rather that it has to be placed on a vascular bed. The only exception to this rule is the "bridging phenomenon,"[70] whereby that portion of a skin graft overlying a small avascular area may survive. This phenomenon is based on the fact that collateral vessels connect the skin graft in the avascular area to the vascularized graft and serve as a network for transporting both an initial plasmatic circulation and a later ingrowth of capillary buds to nourish this area. In ideal circumstances, this collateral circulation will bridge a gap of 0.5 cm from any one margin.

Comparative Vascularity of Recipient Beds. Cortical bone denuded of periosteum, cartilage denuded of perichondrium, and tendon denuded of paratendon are avascular on their external surfaces and cannot be expected to nourish a skin graft placed in contact with them. Neither will any of the body's stratified squamous epithelium support the growth of a skin graft.

Heavily irradiated tissue is a relatively poor recipient bed for skin grafts because it has a poor blood supply. Fat has fewer blood vessels than dermis, fascia, and most other tissues and thus should be considered among the least desirable recipient beds.

Long-standing granulation tissue also serves as a poor bed for skin grafts because it becomes fibrotic, less vascular, and infected, as do the exposed surfaces of chronic ulcers. Arteriosclerotic changes in the blood vessels in the lower extremity of older patients and in diabetic patients make these regions poor recipient beds. In general, recipient beds having limited circulation will require a longer period for the completion of vascularization of a skin graft and consequently require more extended immobilization and aftercare than do grafts placed on beds of greater vascularity.

Thin STSG have a more abundant network of capillaries on their undersurface than do thick STSG or full-thickness grafts. This fine network of terminal vessels is located in the superficial dermis, whereas slightly larger vessels are located in the deep dermis.

Vascularization of Skin Grafts

Several excellent articles on this subject have been written by Smahel and Clodius[71] and Rudolph and Klein.[72]

1. Plasmatic Imbibition. Almost immediately after a skin graft comes into contact with the underlying bed, it begins to absorb a plasma-like fluid from it. This fluid is absorbed into the spongelike structure of the capillary network by capillary action, providing a similar state to *in vivo* tissue culture.[73-76] On microscopic examination, it can be observed that this fluid lying in the endothelium-lined spaces of the graft contains a few erythrocytes. While this process continues, a fibrin network is also being formed between the graft and the recipient bed to hold the graft in place. The plasma-like fluid appears to be absorbed into the graft (plasmatic imbibition) over the first 48 hours, causing its weight to gradually increase (20 per cent increased weight in 24 hours and 30 per cent increased weight in 48 hours).[45] At the 48-hour point, blood flow begins in the graft, and the plasma-like fluid is carried away. The pink color that some grafts attain during the first 12 hours after transplantation probably results from the accumulation of red blood cells drawn into the capillaries of the graft by the plasmatic circulation.[78]

2. Inosculation of Blood Vessels. During the first 48 hours after grafting, vascular buds grow in the intervening fibrin network that binds the skin graft to its recipient site.[45, 77, 79] At this point, two major views exist as to the next step: one is that there is a random inosculation of the vascular buds from the bed with both arteries and veins in the graft. Following this, the blood enters the graft vessels, moving to and fro in a sluggish manner until the fourth to seventh day, when true circulation occurs in the graft. The other view is that vascular buds grow into the graft, even inside some of the old graft vessels, forming an entirely new vascular network.[80] In support of ingrowth of vascular buds, Haller and Billingham[81] found the vascular pattern in the healed grafts of the hamster cheek pouch to be the same as before grafting. They also observed that blockage of the graft vessels occurred by injecting them with silicone rubber solution prior to grafting. This was followed by necrosis of the graft.

The development of anastomoses between bed and graft and the flow of blood into the vessels of the graft have an inhibiting effect on further proliferation of the vascular buds. If a hematoma or seroma separates the graft from its bed, the inhibiting effect will be slower in occurring. Proliferation of granulation tissue will continue, and connective tissue infiltration into the dermis will occur to varying degrees.[80]

Concurrent with those events in the blood circulation, continuity of the lymphatic systems in the bed and graft is being restored. Several investigators have shown that the lymphatic drainage from the graft is established by the fourth or fifth postoperative day, when graft lymphatics connect with recipient bed lymphatics.[82-84]

It is essential that good contact between skin grafts and their recipient beds exists to ensure vascularization and eventual survival of the graft. The thin fibrin network that begins to form almost immediately between the graft and its bed seems to serve as a glue to hold the surfaces together and prevent one from slipping on the other.

Factors Preventing Proper Contact Between the Graft and Its Recipient Bed

These factors include improper adaptation of the graft, a collection of fluid beneath it, and movement between the graft and its bed. It is important that a proper degree of adaptation exists in a skin graft once it has been sutured into place. If the adaptation is insufficient, wrinkles result that never become revascularized because of failure of proper contact with the recipient bed. This same lack of contact results when a graft is stretched too tightly; acting like a drum head, the graft will not dip properly into the recesses of the recipient bed.

Blood, serum, and purulent material may separate the skin graft from its bed, prevent vascularization, and thus cause loss of the graft. If a graft is to be sutured in place the possibility of a hematoma beneath a graft can be greatly decreased by careful hemostasis of even the smallest bleeding points.

Capillary buds "race" against time to revascularize the graft before the cells undergo autolysis with eventual death. When a hematoma only 0.5 mm thick is present, the time required for capillary buds to grow through the added thickness of the clot might be only 12 hours. If the maximal allowable time for vascularization has not been exceeded, the graft will survive in these areas even though it is revascularized 12 hours later in other areas. When, however, the clot is 5 mm thick, the vascularization process will be delayed by 120 hours. At body temperature, most grafts will not survive this length of delay before revascularization and will die from autolysis.

Movement between the graft and its bed damages the capillaries growing into a graft and prevents proper revascularization. This can occur with too much pressure against the graft from a surgical stent, resulting in necrosis and loss of the graft.

Almost all open wounds have a sufficient blood supply to give nourishment to connective tissue and to provide the combined capillaries with granulation tissue. Sanders and McKelvy[85] showed that decortication of bare bone resulted in successful takes of skin grafts. The explanation for success over placement of nondecorticated bone was enhancement of the vascularity of the recipient site by decortication.

Infection, contamination, and the presence of certain bacteria or a disruption in the normal bacterial balance can cause lysis of the graft and dissolution or the lifting of the graft away from the recipient bed, which results in necrosis and loss of the graft. Krizek and Robson[86] have demonstrated that all wounds containing more than 10^5 bacteria per gram of tissue are infected, and skin grafting will not take on such a surface. The evidence available shows the endogenous and not exogenous source of bacteria to be the etiologic agent(s). The endogenous sources are due to (1) direct contact of bacteria from within the body with the edges of the incision, and (2) bacteria present at a distant site in the body entering the wound through the blood stream. As long as there is a normal balance between host resistance and the bacteria, there is no clinical infection. Foreign bodies in the wound enhance wound sepsis.

The removal of bacteria from the wound is best accomplished by mechanical debridement and a pulsating jet lavage. In anticipated procedures prior to grafting, one can use preoperative and intraoperative antibiotics to decrease the number of organisms in the wound and improve the chances of graft survival.

Characteristics of Grafted Skin

Skin that has been transplanted from one region to another will maintain most of its original characteristics, except that sensation and sweating in the graft will more closely resemble that of the recipient site. This was confirmed by Möller and Jölst,[87] who took biopsies from 18 patients in whom skin had been transplanted to the alveolar ridge five years previously. They found that although skin transplanted to the oral cavity undergoes minor changes, it also preserves tissue specificity even after a prolonged period. Only two thirds of the skin graft areas of the biopsies exhibited orthokeratosis, and the keratin layer was not as thick as that of control skin samples. The preservation of the keratinization of the epithelium seemed to indicate that the new graft bed and the moist environment had only a limited effect upon the keratinization process. Dellon and others[88] made similar findings. After 15 years of exposure of STSG and pedicle grafts to the intraoral environment, "mucosalization" of the skin was not evident.

Contraction and contraction relapse are prime considerations in oral tissue transplantation, since all transplanted tissues undergo varying degrees of primary and secondary contraction.

Primary contraction—that is, the contraction that is evident after the skin has been cut and before it is placed on the recipient site—is seen when the elastic fibers of a skin graft cause it to diminish in size as soon as it has been cut. This can easily be overcome by stretching the graft as it is sutured in place. Since elastic fibers are located in the dermis, grafts with a thicker dermis will contract more than thin grafts. Davis and Kitlowski[89] found that full-thickness skin grafts shrank as much as 41 per cent in surface area, whereas thin split-thickness grafts shrank only 9 per cent.

In secondary contraction, maturation of the scar tissue lying between a skin graft and its recipient bed causes the skin graft to contract, permanently decreasing its surface area.[90] This secondary contracture is of greater importance than primary contraction. It is influenced by the following factors: (1) The thicker a skin graft, the less its tendency to undergo secondary contraction; full-thickness skin grafts show little or no evidence of contracture. (2) The more rigid the recipient bed, the less a skin graft contracts; grafts on the periosteum of bone contract less than grafts on more mobile areas and flexor surfaces. (3) Complete take of a skin graft also decreases its degree of contracture; areas of partial loss of a skin graft heal by contraction and epithelialization from the surrounding skin.

Secondary contraction begins about the tenth day after grafting and continues up to six months.[35, 97] The contracting force exerts a steady, unrelenting pull on the wound and can easily overcome even the efforts of strong muscles to prevent it.

Skin grafts and flaps from above the clavicles tend to retain their natural blush shade, while those from below the clavicle take on a yellow or brownish hue with no vestige of red coloration.

Any accessory skin structures (i.e., hair follicles, sebaceous glands, and sweat glands) transplanted with a skin graft will continue to function, but if not included in the graft, these accessory structures do not regenerate. For practical purposes, only in full-thickness and thick STSG will hair grow, sebaceous glands function, and sweating be retained. These are the only grafts thick enough to include pilosebaceous apparatus and sweat glands.[92-94]

Sensation of grafted skin will approximate that of the surrounding skin when there is no dense scarring in the bed to prevent nerve fibers from penetrating the graft.[94, 95] The final return of sensibility in skin grafts placed on a scarred recipient bed, on granulation tissue from bone, or in an area of deep tissue destruction (e.g., full-thickness burns), will always be less than in those skin grafts overlying more favorable recipient sites. The four sensory modalities (i.e., pain, touch, heat, and cold), if they return, follow the pattern of the recipient site. Sensation begins to return three weeks after grafting and must be considered to have reached its maximum after one and a half to two years.[17, 18, 95] At first there is hyperalgesia, but over a period of months a more normal sensation returns. By use of electrophysiologic techniques, it has been shown that initially the sensory fibers to a skin graft are unmyelinated, and they become increasingly myelinated with time.[96]

In general, thick STSG's that have regained sensation are durable. Skin grafts grow in a manner paralleling the growth of the total body surface. Following an initial stage of graft shrinkage, a secondary phase of growth at the same rate as the growth of the total body surface is seen.[80] Tension was shown to have the greatest influence on growth.[97]

Donoff[98] stated that two distinct processes occur in the healing of open wounds: the first is the active process of contraction, which is limited by grafting; the second is remodeling and includes the subgraft, graft, and changes in peripheral tissue (maturation). These processes were applied to vestibuloplasty procedures performed in the oral cavity as well as to oral surgical wounds.

Skin has been used successfully in the oral cavity as a mucosal substitute but not without some disadvantages. These problems include the possible growth of hair from the graft, disagreeable odor and color, and a tendency to excessive keratinization when the skin is functioning under a denture.

Free oral mucosal grafting to the oral cavity, especially keratinized mucosa, has several advantages over STSG. These grafts, since they are taken freehand, are usually thicker or have full thickness and do not undergo significant contracture. Palatal mucosa[99, 100] is masticatory mucosa that closely resembles attached gingiva, which is resilient and very tough as a result of the function it performs. This same attached gingiva forms the gingival scar that overlies the crest of edentulous ridges. Palatal mucosa most clearly resembles this tissue by its resilience, toughness, resistance to traumatic displacement, and comparable color. It is a preferred tissue base for a prosthesis. However, palatal grafts provide a limited amount of tissue and are often not smooth on the recipient site, and the donor site may be painful for a prolonged period. Use of split-thickness mucosa from the lip or cheek for grafts has been suggested by Steinhauser and others,[24, 51, 101-105] especially if the maxillary periphery has not been satisfactory for denture retention. Major disadvantages of split-thickness buccal mucosal graft and full-thickness palatal grafts are limited availability of the tissue and difficulty in procuring the donor tissue and in handling thin split-thickness buccal mucosa, and the poor quality of this tissue for load bearing.

BIBLIOGRAPHY

1. Burwell RG, and Gowland G: Studies in the transplantation of bone. I. Assessment of antigenicity. Serological studies. J Bone Joint Surg (Am) 43B:814, 1961.
2. Burwell RG, and Gowland G: Studies in transplantation of bone. II. The changes occurring in the lymphoid tissue after homografts and autografts of fresh cancellous bone. J Bone Joint Surg (Am) 43B:820, 1961.
3. Burwell RG: Studies in transplantation of bone.

V. The capacity of fresh and treated homografts of bone to evoke transplantation immunity. J Bone Joint Surg (Am) 45B:386, 1963.
4. Burwell RG, Gowland G, and Dexter F: Studies in the transplantation of bone. VI. Further observation concerning the antigenicity of homologous cortical and cancellous bone. J Bone Joint Surg (Am) 45B:597, 1963.
5. Chalmers J: Bone transplantation. In Symposium on Tissue and Organ Transplant. J Clin Pathol 20:540-550, 1967.
6. Enneking WF: Histological investigation of bone transplants in immunologically prepared animals. J Bone Joint Surg 39A:597-615, 1957.
7. Nisbet NW: Antigenicity of bone. J Bone Joint Surg 59B:263-266, 1977.
8. Burwell RG, and Gowland G: Studies in transplantation of bone. III. The immune response of lymph nodes draining components of fresh homogeneous bone treated by different methods. J Bone Joint Surg (Am) 44B:131, 1962.
9. Brooks DB, Heiple KG, Herndon CH, and Powell HS: Immunological factors in homogeneous bone transplantation. IV. The effect of various methods of preparation and irradiation on antigenicity. J Bone Joint Surg 45A:1617, 1963.
10. Bonfiglio M, and Jeter WS: Immunological responses to bone. Clin Orthop Rel Res 87:19-27, 1972.
11. Bonfiglio M, Jeter WS, and Smith CL: The immune concept: In relation to bone transplantation. Ann NY Acad Sci 59:417-433, 1955.
12. Chalmers J: Transplantation immunity in bone homografting. J Bone Joint Surg (Am) 41B:160, 1959.
13. Elves MW: Humoral immune response to allografts of bone. Fut Arch Allergy 47:708-715, 1974.
14. Langer F, Czitrom A, Pritzer KP, and Gross AE: The immunogenicity of fresh and frozen allogeneic bone. J Bone Joint Surg 57A: 216-220, 1975.
15. Muscolo DL, Kawai S, and Ray RD: Cellular and humoral immune response analysis of bone-allografted rats. J Bone Joint Surg 58A:826-832, 1976.
16. Muscolo DL, Kawai S, and Ray RD: In vitro studies of transplantation antigens present on bone cells in the rat. J Bone Joint Surg 59B:342-348, 1977.
17. Halloran PF, Lee EH, Isreal ZF, Langer F, and Gross AE: Orthotopic bone transplantation in mice. Transplantation 27:420, 1979.
18. Halloran PF, Lee EH, Ziv I, and Langer F: Bone grafting in inbred mice: Evidence for H-2K, H-2D and non-H-2 antigens in bone. Transplant Proc XI:1509, 1979.
19. Ray RD: Vascularization of bone grafts and implants. Clin Orthop Rel Res 87:43-48, 1972.
20. Smith RT: The mechanism of graft rejection. Clin Orthop Rel Res 87:15-18, 1972.
21. Fell HB, and Weiss L: The effect of antiserum alone and with hydrocortisone on foetal mouse's bones in culture. J Exp Med 121:551-560, 1965.
22. Hausmann E, Genco R, Weinfeld N, et al.: Effects of sera on bone resorption in tissue culture. Calcif Tissue Res 13:311-317, 1973.
23. Heslop BF, Zeise IH, and Nisbet NW: Studies on transference of bone. I. A comparison of autologous and homologous bone implants with reference to osteocyte survival, osteogenesis and host reactions. Br J Exp Pathol 41:269-287, 1960.
24. Steinhauser EW: Free transplantation of oral mucosa for improvement of denture retention. J Oral Surg 27:955, 1969.
25. Zeiss IH, Nisbet NW, and Heslop BF: Studies on transference of bone. II. Vascularization of autologous and homologous implants of cortical bone in rats. Br J Exp Pathol 41:345-363, 1960.
26. Anderson KJ, Schmidt J, and Clawson DR: The vascularization and cellular response induced by homogeneous deproteinized bone transplants in the anterior chamber of the rats' eye. J Bone Joint Surg 43A:980, 1961.
27. Elves MW, and Pratt LM: The pattern of new bone formation in isografts of bone. Acta Orthop Scand 46:549-560, 1975.
28. Hammack BL, and Enneking WF: Comparative vascularization of autogenous and homogeneous bone transplants. J Bone Joint Surg 42A:811, 1960.
29. Heiple KG, Chase SW, and Herndon GU: A comparative study of the healing process following different types of bone transplantation. J Bone Joint Surg 45A:1593-1616, 1963.
30. Goldberg VM, and Lance EM: Quantitative studies of bone transplantation: The role of the allograft barrier. J Bone Joint Surg 54A:1133, 1972.
31. Nisbet NW, Heslop BF, and Zeiss IH: Studies on transference of bone. III. Manifestations of immunological tolerance to implants of homologous cortical bone in rats. Br J Exp Pathol 41:443-451, 1960.
32. Burchardt H, Glowgewskie FW, and Enneking WF: Allogeneic segmental fibular transplants in azathioprine immunosuppressed dogs. J Bone Joint Surg 59A:881-894, 1977.
33. Emmings FG: Chemically modified osseous material for the restoration of bone defects. J Periodontol 45:385-390, 1974.
34. Kliman M, Halloran PF, Lee E, Esses S, Fortner P, and Langer F: Orthotopic bone transplantation in mice. III. Methods of reducing the immune response and their effect on healing. Transplantation 31(1):34-40, 1981.
35. Cronin TP: The use of a molded splint to prevent contracture after split skin grafting on the neck. Plast Reconstr Surg 27:7, 1961.
36. Esses S, Halloran P, Kliman M, and Langer F: Bone allografts in mice: Determinants of immunogenicity and healing. Transplant Circ XIII:885-887, 1981.
37. Michejda M, Bacher J, Kuwabara T, and Hodgen GD: In utero allogeneic bone transplantation in primates: Roentgenographic and histological observation. Transplantation 32:96-100, 1981.
38. Friedlaender GE: Antigenicity of preserved bone allografts. Transplant Proc 8(Suppl):195-200, 1976.
39. Friedlaender GE: Studies on the antigenicity of bone. I. Freeze-dried and deep-frozen bone allografts in rabbits. J Bone Joint Surg (Am) 58:854, 1976.
40. Friedlaender GE, Strong DM, and Sell KW: The antigenicity of preserved bone allografts. Trans Orthop Res Soc 1:62, 1976.
41. Friedlaender GE, Strong DM, and Sell KW: Donor graft specific anti-HL-A antibodies following freeze-dried bone allografts. Trans Orthop Res Soc 2:219-220, 1977.
42. Kreuz FP, Hyatt GW, Turner TC, et al.: The preservation and clinical use of freeze-dried bone. J Bone Joint Surg 33A:863-888, 1951.
43. Bonfiglio M: Repair of bone-transplant fractures. J Bone Joint Surg 40A:446, 1958.
44. Burchardt H, and Enneking WF: Transplantation of bone. Surg Clin North Am 58:403-427, 1978.

45. Clemmensen T: The early circulation in split-skin grafts. Restoration of blood supply to split-skin autografts. Acta Chir Scand 127:1, 1964.
46. Lundgren G, Moller E, and Thorsby E: In vitro cytotoxicity by human leukocytes from individuals immunized against histocompatibility antigens. II. Relation to HL-A incompatibility between effector and target cells. Clin Exp Immunol 6:671, 1970.
47. Urist MR: Osteoinduction in undemineralized bone implants modified by chemical inhibitors of endogenous matrix enzymes. Clin Orthop 87:132, 1972.
48. Urist MR, Mikulski A, and Boyd SD: A chemosterilized antigen-extracted autodigested alloimplant for bone banks. Arch Surg 110:416-428, 1975.
49. Urist MR, and Iwata H: Preservation and biodegradation of the morphogenetic property of bone matrix. J Theor Biol 38:155, 1973.
50. Urist MR (ed.): Fundamental and Clinical Bone Physiology. Philadelphia, JP Lippincott Co, 1980.
51. Nisbet NW: Immunology of bone transplantation. Clin Orthop Rel Res 47:199-228, 1966.
52. Kramer IR, Killey HC, and Wright HC: The response of the rabbit to implants of processed calf bone (Boplant). Arch Oral Biol 13:1263, 1968.
53. Pieron AP, Bigelow D, and Hamonic M.: Bone grafting with Boplant. Results in 33 cases. J Bone Joint Surg 50B:364-368, 1968.
54. Hancox NM, Owen R, and Singleton A: Cross-species grafts of deproteinised bone. J Bone Joint Surg 43B:152, 1961.
55. Burwell RG: Studies on transplantation of bone. VIII. Treated composite homograft-autografts of cancellous bone. J Bone Joint Surg 48B:532-565, 1966.
56. Bell WH: Current concepts of bone grafting. J Oral Surg 26:118-124, 1968.
57. Bell WH, Buche WA, Kennedy JW, III, et al.: Surgical correction of the atrophic alveolar ridge. A preliminary report on a new concept of treatment. Oral Surg 43(4):485-498, 1977.
58. Danielson PA, and Nemarich AN: Subcortical bone grafting for ridge augmentation. J Oral Surg 34(10):887-889, 1976.
59. Farrell CD, Kent JN, and Guerra LR: One-stage interpositional bone grafting and vestibuloplasty of the atrophic maxilla. J Oral Surg 34(10):901-906, 1976.
60. Fonseca RJ, Nelson JF, Clark PJ, Frost DE, and Olson RA: Revascularization and healing of onlay particulate allogeneic bone grafts in primates. J Oral Maxillofac Surg 41:153-162, 1983.
61. Fonseca RJ, Clark PJ, Burkes EJ, Jr., and Baker RD: Revascularization and healing of onlay particulate autologous bone grafts in primates. J Oral Surg 38:572-577, 1980.
62. Maletta JA, Gasser JA, Fonseca RJ, and Nelson JA: Comparison of the healing and revascularization of onlayed autologous and lyophilized allogeneic rib grafts to the edentulous maxilla. J Oral Maxillofac Surg 41:487-499, 1983.
63. Stroud SW, Fonseca RJ, Sanders GW, and Burkes EJ, Jr.: Healing of interpositional autologous bone grafts after total maxillary osteotomy. J Oral Surg 38:878-885, 1980.
64. Frost DE, and Fonseca RJ: Multiple keratocysts in basal cell nevus syndrome. Oral Surg 40:776, 1982.
65. Marx RE, Snyder RM, and Kline SN: Cellular survival of human marrow during placement of marrow-cancellous bone grafts. J Oral Surg 37:712-717, 1979.
66. Urist MR, Granstein R, Nogami H, et al.: Transmembrane bone morphogenesis across multiple-walled diffusion chambers. New evidence for a diffusible bone morphogenetic property. Arch Surg 112:612, 1977.
67. Urist MR, Mikulski A, and Lietze A: Solubilized and insolubilized bone morphogenetic protein. Proc Natl Acad Sci USA 76:1828, 1979.
68. Burwell RG: Osteogenesis in cancellous bone grafts: Considered in terms of cellular changes, basic mechanisms and the perspective of growth-control and its possible aberrations. Clin Orthop 40:35, 1965.
69. Trueta J: The role of vessels in osteogenesis. J Bone Joint Surg 45B:402, 1963.
70. McGregor IA: Fundamental Techniques of Plastic Surgery. 2nd ed. Edinburgh, Churchill Livingstone, 1962.
71. Smahel J, and Clodius L: The blood vessel system of free human skin grafts. Plast Reconstr Surg 47:61, 1971.
72. Rudolph R, and Klein L: Healing process in skin grafts. Surg Gynecol Obstet 136:641, 1973.
73. Birch J, and Branemark PI: The vascularization of a free full thickness skin graft: II. A microangiographic study. Scand J Plast Reconstr Surg 3:11, 1969.
74. Birch J, and Branemark PI: The vascularization of a free full thickness skin graft: I. A vital microscopy study. Scand J Plast Reconstr Surg 3:1, 1969.
75. Converse JM, Uhlschmid GK, and Ballantyne DL, Jr.: "Plasmatic circulation" in skin grafts. The phase of serum imbibition. Plast Reconstr Surg 43:495, 1969.
76. Clemmensen T: The early circulation in split skin grafts. Acta Chir Scand 124:11, 1962.
77. Converse JM, Ballantyne DL, Jr., Rogers BO, and Raisbeck AP: "Plasmatic circulation" in skin grafts. Transplant Bull 4:154, 1957.
78. Converse JM, and Ballantyne DL, Jr.: Distribution of diphosphopyridine nucleotide diaphorase in rat skin autografts and homografts. Plast Reconstr Surg 30:415, 1962.
79. Smith JW, Ringland J, and Wilson R: Vascularization of skin grafts. Surg Forum 15:473, 1964.
80. Smahel J: The healing of skin grafts. Clin Plast Surg 4:409, 1977.
81. Haller JA, and Billingham RE: Studies of the vascularization in free skin grafts. Ann Surg 166:896, 1967.
82. Oden B: Microlymphangiographic studies of experimental skin autografts. Acta Chir Scand 121:219, 1961.
83. Psillakis JM: Lymphatic vascularization of skin grafts. Plast Reconstr Surg 43:287, 1969.
84. Scothorne RJ: Lymphatic repair and the genesis of homograft immunity. Ann NY Acad Sci 73:673, 1958.
85. Sanders B, and McKelvy B: Split-thickness skin grafts transplanted over exposed maxillary bone in dogs. J Oral Surg 34:510-513, 1976.
86. Krizek TJ, and Robson MC: Evolution of quantitative bacteriology in wound management. Am J Surg 130:579, 1975.
87. Möller JE, and Jölst O: A histologic follow-up study of free autogenous skin grafts to the alveolar ridge of humans. Int J Oral Surg 1:283-289, 1972.
88. Dellon AL, Tarpley TM, and Chretien PB: Histologic evaluation of intraoral skin grafts and pedicle flaps in humans. J Oral Surg 343:789-794, 1976.

89. Davis JS, and Kitlowski EA: The immediate contraction of cutaneous grafts and its cause. Arch Surg 23:954, 1931.
90. Ragnell A: The secondary contraction tendency of free skin grafts. Br J Plast Surg 5:6, 1952.
91. McIndoe AH: The treatment of hypospadeas. Am J Surg 38:176, 1937.
92. Conway H: Sweating function of transplanted skin. Gynecol Obstet 69:756, 1939.
93. Lofgren L: Recovery of nervous function in skin transplants with special reference to sympathetic functions. Acta Chir Scand 102:229, 1951.
94. Pontén B: Grafted skin—observations on innervation and other qualities. Acta Chir Scand (Suppl) 257, 1960.
95. Hutchison J, Tough J, and Wyburn G: Regeneration of sensation in grafted skin. Br J Plast Surg 2:82, 1949.
96. Terzis JK: Functional aspects of reinnervation of free skin grafts. Plast Reconstr Surg 58:142, 1976.
97. Koehnlein HG, and Deitrich EE: Influence of different tensions on growth of skin grafts. Surg Forum 26:562, 1975.
98. Donoff RB: Biological basis for vestibuloplasty procedures. J Oral Surg 34:890-896, 1976.
99. Hall HD: Vestibuloplasty, mucosal grafts (palatal and buccal). J Oral Surg 29:786-791, 1971.
100. Robinson RE: The free mucosal graft in the edentulous mouth. J Calif Dent Assoc 43:552, 1967.
101. Maloney PL, Doku HC, and Shepherd NS: Mucosal grafting in oral reconstructive surgery. J Oral Surg 32:705-710, 1974.
102. Maloney PL, Shepherd NS, and Doku HC: Free buccal mucosa grafts for vestibuloplasty. J Oral Surg 30:716, 1972.
103. Maloney PL, Shepherd NS, and Doku HC: Immediate vestibuloplasty with free mucosal grafts. J Oral Surg 32:343-346, 1974.
104. Maloney PL, Garland SD, Stanwich L, et al.: Immediate vestibuloplasty with fenestrated and intact full-thickness mucosal grafts. Oral Surg 42:543, 1976.
105. Shepherd NS, Maloney PL, and Doku HC: Expanded split thickness mucosal grafts. J Oral Surg 31:687, 1973.

PROSTHODONTIC AND SURGICAL ASPECTS OF TREATMENT PLANNING FOR RECONSTRUCTIVE SURGERY

John Beumer, III, D.D.S., M.S., Howard Landesman, D.D.S., Bill C. Terry, D.D.S., W. Howard Davis, D.D.S., and Christopher L. Davis, D.D.S., M.D.

PROSTHODONTIC ASPECTS OF RECONSTRUCTIVE PREPROSTHETIC SURGERY

A significant number of denture wearers have recurrent complaints regarding their dentures. These difficulties usually are secondary to factors that include unrealistic expectations, obvious anatomic deficiencies such as advanced alveolar ridge resorption, or a combination of both. In the past three decades much progress has been made in alleviating many of the anatomic deficiencies, and much can be offered to the patient if he or she is willing to undergo surgical procedures. Interdisciplinary cooperation among oral and maxillofacial surgeons, general practitioners, and prosthodontists has led to the development of many procedures that may significantly ameliorate anatomic deficiencies. Selected patients with advanced bone resorption of the mandible, poorly keratinized mucosal bearing surfaces of the mandible, acquired jaw defects, and maxillomandibular malrelationships may benefit from a variety of reconstructive preprosthetic surgical procedures. Recently osseointegrated implant systems, in particular, have offered the patient the opportunity to function in a nearly normal fashion.

Criteria for successful conventional complete prostheses are based on the patient's acceptance. Ideal anatomic edentulous structures are rarely encountered. If the patient is satisfied with his or her prostheses with regard to mastication and esthetics, these restorations are usually considered successful. Indeed, it is quite common to see patients with technically deficient complete dentures quite satisfied with the result. Conversely, there are patients with technically adequate dentures who are not satisfied and the prostheses are deemed unsatisfactory.

It is therefore not surprising that a negative attitude prevails among practitioners when fabricating complete dentures. Often, even after lengthy sessions of pretreatment questioning and after evaluating a patient's previous success with dentures, the practitioner fabricates a mechanically perfect set of dentures only to find that after he or she places them in the patient's mouth, the patient cannot tolerate the prostheses, particularly the mandibular prosthesis.

There are two variables that appear to be the determining factors regarding the success the patient will achieve with conventional complete dentures. One is whether the mechanical phases of treatment have been properly executed; namely, the borders of the dentures have been extended properly as a result of good impressions, proper jaw relation records have been made at the correct vertical dimension of occlusion, and the teeth have been properly placed in the record bases to support the musculature while at the same time fulfilling the esthetic and functional requirements of the patient. The second variable is psychological.

Psychological Factors

The reason for acceptance or nonacceptance of removable prostheses must be clearly defined if a surgical procedure is contemplated. In conventional complete dentures surgical procedures are most beneficial when difficulties are anatomic rather than psychological.

The personal interview is the most satisfactory method of identifying patients who will be difficult to treat and to satisfy. Many papers have been written offering suggestions, methods, and devices to use in the interview process in order to identify the patient who will not be successful with treatment. The authors have found the following questionnaire to be a valuable tool in identifying the potentially maladaptive patient (Fig. 3–1).[1] The patient is first asked three simple questions, listed as I, II, and III. If the responses are favorable (e.g., "Got along fine," "Teeth are just loose and worn," or "Never had any difficulties"), no further questions are asked. However, if unfavorable responses are elicited (e.g., "Always had problems" or "Never could chew"), then it is important to determine the nature of the maladaptive response. If the dentures appear to be mechanically acceptable, the dentist must then determine if the maladaptive response can be altered to an adaptive one. This is determined by asking the patient another series of questions (Fig. 3–2). If the responses are negative it is fairly reasonable to assume that the dentist will not be successful in treating the patient without help of a psychologist or therapist. In such patients surgical procedures must be contemplated with great caution.

A psychological assessment of the patient is desirable prior to combined surgical prosthodontic procedures, as the psychologist frequently determines whether the expectations of the patient will be met. Although an initial interview may identify emotional problems, a complete psychological evaluation is beyond the capability of most surgeons or practitioners and therefore referral to a psychologist or social worker may be appropriate.

Anatomic Factors

In addition to psychological factors, the most important anatomic factors when considering fabrication of conventional complete dentures include the configuration of the edentulous bony bearing surfaces of the maxilla and mandible, the nature of mucosa including the amount of attached mucosa and its degree of keratinization, posture of the tongue and floor of the mouth, and the

---

INITIAL INTERVIEW FOR THE DENTURE PATIENT (EDENTULOUS)

Where the patient is requesting a new denture because the present one is not satisfactory, the main purpose of the interview is to determine:
  A. If the denture is adequate or
  B. If the patient is maladaptive

I.   How did you get along with your previous dentures? _____
II. Why do you need new dentures? _____
III. *Expectations of the patient*—What do you expect from the dentures? _____

If the responses are favorable (i.e., "I got along fine," "At first I had trouble, but I got along well later," "The teeth are loose and/or worn so I need new ones," etc.), then usually no difficulties are anticipated.

Less favorable responses (i.e., "I had trouble from the beginning and never was really satisfied," "They changed my appearance," "I cannot chew everything," "They have always felt loose," etc.) indicate a need for an examination of the dentures to determine if they are reasonably satisfactory, and if so, an interview is indicated to determine:
  A. What is the nature of the maladaptive response?
  B. Can the maladaptive response be changed to an adaptive one?
  C. What is the maladaptive response based on?
    1. Fear of dentures prior to tooth loss ⎱ May be altered
    2. Severe anxiety about having had teeth extracted ⎰
    3. Neurotic anxiety or maladaptive behavior that is projected onto dentures } Probably cannot be altered

Figure 3–1. Initial interview for edentulous patient (Part A). (From Levin B, and Landesman HM: A practical questionnaire for predicting denture success or failure. J Prosthet Dent 35:124–130, 1976.)

Figure 3–2. Initial interview for edentulous patient (Part B). (From Levin B, and Landesman HM: A practical questionnaire for predicting denture success or failure. J Prosthet Dent 35:124–130, 1976.)

I. How many dentures have you had? _____
II. How did you get along with your first denture? _____ Second? _____
III. How did you feel about the doctor who made the first denture? _____
IV. Why were your teeth extracted? _____
V. Did you want them extracted? _____
VI. How did you feel about their loss? _____
VII. Did you have removable partial dentures? _____
VIII. Did you have complete dentures immediately? _____
IX. Did you help to choose the front teeth? _____
X. Had you known anyone who had complete dentures? _____
XI. How did they get along with them? _____
XII. *Expectations of the patient*—What do you expect from these dentures? _____

What would you like? _____

Student evaluation: _____

Instructor-student recommendations:
1. Prognosis: Fair ☐ Good ☐ Excellent ☐
2. Refer to Graduate Prosthodontics
3. Refer to Department of Human Behavior

_____ Student
_____ Instructor

---

relationships between the mandible and maxilla.

To the practicing dentist who is concerned with providing a removable prosthesis that is no longer supported by teeth but rather by soft tissue and bone, the preservation of alveolar bone becomes sacred. The reality is that there is a relationship between the success of a removable prosthesis and the amount of alveolar bone present to support the prosthesis. In rare instances, the dentist is limited because of too much bone (e.g., bulbous tuberosities, tori, etc.). Overall, the patient who is in distress with his removable prosthesis is suffering because of alveolar bone resorption and the problem is usually in the mandible. Statistics indicate that bone resorption in the mandible is four times as great as in the maxilla.[2,3] If you add variables such as a tongue and its changing position, a floor of the mouth that is in a constant state of mobility, and an area of bone with much less surface area than the maxilla, the preservation of the mandibular alveolar bone becomes more sacred than ever.

Bone

The process of bone resorption remains unclear. It is presumed that resorption is a direct consequence of osteoclastic activity. It has been postulated that when an imbalance occurs between osteoblastic and osteoclastic activity, resorption also occurs. The significant clinical factors that appear to precipitate bone resorption are excessive lateral movement of the denture base during function and the use of dentures at night during periods of sleep. It has also been suggested that hormonal imbalances may be important, particularly in females[4,5] (see Chapter 1).

Present thinking appears to be directed toward preservation of bone long before resorption begins. Studies utilizing dichloromethylene diphosphonate to inhibit alveolar bone resorption in rats have reported positive results.[6,7] The use of various antibiotics is being studied to override the negative effects of bacteria in plaque. Different dietary agents are being studied, such as calcium and vitamin D.[8,9] Long-term clinical testing has not yet been conducted to confirm the efficacy of systemic therapy in inhibiting resorption of the mandible or maxilla.

It must be noted that the apparent success of osseointegrated implant systems, such as the one proposed and developed by Branemark,[24,25] may change all of the above. It is conceivable that because of these systems complete dentures as we know them today will be reserved only for those patients who are not good candidates to receive osseointegrated implants (see Chapter 7).

Soft Tissue

The size and nature of the denture-bearing area certainly affect the prognosis for the conventional complete denture. In the mandible, the size of this area is determined by the dimension of the mandibular bone, the amount of attached mucosa, the position of muscle attachments, and the posture of the tongue and floor of the mouth. Tongue posture and the size of the mandible are often cited by prosthodontists as the most important prognostic indicators. An overlooked prognostic factor is the nature of the denture-bearing surface mucosa. Following extraction of the remaining mandibular dentition, varying amounts of attached gingiva remain and are usually centrally located on the alveolar ridge. This mucosa is well keratinized and firmly attached to the underlying periosteum and bone via a residual network of gingival fibers. Beyond the mucogingival junction, the epithelium is poorly keratinized and is loosely attached to underlying periosteum and bone. The well-keratinized attached mucosa is obviously better suited to resist the stresses of denture function than is the less well keratinized, poorly attached mucosa beyond the mucogingival junction.

During the years of denture use there is progressive resorption of bone. Accompanying this process is the general deterioration of the quality and amount of attached mucosa that remains. In the face of rapid bone resorption and ill-fitting dentures, the mucosa becomes less well-attached to underlying periosteum and bone, and less keratinized (Fig. 3–3). These factors, combined with loss of alveolar ridge, further compromise complete denture function. In addition, diabetes and reduced salivary flow in some patients lead to increased levels of fungal organisms.[10, 11] Chronic fungal infections often result and adversely affect the degree of keratinization of the attached mucosa. With tongue enlargement and unfavorable tongue and floor of mouth posture, anatomic situations are created wherein surgical intervention may be justified if successful restoration of some form and function is to be achieved with conventional complete dentures. If there is significant compromise of the bearing surface mucosa, serious consideration should be given to resurfacing an area with free autogenous grafts of either skin or palatal mucosa. Skin is preferred because of the ease of harvesting a sufficient amount. In our view, buccal mucosal grafts are considered inappropriate because of their reduced degree of keratinization.

Tongue and Floor of Mouth Posture

The posture and function of the tongue has long been considered a key predictor of denture success or failure. All mandibular dentures move significantly during function and a successful patient can control the denture in the appropriate position on the bearing surface when a force is about to be applied. Consequently, many authors have alluded to the importance of the interface of the mandibular denture with the tongue, the floor of the mouth, and the buccal tissues to enhance the patient's control of the prosthesis.[12–14] Because the lingual musculature is in a state of motion during function, it becomes an almost impossible task for the patient to maintain an effective seal of the mandibular prosthesis while masticating, or more importantly while in the process of parafunctional movements. Probably the most important variable in maintaining this seal is the position of the tongue. This was explained quite effectively by Wright, Swartz, and Godwin.[15] They developed a classification whereby the position of the tongue is a prognostic indicator of whether the mandibular prosthesis will develop maximum retention while the patient is functioning.

Fortunately, approximately 75 per cent of patients have a normal tongue position. In a normal tongue position, as defined by Wright et al.,[15] the floor of the mouth is filled by the tongue. The top surface is round and free of muscular contractions, lateral borders rest on the occlusal surfaces of the lower posterior teeth, and the apex of the tongue rests on the edges of the mandibular incisor teeth or the crest of the ridge just lingual to where the incisors used to reside (Fig. 3–4).

Patients with this normal tongue position have the ability to manipulate their mandibular prosthesis to maintain contact between the lingual flange and the floor of the mouth during function. This helps to maintain a seal between the prosthesis and the tissues.

Wright et al.[15] state that 25 per cent of the population have abnormal tongue positions. They divided them into two classifications.

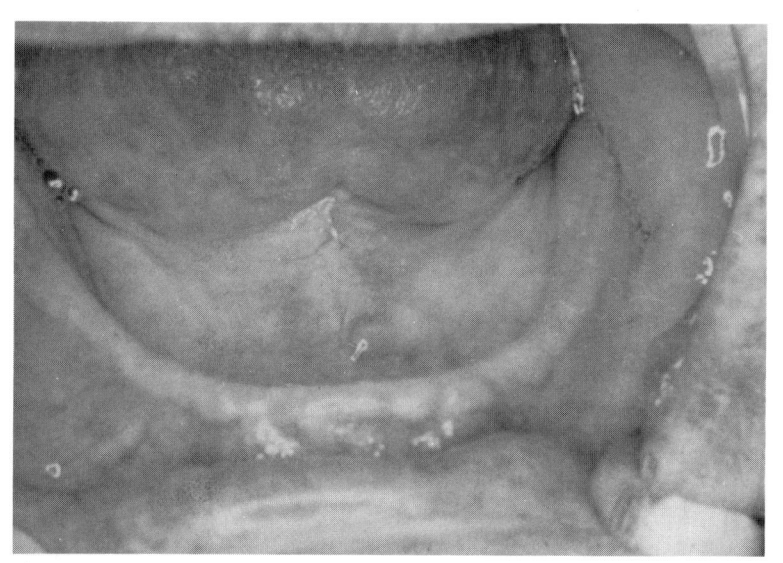

Figure 3–3. Atrophic mandible with a paucity of keratinized attached mucosa.

Generally speaking, these individuals have a tongue whose base is postured posteriorly and maybe superiorly. The apex of the tongue may be postured inferiorly into the floor of the mouth or drawn back into the body of the tongue, losing its complete identity. The lateral borders of the tongue no longer rest on the occlusal surface of the posterior teeth (Fig. 3–5).

The major problem with patients who have this abnormal tongue position is that the seal of the mandibular prosthesis is lost almost immediately because the floor of the mouth is tense and often in a state of constant motion. Accordingly, the prosthesis cannot maintain itself in a nonmobile state.

These abnormal tongue postures preclude the development of adequate retromylohyoid extension posteriorly and impair stability of the mandibular denture. It is not surprising, therefore, to note retruded tongue positions in patients with advanced bony resorption of the mandible accompanied by compromises in the bearing surface mucosa.

Any consideration given to bone augmentation or free grafting should be accompanied by an evaluation of tongue and floor of mouth posture. If tongue posture appears to be a problem, surgical lowering of the floor of the mouth is usually beneficial and should be strongly recommended when free grafting is planned.

Maxillomandibular Malrelations

Severe maxillomandibular malrelationships may compromise conventional complete denture function in the edentulous patient. Osteotomies and ostectomies have usually been reserved for correction of dentulous patients demonstrating severe malocclusions and skeletal discrepancies. However, these procedures can also benefit selected edentulous patients and can improve denture function as well as appearance. Some of the lesser defects can be corrected at the time of tooth extraction or by additional alveoloplasties. However, the removal of teeth and mandibular bone may compromise future function and denture stability, especially for young individuals who will need to wear dentures for many years. Therefore, in selected edentulous patients with prognathism, retrognathism, and apertognathism, a surgical osteotomy may be of value.

A dentulous patient with mandibular prognathism usually has mandibular anterior teeth that are in crossbite or in an edge-to-edge relationship. The patient seldom uses or needs protrusive movements. The dentulous patient who is prognathic is a problem to the prosthodontist, either because of the unusual forces and stresses brought to bear on any prosthesis or because of the difficulty in achieving occlusal harmony. The edentulous prognathic patient continues to be a problem for similar reasons, but some occlusal modifications are possible. In a patient who has recently had extractions, a crossbite ridge or edge-to-edge relationship may actually favor seating the maxillary denture. The occlusion of the mandibular denture would be centralized in crossbite situations, supplementing the stability of both dentures.

An edentulous patient may present with mandibular prognathism because of a developmental deformity or because the normal resorption of the ridges can create a prognathic tendency. In the posterior portion of

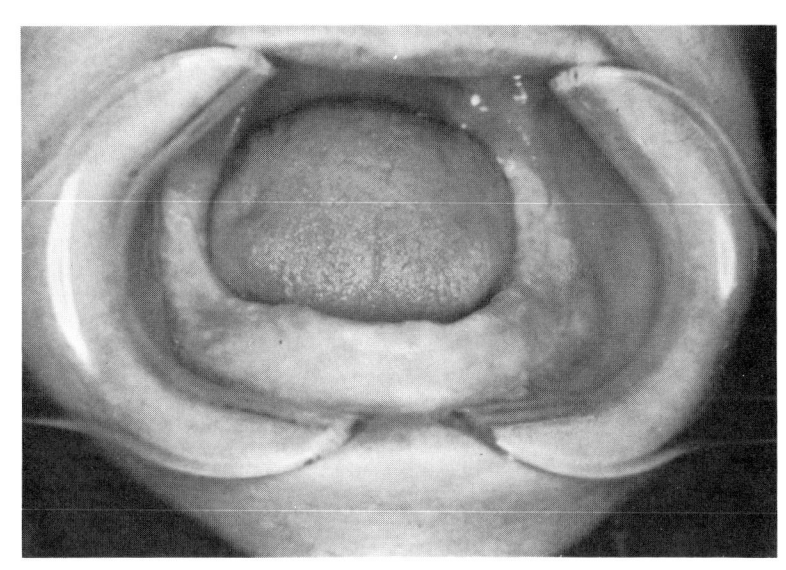

Figure 3–4. Wright's Class I tongue position.

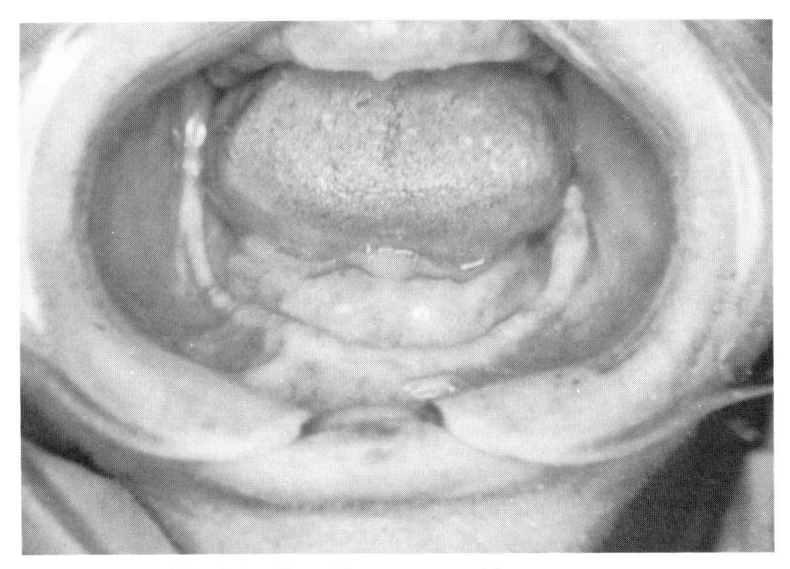

Figure 3–5. Wright's Class II tongue position.

the body of the mandible, the alveolar process is structured lingually relative to the body of the mandible. Thus, as the alveolar portion resorbs vertically, the diameter of the mandible enlarges. A similar but reverse alveolar-to-body relationship occurs in the maxilla. Hence, advanced resorption results in pseudoprognathism and creates vertical and horizontal discrepancies between the ridges.

Esthetics for the prognathic patient are usually determined by the position of the mandibular anterior teeth. Lip contour and tooth visibility in a maxillary denture become a greater problem as ridge resorption progresses and accentuates the mandibular prognathism. Many patients complain of the loss of support of the upper lip. To accommodate esthetics and maintain a normal relationship with the mandibular teeth, the maxillary denture teeth need to be placed in an abnormal anterior position and angle, often creating a levering force on the supporting foundation area during function when the bolus is incised. The effect is more evident in the patient who has maintained mandibular anterior teeth against a maxillary denture, particularly in regard to patterns of bone resorption in the premaxillary segment. Fabrication of conventional complete dentures for such individuals is difficult and their use probably accentuates resorption of both the maxilla and mandible.

In an edentulous patient with a retrognathic mandible, esthetics must often be compromised in order to achieve useful function. The position of the anterior teeth is a delicate compromise between tongue action, lip forces, and occlusion. To obtain an appropriate balance in a protrusive relationship, an increase in horizontal overlap may be necessary to reduce the use of vertical overlap, keeping the compensating curve of the posterior teeth within reasonable limits. In retrognathic patients, it is often difficult to direct occlusal forces over the mandibular ridge.

In patients who present with apertognathia, unsatisfactory vertical and horizontal relationships may be present. Often there is insufficient denture space for placement of posterior denture teeth. When inadequate denture space exists, the usual treatment is to remove soft tissues.

With the above three deformities, surgical correction can greatly aid denture function, as well as afford obvious improvement in facial symmetry and appearance. The risks and potential surgical morbidities must be weighed carefully by both the patient and the clinician before surgery is attempted. It should be noted that osteotomies performed on edentulous patients are more difficult and the chances of relapse greater. The necessary use of intraoral splints anchored to either the mandible and/or the maxilla is uncomfortable, and infection may occasionally occur. Hence, consideration should be given in selected cases to performing such surgical procedures while the patient is in a partially dentulous state, particularly with respect to patients with Class II relationships.

Surgical Options—A Prosthodontic Perspective

Choices available to the surgeon and prosthodontist for patients with anatomic deficiencies are many, and advantages gained by any of the procedures often overlap. When evaluating the needs of a particular patient, this problem is best addressed by considering the issues of stability, support, retention, and esthetics for the future prosthesis and weighing them against the probable surgical morbidities. The issue of the patient's expectations should be considered in regard to comfort, improved masticatory efficiency, improved esthetics, and the price he or she is willing to pay for the possible surgical morbidity.

Soft Tissue

If one looks at the soft tissue procedures (free grafting with skin or palatal mucosa), when considering fabrication of conventional complete dentures, the gains are sufficient for some patients but not for all. Free grafting and lowering the floor of the mouth work well when the primary deficiencies are high muscle attachments and reduced amounts of and compromise of keratinization of attached mucosa. These procedures serve to improve the support available for complete dentures. When combined with surgically lowering the floor of the mouth, stability and control of the mandibular denture are enhanced.[16, 17] Skin graft vestibuloplasties also appear to minimize and in some patients eliminate sensitivity along an exposed inferior alveolar nerve.[18] This may be related to the improved ability of the load-bearing surface to support the denture without loading the mental neurovascular bundle area. However, similar improvements in stability can be effected by the staple implant popularized by Small.[19] Patient acceptance of both procedures appears to be high, and the surgical risks and morbidities are similar. In our view, the choice between these two methods is difficult and at times is determined by the personal preference of the surgeon-prosthodontist team.

Implants

The implant system proposed by Branemark and associates[24, 25] shows great promise. The functional benefits are similar to those achieved with conventional subperiosteal implants. This implant system has been successfully employed in both the mandible and the maxilla. Both removable and fixed partial dentures can be used in association with the osseointegrated fixtures. The forces the patient can bring upon the bolus approaches those possible with the natural dentition. In 15-year follow-up studies the retention rate exceeded 85 per cent in both arches. The surgical morbidities are significantly less and in case of implant removal the mucosal bearing surfaces are not nearly as compromised.

The conventional subperiosteal implant also offers the patient significant improvement in regard to mastication.[20-22] Increased masticatory forces can be brought to bear on the bolus, and stability of the denture can be effectively controlled. According to James,[23] refinements of implant design may result in less bone resorption than previous subperiosteal implant designs and will probably increase success and longevity. However, the above factors must be balanced against the potential surgical morbidities and the frequently encountered postoperative sequelae of pain and infection. Until a means can be developed to prevent epithelial migration along subperiosteal implant frameworks, infection will be a major disadvantage of this approach. Additionally, removal of such an implant may result in significant compromise of the mucosal denture-bearing surfaces.

Indeed, if the early success of Branemark is duplicated by other clinicians and researchers, the osseointegrated system may supplant most other surgical approaches previously applied in patients unable to wear complete dentures because of anatomic deficiencies (see Chapter 7).

Bone Augmentation

In our view, bone augmentation of the severely resorbed mandible is to be considered only in the presence of a risk of pathologic fracture in a patient with reasonable life expectancy. The methods of bone grafting available bring different sets of advantages and disadvantages to the prosthetic-surgical team. Superior border rib grafting techniques have revealed initial rapid resorption rates and have led to the usual prosthodontic problems because of the changing nature of the grafted denture-bearing surfaces.[27] The visor and modification of this technique are not suitable for the patient presenting with a severely resorbed mandible. Additionally, the rate of permanent paresthesia of the lower lip is quite high.[28] In our view, this technique merely succeeds in making an already reasonably sized mandible larger in areas that do not necessarily offer any advantage to the prosthodontist. The iliac crest augmentation method reported by Curtis and Ware, although demonstrating reasonable rates of bone resorption, creates difficult problems for the prosthodontist because of the changing nature of the grafted denture-bearing surfaces.[29]

In recent years, augmentation of the mandible with hydroxyapatite has received much attention. At present, clinical experience indicates that this material is best used in the treatment of unfavorable bone contours and the elimination of undercuts (see Chapter 8). It is possible that the process of bone resorption may also be ameliorated by the use of this material. The effectiveness of hydroxyapatite as a means of bony augmentation has yet to be determined. From a prosthodontic perspective, the current methods suggested for augmentation all have disadvantages and must be undertaken with caution.

If the patient's difficulty in function with complete dentures is basically due to anatomic factors, much can be done surgically to improve the prosthetic prognosis. However, if anatomic factors become intertwined with psychological factors, some caution should be exercised before proceeding with a preprosthetic surgical procedure.

SURGICAL ASPECTS OF RECONSTRUCTIVE PREPROSTHETIC SURGERY

Prior to World War II, surgery to aid the edentulous patient with compromised bony and/or soft tissue was severely limited. Surgical help usually consisted of the removal of bony prominences and excess soft tissue, although in some centers the vestibuloplasty with skin grafting was beginning to evolve,[30-41] as was the maxillary secondary epithelialization procedure.[42-44] There were sparse reports of successful bone or skin grafts for severely damaged jaws.[45] For the most part, there was little predictable help for the patient with moderate to severe edentulous bone loss (EBL) and associated contour defects.

After World War II, major advances in vestibuloplasty procedures began. The predictability of vestibuloplasty procedures was greatly enhanced as the principles governing their success evolved. Several procedures became standard treatment for previously unsolved problems.[46] An excellent solution was attained for the most pervasive problem, the unstable mandibular denture. This solution was the refinement of the vestibuloplasty with skin grafting and the lowering of the floor of the mouth[47-50] and its popularization by Obwegeser. When only the lingual vestibule required altering, the fairly simple repositioning of the mylohyoid muscle by lowering was introduced.[51, 52] When only the mandibular anterior area required vestibular extension, a sulcoplasty was conceived by Fickler and popularized by Edlan.[53] Attention was also directed to the frequent problem of the mandible severely weakened by EBL.[54-56] An interim aid was achieved with autogenous rib or ilium grafting.[57] Then came the addition of nonresorbable hydroxyapatite to the bone graft, which may give a more permanent augmentation.[58] There was also aid attained for the maxilla with EBL and soft tissue problems by various vestibuloplasties,[46, 59] bone augmentation,[60] and alloplastic augmentation using nonresorbable hydroxyapatite.[61]

Considerable effort has been made to provide permanent fixed prostheses for the edentulous mandible and maxilla. In the mandible, reasonable success has been demonstrated by the staple implant.[62, 63] The subperiosteal implant with or without added bone has had variable success,[64-68] as has the ramus frame.[69]

The osseointegrated implants currently provide the possibility of very long-term retention of fixed as well as removable prostheses.[70] It appears now that a breakthrough is at hand with the remarkable results reported by Branemark et al. after a very long-term study (see Chapter 7).

It is thus obvious that today there are many possible surgical aids to help the edentulous patient (Table 3–1), and it has become difficult to decide which procedure is most appropriate. The dilemma is compounded by the lack of long-term objective data on some of these modalities. In evaluating the data that are available, it should be considered that no one is performing all the procedures and therefore no individual can be considered an expert in all of them. Thus, it is not surprising that significant bias is shown by authors reporting on each procedure. Although the editors have attempted to minimize the bias by contributors, some bias understandably remains.

Natural History of the Edentulous Alveolar Process

The alveolar process is formed in response to the developing and erupting teeth. Once the teeth are lost, the remaining alveolar bone undergoes resorption, remodeling, and recontouring.[3] Certain conditions and local factors can increase the rate of these bony changes, as observed in the poorly controlled diabetic patient functioning with ill-fitting dentures. The bony resorption and remodeling pattern may be favorably altered by augmentation with an alloplastic material such as hydroxyapatite, placement of osseointegrated implants, or resurfacing with soft tissue graft of mucosa or skin.

If the edentulous bony anatomy changes, the covering soft tissues may undergo alterations, and the muscle attachments, especially in the mandible, become an important factor in the prosthetic management with conventional dentures. The most common soft tissue problems include excessive crestal tissues and mobility of the remaining covering mucosa. As alveolar bone is lost, the attachments of the mylohyoid and genioglossus muscles on the medial surface of the mandible, and the buccinator and mentalis muscles on the facial surface, become very important, as these attachments may cause shallow vestibules that limit extension of the denture flange. Muscle and mucosal attach-

TABLE 3–1. POSSIBLE PREPROSTHETIC SURGICAL PROCEDURES

I. Augmentations
   A. Onlay
      1. Free submucosal graft
      2. Autogeneic bone
      3. Allogeneic bone
      4. Alloplasts
      5. Any combination of above
   B. Interpositional
      1. Autogeneic bone
      2. Allogeneic bone
      3. Alloplasts
         a. Tricalcium phosphate (TCP)
         b. Nonresorbable hydroxyapatite (HA)
      4. Any combination of above
II. Vestibuloplasties
   A. With soft tissue grafts
   B. With pedicled mucosa grafts
      1. Submucous vestibuloplasty
      2. Crestally pedicled mucosal grafting
   C. Secondary epithelialization
   D. Mouth floor lowering with mylohyoid and portion of genioglossus muscles repositioning
   E. Mylohyoid repositioning
   F. Creation of post-tuberosity (hamular) notch
   G. Any combination of above procedures as appropriate in the mandible or maxilla
III. Implants
   A. Osseointegrated implant (screw, basket, blade)
   B. Ramus frame implant
   C. Subperiosteal implant
   D. Staple implant
   E. Mucosal inserts
IV. Any combination of augmentation vestibuloplasties and implants

ments on the outer surface of the bony deficient maxilla may also present a prosthetic problem in facial flange extension.

Another factor that is important following loss of teeth is an alteration of maxillary and mandibular ridge relationships. Assuming that the patient had a normal occlusion in the dentulous state, as alveolar bone is lost following removal of the teeth, the relative size of the maxilla becomes smaller and that of the mandible larger in the respective sagittal and horizontal dimensions. There is also a continuing increase in intermaxillary vertical distance. These changes must be compensated for in the prosthetic care. If they become severe due to bone loss or if the patient had a preexisting skeletally related malocclusion in the dentulous state, ridge relation corrections may be required before successful prosthetic care can be provided.

Preprosthetic Surgical Goals

The common surgical and preprosthetic goals for rehabilitation of edentulous and partially edentulous patients include restoration of satisfactory esthetics, masticatory and other associated functions (i.e., phonation, etc.), and preservation of the associated hard and soft tissues and motor and sensory nerve function. With implants such as those of Branemark et al. these goals will be frequently attainable.

With conventional dentures or staple implants the specific goals are:

1. Provide a broad, convex ridge form in the maxilla and mandible.
2. Provide fixed tissue over the primary denture support area (residual alveolar ridge).
3. Provide facial and lingual vestibules for denture flange extensions (not critical for staple implants).
4. Provide ideal interridge relationship.
5. In the severely bony deficient mandible, provide bone bulk for strength and protection for neurovascular bundles in bony dehisced mandibular canals.
6. Provide an arched palatal vault form.
7. Provide post-tuberosity (hamular) notching to enhance the posterior border seal and resistance of the denture to anterior dislodging forces.

By fulfilling these goals as nearly as possible, the resultant stable, properly extended conventional prosthesis should allow wide distribution of functionally generated forces. This should reduce the incidence and rate of adverse bone and soft tissue changes and permit satisfactory function and esthetics.

Patient's History with Contraindications and Relative Contraindications

A careful history and clinical examination, including the patient's perspective of his or her problem, can help in choosing a treatment option that will provide predictable and satisfactory results. The final plan must evolve with the consensus of all those concerned—the surgeon, the prosthodontist, and, most importantly, the patient.

First, the patient's complaints and needs are elicited. Chief complaints commonly include unstable dentures, discomfort, and inability to masticate well.

Patients' occupations or life styles may indicate a need for a particular type of prosthesis. A fixed type prosthesis should be considered for patients who play certain wind instruments, actors, and other individuals whose professions or lifestyles dictate a need for temporary or long-term fixed prostheses.

Other patients may object to being without dentures for any period of time. The treatment of these patients must permit almost continuous use of a prosthesis in the immediate postsurgical period. This will provide esthetics and usual speech but will not allow maximum masticatory function.

Most patients who are candidates for preprosthetic surgery are in older age groups and more prone to physical problems. Some systemic problems or habits may contraindicate certain preprosthetic procedures, particularly implant devices. In addition, when patients have notable edentulous bone loss they may have some systemic pathology that contributes to that bone loss. Thus, an appropriate history is necessary.

A good history need not be rigidly structured, but the ADA long form is a good starting point. The evaluation forms in Chapter 1 are designed to provide more detailed information on systemic problems that might affect bone physiology, as well as on possible dietary imbalance.

The general status of the patient may be evaluated by the categories of the American Society of Anesthesiologists as outlined in Table 3–2. Categories I and II, if not impacted by specific diseases, will usually be eligible for most preprosthetic surgical procedures. Category III may allow only minimally stressful procedures. Categories IV and V would contraindicate any elective procedure.

Life expectancy will occasionally play a role in treatment planning. A 30-year-old patient, for example, with severe EBL of the mandible may be a candidate for bone augmentation, whereas a patient of 85 years

TABLE 3–2. AMERICAN SOCIETY OF ANESTHESIOLOGISTS' PATIENT EVALUATION

Class I	A patient who has no organic disease or in whom the disease is localized and causes no systemic disturbances.
Class II	A patient exhibiting slight to moderate systemic disturbance that may or may not be associated with the surgical complaint and that interferes only moderately with the patient's normal activities and general physiologic equilibrium.
Class III	A patient exhibiting severe systemic disturbance that may or may not be associated with the surgical complaint and that seriously interferes with the patient's normal activities.
Class IV	A patient exhibiting extreme systemic disturbance that may or may not be associated with the surgical complaint, that interferes seriously with the patient's normal activities, and that has already become a threat to life.
Class V	The rare patient who is moribund before operation, whose preoperative condition is such that he or she is expected to die within 24 hours even though not subjected to the additional strain of operation.

with the same bone loss might have some lesser procedure suggested.

Patients who are candidates for implant devices offer special medical-legal considerations. Implant devices, in some ways, can be likened to teeth. Like a tooth, they pierce the continuity of the natural defense structure—the mucosa. But unlike teeth, the implants are not placed there by nature, but by man, and in our society, those who place implants are loaded (or overloaded in some cases) with responsibilities. For example, natural teeth may be neglected by the patient and cause significant infection, bone loss, and discomfort, and this is usually regarded as the responsibility of the patient. However, when an implant device is placed, much of this responsibility is shifted to the doctor. The patient should be advised of the possible adverse effects of the implant, specifically the need for scrupulous hygiene, very frequent follow-up observation, and care as required, including removal of the implant if it is deemed nonsalvageable and is adversely affecting the patient's health.

In addition to and apart from the general status of the patient, some diseases and habits affect decisions relative to preprosthetic procedures. The following include most of those specific situations.

Not included in these specific diseases are such conditions as a recent myocardial infarction, acquired immunodeficiency syndrome (AIDS), and debilitating or transmittable hepatitis. These would be covered by following the previously cited ASA guidelines. Specific diseases and conditions will be dealt with in three categories: absolute contraindications; relative contraindications that will primarily be related to the physician's recommendations; and relative contraindications that will primarily be related to the dentist's evaluation of risk vs. benefit. These categories will be applied to soft tissue procedures, hard tissue procedures, and mucosal perforating implant procedures.

The specific diseases will usually be disclosed as a previously diagnosed condition. Less commonly they will be revealed through the current history and physical examination and laboratory tests directed by the history and physical examination form. It is not appropriate to order a "shotgun" approach to laboratory tests.

Table 3–1 delineates the various surgical categories.

Soft Tissue Procedures (Table 3–3). The first surgical category will be vestibuloplasties, including submucosal and secondary epithelialization procedures, lowering of mouth floor with mylohyoid and genioglossus myotomies, and soft tissue grafting procedures of skin and mucosa.

Absolute contraindications to these procedures include pregnancy and untreatable granulocytopenia, pregnancy for the obvious reason of avoiding any elective procedures during a pregnancy period and granulocytopenia because of the abnormal bleeding tendencies with this disease and the fact that unnecessary platelet transfusions are to be avoided. Therefore, an elective procedure in which platelets might be necessary is contraindicated.

Relative contraindications that should be discussed fully with the physician and patient include prolonged corticosteroid usage for any reason, any underlying medical problems that normally require prophylactic antibiotics (for example, subacute bacterial endocarditis), brittle diabetes mellitus, idiopathic thrombocytopenic purpura, thrombotic thrombocytopenic purpura, polymyositis, hemophilias, leukemias, lymphomas and plasma cell dyscrasias, vasculitides, mixed connective tissue disease, rheumatoid arthritis, lupus erythematosus, Sjögren's syndrome, many malignancies, Ehlers-Danlos syndrome, Marfan's syndrome, any history of osteomyelitis in the area to be operated, any history of osteoradionecrosis in the area to be operated, myasthenia gravis, Munchausen's syndrome, personality disorders (especially hysterical, antisocial, paranoid, hypochondriacal, schizoid, dependent, and narcissistic), drug dependence history, psychoses (for example, schizophrenia and bipolar illness), chronic renal failure, im-

TABLE 3–3. CONTRAINDICATIONS TO SOFT TISSUE PROCEDURES (VESTIBULOPLASTIES)*

Absolute	Relative (Physician-Related)	Relative (Patient-Related)
Pregnancy	Prolonged corticosteroid usage	Trigeminal neuralgia
	Required prophylactic antibiotics	
Untreatable granulocytopenia	Brittle diabetes mellitus	Atypical facial pain
	Idiopathic thrombocytopenic purpura	
	Thrombotic thrombocytopenic purpura	Precancerous lesions in operative area
	Polymyositis	
	Hemophilias	
	Leukemias	
	Lymphomas	
	Plasma cell dyscrasias	
	Vasculitides	
	Mixed connective tissue disease	
	Rheumatoid arthritis	
	Lupus erythematosus	
	Sjögren's syndrome	
	Many malignancies	
	Ehlers-Danlos syndrome	
	Marfan's syndrome	
	Osteomyelitis history	
	Osteoradionecrosis history	
	Myasthenia gravis	
	Munchausen's syndrome	
	Personality disorders	
	Drug dependence history	
	Psychoses	
	Chronic renal failure	
	Immune complex renal diseases	
	Chronic glomerular disease	
	Renal tubular acidosis	
	Fanconi's syndrome	
	Major organ transplantation	
	Anticoagulant therapy	
	Chemotherapy	
	Chronic active hepatitis	
	Certain genetic syndromes (e.g., Down's)	

*See Table 3–1.

mune complex renal diseases, chronic glomerular disease, renal tubular acidosis, Fanconi's syndrome, history of renal or other major organ transplantation, anticoagulant therapy or chemotherapy, chronic active hepatitis, and certain genetic syndromes (e.g., Down's).

Chronic corticosteroid therapy may be a relative contraindication because of poor wound healing and an increased susceptibility to infection. Therefore, if elective procedures are to be undertaken, one would wish the patient's primary care physician to be well aware of the proposed surgeries and possible complications thereof. Many diseases are relative contraindications primarily because of possible prolonged steroid usage, including dermatomyositis, benign mucous membrane pemphigoid, pemphigus, Behçet's syndrome, and exfoliative dermatitis.

Other diseases represent possible contraindications because of possible prolonged corticosteroid usage combined with other possible disorders. For instance, idiopathic thrombocytopenic purpura and thrombotic thrombocytopenic purpura may require steroids and may also have associated abnormal bleeding. Many diseases often require steroids but also have involvement of multiple organ systems. These include the vasculitides (e.g., polymyalgia rheumatica, polyarteritis nodosa, Wegener's granulomatosis, and giant cell arteritis), mixed connective tissue disease, rheumatoid arthritis, Sjögren's syndrome, chronic active hepatitis, and lupus erythematosus. Polymyositis involves steroid usage plus possible proximal muscle weakness, which can adversely affect proper oral hygiene (this is very important with regard to implants, discussed later in this chapter).

Those problems that may require prophylactic antibiotics, as in prophylaxis for subacute bacterial endocarditis, warrant discussion with the patient and physician because of the potential need for prolonged antibiotic therapy if delayed healing or chronic infection occurs. This may unnecessarily expose the organ or part to be protected to resistant strains of microbes. However, a history of rheumatic valvular heart disease or cardiac valve replacement may represent more of an absolute contraindication to elective surgery than those problems wherein antibiotic prophylaxis is a bit more debatable, such as mitral valve prolapse.

Patients with marked metabolic or hematologic disturbances like diabetes, leukemias, lymphomas, and plasma cell dyscrasias certainly should have a consultation with the patient's physician.

Ehlers-Danlos syndrome is often associated with markedly fragile tissues that would not respond well to surgery and also is occasionally associated with an abnormal bleeding response that may preclude surgery. The primary problem with Marfan's syndrome is the possibility of an aortic aneurysm because of weakness in the wall of the aorta (tunica media). Therefore, for an elective procedure, the Marfan's patient should be evaluated before being subjected to the increased cardiovascular stress of surgery.

A patient with a past history of osteomyelitis in an area to be operated is a problem. Many people consider osteomyelitis to be a disease that is not cured but rather only controlled and can be exacerbated by trauma to the region.

Patients with osteoradionecrosis have a similar problem. If a bone that has had osteoradionecrosis but has been healed through surgical measures and/or hyperbaric oxygen and antibiotic therapy is re-exposed, one can have a difficult problem with healing of the exposed bone.

Myasthenia gravis can present a problem with elective surgeries, primarily because of potential abnormal responses to anesthesia (particularly neuromuscular blockers) and also because of weakness of respiratory musculature that may result in respiratory embarrassment.

Any psychiatric disorder such as Munchausen's syndrome and personality and psychotic disorders represent relative contraindications to these procedures because of abnormal expectations of the treatment or responses to the treatment. Recovering drug abusers may have postoperative pain requiring medicines that may reincite their abuse.

Patients with chronic renal failure or various renal diseases require consultation with the physician to properly treat the patient as well as to possibly prevent further renal complications.

Transplantation of a major organ represents a nearly absolute contraindication because of the potential of bacteremia infecting the transplant.

Patients on anticoagulant therapy need consultation to find out the reasons for such therapy and whether its discontinuation would be contraindicated for these elective procedures. Chemotherapeutic agents (besides the corticosteroids like prednisone that have been covered previously) require consultation and evaluation to assess their possible adverse effects on various tissue systems, including the bone marrow.

Down's syndrome and other genetic syndromes may require physician consultation to rule out systemic abnormalities (e.g., cardiac anomalies).

Relative contraindications until fully discussed with the patient and general dentist/prosthodontist include trigeminal neuralgia, atypical facial pain, and precancerous lesions (for instance, severe dysplasia) in the area, if not totally cured.

Trigeminal neuralgia and atypical facial pain represent relative contraindications because of the possibility of exacerbating a trigger point and/or of confusing surgical pain with the pain of these problems.

Precancerous lesions in the oral cavity present a relative contraindication to many procedures because of the theoretical possibility of traumatizing and "activating" the lesions.

Hard Tissue Augmentation Procedures (Table 3–4). The second section of procedures includes those hard tissue substances that are placed beneath mucosa. These include alloplastic materials, tricalcium phosphate, hydroxyapatite, and bone grafts, including autogenous and allogeneic grafts.

The *absolute contraindications* include pregnancy and granulocytopenia, as discussed under "Soft Tissue Procedures."

The *physician-dependent relative contraindications* are the same as those for soft tissue procedures.

Relative contraindications that require careful consideration by the surgeon and discussion with the patient and general dentist/prosthodontist include trigeminal neuralgia, atypical facial pain, precancerous lesions in the operative area, disturbances associated with calcium metabolism, bone tumors in the donor or recipient sites, fibrous dysplasia in either site, osteopetrosis, and hypophosphatemic rickets.

Metabolic disturbances associated with calcium metabolism (including vitamin D–related abnormalities—osteomalacia and vitamin D–dependent rickets) may create abnormal or unpredictable responses to grafting. Hypophosphatemic rickets likewise is associated with abnormalities in the metabolism of calcium and phosphate.

Osteopetrosis may also cause unpredictable graft results. Bone tumors (depending on type) and fibrous dysplasia require care-

TABLE 3–4. CONTRAINDICATIONS TO AUGMENTATION PROCEDURES*

Absolute	Relative (Physician-Related)	Relative (Patient-Related)
Pregnancy Granulocytopenia	Prolonged corticosteroid usage Required prophylactic antibiotics Brittle diabetes mellitus Idiopathic thrombocytopenic purpura Thrombotic thrombocytopenic purpura Polymyositis Hemophilias Leukemias Lymphomas Plasma cell dyscrasias Vasculitides Mixed connective tissue disease Rheumatoid arthritis Lupus erythematosus Sjögren's syndrome Many malignancies Ehlers-Danlos syndrome Marfan's syndrome Osteomyelitis history Osteoradionecrosis history Myasthenia gravis Munchausen's syndrome Personality disorders Drug dependence history Psychoses Chronic renal failure Immune complex renal disease Chronic glomerular disease Renal tubular acidosis Fanconi's syndrome Major organ transplantation Anticoagulant therapy Chemotherapy Chronic active hepatitis Certain genetic syndromes (e.g., Down's)	Trigeminal neuralgia Atypical facial pain Precancerous lesions in operative area Calcium metabolism abnormalities Bone tumors Fibrous dysplasia Osteopetrosis Hypophosphatemic rickets

*See Table 3–1.

ful consideration of the risk/benefit ratio.

Transmucosal Implants (Table 3–5). The final category of procedures includes those implants which, in their final form, perforate the oral mucosa. Because of potential complications that are inherent in implants permanently exposed to the oral environment, this group will clearly have the longest list of both absolute and relative contraindications, as shown in Table 3–5. Future research may indicate that osseointegrated devices are likely to have fewer contraindications than other implants. Non-osseointegrated implants are surrounded by soft tissue and are therefore more susceptible to chronic infection.

Absolute contraindications again include pregnancy and granulocytopenia.

Continuous corticosteroid use should be considered an absolute contraindication for this category of procedures because of the increased susceptibility to infection. Diseases that may require intermittent corticosteroid therapy are relative contraindications to be discussed with the patient's physician (as discussed in "relative contraindications" under "Soft Tissue Procedures").

Patients who require prophylactic antibiotics before dental procedures should not have these implants because of the life-threatening periodic bacteremia that may occur. However because there is debate concerning the requirement for prophylactic antibiotics in patients with mitral valve prolapse and total joint replacements, the patient's physician should be consulted in these circumstances.

Other conditions that contraindicate implants include brittle or poorly controlled diabetes mellitus (primarily because of the increased risk of infection and probable short-term "life expectancy" of the implant); hemophilias; Ehlers-Danlos syndrome (because of the easy bleeding and tissue fragility); Marfan's syndrome; previous osteomyelitis in the area (for reasons previously discussed); and previous osteoradionecrosis in the area.

Radiation to the area would be a contraindication depending on total dose. Doses of

TABLE 3-5. CONTRAINDICATIONS TO IMPLANTS*

Absolute (May Be Modified by Special Circumstances)	Relative (Physician-Related)	Relative (Patient-Related)
Pregnancy	Idiopathic thrombocytopenic purpura	Trigeminal neuralgia
Granulocytopenia	Thrombotic thrombocytopenic purpura	Atypical facial pain
Continuous corticosteroid usage	Polymyositis	Precancerous lesions in operative area
Required prophylactic antibiotics	Leukemias	Bone tumors
Brittle or poorly controlled diabetes mellitus	Lymphomas	Erosive lichen planus
Hemophilias	Plasma cell dyscrasias	Osteoporosis
Ehlers-Danlos syndrome	Vasculitides	Osteopetrosis
Marfan's syndrome	Mixed connective tissue disease	Tobacco usage
Osteoradionecrosis history	Rheumatoid arthritis	Bruxism
Radiation therapy	Lupus erythematosus	Poor oral hygiene
Chronic renal failure	Sjögren's syndrome	Poor patient compliance
Major organ transplantation	Many malignancies	
Anticoagulant therapy	Myasthenia gravis	
Hypersensitivity (allergy) to implant material	Munchausen's syndrome	
Fibrous dysplasia	Personality disorders	
Regional enteritis	Drug dependence history	
	Psychoses	
	Immune complex renal diseases	
	Chronic glomerular disease	
	Renal tubular acidosis	
	Fanconi's syndrome	
	Chemotherapy	
	Chronic active hepatitis	
	Certain genetic syndromes (e.g., Down's)	
	Calcium metabolism abnormalities	
	Hypophosphatemic rickets	
	Confusional states (dementia)	
	Chronic antipsychotic medication	
	Multiple sclerosis	
	Parkinson's disease	
	Cerebral palsy	
	Muscular atrophies	
	Muscular dystrophies	
	After splenectomy	
	Gastrointestinal malabsorption	
	Chronic gastric reflux or vomiting	
	Acid-base disturbances	
	Porphyrias	
	Amino acid abnormalities	
	Lipid abnormalities	
	Carbohydrate enzyme abnormalities	
	Amyloidosis	
	Pituitary abnormalities	
	Thyroid abnormalities	
	Adrenal and ACTH hyper- and hypofunction	
	Multiple endocrine neoplasias (Types I, II, III)	
	Pheochromocytoma	
	Carcinoid syndrome	
	Anemias	
	Polycythemia	
	Seizure disorders	

*See Table 3-1.

greater than 5000 rads are known to be associated with increased incidence of osteoradionecrosis.[71] Therefore, one should probably not place implants in bone exposed to more than 5000 rads (and even this may be too great a dose).

Further absolute contraindications include chronic renal failure and renal or any other major organ transplant.

Those patients who require chronic dicoumarol anticoagulant therapy should not receive transmucosal implants for two reasons. First, the risk of bleeding during the operative procedure(s) is great. More important, however, is the added risk of bleeding from the peri-implant mucosa.

Hypersensitivity (allergy) to a component of the implant is obviously an absolute contraindication.

Final contraindications include fibrous dysplasia in the area and regional enteritis. Crohn's disease represents a contraindication because of frequent steroid usage, possible oral involvement, and malabsorption problems.

Relative contraindications that should be discussed with the patient's physician again include idiopathic thrombocytopenic purpura, thrombotic thrombocytopenic purpura, polymyositis, leukemias, lymphomas, plasma cell dyscrasias, vasculitides, mixed connective tissue disease, rheumatoid arthritis, lupus erythematosus, Sjögren's syndrome, many malignancies, myasthenia gravis, Munchausen's syndrome, personality disorders, drug dependence history, psychoses, immune complex renal disease, chronic glomerular disease, renal tubular acidosis, Fanconi's syndrome, chemotherapy, chronic active hepatitis, Down's syndrome and other genetic syndromes as dictated by the underlying abnormalities, abnormalities of vitamin D and calcium metabolism, and hypophosphatemic rickets.

Certain situations and diseases may prevent the patient from physically being able to properly care for their implants. These include confusional states (dementia) if not temporary, and even chronic use of antipsychotic medication (because of potential present or future extrapyramidal reactions). Other neurologic abnormalities that may compromise hygiene include multiple sclerosis, Parkinson's disease, cerebral palsy, and the muscular atrophies and dystrophies.

Another situation that represents a relative contraindication to transmucosal implants is prior splenectomy. Splenectomized patients have a diminished ability to respond to specific bacteria, including *Hemophilus influenzae* and pneumococci.

Gastrointestinal malabsorption diseases that periodically put the patient in a nutritionally imbalanced state are relative contraindications, as is the possibility of gastrointestinal reflux or chronic vomiting, which would bring gastric juices into contact with the implant and peri-implant mucosa.

Acid-base problems that place the patient in periodic metabolic imbalance represent potential contraindications, as do the porphyrias because of the potential for metabolic problems. Amino acid disturbances, lipid abnormalities, and carbohydrate enzymatic abnormalities may be relative contraindications because of metabolic imbalances and an increased risk of infection.

Amyloidosis may cause problems because of its adverse effects on various organs, most particularly the heart and kidneys.

Other endocrinopathies besides diabetes mellitus require careful consideration, including pituitary abnormalities (most particularly panhypopituitarism or growth hormone imbalances), uncontrolled hyper- or hypothyroidism, and adrenal hyper- or hypofunction (including ACTH hyper- or hyposecretion).

The genetic syndromes of multiple endocrine neoplasias Types I, II, and III represent at least relative contraindications to these procedures, as various abnormalities can be seen including mucosal neuromas, medullary thyroid carcinoma, parathyroid abnormalities, pancreatic islet problems, pituitary abnormalities, and adrenal problems including pheochromocytoma. Untreated pheochromocytoma and carcinoid syndrome should also be discussed with the physician.

Anemias that are not treatable or are frequently recurrent may increase the risk of infection and/or implant rejection, and these include the autoimmune hemolytic anemias, sickle cell anemia, and the thalassemias. Polycythemia vera or polycythemia relative to hypoxia may alter graft response via abnormal circulation. (Polycythemia secondary to decreased oxygen concentration as seen at elevated altitudes would not be a problem.)

A seizure disorder would represent a relative contraindication depending primarily on the type of seizure and the frequency of occurrence. Motor seizure activity, as seen in grand mal epilepsy, for instance, may result in excessive trauma to the implants.

Relative contraindications that need to be discussed with the surgeon, the dentist/prosthodontist, and the patient include trigeminal neuralgia, atypical facial pain, and incurable precancerous lesions or benign bone tumors in the region to receive the implant. Erosive lichen planus is thought to be potentially premalignant and thus falls into this category.

Osteopetrosis and osteoporosis may alter bone viability and implant acceptance and thus require consideration.

One should strongly warn the patient to discontinue any tobacco usage, as this may adversely affect implants. Bruxism may also result in abnormal trauma to the implant. Other possible contraindications include present or anticipated poor oral hygiene as well as proven poor compliance with the suggestions of the dental team.

Anatomic Factors and Treatment Planning

After noting the patient's special needs and physical status, the evaluation of the anatomic problems remains.

Before addressing these anatomic problems, consideration should be given to emerging findings about hydroxyapatite (HA) and bone loss that may influence many of our decisions. There is now a hypothesis that the type of bonding of HA to the bone surface may prevent or significantly decrease surface bone resorption (see Chapter 8). If this should prove to be correct, then theoretically nonresorbable HA should be placed on all bony surfaces that will be load-bearing for dentures.

The therapeutic considerations for the following categories of anatomic problems will be discussed. The details of each procedure will be described in subsequent chapters.

Considerations at Time of Tooth Removal. Conservation of bone at the time of tooth removal is important (see Chapter 4).

There is some consideration for implanting fresh sockets with HA in an attempt to preserve the alveolar bone (see Chapter 8). However, long-term data are not available. In the case of vital and nonvital root retention, some long-term data suggest that these procedures are of questionable value, which is contrary to the short-term findings.[72-74]

The Edentulous Mandible

STAGE I. Stage I is characterized by an adequate and well-contoured alveolar ridge, along with the common variables (Table 3–6). The research of Branemark et al. (see Chapter 7) suggests that their osseointegrated implant system may be the first choice in a Stage I mandible. When a conventional denture is considered, localized mucosal or muscle attachments may interfere with denture flange extension and/or result in mobility of tissues covering the residual ridge, and a corrective vestibuloplasty may be appropriate. Concurrent with the vestibuloplasty, any excess tissue such as a mobile crestal scar or reactive fibrous connective tissue should be removed. A crestally pedicled mucosal graft has been successfully used for sulcus deepening when only the anterior mandibular area is involved (see Chapter 5).

When both the labial-buccal and lingual vestibules are inadequate, a complete vestibuloplasty with soft tissue grafting (see Chapter 5) is effective treatment. If only the labial-buccal vestibule is lacking, a soft tissue graft in that area may be considered.

When only the lingual vestibule is at fault, the floor of the mouth can be completely lowered by detachment of the mylohyoid muscles with inferior repositioning along with detachment of the superior fibers of the genioglossus. A less extensive procedure involves release of the mylohyoid muscle attachment, allowing it to retract passively, which provides some lowering of the lingual vestibule in this area (see Chapter 5).

The ultimate goal, of course, is to provide as much fixed tissue as possible over the primary denture support area and provide labial and lingual sulci and as such significantly improve the retention, stability, and support for conventional complete dentures.

If a decision is made to manage the patient's problem with an implant, those with demonstrated osseointegration should be considered first. Since alveolar bone is present in a Stage I mandible, the subperiosteal implant is contraindicated, since alveolar bone is present and resorption beneath such implants occurs. Similarly, the ramus frame implant may resorb excessively in the anterior region if alveolar bone is the supporting structure.

STAGE II. Stage II is characterized by localized alveolar deficiency with variable contour. Here again an osseointegrated device may be the most ideal restorative procedure.

When a conventional denture is to be used and there are localized contour defects of the residual alveolar ridge or when the commonly seen labial or buccal undercut exists, the corrective procedure considered most appropriate today is the onlaying of nonresorbable HA, tricalcium phosphate, or allo-

---

TABLE 3–6. CLASSIFICATION OF THE EDENTULOUS MANDIBLE AND MAXILLA IDENTIFYING BOTH HARD AND SOFT TISSUE PROBLEMS

Stages of edentulous bone loss (EBL)
I. Adequate amount and well-contoured alveolar ridge (usually soft tissue problems)
II. Localized or generalized partial alveolar deficiency with variable contour (as an undercut ridge)
III. Loss of most of the alveolar process usually with poor contour (as a knife edge or no ridge)
IV. Generalized loss of the alveolar process and much of the body (as a very weakened mandible)

Common variables that may be combined with any of the above stages of EBL
A. Shallow facial vestibule
B. Shallow lingual vestibule or palate
C. Mobile tissue covering the ridge
D. Excessive tissue covering the ridge
E. Interarch discrepancy secondary to skeletal malrelation

geneic particulate bone.[75] When contour is acceptable, soft tissue abnormalities or inadequate vestibular extensions may be present and require correction by vestibuloplasty procedures (see Chapter 5).

STAGE III. Stage III is characterized by loss of most of the alveolar process and usually has a poor contour such as the knife edge ridge or a flat ridge. Again, an osseointegrated device may be appropriate.

If a conventional denture is required, augmentation and/or a vestibuloplasty procedure would be helpful. A good choice for augmentation in this circumstance is nonresorbable HA, which may be followed by a vestibuloplasty if needed.

A vestibuloplasty skin graft and lowering of mouth floor alone will usually give a good result if residual ridge contour is reasonably satisfactory. One should keep in mind that the patient might later require an augmentation with a material such as nonresorbable HA, autogeneic or allogeneic bone, or a combination of these. Unfortunately, grafted skin does not provide as viable a flap as normal mucosa, making open augmentation procedures more precarious. Thus, it would appear more beneficial when possible to provide the augmentation before the skin grafting is accomplished. If the augmentation is done after skin grafting, a tunneling approach via selected small vestibular incisions is recommended.

The staple implant, subperiosteal implant, or ramus frame implant may be considered by some for State III patients, but the osseointegrated system may supplant these implant systems.

STAGE IV. Stage IV is characterized by generalized loss of the alveolar process and much of the body. In this circumstance the mandible is in jeopardy of fracture with slight trauma. Ideally the strength of the mandible as well as its function should be restored. The age and physical status of the patient will have some bearing on the need for or feasibility of strength augmentation by increasing cross-sectional bony bulk. Bony restoration can be accomplished by grafts to the superior surface of the body of the mandible or to the inferior surface. Onlay augmentation of the inferior surface, while providing strength, may not contribute to ridge form contour correction or provide protection for an exposed neurovascular bundle in a bony dehisced mandibular canal (see Chapter 6). Recently nonresorbable HA combined with cancellous iliac bone has been advocated, with the hypothesis that the bone will remain surrounding the alloplast particles (see Chapter 8). Because this form of HA does not resorb, it is postulated that the HA-bone augmentation may remain permanently. If this proves to be true, a significant breakthrough will have occurred, as all previous types of bony augmentation eventually undergo significant resorption. Usually the very weak portion of the mandible will be in the premolar-molar areas. Considering the possibility of using an osseointegrated implant system in the anterior area, it may be appropriate to reconstruct only the posterior region. This would be especially true if nonresorbable HA and bone were mixed for the reconstructive material, as HA interspersed in bone may interfere with the use of the osseointegrated system.

If a conventional denture is contemplated after reconstruction, a selected vestibuloplasty procedure with muscle and mucosal repositioning and correction of abnormal covering tissues may be required for a satisfactory final result.

Some advocate placing a subperiosteal implant when as little as 8 mm of mandibular height is present.[76] The implant would add marked functional aid, but the possibility of accelerating the bone loss in an already weakened mandible would appear to be a poor trade-off. The elevated subperiosteal implant with bone grafting was designed to strengthen the mandible as well as provide enhanced function. However, the sparse literature is conflicting with regard to the efficacy of this modality.[65-68]

The anteriorly placed osseointegrated system and the ramus frame implant are advocated by some when the posterior portion of the body of the mandible has severe EBL but a fair amount of bone remains in the anterior region. With the possible exception of the ramus frame, these implants do not add strength to the weakened posterior region, and, ideally, strength augmentation with bone grafting should be considered as discussed.

The Edentulous Maxilla

The factors affecting the treatment plan for maxillary problems differ from those of the mandible. Although the osseointegrated systems appear to provide a rather ideal restoration for the mandible, there are restrictions when considered for the maxilla. In the present state of the art, ideal esthetics may not be achievable and there may not be adequate bone in which to place implants. Bony augmentation is currently being investigated to solve this problem.

In the severely bony deficient maxilla, one does not need to be concerned with a fracture, so strength augmentation does not play a role. Contrary to the mandibular pattern of EBL, the maxillary arch size shrinks as bone is lost. This causes esthetic problems relative to lip and cheek support as well as creating stability problems for the conventional denture. The primary factors affecting the decision-making process are:

1. Denture stability and retention
2. Quality and amount of mucosa over residual ridge
3. Quality of vestibular mucosa
4. Contour of alveolar bone and palate
5. Degree of post-tuberosity (hamular) notching
6. Support for lip and cheeks
7. Interarch size coordination

If the maxillary denture is unstable due to shallow vestibular depth but the alveolar bone has good contour and vestibular mucosa is normal, a submucous vestibuloplasty with excision of any mobile crestal tissue is an appropriate procedure. If the quality of the vestibular mucosa is impaired, and the alveolar size contour is acceptable, a secondary epithelialization procedure may be appropriate if the known relapse is acceptable. When the quantity of mucosa is insufficient or the degree of relapse with a secondary epithelialization procedure is unacceptable, then a skin or mucosal grafting procedure is appropriate (see Chapter 5). However, an augmentation of the maxilla should be done prior to a vestibuloplasty procedure if there is an adequate amount of remaining bone, if there are contour problems, if lip or cheek support is diminished, or if the interridge relationship requires correction by maxillary repositioning and/or augmentation (see Chapters 5 and 8). The specific method chosen to augment the maxilla is based on the identified problem. Nonresorbable HA without bone grafting may be an appropriate modality (see Chapter 8), but bone grafting may occasionally be needed along with the HA if so much alveolar reconstruction is planned that the HA alone would be somewhat mobile (see Chapter 8). Bone grafting without HA is also a valid procedure as long as the long-term results with HA are still unknown (see Chapter 6).

If an absolute increase in vertical dimension is needed to provide a sufficient vestibular depth, the LeFort I downfracturing with interpositional bone grafting may be utilized (see Chapter 6). This approach provides some possibility for limited ridge form correction and has some indication when maxillary repositioning is required for intermaxillary ridge relationship corrections. The use of improved stabilization methods such as rigid fixation with small bone plates may improve the long-term stability of this procedure. The modified LeFort I osteotomy, which includes a portion of the zygomatic arch, often provides stable forward and downward movement with bone grafting.[78]

When the bone loss of the maxilla is so severe that no palatal vault remains, a surgical elevation of the palate may be considered (see Chapter 6). Again this procedure will probably be used less frequently as the ability to augment the alveolar area with nonresorbable ceramic alloplasts to correct the palatal vault problem is improved.

The surgical deepening of the hamular notch (tuberoplasty) is only moderately successful, and this procedure is advocated only when the notch is completely lacking and the tuberosity cannot be rebuilt (see Chapter 4). A post-tuberosity (hamular) notch is important to enhance posterior border seal and resistance of the denture to anterior-posterior dislodging forces.

BIBLIOGRAPHY

1. Levin B, and Landesman HM: A practical questionnaire for predicting denture success or failure. J Prosthet Dent 35:124–130, 1976.
2. Tallgren A: Positional changes of complete dentures: A 7-year longitudinal study. Acta Odont Scand 27:539–561, 1969.
3. Tallgren A: The continuing reduction of the residual alveolar ridges in complete denture wearers: A mixed-longitudinal study covering 25 years. J Prosthet Dent 27:120–131, 1972.
4. Nordin BEC, Horsman A, and Gallagher JL: Effect of various therapies on bone loss in women. In Kuhlencordt F, and Kruse H (eds.): Calcium Metabolism, Bone, and Metabolic Bone Diseases. Berlin, Springer Verlag, 1975, pp 233–242.
5. Zanzi I, Aloia JF, Ellis KJ, and Cohn SH: Combined treatment of primary osteoporosis with oral sodium fluoride, estrogens, and calcium. Calcif Tissue Res (Suppl. 22), 563, 1977.
6. Gotcher JE, and Jee WSS: A study of Cl_2 MDP in the experimental periodontal disease of the rice rat. J Dent Res 58 (Special Issue A):1293, 1979.
7. Leonard EP, Reese WV, and Mandel EJ: The effect of diphosphonates on alveolar bone loss in the rice rat. J Dent Res 58 (Special Issue A):563, 1979.
8. Sorensen RL: A Study of Dietary Calcium and Phosphorus Intakes in Relation to Residual Ridge Resorption. Thesis, School of Health, Loma Linda University, Loma Linda, California, 1977.
9. Wical KE, and Brussee P: Effects of a calcium and vitamin D supplement on alveolar ridge resorption in immediate denture patients. J Prosthet Dent 41:4–11, 1979.
10. Brown LR, Driezen S, Handler S, and Johnson DA: The effect of radiation induced erostomia on human oral microflora. J Dent Res 54:740–745, 1975.
11. Llory H, Damron A, and Frank RM: Changes in the oral flora following buccal-pharyngeal radiotherapy. Arch Oral Biol 16:617–621, 1971.

12. Fish EW: Using the muscles to stabilize the full lower denture. J Am Dent Assoc 20:2163–2169, 1933.
13. Lott F, and Levin B: Flange technique: An anatomic and physiological approach to increased retention, comfort, and appearance of dentures. J Prosthet Dent 16:394–413, 1966.
14. Landesman HM: A technique for the delivery of complete dentures. J Prosthet Dent 43:348–351, 1980.
15. Wright CR, Swartz WH, and Godwin WC: Mandibular denture stability—A new concept. Ann Arbor, MI, Overbeck Co, 1961.
16. Landesman HM, and Levin B: A patient survey of denture tolerance before and after a mandibular vestibuloplasty with skin grafting. J Am Dent Assoc 90:306–310, 1975.
17. Landesman HM, Davis WH, Martinoff J, and Kaminishi R: Resorption of the edentulous mandible after a vestibuloplasty with skin grafting. J Prosthet Dent 49:619–625, 1983.
18. Davis WH, Delo RI, Weiner JR, Kaminishi RM, and Bloom C: Handbook of Mandibular Vestibuloplasty with Skin Grafting. 3rd ed. Southern California Oral and Maxillofacial Surgery Foundation, 400 E Regent St, Inglewood, CA, 1980.
19. Small IA: Survey of experiences with the mandibular staple bone plate. J Oral Surg 36:604–607, 1978.
20. Bodine RL, and Mohammed CL: Implant denture histology: Gross and microscopic studies of a human mandible with a 12-year implant denture. Dent Clin North Am 14:145–159, 1970.
21. Bodine RL, Melrose RJ, and Grenoble DE: Long term implant denture histology and comparison with previous reports. J Prosthet Dent 35:665–673, 1976.
22. Garefis PN: Complete mandibular subperiosteal implants for edentulous mandibles. J Prosthet Dent 39:670–677, 1978.
23. James RS: The support system and pergingival mechanisms surrounding oral implants. Biomater Med Devices Artif Organs 7:147–153, 1979.
24. Branemark P-I, Hansson B-O, Adell R, Breine H, Lindstrom J, Hallen O, and Ohman A: Osseointegrated implants in the treatment of the edentulous jaw. Experience from a 10 year period. Plast Reconstr Surg (Suppl) 16:1, 1977.
25. Branemark P-I: Osseointegration and its experimental background. J Prosthet Dent 50:399–410, 1983.
26. Davis WH, Martinoff JT, and Kaminishi RM: Long-term followup of transoral rib grafts for mandibular atrophy. J Oral Maxillofac Surg 42:606, 1984.
27. Sanders B, and Beumer J: Augmentation rib grafting to the inferior border of the atrophic edentulous mandible: A five year experience. J Prosthet Dent 46:16–22, 1981.
28. Frost DE, Gregg JM, and Terry BC: Mandibular interpositional and onlay bone grafting for treatment of mandibular bone deficiency in the edentulous patient. J Oral Maxillofac Surg 40:353–360, 1982.
29. Curtis T, and Ware W: Autogenous bone grafts for atrophic edentulous mandibles: A review of twenty patients. J Prosthet Dent 49:212–216, 1983.
30. Schnitzler J, and Ewald K: Zur Technik der Hauttransplantation nach Thiersch. Centralbl Chir 21:148, 1894.
31. Moskowicz L: Ueber Verpflanzung Thiersch scher Epidermislappchen in die Mundhohle. Arch Klin Chir Bd 108, 11.2:216, 1915.
32. Esser JF: Neue Wege fur Chirurgische plastiken durch Heranziehung der zahnarztlichen Technik. Beitr Klin Chir 103:547, 1916.
33. Pickerill HB: Intra-oral skin-grafting: The establishment of the buccal sulcus. Proc Soc Med 12:17, 1918.
34. Weiser R: Ein Jahr chirurgisch-zahnarztliche Tatigkeit im Kieferspital. Z Stomat XVI:133, 1918.
35. Dorrance GM: Epithelial inlays versus skin or mucous membrane flaps: For replacing lost mucous membrane in the mouth. JAMA 75:1179, 1920.
36. Gillies HD: Plastic surgery of the face: Based on selected cases of war injuries of the face including burns. London, Henry Frowde and Hodder and Stoughton, 1920, pp 8-12.
37. Waldron CW: In Gillies HD: Plastic Surgery of the Face: Based on selected cases of war injuries of the face including burns. London, Henry Frowde and Hodder and Stoughton, 1920, pp 193–208.
38. Kazanjian VH: Surgical operations as related to satisfactory dentures. Dental Cosmos 66:387, 1924.
39. Pichler H, and Trauner R: Die Alveolarkammplastik. Oest Z Stomatol 28:54, 1930.
40. Wassmund M: Ueber chirurgische formgestaltung des atrophischen kiefers zum zwecke prothetischer versorgung. Vierteljahreschr Zahnheilkd 47:305, 1931.
41. Kazanjian VH: Surgery as an aid to more efficient service with prosthetic dentures. J Am Dent Assoc 22:556, 1935.
42. Ganzer H: Die Weiderherstellung des Vestibulum oris nach Schussverletzungen der Kiefer. Dtsch Mschr Zahnheilkd 34:380, 1916.
43. Rumpel C: Die Weiderherstellung des Vestibulum oris nach Schussverletzungen der Kiefer. Dtsch Zahnarztl Wochenschr 19:262, 1916.
44. Szaba J: Methode zur Verhinderung des Verwachsens der Durchtrennten mundschleimhaut. Oest Vierteljahrschr Zahnheilkd 32:244, 1916.
45. Lexer E: Die freien Transplantationen. Stuttgart, Enke 2:155, 1919.
46. MacIntosh RB, and Obwegeser H: Preprosthetic surgery: A scheme for its effective employment. J Oral Surg 25:397, 1967.
47. Trauner R: Alveoplasty with ridge extensions on the lingual side of the lower jaw to solve the problem of a lower dental prosthesis. Oral Surg 5:340, 1952.
48. Rehrmann A: Beitrag zur alveolar Kammplastik am Unterkiefer. Zahnarztl Rdsch 62:505, 1953.
49. Obwegeser H: Die totale Mundbodenplastik. Schweiz Mschr Zahnheilkd 73:565, 1963.
50. Davis WH, et al.: Mandibular Vestibuloplasty with Skin Grafting. 3rd ed. Southern California Oral Surgery Foundation, 400 E Regent St, Inglewood, CA, 1980.
51. Brown LJ: Surgical solution to a lower denture problem. Br Dent J 95:215, 1953.
52. Downton D: Mylohyoid ridge resection. Dent Pract Dent Rec 74:212, 1954.
53. Edlan A, and Mejchar B: Plastic surgery of the vestibulum in periodontal therapy. Int Dent J 13:593, 1963.
54. Clementschitch F: Cited in Pichler H, and Trauner R (eds.): Mund und Kieferchirurgie II. Berlin, Urban and Schwarzenberg, 1948.
55. Steinhauser E, and Obwegeser HL: Rebuilding the alveolar ridge with bone and cartilage autografts. Trans Int Conf Oral Surg, 2nd Congress, 1965, pp 203–208.
56. Barros-Saint-Pasteur J: Plastia restauradora de la cresta alveolar de la mandibula. Acta Odontol Venezuela 4:3, 1966.

57. Davis WH: Atrophy of the edentulous mandible. In Starshak TJ, and Sanders B (eds.): Preprosthetic Oral and Maxillofacial Surgery. St. Louis, CV Mosby Co, 1980.
58. Zide MF, Misick DJ, Kent JN, and Jarcho M: The evaluation of strength and resorption with different ratios of hydroxyapatite and bone in canine mandibular continuity defects. Unpublished data—see Chapter 8.
59. Obwegeser HL: Die submukose Vestibulumplastik. Dtsch Zahnarztl Z 14:749, 1959.
60. Terry BC, Albright JE, and Baker RD: Alveolar ridge augmentation in the edentulous maxilla with use of autogenous ribs. J Oral Surg 32:429, 1974.
61. Kent JN, Quinn JH, Zide MF, Guerra LR, and Boyne P: Alveolar ridge augmentation using nonresorbable hydroxyapatite with or without autogenous cancellous bone. J Oral Maxillofac Surg 41:629, 1983.
62. Small IA: Survey of experiences with the mandibular staple bone plate. J Oral Surg 36:604–605, 1978.
63. Helfrick JF, Topf JS, and Kaufman M: Mandibular staple bone plate: Long-term evaluation of 250 cases. J Am Dent Assoc 104:318–320, 1982.
64. Bodine RL: Evaluation of 27 mandibular subperiosteal implant dentures after 15 to 22 years. J Prosthet Dent 32:188, 1974.
65. Gershkoff A, and Goldberg NI: Implant Dentures. Philadelphia, JB Lippincott Co, 1957.
66. Kratochvil FJ, and Boyne PJ: Combined use of subperiosteal implant and bone-marrow graft in deficient edentulous mandibles: A preliminary report. J Prosthet Dent 27:645, 1972.
67. Kratochvil FJ, et al.: Rehabilitation of grossly deficient mandibles with combined subperiosteal implants and bone grafts. J Prosthet Dent 35:452, 1976.
68. Bloomquist DS: Long-term results of subperiosteal implants combined with cancellous bone grafts. J Oral Surg 40:348, 1982.
69. Roberts HD, and Roberts RA: The ramus end-osseous implant. J S Calif Dent Assoc 38: 571–577, 1970.
70. Branemark PI, Breine U, Lindstrom J, Adell R, Hansson BO, and Ohlsson A: Intra-osseous anchorage of dental prosthesis. Experimental studies. Scand J Plast Reconstr Surg 3:81, 1969.
71. Marx RE, and Ames JR: The use of hyperbaric oxygen therapy in bony reconstruction of the irradiated and tissue-deficient patient. J Oral Maxillofac Surg 40(7):412–420, 1982.
72. Masterson MP: Retention of vital submerged roots under complete dentures: Report of 10 patients. J Prosthet Dent 41(1):12–15, 1979.
73. Donahue TJ: The case against the edentulous ridge—and an alternative. J Am Dent Assoc 101:781k, 1980.
74. VonWowern N, and Winther S: Submergence of roots for alveolar ridge preservation. Int J Oral Surg 10:247, 1981.
75. Terry BC: Subperiosteal Onlay Grafts. In Stoelinga PJW (ed.): Association of Oral and Maxillofacial Surgeons. Proceedings of Consensus, Conference: The Relative Roles of Vestibuloplasty and Ridge Augmentation in the Management of the Atrophic Mandible. Berlin, Quintessence Publishing Co, Inc, 1984, pp 142–146.
76. Weiss CM, and Judy K: Severe mandibular atrophy—biological considerations of routine treatment with the complete subperiosteal implant. Oral Implantol IV(4):431, 1974.
77. Quinn JH, and Kent JN: Maintenance of human alveolar ridges with hydroxyapatite root implants. Proceedings of the Scientific Session, 65th Annual AAOMS Meeting, Sept 21–25, 1983, p 54.
78. Kaminishi R, Davis WH, et al.: Improved maxillary stability with modified LeFort I technique. J Oral Maxillofac Surg 41:203–205, 1983.

MINOR PREPROSTHETIC PROCEDURES

Richard F. Scott, D.D.S., M.S., and Robert A. J. Olson, D.M.D.

When the natural dentition is lost and prosthetic replacements become necessary, it is of paramount importance that a thorough evaluation of the jaws and contiguous structures be done prior to initiating the fabrication of dentures. As can be deduced from the previous chapters, the problems encountered may affect bone, soft tissue, or any combination thereof. An irregular ridge with bony projections and undercuts may interfere with insertion or adaptation to the ridges. Maxillary and mandibular tori and exostoses may also prevent adequate adaptation and are constantly irritated, causing discomfort. The region of the maxillary tuberosity can cause multiple problems. It is a common site for undercuts that may interfere with the path of insertion; it may grow downward, reducing vertical dimension and freeway space so there is inadequate space in which to construct a denture; a fibrous, mobile tuberosity interferes with stability and may encroach on space. Knifelike alveolar ridges or pronounced mylohyoid ridges are a constant source of irritation and pain and interfere with stability. Enlarged labial or buccal frena and ankyloglossia interfere with stability and retention. Inflammatory papillary hyperplasia is a constant source of irritation and infection, usually candidiasis. Mobile redundant tissue on the maxillary ridge causes loss of stability and retention, while epulis fissuratum of the vestibular sulcus causes pain in addition to lack of stability and retention. Dentures have been made over these conditions, but seldom are they truly satisfactory. These aforementioned conditions all require surgical attention in order to provide the optimum conditions for prosthetic rehabilitation. These corrective procedures constitute the minor reconstructive preprosthetic surgical practice.

The requirements for successful denture function are discussed in Chapter 3. In addition, this chapter will cover the important surgical aspects of the minor preprosthetic procedures.

ALVEOLOPLASTY ALONG WITH TOOTH REMOVAL

The preservation of alveolar bone is a prime concern. To preserve alveolar bone, vital and nonvital root retention has been practiced. Evaluations of the success of these modalities have been mixed. They are now generally considered of questionable value.[1,2]

The placing of alloplastic materials such as hydroxyapatite into fresh extraction sockets is currently being evaluated, but long-term human results are not yet available.

When roots fracture during dental extraction the principle of preserving bone should be considered. The crestal bone should be spared whenever possible. This may mean making a labial or buccal osseous window in the apical area or removing interradicular bone to retrieve the root. Occasionally, a small uninfected root may be left in place if its removal would require significant destruction of the alveolar bone.

When teeth are removed, sharp margins of the sockets are often present. Although the sharp margins may round off within a reasonable time, many times they do not and require trimming secondarily, which presents a dilemma. When the sharp labial or buccal bone is initially removed and no sharp edges remain, it is common to find that the mucosa falls into the socket. This can result in a diminished ridge. Another alternative would be to allow healing of the socket to the point that some organized tissue fills the socket. Then the buccal or labial bone can be removed without unduly diminishing the ridge. Unfortunately, this two-stage process delays or complicates denture construction. A third alternative is the initial use of the muco-osseous flap at the time the teeth are removed. This may be accomplished by removing the interseptal bone and the bone vertically where the margins of the muco-osseous flap will occur. At this point, the mucosa and bony plate can be mobilized intact and partially collapsed lingually, creating a contoured ridge.

Suture Material

If soft tissue does not tend to be displaced, plain gut suture material is ideal. If the soft tissue is subject to being displaced for only a few days, chromic gut suture material is appropriate.

If maintaining soft tissue position is important for a longer period, a slowly resorbable suture material such as polyglycolic acid or a nonresorbable material such as silk, Supramid, Prolene, etc., is appropriate.

SECONDARY ALVEOLAR RECONTOURING

Lateral bony projections, undercuts, or sharp crestal bone (knife-edge ridge) may be deterrents to denture construction and may require surgical modification. The ridge need not be perfectly smooth, and the sharp edges, large prominences, and deep undercuts should be eliminated. Usually, small rounded eminences and slight undercuts are acceptable.

Because the preservation of alveolar bone is important, augmentation rather than reduction of the ridge should be considered when an undesirable ridge contour is present, as discussed in Chapter 6.

When it is appropriate to reduce sharp crestal bone or lateral prominences, a crestal incision is used along with vertical incisions.

After the mucoperiosteal flap is raised, the bone is removed with rongeurs, an osteotome, or a bone file. The flap is then replaced. A secure closure of a mandibular incision is particularly important, as healing will be prolonged if dehiscence occurs.

REDUNDANT CRESTAL TISSUE REMOVAL

Before redundant tissue is removed, it is necessary to decide whether or not ridge augmentation is to be performed. For diagnostic considerations, see Chapter 3. If augmentation is to be accomplished, it is usually best done before the removal of mobile crestal tissue, as discussed in Chapter 6.

When removal of mobile crestal tissue is necessary, one should attempt to preserve some attached mucosa. An elliptical incision is made as narrowly as possible to allow access to the mass of mobile tissue. This incision is V-shaped, with the opening of the V at the mucosal surface. Excessive tissue is removed and the incision margins are tentatively approximated to ensure that adequate tissue has been removed and the edges of the incision approximate evenly. The incision is closed by a running stitch.

MAXILLARY TUBEROSITY REDUCTION

An increase in the vertical dimension of the maxillary tuberosity is frequently encountered. When of sufficient degree, this increase will impinge upon the intermaxillary space required for successful denture construction. It may also be pendulous, inhibiting denture stability, and palatal bony undercuts may be present. Pneumatization of the maxillary sinus may proceed into the elongated tuberosity. To determine the extent of pneumatization, preoperative lateral radiographs are advised, although entry into the antrum does not usually cause a problem. In general, the intermaxillary distance measured from the crest of the tuberosity to the retromolar area of the mandible should equal at least a centimeter when the mandible is placed in a position corresponding to the correct vertical dimension of occlusion. It should be remembered that impingement upon this intermaxillary distance may also be produced by soft tissue and osseous hypertrophy in the mandibular retromolar area. This consideration must be included in the preoperative planning. An additional preoperative aid in determining the amount of reduction required is accurately mounted study models.

Excess tuberosity is removed by wedge resection (Fig. 4–1). Two elliptical incisions are made over the crest of the tuberosity and carried down to bone. The resulting wedge of tissue is grasped with a hemostat and dissected free. The buccal and palatal soft tissues are undermined subperiosteally. Submucous resection of two wedge-shaped blocks of tissue is then accomplished by placing secondary incisions through the submucous portions of each flap paralleling the surface. The buccal and palatal flaps are returned and the margins trimmed to allow closure without overlapping. Both lateral and vertical dimensions of the tuberosity are reduced by this procedure. If bone removal is required, it should be carried out at this time and can be accomplished by utilizing side-cutting bone rongeurs and bone files (Fig. 4–2). No problem should occur when the maxillary sinus is entered if the soft tissue is closed and no antral infection is present. The area should be irrigated with sterile saline and then closed.

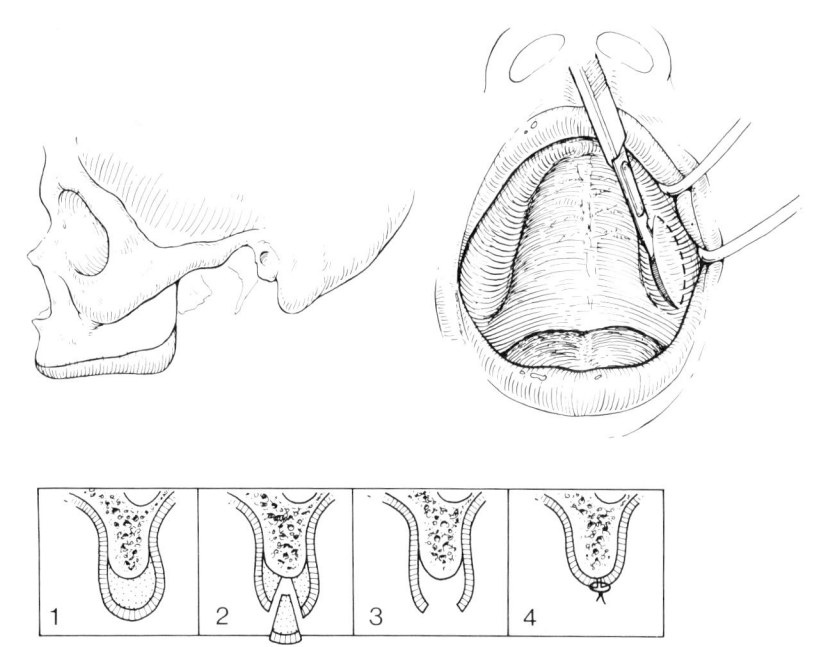

Figure 4–1. Maxillary tuberosity reduction. *Upper left,* Schematic, lateral view of maxilla showing excess tissue over the tuberosity region. *Upper right,* Elliptical wedge incision over the tuberosity. *Box 1,* Frontal view showing excess tissue over the maxillary tuberosity. *Box 2,* Frontal view of wedge excision. *Box 3,* Additional undermining excisions. *Box 4,* Closure.

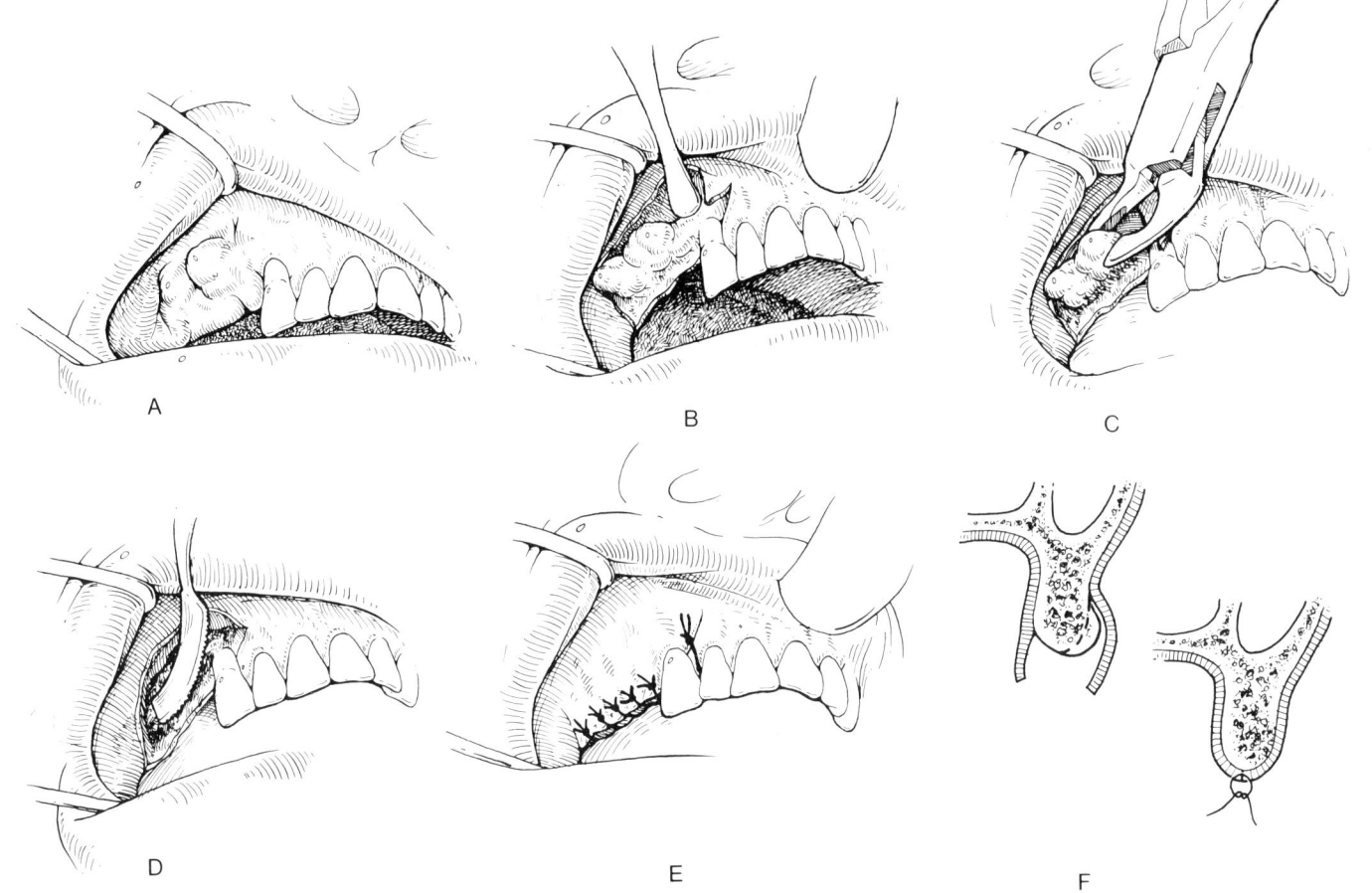

Figure 4–2. Reduction of osseous irregularities in tuberosity region. *A,* Lateral view showing bony irregularity. *B,* Mucoperiosteal flap reflection. *C,* Bony excision. *D,* Final osseous recontouring with bone file. *E,* Closure. *F,* Combination of soft-tissue and osseous tuberosity reduction.

Reduction of the tuberosity should not be carried to the extent that the sulcus depth formed by the hamular notch is obliterated. At least 2 to 3 mm of vertical sulcus height should remain distal to the tuberosity to provide denture stability.

Guernsey[3,4] describes an alternate approach to the tuberosity in which a horizontal incision is made in the buccal vestibule near the inferior border of the malar eminence (Fig. 4–3). The incision is carried through periosteum to bone and extends from the premolar area to the distal aspect of the tuberosity. Anterior and posterior vertical releasing incisions should be made to enhance access. A full-thickness mucoperiosteal flap is reflected inferiorly and includes the thick, fibrous tissue overlying the tuberosity. When the flap is held inferiorly, the thickened tissue can be dissected free. Osseous reductions and removal of undercuts are performed where indicated. The flap can then be returned to its original position. Several millimeters of flap tissue at the margin of the original horizontal incision will result from the removal of the hyperplastic submucosal tissue. This can be trimmed to provide closure without overlapping or local vestibuloplasty can be performed to heighten the depth of the vestibule. This can be done by executing a supraperiosteal dissection superiorly from the original incision and suturing both flaps at this level to the underlying periosteum. Advantages of this lateral approach include good visibility and access, preservation of keratinized soft tissue over the crest of the tuberosity, and the capability of performing concurrent localized vestibuloplasty. When vestibuloplasty is performed with this procedure, a maxillary stent or extended denture is placed to help maintain the vestibular depth gained.

HAMULAR NOTCH DEEPENING (TUBEROPLASTY)

The hamular notch is used as a boundary for the posterior border of the maxillary denture, and the posterior palatal seal is placed through the center of the deepest portion of the notch.[5] The notch may become very shallow in patients presenting with decreased vertical height of the maxillary tuberosity. Poor retention of the denture due to loss of adequate posterior seal and resistance to displacement can result.

A procedure designed to recreate depth of the hamular notch, tuberoplasty[1,6] has limited predictability of success. The area to be operated is infiltrated with a local anesthetic and vasoconstrictor. After the vasoconstrictor has taken effect, a transverse incision is made through the mucosa about 5 mm posterior to the hamular notch and extending from the depth of the buccal vestibule to approximately 2 cm lateral to the midline of the palate. Undermining the mucosa in both an anterior and a posterior direction is then accomplished. Through this incision the posterior aspect of the residual maxillary tuberosity, the notch, and the inferior aspects of the lateral and medial pterygoid plates are then exposed. A curved osteotome is placed in the depth of the notch and lightly malleted until the pterygoid plates are fractured free and displaced in a posterior direction. At this time, hemorrhage may be brisk from the lesser palatine artery or its muscular branches and is usually controlled by packing the site with gauze for several minutes (Fig. 4–4).

Closure may be accomplished in several ways. Obwegeser[7] suggested suturing the undermined tissue to the remnants of soft tissue attached to the tuberosity and then to the pterygoid muscle at the depth of the newly created notch. He also suggested an alternative method. An awl carrying a 3-0 polyglycolic acid–type (Dexon) suture is passed from the inferior aspect of the exposed tuberosity through the maxillary sinus and exited at the depth of the newly created notch. The undermined tissues overlying the fractured pterygoid plates are then pulled into the depth of the notch via this suture. The exposed bone of the maxillary tuberosity is allowed to heal by secondary epithelialization or by grafting with skin or mucosa to the tuberosity in the newly created notch. If

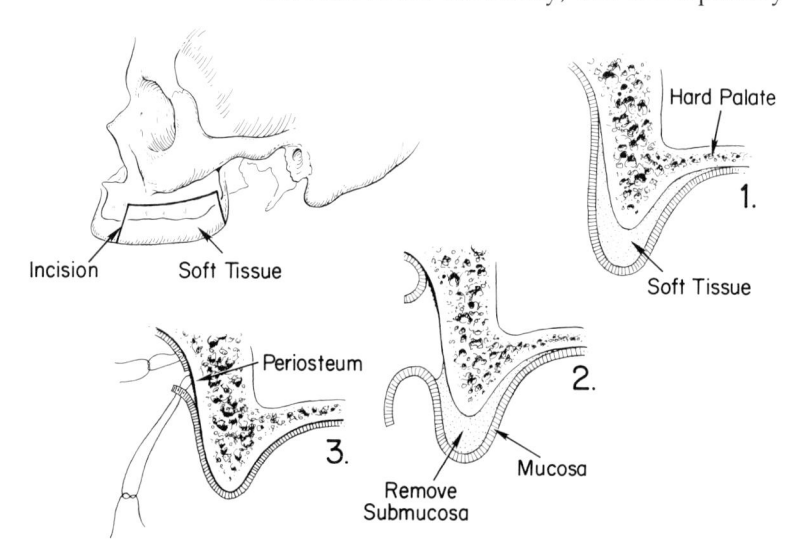

Figure 4–3. Maxillary tuberosity reduction with local vestibuloplasty. *Upper left,* Outline of proposed incision. *Drawing 1,* Frontal view showing hyperplastic tissue over the maxillary tuberosity. *Drawing 2,* Vestibular incision. Note that the superior flap is supraperiosteal while the inferior flap is full-thickness. *Drawing 3,* Closure. Note the reduction in tuberosity height and the superior repositioning of the inferiorly based flap. See text for additional comments.

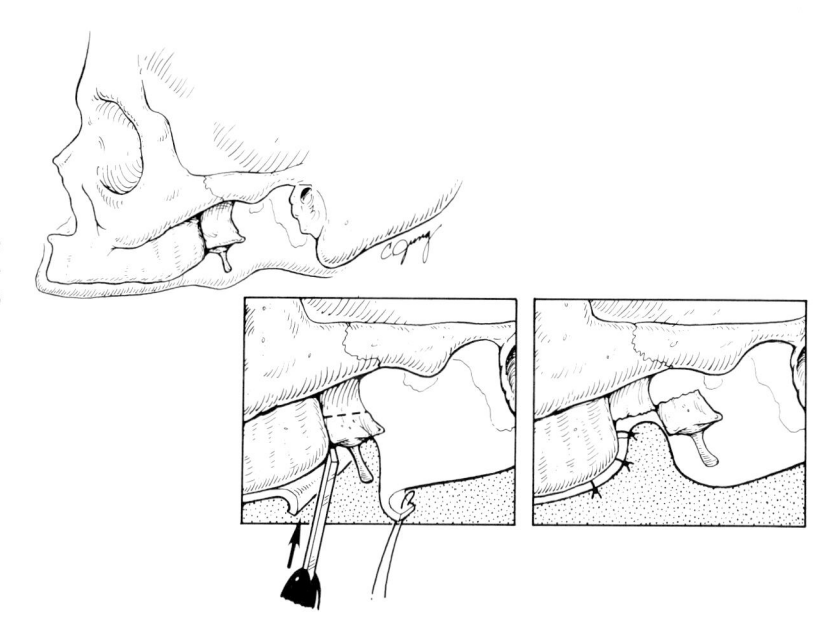

Figure 4-4. Schematic representation of the maxillary tuberoplasty procedure. Note the improved depth of the hamular notch following this procedure. See text for further comments.

the area is grafted, dental compound in a custom tray or modified denture is used to carry the graft into place. The stent is ligated in place for up to 10 days. Denture construction is delayed until the surgical site has healed completely.

ABNORMAL LABIAL OR BUCCAL FRENUM CORRECTION

When a band of tissue attaches close to the crest of the ridge and interferes with denture construction, it should be corrected surgically. The frena may present as a narrow vertical mucosal fold or as a wide band.

Numerous techniques have been advocated for frena removal. They include the Z-plasty, the V-Y advancement flap, and the "diamond" excision. The latter is a simple procedure that produces good results, especially for the maxillary midline frenum. The surgical area is usually injected with local anesthetic and epinephrine for hemostasis. Two curved hemostats grasp the frenum, one from the inferior aspect and one from the superior aspect. A scalpel is then used to excise the frenum by running it along the beaks of the hemostats. With the frenum removed, a "diamond" shaped wound results. The margins of the superior aspect of the wound are undermined with curved scissors or scalpel and closed with absorbable interrupted sutures. The inferior aspect of the wound is allowed to heal by secondary epithelialization (Fig. 4-5). As mentioned above, the Z-plasty may also be utilized. Some authors advocate its use when the base of the frenum is broad.[12] The Z-plasty may produce less scar contraction than the "diamond" technique. In this technique, the middle bar of the Z is placed directly over the midline of the frenum. The two triangles of the mucosa are undermined and then transposed and sutured with interrupted, absorbable suture material (Fig. 4-6).

When the frenum is quite broad, it is best corrected by localized vestibuloplasty. In this procedure, a semilunar incision is made at the junction of the free and attached mucosa around the frenum. A supraperiosteal dissection is performed through this incision with some degree of overcorrection to com-

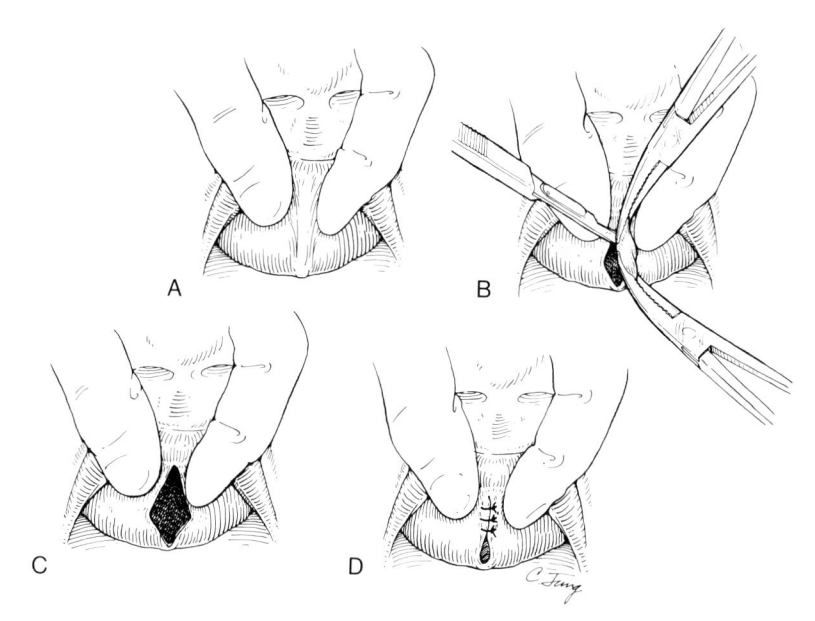

Figure 4-5. Maxillary labial frenectomy via the "diamond" excision. *A,* Eversion of lip to demarcate the labial frenum. *B,* Excision of frenum with scalpel blade following along the beaks of two curved hemostats. *C,* The resulting "diamond" wound. *D,* Closure. The inferior aspect of the wound is allowed to heal by secondary epithelialization.

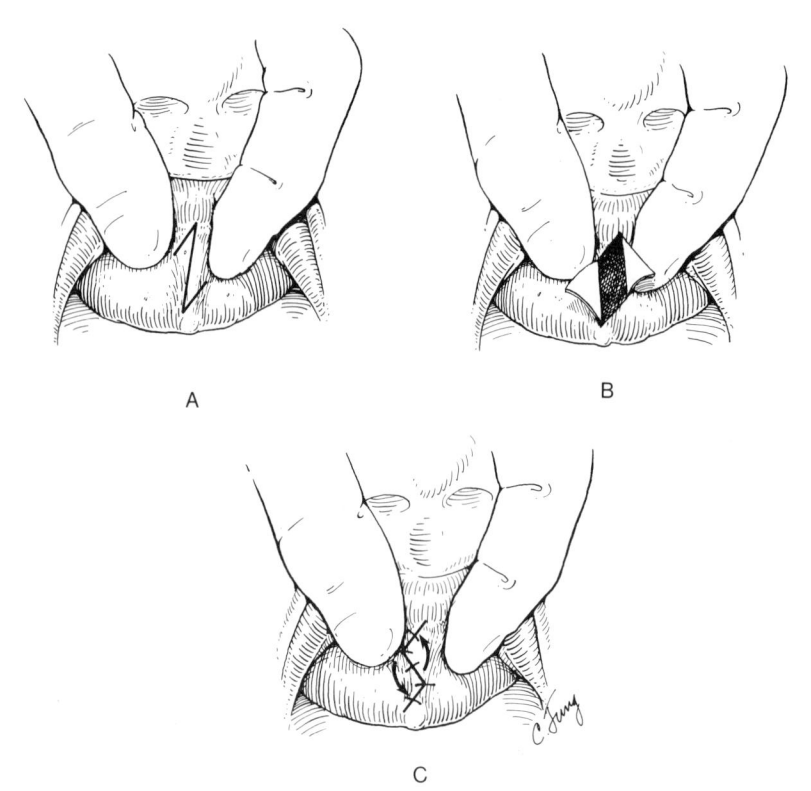

Figure 4–6. Maxillary labial frenectomy via the Z-plasty procedure. See text for details.

pensate for relapse. The flap margin is then sutured to the underlying periosteum as deeply as possible. Absorbable horizontal mattress sutures are placed in an interrupted fashion. The wound is allowed to heal by secondary epithelialization.[8]

ABNORMAL LINGUAL FRENUM (TONGUE TIE, ANKYLOGLOSSIA) CORRECTION

In the edentulous patient, the abnormal lingual frenum may attach at the crest of the ridge. This may create speech defects as well as prevent stability and retention of the denture. This condition requires surgical correction. After the injection of local anesthesia with vasoconstrictor, the tongue tip is elevated with a traction suture. This will stretch the frenum and allow sectioning of the frenum. Cutting the frenum close to the tongue will prevent accidental cutting of the submandibular gland orifice. The cut is directed posteriorly until the tip of the tongue is quite mobile and can reach the palate with the mouth open. It is important that closure is accomplished per primum, as this will prevent readhesion of the frenum. Tongue movement should also be encouraged.

EPULIS FISSURATUM REMOVAL

Submucosal fibrosis secondary to chronic denture irritation, epulis fissuratum, markedly interferes with denture stability and comfort. When first presented, epulides fissurata are usually inflamed and benefit from some treatment before removal. This is accomplished by relieving the denture in the area of irritation, lining the denture with tissue conditioner, and/or leaving the denture out as much as possible. The spontaneous resorption may require many weeks. When the maximum spontaneous resolution has occurred, the remaining epulis is removed. This can be accomplished by surgical excision or by cryosurgery. Cryosurgery may be particularly important if the mental neurovascular bundle is incorporated in the epulis because it can be more conducive to nerve regeneration than is excision. However, because cryosurgery may require several sessions, surgical excision may be the most practical and probably the most efficacious method of surgery.

In surgically removing the epulis, it is desirable to separate the mucosa from the underlying fibrous tissue. However, often the fibrous tissue is so intimately associated with the mucosa that it is impractical to separate the mucosa from the fibrous tissue. Thus, the placement of the mucosal incision will vary and should retain as much mucosa as possible. The fibrous tissue is removed as completely as possible. If there is not enough mucosa to close the incision primarily, secondary epithelialization will occur. Some residual scar will not be unusual.

MYLOHYOID RIDGE REDUCTION

Please refer to Chapter 5.

MANDIBULAR (LINGUAL) TORUS REMOVAL

The mandibular torus is an exostosis located on the lingual surface of the mandible in the molar and premolar region. Tori are usually bilateral and can be singular, lobulated, or multiple. When a mandibular denture is contemplated, these growths often require removal.

The technique for removal is as follows (Fig. 4–7). If the patient is edentulous, an incision is made along the crest of the ridge, long enough to adequately expose the torus. If teeth are present, the incision is modified to an envelope-type flap including the gingival margin. Vertical relaxing incisions should be avoided if possible as they may interfere with blood supply to the very thin mucosa covering the torus. Care should be taken in elevating the flap to minimize the possibility of lacerating the flap. A groove may be cut along the line of intended removal on the superior surface 1 to 2 mm in depth. This cut is not required, but it aids in providing a stable position for the osteotome. The osteotome is stepped along the superior junction of the torus with the mandible to generate a cleavage line. Continued malleting will free the torus from the mandible. After the appropriate amount of bone has been removed and the bone smoothed, the flap is closed. A gauze pack placed under the tongue for an hour or so may help decrease the possibility of hematoma.

PALATAL TORUS REMOVAL

A palatal torus is a sessile mass of bone in the midline of the palate. It affects 20 to 25 per cent of women in the United States, twice the incidence in men.[9] The etiology of these protuberances is unknown. The tori may appear broad and flat or may have a nodular or lobulated configuration. They may be composed entirely of cortical bone or have cancellous bone beneath the overlying cortex.

Not all palatal tori need to be removed prior to denture construction. Indications for removal are (1) the extremely large torus filling the palatal vault; (2) the torus that extends beyond the dam area; (3) the torus with traumatized mucosal coverage; (4) the torus with deep undercuts; (5) the torus that interferes with normal speech; (6) the torus that poses a psychological problem for the patient (e.g., malignancy phobia).[10]

Before removing a palatal torus, the patient should be informed of the remote possibility of an oral-nasal fistula because of the very thin palatal bone that is sometimes present adjacent to the torus.

Prior to surgery a maxillary impression should be made and a study model poured. The surgeon should trim the torus from the model and use this modified model for construction of a maxillary palatal splint to be placed at the time of surgery. The splint will aid in postoperative comfort, protect the surgical site from trauma, and prevent hematoma development beneath the palatal tissues. It is not necessary to remove the torus completely, minimizing the possibility of an oral-nasal fistula.

A local anesthetic with epinephrine is injected around the base of the torus to aid hemostasis. An incision is placed directly over

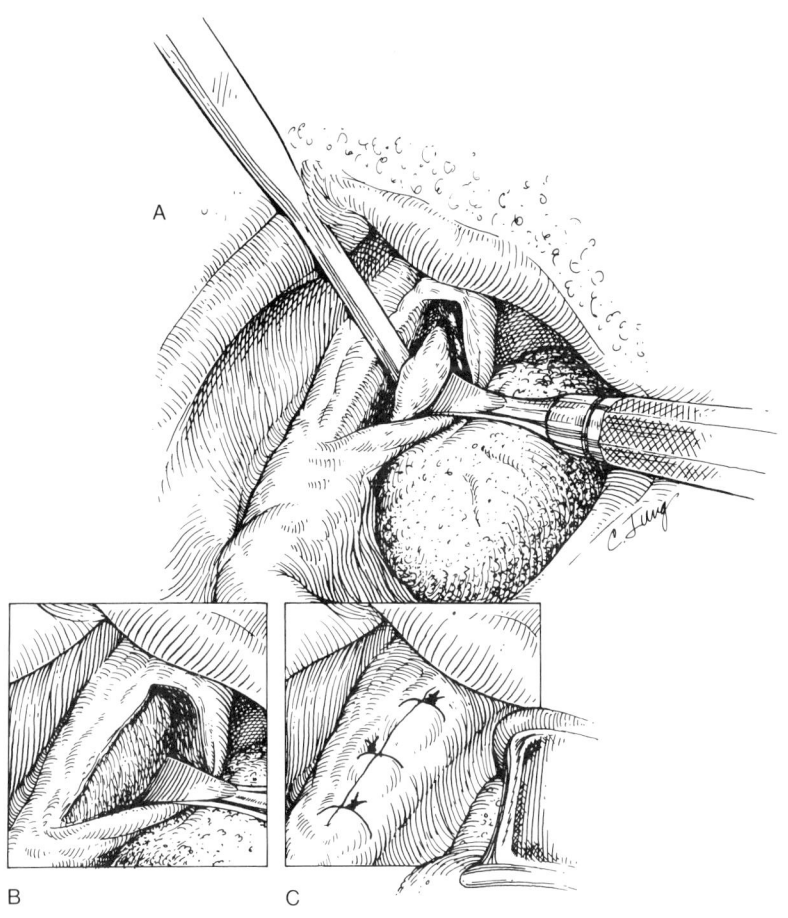

Figure 4–7. Removal of mandibular lingual torus. *A*, Crestal incision and reflection of mucoperiosteal flap. Note placement of elevator while using osteotome. *B*, Appearance of bone after final smoothing. *C*, Closure.

the midline of the torus. Releasing incisions are placed at the anterior and posterior limits if necessary. The result is an incision with a Y at each end. This provides adequate access and preserves the blood supply. Reflection of these flaps is done as carefully as possible to minimize the possibility of laceration of the very thin mucosa. Retraction sutures may be placed to maintain access and visibility. The palatal torus does not lend itself to removal in one piece because the thin bone adjacent to the torus may fracture before the more dense torus bone. If a chisel technique is used, it is appropriate to remove the bone in layers, which often leaves a small, smooth residual portion of the torus. If the bone is to be removed with a bur, it is often helpful to make scoring bur cuts in the torus to delineate the amount of bone to be removed. After the bone is removed and smoothed with a bone file, the area is irrigated and the flaps repositioned. Horizontal mattress sutures help take up the slack of the excess soft tissue, leaving the edges of the flaps everted. The excess tissue may be trimmed as needed and if a splint has been constructed, it may be placed. Relining with a "soft" tissue conditioner may be needed before securing the stent.

PALATAL PAPILLARY HYPERPLASIA REMOVAL

Papillary hyperplasia of the tissues of the palatal vault is a condition of unknown etiology and is generally seen in edentulous patients who are wearing ill-fitting dentures. Wearing the dentures on a 24-hour per day basis may be associated with a higher incidence of papillary hyperplasia, but the condition will occasionally occur in non–denture wearing patients. It may exhibit associated inflammation and edema of the palatal tissues. It presents as numerous papillary projections that cover part or all of the hard palate. These projections are usually small, imparting a pebble-strewn appearance to the palate. Small food particles and bacteria may be lodged between these projections, increasing the inflammatory response. The lesion was at one time thought to be premalignant but now is considered no more premalignant than other areas of hyperplastic mucosa. Initial conservative therapy may be indicated in those patients exhibiting unusual inflammation and edema of the hyperplastic tissue. This entails removing the ill-fitting denture or relining it with a tissue conditioner. Any existing candidal infection should be eliminated with appropriate fungicides. Oral hygiene should be reemphasized to the patient. The palatal tissues should be brushed lightly with a soft-bristled toothbrush on a daily basis. The relined denture should be thoroughly cleaned after each meal. Such measures will significantly reduce the inflammation and edema in the palatal tissues.

Numerous techniques are advocated for removing the hyperplastic palatal tissues.[11] An antral curette may be used to remove the affected tissue, leaving the periosteum and a little adjacent soft tissue. Electrocauterization, mucoabrasion with a slow-moving acrylic bur, and cryosurgery can also be used to produce similar results.

Following removal, the patient's relined denture or a maxillary stent should be inserted to help stop hemorrhage and protect the wound. Healing takes place by secondary epithelialization and is usually complete within three to five weeks.

BIBLIOGRAPHY

1. Masterson MP: Retention of vital submerged roots under complete dentures. J Prosthet Dent 41 (1):12, 1979.
2. VonWowern N, and Wintern S: Submergence of roots for alveolar ridge preservation. Int J Oral Surg 10:247, 1981.
3. Guernsey LH: Preprosthetic surgery. Dent Clin North Am 15:455, 1971.
4. Guernsey LH: Preprosthetic Surgery. *In* Kruger G (ed.): Textbook of Oral and Maxillofacial Surgery. 5th ed. St. Louis, CV Mosby Co, 1979.
5. Boucher CO: Swenson's Complete Dentures. St. Louis, CV Mosby Co, 1970.
6. Celesnik F: La plastique tuberosite dans le cas d'atrophi du maxillaire superieur. Arch Stoma Liege 9:82, 1954.
7. Obwegeser HL: Surgical preparation of the maxilla for prosthesis. J Oral Surg 22:127, 1964.
8. Birn H, and Winther JE: Manual of Minor Oral Surgery, Philadelphia, WB Saunders Co, 1975.
9. Kolas S, Halperin V, Jefferis K, Huddleston SD, and Robinson H: The occurrence of torus palatinus and torus mandibularis in 2,478 dental patients. Oral Surg 6:1134, 1953.
10. Shafer W, Hine M, and Levy B: A Textbook of Oral Pathology. Philadelphia, WB Saunders Co, 1974.
11. Guernsey LH: Reactive inflammatory papillary hyperplasia of the palate. Oral Surg 20:814, 1965.
12. Hooley J, and Steinhauser E: Preprosthetic surgery. *In* Hayward JR (ed.): Oral Surgery. Springfield, IL, Charles C Thomas, Publisher, 1976.

5

SURGICAL MANAGEMENT OF SOFT TISSUE PROBLEMS

*W. Howard Davis, D.D.S.,
and
Christopher L. Davis, D.D.S., M.D.,
with contributions by
Richard Delo, D.D.S.,
Jay R. Weiner, D.D.S.,
Ronald Kaminishi, D.D.S.,
Craig Bloom, D.M.D.,
Paul V.W. Stoelinga, D.D.S., M.D., Ph.D.,
Raymond J. Fonseca, D.M.D.,
Bill C. Terry, D.D.S.,
and Glenn Minsley, D.M.D.*

There are two primary reasons for altering the soft tissue of the denture-seating area. One is to allow deepening of the flange area so that increased resistance to displacement forces is provided. The second is to provide stable soft tissue upon which dentures can rest. The provision of improved load-bearing tissue and decreasing resorption of the underlying bone are other secondary reasons for altering the soft tissue of the denture-seating area. For specific indications for each procedure, the reader is referred to Chapter 3.

This chapter will deal with soft tissue alteration in two broad categories, mandibular procedures and maxillary procedures.

MANDIBULAR PROCEDURES

VESTIBULOPLASTY WITH SKIN GRAFTING AND LOWERING OF THE FLOOR OF THE MOUTH

History

According to an article by McDowell,[1] Reverdin, a 27-year-old intern, presented a paper on skin grafting to the Imperial Surgical Society of Paris in 1869.[2] Although it was poorly received, the paper was automatically published in the Proceedings of the Society. In this paper, Reverdin reported the success he had found when bits of skin (pinch grafts) were applied to wounds.

After the Franco-Prussian War of 1870-71, Carl Thiersch[3] began work on epidermal grafting and proved that thin grafts are most easily vitalized. His paper appeared in 1874 and described microscopic findings. Ollier was also doing similar experiments and published his results in 1872.

According to Slanetz and Rankow in the American Journal of Surgery, Schnitzler and Ewald successfully applied a Thiersch graft to a granulating defect of the buccal mucosa in 1894.[4,5] According to this article, their technique fell into disrepute because they did not realize the importance of immobilizing the graft on the recipient site.

Pichler and Trauner[6] cited Moskowicz in 1915 as the first to create a buccal vestibule with a Thiersch graft.[7] This was done by making a percutaneous pocket close to the mucosa, inserting the epidermal graft, and allowing it to heal. Secondarily, the mucosa and underlying skin graft were opened to provide a new sulcus.

According to Pichler and Trauner,[6] Esser,

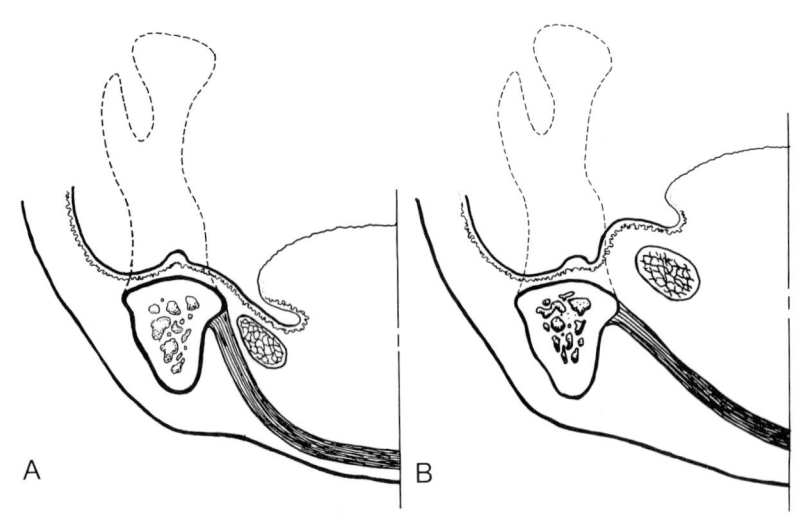

Figure 5–1. *A,* Floor of the mouth with mylohyoid relaxed. *B,* Elevation of the floor of the mouth by contraction of the mylohyoid muscle.

in 1916, was the first to demonstrate placement of a plastic material (dental compound) in the percutaneous pocket with the skin fixed to the compound with glue made from egg yolk.[8]

Weiser[9] was probably the first to apply skin perorally to the buccal vestibule. Many others published on this procedure, including Waldron as cited in Gillies,[10] Pickerill,[11] Kilner and Jackson,[12] and Kazanjian.[13]

In 1930, Pichler and Trauner[6] published a very comprehensive article delineating many of the present principles of this procedure, including the need for dissection close to the periosteum, the use of the hip as a donor site, and the desirability of dry crust on the donor site (although, they pointed out, this was not essential).

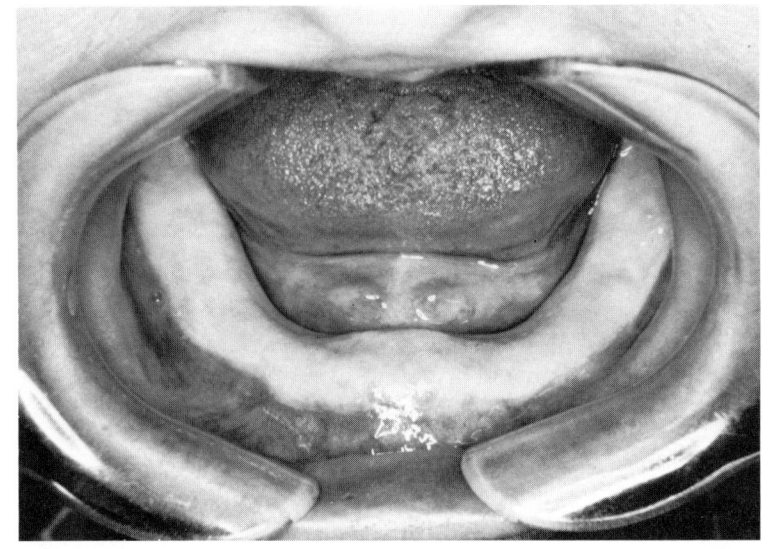

Figure 5–2. Note that traction on the lips and cheeks does not disturb the skin grafted to the periosteum, giving a nondisplaceable denture-seating area.

In 1931 Wassmund introduced the lowering of the genioglossus attachment.[14] In 1952, Trauner reported the lowering of the mylohyoid muscle on each side from the canine region posteriorly.[15] According to Obwegeser,[16] in 1951 Mathis[17] demonstrated a technique for lowering of the mental foramen.

The skin grafting of the labiobuccal surface of the mandible only, without creating a skin-lined pouch, was reported by Schuchardt in 1952.[18] In 1953, Rehrmann[19] described the currently used method for submandibular suturing to hold the buccal and lingual mucosal margins in the depressed position and closely adapted to the bone surface.

In 1963, Obwegeser[16] reported sectioning of the mylohyoid as far forward as possible plus sectioning parts of the genioglossi. This created a total lowering of the floor of the mouth. Obwegeser was primarily responsible for popularizing this procedure.

Objectives

1. **Mechanical resistance to displacement forces.** The vestibuloplasty with skin grafting (VSG) and lowering the floor of the mouth (LFM) provide increased sulcus depth, especially in the lingual flange area, which materially helps control lateral displacement.

2. **Stable denture-seating area.** The atrophic mandibular ridge has only a small line of attached mucosa forming the "crest of the ridge." All the remaining mucosa of the denture-seating area can be elevated by movement of the lip, cheeks, and tongue (Fig. 5–1).

The vestibuloplasty with skin grafting and lowering of the floor of the mouth (VSG and LFM) produce a nondisplaceable tissue covering the entire denture-bearing area. The skin's firm attachment to the periosteum permits denture stability even in the severely atrophied mandible when no significant "ridge" height can be created. This is exemplified in Figure 5–2.

3. **Skin as a load-bearing tissue.** Whereas mucosa tends to ulcerate in response to pressure, skin tends to form a benign hyperkeratosis similar to the callus response on the hand. These hyperkeratoses are rarely painful. The pain threshold of grafted skin is higher than that of mucosa, and touch perception is somewhat diminished (Fig. 5–3). Patients are usually more comfortable with skin than mucosa as a load-bearing tissue.

Both skin and mucosa will rarely exhibit problems with candidiasis.

4. Probable slower mandibular resorption beneath skin.[20]

Long-term Evaluation of the VSG and LFM

In 1975, Landesman and Levin published an evaluation of 36 VSG and LFM patients who had been edentulous 16 years (mean) prior to VSG and LFM.[21] They found that these procedures dramatically improved denture function related to looseness, chewing problems, and pain ($p < 0.001$). Similar favorable findings were reported by Steinhauser in 1969.[22] He found 87 per cent of 282 VSG and LFM patients were pleased with the results of their surgery.

Although the VSG and LFM have proved of functional benefit to patients, it is important to assess the effect these procedures have on the natural resorption of the edentulous mandible. To determine this, Landesman et al.[20] examined patients who had returned for serial panoramic radiographs 5 to 12 years after surgery (8 years mean). Twenty-nine patients were thus evaluated. The mandibular height was measured 1 cm posterior to the mental foramina. The rate of resorption was variable, but most patients had very little resorption; 17 of the 29 had none. The percentage of resorption of the height of the mandible varied from 0 to 1.9 per cent per year, with an average of 0.42 per cent per year (at that rate it would take 100 years to resorb one half of the mandible). Thus, it appears that the VSG and LFM do not tend to increase the rate of resorption and probably actually diminish the rate of resorption. Possible explanations are the distribution of the denture load over a larger area and better denture stability.

Fifteen years of experience (W.H.D.) with the use of VSG and LFM also indicate that the highly important fixation of the skin to the mandible does not materially change with time. Thus, the beneficial effects of these procedures are apparently lifelong.

The predictable beneficial results of the VSG and LFM have made these procedures a source of gratification to the patient, the surgeon, the prosthodontist, and the general dentist. They could logically serve as a benchmark for evaluating other denture-stabilizing procedures.

Preliminary Details

Points to Discuss with the Patient

There are several points to discuss with the patient prior to VSG and LFM. The pa-

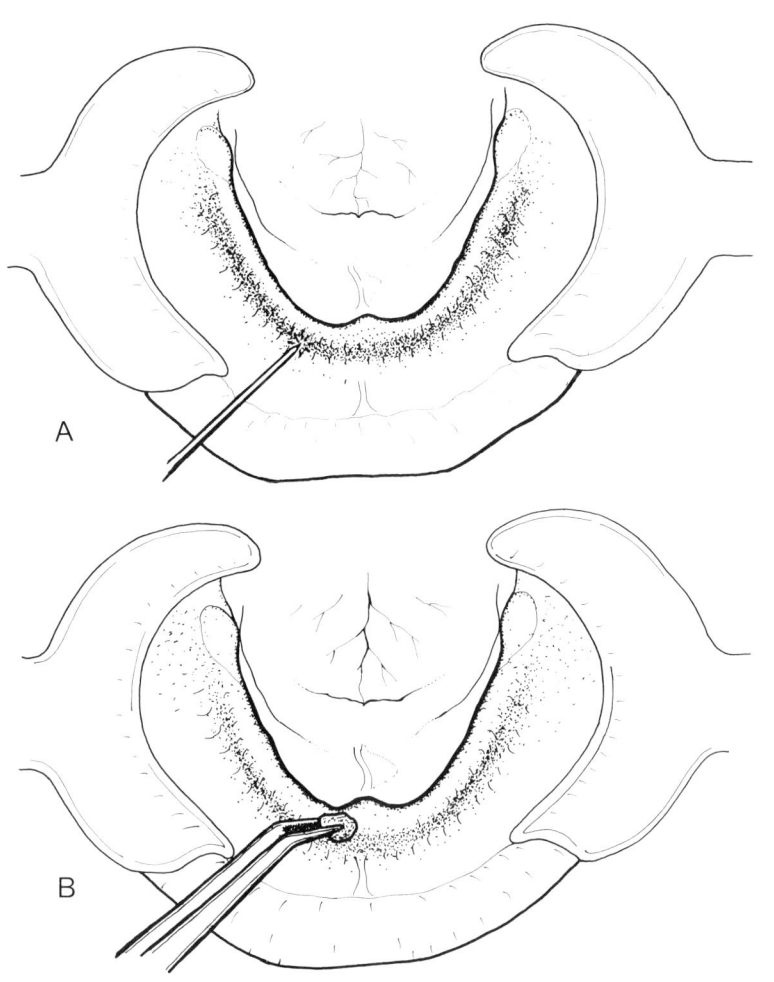

Figure 5–3. *A*, Pain is perceived slightly less than in mucosa. *B*, Touch sensation is notably less than in mucosa at first but approaches mucosal response in time.

tient should be informed of the significant probability of a beneficial result and the probable lifelong benefit of the procedures. There is also evidence of a possible diminution of the rate of mandibular resorption. A probable paresthesia of the lower lip with a probable return to normal or close to normal function should be discussed with the patient.

The patient should be aware of postoperative discomfort of both the donor and recipient sites. Discomfort at the donor site usually resolves in about two weeks but can be prolonged. Donor site color and texture will be changed but is usually close to normal after several months. However, this may dissuade the patient from wearing a bikini-type bathing suit.

Usually the combined vestibuloplasty and mouth floor plasty will require two to three hours of surgery time, and the hospital stay may vary from three to five or more days. Impressions can be made after one week, but most patients wish to wait about three weeks because of the tenderness of the mouth.

The possible need for blood transfusions and other usual sequelae of surgery should be discussed with the patient.

Preoperative Evaluation

General History and Physical Evaluation. See Chapter 3.

Oral and Maxillofacial Evaluation. The chief complaint is usually an inability to function satisfactorily with a mandibular denture. This is usually concomitant with a degenerated mandibular ridge. However, if the patient has a reasonably good ridge, a psychological problem may exist and should be evaluated before further treatment is considered. In the authors' experience, patients with psychological problems usually report improvement after VSG and LFM. Even patients who are known psychotics have had notable functional improvement with the VSG and LFM. The evaluation of the need for a VSG and LFM as related to other procedures is discussed in Chapter 3.

Panoramic Radiograph. Generally 15 mm or more of body height will provide good vestibular depth after the VSG and LFM procedures (Fig. 5–4). In cases of more severe degeneration, the VSG and LFM procedures will produce only a slight vestibule. However, the broad, immobile area of good stress-bearing tissue and the increased lingual and lateral throat form will produce a marked improvement.

Management of Epulis Fissuratum. Large epulides regress slowly but significantly when the denture flange is removed in the area of the epulis. The remaining portion is removed by excision, cryotherapy, or electrocautery. This is done several weeks before the VSG and LFM to allow regeneration of mucosa and softening of the scar tissue. Small epulides may be removed at the time of the VSG and LFM and the denuded area covered by skin.

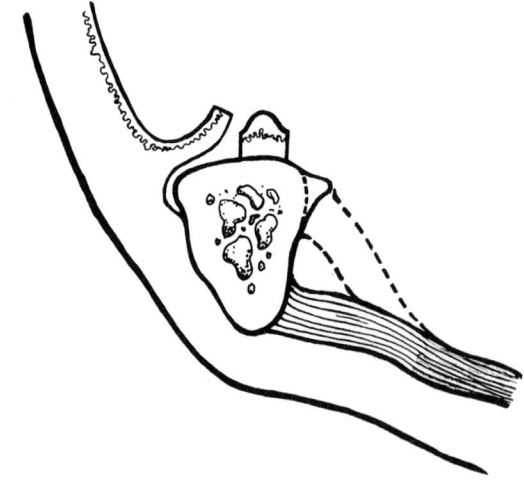

Figure 5–5. Lightly dotted line indicates the approximate amount of resorption of the mylohyoid ridge that will occur after detachment and relocation of the mylohyoid muscle.

Management of the Mylohyoid Ridge. The undercut of the mylohyoid ridge need not be removed unless the prosthodontist feels it should be. A sharp mylohyoid ridge can be removed at the time of grafting but will usually atrophy after detachment of the mylohyoid muscle during lowering of the floor of the mouth (Fig. 5–5). A modified technique for mylohyoid muscle lowering is discussed elsewhere in this chapter.

Management of the Genial Tubercles. Any sharpness of the genial tubercle will usually atrophy after the superior portions of the genioglossi are removed. Significant recontouring of the genial tubercle is ideally performed at least two months prior to skin grafting.

Fixation Methods for the Graft

At this point, a decision should be made regarding whether the skin will be applied with a stent or sutured in place.

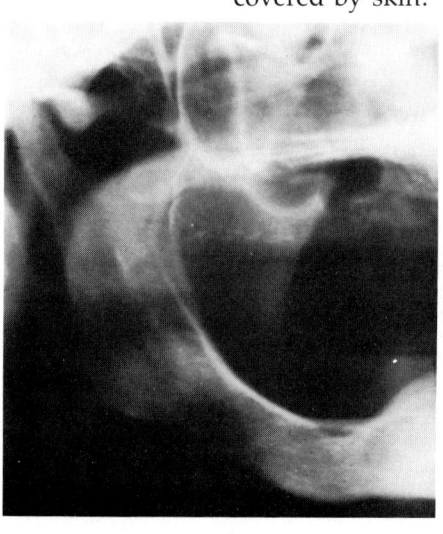

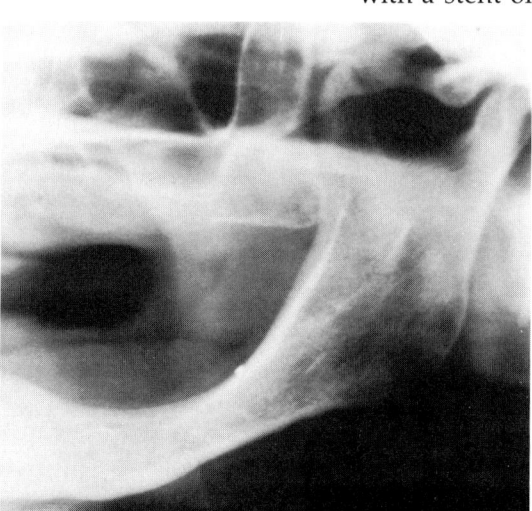

Figure 5–4. The typical amount of bone that will allow a good postoperative ridge as well as nondisplaceable tissue.

Advantages of the Stent. The stent is more versatile because the skin can be adapted with accuracy to any contour of the labial-buccal area, whereas, with the suturing method, there should be minimal depressions in the labial-buccal contour. With the stent technique, the skin can be adapted to the lingual undercut via the Protaform type wash, and poor crestal soft tissue or sharp crestal bone can be dealt with at the time of grafting. With the suturing method, these problems need to be dealt with in a separate procedure.

A graft with voids can be tolerated using the stent method, as it can be manipulated on the stent to give proper coverage. This allows a thinner graft than may be used in the suturing method, thus predisposing to better donor site healing.

Advantages of the Suturing Method. Without the stent the patient is more comfortable for the first week postoperatively. In addition, no stent construction or adaptation materials are required.

Technique Alterations for the Suturing Method. The following parts of the text describing the stent technique can be ignored or altered if the suturing technique is decided upon.

1. The models, stent, and stent construction materials are not required.
2. 4-0 chromic gut or Dexon-type suture material on a small 3/8-circle cutting needle (such as an Ethicon FS-2) will be required.
3. The graft can be somewhat narrower, i.e., 3 cm to 4 cm (because coverage of the lingual side is usually not attempted).
4. It is probably desirable to take the graft a little thicker to provide a graft without voids. A thickness of about 0.014 inch (0.35 mm) is appropriate.
5. Eliminate steps involving stent construction.
6. Eliminate the circummandibular suture that would be used to hold the stent in place.
7. Keep the crestal soft tissue intact to allow suturing to it.
8. Eliminate steps relating to stent removal.

Acrylic Tray Construction (for the stent method). An edentulous tray is used with alginate or compound as the impression material. Compound will give a more displaced periphery, but its use is not essential. One may outline the desired extent of the periphery with indelible pencil marking on the mucosa. The impression can then be replaced to transfer the mark to the impression (Fig. 5–6), or the mark can be made directly on the impression after correlating the impression with the mouth.

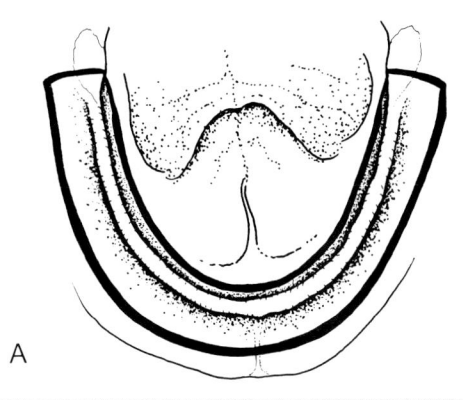

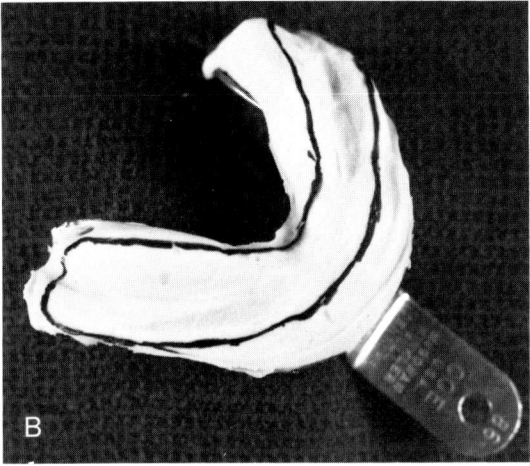

Figure 5–6. *A,* Indelible pencil marking of the mucosa to designate the projected peripheral extension of the acrylic tray. *B,* Alginate impression showing projected extension of the acrylic tray.

Buccally and labially, the periphery of the stent should extend approximately to the lateral extent of the bone. The flange of the stent should be extended lingually just to the undercut or the horizontal lingual extent of the bone, stopping just short of the retromolar pad. If the stent is extended too far posteriorly, the end of the stent will be elevated and contact the maxillary tuberosity when the patient closes. It is very important that this does not occur, as movement of the stent will prevent take of the graft. A wire handle can be incorporated in the anterior area of the tray to allow grasping (Fig. 5–7).

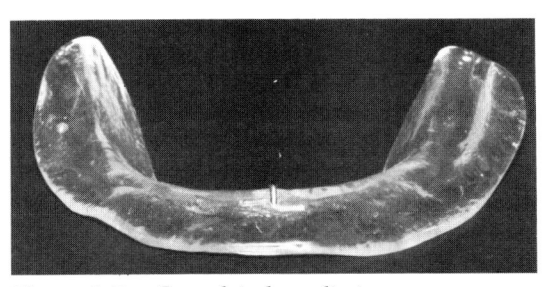

Figure 5–7. Completed acrylic tray.

The Surgical Procedure

Preoperative Considerations

Blood replacement is rarely required; however, obtaining one unit of autologous blood is recommended rather than using homologous blood. Antibiotics are desirable and are usually begun intravenously just before surgery. They are continued until oral administration can be substituted. When not contraindicated, a corticosteroid to decrease swelling is begun just before surgery and is continued for one or two days postoperatively. Also, 1 per cent hydrocortisone cream may be applied to the lips during surgery and postoperatively.

Discussion with the Anesthesiologist

Nasal intubation is needed. A low profile exit of the tubing is preferable so the operator can see easily into the mouth while sitting midsagittally to the patient. An acute-angle adapter (60 degrees) or an endotracheal tube with an acute angle incorporated is helpful for this purpose (Fig. 5–8).

The anesthesiologist should be at the side of the table during the mouth surgery. This gives the surgeon and assistant better access to the head area. It is desirable to use a vasoconstrictor such as 1/200,000 epinephrine for hemostasis. Less than 10 ml would generally be used at one time.

Instruments and Setup

Instruments required for graft-taking, grafting, and vestibuloplasty are listed in Tables 5–1, 5–2, and 5–3, respectively.

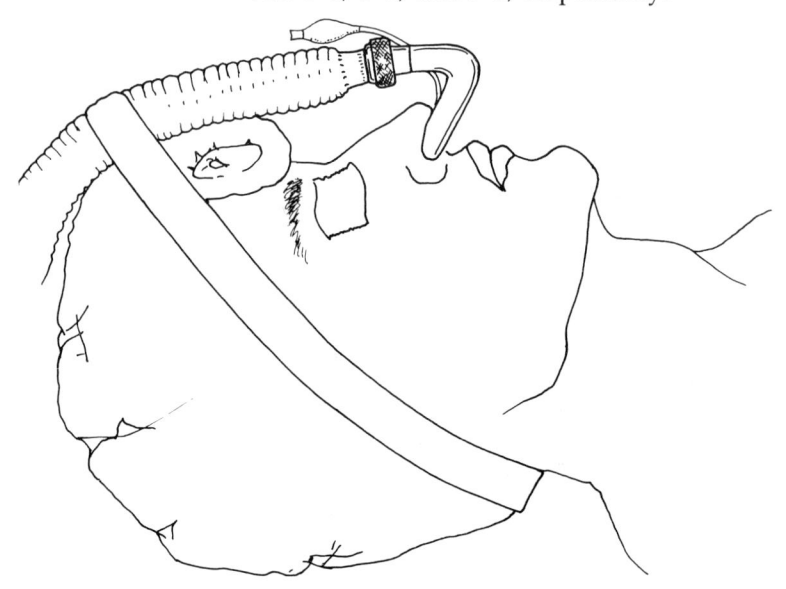

Figure 5–8. Note that the intubation connection is kept close to the patient so that it will minimally obstruct the vision of the surgeon, who will sit at the head of the table.

TABLE 5–1. GRAFT-TAKING SETUP

1. Dermatome—Stryker, Brown, etc.
2. Stainless steel ruler—at least 16 cm long.
3. Mineral oil in medicine cup.
4. Wooden tongue blade—to spread mineral oil and, if desired, to flatten the skin ahead of the dermatome.
5. Two mosquito hemostats to hold the graft as it is being taken.
6. If a test cut is used:
   a. 5-0 nylon or equivalent on a small needle and a needle holder.
   b. Scissors
7. Donor site dressing, such as Opsite or Owen's, Vaseline, Betadine, scarlet red, Xeroform gauze, etc.
8. An absorbent dressing such as an ABD pad if gauze is used.
9. Tape to cover the edges of the dressing.

TABLE 5–2. GRAFT TABLE SETUP

1. Two mosquito hemostats (from graft-taking set-up).
2. One pair of straight scissors.
3. One tissue forceps (Adson).
4. A skin board or a piece of plastic about 5 × 8 × 0.5 inch that can be autoclaved.
5. One 12 × 12 inch gauze (single layer as an opened 4 × 4 inch).
6. Six 4 × 4 inch gauzes.
7. One medicine cup for dermal glue.
8. Two small basins
   a. One for physiologic saline
   b. One for storage of the skin
9. Physiologic saline.
10. Four cotton tipped applicators—to apply glue and adapt skin to stent.

Technique for Donor Site Surgery

The patient is placed in the supine position with the donor site elevated with sand bags for access. The donor site and facial area are prepared with hexachlorophene or an equivalent. Iodophor is contraindicated, since it may inhibit the viability of the graft. One entire hip area should be exposed by the draping.

The dermatome should be assembled while the donor site is being prepared and draped. The blade is carefully placed in the dermatome, protecting the cutting edge.

The width of the graft depends on the height of the body of the mandible. The graft width will usually vary from 5 to 6 cm. The thickness can be minimal, about 0.012 inch (0.3 mm). The area of the donor site is not critical. Most commonly it is parallel and just caudal to the iliac crest. However, one should ask the patient if he or she has a preferred site. With most dermatomes it is advisable to spread mineral oil liberally over the donor area.

A test cut can be made, although it is rarely needed (Fig. 5–9). One should begin adjacent to the donor site, starting the der-

SURGICAL MANAGEMENT OF SOFT TISSUE PROBLEMS / 75

TABLE 5–3. VESTIBULOPLASTY INSTRUMENTS

1. Facial and donor site preparation solution. (Hexachlorophene seems preferable to iodophor, as iodophor may interfere with the viability of the graft.)
2. Adhesive drape approximately 24 × 30 inches with adhesive covering most of the drape (Vidrape or Steridrape, etc.).
3. A set of plastic instruments.
4. Pharyngeal gauze pack.
5. Ten ml syringe with 1.5-inch, 25-gauge needle.
6. Epinephrine 1/200,000 or 1/400,000—usually obtained by diluting lidocaine with 1/100,000 epinephrine with lidocaine without epinephrine.
7. Three Davis nested double-L retractors (or equivalent).
8. Tongue retractor.
9. No. 15 blades and two No. 7 Bard-Parker handles.
10. Single skin hook.
11. Double skin hook.
12. Sharp, small osteotome and mallet.
13. Two sponge sticks of gauze rolled to 2 × 2 × 3 cm size on gauze-holding forceps or Allison forceps.
14. Two 3/4-inch 3/8 circle cutting needles (or similar).
15. Ten pieces (two extra) of 2-0 plain gut or 2-0 black Supramid, 12 inches long.
16. Two or more mandibular awls—one with a fairly tight curve.
17. Three pieces (one extra) of No. 1 white Supramid or equivalent, 22 inches long.
18. Saline solution or sterile water to half fill the heater container.
19. Two cakes (one extra) of grey compound—sterilized in nonalcoholic, nonirritating solution such as hexachlorophene.
20. Irrigating syringe.
21. No. 15 blade, preferably in a regular (3) handle.
22. Two pieces (one extra) of Protaform—sterilized in hexachlorophene.
23. 500 ml of saline solution.
24. Hanau water bath heater—the water container is sterilized.
25. Dermal glue (not on sterile setup).

matome at a steep angle until the skin is engaged, then flattening it so that the bottom of the dermatome is parallel to the skin. An assistant picks up the corners of the graft with hemostats. After 1 cm, the dermatome

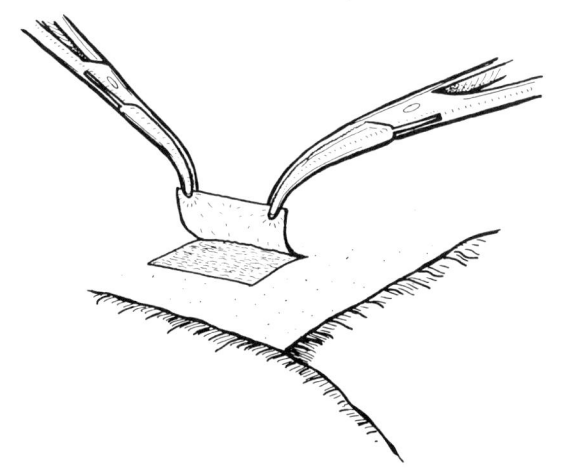

Figure 5–9. The thickness and character of the test cut is inspected.

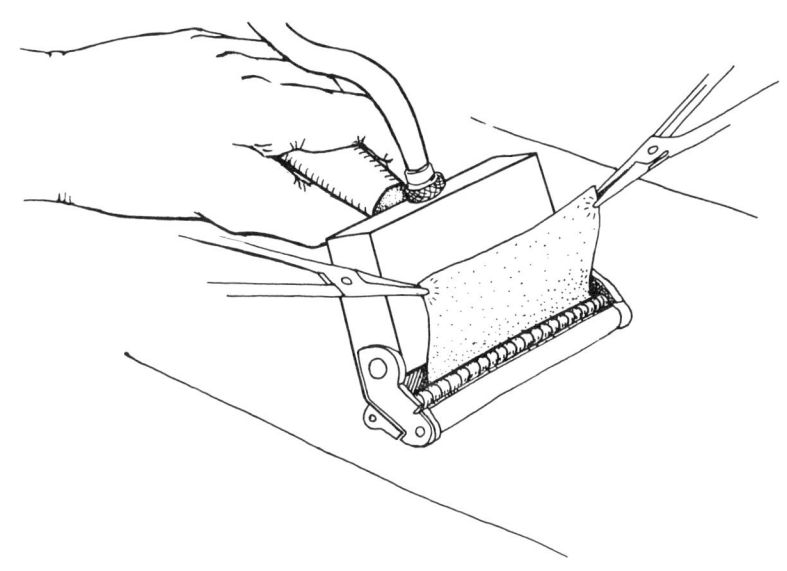

Figure 5–10. Assistants holding skin with passive tension as it is being removed.

is stopped and withdrawn without excising the test cut. The graft is examined for any pattern of irregularities that would indicate a defective blade. The thickness may vary from translucent (Thiersch) to opaque (medium split thickness). No fat should be present on the graft. The dermatome is adjusted if necessary, and excision is begun just beyond the test cut.

Variables that will affect the depth of the cut are: (1) The tension that the assistant applies to hold the graft as it is being cut. The more tension, the thicker the cut (Fig. 5–10). (2) The pressure on the dermatome. The heavier the pressure, the thicker the cut. (3) The angle of the dermatome. The steeper the angulation, the thicker the cut. (4) The resistance of underlying tissue. Cutting over bone will give a thicker cut.

The dermatome may be stopped in place to make adjustments. The length of the graft should be about 16 cm. The cut is stopped by depressing the handle to elevate the leading edge while the dermatome is operating. If a test cut was made, the skin pedicle is sutured back into place. Exact replacement of margins is not necessary.

Dressing the Donor Site

The production of a dry crust was formerly considered the best management of the donor site. However, the advent of Opsite has changed this concept. The donor site can be treated in a variety of ways.

First, a thrombin dressing may be applied to give hemostasis and the donor site may be dressed at this point or at the end of the procedure. There are basically two types of donor site dressings, Opsite or an equivalent

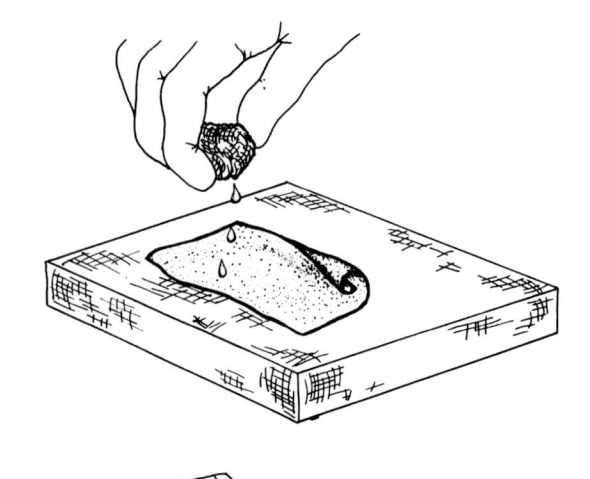

Figure 5–11. Moistening the skin with saline helps to prevent curling of the edges as the skin is laid flat.

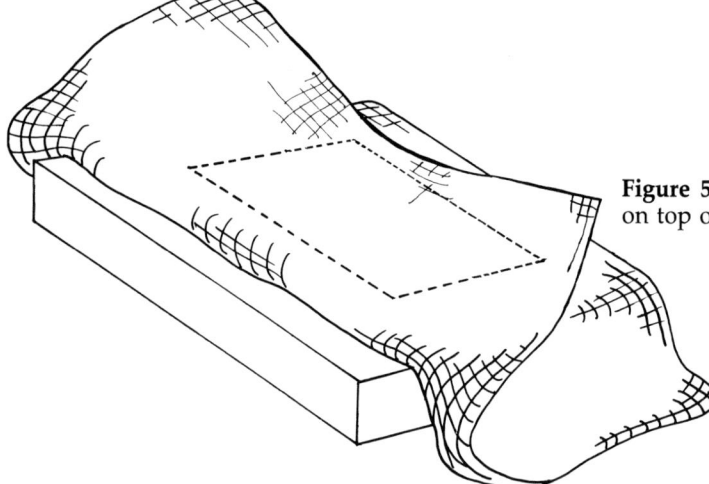

Figure 5–12. Part of the excess gauze is folded on top of the skin.

microporous dressing and various gauze dressings. Opsite (or equivalent) provides a comfortable donor site dressing that allows moisture to escape. However, it does not allow drainage if suppuration develops. Various gauze dressings such as Owens, Betadine, Xeroform, and scarlet red provide some porosity for drainage but are not as comfortable.

The Opsite-type dressing is adhesive and should extend about 5 cm beyond the wound edges for the adhesive to adhere properly. It is recommended that the skin surrounding the donor area be defatted with acetone. To keep blood away from the area where adhesion is desired, the patient can be placed so that the donor site is horizontal.

Postoperatively serosanguinous exudate will collect under the Opsite if the periphery is completely sealed. This fluid can be aspirated if desired, although it may evaporate with time. The dressing can be left in place for two to three weeks unless suppuration is suspected.

Storing the Graft

The graft is stretched on a gauze-covered board or pan. The internal surface of the graft is exposed. The graft is kept moist with saline, which helps prevent curling of the margins (Fig. 5–11).

The margins of the gauze are freed from the board or pan, and one layer of the excess gauze is folded over the graft (Fig. 5–12).

Both layers of the gauze are cut close to the graft, leaving one layer of gauze below and one layer of gauze covering the graft (Fig. 5–13). The graft and gauze are then rolled with the dermal surface inward. The graft is placed in a container with a saline-soaked gauze sponge beneath and one covering the graft. Ideally the container should be covered to prevent evaporation, but this is not critical.

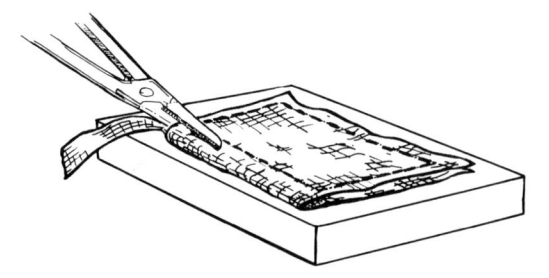

Figure 5–13. Both layers of gauze are cut adjacent to the graft.

Figure 5–14. The adhesive drape is adapted first over the nose and upper lip while the assistants elevate the margins of the drape.

Technique for Preparation of the Oral Cavity

The facial area should be scrubbed with aqueous hexachlorophene if a prep was not done when the donor site was prepped. The face may be draped with towels, body drape, and apron around the head of the table. The draping may be completed with adhesive Vi-drape or Steridrape (24 × 30 inches). This replaces towel clips and minimizes bulkiness of the usual head drape (Fig. 5–14).

The pharynx should not be packed too fully because it will cause excessive elevation of the tongue. (A hemostat clipped to the cover of the Mayo stand may be used as a reminder of the pharyngeal pack. Using a Raytec sponge for the throat pack will also be a reminder.)

Buccolabial Dissection

A solution of 1/200,000 or 1/400,000 epinephrine is used. Usually a solution of 1/100,000 epinephrine is diluted with plain 1 per cent lidocaine to obtain the desired dilution. Four to ten ml are used to balloon the submucous tissue in each quadrant prior to incision. A limited trial of phenylephrine (Neo-Synephrine) suggested that it is not as effective as epinephrine for hemostasis.

Double-ended, wide-blade retractors (Davis) and a tongue retractor are used for access (Fig. 5–15). The length and shape of the retractors should be such that the retractors do not interfere with the operator's access and conform to lip contour to minimize trauma to the lips.

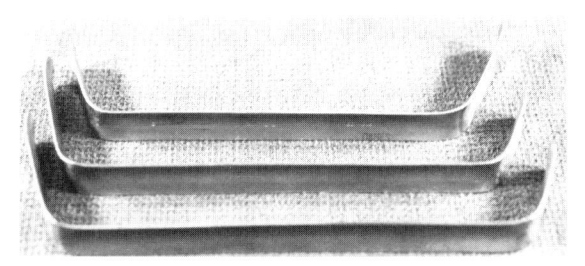

Figure 5–15. Davis nested retractors with curvatures to conform to lip contour and length of shank to allow assistant's hand to be out of the operative field.

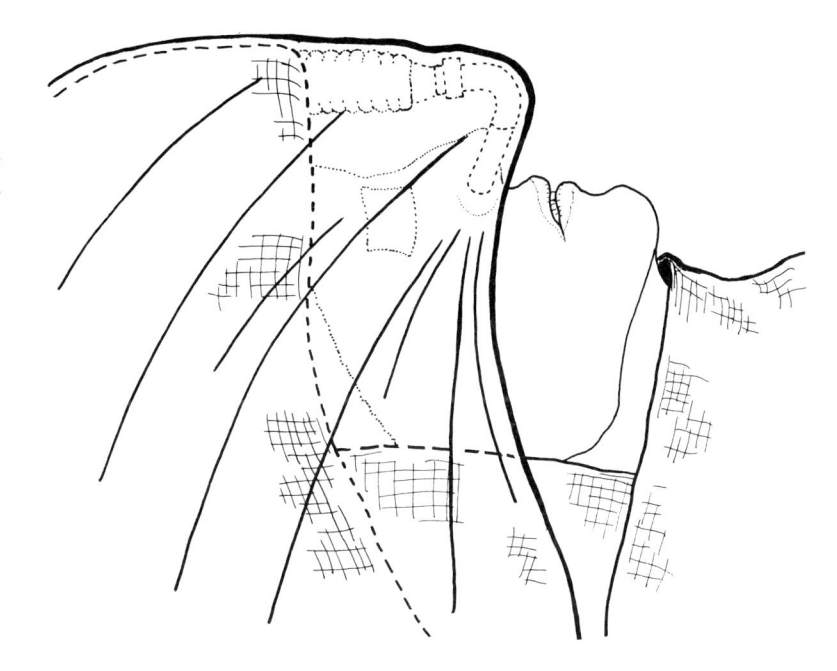

A suction tip with a bright fiberoptic light source attached is helpful, although a headlight or overhead light is satisfactory.

The crestal incision is made with a No. 15 blade on a long handle (No. 7). The incision is begun at the lateral margin of the retromolar pad just distal to the beginning of the pad (Fig. 5–16). The incision should be deep enough to contact bone occasionally (this gives a tactile sense to be sure the incision is at the supraperiosteal plane). One proceeds anteriorly, *staying at the lateral junction of the free and attached mucosa*. This should place the incision medial to the mental nerve. The incision is continued past the midline to the opposite cuspid region.

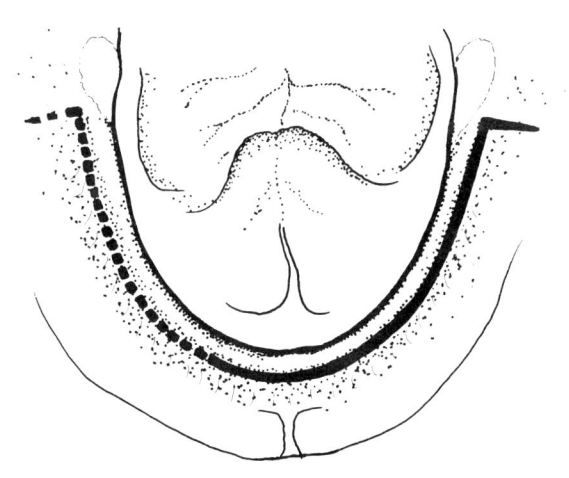

Figure 5–16. The continuous heavy line shows the initial incision for the first phase of the dissection. The dotted line indicates the completion of the incision for the second phase of the dissection.

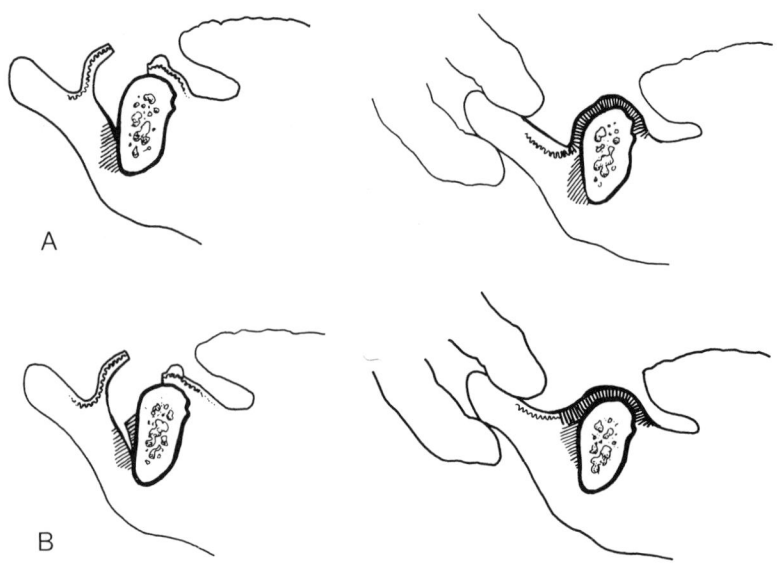

Figure 5–17. *A*, Muscle attachments properly dissected from the periosteum, resulting in no relapse of completed case. *B*, Muscle not completely detached from periosteum, causing a relapse in the completed case as shown.

err by removing too much soft tissue and exposing bone in small areas than to allow excess soft tissue over the periosteum. Experience has shown that the graft will usually remain vital and attach to the bone if the area of denuded bone is less than 1 sq cm.

In making the supraperiosteal dissection, tension should be maintained on the margin of the wound with a skin hook (a double skin hook is a good instrument). This greatly aids visualization and recognition of the supraperiosteal plane. The No. 15 blade should be used in a plane almost parallel to the periosteum. The blade can be used to gauge tactilely the thickness of the periosteum. Dissection should be carried laterally in progressive increments parallel to the incision plane. Dissecting to the full lateral extension in one spot restricts visibility and does not take advantage of the self-separating tendency of the retracting tension. After the initial separation of the margins of the flap, dissection should be carried anteriorly and posteriorly relative to the mental neurovascular (N-V) region. As the mental N-V bundle is approached, it is easily visualized because its white fibers can be seen through some overlying tissue.

In the most posterior area, the dissection should end at, or just clear of, the external oblique line but should be no deeper than about 2 mm on the lateral side (Fig. 5–18*A*). Further lateral dissection tends to heal with an acute angle that would be difficult for the patient to keep clean.

The transverse incision at the retromolar pad is begun at the posterior origin of the crestal incisions. The incision is carried laterally about 1 cm to the lateral margin of the mandible. This incision prevents a band type of scar contraction.

A supraperiosteal plane of dissection is used, and it is important to clear virtually all of the soft tissue from the periosteum. Wherever there is soft tissue in excess of the periosteum, the skin will not be fixed to the bone and the graft will be mobile (Fig. 5–17). Such mobility would defeat the major benefit of the procedure. It is therefore better to

From the most posterior area, the dissection is progressively deepened to the first molar region. At this point, the depth can be almost to the inferior border, if necessary

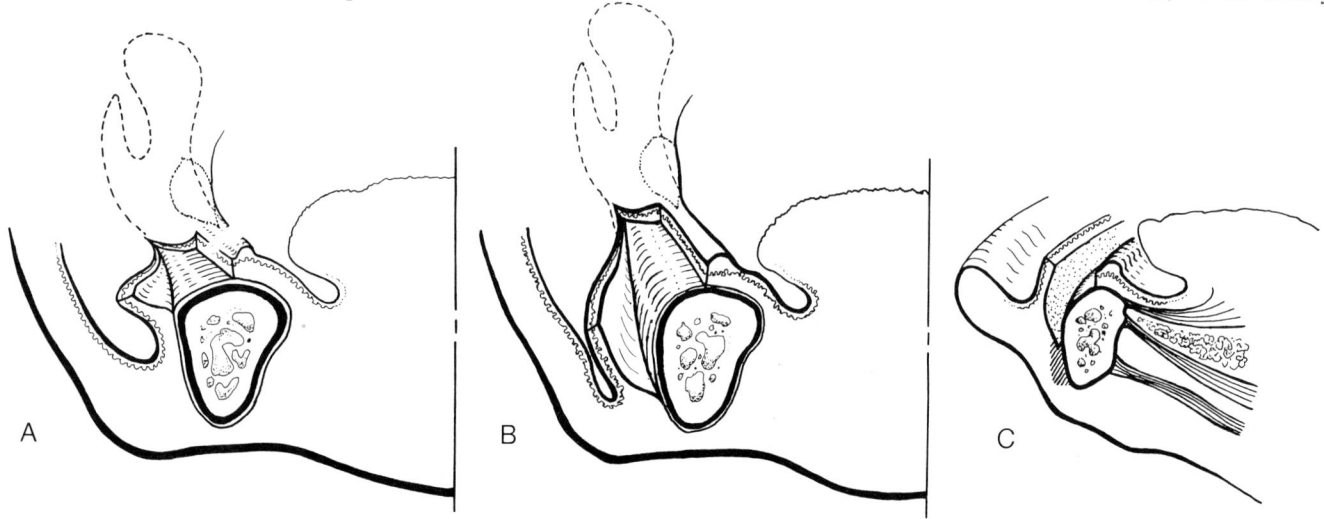

Figure 5–18. *A*, Dissection is carried just slightly past the external oblique line in the third molar region. *B*, This diagram depicts the first molar area where the buccal dissection can be carried almost to the inferior border of the mandible if needed. *C*, Dissection of only part of the mentalis muscle from the mandible to prevent drooping of the chin.

(Fig. 5–18*B*). In the mental N-V area, the dissection is shallow to minimize trauma to the N-V bundle. Anterior to the mental nerve, the dissection can again be deepened.

Around the midline of the mandible, the dissection should terminate at least 1 cm above the inferior border of the mandible. This prevents drooping of the chin. The depth of vestibule in this region is not critical. Therefore, the dissection at the midline should not be carried to the inferior border— a great temptation (Fig. 5–18*C*). Supraperiosteal dissection in the anterior area is difficult because there is usually no recognizable periosteal plane. A similar dissection is then carried out on the opposite side.

Experience suggests that minimal vestibular depth in the N-V bundle area is almost always tolerable. When a sharp bone ridge or prominence is present on the caudal margin of the mental foramen, it may be desirable to remove this sharp margin. However, the dissection of the N-V bundle needed to do this will often incur some significant paresthesia of the mental nerve. If the sharp bony margin is to be removed, the N-V bundle is separated from the periosteum by blunt and sharp dissection, enough to allow access beneath the nerve. A chisel is placed in the anterior margin of the foramen with the edge directed laterally, and the cut is made directly laterally and caudally (Fig. 5–19*A* and *B*). An identical cut is made laterally at the posterior edge of the foramen (Fig. 5–19*A* and *B*). With elevation of the nerve fibers, a chisel is placed in the anterior cut with the blade directed caudally and distally to release the bone between the vertical cuts (Fig. 5–19*C*). This bone is then grasped and removed, leaving the channel for the N-V bundle.

Lingual Dissection

Before the lingual dissection is made, a vasoconstrictor is infiltrated. The epinephrine solution is deposited in the submucous, mylohyoid, and genioglossus regions adjacent to the mandible.

A bolus of gauze, about 2 × 2 × 3 cm is placed firmly in a gauze-holding forceps. If a second instrument is available, delay is avoided in changing the gauze. This gauze retractor is placed in the posterior sublingual region. A rotation of the gauze away from the crest of the ridge will provide good visibility and retraction (Fig. 5–20). The main retraction should be directed medially. If the retraction is directed caudally, very poor access and visibility will result.

The incision is begun on the lingual side of the retromolar pad near the pad's anterior margin (Fig. 5–21). The incision should be placed at the lingual junction of the free and the attached mucosa, slightly in the free mucosa. The incision should just penetrate the mucosa along the retromolar pad (to protect

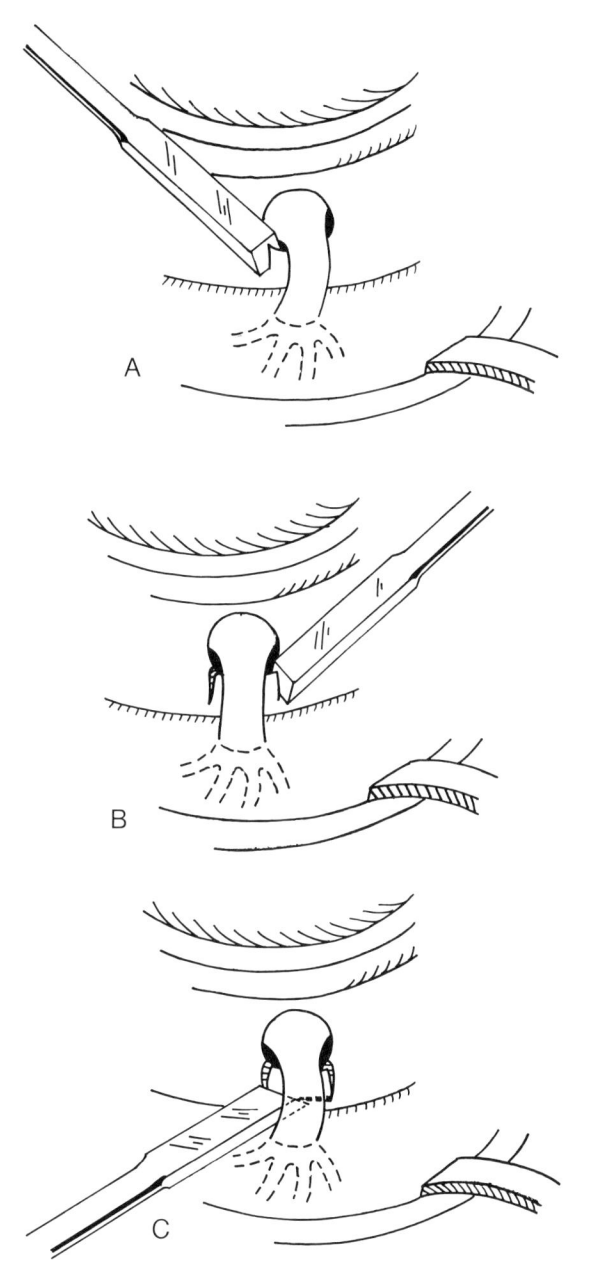

Figure 5–19. *A*, The edge of the chisel engages the anterior inferior margin of the mental foramen and is directed inferiorly and laterally. *B*, View from the posterior aspect showing both vertical limiting cuts and the inferior cut which, in effect, scoops out the sharp inferior margin of the mental foramen. *C*, With elevation of the neurovascular bundle, the small osteotome makes the final connecting cut.

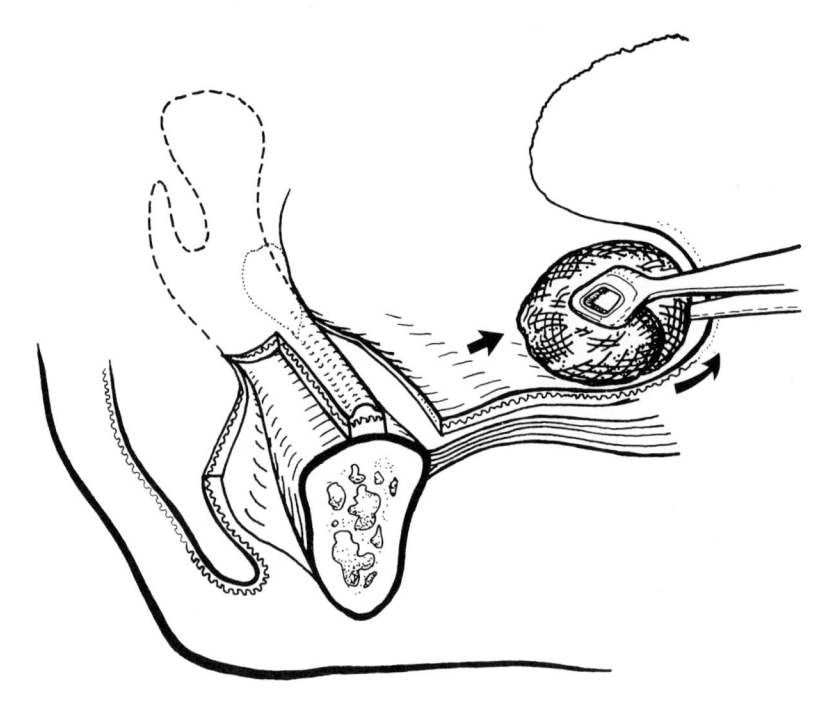

80 / SURGICAL MANAGEMENT OF SOFT TISSUE PROBLEMS

Figure 5–20. Note that retraction exposes the mylohyoid muscle after the mucosa has been completely incised.

the lingual nerve). Anterior to the retromolar pad, the incision should be made completely through mucosa with the blade occasionally contacting bone. The incision is continued past the midline to the opposite cuspid region.

If the suturing method of graft placement is to be used, the skin may not cover the lingual area. It is then desirable to be careful in the lingual dissection to maintain a periosteal covering of the bone. If the periosteum is intact, rapid secondary epithelialization will occur (usually within two weeks).

In sectioning the mylohyoid muscle, one should recall that the anterior portion of the mylohyoid is hidden by the genial muscles. This portion is left intact. With medial retraction, the accessible fibers of the mylohyoid are sectioned at the mandible with a No. 15 blade. As the dissection continues caudally along the lingual surface of the mandible, it flares laterally to a marked degree, and the remaining attachment of the posterior portion of the mylohyoid muscle is not easily visualized. A curved Kelly hemostat may be placed caudal to the muscle fibers near the mandible to elevate the muscle. This allows easier sectioning of the muscle with a blade or curved Metzenbaum scissors (Fig. 5–22). Some extreme posterior muscle fibers may remain. These fibers may be cut if desired, but care must be taken to section the muscle fibers close to the mandible to avoid the lingual nerve. The index finger is used to continue the dissection to the inferior border of the mandible in the region of the submandibular gland. This finger dissection should not be carried beneath the mandible (Fig. 5–23). The same procedure is carried out on the opposite side. The sharp edge of the mylohyoid ridge, having been denuded of its muscular attachment, will resorb and need not be trimmed unless it is very sharp or the prosthodontist does not wish an undercut. A bone file easily smoothes a sharp edge.

One may note that the separation between the genioglossi and geniohyoids can often be

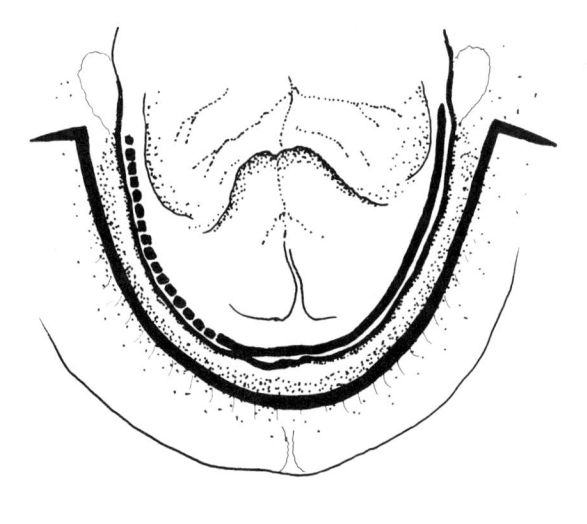

Figure 5–21. The heavy line on the lingual side indicates the initial incision to allow the first phase of the lingual dissection. The dotted line indicates the completion of the incision to allow the remaining lingual dissection.

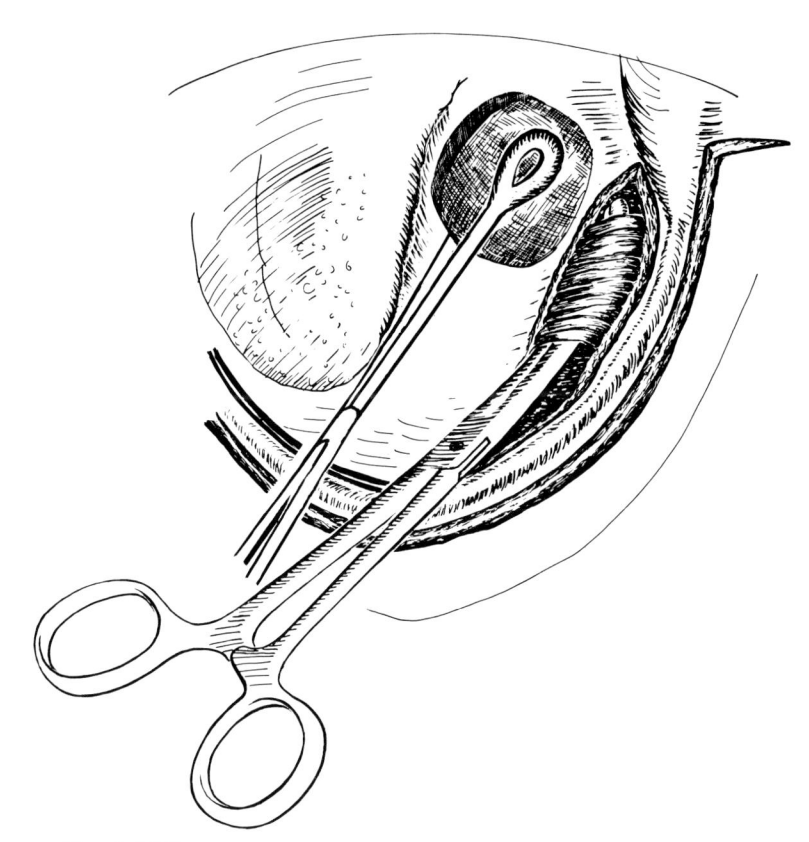

SURGICAL MANAGEMENT OF SOFT TISSUE PROBLEMS / **81**

Figure 5–22. An instrument such as curved Kelly forceps placed beneath the fibers of the mylohyoid muscle facilitates dissection of the muscle from the mandible.

identified by a layer of fat between these muscles, but it is not critical that this separation be visualized. Approximately one half or less of the genioglossi are sectioned at the genial tubercle on the superior and lateral portions (Fig. 5–24). Obwegeser reports that difficulty in swallowing will occur for several months if the genioglossi are completely sectioned. The dimensions of the genial tubercle are highly variable. Like the mylohyoid ridge, sharp edges may be trimmed but do not require trimming, as they will usually resorb.

Crestal Tissue

If the suturing technique for graft placement is utilized, it is necessary to leave the crestal tissue in place to permit suturing of the graft to this tissue.

If the stent method is used, the following steps apply. Firm, fixed tissue on the crest of the ridge and over smooth bone may be left, but any flabby crestal tissue should be removed. The crestal tissue should be removed over any sharp edges of bone so that the sharp edges themselves can be removed.

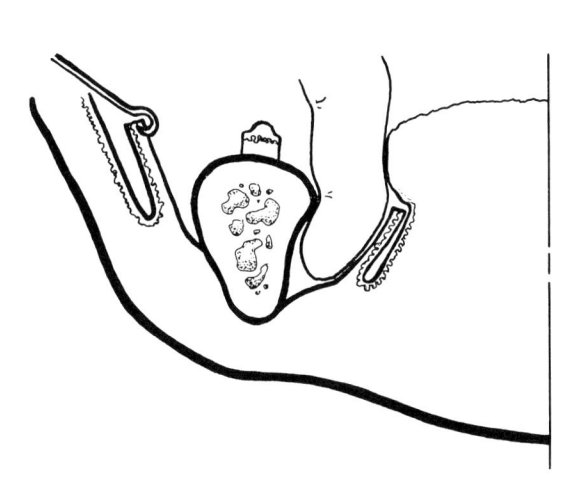

Figure 5–23. The index finger is used to bluntly dissect any remaining soft tissue attachments in the posterior area of the lingual dissection.

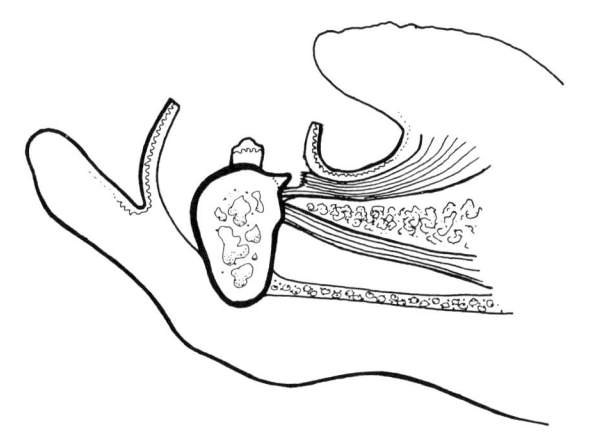

Figure 5–24. Note the layer of fat that usually separates the genioglossus muscles from the geniohyoid muscles. The dotted line indicates the resorption that usually takes place when parts of the genioglossi are severed.

A rongeur is effective in removing this bone. However, the periosteum may not be severed by the rongeur, and a scalpel can be used to cut the periosteum before the rongeur is removed. This will prevent unnecessary loss of periosteum. Occasionally the anterior portion of the crestal soft tissue will lie folded lingually, requiring removal before the lingual incision and dissection.

The Submandibular Sutures

Before the submandibular sutures are placed, the dissected area on the lingual should be inspected for persistent bleeding and appropriate hemostasis applied. Bleeding from the lingual area can cause significant tongue swelling and rapid airway embarrassment.

A monofilament material will probably afford the least risk of infection, but it requires removal. Plain catgut material carries a slightly higher risk of infection, but not having to remove it makes catgut probably the most desirable material. If a monofilament material is selected, Supramid is a good choice. It is actually a woven material that is covered to act as a monofilament. A limited trial of polyglycolic acid (Dexon) suture material produced one case in which two of the sutures did not resorb and abscesses occurred. Similar experiences have been reported by others. However, Dexon can be used if it is treated as a nonabsorbable material that must be removed. A nonabsorbable suture material is desirable if the graft is placed by suturing. It is critical that the sutures remain stable for at least one week. Eight pieces of 2-0 size are usually used. Figure 5–25 shows the position of each suture, although they are not placed through the lingual tissue at one time, but individually as described below.

The suture material is threaded on a 3/4-inch, 3/8-circle needle. The needle and suture material are passed through the lingual mucosa in the anterior region about 1 cm from the midline for the first pair of sutures, care being taken to avoid the submandibular ducts. The awl that is used for each anterior suture is best started in the skin toward the anterior portion of the inferior border of the mandible (about 1 cm from the midline). This facilitates the later completion of the labial portion of the pass (Fig. 5–26). The awl is kept close to the mandible and directed toward the lingual side of the mandible. When the tip of the awl is presented on the lingual side of the mandible, the two ends of the suture are passed through the concave side of the awl. Passing the suture ends into the hole in the awl is facilitated if the ends are grasped for introduction with one end longer than the other. The ends of the suture are pulled through about 4 cm and released (Fig. 5–27). The awl is withdrawn,

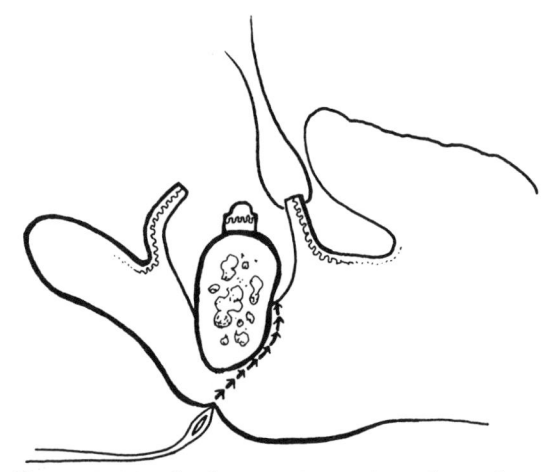

Figure 5–26. In the anterior region, the awl engages the skin toward the anterior inferior border of the mandible.

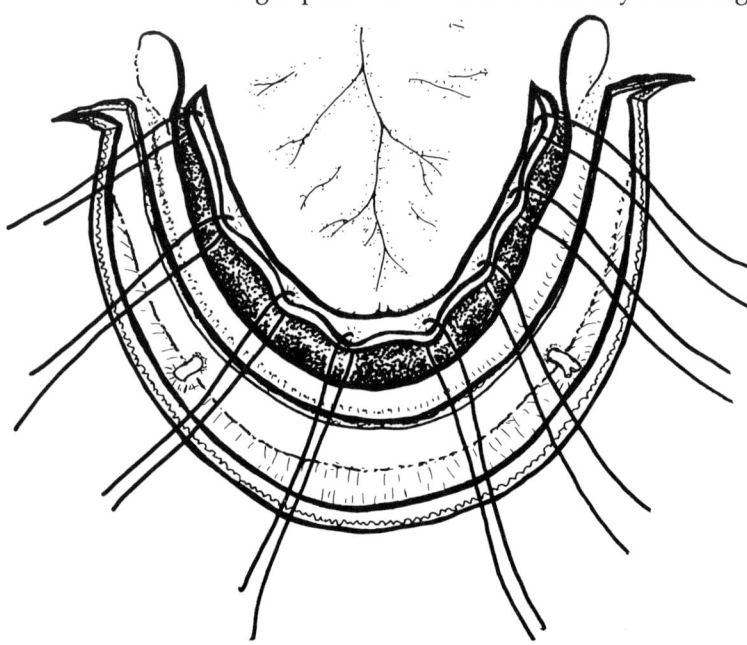

Figure 5–25. The position of the sutures as they would be if passed through the lingual mucosa at the same time.

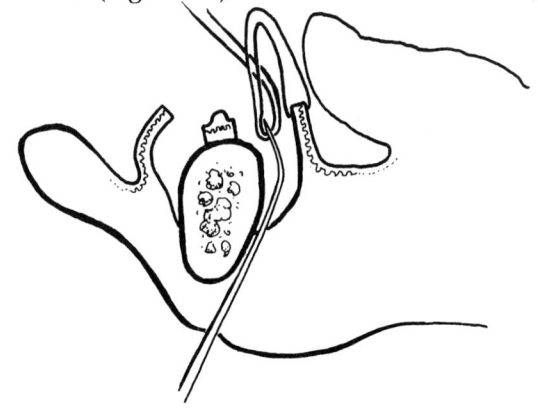

Figure 5–27. Both ends of the suture are passed through the eye of the awl approximately 1.5 inches and then released from the hemostat.

SURGICAL MANAGEMENT OF SOFT TISSUE PROBLEMS / **83**

keeping it in contact with the mandible. After reaching the inferior border of the mandible, it is kept in contact with the bone and introduced into the labiobuccal dissection area. It is important that the point of the awl emerge adjacent to the periosteum, because the margin of the mucosa will later be brought to this point (Figs. 5–28 and 5–29).

When the eye of the awl is presented, one of the ends of the suture is removed. The material should always be grasped from the same side (concave) from which the material was introduced to avoid confusion in pulling (Fig. 5–29). The point is then introduced through the labiobuccal mucosa about 3 mm from the edge of the mucosa (Fig. 5–30). The

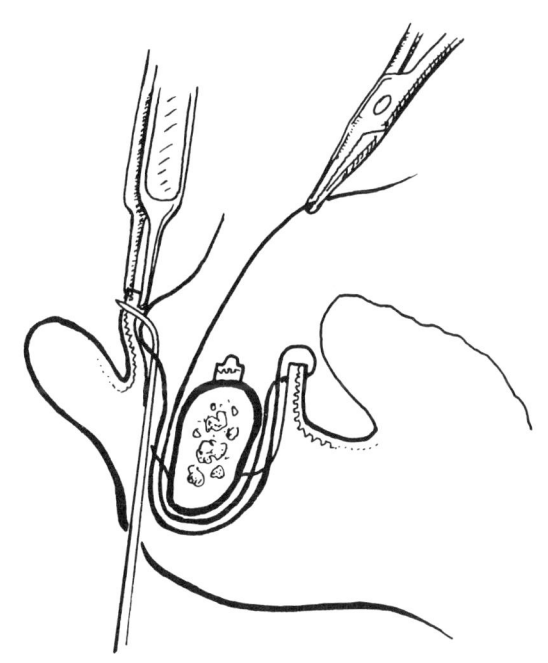

Figure 5–30. The awl with one suture remaining is passed through the labial tissue near the margin of the incision.

remaining end of the suture is removed from the awl (Fig. 5–31). The two ends are clipped together with a hemostat. The awl is removed and wiped with iodophor (or equivalent) before each pass.

The second pair of sutures is placed just anterior to the mental neurovascular bundle. The third pair of sutures is placed about 1 cm distal to the bundle. The most distal pair of sutures is placed at the distal ends of the incision. The awl should enter the skin at the inferior border of the mandible just anterior to the angle of the mandible (Fig. 5–32) rather than in the plane of the suture. Otherwise, it will be difficult to keep the sutures far enough posterior. A fairly tightly curved awl should be used for this pass. One

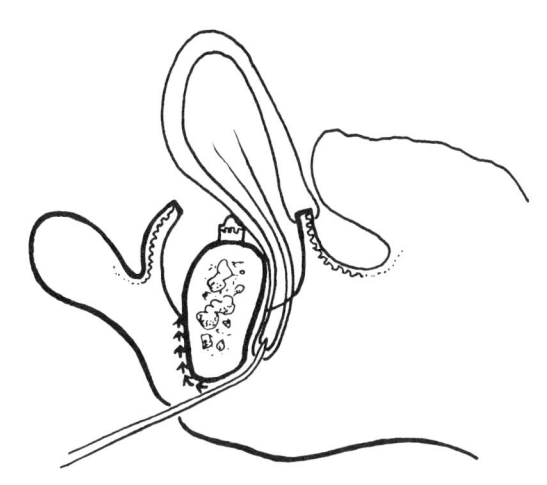

Figure 5–28. The awl is withdrawn adjacent to the mandible.

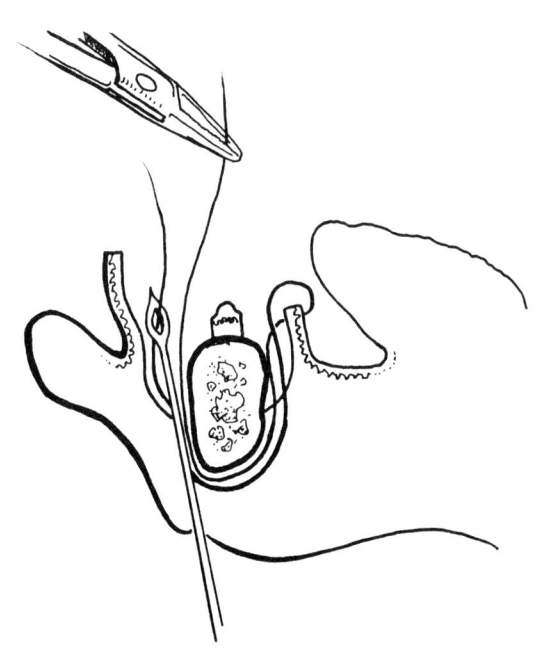

Figure 5–29. The awl is passed adjacent to the mandible without exiting the skin and then is projected in the labiobuccal dissection adjacent to the periosteum.

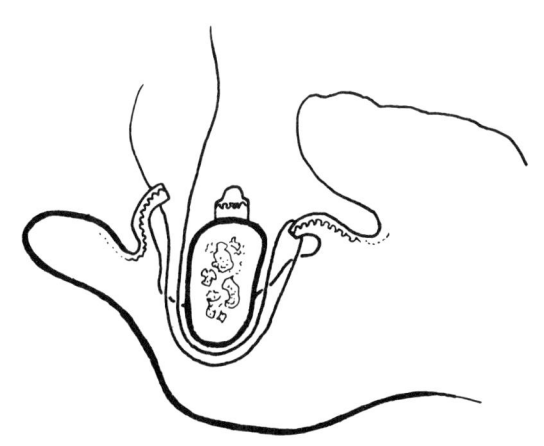

Figure 5–31. Diagrammatic representation of the suture before it is tied.

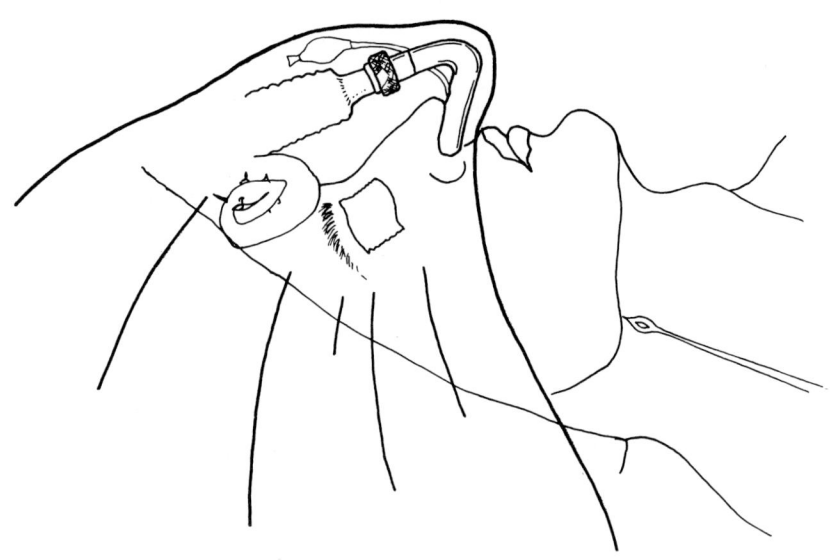

84 / SURGICAL MANAGEMENT OF SOFT TISSUE PROBLEMS

Figure 5–32. The awl penetrates the skin for the most distal submandibular suture, just anterior to the angle of the mandible.

should proceed as before but should penetrate in the corner made by the crestal and lateral incisions when entering the buccal mucosa (Fig. 5–33). To facilitate removal of nonabsorbable suture material (including Dexon), the ends of the suture should be left long enough to be grasped.

Tying the Submandibular Sutures (Fig. 5–34). Again, the lingual area should be inspected for bleeding with appropriate hemostasis before the sutures are placed. Before each suture is tied, tension should be applied so that the lingual tissue can be felt to

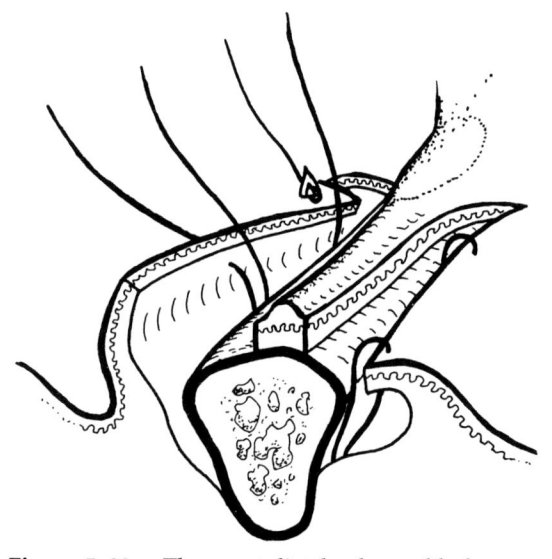

Figure 5–33. The most distal submandibular suture penetrates the buccal mucosa at the angle made by the buccal and lateral incisions.

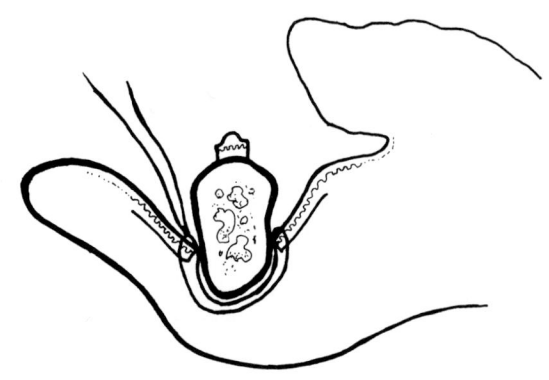

Figure 5–34. Final appearance of a submandibular suture when tied.

be drawn snugly to the mandible. Great force should not be used, as the lingual tissue should not be drawn under the mandible. The index finger is used to snug the throws of the knot, rather than just pulling on the ends of the suture. This allows greater tactile sense and prevents tying the suture too tightly. Four throws are used. The sutures are not cut, as the ends could become entrapped beneath the skin graft. The sutures also aid in retraction.

Circummandibular Ligatures
(Fig. 5–35)

Two No. 1 white Supramid sutures (or their equivalent) are used. Wire is probably not as desirable as Supramid because wire lacks the resiliency to help prevent excessive pressure on the graft. Size 1-0 nylon monofilament may be substituted if necessary. One ligature is passed just anterior to the mental nerve on one side, and one is placed just posterior to the mental nerve on the opposite side. These ligatures can be placed along with the corresponding submandibular sutures. The lingual ends of the two sutures are clipped together with a hemostat and allowed to rest on the forehead. The lateral ends are clipped separately with hemostats and allowed to rest on the outside of the face with the submandibular suture ends.

Making the Stent

The plastic stent tray is placed in the compound heater. The compound is formed into a roll and placed in the tray, with the bulk of the compound toward the labiobuccal side. With assistants providing good retraction of the corners of the mouth, the tray and compound are placed in the mouth and adapted with finger pressure to the labiobuccal vestibule. When it is hard, it is removed and the excess trimmed with a No. 15 blade (a No. 10 blade may cut the thumb). All material engaging undercut areas of the lingual re-

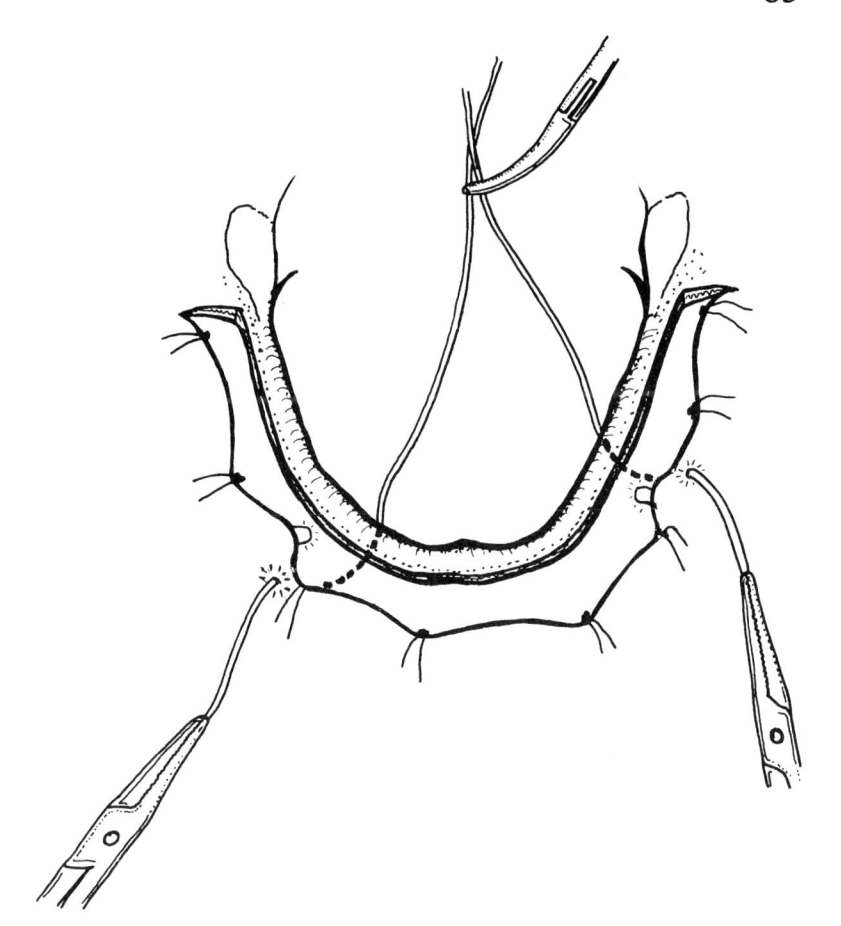

Figure 5–35. One circummandibular suture is placed anterior and one posterior to the mental nerve.

gion should be removed. Excess in the retromolar pad area should be removed to allow the patient to close without contacting the stent.

Refrigerated saline is added to the heater solution to cool it to 110° F. A piece of Protaform is folded lengthwise and waved through the water bath. The material melts quickly, so if the water is warmer than 110° F, it should be held in the water only momentarily. The material is placed on the entire surface of the compound. The assistants provide good retraction of the corners of the mouth and the tray with compound and Protaform is placed in the mouth. The Protaform is cooled in the mouth with refrigerated saline solution if desired, and the stent is then removed from the mouth with a hemostat. Using the Protaform as the material next to the graft helps eliminate areas of excessive pressure on the graft during the immobilization period and allows the skin to be carried into the lingual undercut.

Placing the Skin on the Stent

The stent is dried. A small amount of dermatome glue (Reese or comparable) is placed in a medicine cup. The glue is applied to the Protaform with a cotton-tipped applicator while the stent is held with a hemostat. The skin is unrolled with external surface upward and the top layer of gauze is removed. The *external* surface of the skin is adapted to the stent starting at one retromolar area. (Thus the dermal [internal] side of the graft will be in contact with the periosteum.) The assistant holds one end of the skin above the stent with two hemostats. Adaptation of the skin to the stent is accomplished with wet cotton applicators. Proper identification of the external and dermal surfaces is assured by the fact that the skin edge always rolls toward the dermal (inner) surface. The remaining layer of gauze is removed by pulling the gauze back on itself. The folded skin in the anterior lingual area may be trimmed, but once healing is complete it is not possible to detect where overlapping occurred.

Placing and Securing the Stent

The mouth is irrigated with saline. Assistants provide good retraction of the corners of the mouth, and the stent is carried into the mouth with a hemostat. The circummandibular ligatures are tied, using a double throw first, pulling snugly, and grasping the knot with a hemostat. A second throw is made and the hemostat is removed. Two more throws are made and the ligature is cut.

The submandibular sutures are cut, leaving the ends long (about 1 cm) if Supramid is used. If 2-0 catgut is used, the ends can be shorter.

With a periosteal elevator or finger tip, the excess labial and buccal Protaform is displaced caudally to fill any void in adaptation of the stent to the margin of the dissection

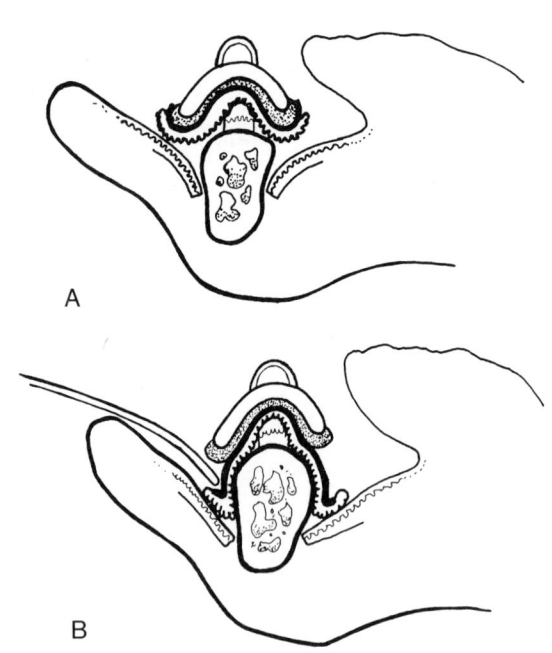

Figure 5–36. By fingernail or instrument, the Protaform material is displaced inferiorly into any passive voids between the compound and the depth of the dissection. This causes the skin to cover any dissected area where the compound is not sufficiently extended on the labiobuccal and into the lingual undercut.

(Fig. 5–36). The Protaform is also displaced caudally on the lingual side to carry the skin into the lingual undercut area.

The pharyngeal pack is removed and a gastric tube (18-gauge Salem sump) may be used to evacuate the stomach, which helps prevent postoperative nausea. A pressure dressing is applied in the submandibular area with elastic tape such as 4-inch Elastoplast or Conform. After extubation, the patient may be placed on his or her side to allow dependent drainage of the mouth until he or she is completely conscious.

Immediate Postoperative Care

In addition to the routine postoperative orders, it appears helpful to have hydrocortisone cream 1 per cent applied to lips. (It should be used for no more than three days to avoid Candida superinfection.) Parenteral corticosteroids are also helpful, if not contraindicated, for a day or two postoperatively. Considering the various portals for infection, it is probably appropriate to continue antibiotic therapy until just after the stent is removed. If the patient wishes to use a maxillary denture, one must be sure that the posterior teeth do not contact the stent. Any movement of the stent during the time that it is in place may interfere with the take of the graft.

Stent Removal

The stent is usually removed seven to ten days after the initial surgery. As noted, antibiotic coverage is usually continued until the stent is removed. In any case, antibiotics should be used before and after stent removal. Sedation may be desirable during stent removal. All the debris is cleaned away from the labiobuccal portions of the sutures with antiseptic-soaked cotton swabs and aspiration. The loose skin is peeled away from the stent. Otherwise the excess skin that is adapted to the stent, especially in the retromolar area, may cause separation of the graft from the host bed as the stent is removed. The circummandibular ligatures are cut on the labiobuccal side and removed from the lingual side, and the stent is removed. If nonresorbable submandibular sutures were used, these are also cut and removed. The excess unattached skin may be cut away or left to slough spontaneously. Gross amounts of excess tissue are often an annoyance to the patient and are generally removed.

Follow-Up

In the first few days after stent removal, granulations sometimes occur at the junction of the skin and mucosa. These may be easily and painlessly removed with a cotton forceps. Any exposed bone on the lingual side will cover with granulation and epithelialize or will slough off as a thin layer and granulate as expected. The denture may be constructed when the patient is ready, as there is little tendency for shrinkage or scar contraction with this procedure. The initial denture should have the flanges a little short of the full extension. Excessive contact with the junction of the skin and mucosa will usually cause persistent granulation tissue and resultant scarring. Once this area has matured (about six months), the flanges can be extended to the normal length. Excess pressure of the denture often causes focal nonpainful keratoses rather than the painful ulcers that occur on normal mucosa. Patients should therefore be advised to have routine postoperative evaluations at least every six months. A typical result of this procedure is shown in Figure 5–37.

Complications

Mental nerve paresthesia or anesthesia is usually in direct proportion to the degree of dissection of the mental N-V bundles. A shallow vestibule can be tolerated in the mental foramen area, and little anesthesia will be produced. Initially, one of us (W.H.D.) grooved the mandible as previously described for the mental nerve. This required extensive dissection of the nerve and paresthesia was frequent. As time passed, it was noted that patients did not complain of the prominence of the mental nerve. Thus, it appears that channeling for the mental nerve is rarely necessary. Lingual nerve paresthesia is very uncommon.

Lingual and sublingual swelling rarely occurs to the point of difficulty in making and placing the stent. In the authors' experience two cases of swelling of the tongue and the floor of the mouth seemed a possible threat to respiration. An elective tracheostomy was needed in one case and immediate evacuation of a sublingual hematoma (and Penrose drain placement) was required in the other. It is probable that hemostasis in the lingual dissection area is the most important factor in minimizing lingual swelling. This can be accomplished by direct hemostasis during surgery by tying or cauterizing bleeding points. If bleeding occurs postoperatively, it will usually be in the sublingual area. A 3 × 3 inch gauze rolled to fit beneath the lateral portion of the tongue and under the stent flange will usually stop postoperative bleeding. Blood loss at surgery is usually 100 to 500 ml. As previously mentioned, use of corticosteroids at surgery and postoperatively is also helpful for swelling.

Occasionally bone will be exposed on the lingual of the mandible, but this is not a significant problem. The denture may be constructed without waiting for soft tissue covering of the bone if slight relief of the denture is provided in the exposed area.

If significant vestibular depth is required in the genioglossi areas, the attachments may be released before or after the grafting procedure when the mylohyoid muscle is attached to the mandible. If, by accident, the genioglossi are completely detached at the time of the grafting procedure, difficulty in swallowing may occur. If complete detachment does occur it is undoubtedly best to try to reattach the genioglossi if possible.

The sulcus depth may be too great in the buccal retromolar area if one does not resist the temptation to dissect too deeply in area.

A suture abscess may occur rarely. Catgut probably will have a slightly higher incidence of abscess than Supramid. Dexon may

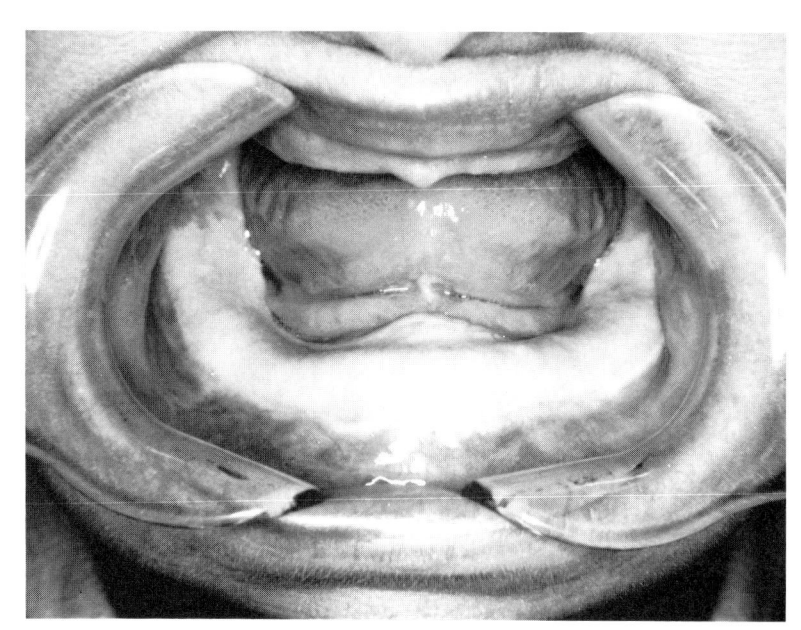

Figure 5-37. This illustration exemplifies the typically good result obtained by the procedure.

be a significant problem due to lack of resorption if infection occurs. Percutaneous incision and drainage seem to resolve suture abscesses quickly. This complication can be minimized by antibiotic coverage prior to suture removal and cleaning the mouth well before suture removal.

A small area of periosteum may be exposed if a small portion of the graft does not revitalize. This will cover by secondary epithelialization. Failure of a significant portion of the graft to revitalize rarely occurs and is probably related to movement of the graft during the first week. After a prolonged period of granulation, mucosa will cover this area, but loss of vestibular depth may occur.

Drooping of the chin related to this procedure is caused by excessive dissection in the labial area. At least 1 cm of soft tissue should be left untouched in the mentalis area.

Occasionally, prolonged weeping of the donor site will occur. Cleaning with soap and water by the patient at least twice daily is usually all that is necessary. It is also important to minimize local trauma from clothing.

Hair in the graft is usually related to the thickness of the graft but is uncommon and of no real significance. If desired, the hair can be removed by cautery of the base of the follicle.

Suturing Technique in the Application of the Skin Graft (Bloom)

In 1970, Walker[23] advocated the suturing of the skin graft as an alternative to the stent

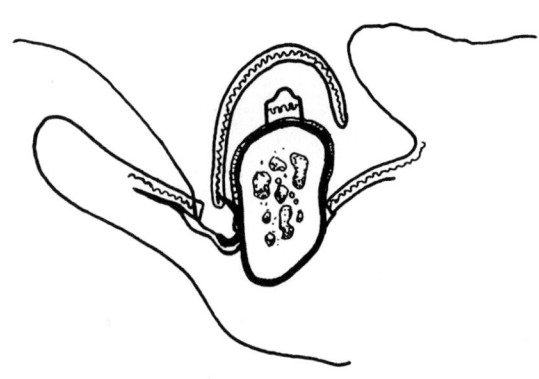

88 / SURGICAL MANAGEMENT OF SOFT TISSUE PROBLEMS

Figure 5-38. The suture is passed through the labiobuccal mucosa 3 mm from the incised edge and the exposed periosteum is engaged as inferiorly as possible. Then the suture is passed through the skin graft within 2 to 3 mm of its inferior margin.

method of placing the skin graft. Alexander and Bloom have evolved the following technique, which has proven successful.

Intra-oral Placement of Graft

With the suturing technique, the submandibular sutures are cut, leaving enough of the free ends to facilitate removal. The mouth is irrigated with saline and examined to be sure that hemostasis is accomplished. The skin is unrolled and positioned with its external surface facing up. The layer of gauze on the dermal (inner) surface is removed. The gauze on the external surface is kept in place to help transport the skin into the mouth. With two tissue forceps (Adson), the skin is grasped lengthwise at what will be its superior margin and about 2.5 cm from the midline bilaterally. To facilitate introduction of the graft, assistants retract the corners of the mouth and lower lip. The graft is placed intra-orally with its internal surface facing the buccolabial periosteum and the final layer of gauze is removed. The graft is centered to assure bilateral distal coverage. Beginning at the midline, the tissue forceps and/or the index fingers are used to unfold and unroll the inferior margin of the graft and place it at the mucoperiosteal junction. With the inferior margin of skin held in place with finger pressure, the superior margin of the graft may then be draped over the alveolar crest and will hang passively toward the lingual area.

Suturing the Graft

Suturing of the inferior skin margin is begun in the midline. The inferior margin is sutured with 4-0 chromic gut on a small 3/8-inch circle cutting needle, such as an Ethicon FS-2. The suture is passed through the labiobuccal mucosa 3 mm from the incised edge (Fig. 5-38) and continued in the same pass to engage the exposed periosteum as inferiorly as possible. Then the suture is passed through the skin graft within 2 to 3 mm of its inferior margin. In order to pass the needle accurately near the skin margin and not displace the graft, the edge of the skin is slightly elevated and stabilized with a tissue forceps while the needle is passed. The suture is tied and cut, thus securing the graft to the mucoperiosteal interface. Critical to the proper adaptation of the graft inferiorly, the skin must be stretched distally and held taut with gentle finger pressure as each suture is passed and tied (Fig. 5-39). The inferior sutures are positioned 0.5 cm apart in the parasymphysis region, and care is taken to place sutures just anterior and posterior to the mental neurovascular bundle. Distal to the mental N-V bundles the sutures are placed 1 cm apart. After three or four sutures have been placed bilaterally in the inferior margin, superior sutures may be placed. The graft is gently stretched over the alveolar crest in a lingual and inferior direction and this tension is maintained during passage for each superior suture. Size 3-0 chromic gut is used for the superior line of sutures, which are placed at 1-cm intervals along the alveolar crest. Finger tension is maintained on the graft in a lingual and inferior direction as the suture is placed through the graft, through crestal tissue, and then through the lingual drape of the graft (Fig. 5-40).

The suture is tied, with finger tension released when the superior line of sutures is tied but maintained during suture passage. The superior sutures are placed so that the inferior suture line is advanced 1 cm ahead

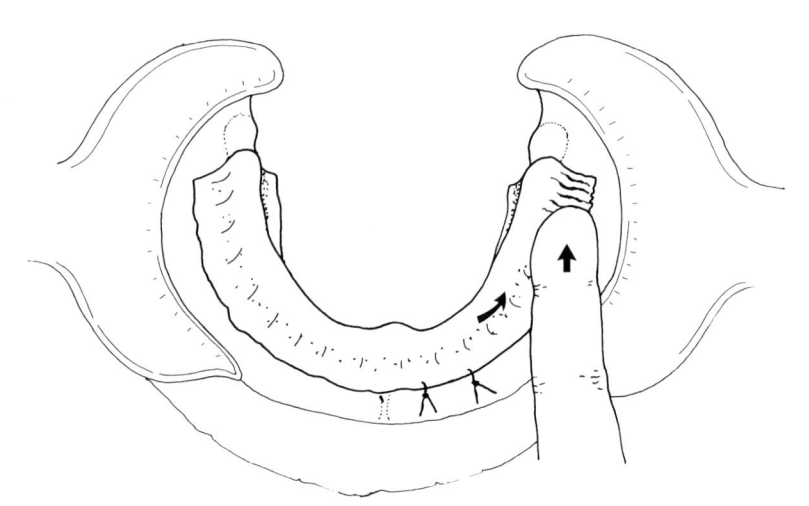

Figure 5-39. Critical to the proper adaptation of the graft inferiorly, the assistant must stretch the skin distally with gentle finger pressure as each suture is passed and tied.

of the superior sutures. This alternating technique (inferior then superior) is continued distally and bilaterally. When excesssive skin makes suturing difficult in the distal and retromolar regions, the tissue is trimmed prior to suturing.

After the graft has been completely secured, excessive skin is carefully trimmed at the most inferior and distal suture line and lingual to the superior suture line (Fig. 5–41). This trimming procedure can be facilitated by grasping the free margin of the excessive skin under light tension with a tissue forceps and excising the excessive tissue with a small Metzenbaum or iris scissors. The trimming is begun distolingually and advanced around the anterolingual curvature of the mandible to the contralateral distolingual extent. Occasionally, one or two 4-0 sutures are necessary at the distal portion of the recipient bed at the angular incision of the retromolar pad. If there is concavity in the anatomy of the mandibular buccal surface, and there appears to be poor adaptation of the graft to the periosteum (tenting), 4-0 chromic catgut sutures may be placed through the skin and periosteum. This is done in the area of the concavity and at 1- or 2-cm intervals, or as necessary to more effectively adapt the skin to its recipient bed (Fig. 5–42).

In order to prevent blood or serum accumulation under the skin, several small stab incisions are made 1 to 2 cm apart along the midportion of the graft (Fig. 5–43). The mouth is irrigated with saline and inspected for hemostasis under the graft and in the floor of the mouth, and the pharyngeal pack is removed. A pressure dressing is applied over the anterior and lateral surface of the mandible.

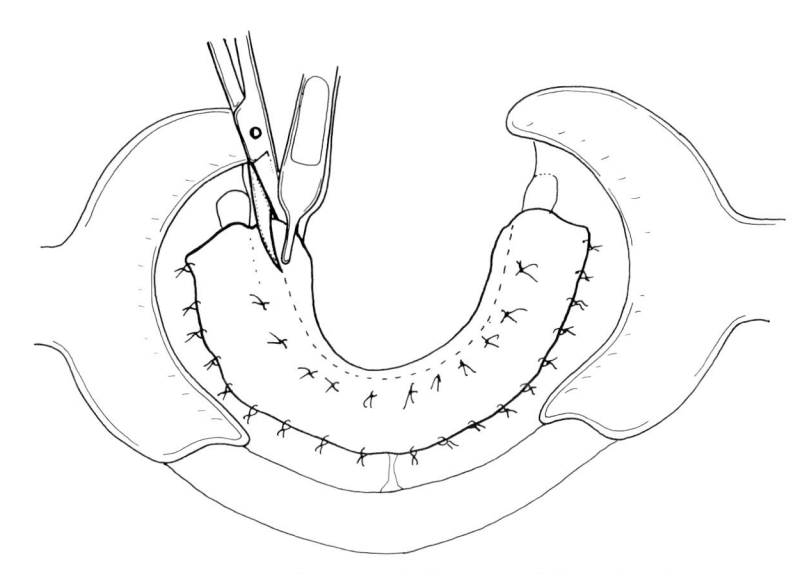

Figure 5–41. Excessive skin is carefully trimmed lingual to the superior suture line. The free margin of the excessive tissue is grasped under light tension and excised with a small scissors.

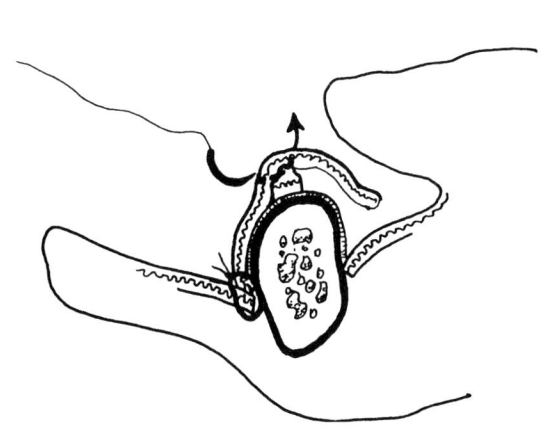

Figure 5–40. With finger tension maintained on the graft in a lingual and inferior direction, the suture is placed through the graft, through crestal tissue, and then back out through the graft.

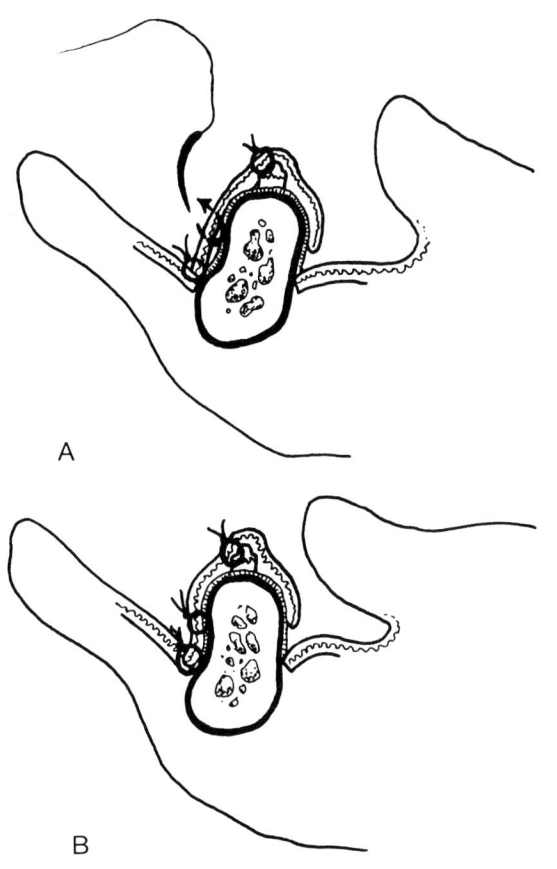

Figure 5–42. *A*, With a marked concavity in the anatomy of the mandible's buccal surface, there may be poor adaptation of the graft to the periosteum (tenting). *B*, Sutures are placed through the skin and periosteum in the area of the concavity to more effectively adapt the skin to its recipient bed.

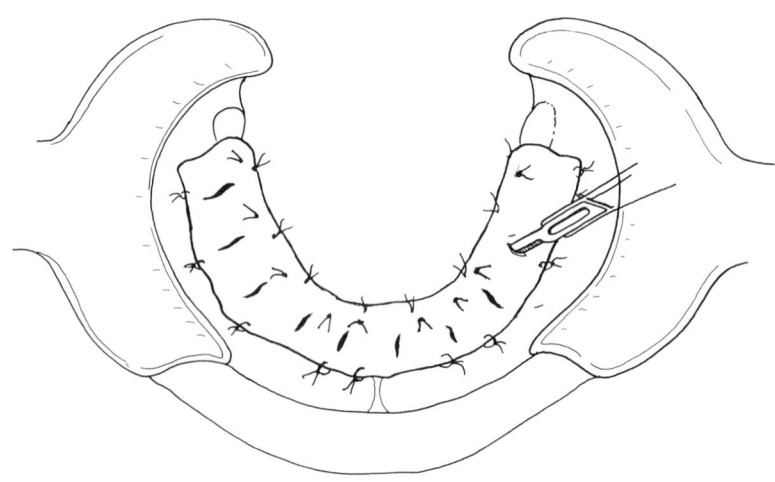

Figure 5–43. In order to prevent blood or serum accumulation under the skin, several small stab incisions are made along the midportion of the graft.

Postoperative Care

The pressure dressing is removed on the first postoperative day. Intra-oral warm saline irrigations are suggested every two hours while the patient is awake during hospitalization and during the first two weeks postoperatively.

The graft should be inspected for excessive fluid accumulation. It can be evacuated by milking it out to the edges, or, if necessary, a small stab incision can be made in the skin directly over the collected fluid to allow evacuation. Debris should be cleaned away from labiobuccal surfaces. This can be done with irrigation or moistened cotton swabs.

Follow-Up

Excess unattached skin at the superior margin may be removed as desired; it will slough eventually, as will a very thin external surface layer.

Suture removal should be performed 7 to 10 days after the initial surgery. Several of the graft sutures in the inferior and superior margins will have loosened and can be easily removed. Some sutures may have been exfoliated. Buccolabial granulations often occur over the tied knot of the submandibular sutures and at the junction of the skin and mucosa. These granulations are easily and painlessly removed with a cotton forceps or fine scissors, thus exposing the submandibular suture. The free ends of the submandibular suture are grasped with a small hemostat and slightly elevated above the mucosa. One portion of the loop is cut below the knot and the suture removed in a buccal and superior direction.

Excessive granulation tissue may also form over the lingual periosteum. This is easily and painlessly excised. The optimum time for removal of this tissue is 10 to 14 days after the initial surgery.

Denture construction may begin one week or later after the initial surgery. There is no tendency for shrinkage or scar contraction of the skin graft when this procedure is performed properly.

LOWERING OF THE FLOOR OF THE MOUTH ONLY

Occasionally, one will encounter an edentulous mandibular ridge that has adequate labial and buccal vestibular depth but inadequate lingual depth. This situation lends itself to an isolated procedure on the mouth floor because secondary epithelialization is so predictable on the lingual side of the mandible that no skin graft is necessary. The possibility of an office procedure should be considered if the patient's health status will allow it.

The procedure is exactly as discussed previously with the skin grafting procedure. Once the dissection has been accomplished the mobilized lingual flap has to be fixed in an inferior position against the mandible. This can be accomplished in either of two ways, both of which require passing awls. Also, in both cases, nonresorbable sutures should be used; 2-0 Supramid is chosen by the authors.

The procedure for passing the sutures is followed as discussed previously. The suture ends are either brought out through the submandibular skin or are carried through into the labiobuccal vestibule. If taken extraorally, they can be tied to sewing buttons approximating the patient's skin color (Fig. 5–44) or can be tied over Silastic (or similar) tubing (Fig. 5–45). If taken into the labiobuccal vestibule, they are best sutured over Sil-

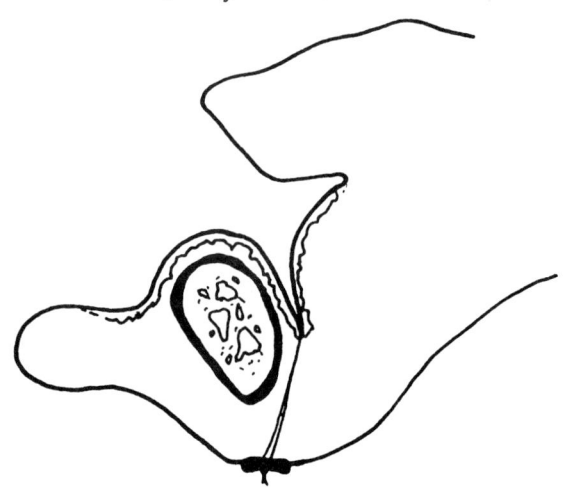

Figure 5–44. The suture is passed extraorally and ligated to a button.

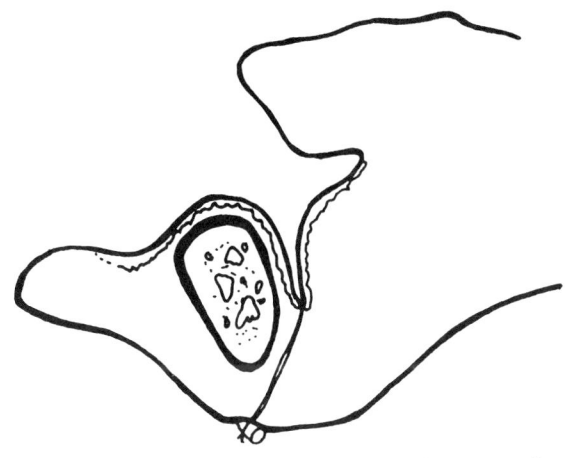

Figure 5-45. The suture is passed extraorally and ligated to Silastic tubing. (Note: Silastic tube is one continuous tube with all sutures tied to it.)

astic tubing (Fig. 5-46). Whichever method is chosen, the idea is to "snug" the lingual flap into an inferiorly displaced position against the mandible. The sutures are removed after one week and the denture can be made at any time thereafter. In order to prevent hypertrophic scarring, the lingual flange should not cause irritation during healing.

LABIOBUCCAL GRAFT WITHOUT LOWERING THE FLOOR OF THE MOUTH

Just as the floor of the mouth may be the only site that requires extension, the labiobuccal vestibule may be the only area that requires more "depth" and better fixed tissue. In this case, an isolated vestibuloplasty with skin grafting is an appropriate treatment. This allows the possibility of an office procedure if desired.

The soft tissue dissection is accomplished as discussed previously. The flap margin is

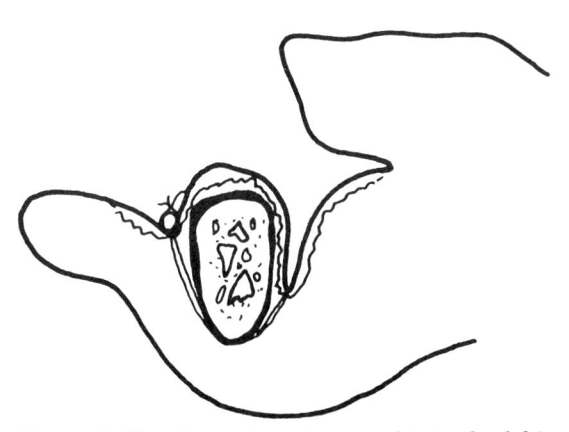

Figure 5-46. The suture is passed into the labiobuccal vestibule and ligated to Silastic tubing. (Note: Silastic tube is one continuous tube.)

then sutured to the periosteum. This is done at the depth of the dissection with multiple (8 to 10) interrupted 3-0 chromic sutures or with a continuous chromic suture. The graft is sutured in place as previously described.

The denture may be placed after one week but should not irritate the skin-mucosal junction.

THE CRESTALLY PEDICLED MUCOSAL GRAFT (LIP SWITCH)

Preliminary Considerations

The diagnostic criteria that suggest the use of this procedure are discussed in Chapter 3. They are essentially the same as those used for mandibular vestibuloplasty (*not including* *mouth floor lowering*) with skin grafting. However, the pedicled mucosal graft is a compromise because it does not produce predictably good results, as does the skin grafting procedure. It is usually limited to a smaller portion of the ridge, i.e., the anterior area.

History

Kazanjian presented in 1922, and published in 1924, the use of a crestally based mucosal flap for a vestibuloplasty.[24] He described placing the mucosal flap on a periosteal bed. This was modified by Godwin in 1947[25] by elevating the periosteum and allowing the mucosa to be grafted directly to bone. Many other authors have subsequently made important minor variations.[26-29]

Discussion with the Patient

A sharp, rather rounded vestibular sulcus may be present initially, and there may be a scar at the margins of the vestibuloplasty which tends to partially resolve with time. If the vestibuloplasty involves the area of the mental neurovascular bundle, there is the possibility of temporary or permanent paresthesia. The patient should be informed that further surgery to modify scar bands may be necessary.

Technique Under Intravenous Sedation

Local anesthesia with epinephrine is injected. The desired vestibular depth is visualized in the operator's mind. A mucosal in-

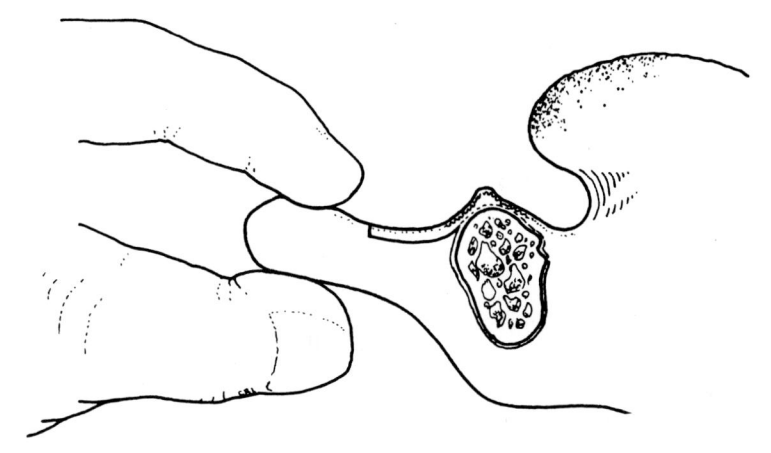

Figure 5-47. A mucosal flap is outlined. The length to be raised from the lip vestibule is somewhat longer than the projected depth of the vestibule.

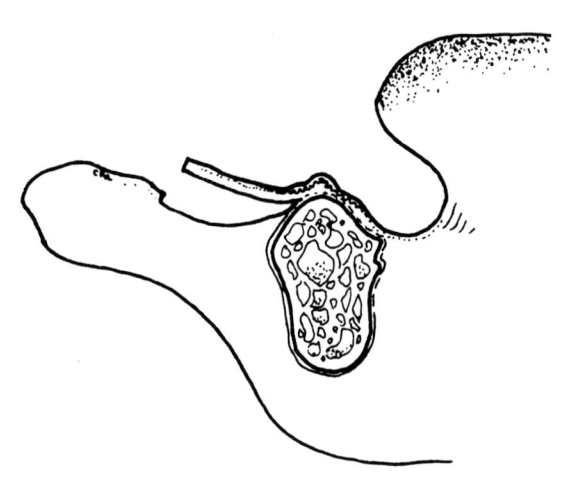

Figure 5-48. A thin mucosal flap is elevated, pedicled on the crest of the ridge.

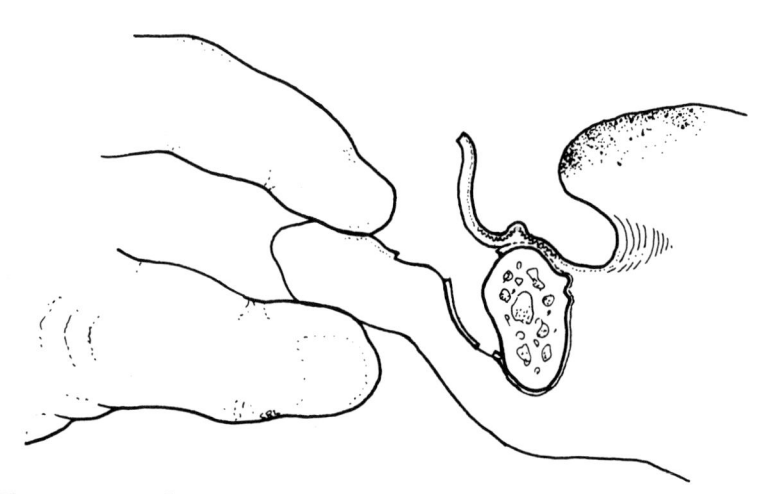

Figure 5-49. The periosteum is incised at the base of the pedicle. This is followed by elevation of the periosteum somewhat beyond the projected depth of the vestibule. The reflected periosteum is again incised just above the depth of the dissection of the periosteum. This provides a purchase layer to which the mucosa can be sutured.

cision is made 1.5 times farther away from the attached tissue than the proposed vestibular depth would indicate (Fig. 5-47). A mucosal flap is elevated, being pedicled at the attached mucosa (Fig. 5-48).

An incision is made through the submucosa and periosteum at that level, and the periosteum is dissected off the bone to the desired vestibular depth (Fig. 5-49). The free periosteal margin is sutured as close to the incised lip mucosal margin as possible using interrupted sutures of choice (Fig. 5-50). The free mucosal flap margin is sutured to the periosteum at the depth of the dissection with interrupted 4-0 chromic sutures (Fig. 5-50). A pressure dressing may be quite important to adapt the mucosal flap close to the bone. This can be accomplished by using 1/2-inch stretchable tape such as Dermaclear and placing it so that a fold is created in both cheek areas (Fig. 5-51). This should be kept in place at least two days, or longer if possible.

Prophylactic antibiotics of choice are generally prescribed, and routine postoperative oral hygiene is used. This includes a liquid diet and saline mouth rinses. Denture construction may begin from one week postoperatively as with the skin graft/vestibuloplasty, including denture construction at that time. Again, the labiobuccal flange must be slightly underextended for a minimum of three months.

MANDIBULAR ANTERIOR VESTIBULOPLASTY WITH FREE MUCOSAL GRAFT (STOELINGA)

Preliminary Considerations

Vestibuloplasties that involve dissection of the mental nerve tend to cause some loss of sensation in the distribution of the mental nerve.[30, 31] Whether this is due to actual damage of the fine nerve endings caused by the supraperiosteal dissection or is the result of local ischemia of the mental nerve when dissected free remains unresolved. Both mechanisms probably play a role.

Although follow-up studies have shown that a gradual improvement may be expected over the years, some patients still consider this inconvenience to be a drawback of the procedure. In a study of 87 patients, 9 considered their surgery unsuccessful because of this side effect.[30]

Another displeasing effect of vestibuloplasties can be the creation of a sagging chin. It is well documented that complete dissection of the mentalis muscle causes this phenomenon. One should bear in mind, however, that many patients with severe edentulous bone loss (EBL) of the mandibular ridge may have already lost soft tissue support of the chin. A vestibuloplasty could aggravate this pre-existing condition. At least 5 mm of muscle tissue above the lower border should be left attached* (Fig. 5–52).[32] This, in turn, raises the question of whether an anterior vestibuloplasty is still indicated in mandibles that are less than 15 mm high, measured at the symphysis.

In a medically compromised patient or one in whom only the anterior mandible has some EBL, the more limited procedure of an anterior vestibuloplasty with free mucosal graft[33] may be considered.

Technique

The surgery may be done under local or general anesthesia, depending on the condition of the patient and the preference of both patient and surgeon. The area between the mental foramina is injected supraperiosteally with lidocaine with 1:200,000 epinephrine (Fig. 5–53). An incision is made from first premolar to first premolar at the junction of the free and attached mucosa. A supraperiosteal dissection is then carried out with a sharp blade. Care is taken not to expose the mental foramina and to preserve greater than 5 mm of muscle tissue attachment

---

*It may be best to leave at least 10 mm of soft tissue attached above the inferior border of the mandible as the mentalis muscle originates well above the inferior border of the mandible.

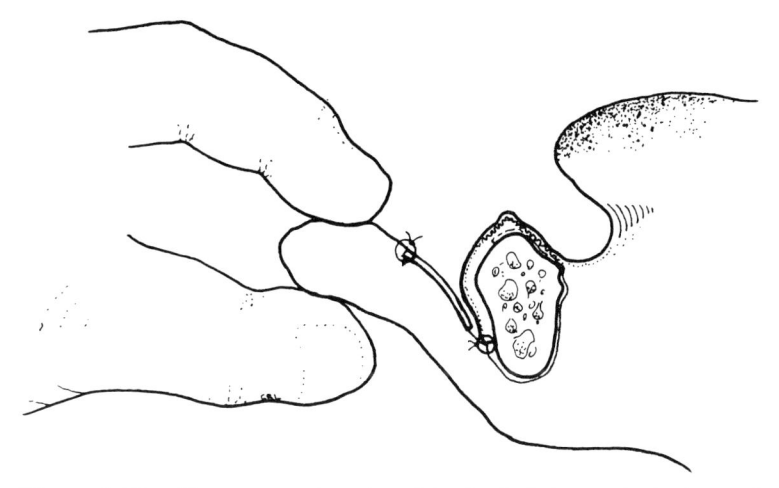

Figure 5–50. The mucosa is sutured to the inferior periosteal margin. The superior periosteal margin, now on the lip surface, is sutured as closely as possible to the margin of the mucosa on the lip.

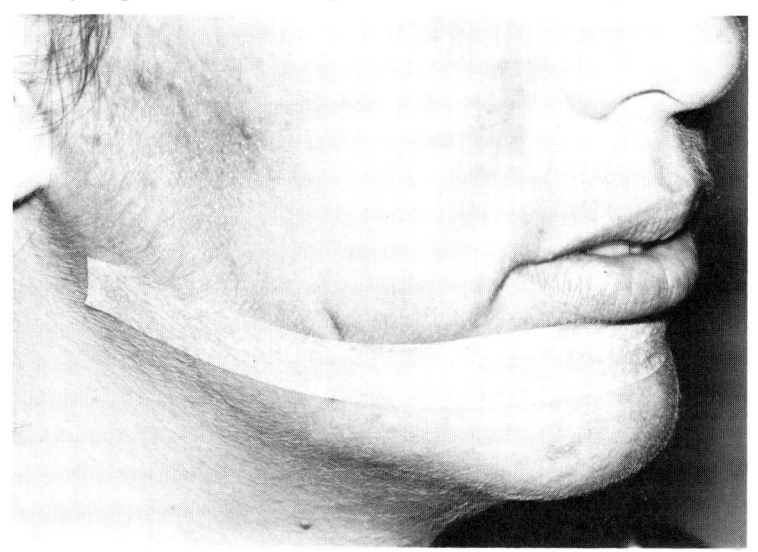

Figure 5–51. A one-half inch layer of tape is applied across the lip with tension to adapt the mucosa firmly to the bone.

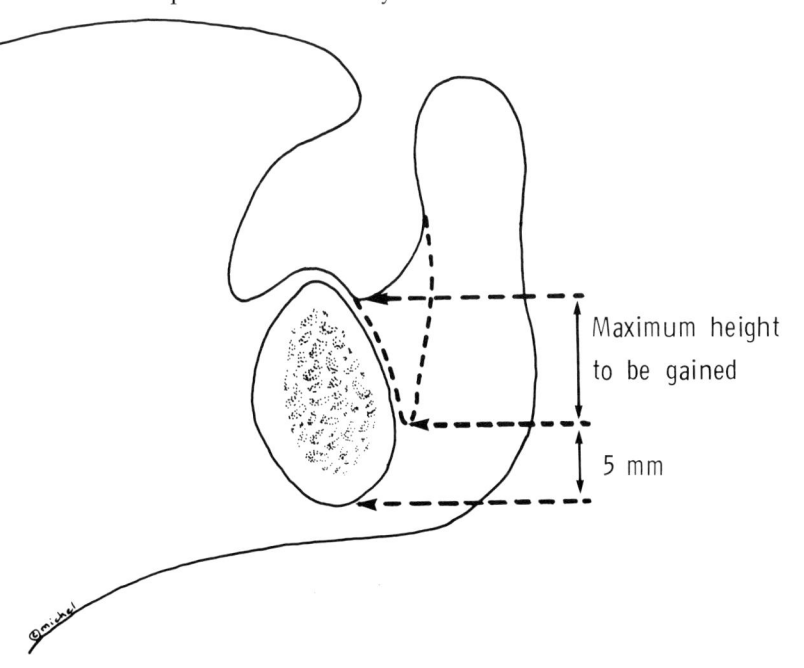

Figure 5–52. Diagram illustrating the maximum height to be gained in order to avoid a sagging chin. Approximately 5 mm of muscular tissue (or 10 mm of soft tissue) needs to be left attached to the vestibular periosteum. (From Huybers TJM, Stoelinga PJW, deKoomen HA, and Tideman H: Mandibular vestibuloplasty using a free mucosal graft (2–7 year evaluation). Int J Oral Surg 14:11–15, 1985.)

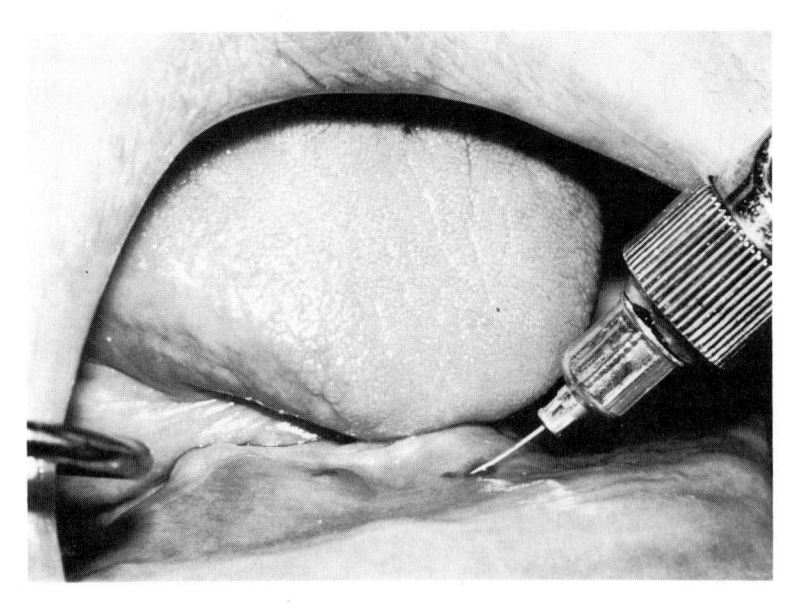

Figure 5–53. Buccal vestibule injected with local anesthetic to facilitate the supraperiosteal dissection.

(probably 10 mm of soft tissue) above the inferior border of the mandible (Fig. 5–54). The labial mucosa is then secured with submandibular sutures. The sutures are attached to the crestal tissue, passed beneath the mandible, and exit about 5 mm from the mucosal margin (Fig. 5–55). This causes the scar between the mucosal graft and the replaced labial mucosa to be within the limits of the new denture base and avoids scar tissue in the depth of the new vestibule.

The mucosal graft is taken from the inner side of the cheek using a retractor (Fig. 5–56). To facilitate cutting the graft, the mucosa may be injected with saline, which helps to define the lamina propria from the underlying muscle. A spindle-shaped graft measuring approximately 4 × 2 cm is usually sufficient to cover the recipient site. The donor site is closed with resorbable suture. Care is taken not to include any muscular tissue in the graft, and the suturing is done in a very superficial fashion in order not to entrap any muscular tissue in the scar (Fig. 5–57). This will minimize the possibility of trismus caused by excessive scarring of the cheek.

The graft is carefully thinned by cutting away as much of the lamina propria as possible, rendering a very thin mucosal graft that can be stretched about 1.5 times its original length in both directions. The graft is secured to the free margin of the labial mucosa with a fine running suture. The superior margin of the graft is attached to the crestal mucosa with a few interrupted sutures. The graft should be maximally stretched when sutured (Fig. 5–58). A stent is used to hold the graft in place and to prevent hematoma formation beneath it. The stent is secured with three circummandibular sutures and removed after seven days (Fig. 5–59). The fab-

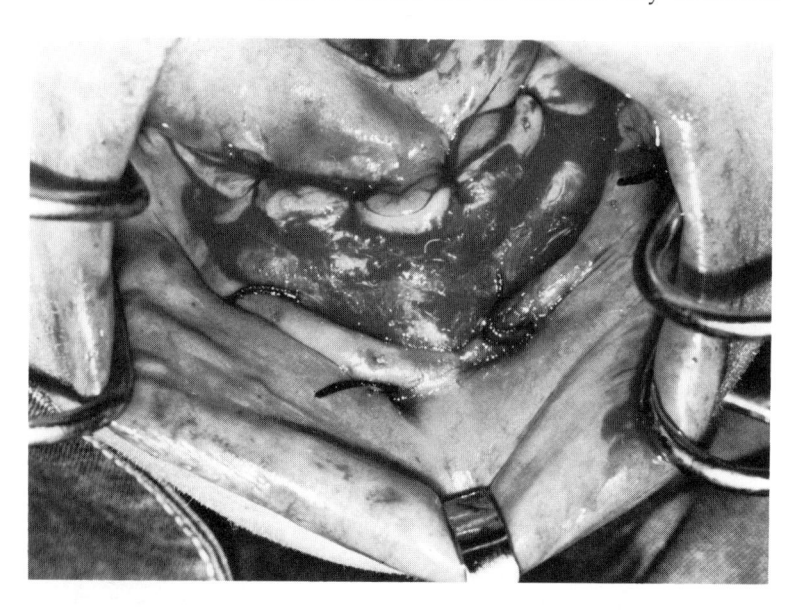

Figure 5–54. Supraperiosteal dissection completed. The arrow points to the area where the mental nerve can be seen through the overlying tissue. Note the mentalis muscles in the inferior portion of the dissection still attached to the periosteum.

Figure 5–55. Labial mucosa secured with four 1-0 resorbable sutures, leaving a free margin of approximately 5 mm folded against the periosteum.

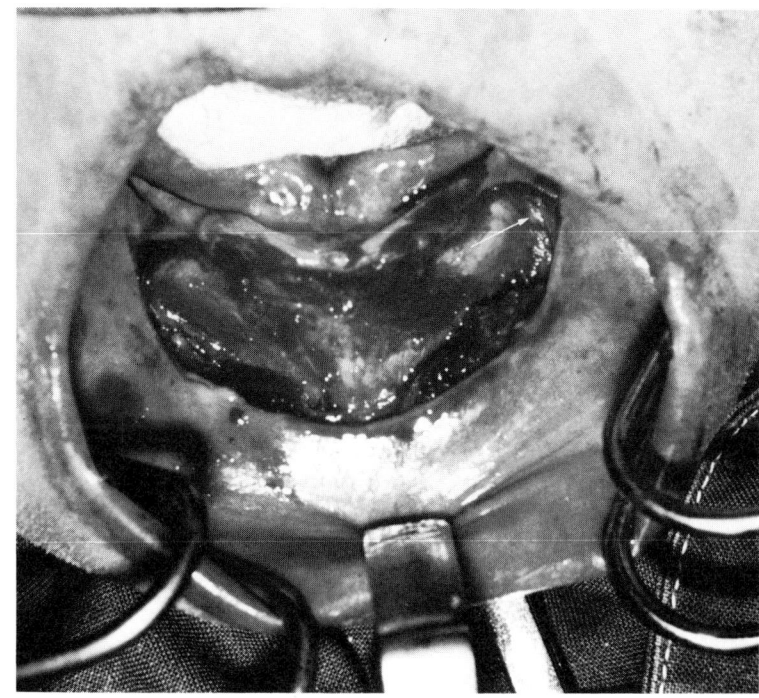

Figure 5–56. Retractor according to "Arnhem" design used to expose inner side of the cheek. Injection with saline helps to differentiate the lamina propria from the underlying muscles.

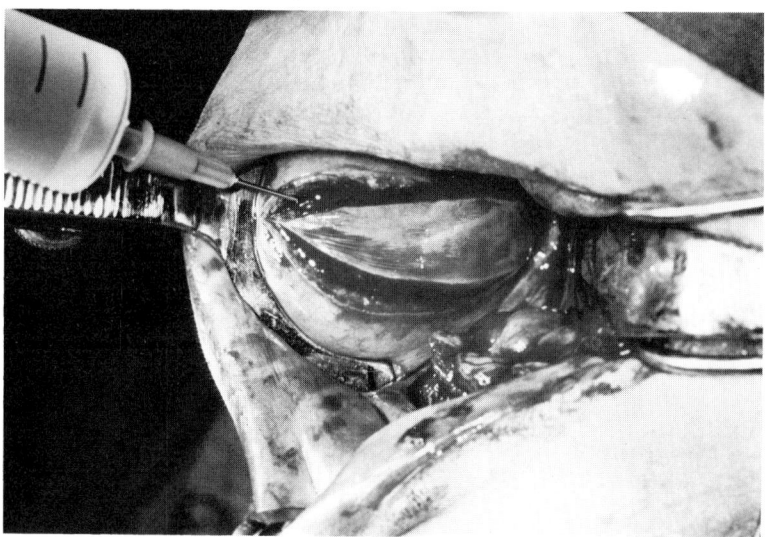

Figure 5–57. Superficial suturing with a running 2-0 resorbable suture should be done without entrapping muscular tissue in order to avoid scarring and subsequent limitation of opening of the mouth.

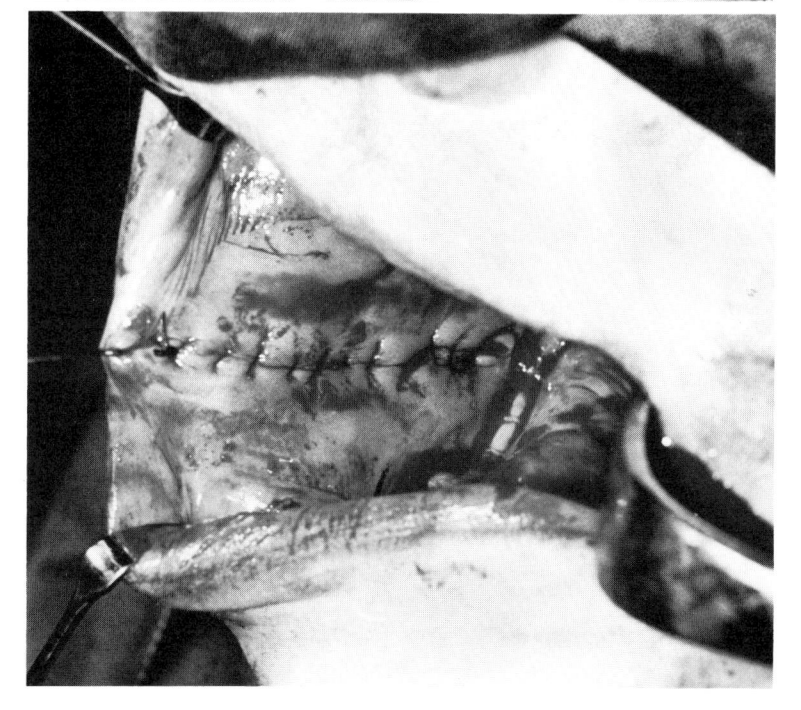

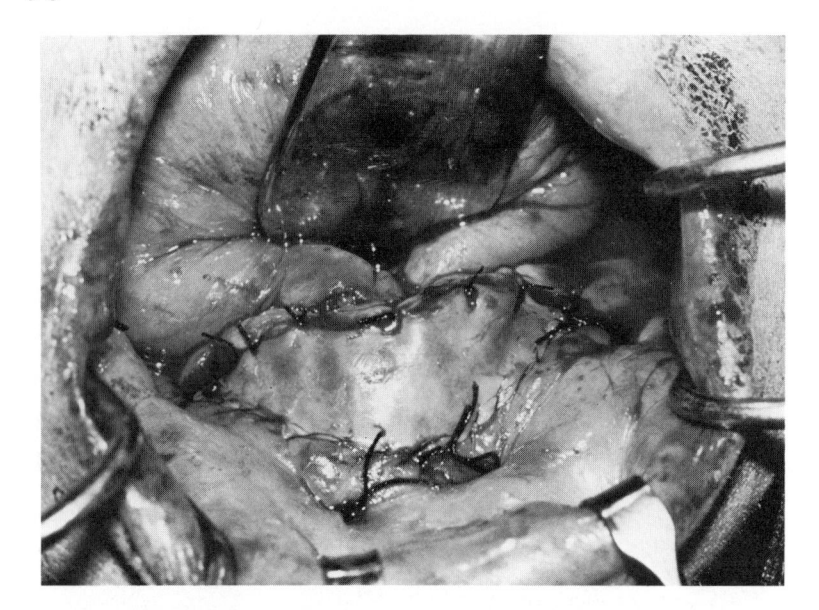

96 / SURGICAL MANAGEMENT OF SOFT TISSUE PROBLEMS

Figure 5–58. Thinned mucosal graft secured in place by 6-0 silk running suture to the free margin of the labial mucosa and a few interrupted sutures on top of the crest. The graft is maximally stretched.

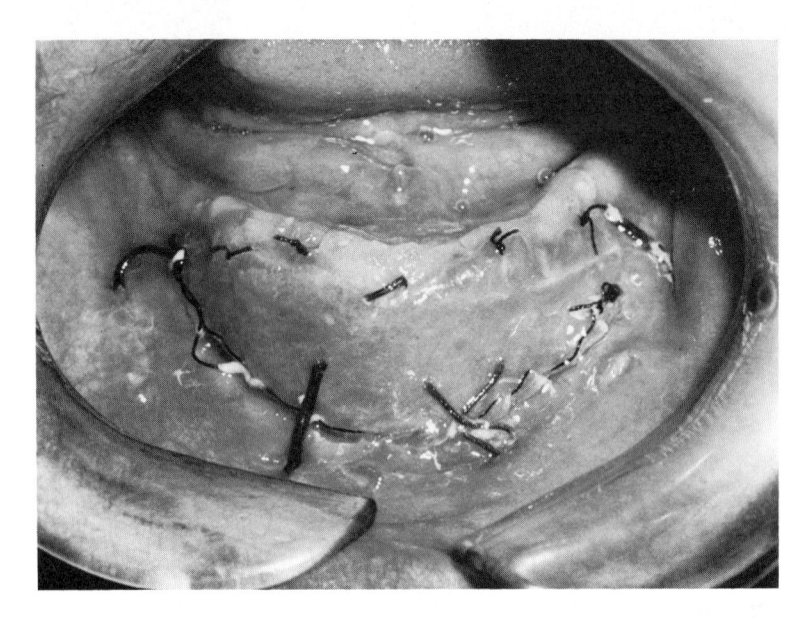

Figure 5–59. Condition of the graft after stent removal seven days postoperatively.

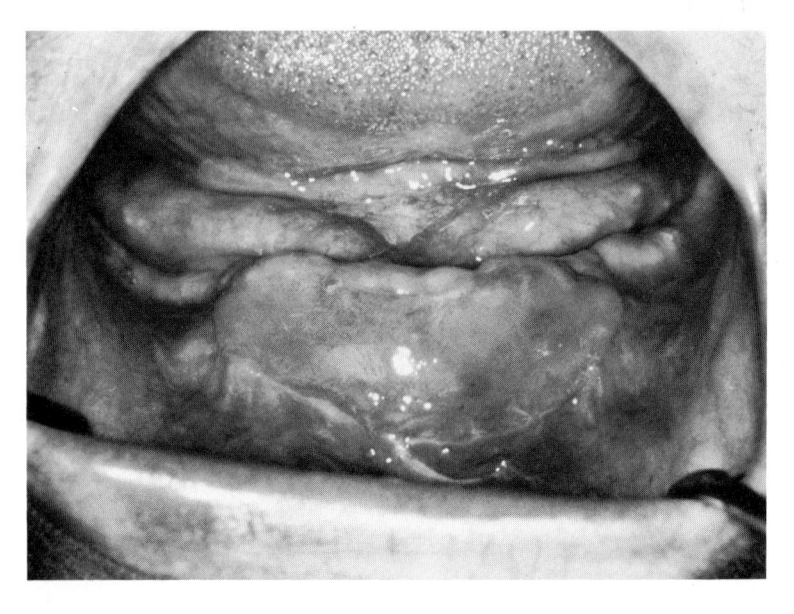

Figure 5–60. Condition of the graft three months postoperatively. The scar is within the limits of the new denture base. Note the ingrowth of capillaries from the periphery toward the center of the graft.

rication of a denture is usually begun about three weeks after removal of the stent. In six weeks the graft should be tight and adherent to the periosteum (Fig. 5–60).

MYLOHYOID AREA VESTIBULOPLASTY
(Stoelinga)

Preliminary Considerations

When the depth of the vestibule is lost in the mylohyoid origin area (Fig. 5–61), stability of the mandibular denture is significantly compromised. Thus the restoration of the vestibule in this area is critical. The technique described by Trauner-Obwegeser renders excellent results with respect to sulcus depth.[34] However, there may be more morbidity associated with this procedure as compared to the Brown-Downton-Caldwell procedure.[35-39] Bleeding from the mylohyoid muscle occasionally gives rise to considerable swelling in the floor of the mouth and rarely may cause the tongue to become dangerously swollen, necessitating prolonged intubation or even tracheotomy. In the authors' experience with over 200 floor of the mouth procedures, this has happened three times and at least two additional cases have been reported.[40, 41] The Brown-Downton-Caldwell procedure gives less sulcus depth but is much less likely to endanger the airway, and it may easily be carried out under local anesthesia.

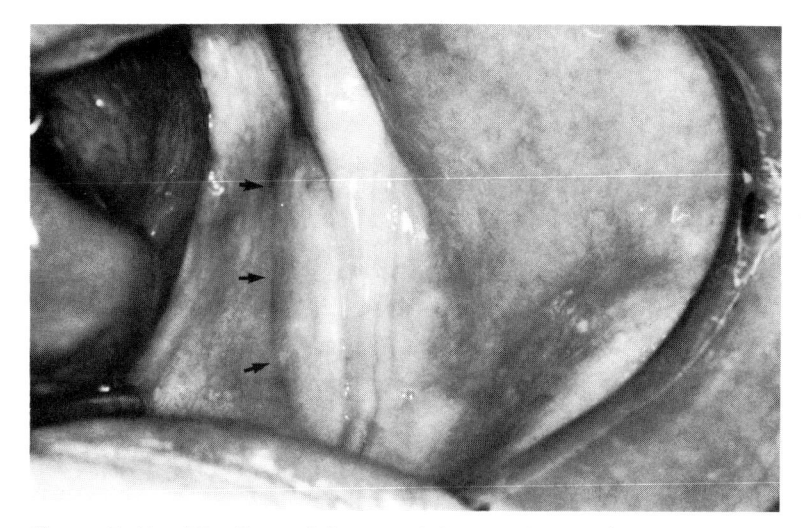

Figure 5–61. The floor of the mouth in a patient with prominent mylohyoid crest (arrows).

Technique

The operation starts with an incision on top of the crest (Fig. 5–62). The flap is reflected lingually beneath the periosteum, thus exposing the fibers of the mylohyoid muscle (Fig. 5–63). The subperiosteal dissec-

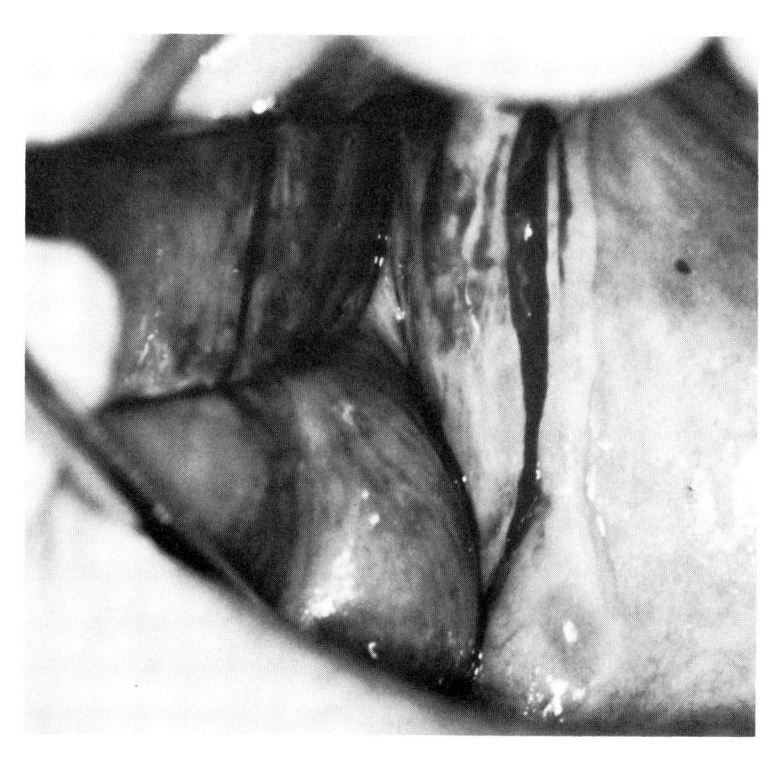

Figure 5–62. Incision on top of the crest of the posterior alveolar ridge through the periosteum.

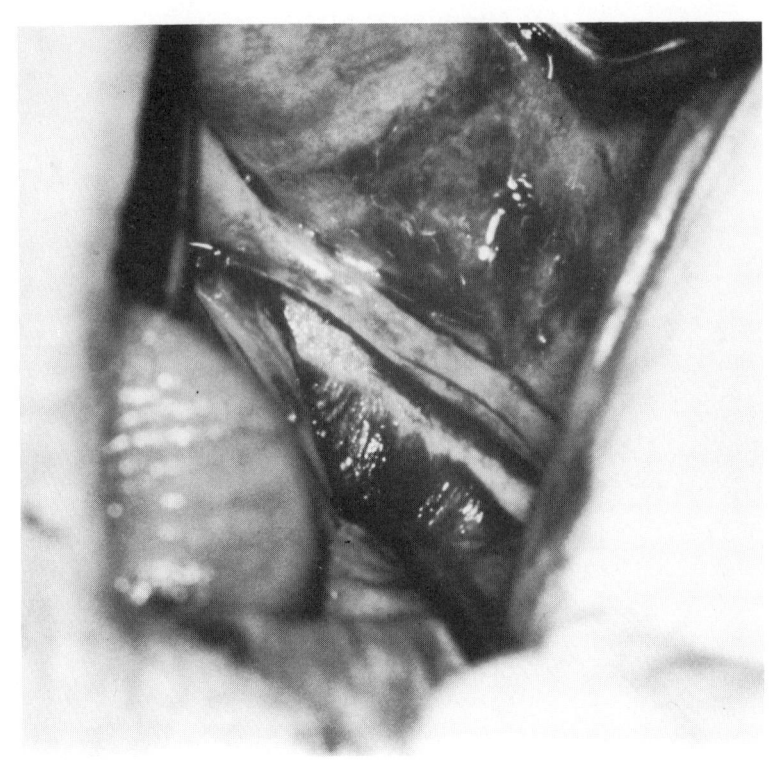

Figure 5-63. Subperiosteal dissection exposes the mylohyoid muscle.

tion protects the mylohyoid artery and its branches and thus prevents an excessive hematoma. The muscle is sharply detached from the ridge. With an acrylic bur, the ridge is then reduced (Figs. 5–64 and 5–65). Since

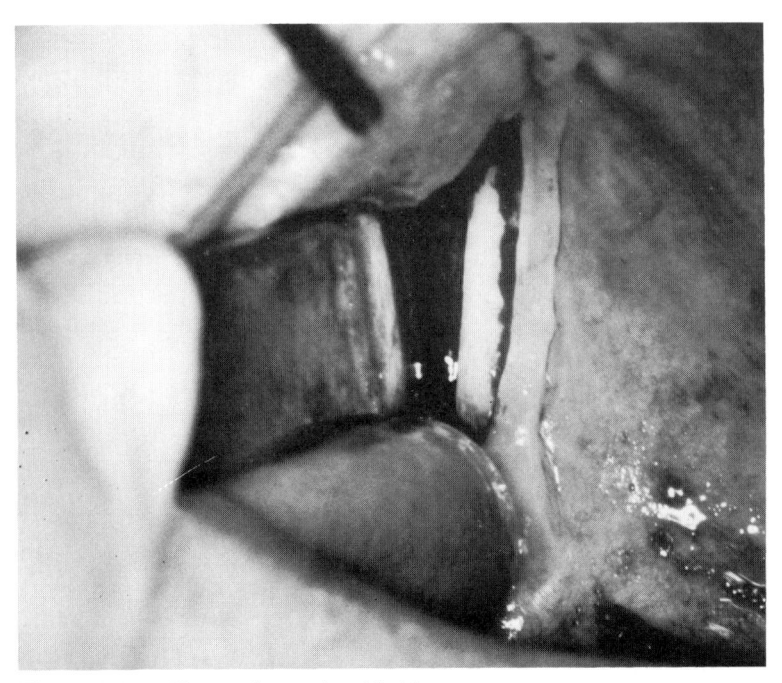

Figure 5-64. Exposed mylohyoid ridge.

fibers of the mylohyoid muscle are often attached to the mucosa of the floor of the mouth, these should be dissected free. This allows the mucosa to be resutured to the crest of the ridge while the mylohyoid muscle may reattach inferiorly.[39] The mucosa is repositioned and sutured with resorbable suture (Fig. 5–66). After completion of the vestibuloplasty, the denture should be adapted to the new morphology by extending the lingual flanges with compound to help the mucosa attach to the lingual periosteum.[41] After seven days the stent may be removed and sufficient sulcus depth is usually gained (Fig. 5–67).

MAXILLARY PROCEDURES

Maxillary Vestibuloplasty with Skin Grafting

Preliminary Considerations

The diagnostic criteria suggesting a vestibuloplasty with skin grafting are discussed in Chapter 3. See also the preliminary considerations discussed in the section on mandibular vestibuloplasty with skin grafting and lowering of the floor of the mouth.

History

MacIntosh and Obwegeser[42] cite Weiser[9] as the first to have described the maxillary vestibuloplasty with skin grafting in 1918. This was later modified by Schuchardt.[18]

Discussion with Patient

Discussion with the patient is essentially the same as for the mandibular vestibuloplasty with skin grafting.

Plastic Stent Construction

The model from which the stent is constructed need not have exaggerated vestibular extensions. The compound and Protaform will compensate easily for any underextension. The stent should have an appropriate palatal extension to accommodate the method of fixation of the stent. It is usually held in place with circumnasal floor wiring, a palatal screw, alveolar pins, or a perialveolar wire. The stent for the circum-

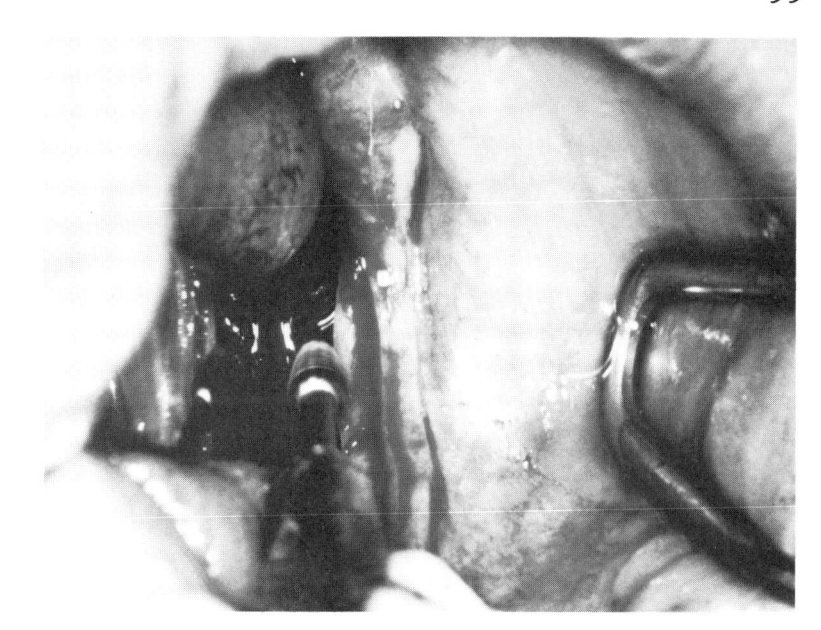

Figure 5–65. Mylohyoid ridge reduced with acrylic bur.

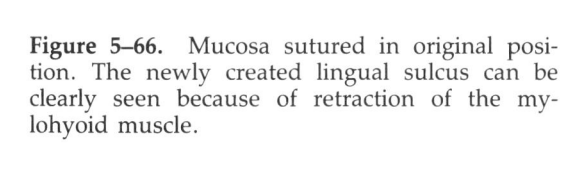

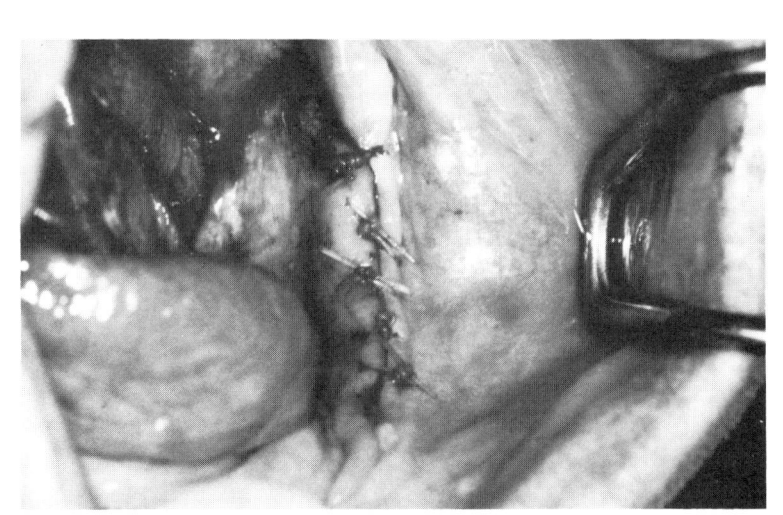

Figure 5–66. Mucosa sutured in original position. The newly created lingual sulcus can be clearly seen because of retraction of the mylohyoid muscle.

Figure 5–67. Lingual sulcus as created by the Brown-Downton-Caldwell procedure 10 days postoperatively.

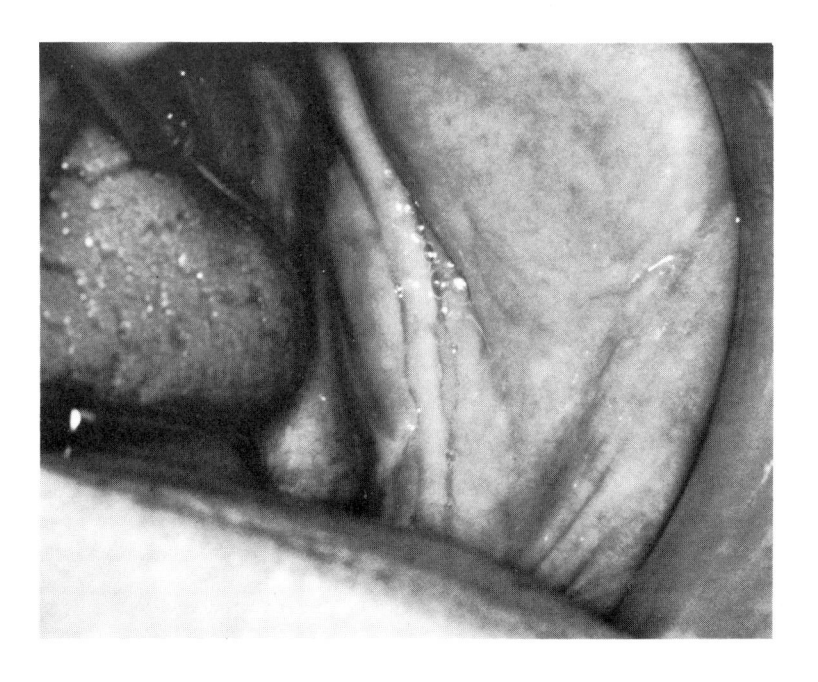

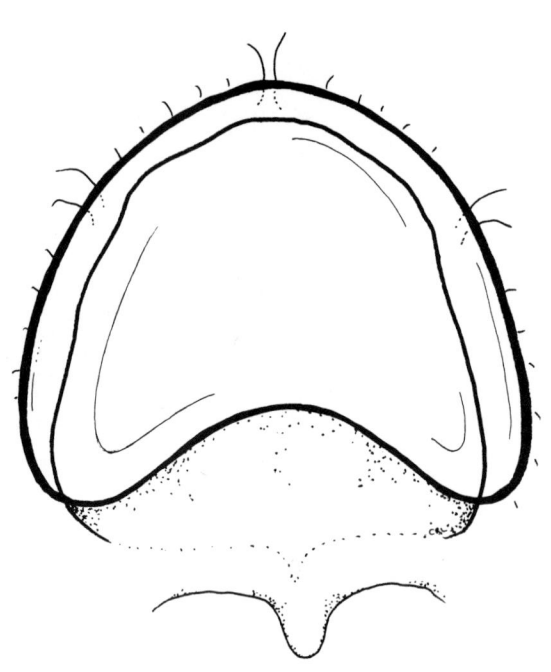

Figure 5–68. Outline of the stent to be used in the area of circumpalatal fixation. Note that the outline for the stent is shortened in the post-dam area. The edge of the stent in this area should be well anterior to the posterior margin of the bony palate.

nasal floor wiring, palatal screw fixation, or alveolar pins can have the same configuration. For the circumnasal method, it is important that the palatal extension of the stent be shorter than the posterior extension of the hard palate (Fig. 5–68). This allows posterior tension on the stent as the wire is tightened.

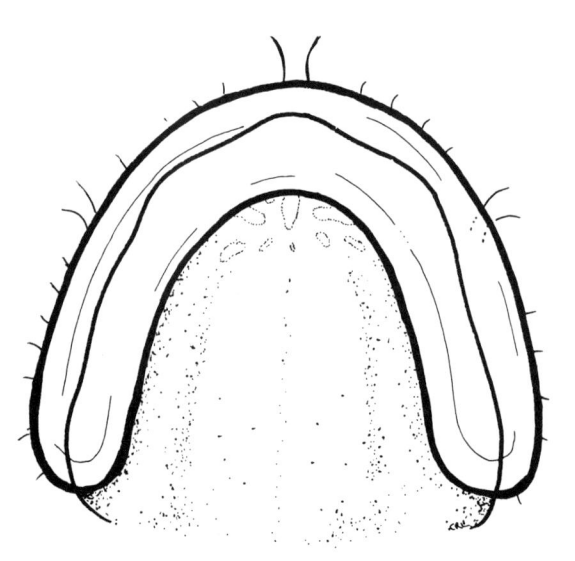

Figure 5–69. Outline of the stent to be used in the area of circumalveolar fixation.

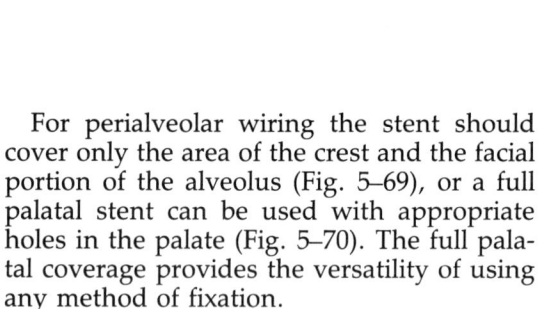

Figure 5–70. Outline of the stent to be used in the area of circumalveolar or palatal screw fixation.

For perialveolar wiring the stent should cover only the area of the crest and the facial portion of the alveolus (Fig. 5–69), or a full palatal stent can be used with appropriate holes in the palate (Fig. 5–70). The full palatal coverage provides the versatility of using any method of fixation.

Operative Procedure

The vestibular mucosa adjacent to the crest of the ridge is ballooned with a local anesthetic solution that contains a dilute vasoconstrictor such as 1:200,000 epinephrine. An incision is begun near the hamular notch and the incision is carried anteriorly at the junction of free and attached mucosa. It finishes near the opposite hamular notch. At each end of the incision, a lateral incision of about 6 mm is made (Fig. 5–71). The soft tissue is then sharply dissected from the labiobuccal area, leaving the periosteum intact on the bone. Vision and access are most easily gained by progressively elevating a few millimeters at a time all along the incision. The superior extension of the dissection is usually limited by the floor of the nose and the zygomatic process. Any soft tissue other than periosteum should be excised.

The edge of the mucosal flap is sutured to the periosteum as far superiorly as possible.

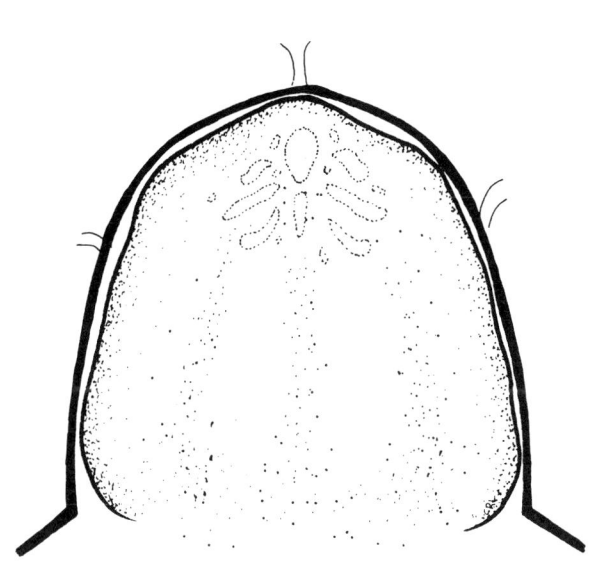

Figure 5–71. Diagram of mucosal incision where secondary epithelialization vestibuloplasty is required for the entire arch.

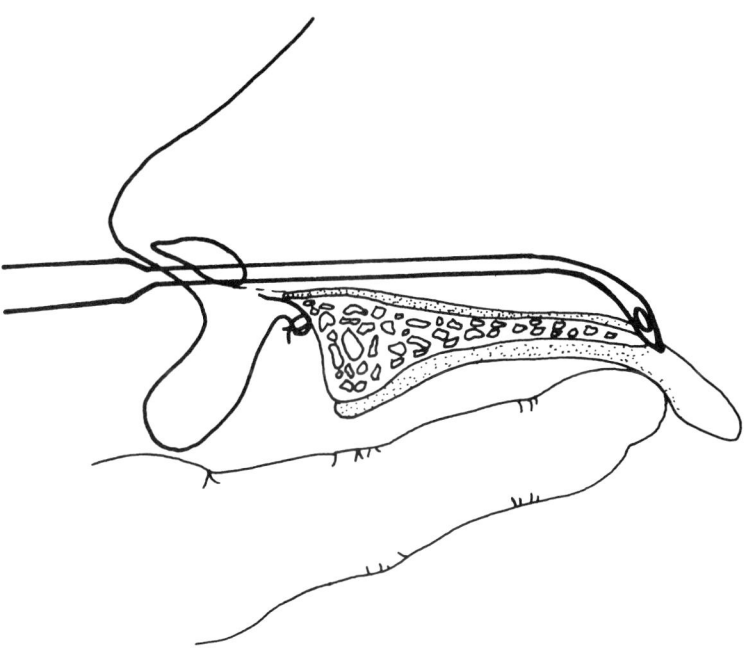

Figure 5–73. Diagram of the awl passed through the nares and about to penetrate the soft palate just posterior to the posterior margin of the hard palate.

4-0 or 5-0 chromic suture material is appropriate, with mattress type stitches placed about 1 cm apart (Fig. 5–72).

Softened grey compound is placed in the preconstructed acrylic tray and an impression of the area covered by the tray is obtained. A layer of Protaform is added to give good adaptation and to provide a soft, pliable material upon which the skin is placed.

The method of fixation previously decided upon is now implemented. The circumnasal floor method has been found to be positive and is the procedure of choice in the hospitalized patient. A long awl with a fairly tightly curved tip is needed. The awl is passed through one nasal vestibule and just above the mucosa of the floor of the nose. In the region of the posterior margin of the hard palate, the awl is made to penetrate the soft palate. This maneuver is guided by the finger elevating the soft palate and palpating the tip of the awl (Fig. 5–73).

When the eye of the awl is visualized in the mouth, two long wires (0.016 inch) are passed through and the ends are folded back on the awl (Fig. 5–74). The awl is withdrawn back out through the nose, the wires are removed from the awl, and the ends of the wires are clamped (Fig. 5–75). A smaller awl is then passed from the labial vestibule into the nasal vestibule. The ends of the wires

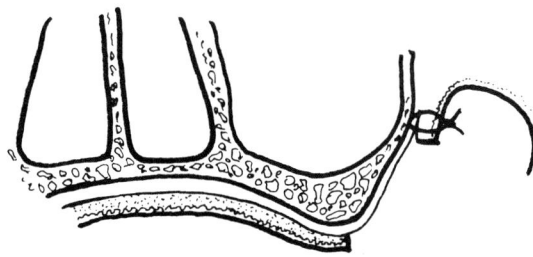

Figure 5–72. Appearance of the vestibule at the completion of secondary epithelialization. Mattress sutures place the mucosal margin as high as possible in the vestibule.

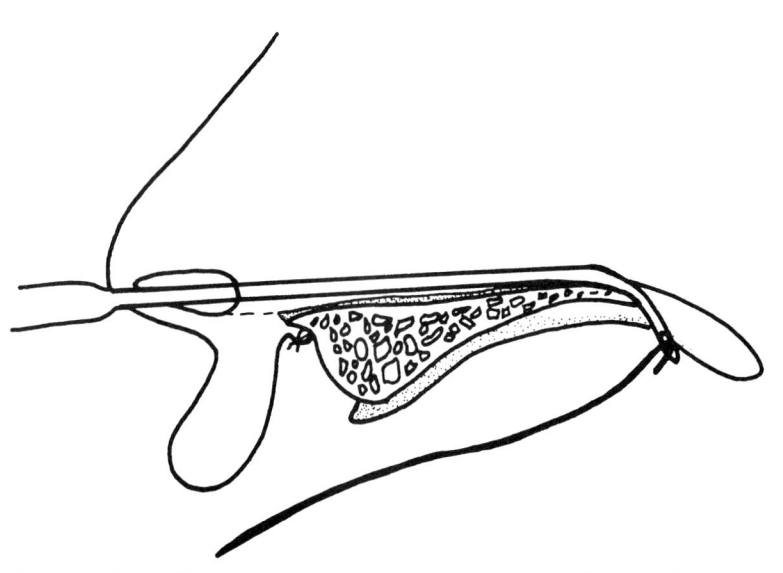

Figure 5–74. Wires have been passed through eye of the awl and are ready to be withdrawn through the nose.

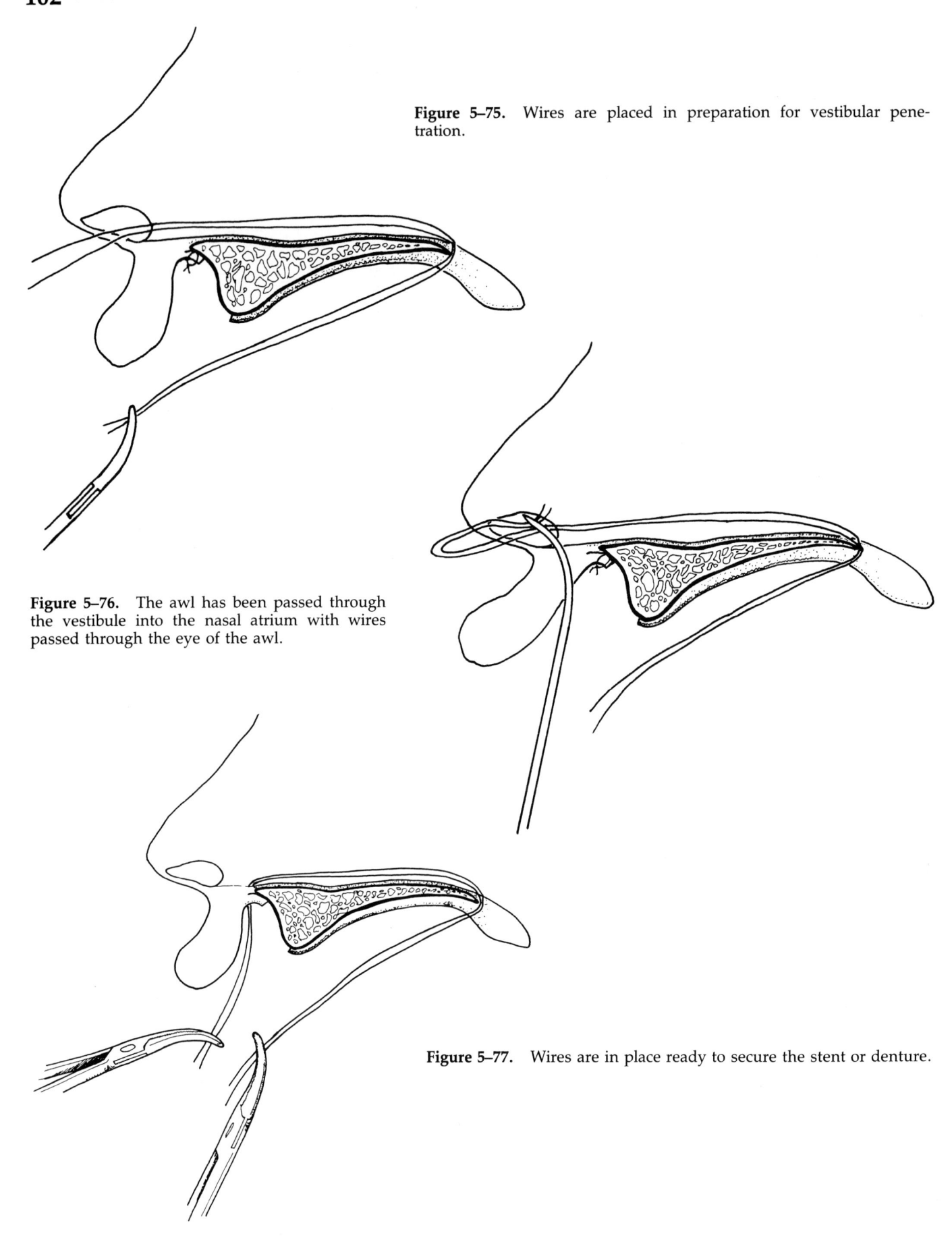

102 / SURGICAL MANAGEMENT OF SOFT TISSUE PROBLEMS

Figure 5–75. Wires are placed in preparation for vestibular penetration.

Figure 5–76. The awl has been passed through the vestibule into the nasal atrium with wires passed through the eye of the awl.

Figure 5–77. Wires are in place ready to secure the stent or denture.

protruding from the nose are passed through the eye of the awl (Fig. 5–76). The awl is withdrawn into the mouth and the wires are removed from the awl (Fig. 5–77). A piece of plastic tubing about 2.5 cm long can be threaded over the oral part of the wires to minimize tongue irritation. The previously excised skin is adapted to the stent and carried to the mouth. The wires are then tightened separately (in case one breaks). Owing to the short palatal extension, tightening the wires will seat the stent in the desired posterior and superior direction (Fig. 5–78).

If the surgery is to be performed where the airway is not controlled by intubation, and excessive nasal bleeding could present an airway hazard, then alternative methods of stent fixation may be preferable. A useful stent design is shown in Figure 5–79. This design allows use of the submucosal transpalatal method, a septal screw, or perialveolar ligation.

An alternative to the transpalatal fixation is that reported by Smylski.[43] Instead of passing the wire completely around the hard palate, the awl penetrates the hard palate just posterior to the alveolus. A sharp curved awl is passed through the soft tissue high in the vestibule and then over the inferior border of the piriform aperture. The tip of the awl is kept beneath the mucosa of the floor of the nose and progresses well past the alveolus. With firm pressure and slight motion the awl is made to penetrate the hard palate just lateral to the midline. A wire is fed into the eye of the awl and the awl withdrawn. The same procedure is performed on the opposite side of the palate. The stent shown in Figure 5–79 or a denture similarly trimmed plus the adaptation material is placed. The wires are passed through the palatal holes and twisted to fix the stent or denture to the maxilla. Because this procedure can be performed with no nasal bleeding, it is more practical as an office procedure than is the circumpalatal method.

If a septal screw method is used, a midline hole should be placed in the denture larger than the diameter of the screw. The stent is placed and a pilot hole, slightly smaller than the outside diameter of the thread, is drilled in the palate. A lag-type screw is inserted. A fine silk suture may be tied to the screw to prevent its aspiration should it become dislodged.

If the perialveolar method is desired, the stent is positioned. An alveolar awl is passed through the buccal mucosa above the buccal flange, piercing the lateral sinus wall, the sinus, the palatal bone, palatal soft tissue, and the cutout in the stent. Two fine wires are passed through the eye of the awl as described, and the awl withdrawn. The identical procedure is used on the opposite side. The wires of one side and then the other are tightened, while the stent is held in the desired position.

It may be appropriate to keep the patient on antibiotic medication until just after the wires are removed.

The stent is usually kept in place for one week. Just before removal of the stent, the

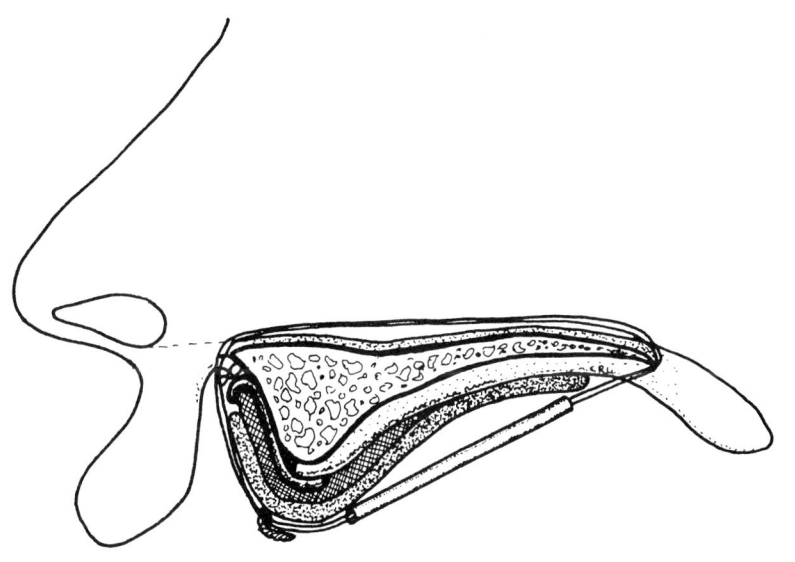

Figure 5–78. Diagram of transpalatal fixation of the stent.

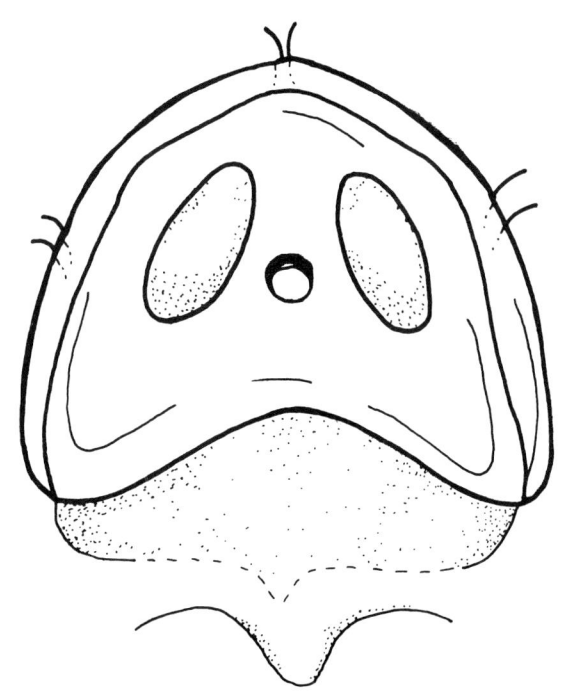

Figure 5–79. Diagram of the stent is useful for transpalatal fixation with either a septal screw or perialveolar ligation.

edge of the graft should be freed from the stent. This will remove the friction of the skin on the stent which might cause the skin to adhere to the stent as it is being removed. Excess skin will soon slough.

The denture can be constructed when the patient feels ready for the process.

Submucous Vestibuloplasty

Introduction

In Chapter 3, the indications and contraindications for submucous vestibuloplasty are explained. Illustration of results of this procedure are shown in Figures 5–80 and 5–81.

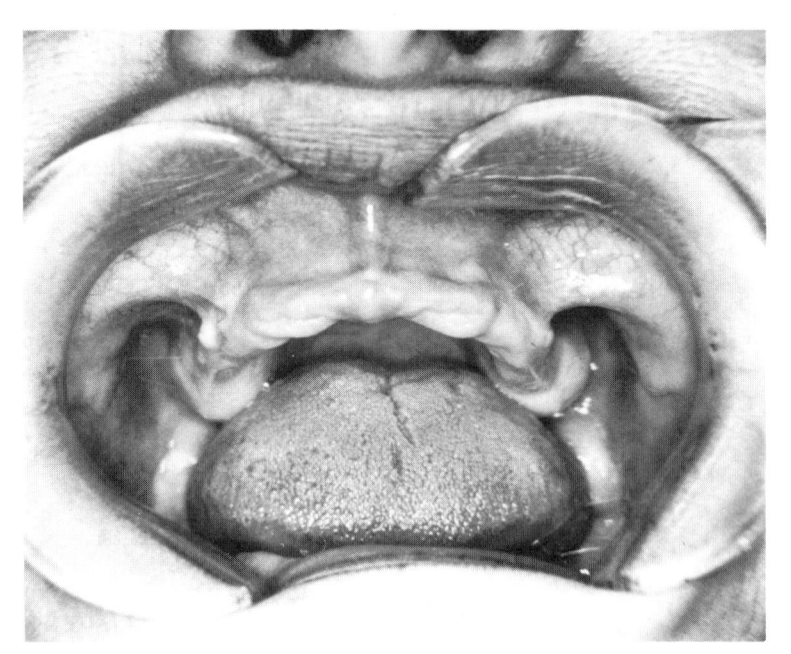

Figure 5–80. Preoperative photo. All of the apparent ridge is flabby tissue. Note low soft tissue attachment in the bicuspid regions.

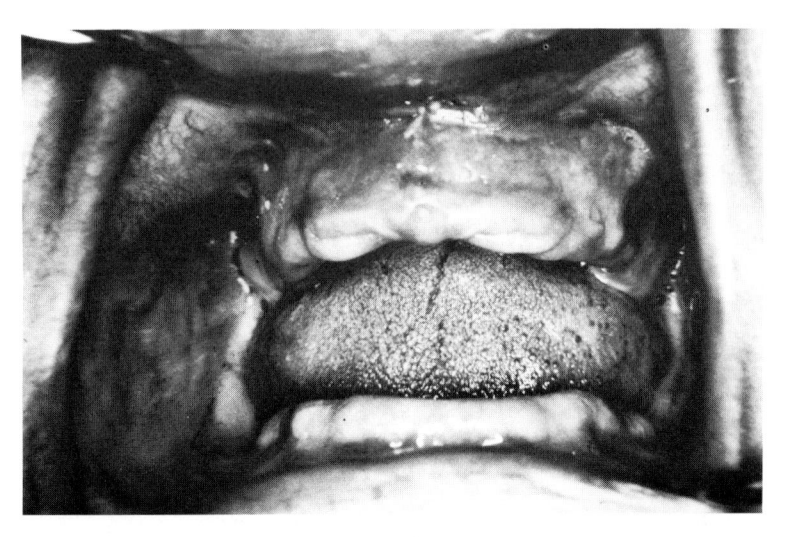

Figure 5–81. Postoperative result after submucous vestibuloplasty.

History

Submucosal vestibuloplasty was advocated for the mandible by Kazanjian[13] but was not notably successful. The submucous vestibuloplasty for the mandible was described as unsuccessful by Obwegeser and thus was recommended only for the maxilla. This was described by Obwegeser in 1959.[44]

Discussion with the Patient

Patients should be advised of the need to be without a denture for two weeks or more. Discussion about the fullness of the cheeks postoperatively may be appropriate. This can be adjusted as noted in the Procedure section that follows. Numbness of the upper lip is a remote possibility.

Procedure

The essence of the submucous vestibuloplasty procedure is the direct grafting of a thin mucosal flap to periosteum, as illustrated in Figures 5–82 and 5–83. Local or general anesthesia may be utilized. Antibiotics or corticosteroids may be instituted pre-

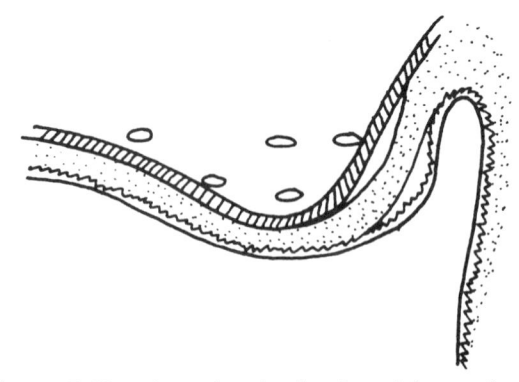

Figure 5–82. A pocket is developed by undermining the mucosa and another pocket is developed supraperiosteally.

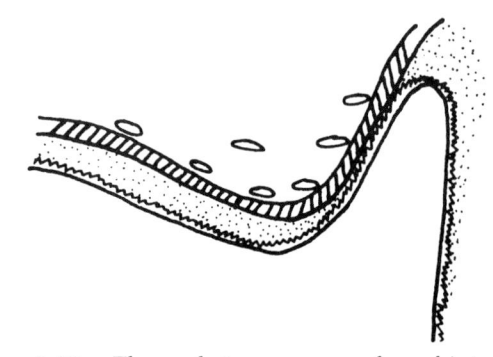

Figure 5–83. The pockets are now coalesced into one and the mucosa is collapsed against the periosteum. This allows grafting of the mucosa to the periosteum.

operatively if desired. A vasoconstrictor solution such as 1:200,000 epinephrine with local anesthesia is instilled submucosally in the area to be dissected, ballooning the mucosa in that area.

A midline incision is made through the mucosa to bone from the crest of the ridge proceeding superiorly approximately 15 mm. Small curved Metzenbaum scissors easily separate the mucosa from the submucosa (Fig. 5–84). The mucosal layer should be quite thin. This can be evaluated by being able to see the scissors beneath the translucent mucosa. The mucosa is most effectively separated when the dissection starts at the area adjacent to the attached mucosa and proceeds superiorly to about 1.5 cm from the "crest" of the ridge. Anteroposteriorly, the mucosal dissection is carried posteriorly to the region where the vestibular depth is already adequate. Supplementary vertical incisions may rarely be needed to gain access to the posterior part of the mandible.

A second plane of dissection is developed parallel to the submucosal plane. This new plane separates the periosteum from the soft tissue lateral to it (Fig. 5–85). Thin scissors, or periosteal elevators, are effective for this purpose. It is important to remember that any soft tissue left on the periosteum invites relapse of the vestibular depth or excessive thickness of the mucosa in the denture-seating area.

After these layers are developed, a scalpel is introduced in the supraperiosteal pocket and used to free the "crestal" attachment of the soft tissue between the mucosa and the periosteum. This intermediate layer is elevated superiorly so that the mucosal flap can be adapted directly to the periosteum. The esthetic effect of the superior positioning of this intermediate tissue should be noted and if the patient can benefit from this increased fullness, it should be left. However, if increased fullness of the cheek is undesirable, a "wedge" of submucosal tissue can be excised and removed.

Usually the "crestal" margin of the mucosal flap is left attached, but if increased visibility or access is needed, the crestal edge of the flap can be freed. After the periosteal area is explored and the intermediate tissue removed, the mucosal edge can be sutured to the attached mucosa.

Before the midline incision is closed, the bone of the anterior nasal spine in the vestibule area can be rongeured away. Use of a figure-eight suture to draw the mucosa toward the nasal septum to gain increased elevation of the vestibule is an important step. Any remaining mucosal incision areas are then closed.

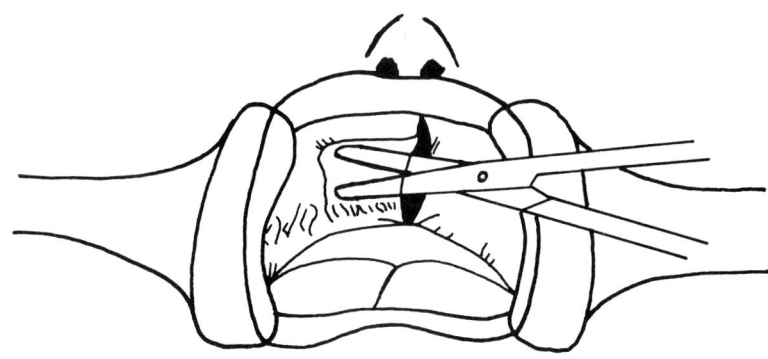

Figure 5–84. Scissors are used to separate a thin layer of mucosa from the submucosa.

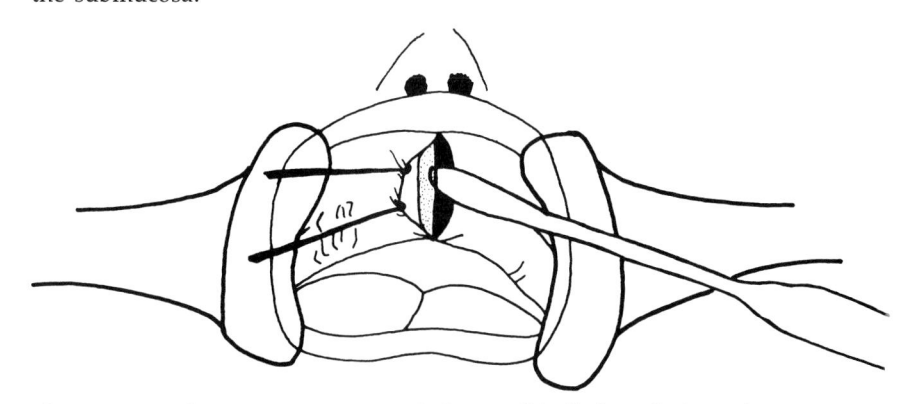

Figure 5–85. Scissors or a periosteal elevator lift all the soft tissue from the periosteum.

Grey compound is warmed and added to the preconstructed acrylic splint. The compound is molded into the depth of the vestibule. Protaform can be added over the compound, if desired.

An effective method of retention is the passage of wires around the nasal floor and the stent (Fig. 5–86). For the details of placement and other methods, see the section on Maxillary Vestibuloplasty with Skin Grafting.

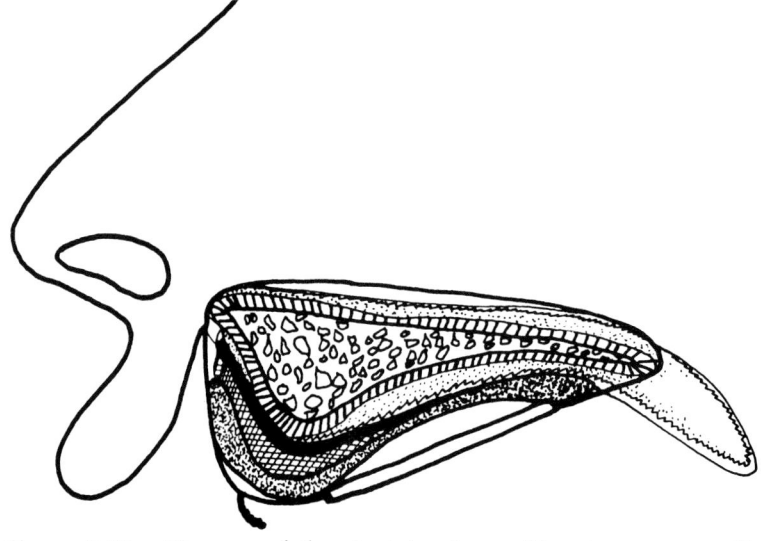

Figure 5–86. Diagram of the stent in place with submucous vestibuloplasty.

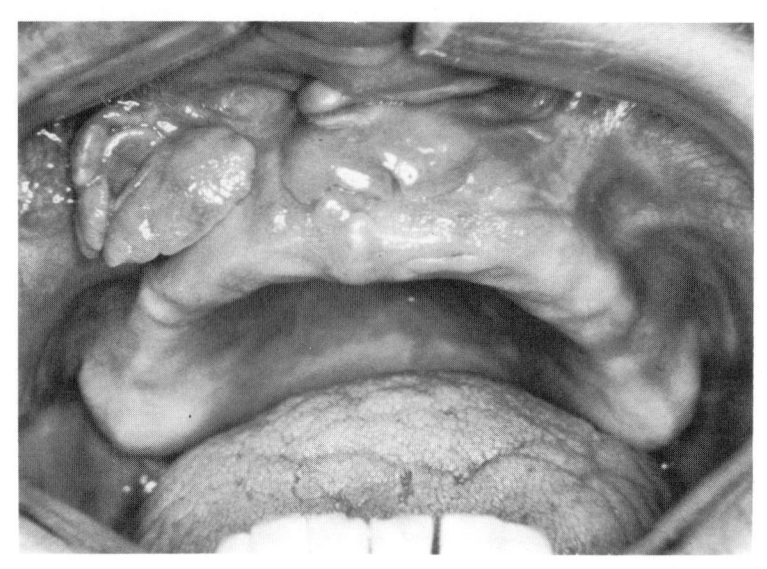

Figure 5–87. Preoperative photo of a patient with loss of some alveolar bone with marked epulides.

Postoperative Considerations

To allow the mucosa to "take," the stent should remain in place for about one week. No movement of the stent should occur during this period. A denture can be constructed as soon as the patient wishes. It is not necessary or desirable to overextend the flange of the denture to preserve the elevation of the vestibule.

SECONDARY EPITHELIALIZATION

Introduction

The secondary epithelialization procedure is effective in dealing with the maxillary epulis fissuratum accompanied by some degree of alveolar loss, as illustrated by Figures 5–87 and 5–88 and discussed in Chapter 3.

History

Obwegeser,[45] Rumpel,[46] Szaba,[47] and Ganzer[48] described the procedure of vestibuloplasty by secondary epithelialization as illustrated in this chapter. Other secondary epithelialization procedures, as described by Kazanjian,[24] Smedley,[49] Godwin,[25] Clark,[50] Edlan,[26] and Howe,[27] do not provide predictably satisfactory results and therefore are not described here.

Discussion with the Patient

A denture with virtually no flange will be required for several weeks. During this period, only limited function and stability will be provided. The patient should be informed that some relapse is anticipated.

Technique

The exophytic scar tissue, which is present in the buccal labial tissue, may be removed before or at the time of the secondary epithelialization procedure. If ridge augmentation is done (as with hydroxyapatite) as part of the treatment plan, it will usually be done before the removal of the excess tissue, as some of this tissue may be usable in constructing the augmentation pocket. Otherwise the removal of this excess tissue is ideally performed several weeks before the secondary epithelialization procedure. If this is impractical, the full thickness of mucosa that contains the epulis fissuratum lesion is removed at the time of the secondary epithelialization.

The instillation of a dilute vasoconstrictor solution, such as 1:200,000 epinephrine with 1 per cent lidocaine, in the submucosa of the vestibule will facilitate dissection.

An incision is made at the crest of the ridge and at the junction of the free and attached mucosa. The incision is begun posteriorly, from where the vestibuloplasty is required, and proceeds anteriorly and around to the corresponding area of the opposite side (Fig. 5–89). This figure also illustrates the oblique vertical incision that is made at the termination of the crestal incision, allowing superior repositioning of the flap in the posterior areas. The mucosal-submucosal flap is elevated, leaving only the periosteum remaining on the bone. Keeping tension on the flap with double skin hooks facilitates dissection. The elevation is carried superi-

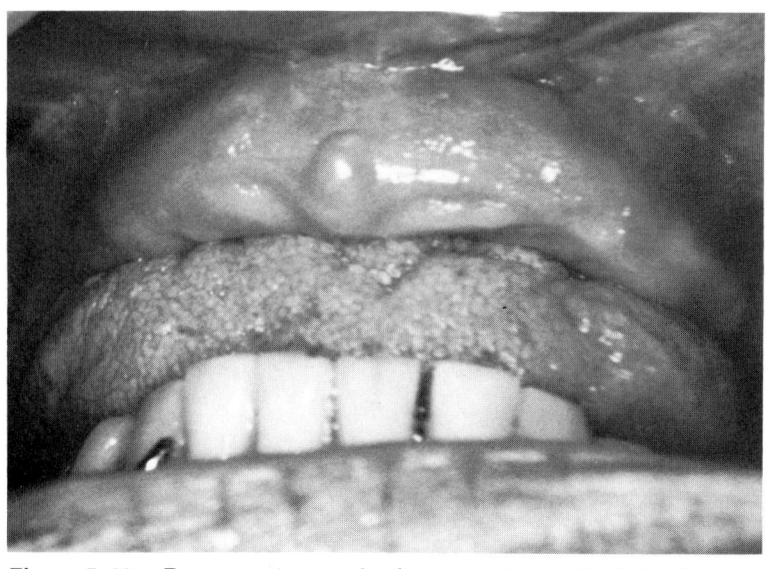

Figure 5–88. Postoperative result after secondary epithelialization.

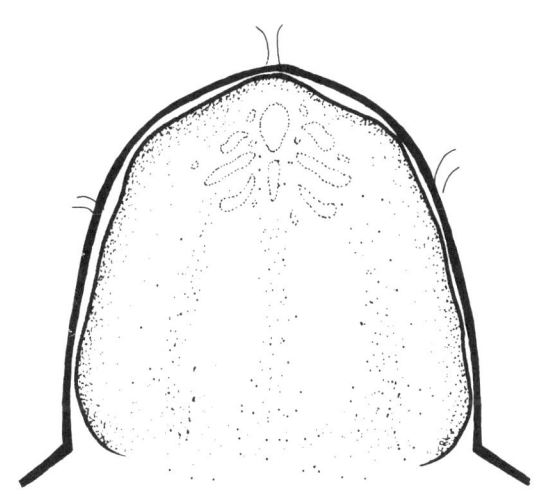

Figure 5–89. Diagram of mucosal incision where secondary epithelialization vestibuloplasty is required for the entire arch.

orly to the floor of the nose anteriorly, and slightly up the zygomatic buttress posteriorly. If epulis fissuratum tissue is still present, it is removed, preserving as much pliable mucosa as possible.

The portion of the anterior nasal spine adjacent to the crest of the ridge is removed if needed. The edge of the mucosa is sutured as far superiorly as possible, as shown in Figure 5–90.

If a small 1/2-round needle is used, it will help engage the delicate periosteum. The type of stitch is probably not critical. Horizontal mattress stitches with 4-0 chromic catgut are used most commonly, spaced about 1 cm apart. It is helpful to leave the stitch untied until the adjacent one has been placed. In the midline, the stitch can engage the septal cartilage if some of the anterior nasal spine has been removed. This can be the end of the procedure if a splint is not used.

If the bone has not been exposed, a pseudomembrane will soon form followed by secondary epithelialization.

If a stent is to be used, see Maxillary Vestibuloplasty with Skin Grafting in this chapter.

Dentures should not contact the open wound until some epithelialization has taken place, as movement of a denture will stimulate granulation tissue. If a stent has been placed (as discussed in the submucous vestibuloplasty section), it should remain fixed in place for one week. Miller[51] reports favorable results using a stent without suturing. The stent is adapted to the depth of the dissection beneath the soft tissue flap. It is allowed to remain there fixedly for two weeks.

Secondary epithelialization will usually occur nicely over exposed mature areas of hydroxyapatite augmentation (i.e., three months or more after augmentation).

Sharp junctional areas will usually be present initially at the area of the flange margin, after secondary epithelialization. This usually softens and rounds over after many months.

PALATAL MUCOSAL GRAFTS (Fonseca)

Although skin grafts placed over mandibular and maxillary vestibuloplasties are useful in decreasing the migration of mobile tissue toward the crest of the ridges, these grafts are not without complication. Discoloration, hair growth, and donor site tenderness are some of the complications associated with the use of split thickness skin grafts. The use of palatal mucosa grafts as an alternative can help eliminate some of these problems, although palatal mucosa has its own problems such as donor site discomfort and lack of material.

Surgical Technique

A hemostatic agent is injected into the donor region supraperiosteally (Fig. 5–91). The donor site is then outlined with a No. 15 blade (Fig. 5–92). This outline is extended

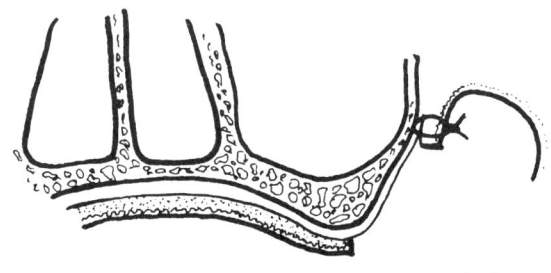

Figure 5–90. Appearance of the vestibule at completion of secondary epithelialization. Mattress sutures place the mucosal margin as high as possible in the vestibule.

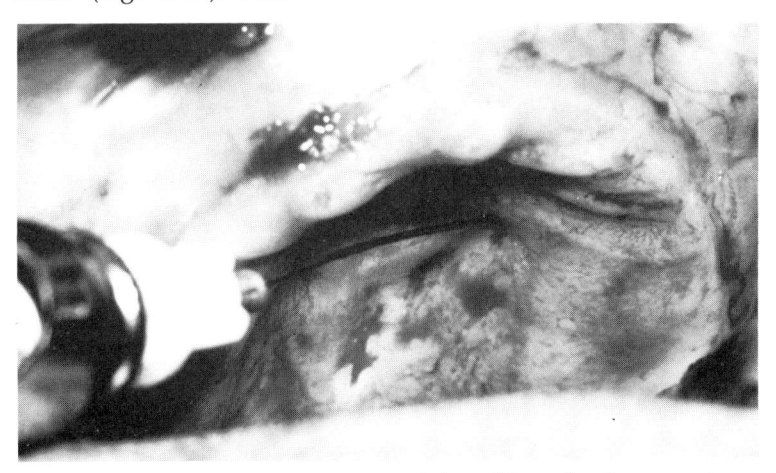

Figure 5–91. A hemostatic agent is injected into the donor region supraperiosteally.

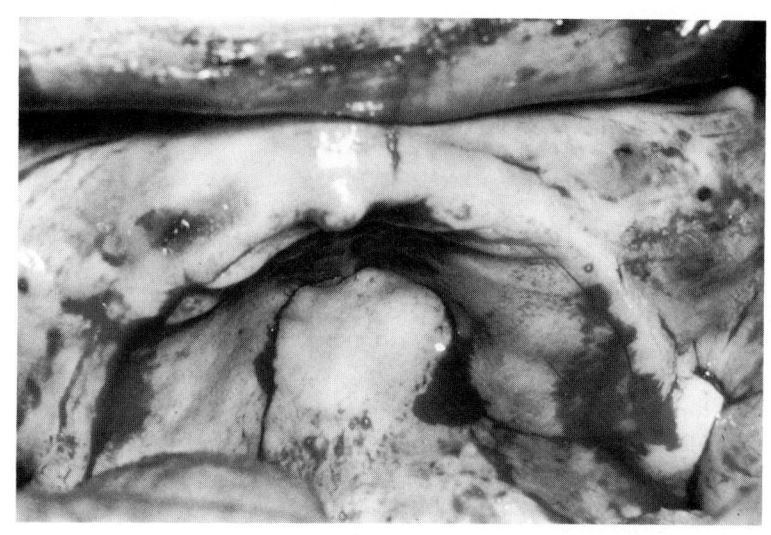

Figure 5–92. The donor site is outlined with a No. 15 blade, and small Metzenbaum scissors are used to dissect sharply between the lamina propria and the submucous tissues.

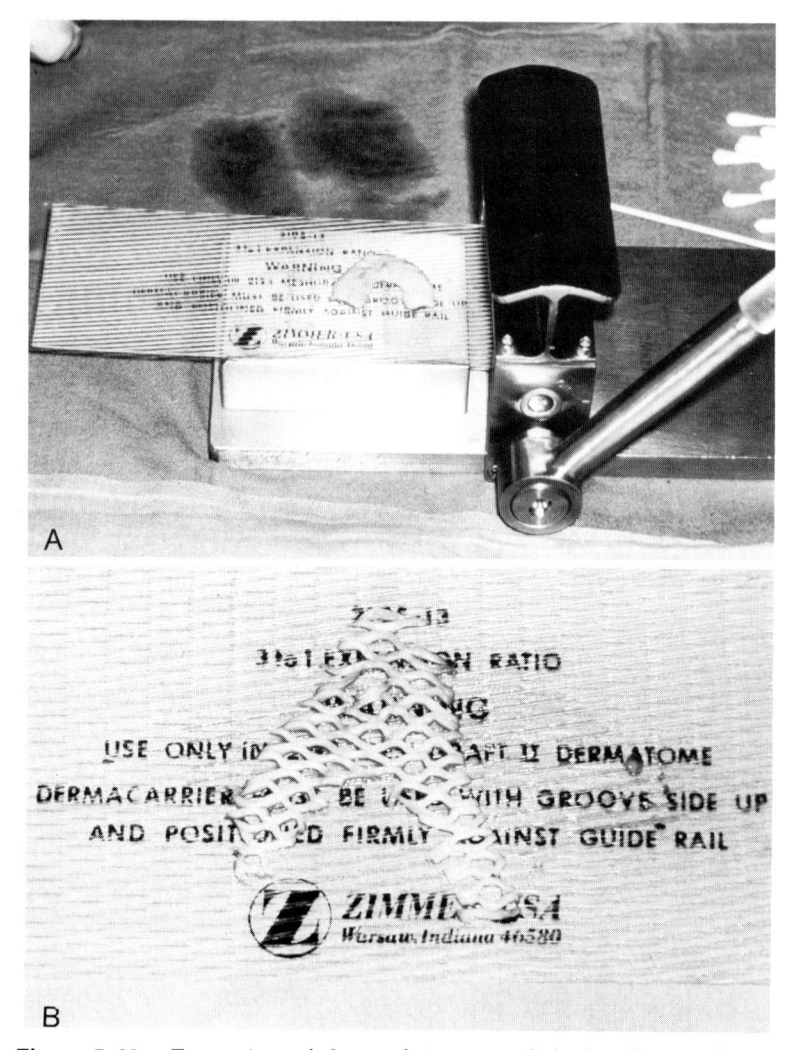

Figure 5–93. Expansion of the graft is accomplished with a graft expander using a 3 to 1 mesh.

superficial to the periosteum. The No. 15 blade or small Metzenbaum scissors is used to dissect sharply between the lamina propria and the submucous tissues. Once the graft is completely excised it is brought to a sterile back table. The graft is then placed mucosal side down, and the fat and minor salivary glands are removed with small iridectomy scissors.

Expansion of the graft can now be accomplished with a graft expander using a 3 to 1 mesh (Fig. 5–93). Once the graft is expanded it is ready for delivery to the splint as previously described in the skin graft section of this chapter. If the quantity of tissue is inadequate the graft should be placed on the periphery of the splint to help prevent relapse (Fig. 5–94). The splint should be removed at approximately seven days and necrotic tissue excised. The long-term result of this technique will provide attached tissue that is very similar to the tissue that normally inhabits this area of the mouth (Fig. 5–95).

Donor site care is usually accomplished by placing one layer of Protaform into a maxillary splint or denture. The splint may be fixed to the maxilla in the midpalatal area. The screw is removed at seven days with minimal discomfort to the patient. The Protaform is removed at this time and a soft liner is substituted.

The *advantages* of the palatal grafting technique are (1) similarity to the adjacent recipient site tissue, (2) ease of procurement of the graft, (3) lack of hair and other skin appendages, and (4) proximity of the donor site to the recipient site, thereby limiting morbidity to a specific region of the body.

The *disadvantages* of palatal mucous grafts are (1) limited tissue available, and (2) prolonged donor site morbidity if the dissection is too deep.

Skin-Lined Pockets

A system of denture retention was described by Wallenius and Owall in 1966.[52] To improve retention of the mandibular denture, skin-lined pouches project beneath the anterior portion of the mandible and accept prongs that project from the denture. Similarly, skin-lined tubes are created from the anterior vestibule of the maxilla into the floor of the nose. The need for these procedures has for the most part been supplanted by other vestibuloplasty procedures. However, they do enhance conventional retention and may be utilized in some situations in which ablation has occurred.

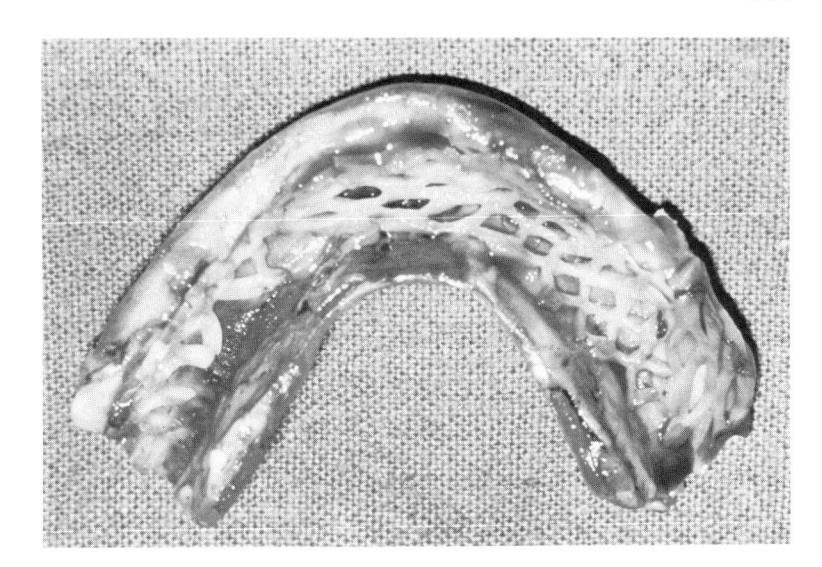

Figure 5–94. If the quantity of tissue is inadequate, the graft should be placed on the periphery of the splint to help prevent relapse.

Maxillary Buccal Inlay Vestibuloplasty (Terry and Minsley)

MacIntosh and Obwegeser described four basic maxillary vestibuloplasties including specific indications for each procedure and expected results.[42] Of the four—submucous vestibuloplasty, secondary epithelialization vestibuloplasty, ridge skin grafting vestibuloplasty, and buccal sulcus skin grafting (buccal inlay)—the latter procedure remains the most controversial. Not only does the buccal inlay based on the original work as described by Gillies[10] depend on the surgical technique for ultimate success, but it also requires expert prosthetic care as well as the utmost in patient cooperation. These variables have caused problems for many surgeons, resulting in limited use of the buccal inlay. Certain technical modifications in the surgery and postsurgical care have improved the overall success of this maxillary vestibuloplasty procedure, making it the method of choice in carefully selected patients.

The maxillary buccal inlay procedure is specifically indicated when there is an absolute deficiency of facial mucosa because of tissue loss related to previous trauma (Fig. 5–96), ablative surgery for pathology, or any other reason, such as a naturally occurring short upper lip in an edentulous patient. The procedure is also indicated when there is severe hard tissue loss that cannot easily be corrected by grafting with bone or a nonresorbable hydroxyapatite material.

The success of the buccal inlay depends on the creation and maintenance of a split thickness skin–lined facial pouch with the

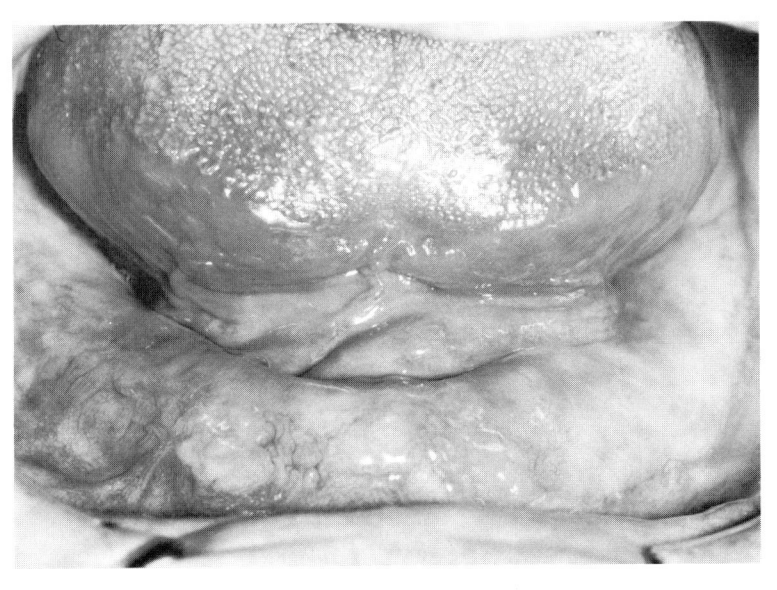

Figure 5–95. The long-term result of the technique will provide attached tissue that is similar to the normal attached tissue.

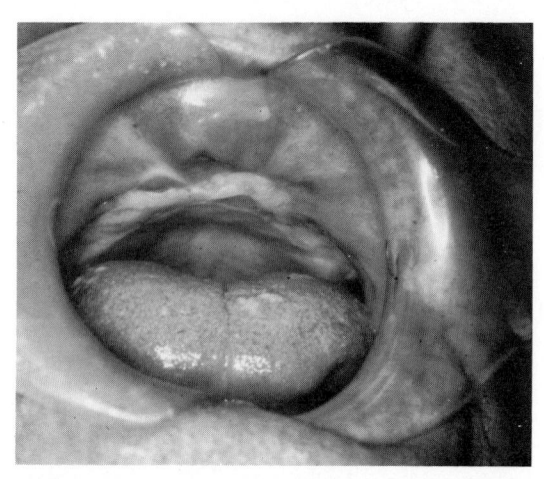

Figure 5–96. Patient after bone graft reconstruction following traumatic hard and soft tissue avulsion of the anterior half of the maxilla. There is an absolute deficiency of facial mucosa that is attached into the crestal area of the reconstructed ridge.

graft extending from the residual ridge well out into the facial sulcus. As postsurgical healing occurs, a sphincter develops in the vestibule at the mucosa–skin graft juncture. This sphincter will encompass an exaggerated denture flange with an undercut just below the flange, thus providing greatly increased mechanical retention. The greater area of fixed tissue over the residual ridge also provides increased denture stability.

Presurgical Phase

The presurgical phase involves the preparation and fabrication of the surgical stent. It is important that the immediate transitional splint also be made before the one-week postsurgical appointment. When the surgical stent is removed, the transitional splint can be immediately inserted.

There are two methods that can be used in the construction of the immediate transitional splint. In the first method, a heat-cured methyl methacrylate resin base covering primarily the palate and the fixed tissue over the residual ridge is made presurgically. Immediately upon removal of the surgical stent seven to ten days postsurgically, the prepared base is attached to an autopolymerized resin flange made at surgery from an impression of the surgical stent.

The second method involves making a complete immediate transitional splint at the time of surgery, which again is inserted at the first postsurgical appointment. Regardless of the method selected for the fabrication of the immediate transitional splint, a definitive transitional splint is made for insertion at the third postsurgical appointment, usually 7 to 14 days after removal of the surgical stent.

An impression of the patient's maxilla is made prior to surgery, allowing sufficient time for the required laboratory procedures for stent fabrication. This impression should be made as accurately as possible. A customized impression compound is preferred for making the impression. A suitable impression material should be used with the custom tray. The impression should be boxed and poured in dental stone to produce a master cast. The master cast is then duplicated using reversible hydrocolloid. The master cast can be used to fabricate the immediate transitional base. The duplicate cast will be used to fabricate the surgical stent.

Surgical Stent

The surgical stent is formed from the duplicate master cast using heat-curing methyl methacrylate resin. Since it is impossible to get a sufficiently tissue-displaced impression to construct a surgical stent with adequately extended flanges, it is necessary to incorporate wire loops into the flange of the prepared stent to engage the thermoplastic material used to accurately record the wound bed, which includes the periosteally covered residual alveolar ridge and the facial pouch. The thermoplastic materials commonly used for this are red compound initially, then a final lining with Protaform. Protaform is a material that provides very exact detail of the impressed surfaces and will continue to flow at body temperature under light forces, which reduces the danger of pressure-related ischemia and resultant tissue necrosis.

The surgical stent must also include a series of embedded wire loops placed toward the palatal side of the residual ridge (Fig. 5–97). These loops are used to support a series of equally spaced sutures that are placed through the edges of the mucosal flap. When the stent has been modified with the thermoplastic materials, the area adjacent to the periosteum and facial wound bed covered with split thickness skin, and the stent secured into position, the sutures are passed through the wire loops and tied. This pulls the mucosal edges over the modified stent and stabilizes the wound bed over the skin graft.

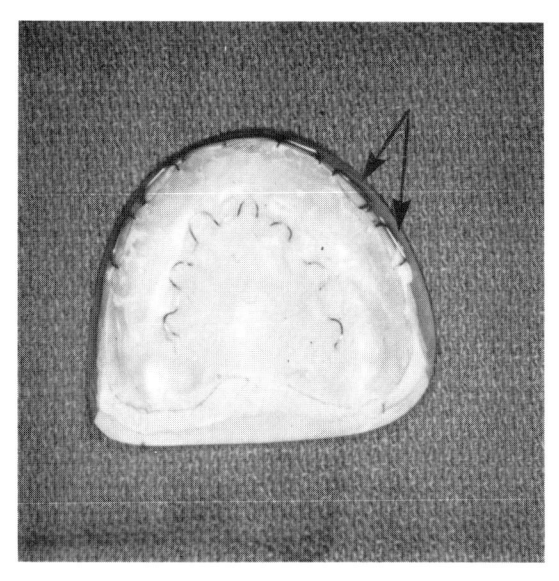

Figure 5–97. Surgical stent with wire loops in the flange periphery (arrows) to engage the compound during modification at surgery and loops just medial to the ridge crest to support the tethering sutures.

Surgical Technique

The surgical technique includes a primary incision at the juncture of the attached and unattached mucosa around the facial aspect of the residual ridge. A supraperiosteal dissection is carried out well into the entire facial sulcus, keeping in mind that a skin-lined pouch is to be created with sufficient width and depth to encompass an exaggerated, undercut denture flange. If possible, this dissection should extend for at least a centimeter or more (Fig. 5–98). It may be necessary to remove the bony nasal spine, and care must be taken not to perforate the nasal mucosa or injure the infraorbital nerves. After completion of the dissection an accurate impression of the wound bed must be recorded in the surgical stent.

Prosthetic Care at Surgery

As soon as the surgical stent has been properly extended with red compound at surgery (Fig. 5–99), it is given to the prosthodontist. The modified surgical stent is duplicated using irreversible hydrocolloid. If the transitional base was previously fabricated from the original master cast, only the flange needs to be duplicated. However, if the complete transitional splint is to be fabricated at this time, then the entire tissue surface of the stent is duplicated.

The irreversible hydrocolloid is mixed in sufficient amounts in a rubber bowl. The entire flange of the stent is submerged in the material. The stent should be loaded with the irreversible hydrocolloid before inverting into the larger mass to ensure complete duplication (Fig. 5–100). Once the material has set, the stent is recovered and the impression inspected for accuracy. If there are flaws or inaccuracies, the process can be repeated. Otherwise the stent is placed in a germicidal solution and, after a sufficient time for disinfection, it is thoroughly washed with sterile water and modified for final detail with Protaform. The split thickness skin graft is at-

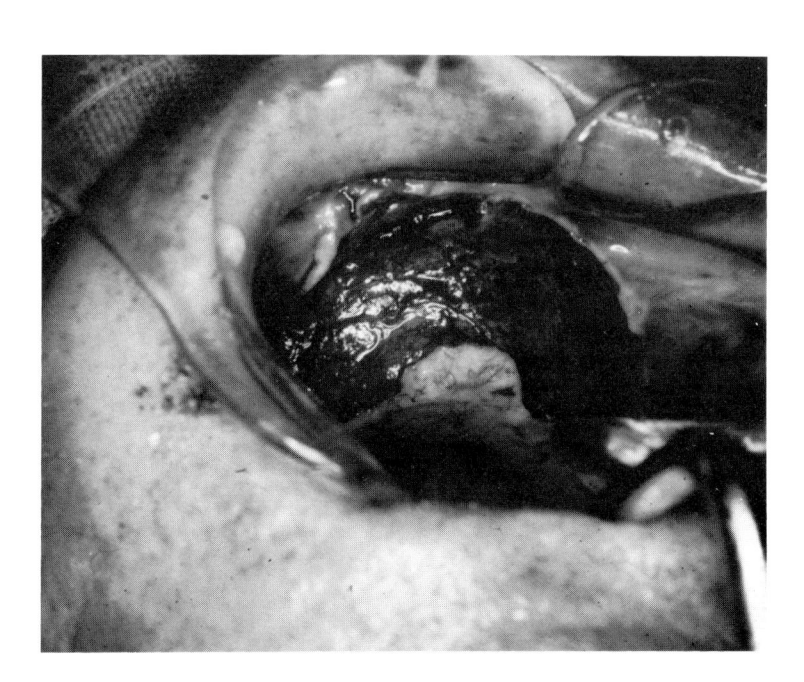

Figure 5–98. Primary incision line at the juncture of the attached and unattached mucosa can be seen, as well as the extent of the dissection.

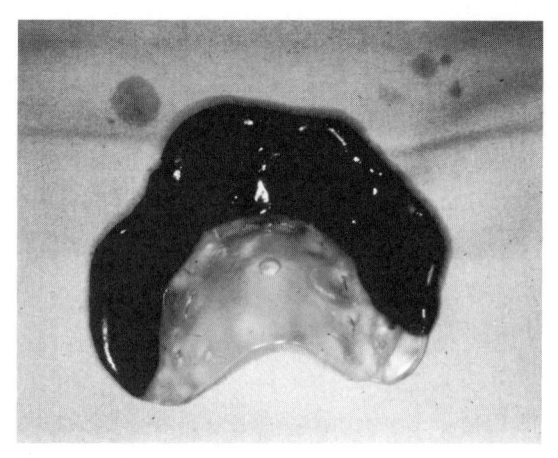

112 / SURGICAL MANAGEMENT OF SOFT TISSUE PROBLEMS

Figure 5–99. Stent extended at surgery with compound.

tached to the stent with a biologically acceptable adhesive and the procedure completed as described (Fig. 5–101). The stent is usually held in place with a single midpalatal screw (Fig. 5–102).

Autopolymerizing methyl methacrylate resin is mixed to a free-flowing consistency. The mixture is poured into the impression and allowed to cure. When cured, the duplicate of the flange or the entire stent is recovered from the impression material. Any excess is removed and the flange or stent is lightly polished.

Approximately seven to ten days after the surgery, the surgical stent is removed. If the immediate transitional base was made previously, the duplicate flange is placed into po-

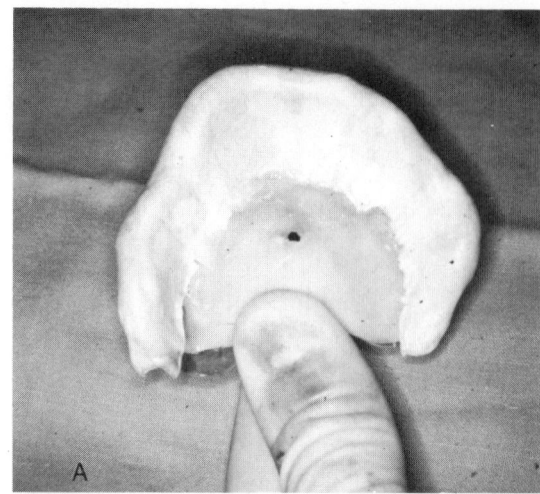

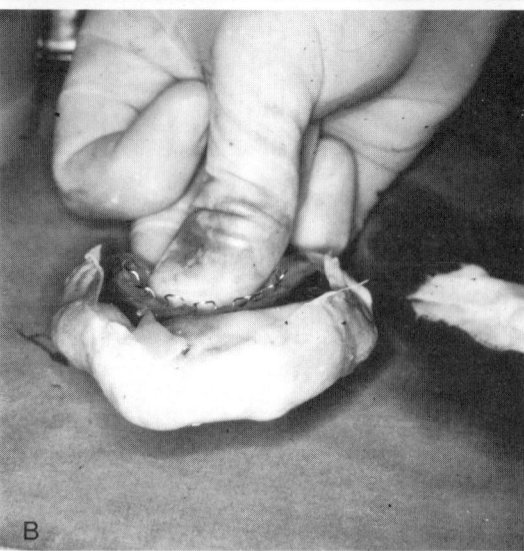

Figure 5–101. Surgical stent modified with one layer of Protaform to which the split thickness skin graft has been attached with adhesive. The graft will cover the entire surgical wound. *A,* Palatal view; *B,* facial view.

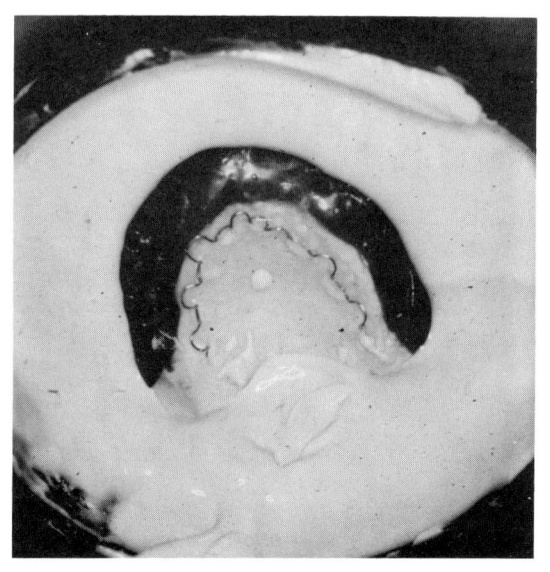

Figure 5–100. Modified stent seated into the irreversible hydrocolloid material.

sition within the newly formed pocket. The transitional base is then positioned over the palate and the portion of the ridge unaffected by the surgery. The borders of the base may have to be reduced to allow for complete seating of the base and to provide clearance between the borders of the base and the duplicate flange. The tissues adjacent to the space between the flange and the base are protected by the application of petroleum jelly. The base is reseated and the two sections are secured with autopolymerizing methyl methacrylate resin. When the resin has completely cured, the splint is removed. The surgical stent is repositioned in the mouth while the transitional splint is trimmed of any excess material. The flange

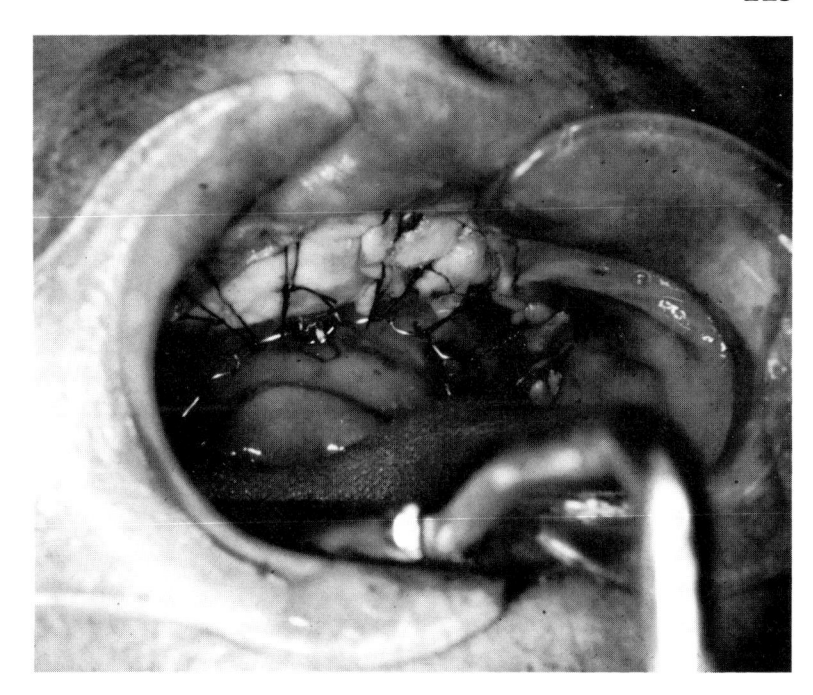

Figure 5–102. Surgical stent with attached split thickness skin graft. The stent is held in place with one palatal screw. Tethering sutures through the mucosal flap edges stabilize the soft tissue wound against the graft.

is then undercut just below the periphery to allow for the creation of a retentive undercut within the grafted pocket. The splint is polished and reinserted into the mouth. Usually adequate retention and stability are achieved at this time. As healing progresses, any discrepancies between the graft and the splint can be corrected with the addition of tissue-conditioning material.

If a complete transitional splint is made from the duplication of the stent at the time of surgery (Fig. 5–103), it can be inserted as soon as the surgical stent is removed (Fig. 5–104). The splint is relined with a tissue-conditioning agent to provide better adaptation to the palatal tissues. Again, the flange is *undercut* just below the periphery.

While the patient wears the immediate transitional splint, the surgical stent can be duplicated again to form a custom tray that is used to make a more detailed impression of the maxilla and surgical site (Fig. 5–105). From this impression, a definitive transitional splint can be made to replace the immediate one.

This immediate insertion of the transitional splint following removal of the surgical stent is considered critical, as the soft tissue wound bed will contract dramatically, sometimes within minutes to several hours, if left without a retention splint. Having this temporary retention splint ready for immediate insertion also makes it unnecessary to excessively manipulate the healing wound in taking an impression to prepare such a splint, thus reducing potential patient discomfort as well as the length of the office visit.

The surgical stent, which has adapted exactly to the residual ridge form and created vestibule, can be used as the final impression to construct either a more permanent heat-processed acrylic splint or to make a tray for an impression to accomplish this at a later time, including denture fabrication. Denture construction can usually begin six to eight weeks after surgery.

The acrylic splint and/or denture with the

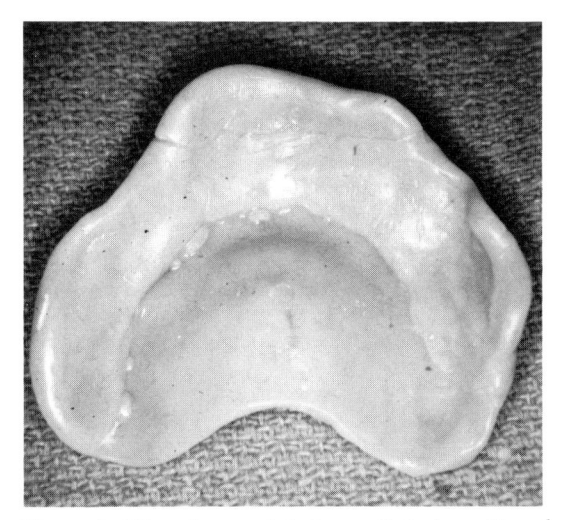

Figure 5–103. A complete immediate transitional splint after trimming and polishing.

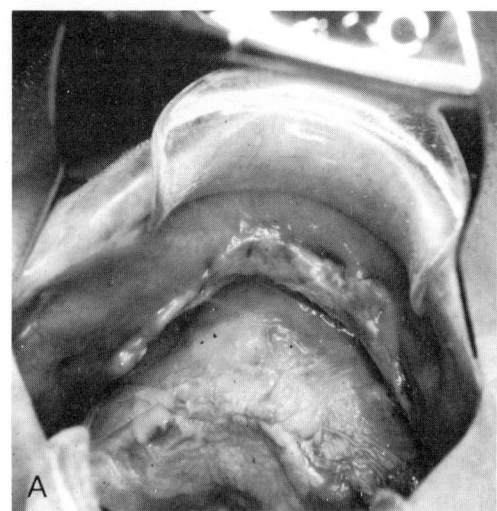

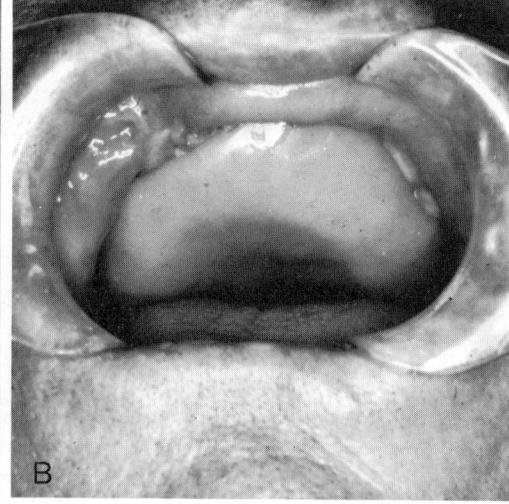

114 / SURGICAL MANAGEMENT OF SOFT TISSUE PROBLEMS

Figure 5–104. *A,* View of the anterior maxilla seven days after surgery immediately following removal of the surgical stent. Note the skin graft extending from the residual ridge and completely lining the vestibule to the mucosal flap edge. *B,* Transitional acrylic splint in position.

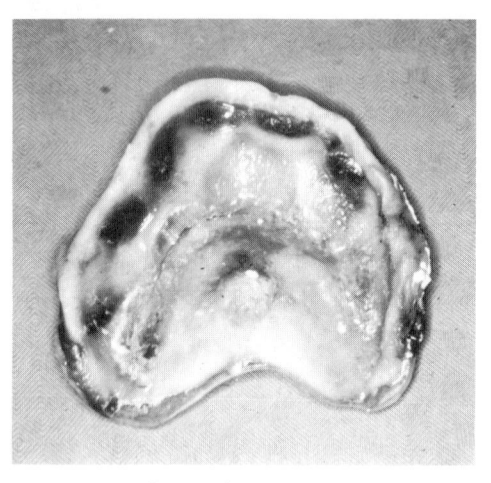

Figure 5–105. Surgical stent used to construct impression tray for making the definitive acrylic resin transitional splint. Note how the Protaform has continued to flow and adapt to the underlying tissues.

exaggerated, *undercut* flange maintains the vestibular form and reduces and/or limits wound contracture. It is imperative that the patient wear the acrylic splint and then the denture constantly day and night for 12 to 18 months following surgery, removing the appliance only for a few minutes at a time for cleaning (Fig. 5–106). After this period maximum healing, including wound contracture, has occurred and the patient can resume a more usual denture-wearing pattern, including removal at night during sleep.

In summary, this modified buccal inlay technique has provided predictable and consistently acceptable results. The procedure does require very close cooperation between the prosthodontist and surgeon preoperatively in preparing the basic surgical stent, intraoperatively in reproducing the modified

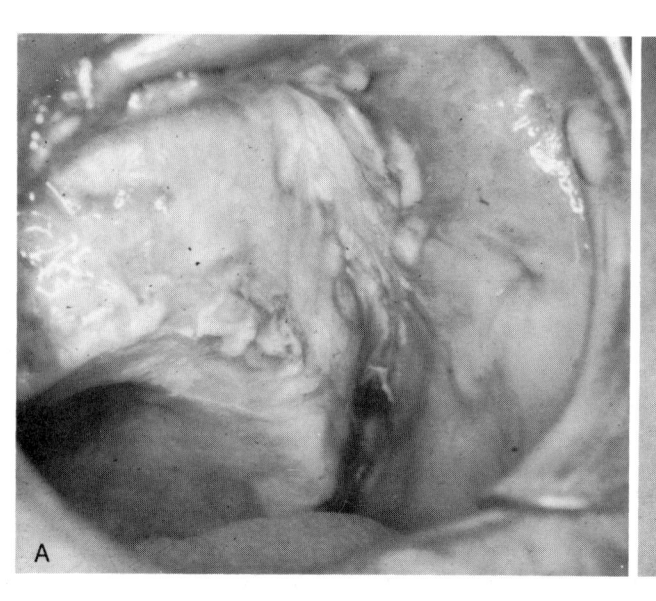

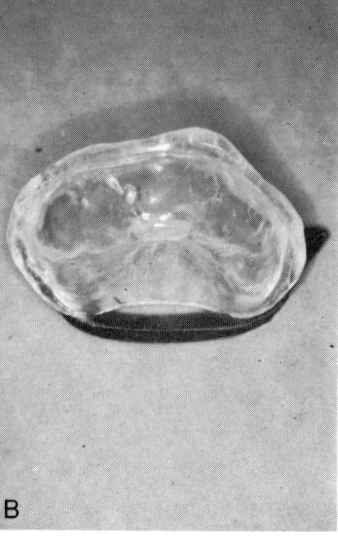

Figure 5–106. *A,* Three weeks after surgery showing graft maturation and maintenance of the sulcus form. *B,* Definitive transitional acrylic resin splint. The exaggerated undercut denture flange will be duplicated in the denture.

surgical stent for fabrication of the initial acrylic splint to be inserted seven to ten days following surgery, and postoperatively in producing an accurate acrylic splint and finally a denture that allows retention of the vestibular form achieved by the surgery.

BIBLIOGRAPHY

1. McDowell F: Carl Thiersch, microscopy and skin grafting. Plast Reconstr Surg 41:369, 1968.
2. Reverdin JL: Greffe epidermique. Arch Gen Med 19:277, 555, 703, 1872.
3. Thiersch C: Ueber die feineren anatomnischen Veranderungen bei aufheilung von Haut auf Granulationen. Arch Klin Chir 17:318, 1874.
4. Slanetz CA, and Rankow RM: The intra-oral use of split-thickness skin grafts in head and neck surgery. Am J Surg 104:721, 1962.
5. Schnitzler J, and Ewald K: Zur Technik der Hauttransplantation nach Thiersch. Centralbl Chir 21:148, 1894.
6. Pichler H, and Trauner R: Die alveolarkammplastik. Oest Z Stomatol 28:54, 1930.
7. Moskowicz L: Ueber Verpflanzung Thiersch scher Epidermislappchen in die Mundhohle. Arch Klin Chir Bd 108: 216, 1915.
8. Esser JFF: Neue Wege fur Chirurgische plastiken durch Heranziehung der zahnarztlichen Technik. Beitr Klin Chir 103:547, 1916.
9. Weiser R: Ein Jahr chirurgisch-zahnarztliche Tatigkeit im Kieferspital. Z Stomatol XVI:133, 1918.
10. Gillies HD: Plastic Surgery of the Face. London, Henry Frowdz and Hodder and Stough, 1920, pp 8–12, 193–208.
11. Pickerill HB: Intra-oral skin-grafting: The establishment of the buccal sulcus. Proc R Soc Med 12:17, 1918.
12. Kilner TP, and Jackson T: Skin grafting in the buccal cavity. Br J Surg 9:148, 1921.
13. Kazanjian VH: In Blair VP et al. (eds.): Essentials of Oral Surgery. 3rd ed. St. Louis, CV Mosby Co, 1944.
14. Wassmund M: Ueber chirurgische Formgestaltung des atrophischen Kiefers zum zwecke prothetischer Versorgung. Vierteljahreschrift Zahnheilkd 47:305, 1931.
15. Trauner R: Alveoloplasty with ridge extensions on the lingual side of the lower jaw to solve the problem of a lower dental prosthesis. Oral Surg 5:340, 1952.
16. Obwegeser H: Die totale Mundbodenplastik. Schweiz Mschr Zahnheilkd 73:565, 1963.
17. Mathis H: Einfache chirgische Massnahmen zur Sicherung von Halt und Stabilitat der prothesen in der Alltagspraxis. Dtsch Zahnarztl Z 6:44, 1951.
18. Schuchardt K: Die Epidermistransplantation bie der Mundvorhofplastik. Dtsch Zahnarztl Z 7:364, 1952.
19. Rehrmann A: Beitrag zur Alveolarkammplastik am Unterkiefer. Zahnarztl Rdsch 62:505, 1953.
20. Landesman HM, Davis WH, Martinoff J, and Kaminishi R: Resorption of the edentulous mandible after a vestibuloplasty with skin grafting. J Prosthet Dent 49:619, 1983.
21. Landesman HM, and Levin B: A patient survey of the denture tolerance before and after a mandibular vestibuloplasty with skin grafting. J Am Dent Assoc 90:806, 1975.
22. Steinhauser E: Free transplantation of oral mucosa for improvement of denture retention. J Oral Surg 27:955, 1969.
23. Walker RV: Personal communication.
24. Kazanjian VH: Surgical operations as related to satisfactory dentures. Dental Cosmos 66:387, 1924.
25. Godwin JG: Submucous surgery for better denture service. J Am Dent Assoc 34:678–686, 1947.
26. Edlan A, and Mejchar B: Plastic surgery of the vestibulum in periodontal therapy. Int Dent J 13:593, 1963.
27. Howe GL: Preprosthetic surgery in the lower labial sulcus. Dent Pract 16:119–124, 1965.
28. Kethley JL, and Gamble JW: The lipswitch: A modification of Kazanjian's labial vestibuloplasty. J Oral Surg 36:701–705, 1978.
29. Wessberg GA, Hill SC, and Epker BN: Transpositional flap technique for mandibular vestibuloplasty. J Am Dent Assoc 98:929–933, 1979.
30. Huybers TJM, Stoelinga PJW, deKoomen HA, and Tideman H: Mandibular vestibuloplasty using a free mucosal graft (2–7 year evaluation). Int J Oral Surg. 14:11–15, 1985.
31. Hjøring-Hansen E, Adawy AM, and Hillerup S: Mandibular vestibulolingual sulcoplasty with free skin-graft: A five year clinical follow-up study. J Oral Maxillofac Surg 41:173–176, 1983.
32. Hillerup S: Mandibular vestibuloplasty using oral mucosa. In Stoelinga PJW (ed.): Proceedings of the Consensus Conference on the relative roles of vestibuloplasty and ridge augmentation in management of the atrophic mandible. Eighth International Conference on Oral Surgery. Chicago, Quintessence, 1984, p 17.
33. Tideman H: A technique of vestibuloplasty using a free mucosal graft from the cheek. Int J Oral Surg 1:76–80, 1972.
34. deKoomen HA: A prosthetic view on vestibuloplasty with free mucosal graft. Int J Oral Surg 6:38–41, 1977.
35. Obwegeser H: Eine Modification der Lingualen alveolar Kammplastiek nach R. Trauner. Schweiz Mschr Zahnheilkd 63:788–799, 1953.
36. Brown LJ: A surgical solution to a lower denture problem. Br Dent J 95:215–216, 1953.
37. Caldwell JB: Lingual ridge extension. J Oral Surg 13:287, 1955.
38. Downton D: Mylohyoid ridge resection. Dent Rec 74:212–214, 1953.
39. Hopkins R, Stafford GD, and Gregory ME: Preprosthetic surgery of the edentulous mandible. Br Dent J 148:183–188, 1980.
40. Hull, M: Life threatening swelling after mandibular vestibuloplasty. J Oral Surg 35:511–514, 1977.
41. Popwich L, and Sanit A: Respiratory obstruction following vestibuloplasty and lowering of the floor of the mouth. J Oral Maxillofac Surg 41:255–257, 1983.
42. MacIntosh R, and Obwegeser H: Preprosthetic surgery: A scheme for its effective employment. J Oral Surg 25:397–413, 1967.
43. Smylski PT: Closed transpalatal method of wiring a maxillary splint or denture. Int J Oral Surg 2:200–202, 1973.
44. Obwegeser HL: Die submukose Vestibulumplastik. Dtsch Zahnarztl Z 14:629, 749, 1959.
45. Obwegeser H: Co-report: Surgical preparation of the mouth for full dentures. Int Dent J 8:252–253, 1958.
46. Rumpel C: Die Wiederherstellung des Vestibulum oris nach Schussverletzung der Kiefer. Dtsch Zahnarztl Wochenschr 19:262, 1916.
47. Szaba J: Methode zur Verhinderung des Verwachsens der durchtrennten Mundschleimhaut. Oester Vierteljahrsschr Zahnheilkd 32:244, 1916.

48. Ganzer H: Die Wiederherstellung des Vestibulum oris nach Schussverletzungen der Kiefer. Dtsch Mschr Zahnheilkd 34:380, 1916.
49. Smedley VC: Increasing the possible denture foundation area by surgical means. J Am Dent Assoc 28:1616–1623, 1941.
50. Clark HB: Deepening of labial sulcus by mucosal flap advancement: Report of case. J Oral Surg 11:165, 1953.
51. Miller E: Personal communication, 1984.
52. Wallenius K, and Owall B: Retention of dentures by skin-folded pockets. Odont Revy 17:222, 1966.

6

OSSEOUS RECONSTRUCTION OF EDENTULOUS BONE LOSS

*by Raymond J. Fonseca, D.M.D.,
David Frost, D.D.S.,[*]
Deborah Zeitler, D.D.S., M. S.,
and Paul J.W. Stoelinga, D.D.S., M.D., Ph.D.*

The basic goal of dentistry is to preserve and restore dental function, phonetics, and esthetics. With this in mind, the adequate restoration of the edentulous maxilla and mandible is usually well within the capabilities of the general dentist or prosthodontist. However, there is a population of patients with EBL (edentulous bone loss) severe enough to make conventional prosthetics impossible. These patients, as well as those rendered totally or partially edentulous secondary to trauma or surgical resection, would benefit from one or more of various surgical procedures designed to return the anatomy to a normal state. The edentulous maxilla and mandible present challenges in surgical management that often relate directly to characteristic patterns of EBL. Without the repetitive stimuli of loading stresses on natural teeth, the alveolar bone is prone to EBL. This EBL occurs at various rates in different patients and may or may not occur uniformly around the edentulous ridge.

Ridge extension procedures are discussed in Chapter 5. Procedures to be discussed in this chapter include onlay augmentation with bone and bone substitutes, osteotomies for repositioning the maxilla or parts thereof either with or without bone grafting and combinations of these procedures.

MAXILLARY PROCEDURES

Surgical prosthetic reconstruction of the maxilla is complicated by several problems unique to the area. Anatomic proximity to the maxillary sinus and nasal cavity, the contour of the zygomatic buttress, the position of the hamulus, and the nature of the alveolar bone of the maxilla make surgical augmentation difficult. The differential diagnosis and treatment planning of maxillary bony EBL are discussed in Chapter 3. Three types of maxillary EBL and their surgical management will be presented: (1) those due to the early loss of the dentition with physiologic EBL, (2) traumatic loss of bone, and (3) surgical resections secondary to pathologic states. This chapter deals only with the osseous management of physiologic EBL (Table 6–1).

Surgical procedures have been devised to correct all recognized deficiency states of the maxilla; however, this is not to say that further modifications or newly developed procedures might not be more beneficial to an individual patient (Tables 6–1 and 6–2). Each surgeon is advised to evaluate his or her patient closely for possible individualization of surgical procedures that would better serve the patient.

TABLE 6–1. BONY DEFICIENCY STATES OF THE MAXILLA

1. Total maxillary atrophy with poor palatal vault form
2. Total maxillary atrophy with acceptable palatal vault form
3. Regional problems
   a. Anterior atrophy
   b. Posterior segmental atrophy
   c. Undercut regions

---

[*]Dr. David Frost's contribution to this chapter, including the illustrations, has been published with the permission of the United States Air Force.

TABLE 6–2. SURGICAL PROCEDURES FOR MAXILLARY BONY DEFICIENCY

1. Onlay bone graft—total
2. Onlay bone graft—segmental
3. Total interpositional bone graft
4. Segmental interpositional bone grafts
5. Segmental osteotomies without grafts
6. Palatal osteotomies
7. Combination procedures
8. Maxillary sinus floor graft

Preoperative Evaluation

Preoperative evaluation should include a detailed history for possible contributing reasons for the advanced state of EBL. Contributing aspects such as periodontal disease, malnutrition, menopause and systemic disease states such as osteoporosis should be evaluated and corrected preoperatively whenever possible (see Chapter 1).

The majority of treatment plans require two major surgical procedures with two general anesthetics. Patients with significant systemic disease may not be able to tolerate this. Furthermore, since grafting of bone (whether it is autogenous or allogeneic) requires prolonged healing and the re-establishment of blood supply, conditions that interfere with the normal healing process may contraindicate this type of surgery. Such conditions may include diabetes mellitus, previous radiation therapy, and autoimmune disorders.

Clinical examination should be conducted systematically. Radiographs, models, diagnostic mountings, and clinical examination will need to be combined into a coordinated evaluation to arrive at a complete diagnosis and to allow for formulation of a total treatment plan. The coordinated effort between surgeon and prosthodontist will eventually result in the best treatment.

Oral and maxillofacial surgeons will require panoramic radiographs to evaluate the jaws for pathology, sinusitis, retained teeth, residual bony height of the mandible, proximity of the maxillary antrum to the alveolus, and position of the inferior alveolar neurovascular bundle. Lateral cephalograms with the head in natural position and the lips in an unstrained position will allow for evaluation of the anteroposterior relationship of the maxilla and the mandible. Vertical height, position of the genial tubercles, and proximity of the sinuses and nasal floor can also be evaluated. An occlusal radiograph of the mandible can permit evaluation of mandibular width.

Mounted models are probably best evaluated by the prosthodontist in conjunction with his clinical evaluation. Specific concerns with this evaluation are interarch space, adequacy of the tuberosity, character and nature of the ridge mucosa, negative ridge form in the mandible and undercuts in the maxilla, palatal vault form, face height, and lip support and relation to occlusal rims.

Clinical evaluation includes examination of the health of the mucosa, morphology of the alveolar ridges, width of the ridges, position of the neurovascular bundles, anterior nasal spine in relation to the alveolar crest, tuberosity shape, and maxillomandibular relationships.

Onlay Bone Grafting

Background

Severe EBL of the edentulous maxilla is common. MacIntosh and Obwegeser[1] noted that when a nearly flat surface exists between the palate and the vestibule, replacement of the supportive bone should be undertaken. Terry et al.[2] first described the use of autologous ribs to be placed in an onlay fashion on the bony-deficient maxilla. The rib was stabilized in these early cases with a Vitallium strip and stainless steel wires. Particulate bone was packed on the facial and palatal aspects of the primary rib strut. Closure was accomplished after adequate relaxation of the flaps was achieved. This procedure was followed between four and six months later with a soft-tissue procedure to allow for utilization of the grafted bone.

Baker and Connole[3] reported on the follow-up results of the first group of patients treated with maxillary autologous onlay rib grafts. Of a series of seven, at least two had protracted periods of sequestration. To date, there have been no well-documented long-

TABLE 6–3. TOTAL MAXILLARY ATROPHY WITH POOR PALATAL VAULT FORM

Treatment:	Autologous onlay bone graft (rib)
Indications:	1. Severe maxillary alveolar atrophy
	2. Flat palatal vault form
	3. Mild to moderate anteroposterior ridge relation discrepancy
Contraindications:	Compromised pulmonary status
Advantages:	1. Augments alveolus
	2. Improves vault form
	3. Anteroposterior relations improved
	4. Remodeling leaves good ridge form
Disadvantages:	1. Slow to revascularize
	2. Thoracotomy required
	3. Resorption variable with no long-term studies
	4. Secondary soft tissue procedure required
	5. Must be without prosthetic replacement for approximately six to seven months

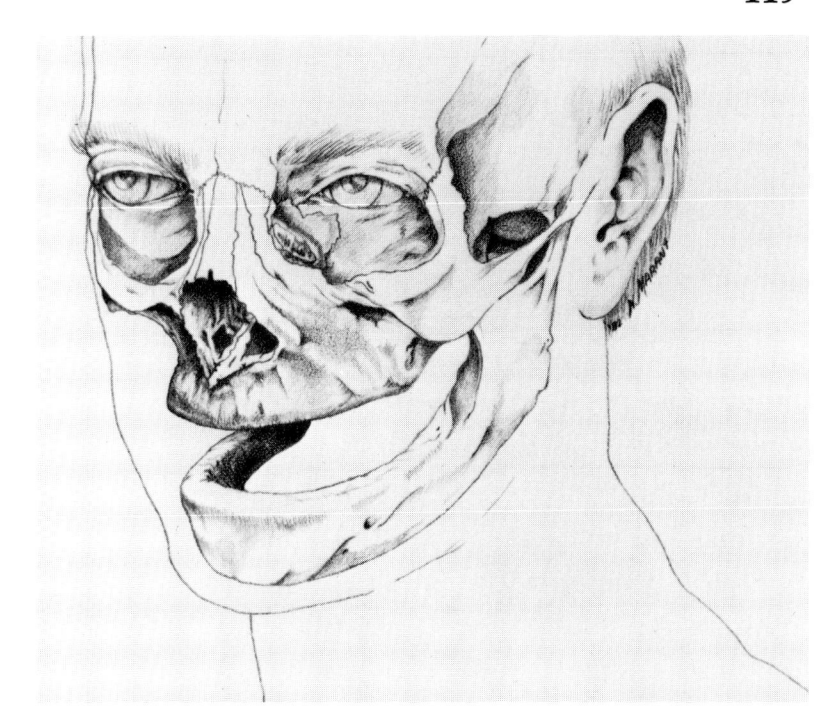

Figure 6–1. Resorption of the edentulous maxillary ridge, reducing the maxilla to a nearly flat surface.

term studies of onlay rib grafting procedures to the maxilla. Wolford and Epker[4] reported on the preliminary results of ridge augmentation with freeze-dried bone cribs. It appears from the data that one patient was treated with this technique and a soft-tissue breakdown occurred 10 days postoperatively, with loss of approximately one third of the graft. Studies have shown, in an experimental model, that autologous onlay bone grafts to the atrophic maxilla are more acceptable, are more readily revascularized, and heal with less difficulty than do allogeneic onlay grafts to the same defect.[5] Therefore, only the clinically useful autologous onlay rib graft will be discussed further.

When resorption of the edentulous maxillary ridge is symmetrical, and the alveolar bone loss has been so extreme as to reduce the maxilla to a nearly flat surface between the palate and the vestibule, an onlay bone grafting procedure should be considered (Fig. 6–1, Table 6–3). Other indications for onlay bone grafting of the maxilla include mild anteroposterior discrepancies of ridge relationship, or severe anterior EBL that extends to but does not include the tuberosities (Fig. 6–2). In these instances, the crest of the maxilla is so close to the piriform aperture that soft tissue procedures exposing more usable maxilla are highly impractical.[1, 2] Clinically, these patients will have redundant gingival tissue that is flabby and unsupported. This tissue is generally unsuitable for prosthetic support; however, it should be maintained for use over the bone graft. Secondary soft-tissue procedures will correct the soft-tissue problems.

Surgical Procedure

Low-profile naso-endotracheal intubation is recommended for the administration of anesthesia. Once the ribs have been harvested (the technique is described elsewhere

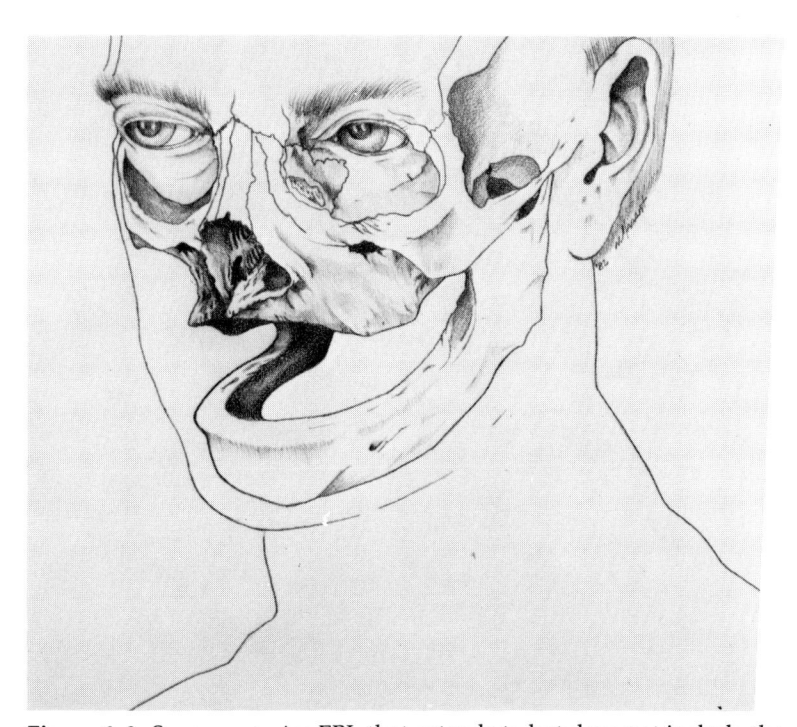

Figure 6–2. Severe anterior EBL that extends to but does not include the tuberosities.

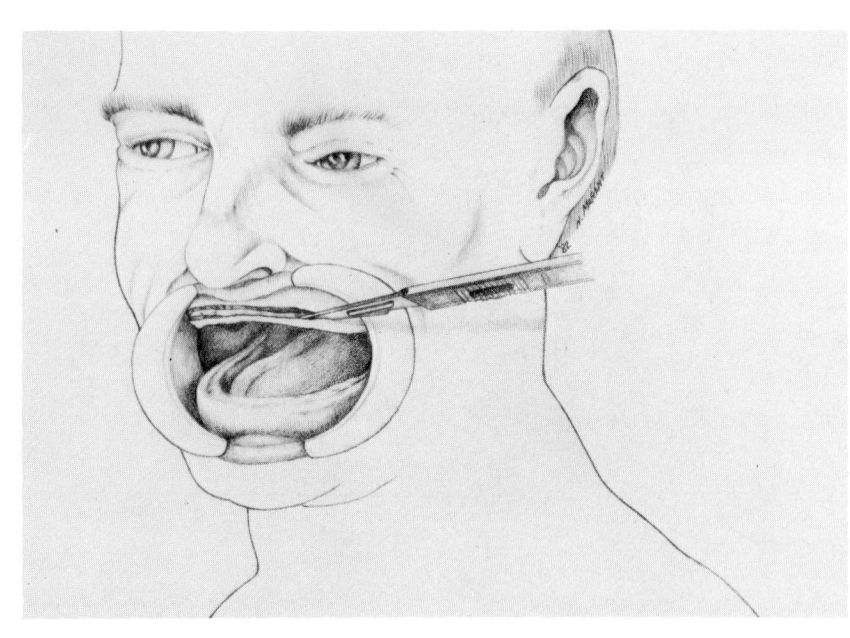

120 / OSSEOUS RECONSTRUCTION OF EDENTULOUS BONE LOSS

Figure 6–3. An incision is made through the crestal tissue from tuberosity to tuberosity region.

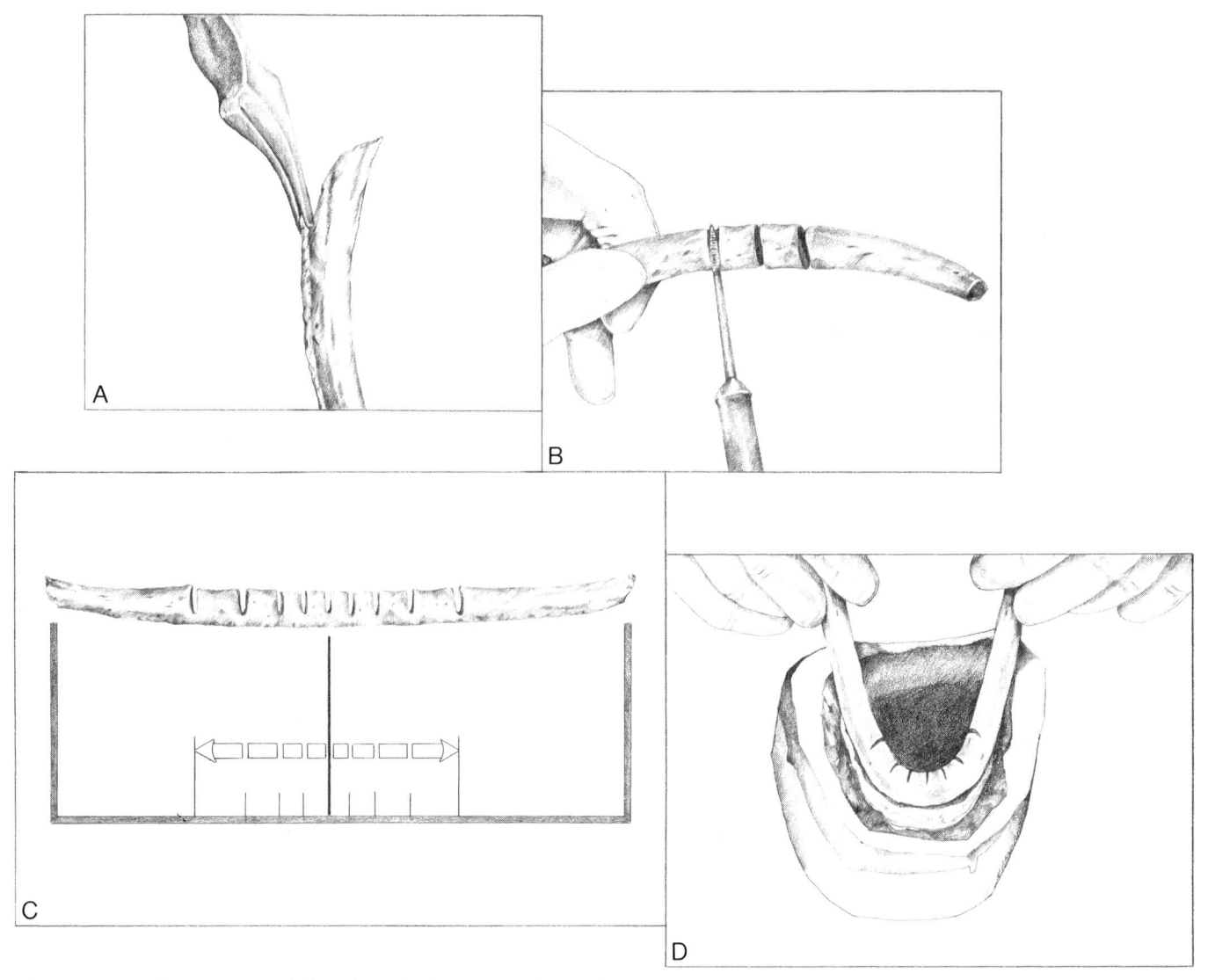

Figure 6–4. *A,* Preparation of the rib with despining of the rib. *B–D,* The notching of the rib should extend 270 degrees around the rib cortex to allow for ease of contouring.

in this chapter), the orofacial region is approached. A standard throat pack is placed and an intra-oral facial preparation with an antiseptic solution is performed. The tissues around the maxillary crest are infiltrated with 10 to 15 ml of a dilute mixture of lidocaine and epinephrine (0.5 per cent with 1:400,000 or 0.25 per cent with 1:200,000). This gives the added benefit of hemostasis as well as demarcation of the mucogingival junction.

An incision is made through the crestal tissue from tuberosity to tuberosity (Fig. 6–3). A facial mucoperiosteal flap is reflected, exposing the zygomatic crest of the maxilla, the piriform apertures, and, if necessary, the infraorbital foramen. As originally described by Terry and others,[2] a full palatal flap may be elevated. Depending on the amount of facial tissue available for closure, a limited palatal flap may be developed. This limited flap eliminates the potential dead space on the palate as well as the need for a palatal pack. The rib graft may be fixed by a variety of techniques, including Vitallium strip,[2] stainless steel wire,[2,3] and miniplates. Preparation of the rib for grafting is performed on a separate back table while the maxilla is prepared. The technique of preparing the rib is similar to that described by Davis and others.[6] Using a cast of the maxilla, poured in acrylic and gas sterilized for use in the surgical field, one rib is despined (Fig. 6–4A) and kerfed (notched) on the inner aspect (lesser curvature), allowing it to bend to the contour of the residual maxilla. The notching of the rib should extend 270 degrees around the rib cortex, allowing for ease of contouring (Fig. 6–4B-D). The rib is cut to the appropriate length and shaped in the posterior region to conform to the tuberosity (Fig. 6–5). Should the atrophy extend the total length of the alveolar ridge, the rib is contoured to the ideal tuberosity shape (Fig. 6–6). Holes are placed in the rib at appropriate points to allow for transosseous stabilization (Fig. 6–7).

A second rib is split, the marrow is removed with a curette, and the cortical bone layers are particulated. These bone chips and marrow are stored and will be used later in the procedure. The marrow and particulate bone, along with the rib, should be stored in either normal saline or 5 per cent dextrose in water (D5W) until the recipient bed is prepared.[7] This will enhance survival of the marrow cells.

Ideally, the preparation of the recipient site and the donor bone will be completed simultaneously and there will be no delay in grafting. Once both the graft and the bed are prepared, the rib strut is tried in the mouth.

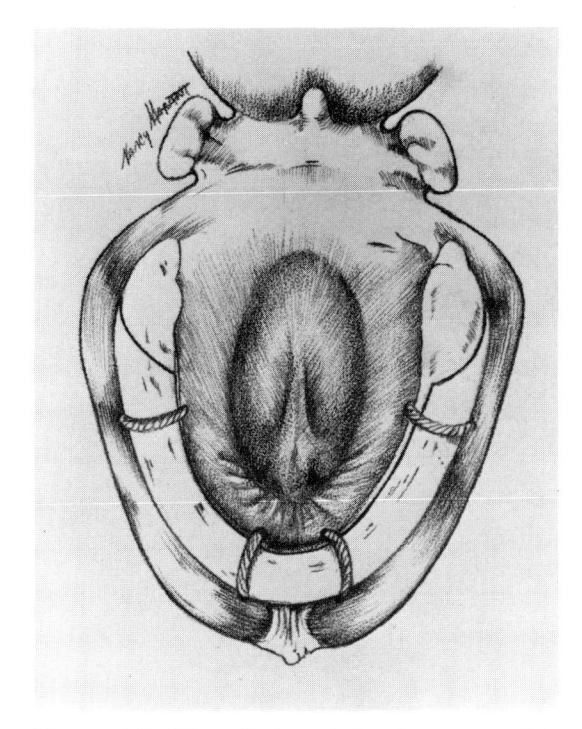

Figure 6–5. The rib is cut to the appropriate length and shaped in the posterior region to conform to the tuberosity.

Some final adjusting of the contour and length may be required. Once the graft is adequately adapted, stainless steel wires may be passed through the rib and the piriform anteriorly, or the tuberosity or zygomatic

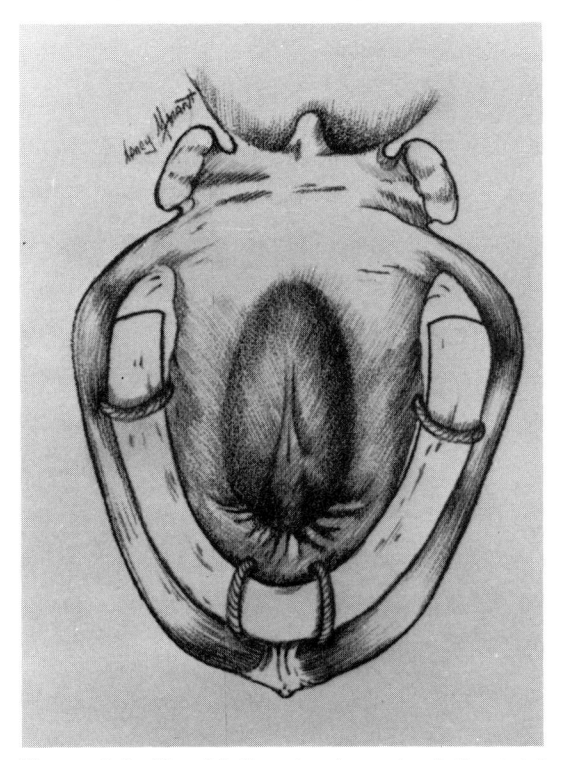

Figure 6–6. Should the atrophy extend the total length of the alveolar ridge, the rib is contoured to the ideal tuberosity shape.

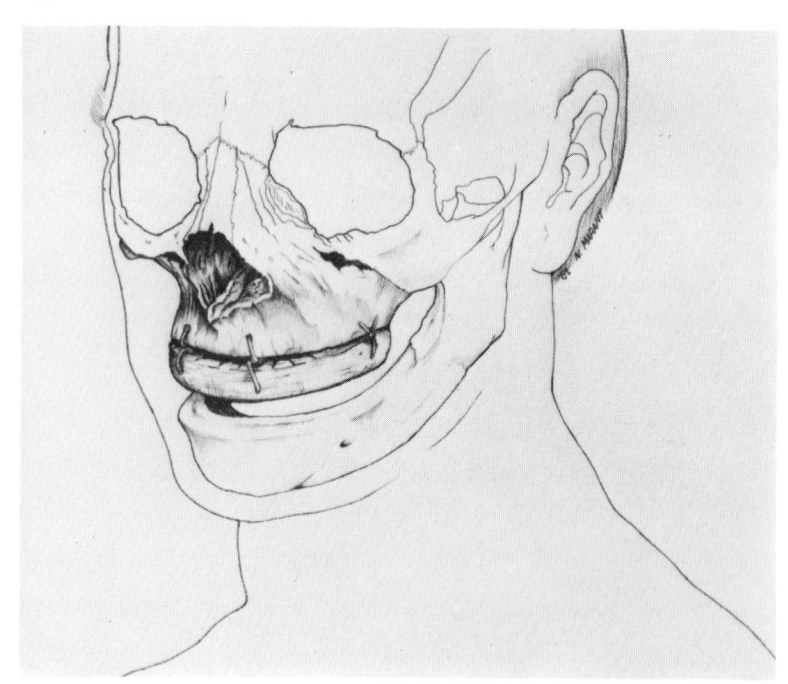

Figure 6–7. Holes are placed in the rib at appropriate points to allow for transosseous stabilization.

process of the maxilla posteriorly. These wires will firmly secure the rib to the maxilla. Should the continuity of the major strut be lost, especially in the anterior region, these wires will tend to displace the rib laterally; therefore, every effort should be made to maintain continuity of the primary rib strut around the arch. If the rib cannot be maintained in one piece, a stainless steel wire at the split may restore continuity and stability. If not, the rib can be stabilized in one of the other ways mentioned above.

Once the rib strut has been stabilized, the flaps are mobilized and evaluated to assure adequate relaxation for closure. If necessary, periosteal releasing incisions can be made in the facial flap. Right angle scissors can be used to dissect into the lip and cheek for a short distance for adequate relaxation to occur, and the palatal tissue can be left attached. However, if relaxation is still inadequate, a complete palatal flap will give sufficient soft-tissue release. The particulate rib and marrow can be packed around the rib on the facial and palatal aspects. If suturing is begun prior to placing the particulate bone, a tunnel can be formed which will allow a more controlled placement of the particulate bone (Fig. 6–8). Closure is accomplished with a horizontal mattress suture and followed by oversewing with a continuous suture for good wound edge eversion and a "belt and braces" closure (Fig. 6–9). A monofilament nonresorbable suture is recommended for this closure.

Anterior Bone Loss Only. If the atrophy is such that the anterior maxilla is grossly deficient and the tuberosities are still acceptable, the rib strut can be contoured to onlay the tuberosity laterally and inferiorly, while resting off the ridge anteriorly and being stabilized with a "figure-eight" wire.[3] The area is then packed with particulate graft material as noted above.

Forward (anterior) positioning of the rib on the maxilla or anterior nasal spine will aid in correction of minor anteroposterior (A-P) arch discrepancies but should not be used to correct a significant A-P deficiency of the maxilla. These are best treated in the maxilla at the LeFort I level, or in the mandibular ramus.

Correction of severe anterior bone loss has been reported and discussed using autologous ilium in an onlay fashion.[8,9] The use of onlayed allogeneic bone[8] has also been described. Fonseca and others[10] have found onlayed allogeneic bone to be unacceptable in the experimental model. No well-documented case or series of patients has been presented in the literature to substantiate the use of freeze-dried bone onlayed to the maxilla.

TOTAL MAXILLARY OSTEOTOMY WITH INTERPOSITIONAL GRAFTING

The patient with an edentulous, bony-deficient maxilla with adequate palatal vault

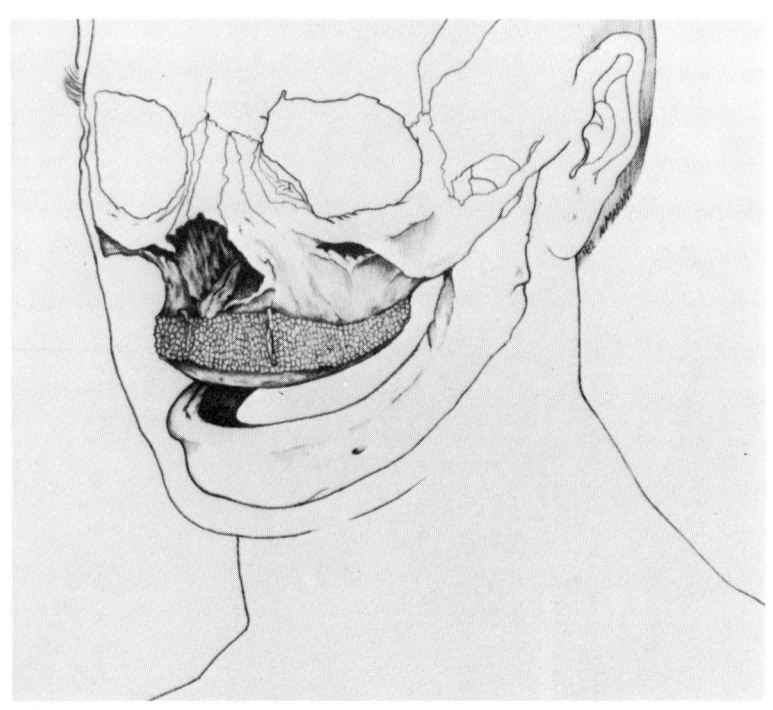

Figure 6–8. Suturing is begun prior to placing the particulate bone, providing a tunnel that allows a more controlled placement of the particulate bone.

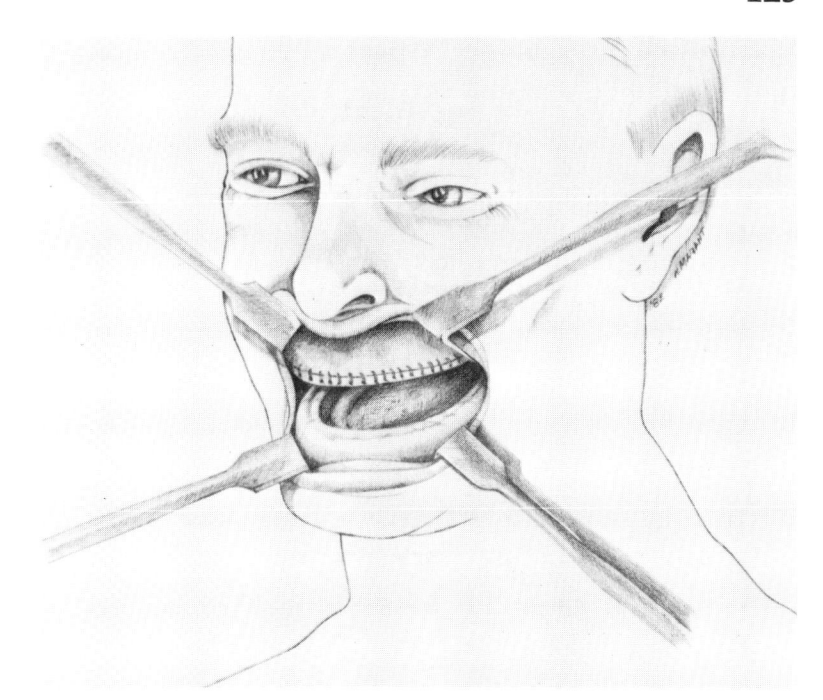

Figure 6–9. Closure is accomplished with a horizontal mattress suture and followed by oversewing with a continuous suture for good wound edge eversion.

form is the primary candidate for the total maxillary osteotomy with interpositional grafting. Patients with Class III relationships, usually secondary to the EBL of both the maxilla and mandible, can also be helped with anterior repositioning of the mobilized segment (Table 6–4). Not until Farrell and coworkers[11] described the use of autologous bone grafting in an interpositional fashion, with the LeFort I osteotomy, was this advocated for treatment of maxillary bone atrophy. Owing to the rapid resorption of the onlay bone graft system, they preferred the interpositional bone graft for the atrophic maxilla with good palatal vault form.

TABLE 6–4. TOTAL MAXILLARY ATROPHY WITH GOOD PALATAL VAULT FORM

Treatment:	Total maxillary osteotomy with interpositional bone grafting
Indications:	1. Severe bony deficiency with good to adequate palatal vault form
	2. Mild to moderate anteroposterior discrepancy
	3. Transverse discrepancies between maxilla and mandible
Contraindications:	1. Poor vault form
Advantages:	1. Stable, predictable movements
	2. Allogeneic bone is acceptable
	3. May not require soft tissue procedure
	4. Changes of ridge relation possible in three dimensions
Disadvantages:	1. Used alone will require good vault form
	2. May require secondary bone donor site
	3. May require soft tissue procedure

Bell and coworkers[7] reported in 1977 on the use of interpositional bone grafting procedures for correction of maxillary atrophy. Originally they reported using dumbbell-shaped blocks of corticocancellous bone from the iliac crest. However, Bell and Buckles[12] reported in a later article on the use of a "large block of corticocancellous bone" interposed between the mobilized portions of the maxilla, the medial and lateral antral walls, and the nasal septum to "decrease the amount of vertical relapse, provide additional stability to the repositioned maxilla and obliterate dead space." In their follow-up of 3 to 14 months, they reported resorption of 0 to 1 mm with no significant surgical complications.

The biologic acceptance of the interpositional graft system to the LeFort I site was investigated by Stroud et al.[13] and Frost and Fonseca[14] using autologous iliac grafts and allogeneic grafts, respectively. Their animal studies verified the acceptance of allogeneic bone and the increased osteoinduction of autologous bone in the LeFort I site of monkeys. Frost and Fonseca[14] concluded that allogeneic bone was acceptable but was incorporated much more slowly. The currently accepted and recommended bone grafting technique for total arch EBL of the maxilla, with adequate palatal vault, is total maxillary osteotomy with inferior repositioning of the desired distance. It is followed by interpositional bone grafting with an allogeneic strut of bone between the lateral antral walls. This technique gives a stable result with minimal insult to the patient and soft-tissue procedures follow three to five months later.

Surgical Technique

The surgical procedure is similar to those described in many previous publications.[7, 11, 12] A circumvestibular incision from zygomatic buttress to zygomatic buttress is employed. The incision should be placed in the vestibule and short of the mucosal reflection to avoid placing the scar at the periphery of the prosthesis (Fig. 6–10). Subperiosteal dissection, with elevation of the mucoperiosteal flap superiorly to the area of the infraorbital foramen, is followed by the release of the nasal mucoperiosteum from the piriform aperture. The dissection extends posteriorly along the lateral nasal wall. Tunneling below the mucoperiosteal flap and posteriorly around the tuberosity to the pterygoid plate region completes the soft tissue dissection and adequately exposes the atrophic maxilla.

Vertical reference lines are placed in the canine fossa region and at the zygomatic buttress if anteroposterior movements are planned. If only vertical movements are planned, bur holes, to act as reference markers and later to serve as transosseous wire stabilization points, are placed in the canine fossa and zygomatic buttress regions. Now the osteotomy can be completed above the level of the nasal floor from the tuberosity region to the piriform aperture bilaterally. These osteotomies should be directed parallel to the nasal floor. Careful retraction of the nasal soft tissues will prevent needless penetration of these tissues.

Finally, the maxilla is separated from the pterygoid plates using a curved osteotome. The osteotome should be malletted medioanteriorly, with the surgeon's finger on the palatal mucosa to palpate the bony penetration of the osteotome. Digital pressure applied bilaterally in the canine fossa area of the maxilla will aid in mobilization and downfracturing of the maxilla. Additionally, wide straight osteotomes should be placed along the lateral wall of the nose (medial wall of the sinus) posteriorly just in front of the greater palatine vessels. The downfracturing forces can be transmitted over a greater surface area to prevent multiple fractures of the maxilla. Care should be taken to assure that the nasal mucosa is elevated from the nasal floor when the downfracturing is completed (Fig. 6–11). The maxilla is thoroughly mobilized with disimpaction instruments.

Any tears in the nasal mucosa should be carefully repaired at this time. When allogeneic bone is used for interpositional grafting, the exposure via a nasal mucosal tear can adversely affect the bone graft.[14]

The bone graft, which has been shaped to the proper height and dumbbell mortised for insertion along the lateral antral wall, is positioned and retained in place with transosseous wires through the previously placed reference holes (Fig. 6–12). The exact amount of inferior movement can be verified at this time. If anteroposterior movement is planned, a bone block can be inserted between the posterior aspect of the maxilla and

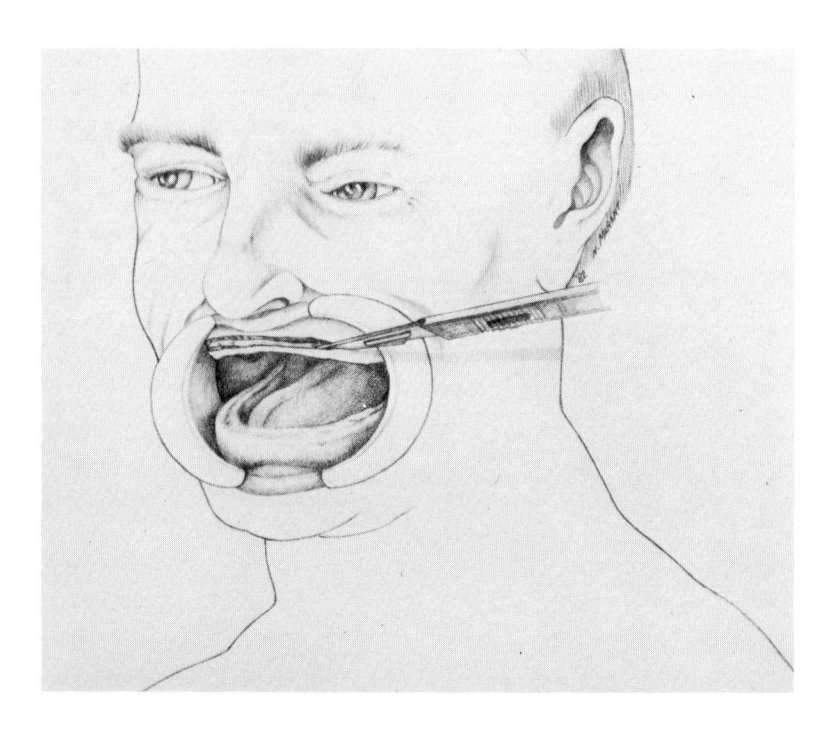

Figure 6–10. The incision should be placed in the vestibule and short of the mucosal reflection to avoid placing the scar at the periphery of the prosthesis.

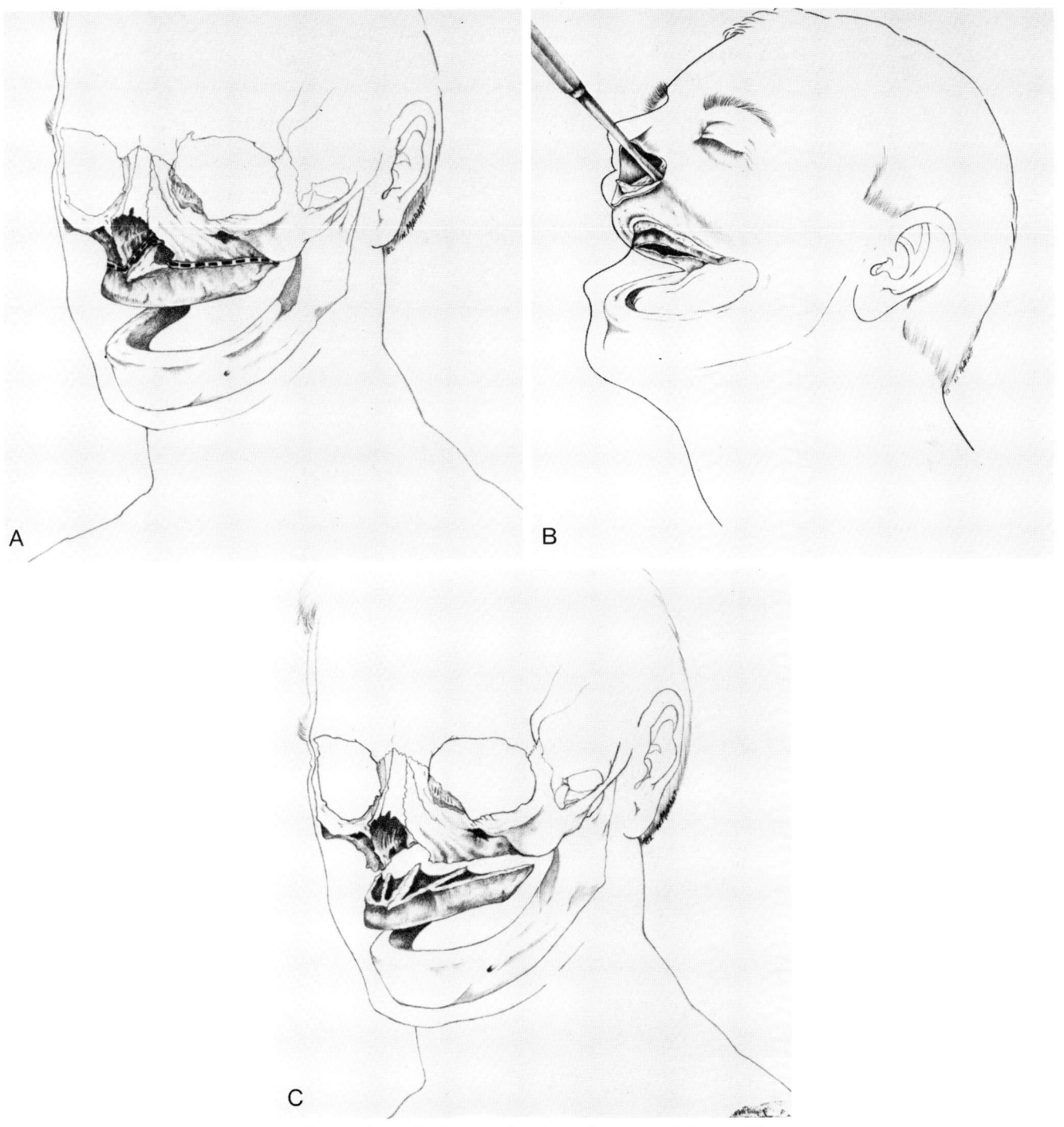

Figure 6–11. Technique for downfracture of the maxilla.

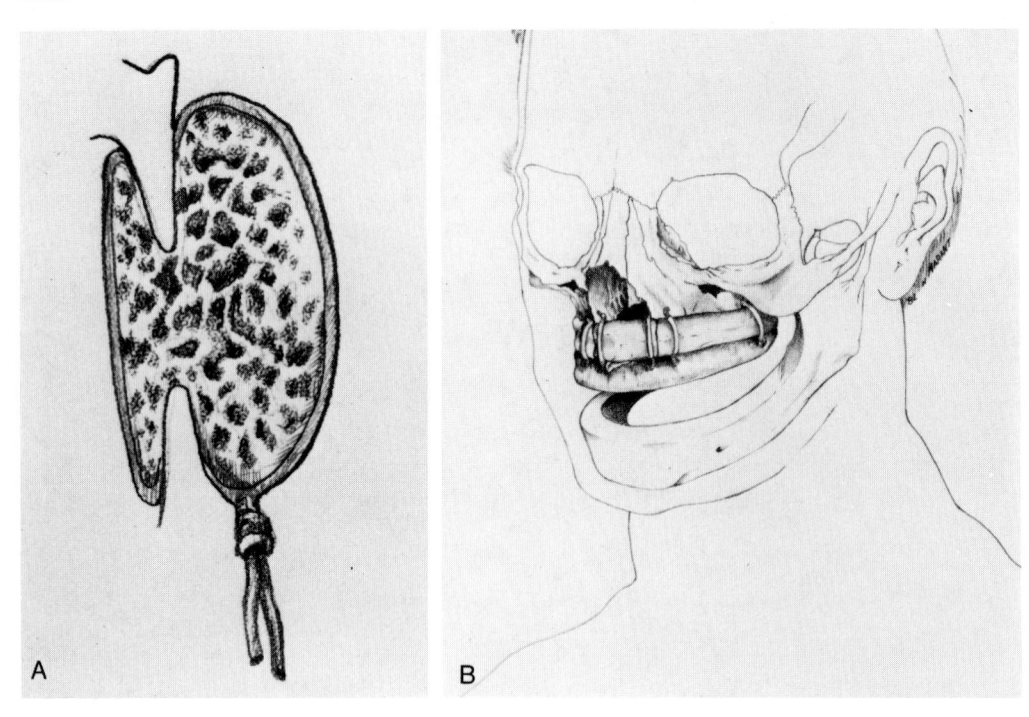

Figure 6–12. The bone graft, which has been shaped to the proper height and dumbbell mortised (*A*) for insertion along the lateral antral wall, is positioned and retained in place with transosseous wires placed through the previously placed reference holes (*B*).

the pterygoid plates[15] (Fig. 6–13). This is generally unnecessary for movements of less than 5 mm.

If allogeneic bone has been used for the interpositional graft, the autologous cancellous bone can be overlayed on the lateral aspect of the graft. This composite graft system will aid in stabilization via the allogeneic strut and in rapidity of consolidation via the autologous cancellous bone.[13, 14] A description of donor site surgery will be presented elsewhere in this chapter.

For closure it has been recommended by some to use a continuous horizontal mattress suture followed by an over-and-over stitch. However, this leaves a prominent scar in the vestibule. If close attention is paid to wound edge eversion, either a horizontal mattress suture or a continuous over-and-over stitch should be satisfactory (Fig. 6-14).

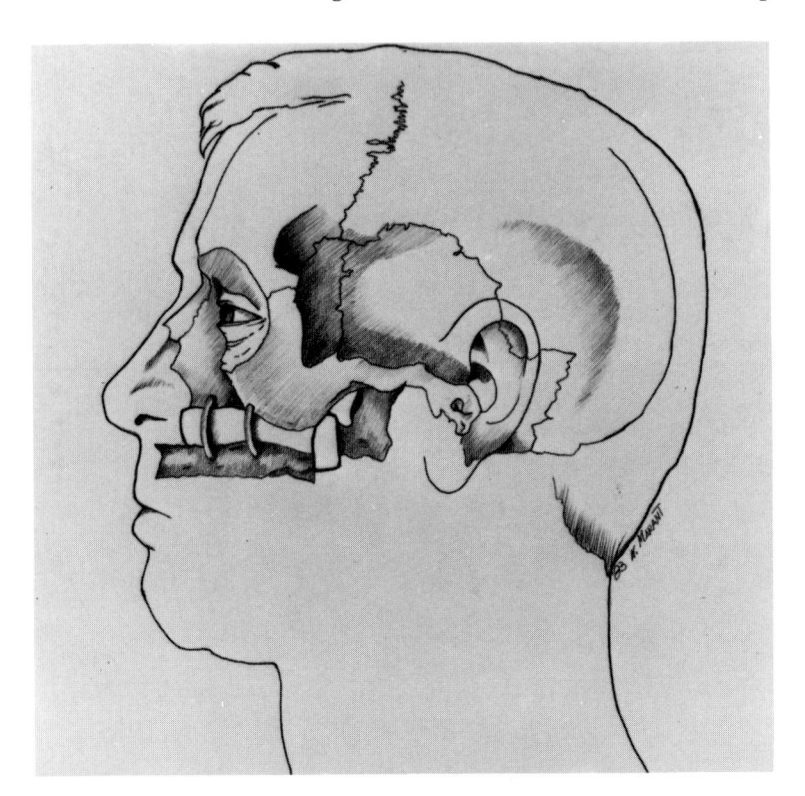

Figure 6–13. If anteroposterior movement is planned, a bone block can be inserted between the posterior aspect of the maxilla and the pterygoid plates.

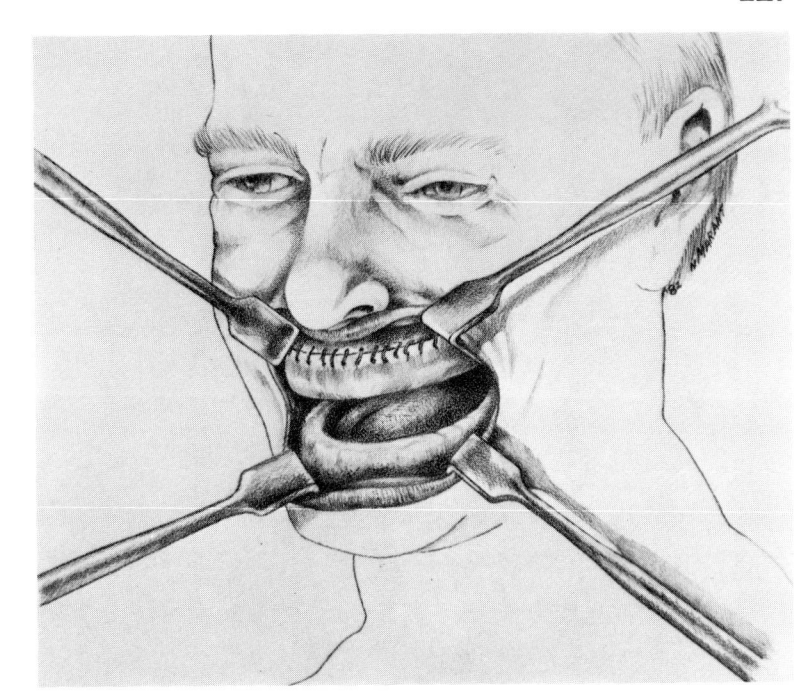

Figure 6–14. Either a horizontal mattress suture or a continuous over-and-over stitch should be satisfactory.

TOTAL MAXILLARY OSTEOTOMY WITH ADVANCEMENT

The natural tendency is for the maxilla to resorb to a smaller, more posterior position while the mandible seems to become more prominent with EBL. This, combined with vertical overclosure, gives the appearance of mandibular prognathism. If, after thorough preoperative evaluation, the patient is deemed to have a deficiency in the anteroposterior relationship or in the transverse dimension, this can be corrected at the time of vertical augmentation with interpositional bone grafting.

The maxilla can be positioned forward for a predetermined distance and stabilized with the transosseous wires and interpositional bone graft. It is advisable to graft the pterygoid plate region if movement is greater than 5 mm or if there is an anamoly that would increase the chances of relapse (cleft palate).[15] This amount of movement is generally unnecessary.

Wolford[4] has adapted the high maxillary osteotomy as advocated by Davis. A high to low osteotomy is made from high posteriorly to low anteriorly. The mobilization and advancement of the maxilla along this inclined plane will thus accomplish correction of true maxillary atrophy as well as the pseudo-class III relationship. There is a necessary limit to the amount of true inferior augmentation possible with this adaptation within the confines of the required advancement. It is still believed by this author that interpositional grafting in conjunction with this modification will be necessary in a majority of patients.

The transverse deficiency can be corrected by segmentalization of the downfractured maxilla. This is most easily completed by sectioning in a parasagittal fashion from the posterior nasal spine region to the anterior maxilla. Care is taken to assure that the palatal mucosa is not injured (Fig. 6–15). Once the osteotomy is completed, the two hemi-

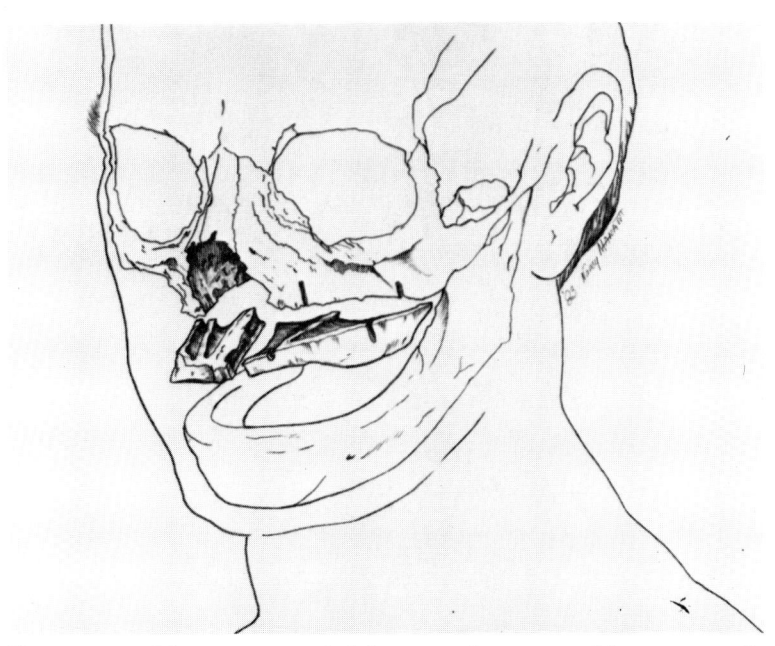

Figure 6–15 The transverse deficiency can be corrected by segmentalization of the downfractured maxilla in a parasagittal fashion from the posterior nasal spine region to the anterior maxilla.

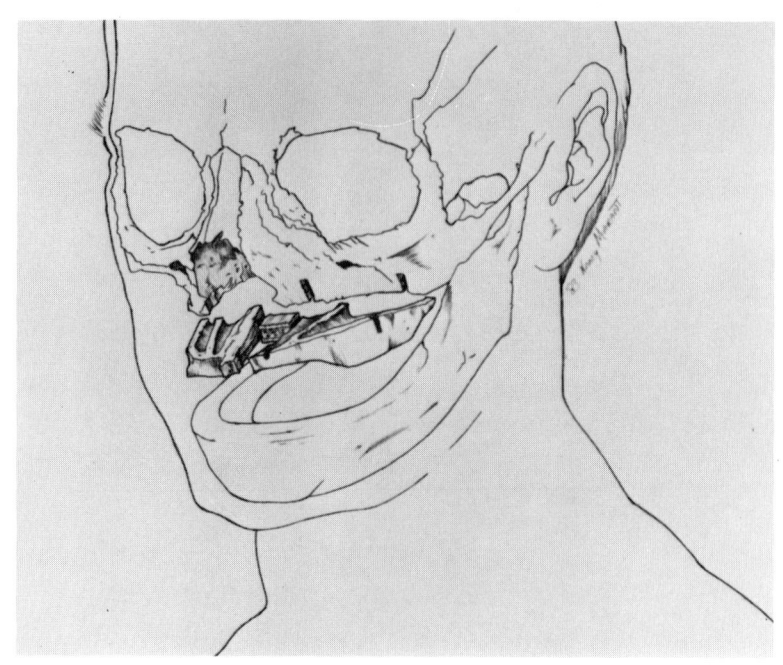

Figure 6–16. Stabilization is easily accomplished with a block of allogeneic bone placed in the posterior section to wedge the posterior aspects of the maxilla apart.

maxillary segments can be separated by rotation, and a moderate amount of palatal mucoperiosteum can be reflected from the superior aspect. This allows adequate "stretching" and lateral movement of the bony segments. Stabilization is easily accomplished by placing a block of allogeneic bone in the posterior section and wedging the posterior aspects of the maxilla apart (Fig. 6–16). The final stabilization of the maxilla can then be completed as discussed above.

TOTAL MAXILLARY OSTEOTOMY WITH PALATAL VAULT ELEVATION

The patient with severe bony deficiency in the maxilla and mild to moderate palatal vault deficiency can be treated with a total maxillary osteotomy in conjunction with a palatal vault osteotomy. The total maxillary osteotomy is completed as described above. Once in the downfractured position, a palatal osteotomy is completed from the superior aspect. The bony cuts run along the lateral aspect of the nasal palate, medial to the medial antral wall, extending from the posterior aspect of the hard palate to the canine region. The osteotomy then curves toward the midline to connect with an osteotomy of similar design from the opposite side (Fig. 6–17). This nasal floor segment is then elevated in the anterior aspect to allow for superior repositioning while the maxilla is moved inferiorly (Fig. 6–18). The nasal floor can be blocked superiorly by allogeneic bone grafts and placed anteriorly. It can be moved anteriorly and onlayed over the cut edge of maxillary bone. Generally, no resection of nasal septum is necessary when the total maxilla is repositioned inferiorly. The remainder of the procedure is as described above.

PALATAL VAULT OSTEOTOMY

Adequate stability of the maxillary prosthesis is usually not difficult for the prosthodontist to achieve; however, when anteroposterior stability cannot be achieved, the palatal vault osteotomy, as described by Charest and Goodyear[16] and modified by Leonard and Howe,[17] adds depth to the hard palate and causes a pseudoaugmentation of the alveolar ridge (Table 6–5). As described by Charest and Goodyear,[16] the palatal vault osteotomy requires a full palatal flap followed by downfracture of the palate and removal of septal bone. The palate is then moved superiorly. Poor blood supply to the palatal bone is a hazard. Charest and Goodyear found gains in the palatal vault depth of 8 to 10 mm. Leonard and Howe[17] used a similar procedure and reported their results in five patients. They used a stent lined with gutta-percha to maintain the height over a three- to four-week period.

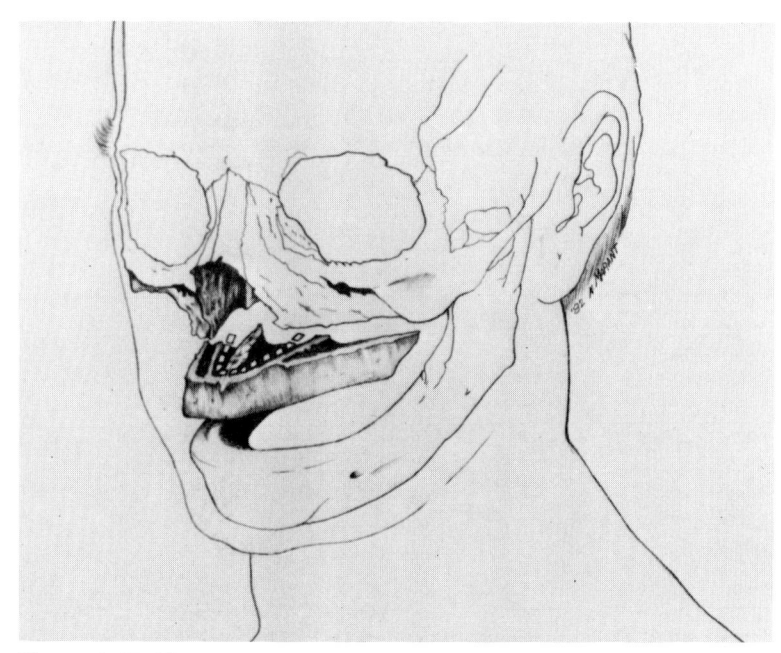

Figure 6–17. The osteotomy curves toward the midline to connect with an osteotomy of similar design from the opposite side.

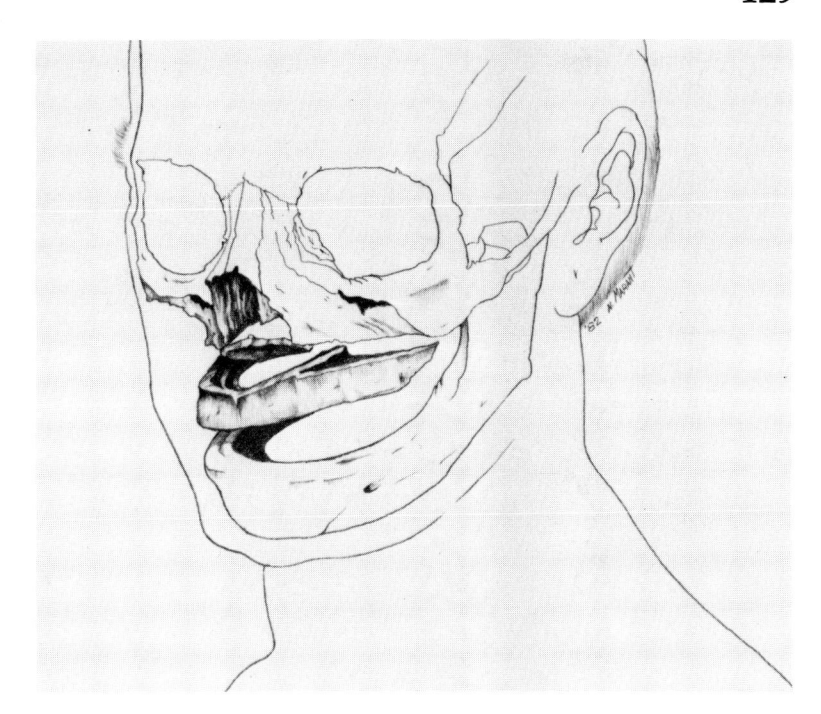

Figure 6–18. This nasal floor segment is then elevated in the anterior aspect so as to allow for superior repositioning while the maxilla is moved inferiorly.

The results were stable over a brief follow-up period and compared favorably in vault depth to a group of patients who had recently had all their teeth removed.

Indications for this procedure include adequate maxillary height and proper position. Poor vault form causes instability of the prosthesis or requires an interpositional graft to improve vault form. Advantages of the procedure are relative ease of operation, creation of a new vault form with increased resistance to prosthetic displacement, and pseudoaugmentation of the alveolar ridge. Disadvantages are the danger to the blood supply with the Charest technique[16] and the unknown stability of the procedure. There are only two reported series, both quite small.

TABLE 6–5. ISOLATED POOR PALATAL VAULT FORM

Treatment:	Palatal vault osteotomy
Indications:	1. Adequate ridge height and position but poor vault form
	2. In conjunction with interpositional grafts to improve vault forms
Contraindications:	1. Scarred palate of cleft patient
Advantages:	1. Creates new vault form
	2. Stability of prosthesis is improved
	3. Pseudoaugmentation of the atrophic ridge
Disadvantages:	1. Poor blood supply to palatal segment
	2. Stability and long-term results unknown

Surgical Technique

The surgical procedure requires general anesthesia with nasal intubation. The original description involved a complete palatal mucoperiosteal flap just to the palatal aspect of the ridge crest (Figs. 6–19 and 6–20). Care must be taken to preserve the greater palatine vessels. The osteotomy is completed with a round bur, in a U shape along the base of the residual alveolar ridge on the palatal aspect. Once the osteotomy is completed to the posterior aspect of the palate and medial to the palatine vessels, the bone section is slightly downfractured in the anterior to expose the nasal mucosa and septum. The nasal septum is sectioned and the hard palate becomes completely free (Fig. 6–21). Cartilage and bone are removed from the nasal septum to allow for superior repositioning of the palatal bone (Fig. 6–22).

The palatal bone is pushed superiorly to maintain contact with the nasal mucosa. The bone is raised higher anteriorly to give a favorable slope to the palate for retention of the prosthesis as well as nasal drainage[17] (Fig. 6–23).

Closure is accomplished after mobilization and advancement of the palatal flap. Closure using vertical mattress sutures is recommended (Fig. 6–24). The patient's prosthesis can be modified with compound added to the palatal side of the prosthesis to maintain flap position. Pressure should not be placed over the palatal vessels or the mucosa. Stabilization is usually unnecessary and the device is treated like an immediate prosthesis, removed after 48 hours for cleaning only.

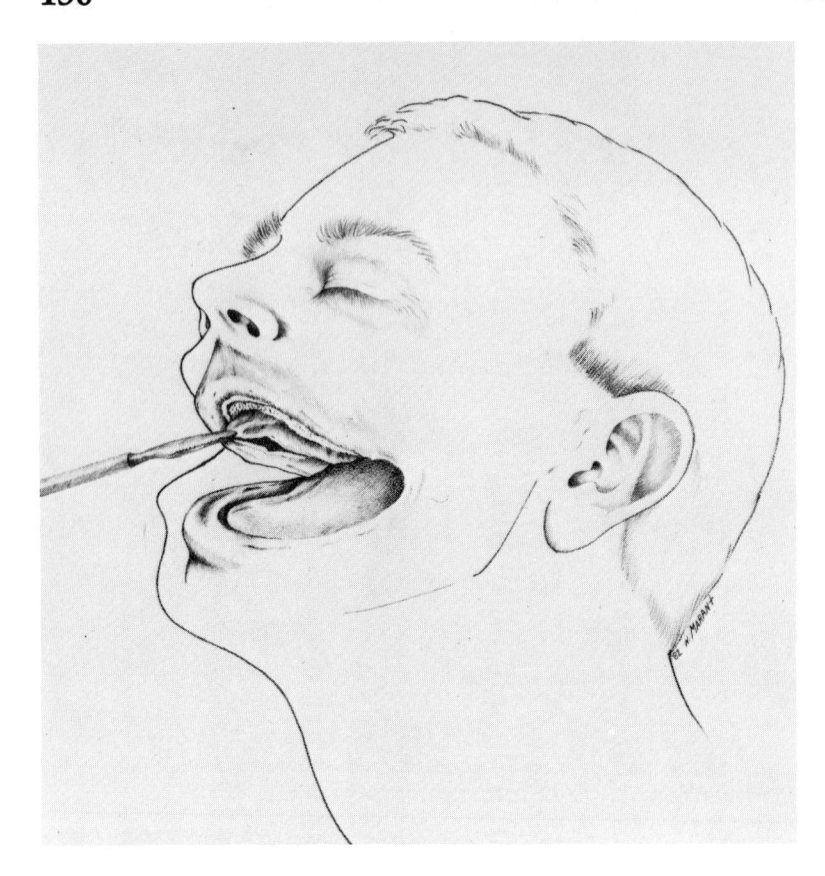

Figure 6–19. The original description involved a complete palatal mucoperiosteal flap just to the palatal aspect of the ridge crest.

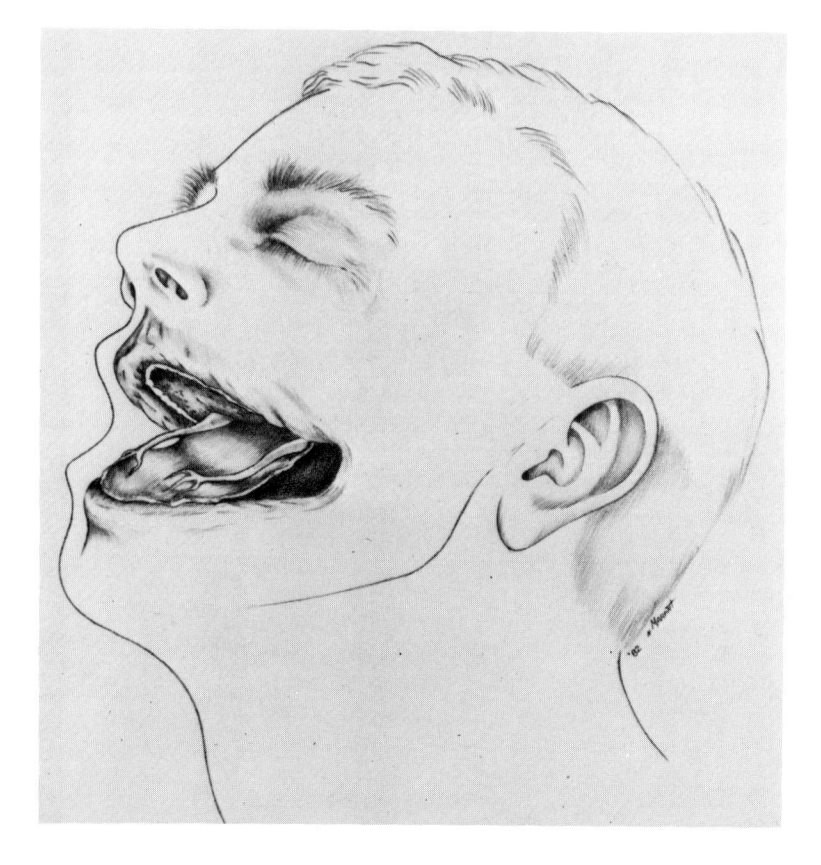

Figure 6–20. Care must be taken to preserve the greater palatine vessels.

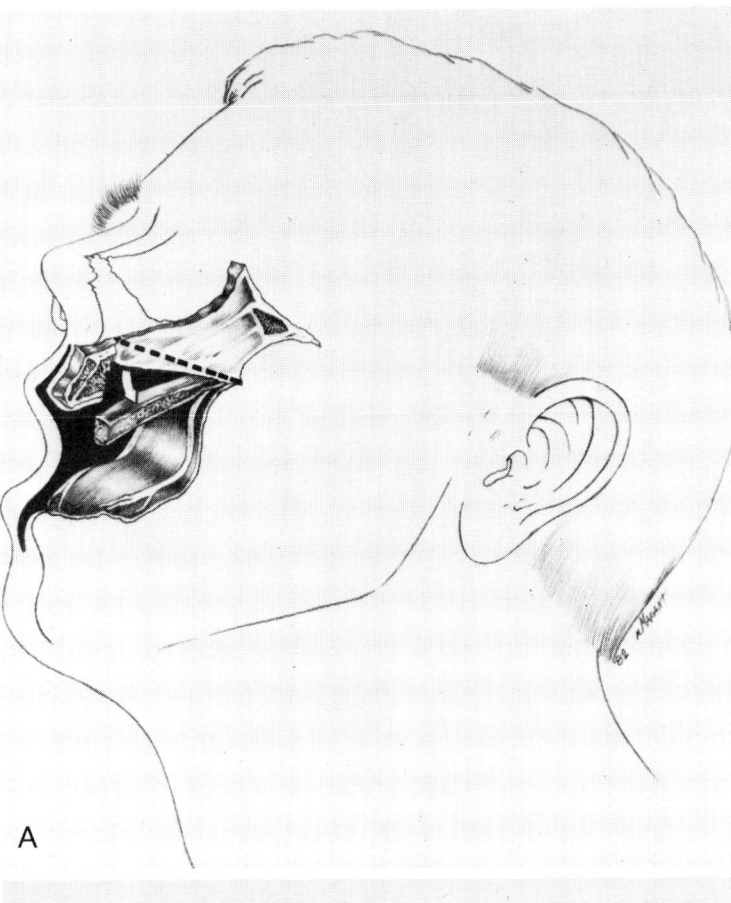

Figure 6–21. The nasal septum is sectioned (*A*) and the hard palate becomes completely free (*B*).

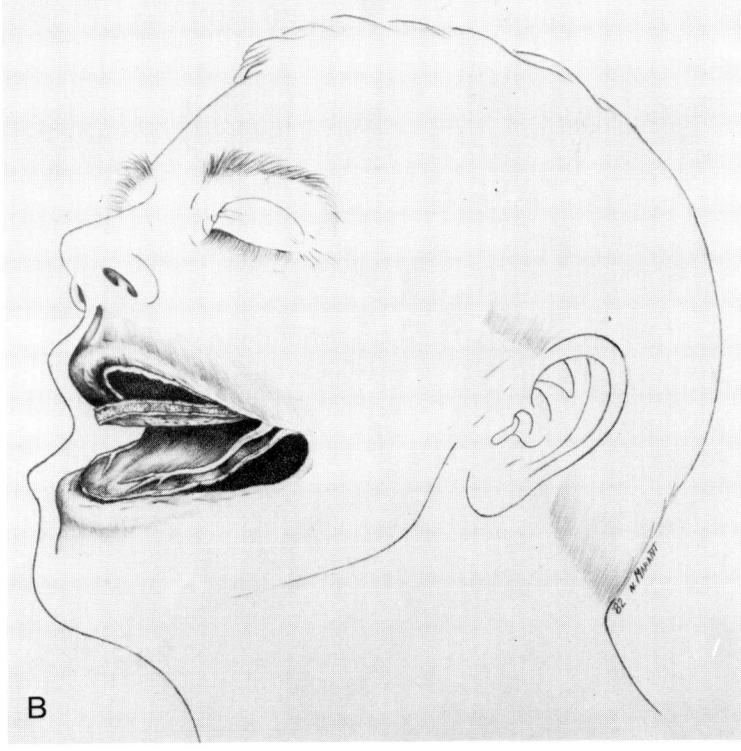

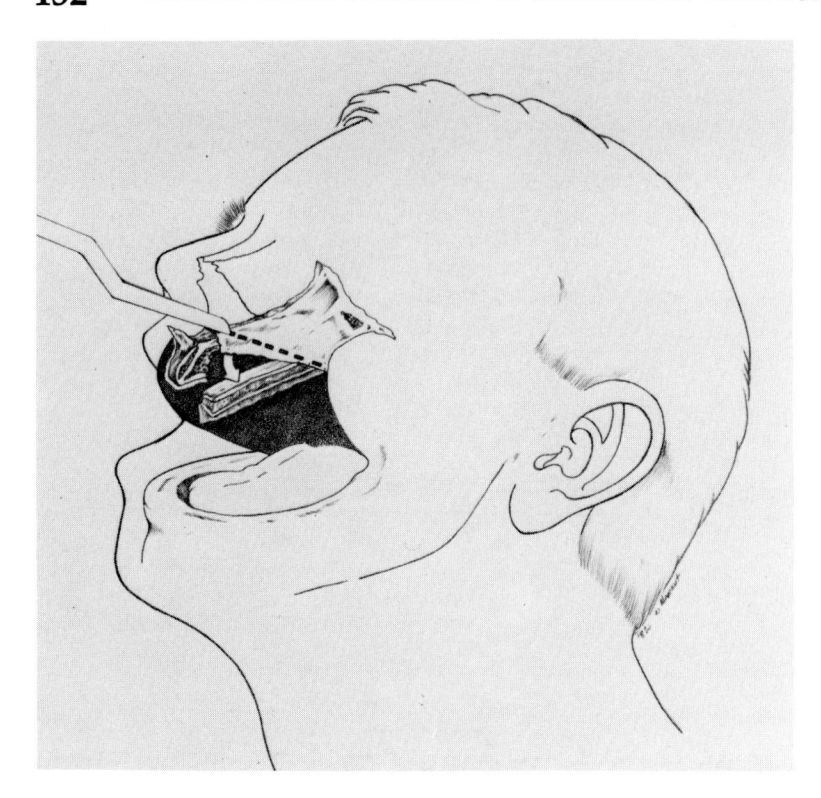

132 / OSSEOUS RECONSTRUCTION OF EDENTULOUS BONE LOSS

Figure 6–22. Cartilage and bone are removed from the nasal septum to allow for superior repositioning of the palatal bone.

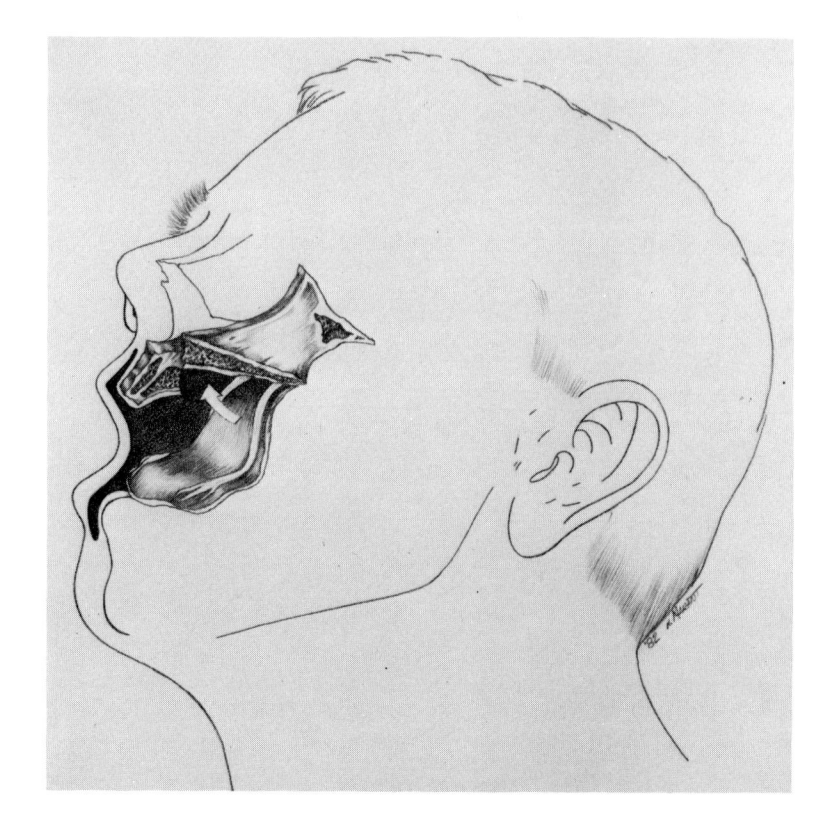

Figure 6–23. The bone is raised higher anteriorly to give a favorable slope to the palate for retention of the prosthesis as well as for nasal drainage.

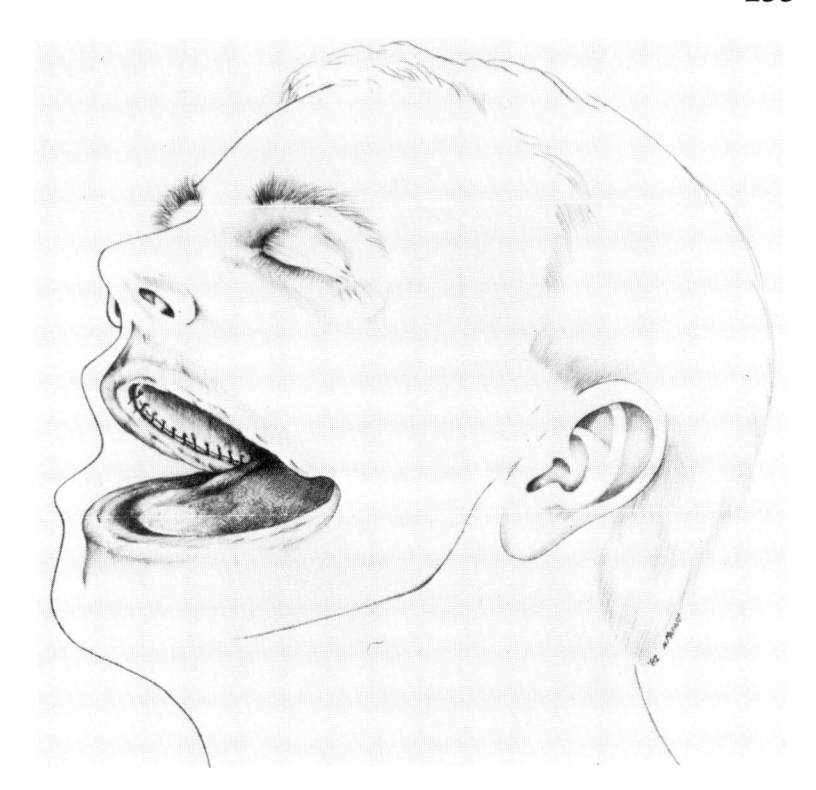

Figure 6–24. Closure is accomplished after mobilization and advancement of the palatal flap using vertical mattress sutures.

ANTERIOR MAXILLARY OSTEOTOMIES

Anterior maxillary osteotomies are generally well accepted in orthognathic surgery to correct localized deformities in the anterior maxilla (Table 6–6). There has been only one report in the English literature of an adaptation of these procedures for the edentulous patient. These patients may have anterior EBL that is more severe than the posterior EBL[18] and lends itself to anterior correction. It is usually a result of occlusion between natural mandibular anterior teeth and an edentulous maxilla. The abnormal and excessive forces applied to the anterior maxilla will result in early and excessive atrophy.

Indications for maxillary anterior osteotomies to correct EBL include those commonly seen in patients who require onlay bone grafting procedures. Inadequate basal bone to permit a satisfactory maxillary vestibuloplasty, with adequate tuberosities and a poor palatal vault form, could be corrected by one of the following procedures. Contraindications would be a redundant soft-tissue ridge with a good basilar bone level. Advantages of the anterior maxillary procedures are rapid healing, localized procedure with minimal surgical difficulty, and relatively rapid (vs. onlay bone grafts) prosthetic completion. Unfortunately, the long-term results using this technique are not yet known.

Liposky reported in 1979 on the combined use of a vestibuloplasty and osteotomy for correction of anterior maxillary EBL.[18] His procedure was a stepped osteotomy that allowed for telescoping of the pedicled osseous segment inferiorly while still maintaining bony contact at the lateral piriform margins and at the posterior contact points (Fig. 6–25). The osteotomy was stabilized with wire osteosynthesis. If necessary, a bone graft can be placed in the nasal septum area. Vertical cuts of the osteotomy should parallel the planned movement in order to aid in immobilization. Liposky recommended harvesting the bone graft from the malar eminence.

One inherent problem with this procedure without interpositional grafting is the increase in size of the piriform aperture and

TABLE 6–6. ANTERIOR MAXILLARY ATROPHY

Treatment:	Anterior maxillary osteotomy with or without bone grafting
Indications:	1. Severe anterior atrophy 2. Poor anterior palatal form
Contraindications:	1. Total ridge atrophy 2. Redundant soft tissue over adequate basilar bone
Advantages:	1. Corrects localized atrophy 2. Creates better vault form 3. May not require secondary soft tissue procedure
Disadvantages:	Stability unknown

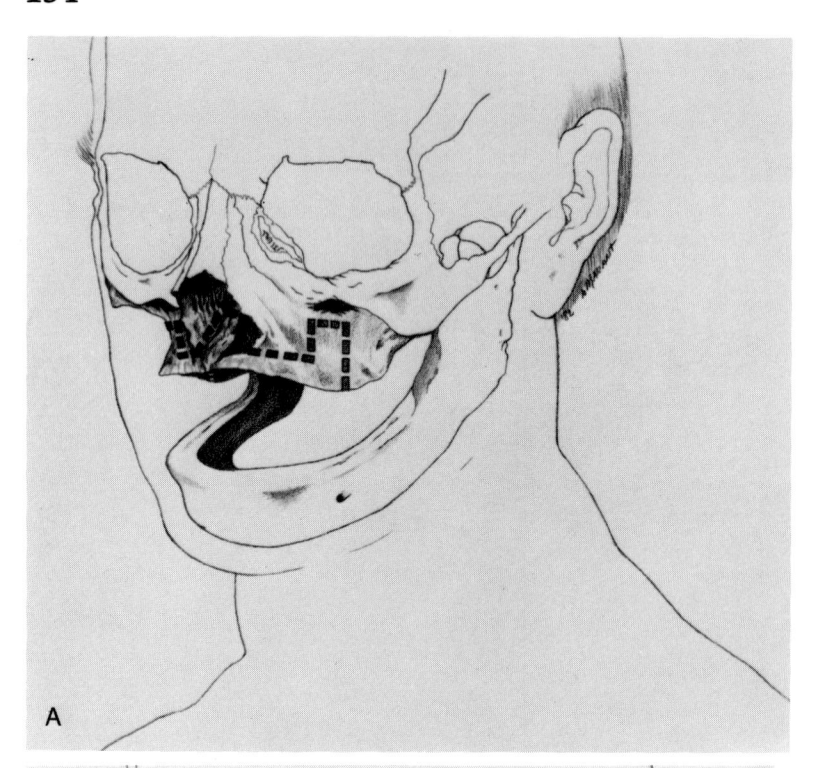

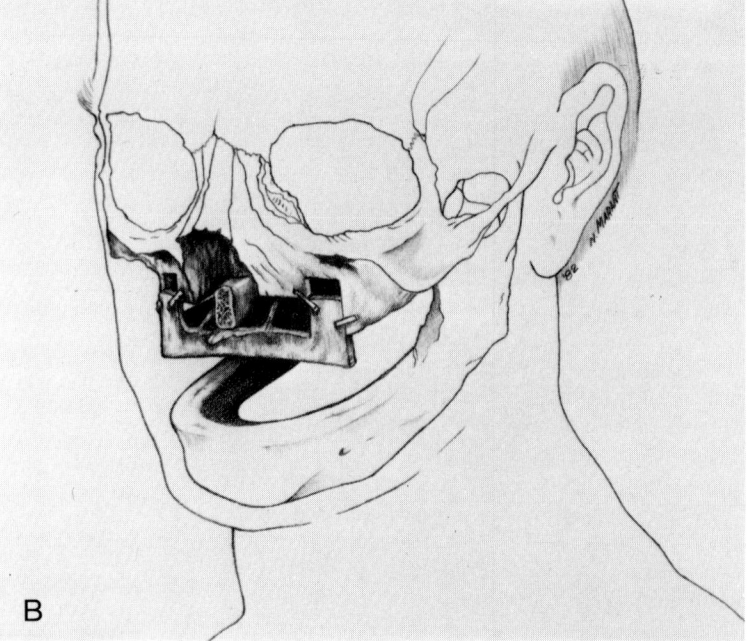

134 / OSSEOUS RECONSTRUCTION OF EDENTULOUS BONE LOSS

Figure 6–25. Telescoping of the pedicled osseous segment inferiorly while still maintaining bony contact at the lateral piriform margins and at the posterior contact points.

the unsupported soft tissue that overlies it. Continued resorption, which can be expected, would not be managed by this technique. Adaptation of this osteotomy to follow the well-accepted concept of interpositional bone grafting is suggested.

Surgical Technique

An anterior segmental osteotomy with downfracture is performed. Bone cuts are made at the juncture of the posterior maxilla with the anterior EBL (Fig. 6–26) and extend vertically 8 to 12 mm. Then a horizontal osteotomy is completed through the lateral maxillary wall into the piriform aperture. Adequate protection and retraction of soft tissues in the nose are performed. Next, with digital palpation of the palate a palatal osteotomy is completed in the midline. Protection of the palatal mucosa from damage is of great importance, as this is the major blood supply to the segment. Finally, the nasal septum is released with an appropriate osteotome. This allows for downfracturing of the anterior maxilla (Fig. 6–27). Using digital manipulation of the segment, as well as

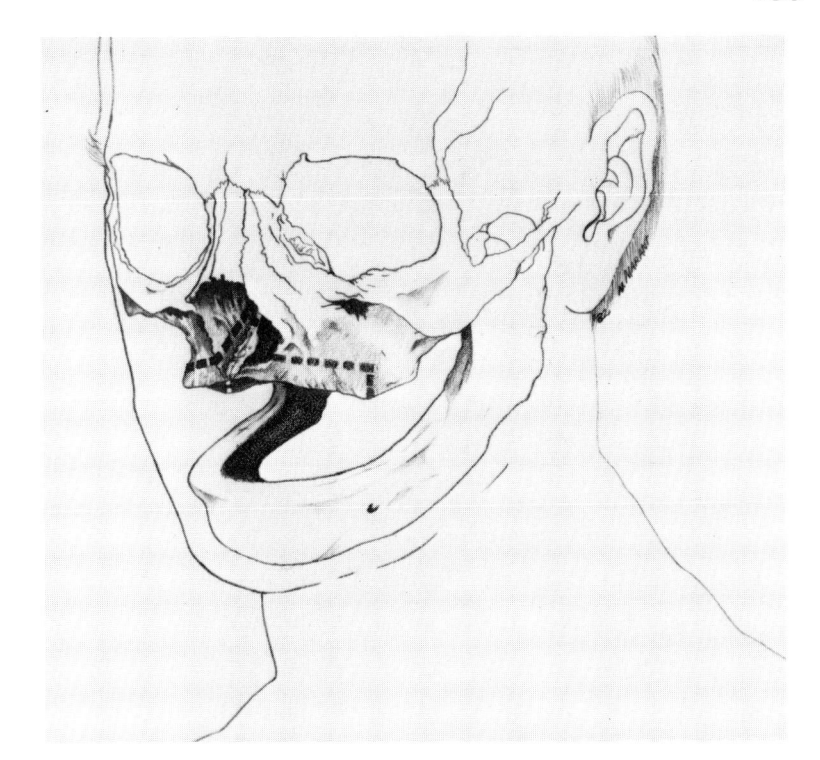

OSSEOUS RECONSTRUCTION OF EDENTULOUS BONE LOSS / **135**

Figure 6–26. Bone cuts are made at the juncture of the posterior maxilla with the anterior EBL and extend vertically 8 to 12 mm.

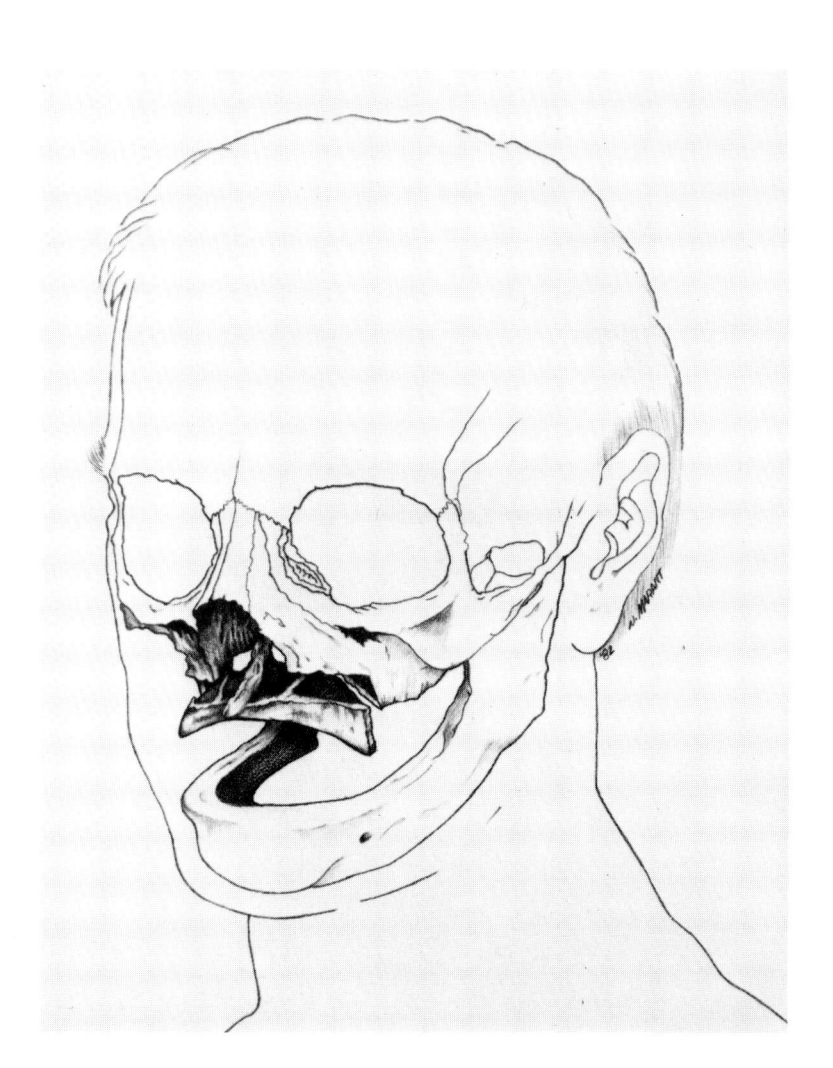

Figure 6–27. The nasal septum is released with an appropriate osteotome, allowing for downfracturing of the anterior maxilla.

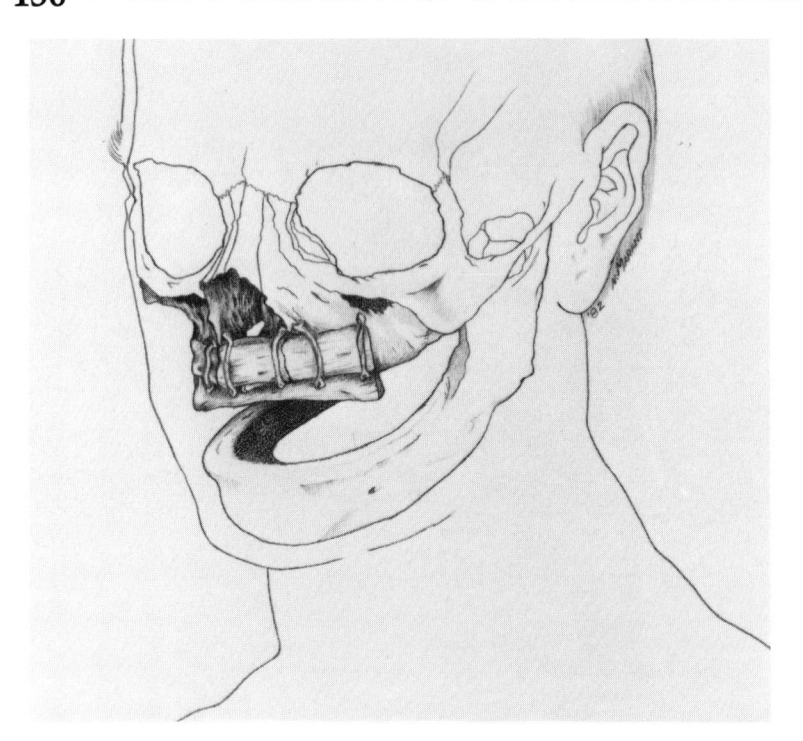

Figure 6-28. Interpositional bone grafts of an appropriate material can be fashioned to stabilize the anterior maxilla in its new inferior position.

subperiosteal dissection of the stable posterior maxilla, the segment can be mobilized to allow for inferior repositioning. This is accomplished by dissecting the palatal mucosa and alveolar ridge mucosa off the stable segment from the downfractured position.

Interpositional bone grafts of an appropriate material can be fashioned to stabilize the anterior maxilla in its new inferior position (Fig. 6-28). Allogeneic bone with autologous marrow can be used for this procedure; however, there is no clinical reason to avoid allogeneic bone solely. The graft should be "dumbbelled" to stabilize the segment without danger of slipping. It is then wired in place. It should cross the entire labial length of the osteotomy. This gives support to the labial soft tissue as well and allows for less change in the piriform aperture.

Postoperative Management for Maxillary Procedures

Dietary considerations are managed as in all postoperative patients. Special attention to the suture line includes the use of a clear liquid diet for the first 48 hours postoperatively to prevent accumulation of milk products and food particles on the incision until initial sealing has occurred. After 48 hours, a soft pureed diet should be prescribed. It is desirable to discourage the patient from chewing or performing functions that would place stress on the graft or suture lines.

Frequent saline rinses and cleaning of the suture line with cotton-tipped applicators mechanically remove debris and food particles. This should be done frequently after the first 48 hours.

Antibiotics are given parenterally beginning immediately preoperatively and continuing until the intravenous line is removed, usually at 48 hours. Then the antibiotics are administered orally for 10 days. For operations that have involved the maxillary antrum, systemic decongestants and local, topically active decongestants and antihistamines are used to maintain patency of the osteum and decrease nasal mucosal engorgement.

Steroids, in a regimen similar to that employed for orthognathic surgical cases, have routinely been used for these osteotomies and bone grafts over the past five years without any appreciable deleterious effects and without any contraindications to steroids. Methylprednisolone, 500 mg intravenously when the procedure begins and then 250 mg every four hours until the intravenous fluids are stopped, has reduced edema and improved patient comfort. A slow-release intramuscular steroid is administered once when the final dose of intravenous steroids (80 mg methylprednisolone) has been administered.

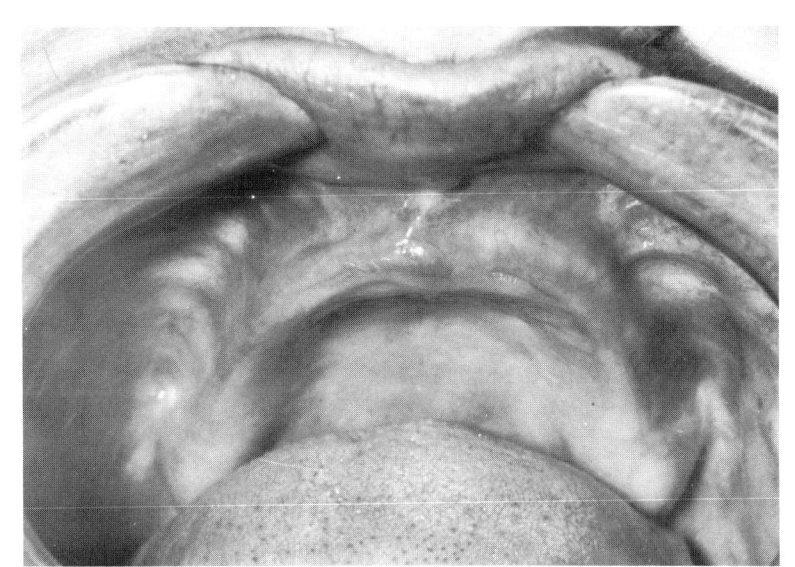

Figure 6–29. Clinical appearance of the vertically deficient maxilla.

CASE I—MAXILLARY ATROPHY WITH ADEQUATE PALATAL VAULT FORM

B.F. presented with a chief complaint of inability to adequately tolerate upper and lower prostheses. She had been edentulous for over 25 years and had had multiple prosthetic replacements. She was evaluated by the prosthetic and oral/maxillofacial services for reconstruction of the atrophic maxilla and mandible. The maxilla will be discussed here.

Clinically there was adequate palatal vault shape and depth but moderate to severe vertical bony deficiency and mild horizontal deficiency. The transverse arch size was acceptable. The soft tissue was of adequate character; however, the depth of the labial vestibule was minimal. A mirror test verified that the soft tissue was adequate but the bony base was deficient (Fig. 6–29)

Radiographically the lateral cephalogram, posterior cephalogram, and panoramic views showed severe maxillary atrophy vertically and mild horizontal hypoplasia (Fig. 6–30).

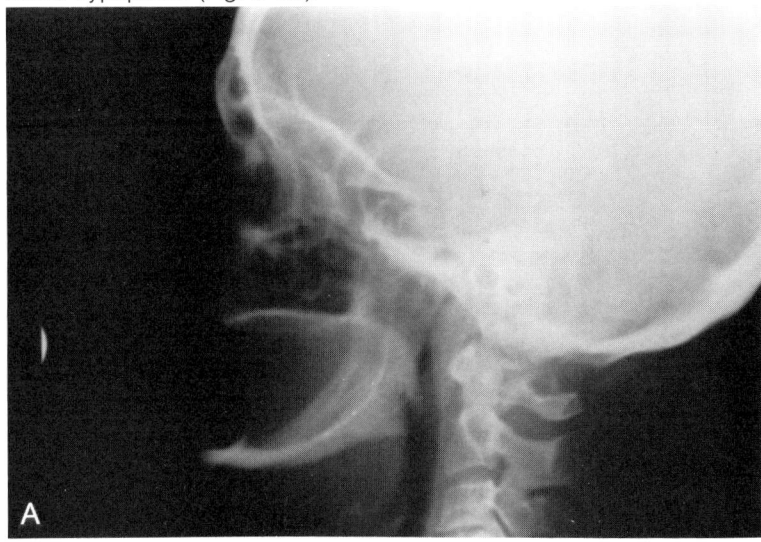

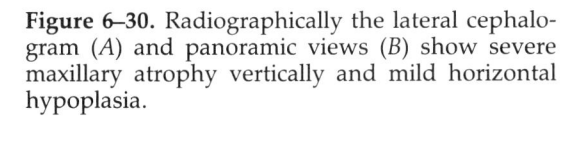

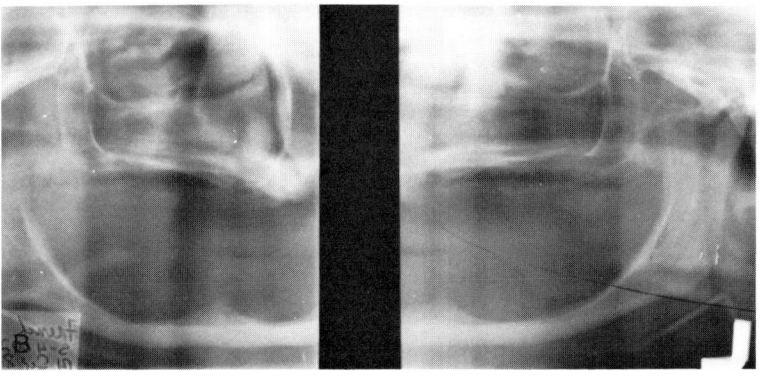

Figure 6–30. Radiographically the lateral cephalogram (A) and panoramic views (B) show severe maxillary atrophy vertically and mild horizontal hypoplasia.

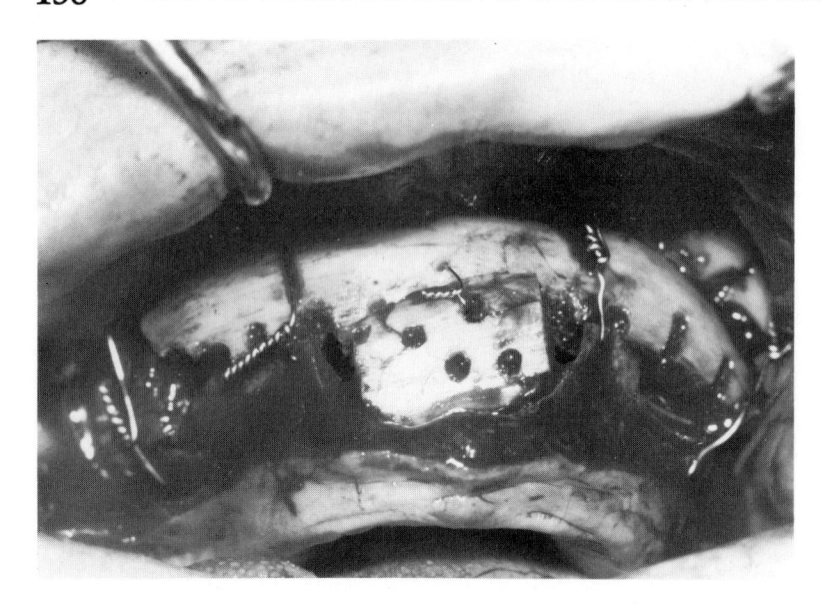

Figure 6–31. The graft was stabilized with transosseous stainless steel wire.

A problem list and treatment plan were developed.
Problems
 1. Maxillary vertical atrophy
 2. Maxillary horizontal deficiency
 3. Mandibular problems (discussed previously)
Treatment Plan
 1. Total maxillary osteotomy; interpositional bone graft with allogeneic rib and particulate cancellous marrow (composite graft)
 2. Mandibular procedures (discussed previously)

Under general anesthesia the total maxillary osteotomy with interpositional bone grafting was performed as previously described. The graft was stabilized with transosseous stainless steel wire (Fig. 6–31). Healing was uneventful and the prosthetic department completed removable denture fabrication. The patient is shown two years postoperatively (Fig. 6–32) with excellent vestibular depth and good vertical height of the maxillary alveolus.

Radiographs immediately postoperatively (Fig. 6–33A) and two years postoperatively (Fig. 6–33B) show good horizontal and vertical position to the maxilla. The grafts of allogeneic bone are still evident.

CASE II—ANTERIOR MAXILLARY ATROPHY WITH ADEQUATE TUBEROSITY

G.A., a 53-year-old white female, was referred by her prosthodontist for correction of severe maxillary anterior atrophy. The mandibular problems were also treated and will be discussed elsewhere. She had been totally edentulous for some 20 years and had worn some form of prosthesis for 25 years. She had undergone multiple recent attempts at prosthetic rehabilitation, all of which were unsuccessful. She and her prosthodontist desired bony reconstruction of the maxilla to facilitate normal prosthetic management.

Clinically there was an anterior deficit of bone

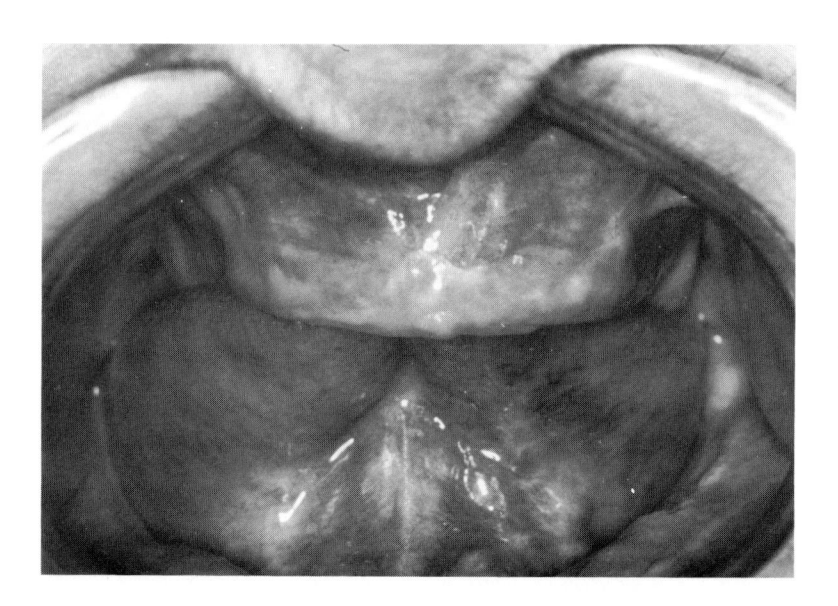

Figure 6–32. The patient is shown two years postoperatively with excellent vestibular depth and good vertical height of the maxillary alveolus.

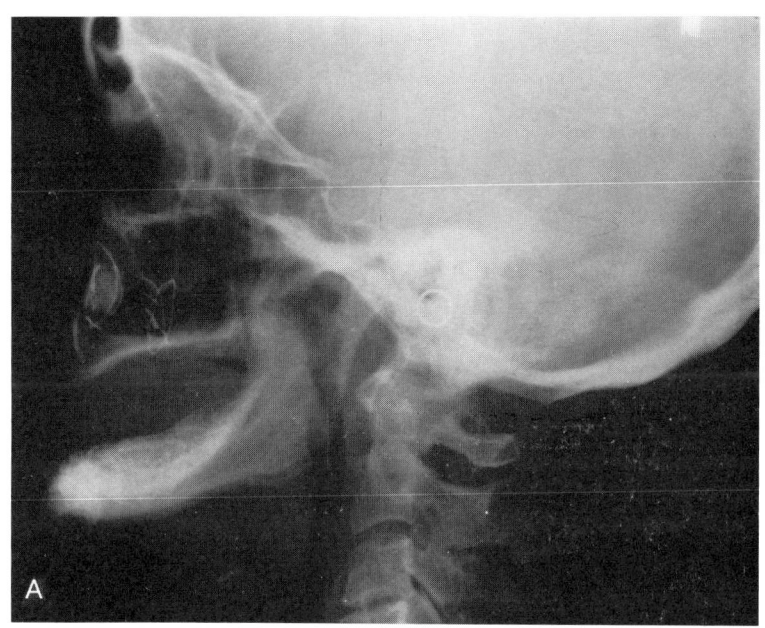

OSSEOUS RECONSTRUCTION OF EDENTULOUS BONE LOSS / **139**

Figure 6–33. Radiographs immediately postoperatively (*A*) and two years postoperatively (*B*) show good horizontal and vertical position to the maxilla. The grafts of allogeneic bone are still evident.

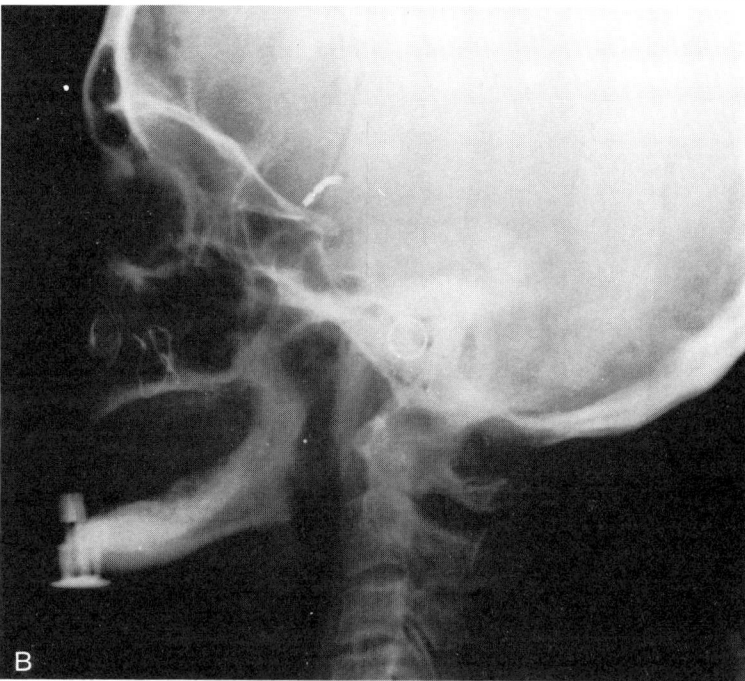

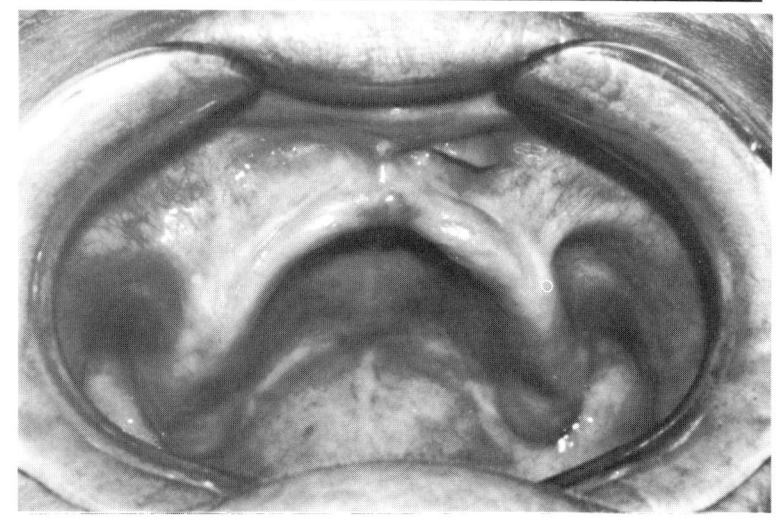

Figure 6–34. Clinically there was an anterior deficit of bone with poor palatal vault form. Posteriorly the tuberosities were acceptable and the palatal form was good.

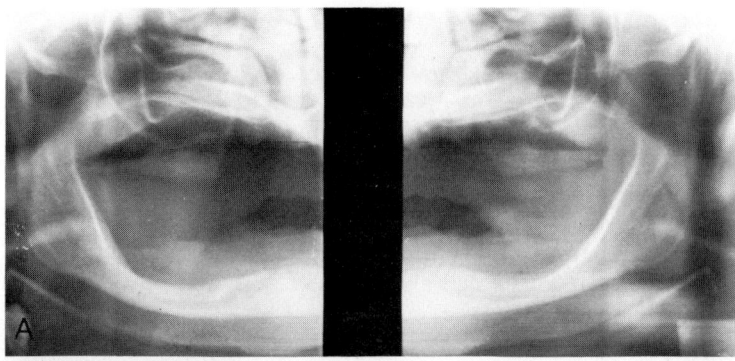

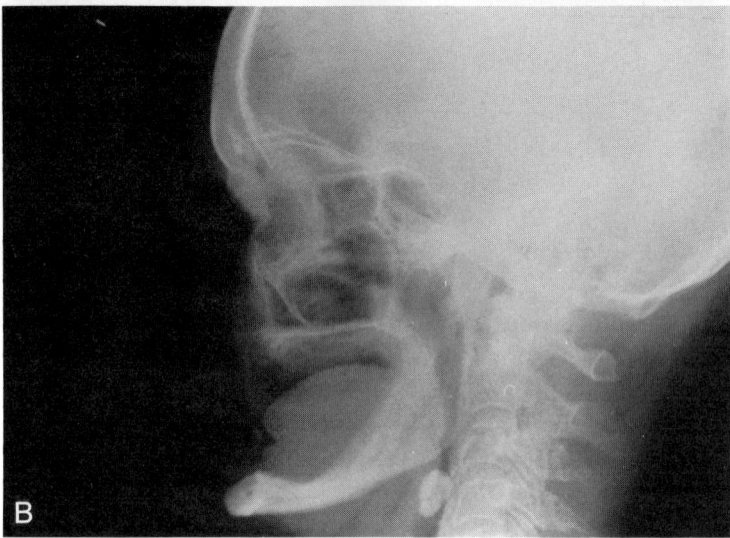

140 / OSSEOUS RECONSTRUCTION OF EDENTULOUS BONE LOSS

Figure 6–35. Radiographically there is a marked vertical slant to the anterior maxilla while the posterior maxilla appears relatively normal.

with poor palatal vault form. Posteriorly the tuberosities were acceptable and the palatal form was good (Fig. 6–34). There was no horizontal deficit to the maxilla.

Radiographically there was a marked vertical slant to the anterior maxilla (Fig. 6–35), whereas the posterior maxilla appeared relatively normal. The defect started in approximately the premolar region bilaterally.

A problem list and treatment plan were developed.

Problems
1. Maxillary anterior vertical atrophy
2. Mandibular atrophy (discussed previously)

Treatment Plan
1. Anterior maxillary osteotomy with interpositional bone graft
2. Mandibular procedures (discussed previously)

Under general anesthesia the maxilla was approached with a vestibular incision from the pre-

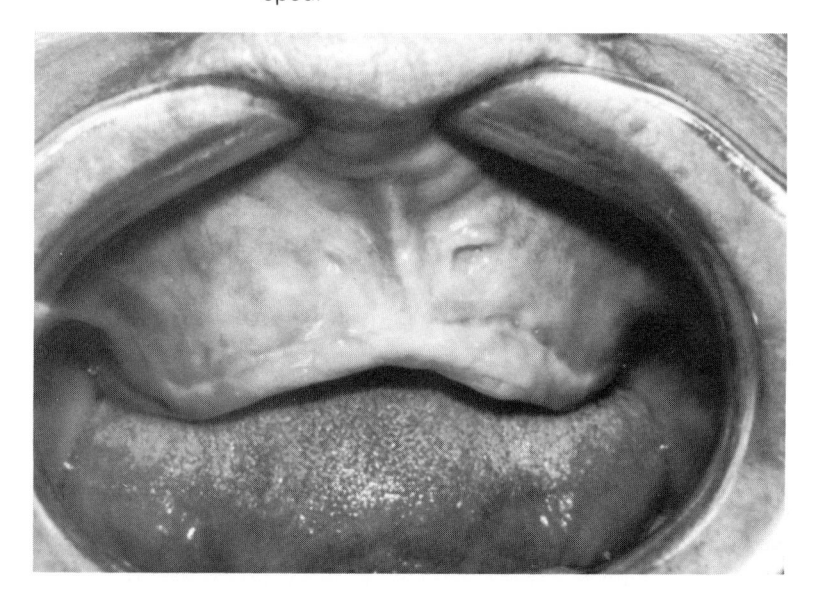

Figure 6–36. The postoperative result is excellent, and prosthetic replacement was completed without complications.

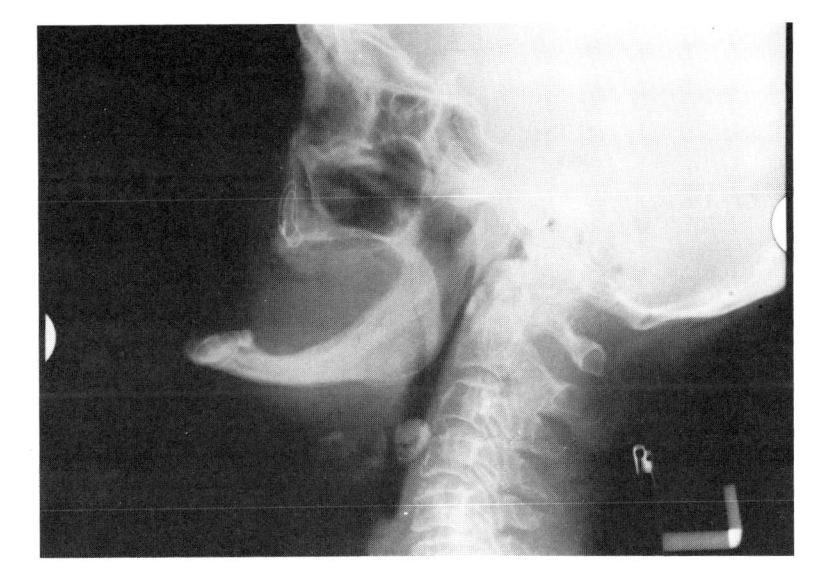

Figure 6–37. Radiographic evaluation of the graft two years postoperatively shows the stable result.

molar region on the right to the premolar region on the left. After elevation of the flaps an anterior maxillary osteotomy was performed, as previously described in the text. The area was inferiorly repositioned and stabilized with an interpositional graft of allogeneic rib. The graft was held in position with stainless steel wire and the incision closed.

The postoperative result was excellent, and prosthetic replacement was completed without complications (Fig. 6–36). Radiographic evaluation of the graft two years postoperatively shows the stable result (Fig. 6–37).

CASE III—TOTAL MAXILLARY OSTEOTOMY WITH PALATAL VAULT EXTENSION

A 50-year-old white female presented to the University of Iowa oral surgery clinic with a chief complaint of inability to wear her upper denture. She was referred by her prosthodontist, who had requested a ridge augmentation procedure to increase the denture-bearing area of the maxilla. Clinical and radiographic examination revealed an atrophic maxilla with very little basilar bone left to the maxilla and a very shallow palatal vault (Fig. 6–38). Her buccal and labial vestibules were confluent with the crest of the ridge. It was felt that a total maxillary osteotomy with a palatal vault extension would be the procedure of choice to correct her problem.

In May of 1979, under general anesthesia, she underwent a total maxillary osteotomy with a horizontal incision from the buttress area on the one side to the buttress area on the opposite side. Once the maxilla was downfractured, a palatal vault osteotomy was performed at the junction of the alveolar and palatal portions of the maxilla in a horseshoe-shaped fashion (Fig. 6–39). Allogeneic bone grafts were placed between the palatal and alveolar portions of the palatal osteotomy and along the lateral wall of the maxilla and wired into place with 25-A stainless steel wire at the buttress and piriform aperture areas (Fig. 6–40). A small bone graft was placed across the base of the piriform aperture connecting the two lateral bone grafts. The patient's immediate postoperative course was uneventful and she was discharged on the fourth postoperative day.

Approximately five months after the ridge augmentation procedure a maxillary vestibuloplasty utilizing palatal mucosa as donor tissue was performed. Approximately two months after that the patient's dentures were fabricated. A two-year follow-up of her result revealed good retention of

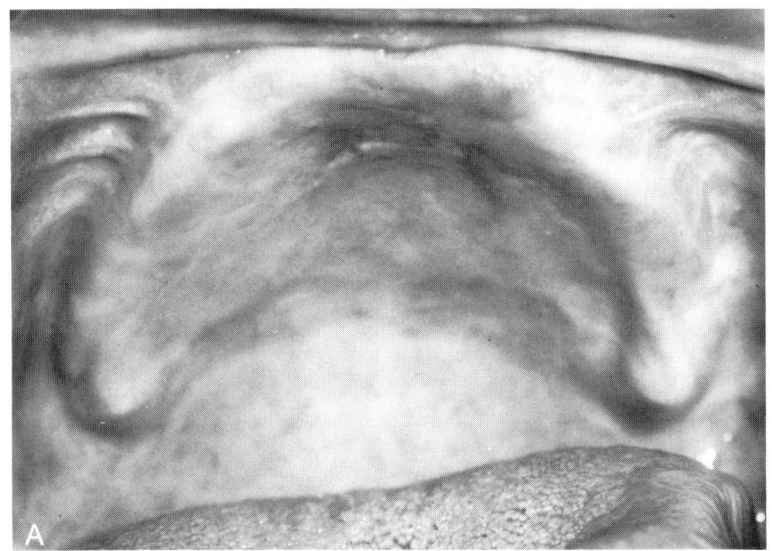

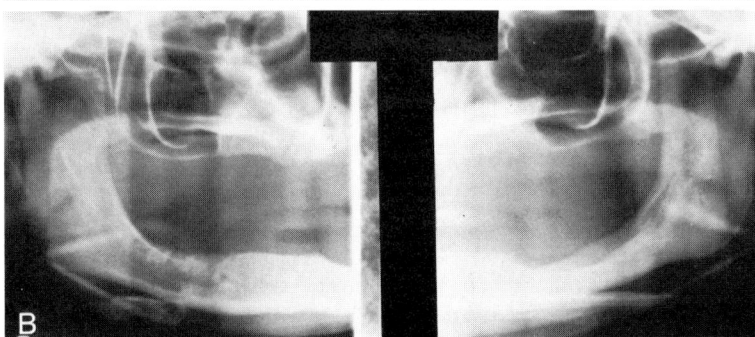

Figure 6–38. Clinical (*A*) and radiographic (*B*) examination revealed an atrophic maxilla with very little basilar bone left to the maxilla and a very shallow palatal vault.

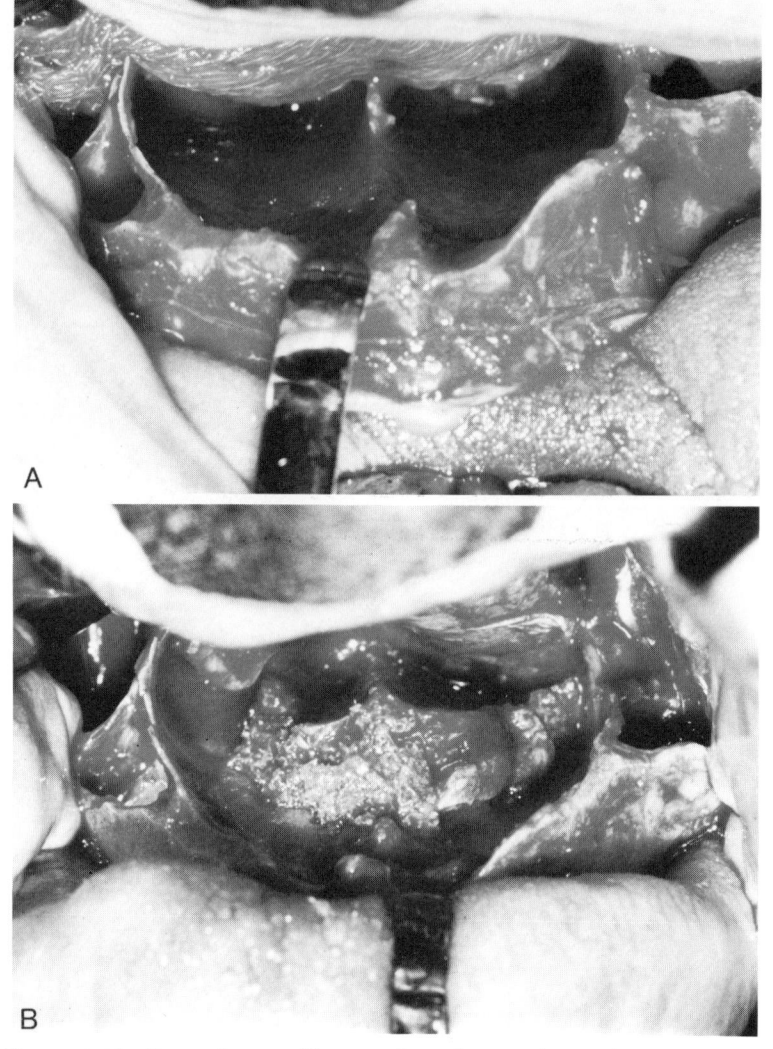

Figure 6–39. Once the maxilla was downfractured, a palatal vault osteotomy was performed at the junction of the alveolar and palatal portions of the maxilla in a horseshoe-shaped fashion.

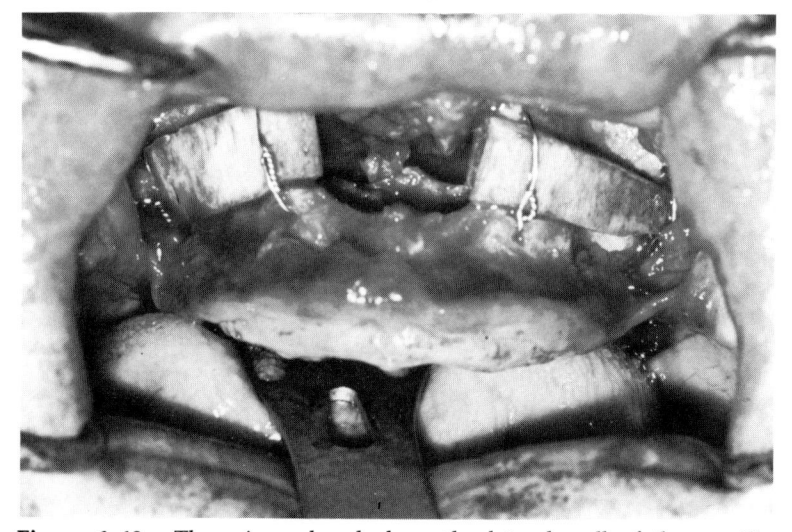

Figure 6–40. The wires placed along the lateral wall of the maxilla were fixed in place with 25-A stainless steel wire at the buttress area and the piriform aperture area.

bone augmentation and an adequate amount of fixed tissue allowing for continued denture function (Fig. 6–41).

MANDIBULAR PROCEDURES

A common pattern of mandibular EBL involves a generalized loss of alveolar bone, fairly uniform around the arch. This tends to produce a mandible in which the genial tubercles and mylohyoid ridges remain elevated and the rest of the ridge is flat. The basal bone is all that remains, leaving a mandible that may appear pencil-thin on a panoramic radiograph. Clinically, a "negative ridge" exists where the muscle attachments are actually elevated above the region available for denture bearing.

Occasionally, the process of alveolar bone loss appears to occur more rapidly in the posterior areas than in the anterior, leaving a clinical ridge that is of inadequate height and contour. In the posterior, the bone loss leaves a depressed area between the external oblique line and the mylohyoid ridge. This gives the clinical impression of a negative ridge form localized to the posterior mandible.

In some patients, the loss of bone may result in a mandible so thin that a fracture may occur after a minimally traumatic insult. In others, the points of muscle attachment on the lingual may become so prominent that a bizarre appearance results. Patients with localized defects (i.e., trauma, infection, neoplasm) require an individualized approach.

Once it is determined that the patient is a candidate for surgical reconstruction of the mandible, a thorough intra-oral examination should be performed. Examination of the mandibular arch should be both visual and bimanual. The arch should be evaluated for height and width. The relationship of the genial tubercles, and of the mylohyoid ridge to the remainder of the mandibular ridge, must be identified. The soft tissues in the denture-bearing area must be evaluated for ulceration, epulis, previously grafted tissue, and other conditions that might compromise healing.

The radiographic examination should begin with a panoramic radiograph. The height of the remaining mandibular bone can be measured at the mental foramen region. The presence and configuration of localized defects will be apparent on this radiograph. A cephalometric radiograph, or a conventional lateral view of the jaws, will aid in determining the shape of the symphysis region. A true occlusal view may occasionally be useful in determining the width of the mandible in the anterior and posterior regions. Of course, other views may be indicated for specific situations.

The radiographs are important not only for the preoperative evaluation but also for postoperative assessments. The height of the augmented mandible can be followed in serial radiographs. Replacement of grafted bone by new bone fill can be seen over long periods of time. Thorough follow-up will provide data to evaluate procedures.

The goals of surgical treatment to augment the mandible include (1) provision of optimum ridge form for the support of a denture, (2) improvement of maxillomandibular relationships, and (3) increase in bony bulk of the mandible. The surgery should ultimately result in a stronger mandible that can support a functional and esthetic prosthesis.

There are several procedures available for augmentation of the edentulous mandible. Many of the procedures involve the grafting of bone (autogenous and/or allogeneic) to the patient's mandible. These surgical procedures include total onlay grafts, modifications of the visor osteotomy, and the anterior interpositional and posterior onlay graft.

Choice of the type of bone graft is an important decision. Generally, the choice involves either autogenous bone, allogeneic bone, or a combination of the two. Autogenous bone has several advantages. The patient's own bone has no potential for rejection. Its osteogenetic ability results in relatively rapid incorporation into the grafted site. Autogenous bone is available from various sites for different uses. There may be less chance for infection in an autogenous bone graft because of the rapid healing.

Allogeneic bone that has been freeze-dried has the advantage of not requiring a surgical procedure to procure the graft material. It has an indefinite shelf life. It is incorporated into bone more slowly than an autogenous graft, which may be advantageous in selected procedures. Occasionally it may be useful to combine the two types of bone (autogenous cancellous bone with allogeneic rib, for example) to take advantage of some qualities of each.

Surgical Procedures

Total Onlay Grafts

For the mandible with generalized atrophy that measures less than 5 or 6 mm at the mental foramen region, there are few treatment alternatives. The patient usually is unable to wear a lower denture, has a Class III ridge relationship, and is at risk for injury from minor trauma. The total onlay graft is one of few surgical options feasible for these patients. The contraindications to this procedure include the ability to do any other augmentation procedure and any medical contraindication to general anesthesia. Pulmonary disease is a relative contraindication for removal of an autogenous rib for use as a graft.

Surgical Technique

The soft tissue dissection begins with an incision over the crest of the ridge through the remaining attached gingiva. This incision should extend from one retromolar area to the other (Fig. 6–42). A releasing incision extending laterally to the external oblique ridge

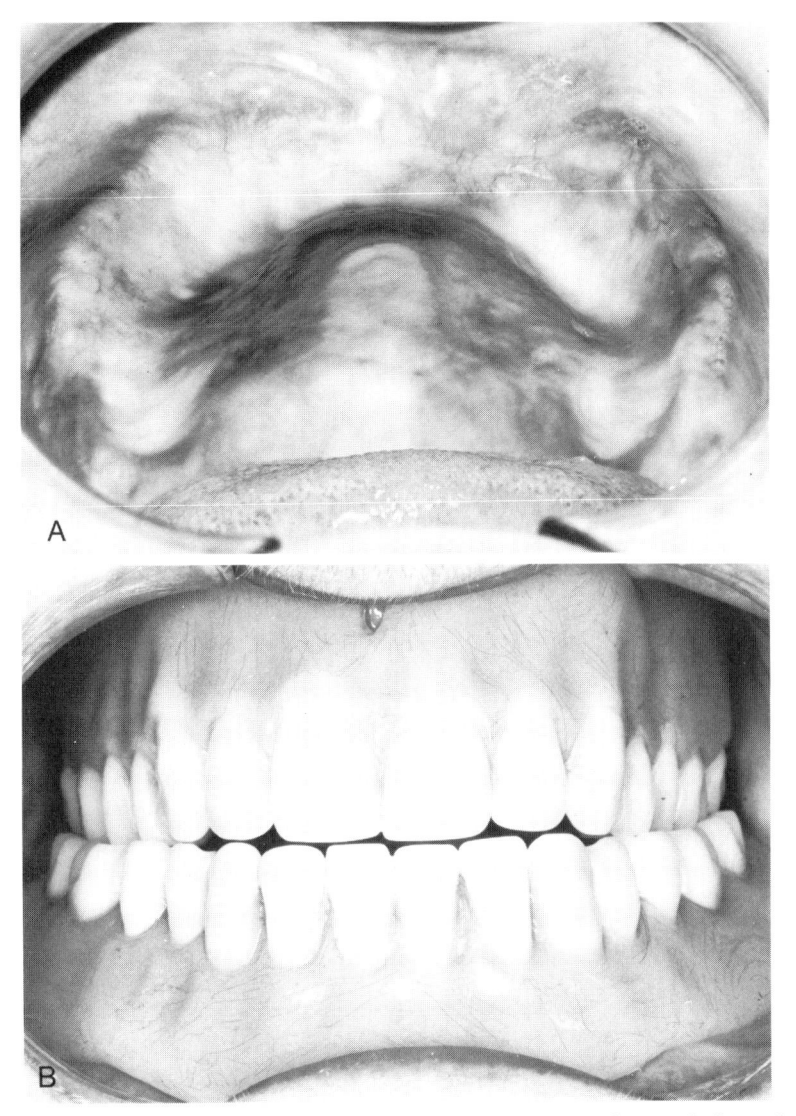

Figure 6–41. A two-year follow-up of the patient's result revealed good bony retention of augmentation and an adequate amount of fixed tissue, allowing for continued denture function.

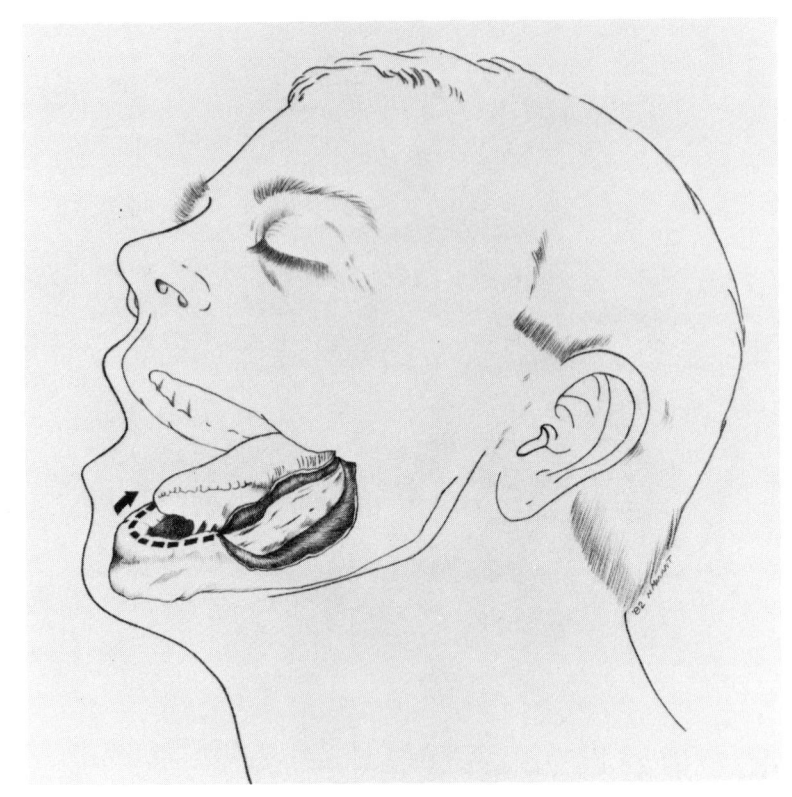

Figure 6–42. This incision should extend from one retromolar area to the other.

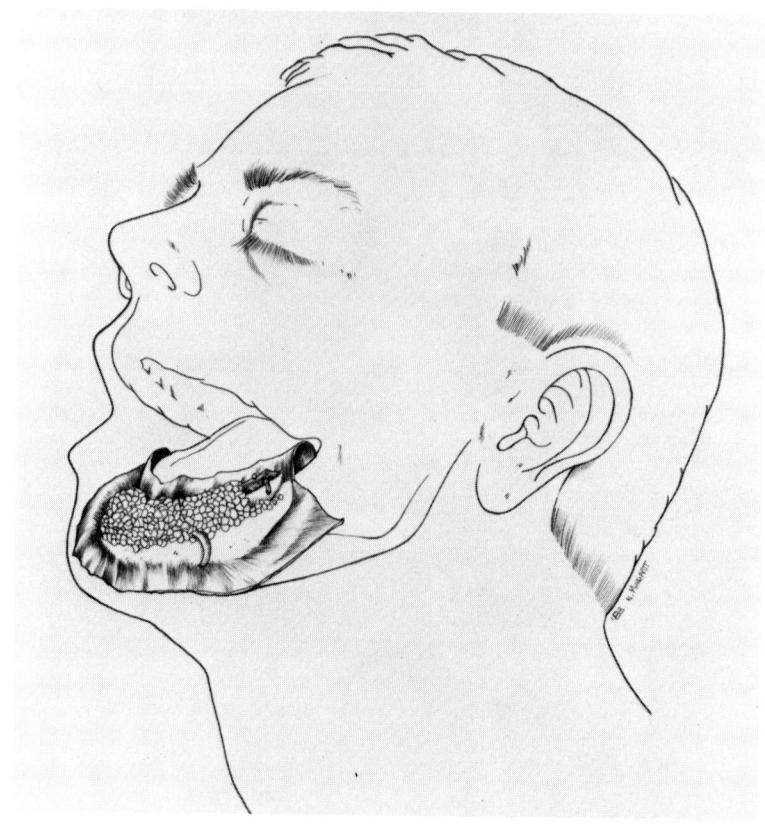

Figure 6–43. Chips of rib and cancellous bone can be packed on the buccal surface of the rib and into the void between the rib and the mandible.

on each side at the posterior extent will facilitate the dissection. The bone is then exposed by developing full-thickness mucoperiosteal flaps on the buccal and lingual surfaces of the mandible. The buccal dissection should extend to the external oblique ridge but need not be carried further inferiorly. On the lingual surface, the genial tubercles should be identified. The dissection should expose the lingual surface where the ramus begins to ascend.

The graft material of the total onlay graft should be autologous bone. The most common method, previously described in the section in this chapter on maxillary onlay rib grafting, involves using two 15- to 20-cm lengths of autogenous rib. The ribs are removed by a thoracic surgeon before the intra-oral procedure is begun. The ribs are prepared by removing all adhering pieces of soft tissue. The sharp spine on the superior edge of the rib is removed using a rongeur. One rib is split lengthwise; the cancellous bone is removed, and the cortical bone is made into chips approximately 5 cm in each dimension. The remaining rib is kerfed by placing vertical grooves through the inner cortex and the superior and inferior surfaces at 5- to 10-mm intervals. These grooves allow the rib to be curved into the shape of the mandibular ridge.

If an acrylic model of the patient's mandibular ridge has been made and gas sterilized, the rib may be accurately curved and its length adjusted outside of the mouth. Alternatively, a strip of aluminum can be used as a template. The placement of the rib should be slightly toward the lingual surface of the mandible. This is in an attempt to reproduce the position of the resorbed alveolar bone. The ends of the curved rib should be adjusted to fit just medial to the ascending ramus. Anteriorly, the rib should rest on the mandible, toward its lingual surface. The contour of the mandible is usually such that a void will be present in the midbody region between the rib and the mandible.

The rib should now be wired into position. In the posterior, the wires should pass through the rib and the anterior border of the ascending ramus on each side. In the anterior, the wires may be circummandibular or transosseous, and they may pass over or through the rib. The placement of the wires will depend on the anatomy of the mandible and the surgeon's preference. One wire in the midline may be sufficient, but two wires in the canine regions provide more positive stabilization. Soft tissue closure is begun once the rib is stabilized. At that time, chips of rib and cancellous bone can be packed on the buccal surface of the rib and into the void between the rib and the mandible (Fig. 6–43).

The soft-tissue closure must be water-tight and without tension. Undermining is usually necessary in the anterior portion of the labial flap and into the lip to provide adequate release. This should be avoided in the small lingual flap to avoid damage to the structures located immediately deep to the periosteum. The soft tissues may be closed with a nonresorbable suture such as Supramid. A running horizontal mattress suture is placed, and care is taken that all edges of the flaps are everted. Then a simple running suture is placed to lightly approximate the edges.

An alternate method may be used for grafting autogenous rib to the mandible by splitting both ribs and removing the cancellous bone. Four sections of rib are placed so that each inner surface is next to an outer surface (Fig. 6–44). Resorbable sutures are then used to tie sections together (Fig. 6–45). The bundle is contoured and placed as in the previous description (Fig. 6–46). The cancellous bone and any chips from the excess length of rib may be packed around the rib.

The total onlay graft to augment the mandible can achieve an immediate increase in the mandibular height equal to the height of the graft placed. This height will show rapid resorption. Studies have shown that rapid vertical resorption occurs in the initial two years after augmentation to the extent of one half to two thirds of the augmentation. The rate of resorption then decreases dramatically.[19] This is true for both rib and iliac crest onlay grafts.[20] Clinically, however, the healed ridge has a broader base and better contour for denture stability. While this improvement is difficult to quantitate, patients report an improvement in function and are generally satisfied with the procedure.[3, 19-21] This procedure requires a vestibuloplasty after initial healing and, when autologous bone is used, can be performed six months to one year after the bone-grafting procedure.

Interposed Bone Graft Augmentation of the Atrophic Mandible

In an attempt to overcome the main disadvantage of subperiosteal onlay grafting, i.e., rapid resorption, interposed bone graft techniques have been developed. Barros Saint-Pasteur,[22, 23] a pioneer in the field, initially described a two-stage procedure. This involved mobilization of the alveolar part of the mandible via a horizontal osteotomy be-

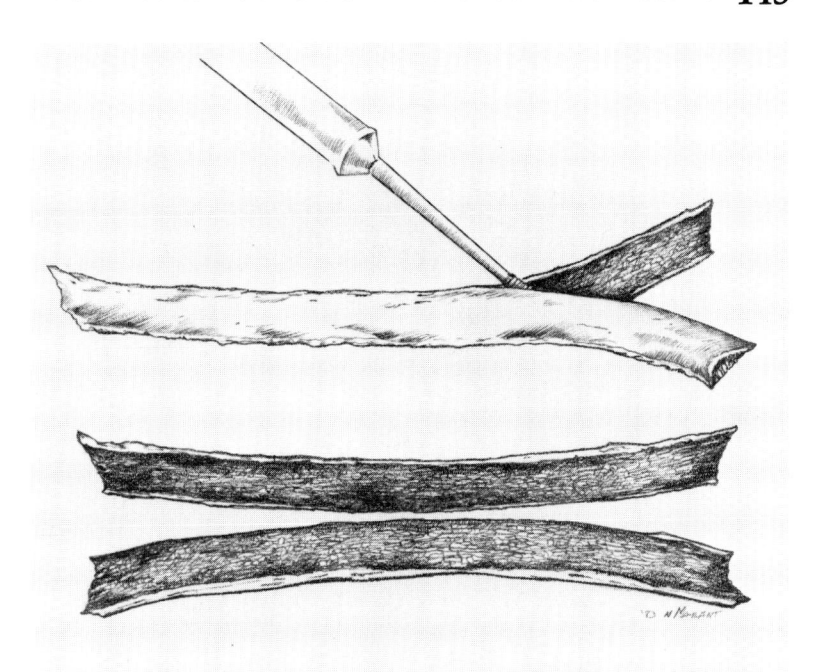

Figure 6–44. Four sections of rib are placed so that each inner surface is next to an outer surface.

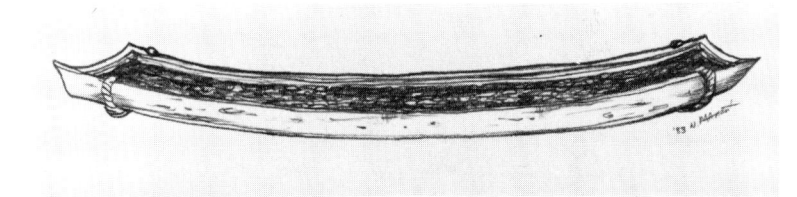

Figure 6–45. Resorbable sutures are used to tie sections together.

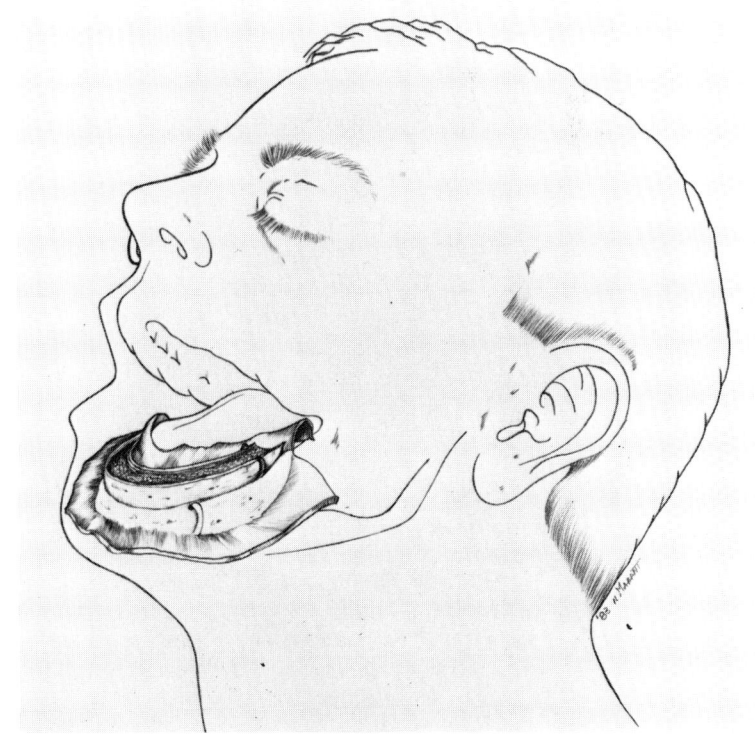

Figure 6–46. The bundle is contoured and placed as in the previous description.

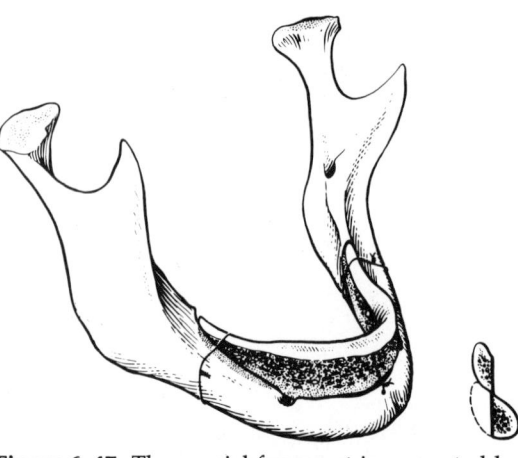

Figure 6–47. The cranial fragment is separated by a sagittal osteotomy and moved vertically, i. e., the sliding "visor" osteotomy.

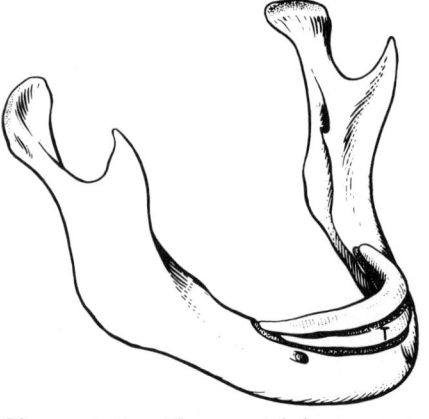

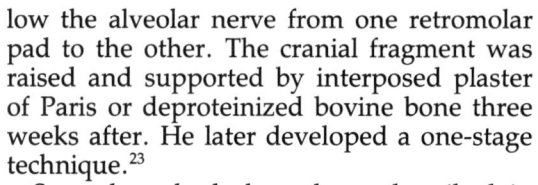

Figure 6–48. The cranial fragment is separated by a horizontal osteotomy and carried out between the two mental foramina. Thus, it lifts only the anterior fragment, i. e., the "sandwich" technique.

low the alveolar nerve from one retromolar pad to the other. The cranial fragment was raised and supported by interposed plaster of Paris or deproteinized bovine bone three weeks after. He later developed a one-stage technique.[23]

Several methods have been described in which the mandible or part of it was split in a horizontal, oblique, or vertical fashion. Then the cranial fragment was raised and in most cases supported by interposed grafts such as autogenous bone or cartilage, freeze-dried bone, alloplastic material, or combinations of these grafts.[21, 24–26] Follow-up studies on several of these techniques show that a fairly stable result can be expected after initial loss of height in the first six months. The loss of augmented height after two years ranged from 28 to 49 per cent.[25, 27–29] After that period, follow-up studies show that average resorption is much in accordance with the normal resorption pattern found in edentulous mandibles.[25, 27, 30]

There are basically three techniques designed to achieve interposed bone graft augmentation:

1. The cranial fragment is separated by a sagittal osteotomy and moved vertically, i.e., the sliding "visor" osteotomy[31–34] (Fig. 6–47).

2. The cranial fragment is separated by a horizontal osteotomy and carried out between the two mental foramina. Thus, it lifts only the anterior fragment, i.e., "sandwich" technique[24, 35] (Fig. 6–48). This procedure has also been extended beyond the mental foramina and below the nerve, although some authors have recommended that the inclination of the osteotomy be oblique.[7, 36, 37]

3. The "visor" and "sandwich" techniques are combined. The osteotomy posterior to the mental foramina is in a vertical plane, changing to 45 degrees in the anterior region (Fig. 6–49).[27, 38, 39]

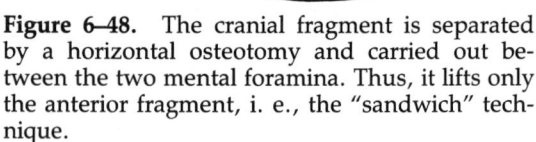

Although good success has been reported with the "visor" osteotomy, inherent limitations exist. Because the mandible is vertically split, its width will be reduced to half the original size. Furthermore, not more than twice its original height can be gained, unless one modifies the technique according to Hopkins.[33] The main drawback of this technique, however, appears to be potential damage to the nerve. In many atrophic mandibles, the alveolar nerve will be located lingually, not allowing sufficient space to make a bone cut lingual to the foramen. In an attempt to compromise, one easily damages the alveolar nerve, causing sensory disturbances.

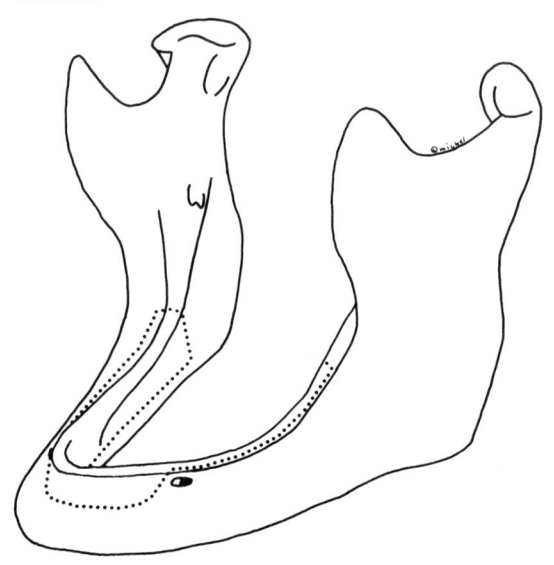

Figure 6–49. The "visor" and "sandwich" techniques are combined. The osteotomy posterior to the mental foramina is in a vertical plane, changing to 45 degrees in the anterior region.

The "sandwich" osteotomy is limited by the anatomy of severely atrophic mandibles. In most cases, there is not enough space between the foramina and the crest to make a bone cut. If one stays between the foramina, the area posterior to the foramina will still be deficient. This is very often the area that needs the most augmentation.

Horizontal osteotomies that are done below the alveolar nerve and extend posterior to the mental foramen put the mandible at risk. Fractures of the thin mandibular lower border have occurred, and the mental nerve, lifted up in the cranial fragment, is not protected by this osteotomy design.[37, 38]

Modified "Visor" Osteotomy

The combination of the "visor" and "sandwich" techniques was designed to overcome the aforementioned disadvantages of both methods. A modification of the visor osteotomy may be considered for the patient with at least 8 mm of bone height as measured at the mental nerve region. This procedure involves a parasagittal split of the mandible from midbody on one side to the same position on the opposite side. The lingually pedicled segment is raised in visor fashion and wired into position. This procedure has been modified in various reports. Peterson and Slade[34] raised the lingual segment along a greater length of the mandibular body and added free chips of bone to the lateral aspect of the raised bony segment.

Frost and colleagues[40] use a sagittal cut in the body regions of the mandible but change to a horizontal cut anteriorly. This allows use of a block of grafted bone in an interpositional fashion in the anterior region and for easy mobilization of the pedicled segment, firm stabilization with a corticocancellous block of bone in the anterior, and maintenance of the full width of the anterior ridge.

Surgical Technique

An incision is made from the lateral aspect of the anterior ramus, splitting the fibrous crestal tissue to the opposite ramus. A facial mucoperiosteal flap is reflected to the inferior borders of the mandible anterior to the rami (Fig. 6–50). The mental neurovascular bundles are identified and dissected free for a few millimeters at their soft-tissue interface. Then a full-thickness lingual mucosal flap is developed for several millimeters medially by reflecting the crestal attachment down to the underlying mylohyoid and genioglossus muscles.

Decompression of the inferior alveolar neurovascular bundle is completed by removing the overlying bone from the mental foramen to the anterior aspect of the ramus-body juncture. The incisal continuation to

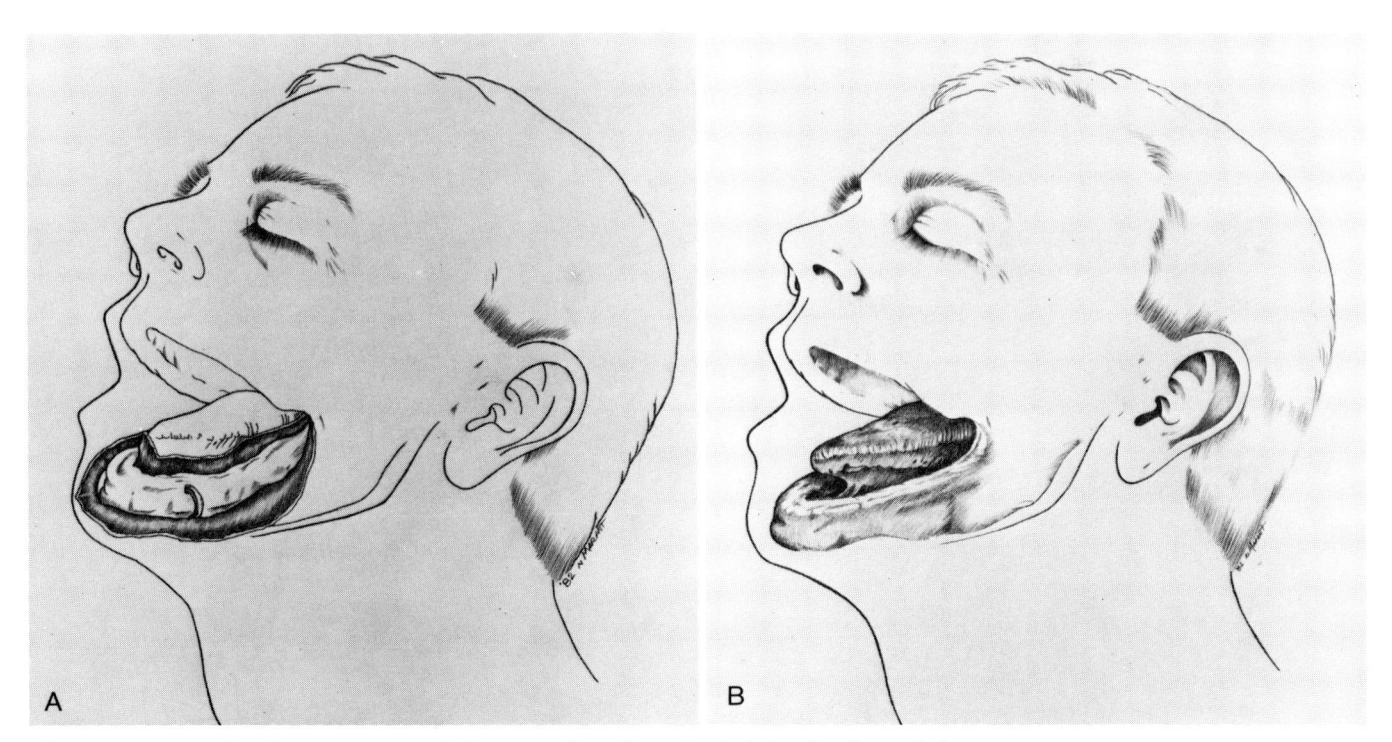

Figure 6–50. A facial mucoperiosteal flap is reflected to the inferior borders of the mandible anterior to the rami.

the anterior mandible is severed after the neurovascular bundle is exposed. The proximal bundle is lifted from the canal posteriorly to the ramus body juncture. Careful retraction protects the neurovascular bundle and maintains the integrity at the soft-tissue interface as well as the continuation in the proximal bony canal (Fig. 6–51).

Short-term follow-up studies have shown that relatively stable results can be expected using this technique.[25, 27] The gain in height is better than with onlay grafting.[2, 19, 41] Re-

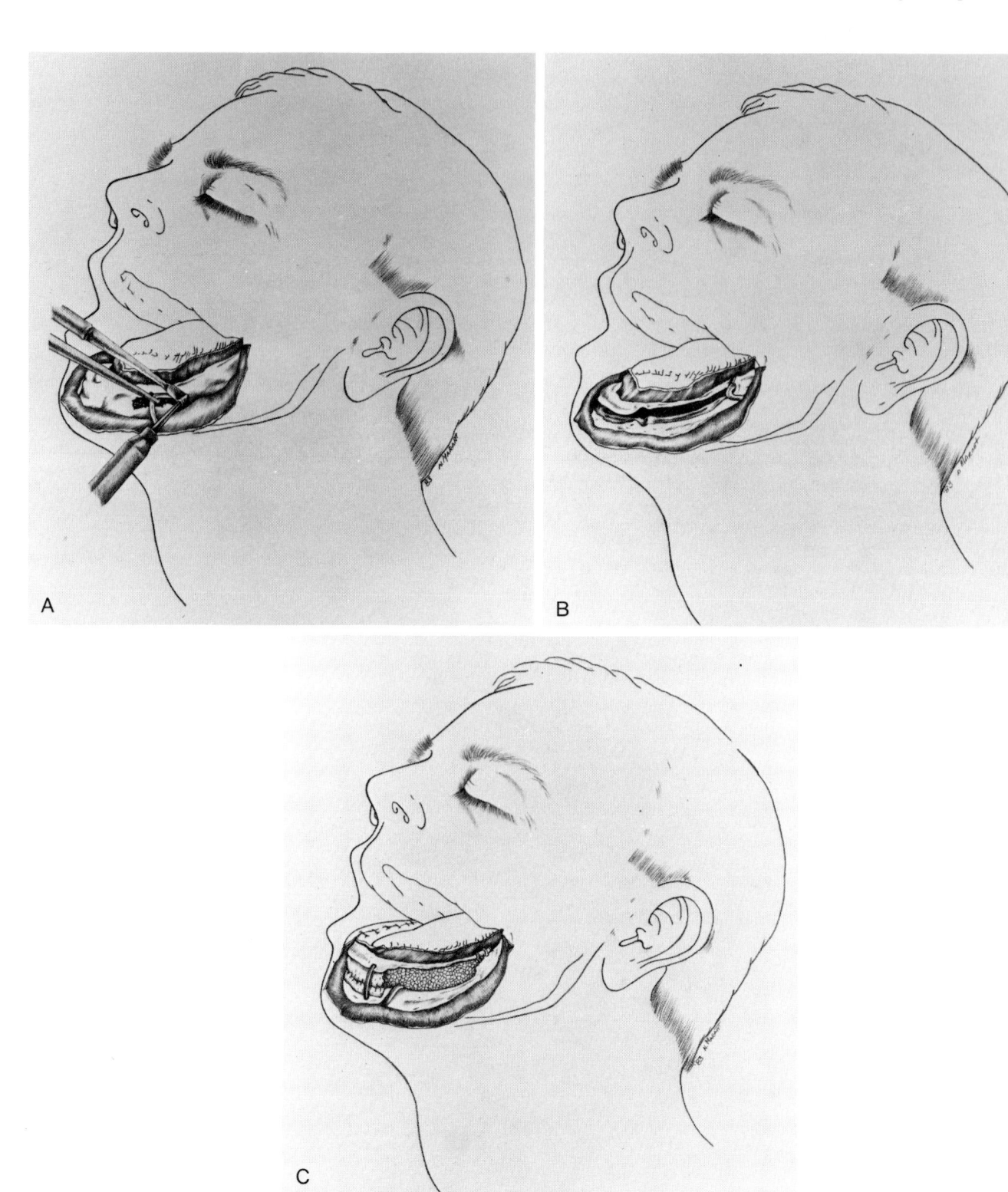

Figure 6–51. Decompression of the inferior alveolar neurovascular bundle.

sorption, however, will continue to occur not only from the top but also on the osteotomy side of the cranial fragment. The latter can be prevented by ensuring that the cranial fragment is brought forward and secured directly above the caudal fragment. In this way, unfavorable loading from the denture can be prevented, and less resorption of the grafted bone occurs. The postponement of denture wearing as well as the delay of the vestibuloplasty probably leads to better results with regard to resorption.[25, 42] If the initial vestibular incision is carried a bit more into the vestibule, healing after the bone graft might leave a sulcus depth. It is our current practice to fabricate dentures approximately two months postoperatively and evaluate the situation again after one year. A vestibuloplasty then will be carried out if necessary and the denture extended and relined. Even though a two-month period without a lower denture seems lengthy, patients seldom complain. The improvement in esthetics as a result of their newly built-up mandible dominates their feelings.

The main drawback of this procedure, along with the "visor" and "sandwich" techniques, is the relatively high incidence of persistent sensory disturbances in the chin and lower lip.[25, 27–29, 32, 40] Even though certain improvements have been noted over the years, approximately 65 per cent of the patients have some type of persistent sensory disturbance.[25, 27] The dissection of the nerve out of its canal prior to the vertical bone cuts does not appear to be beneficial.[25, 28] The results with regard to sensory disturbances remain highly unsatisfactory. Although the denture base and functioning of the denture have improved quite considerably, approximately 20 per cent of the patients regret their surgery.

Another part of the operation that is not completely predictable is the manipulation of the posterior part of the cranial fragment. If this fragment is fractured, usually at the mental foramen, the posterior fragment then becomes a free graft. The posterior fragment slips back into its original position or is displaced so that no graft can be interposed. In some cases, the posterior cranial fragment is merely a lingual cortical plate whereby bone is grafted instead of being interposed. This leads to rapid resorption, as in subperiosteal onlay grafts. In order to avoid these disadvantages, a modification has been developed for those mandibles which, because of a lack of space between the mental foramen and the lingual plate, do not allow for a one-piece bone. The nerve is left in its canal and

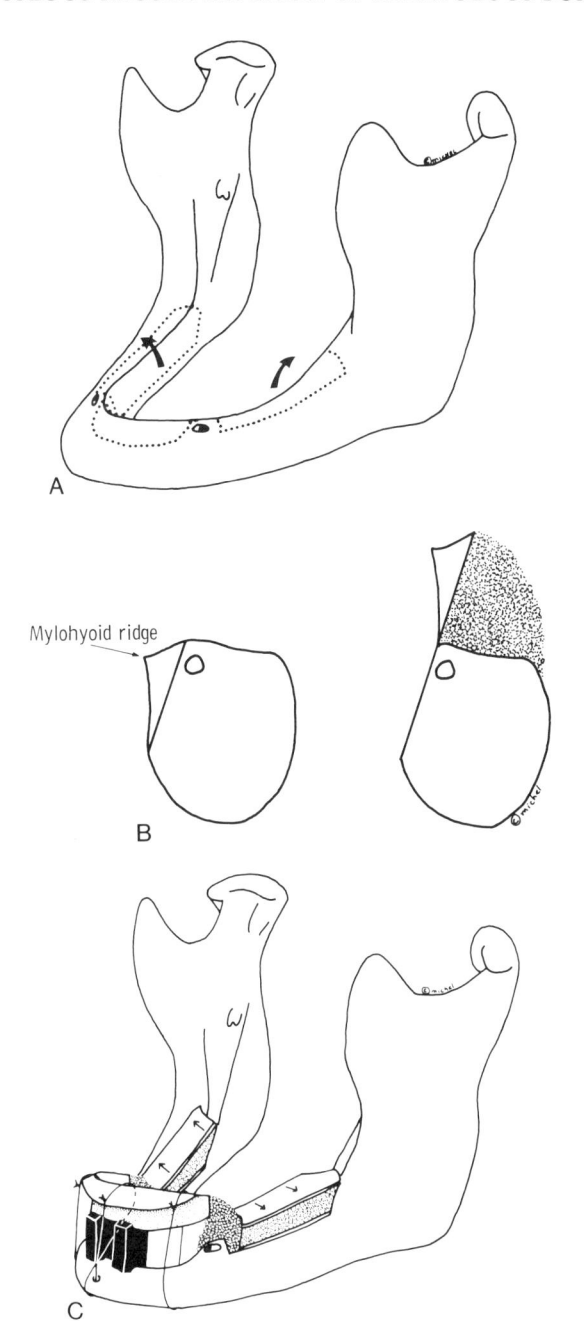

Figure 6–52. The osteotomy redesigned to create three fragments ("three-piece augmentation").

the osteotomy is redesigned to create three fragments ("three-piece augmentation") (Figs. 6–52 and 6–53). The anterior cranial fragment is secured with a figure-of-eight wire passed through a hole in the symphysis. The thin posterior cranial fragments are lifted up and rotated 90 degrees to cover the interposed lingual cortical plates and become the occlusal surfaces of the alveolar ridge. Soft-tissue attachments to this previously lingual fragment are not disturbed. Since only minimal muscle pull is involved, fixation can usually be achieved by suturing the mucosa

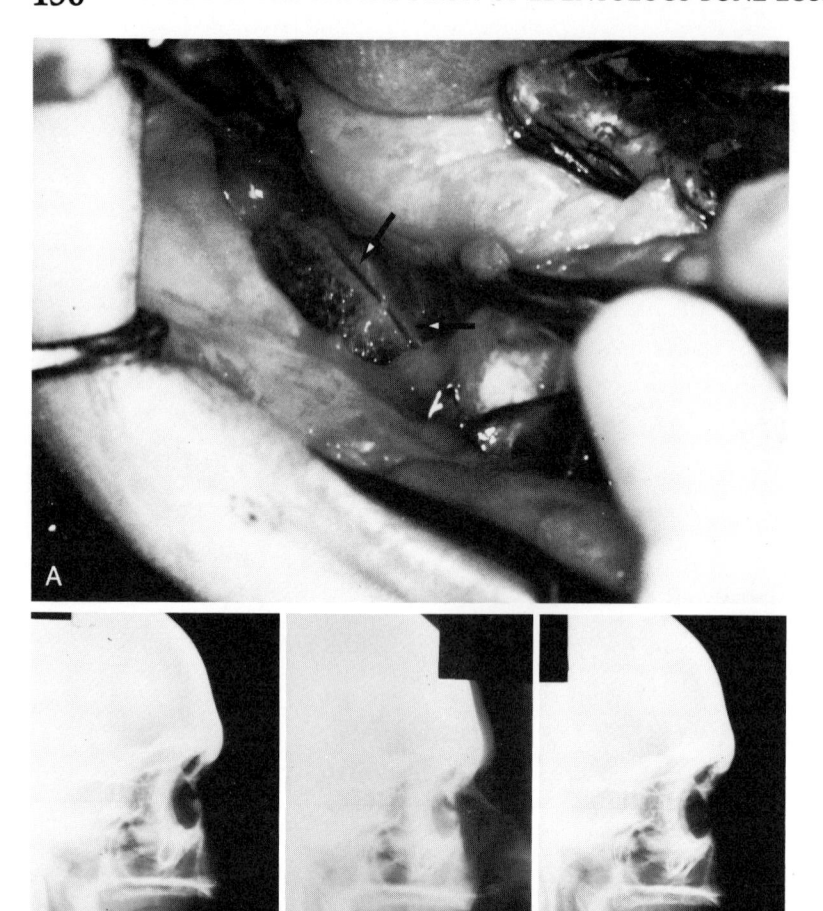

150 / OSSEOUS RECONSTRUCTION OF EDENTULOUS BONE LOSS

Figure 6–53. Intra-oral (A) and lateral (B) radiographic views of the three-piece augmentation.

TABLE 6–7. NERVE SENSIBILITY TESTING RESULTS IN 54 PATIENTS (108 SITES)

Pattern	Brush Contact Sense (%)	Movement Appreciation and Directional Sense (%)
Normal	80	50
Anesthesia	6	6
Paresthesia	10	36
Hypoesthesia	0	2
Hyperesthesia	4	6
	100%	100%

The augmentation and the contour of the posterior ridge also appeared to be better. It appears that the three-piece technique has eliminated many of the disadvantages of the previous methods.

Anterior Osteotomy with Posterior Onlay Graft

In an attempt to achieve results similar to the modified visor osteotomy with less nerve trauma, the procedure combining an anterior osteotomy with posterior onlay grafts was developed. The indications and contraindications for this procedure are the same as for the modified visor osteotomy.

Surgical Technique

The soft-tissue dissection begins with an incision over the crest of the ridge, with the posterior extent approximately 1 cm posterior to the mental foramina on each side (Fig. 6–54). A full-thickness dissection is carried out on the labial surface of the mandible, and the mental nerves are identified on each side. Just enough dissection should be carried at the mental foramen area to allow retraction of the mucoperiosteal flap without tension on the nerves. Posteriorly, a subperiosteal tunnel is developed between the external oblique ridge and the mylohyoid ridge. This tunnel should extend to the retromolar region. The soft tissues on the lingual side of the incision are minimally reflected for ease in closure.

After this, an anterior segmental osteotomy is performed. The vertical cuts are made with a fissure bur just anterior to the mental foramina on each side to prevent penetration of the lingual mucosa. These cuts are carried through approximately one half the vertical height of the mandible and, using a saw, are connected with a horizontal osteotomy (Fig. 6–55). The osteotomy may be inclined slightly down toward the lingual soft tissues. When the osteotomies are complete, the segment may be raised superiorly,

attached to these lingual plates to the buccal mucosa. If the mylohyoid muscle becomes prominent, causing the lingual space to be eliminated, a simple dissection may be done, according to Brown[43] and Downton,[44] about ten weeks later.

The chances of damaging the neurovascular bundle are greatly reduced, since the area of the mental foramen is not disturbed. The build-up of the posterior part of the mandible is also much more substantial and certainly more predictable.

A group of 54 patients, who underwent an augmentation in which the selection for the use of the one- or "three-piece" technique was based on the width between the mental foramen and the lingual plate, has been followed.[42] Generally, a width of less than 5 mm was considered to be insufficient to carry out the one-piece technique. The results of this study show far better scores in relation to nerve disturbances (Table 6–7).

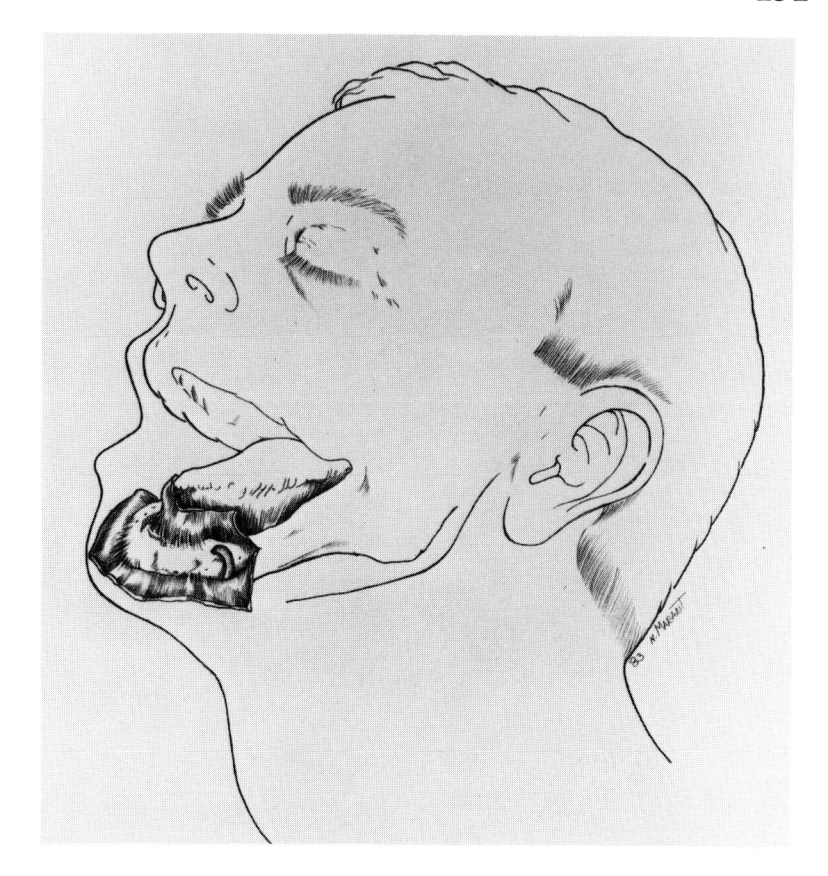

Figure 6–54. The soft tissue dissection begins with an incision over the crest of the ridge with the posterior extent approximately one centimeter posterior to the mental foramina on each side.

taking care to maintain the soft-tissue pedicle on the lingual surface.

The segment is maintained in a superior position by wedging a corticocancellous block of bone into the osteotomy site. It should measure approximately 1 cm square in cross-section and the exact length of the anterior segment. The graft and mobilized section of bone can be easily stabilized with two circummandibular wires. Posteriorly, onlay grafts or hydroxyapatite particles are placed which extend from the ascending ramus to the edge of the superiorly positioned anterior segment. The onlay grafts are approximately 1 cm in cross-section and must lie between the external oblique line and the mylohyoid ridge. The onlay graft may be held in place with a single circummandibular wire.

The anterior interpositional graft may be either autologous or allogeneic. Allogeneic bone is the preferred graft material for this operation because it is more slowly incorporated than autogenous bone. This maintains more of the augmentation than would occur with autogenous bone. The material of choice for the posterior region is hydroxyapatite. Once the grafts are positioned, voids or irregularities may be contoured by the placement of particles of hydroxyapatite.

The incision should be closed with a dou-

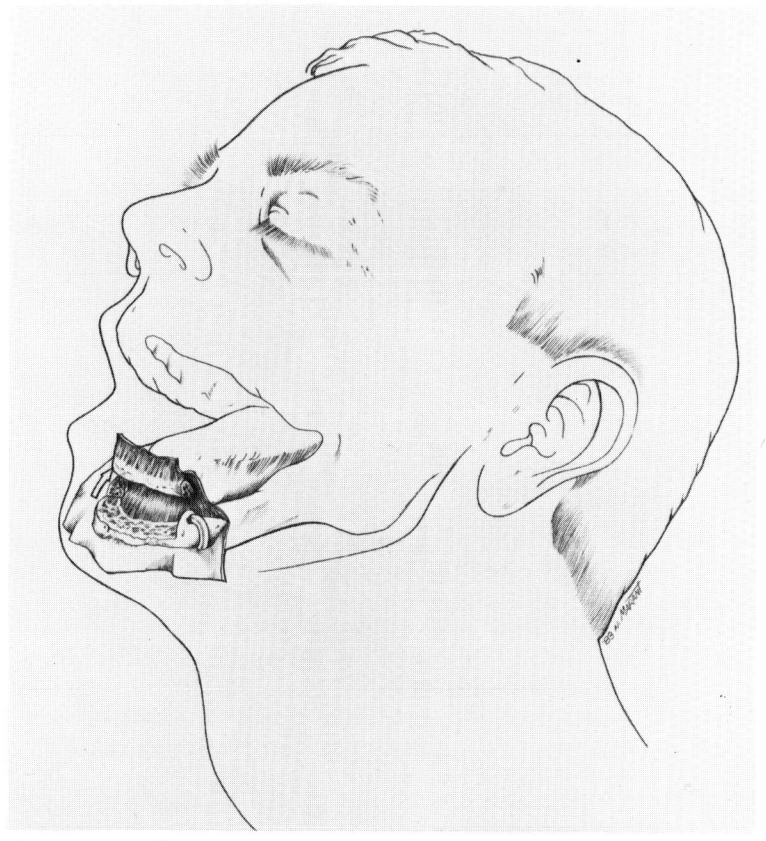

Figure 6–55. These cuts are carried through approximately one half the vertical height of the mandible and, using a saw, are connected with a horizontal osteotomy.

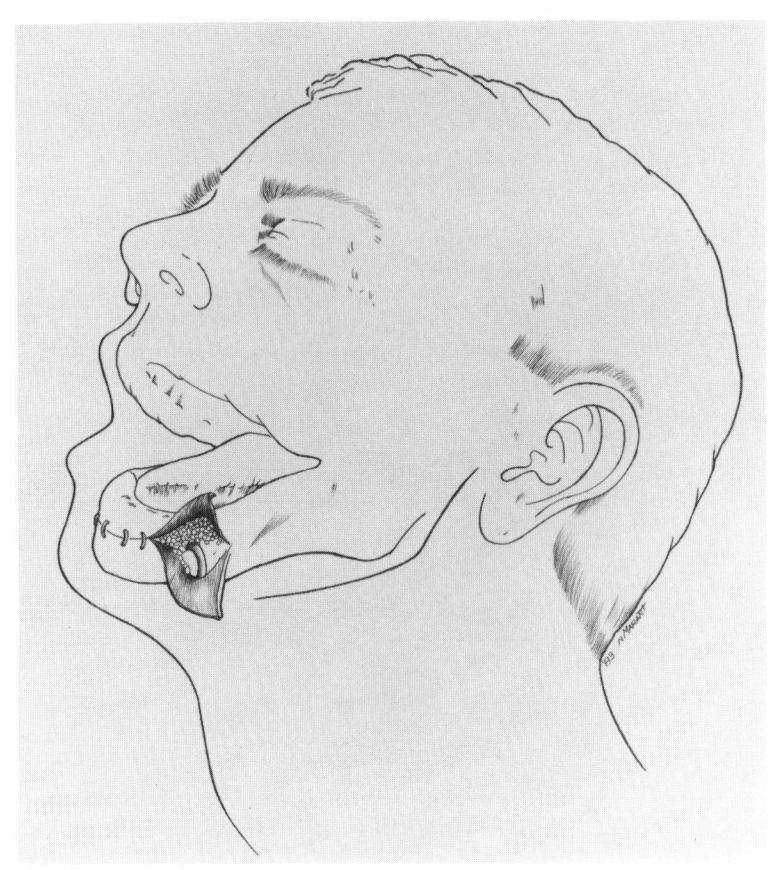

Figure 6–56. The incision should be closed with a double-layer technique as previously described.

ble-layer technique, as previously described (Fig. 6–56). If the graft is of allogeneic bone, it should be allowed to heal for approximately six months prior to any soft-tissue procedure. Six weeks before the vestibuloplasty, the circummandibular wires should be removed and bony irregularities may be conservatively smoothed. Frequently, the genial tubercles will need reduction after this procedure. The vestibuloplasty, combined with a floor of mouth procedure, is performed in the standard fashion.

The long-term results of this procedure are still uncertain. Because this procedure has been a fairly recent innovation, further follow-up studies will be forthcoming. The short-term results are encouraging, with good maintenance of contour both anteriorly and posteriorly. When the vestibuloplasty and alveoloplasties have been done, the onlay bone has been stable and vascular. The most encouraging advantage of this procedure, when compared to the modified visor osteotomy, is the decreased incidence of long-lasting mental nerve paresthesia. While paresthesia often results from the handling the mental nerve receives in this operation, the altered sensation is usually transient and rarely noxious.

Soft-Tissue Procedures

After the graft procedures, a vestibuloplasty is usually performed prior to fabrication of a prosthesis. The healing of allogeneic grafts usually takes approximately one year, while autologous bone may be sufficiently healed for the secondary soft-tissue surgery after six months. The soft-tissue procedures are similar to vestibuloplasties performed on mandibles without prior grafts. Several important considerations should be discussed.

After a grafting procedure, there are occasionally irregularities in contour that would compromise denture fit if allowed to remain. It may be necessary to perform an alveoloplasty prior to the vestibuloplasty. When performing such a procedure, care should be taken in reflecting periosteum to expose the smallest possible area of bone; it should be done approximately six weeks prior to the vestibuloplasty. At that time, circummandibular wires should be removed while transosseous wires remain in place.

The vestibuloplasty dissection should be done so as to avoid interrupting the periosteum. In areas where the periosteum has been incised during the grafting procedure, the tissue covering the bone may be thicker and more fibrous than normal. It is in these areas that accidental exposure of the underlying bone may result in a persistent dehiscence requiring many months to heal.

While a split thickness skin graft may be acceptable for use in a vestibuloplasty on an ungrafted mandible, the authors use meshed palatal mucosa exclusively for grafting over interpositional allogeneic bone grafts. The thicker palatal mucosa appears to give a better quality graft. The vestibuloplasty should include both a buccal dissection and a lowering of the floor of the mouth procedure. This, with placement of a palatal mucosal graft that has been meshed (3:1), will ensure the best possible ridge for fabrication of a prosthesis.

Postoperative Considerations

After a grafting procedure to the mandible, a steroid and antibiotic regimen is continued. The authors generally use a preoperative intravenous dose of 500 mg methylprednisolone followed by 250 mg every four hours until the intravenous line is discontinued. At that time, 80 mg methylprednisolone in a sustained-release form is given intramuscularly. Any steroid regimen that will prevent excessive soft tissue edema is acceptable.

Penicillin is the preferred antibiotic for use with bone grafting and may be given intravenously until the patient takes fluids well. Oral antibiotics should be continued until the intraoral incisions are well healed. Since suture removal is usually delayed until three weeks after surgery, antibiotics may be continued until then but should be given again for procedures such as removal of circummandibular wires and alveoloplasty.

Oral hygiene should include avoidance of any mandibular prosthesis until after the vestibuloplasty procedure. Frequent mouth rinsing to clean the sutures and incision line of food debris should be encouraged. Diet may be advanced from clear liquids to a full liquid diet. After ten days, a soft diet should be well tolerated; however, the patient should not be permitted to chew foods or put pressure on the grafted ridge until after the vestibuloplasty and fabrication of dentures.

Potential complications of these procedures include paresthesia of the inferior alveolar nerve, infection, exposure of the grafted bone, and fracture of the mandible. Paresthesia of the inferior alveolar nerves is very common, especially following the modified visor osteotomy. Frost and coworkers[40] have found an incidence of altered sensations in 9 of 16 patients after the modified visor osteotomy. After other procedures, the occurrence of paresthesia appears to be less frequent and less profound, but still common. In all the procedures, the neurovascular bundle is in a position where accidental trauma could occur.

When infections occur, they are usually localized and associated with an incisional dehiscence.[45] This type of infection is usually easily managed with antibiotics and careful irrigation of the infected region. The authors have seen three cases of more severe infections involving patients who had modified visor osteotomies with allogeneic bone grafts. The three patients had unilateral submandibular and buccal swelling and increased pain in the region. The incisions were intact and no purulence was identified. In all three instances, the allogeneic bone had been reconstituted without using antibiotics. These patients were treated with antibiotics, two as inpatients with intravenous antibiotics, and incision and drainage were avoided. All three infections resolved, but one patient showed severe resorption of the grafted bone. Because no severe infections have occurred in patients whose allogeneic bone grafts had been reconstituted with an antibiotic solution, it is recommended that antibiotics be included in the solution used to reconstitute the allogeneic bone.

Occasionally, the grafted bone may become exposed to the oral cavity through breakdown of an incision or by erosion through previously intact mucosa. Similarly, a wire may occasionally break through the overlying mucosa. If the graft is sufficiently stable, the wire may simply be removed. Otherwise, conservative management with antibiotics and good oral hygiene is indicated for exposed wires until they can be removed. Exposed grafted bone should also be treated conservatively. Small exposures should be treated with antibiotics and gentle frequent irrigations. The temptation to mobilize soft tissue and attempt primary closure should be suppressed. This intervention almost always results in a second breakdown that exposes more grafted bone than the first. With time, the surface of the grafted bone will slough, leaving a granulated surface that will epithelialize. The problem of graft exposure seems to occur more frequently with the use of allogeneic bone and is probably due to the slower development of its blood supply.[46] Exposure of the graft will result in slower healing prior to the vestibuloplasty. Unless a large proportion of the graft becomes exposed, it does not usually result in a major loss of ridge height.[45]

Fracture of the mandible, or of the mobilized segment, is a potential complication of the modified visor osteotomy. To a lesser extent, the anterior osteotomy with posterior onlay grafts is a potential complication. In the modified visor osteotomy, the mobilized segment of bone is prone to fracture at the mental foramen region where the osteotomy turns from vertical to horizontal. Care must be taken when the segment is mobilized superiorly to avoid fracture at this time. If a fracture of this segment occurs, it should be stabilized in its new position by wedging a block of grafted bone into the osteotomy site and holding the graft and fractured segment in place with the circummandibular wire. This type of complication usually heals well unless the lingual pedicle of soft tissue becomes stripped from the mobilized segment.

Fracture of the mandible itself may occur in the mental foramen region during either type of osteotomy but is uncommon. The fracture should be reduced and directly wired if possible. Then a strip of graft bone (either autogenous or allogeneic) should be placed in onlay fashion across the fracture site and stabilized with transosseous wires. Usually the best stability will result when the bone is placed on the facial surface of the mandible. The procedure is completed as if the fracture were not present. All patients who have undergone an osteotomy and graft to an atrophic mandible should understand that the jaw will actually be weaker until healing of the graft is complete. Patients who have had visor or sandwich procedures should avoid activities that might cause injury, as the mandible is more susceptible to fracture during the healing period. If fracture does occur, treatment is conservative, avoiding open reduction, and usually involves observation and a pureed diet. A fracture in this circumstance will usually result in severe resorption of the graft and may require a second augmentation procedure.

CASE IV

These two cases represent patients who underwent onlay superior border rib grafts with subsequent split thickness skin graft vestibuloplasties.

The first illustrations represent the clinical and radiographic condition of one of the patients preoperatively (Fig. 6–57). The next set of illustrations represents a two-year radiographic and clinical follow-up (Fig. 6–58). Lastly, a ten-year follow-up is presented to show a good clinical result with a broad-based ridge (Fig. 6–59).

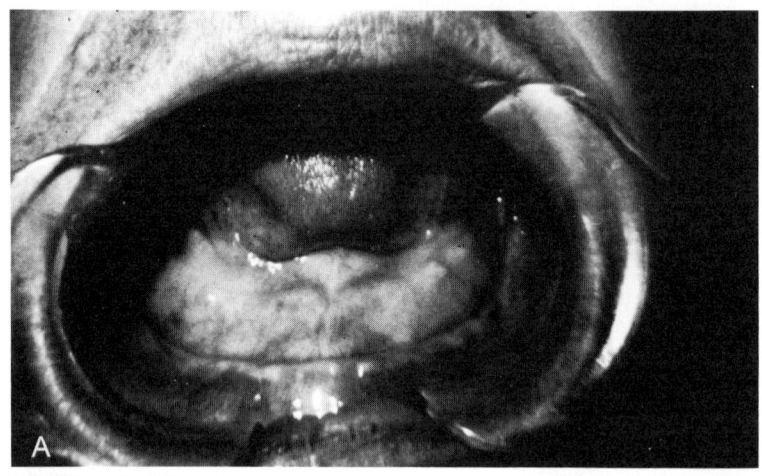

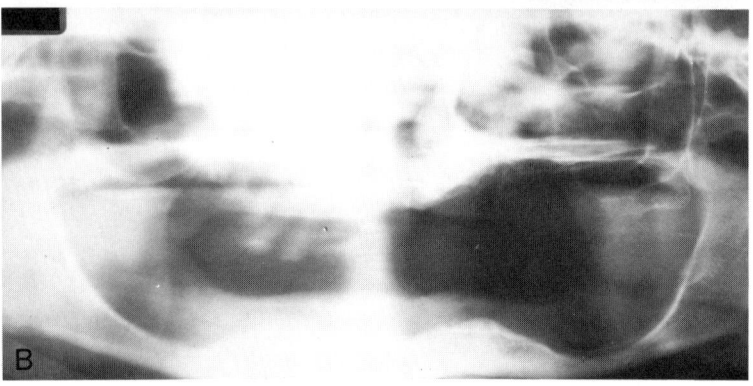

Figure 6–57. The clinical (*A*) and radiographic (*B*) condition of the patient preoperatively.

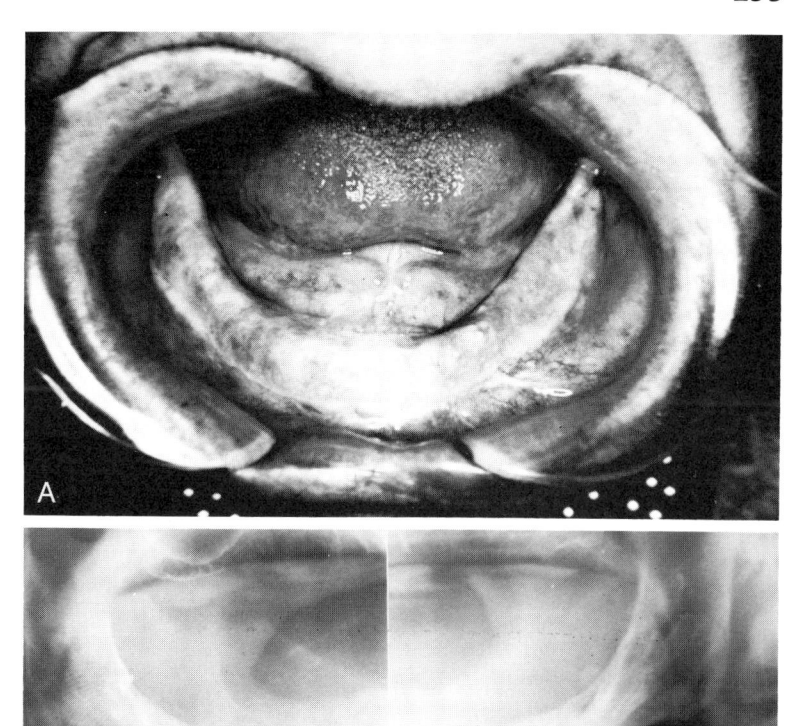

OSSEOUS RECONSTRUCTION OF EDENTULOUS BONE LOSS / **155**

Figure 6–58. Two-year clinical (*A*) and radiographic (*B*) follow-up.

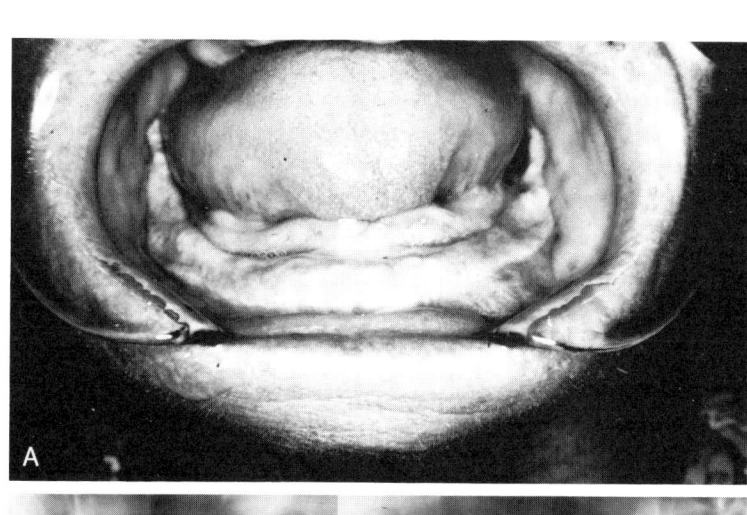

Figure 6–59. A ten-year follow-up showing a good clinical result with a broad-based ridge.

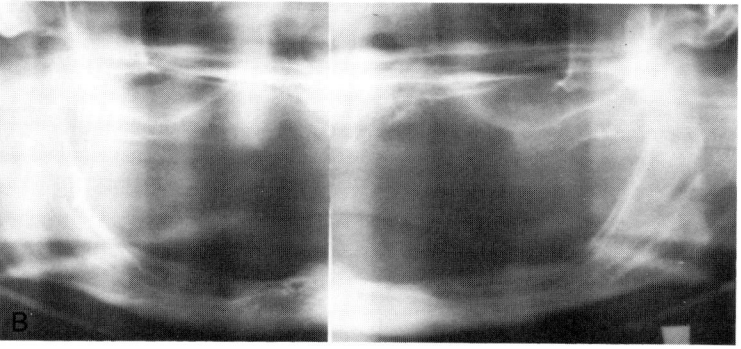

156 / OSSEOUS RECONSTRUCTION OF EDENTULOUS BONE LOSS

CASE V

This patient represents another example of extreme edentulous bone loss (Fig. 6–60). The patient had an onlay bone graft followed by split thickness skin graft. The two-year follow-up shows an adequate buccal and labial vestibule with some resorption of the bone graft (Fig. 6–61). Long-term (11-year) follow-up reveals a progressive resorption of the graft, but prosthetic function is still improved (Fig. 6–62).

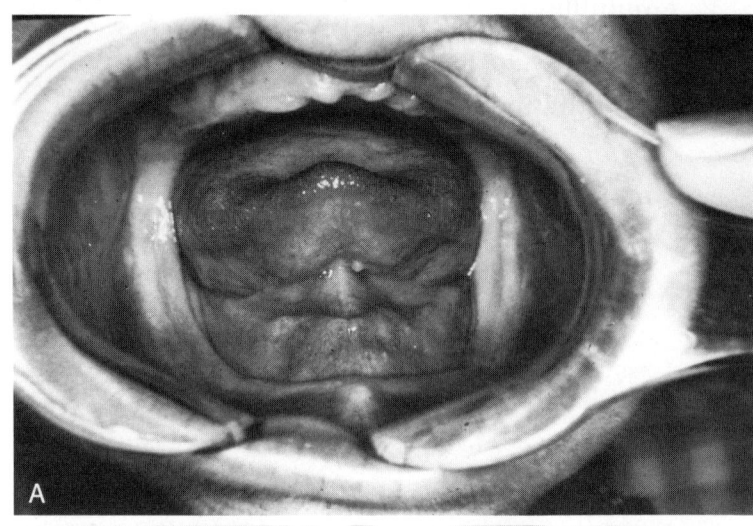

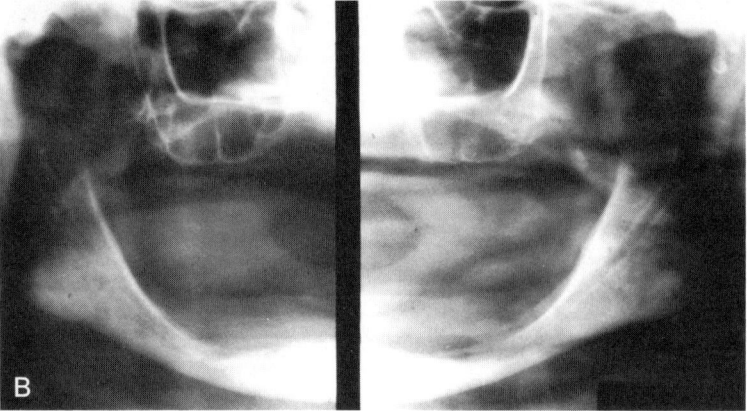

Figure 6–60. Another example of extreme edentulous loss.

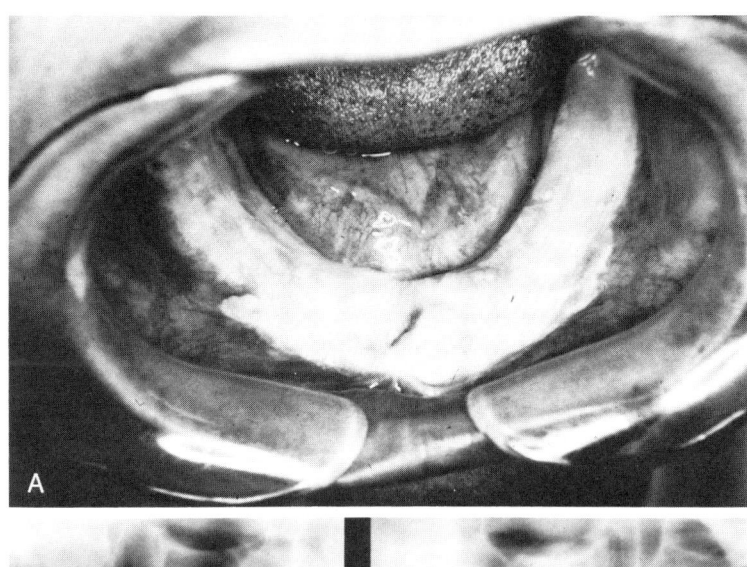

OSSEOUS RECONSTRUCTION OF EDENTULOUS BONE LOSS / **157**

Figure 6–61. The two-year follow-up shows an adequate buccal and labial vestibule with some resorption of the bone graft.

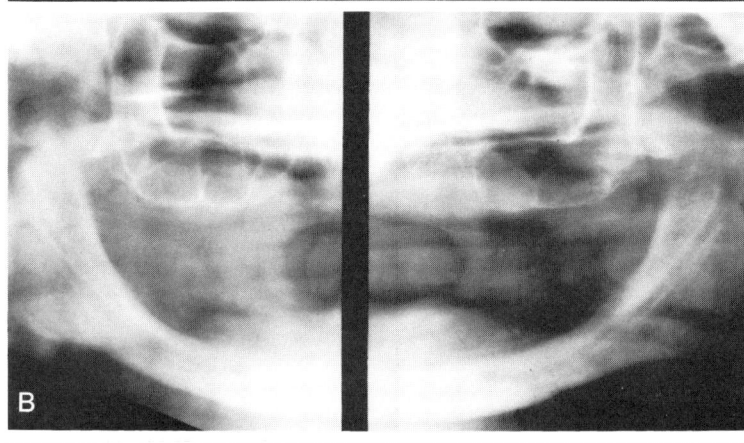

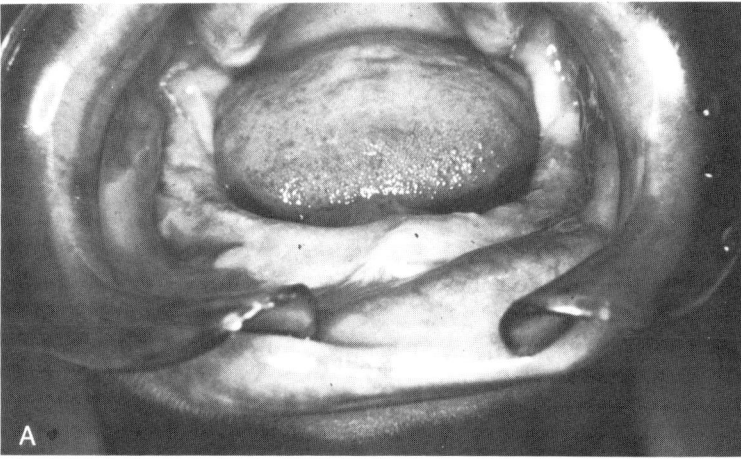

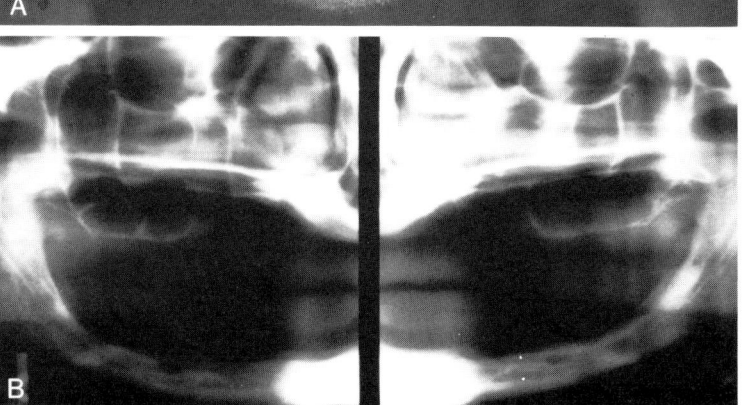

Figure 6–62. Long-term (11 year) follow-up reveals a progressive resorption of the graft, but prosthetic function is still improved.

CASE VI

This 44-year-old white woman presented with a chief complaint of an inability to wear her lower denture.

Clinical radiographic evaluation revealed moderate anterior edentulous bone loss and severe posterior loss (Fig. 6–63).

The patient was considered to be an excellent candidate for an anterior horizontal osteotomy with an interposed allogeneic block graft and posterior tunnelling using hydroxyapatite particles.

A crestal incision from one first molar area to the other was made. Labial and buccal dissection to expose the anterior mandible and mental foramina was performed. Bilateral vertical osteotomies were made just anterior to the mental foramina, extending inferiorly approximately one third the distance toward the inferior border (Fig. 6–64). These two vertical cuts were connected by a horizontal cut extending through the lingual plate of bone (Fig. 6–65). Care was taken to not violate the lingual soft tissue pedicle. Once the cuts were complete the pedicle was mobilized superiorly (Fig. 6–66). The bone graft was wired using two circummandibular wires.

The posterior tunnels were then developed bilaterally (Fig. 6–67). The hydroxyapatite particles were injected into the tunnelled dissection (Fig. 6–68). Closure was performed by advancing the sutured area and injecting additional particles as the closure proceeded anteriorly (Fig. 6–69).

Six months postoperatively a palatal mucosal graft procedure was performed. Two years postoperatively the patient has good prosthetic function and ridge form (Fig. 6–70).

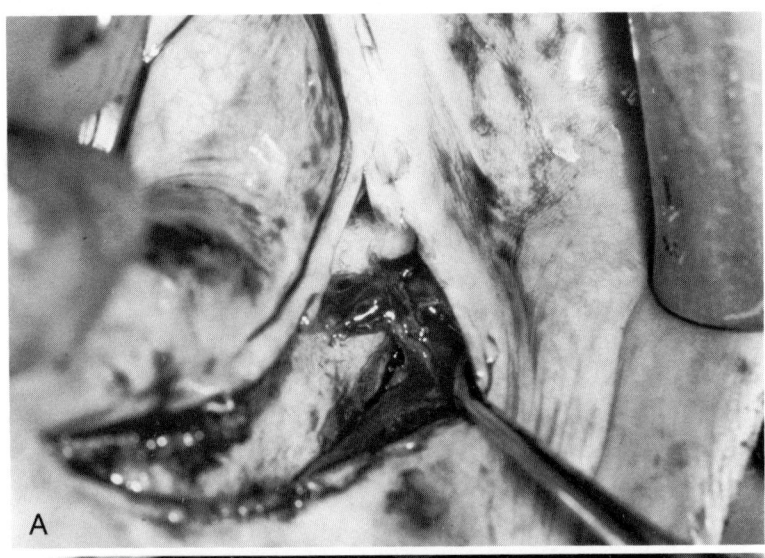

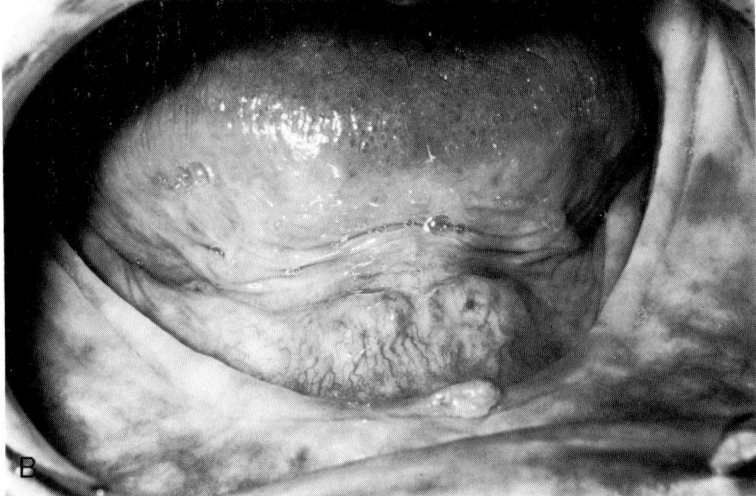

Figure 6–63. Clinical evaluation reveals moderate anterior edentulous bone loss and severe posterior loss.

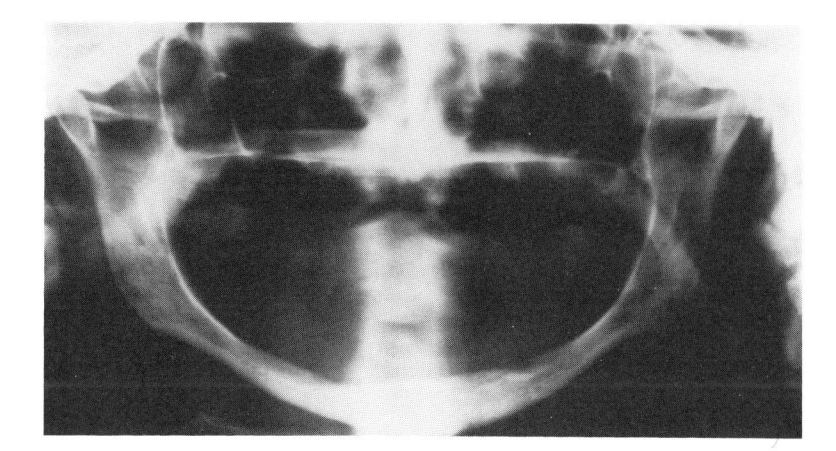

Figure 6–64. Bilateral osteotomies were made just anterior to the mental foramina extending inferiorly approximately one third the distance toward the inferior border.

Figure 6–65. These two vertical cuts were connected by a horizontal cut extending through the lingual plate of bone.

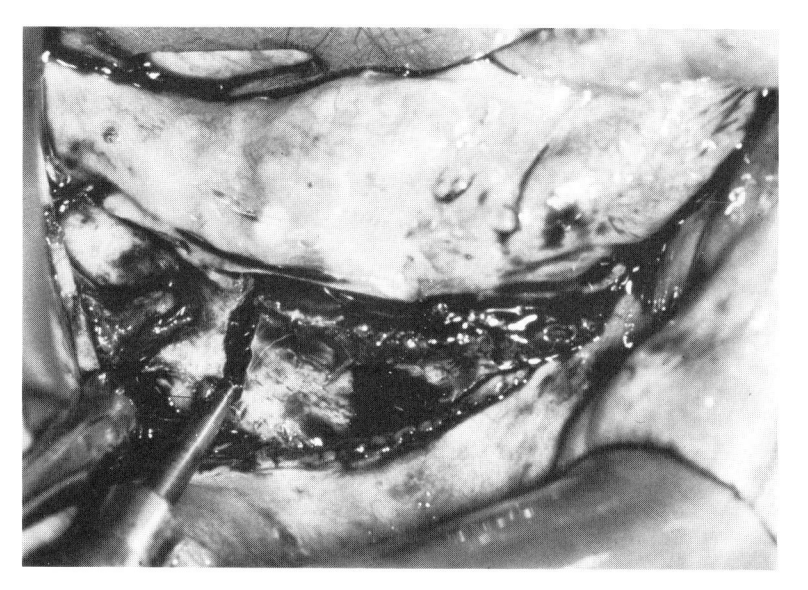

Figure 6–66. Once the cuts were complete, the pedicle was mobilized superiorly.

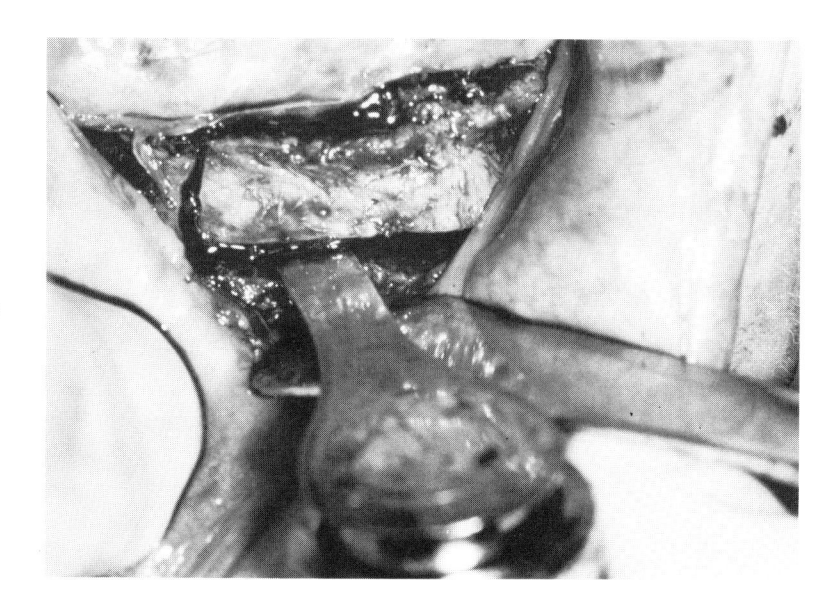

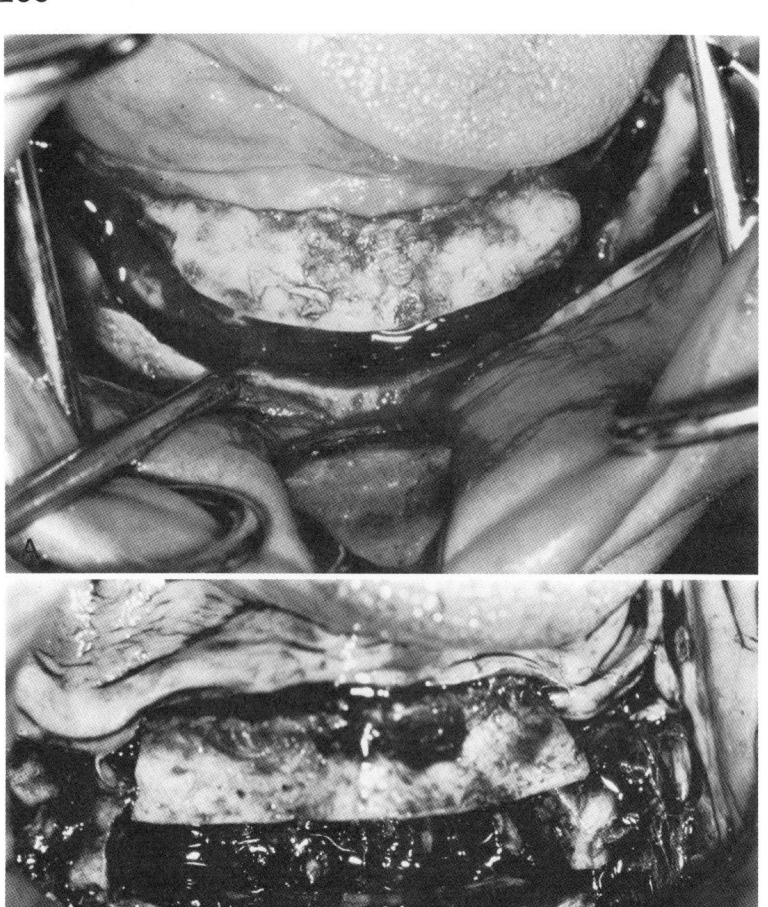

160 / OSSEOUS RECONSTRUCTION OF EDENTULOUS BONE LOSS

Figure 6–67. The posterior tunnels were developed bilaterally.

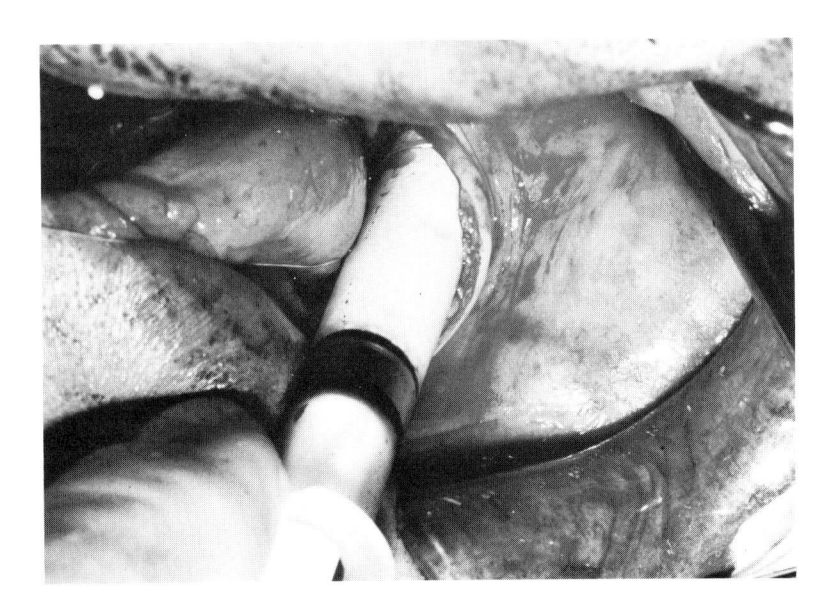

Figure 6–68. The hydroxyapatite particles were injected into the tunnelled dissection.

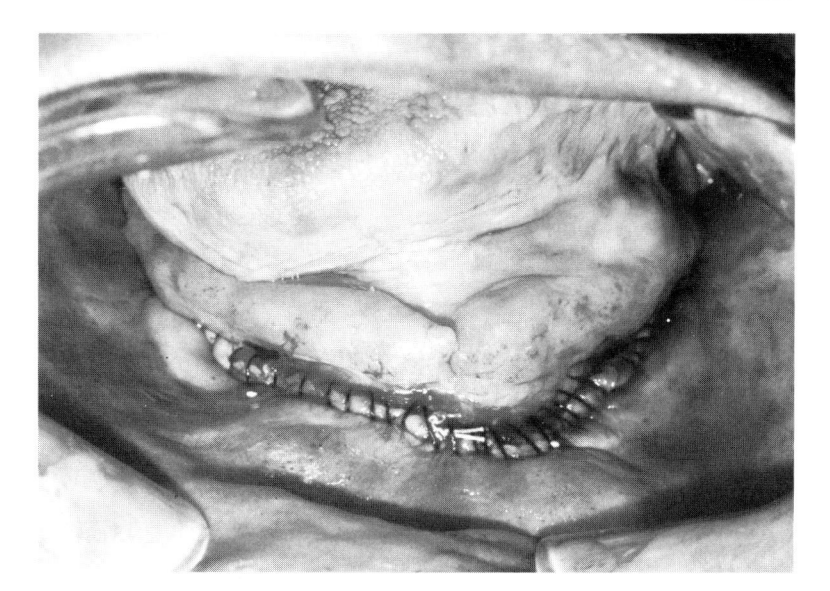

OSSEOUS RECONSTRUCTION OF EDENTULOUS BONE LOSS / **161**

Figure 6–69. Closure was performed by advancing the sutured area and injecting additional particles as the closure proceeded anteriorly.

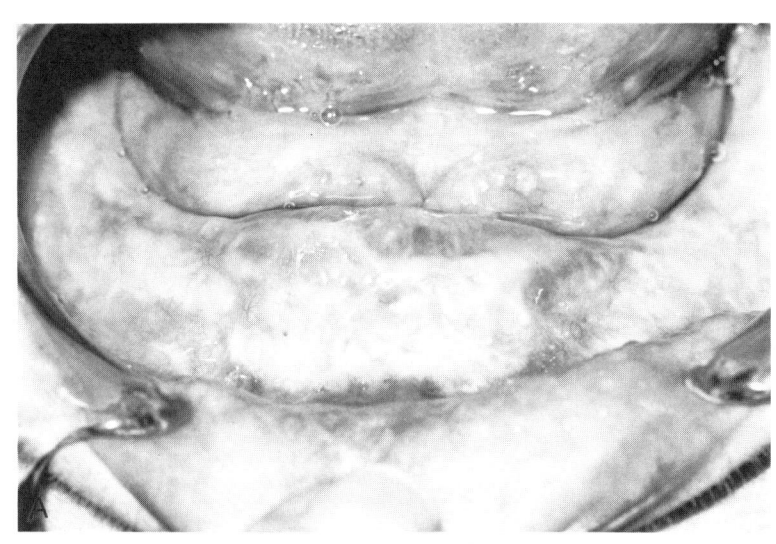

Figure 6–70. Two years postoperatively, the patient has good prosthetic function and ridge form.

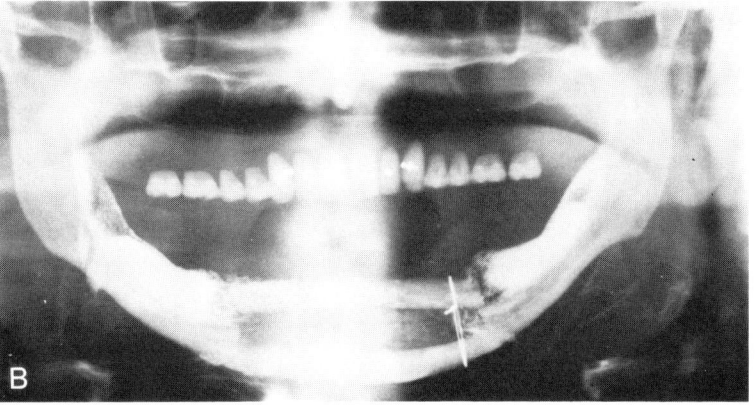

Donor Site Surgery

Iliac Crest

The iliac crest is a widely used source of both cancellous and corticocancellous bone for use in autogenous grafting. The bone is easily accessible, can be obtained in adequate quantities for most purposes, and may be obtained at the same time that the recipient site is prepared. The morbidity of bone removal from the anterior iliac crest is low. A standard approach to the anterior iliac crest will be described, with modifications for specific situations.

The ala of the ilium is the large expanded portion that bounds the greater pelvis laterally. The ala is smoothly concave on the pelvic surface, and ventrally is convex on the gluteal surface. The anterosuperior and posterosuperior iliac spines form the boundaries of the crest. Approximately 5 cm dorsal to the anterosuperior spine is a prominent tubercle. The crest is thinner in the central portion than near the spines. Because the ilium is thickest between the anterosuperior spine and the tubercle, these are important landmarks.

The patient is positioned with sand bags elevating the hip and shoulder. Following preparation of the skin and isolation of the field, the anterosuperior iliac spine, crest, and tubercle are palpated. By firmly pressing medial and superior to these landmarks, the skin may be pulled over the crest. The skin incision may be made beginning 1 cm dorsal to the spine and should be approximately 5 cm in length. Once the skin relaxes, this incision will be located away from the bony prominences and belt line and in an area within swimsuit lines. The initial incision is carried through skin and subcutaneous tissues to the fascia lata. The tissues should be undermined at this time.

The crest is again palpated and the incision is continued through fascia lata, muscle, and periosteum. Again, it is important to remain 1 cm dorsal to the spine in order to avoid the lateral femoral cutaneous nerve, which may take a variable path in this region. This is the only major vascular or neural structure in the dissection field. The periosteum is elevated along the incision and over the crest for a distance varying with the amount of bone required.

At this point, the technique will vary depending on the type of graft required and operator preference as to approach. The simplest and most direct method will use a lateral approach that divides the iliac crest. When only cancellous bone is required, the periosteum need be undermined only enough to identify the crest. An osteotome is then directed vertically to outline the bone flap at its anterior and posterior extents. The osteotome is used to cut through the lateral cortex for a distance of 2 to 3 cm. Between these vertical cuts, the osteotome is used to make a cut midway along the crest. Using a large osteotome, this flap is now outfractured to expose the cancellous bone, which may be carefully removed with curettes. Perforation of the medial cortical plate is to be avoided. This bone, as removed, should be stored in sterile saline.

Following removal of all cancellous bone, the wound is irrigated and the bone flap is replaced by digital pressure.

When a corticocancellous graft is to be obtained, the periosteum is elevated over the lateral surface to expose an area slightly larger than the proposed graft. The outline of the graft may be made with osteotomes or a drill. Again this flap may be fractured out with large osteotomes. Once the flap is removed and stored in saline, the remaining cancellous bone is removed with curettes.

Following wound irrigation and after establishing hemostasis, the periosteum and muscles are reapproximated. If a drain is necessary, it is inserted superficial to the periosteal closure and may exit through the dorsal end of the incision or through a stab wound. The drain must be placed so that it exits in a region that is dependent while the patient is supine. The following layers are closed in order: fascia lata, Scarpa's fascia and subcutaneous tissues, and skin. A pressure dressing is placed and maintained for 48 hours.

Modifications of the above methods have been described which include the medial approach to the ilium. This approach is essentially the same as that described but involves exposing the medial surface and there developing the bone flaps. The medial ap-

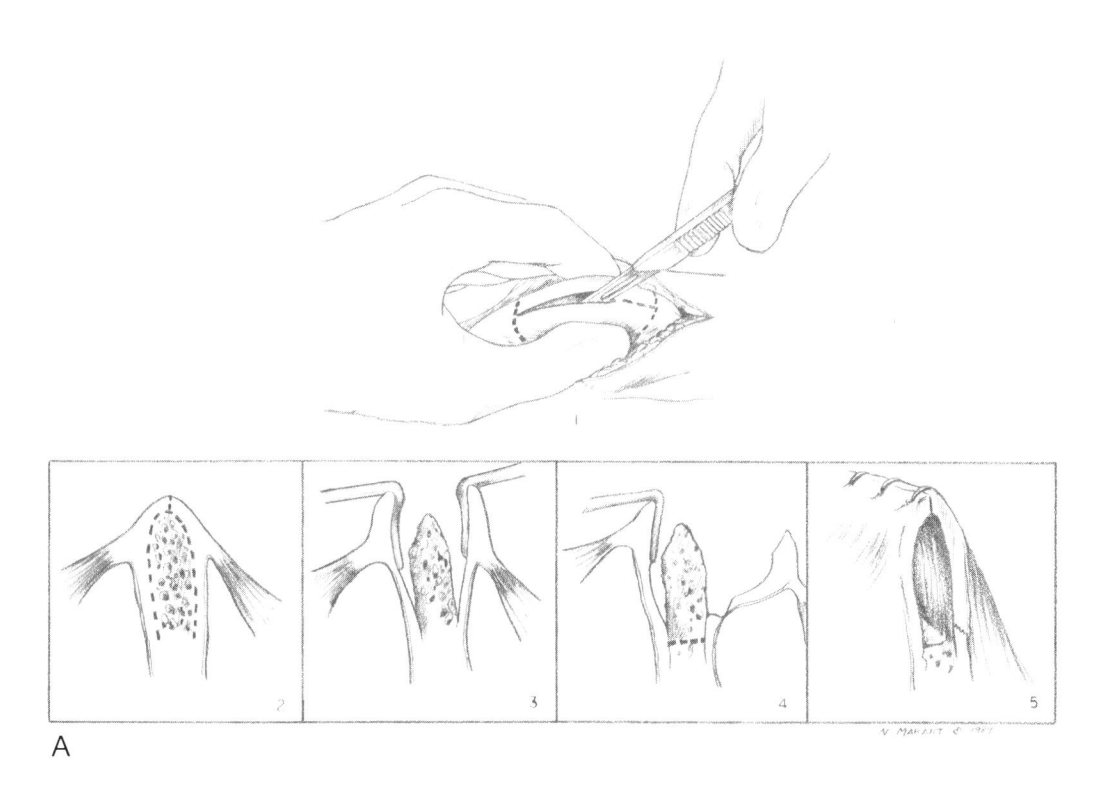

OSSEOUS RECONSTRUCTION OF EDENTULOUS BONE LOSS / **163**

Figure 6–71. A medial approach to the ilium. This approach is essentially the same as what is described in the text, but involves exposing the medial surface and there developing the bone flaps. It is claimed that the medial approach provides easy access for all types of grafts while avoiding gait disturbances and inadvertent perforation of the peritoneum.

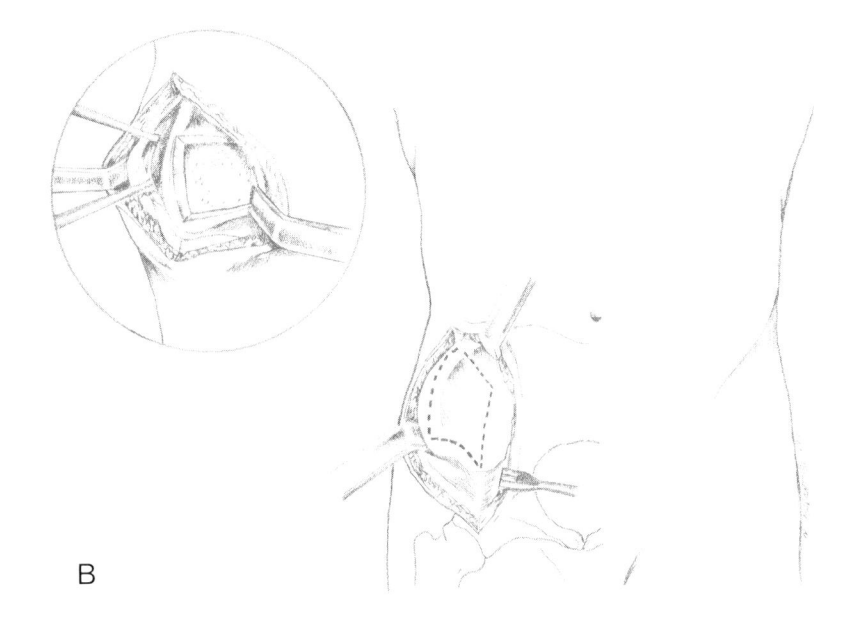

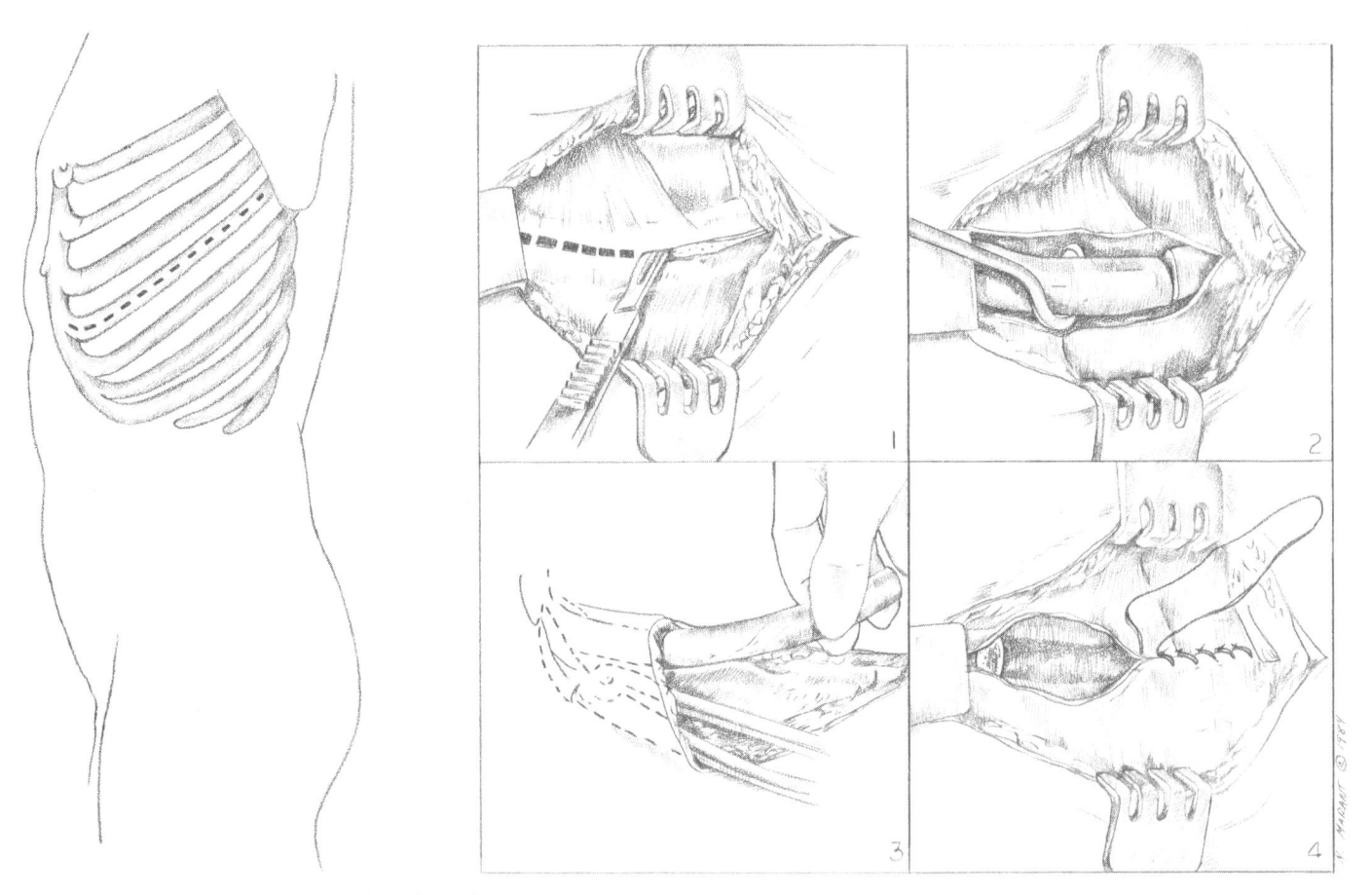

Figure 6–72. Surgical technique for rib grafting.

proach is stated to provide easy access for all types of grafts while avoiding gait disturbances and inadvertent perforation of the peritoneum (Fig. 6–71).

The iliac crest functions as an epiphysis until fusion occurs at age 20 to 25. Because of this, some experts advocate avoiding the iliac crest and using a subepiphyseal approach.

Rib

Because most oral and maxillofacial surgeons are not proficient in thoracic surgery, it is important that a thoracic surgeon perform the surgery to procure a rib graft. A common approach to resect one or more ribs will be discussed (Fig. 6–72).

The patient is positioned in a lateral decubitus position. The skin incision is made along the line of the rib in the region of ribs 5 to 7. The length will be dictated by the required graft size. The muscles are sharply divided and the periosteum of the rib exposed. Vertical incisions are made through periosteum at the anterior and posterior extent of the graft. A curved elevator is used to dissect first to the superior edge of the rib and then to the inferior edge. A sharp, curved raspatory is carefully used to separate the periosteum from the rib's inner surface. This separation should be performed carefully and cleanly to avoid perforating the pleural cavity.

Without removing the raspatory, a rib forceps is inserted and the rib is cut and removed and should be stored in saline. Bleeding is usually slight, but should be controlled by cautery or ligation. Careful examination for pneumothorax must be made, and a chest tube is inserted if necessary. The wound is closed in layers: periosteum, muscle, subcutaneous tissues, and skin. A postoperative chest radiograph is mandatory. Chest physiotherapy must be prescribed postoperatively.

BIBLIOGRAPHY

1. MacIntosh RB, and Obwegeser HL: Preprosthetic surgery: A scheme for its effective employment. J Oral Surg 25:397, 1967.
2. Terry BC, Albright JE, and Baker RD: Alveolar ridge augmentation in the edentulous maxilla with use of autogenous ribs. J Oral Surg 32:429–434, 1974.

3. Baker RD, and Connole PW: Preprosthetic augmentation grafting—autogenous bone. J Oral Surg 35:541, 1977.
4. Wolford LM, and Epker BN: The use of freeze-dried bone as a biologic crib for ridge augmentation. A preliminary report.
5. Male AJ, Gasser J, Fonseca RJ, and Nelson J: Comparison of onlay autologous and allogeneic bone grafts to the maxilla in primates. J Oral Maxillofac Surg 42:487–499, 1983.
6. Davis WH, Delo RI, Weiner JR, et al.: Transoral bone graft for atrophy of the mandible. J Oral Surg 28:760–765, 1970.
7. Bell WH, Buche WA, Kennedy JW, and Ampil JP: Surgical correction of the atrophic alveolar ridge. A preliminary report on a new concept of treatment. Oral Surg 43:485–498, 1977.
8. Wessberg GA, Jacobs MK, Wolford LM, and Walker RV: Preprosthetic management of severe alveolar ridge atrophy. J Am Dent Assoc 104:464–472, 1982.
9. Breine U, and Branemark P: An experimental and clinical study of immediate and preformed autologous bone grafts in combination with osseointegrated implants. Scand J Plast Reconstr Surg 14:23–48, 1980.
10. Fonseca RJ, Nelson JF, Clark PJ, Frost DE, and Olson RA: Revascularization and healing of onlay particulate allogeneic bone grafts in primates. J Oral Maxillofac Surg 41:153, 1983.
11. Farrell CD, Kent JN, and Guerra LR: One-stage interpositional bone grafting and vestibuloplasty of the atrophic maxilla. J Oral Surg 34:901–906, 1976.
12. Bell WH, and Buckles RL: Correction of the atrophic alveolar ridge by interpositional bone grafting: A progress report. J Oral Surg 36:693–700, 1978.
13. Stroud SW, Fonseca RJ, Sanders GW, and Burkes EJ, Jr.: Healing of interpositional autologous bone grafts after total maxillary osteotomy. J Oral Surg 38:878–885, 1980.
14. Frost DE, Fonseca RJ and Burkes EJ, Jr: Interpositional homologous grafts to the maxilla. J Oral Surg 40:776–784, 1982.
15. Araujo A, Schendel SA, Wolford LM, and Epker BN: Total maxillary advancement with and without bone grafting. J Oral Surg 36:849–858, 1978.
16. Charest A, and Goodyear V: Palatal osteotomy: A simple approach to maxillary alveolar atrophy. J Oral Surg 34:442–444, 1976.
17. Leonard M, and Howe GL: Palatal vault osteotomy. Oral Surg 46(3):344–348, 1978.
18. Liposky RB: Maxillary osteotomy and vestibuloplasty for the correction of maxillary anterior atrophy: Preliminary report. Oral Surg 48(2):101–107, 1979.
19. Wang JH, Waite DE, and Steinhauser E: Ridge augmentation: An evaluation and follow-up report. J Oral Surg 34:600, 1976.
20. Fazilli M, vanOvervest-Eerdman GR, Vernooy AM, Visser WJ, and vanWaas AJ: Follow-up investigation of reconstruction of the alveolar process in atrophic mandible. Int J Oral Surg 7:400–404, 1978.
21. Davis WH, Delo RI, Ward WB, Terry B, and Patakas B: Long term ridge augmentation with rib graft. J Maxillofac Surg 3:105–106, 1975.
22. Barros Saint-Pasteur J: Plastia restauradora de la cruesta alveolar de la mandibula. Acta Odont Venez 4:3–21, 1966.
23. Barros Saint-Pasteur J: Plastia reconstructiva del reborde alveolar. Nuestra investigacion clinicoguirugica. Acta Odont Venez 8:168–182, 1970.
24. Schettler D: Sandwich Technique mit Knorpeltransplantat zur Alveolarkamm erhöhung im Unterkiefer. Fortsch Kiefer Gesichtschir XX:61–63, 1976.
25. Stoelinga PJW, deKoomen HA, Tideman H, and Huybers TMJ: A reappraisal of the interposed bonegraft augmentation of the atrophic mandible. J Maxillofac Surg 11:107–112, 1983.
26. Bunte M, and Strunz V: Ceramic augmentation of the lower jaw. J Maxillofac Surg 5:303–309, 1977.
27. deKoomen HA: De verhoging van de geresorbeerde mandibula. Thesis. Catholic University of Nijmegen. The Netherlands, 1982.
28. Härle F: Long-term results with the visor-osteotomy. Int J Oral Surg (Suppl)1:83–87, 1981.
29. Sugar A, and Hopkins R: A sandwich mandibular osteotomy: A progress report. Br J Oral Surg 20:168–174, 1982.
30. Tallgren A: The continuing reduction of the residual alveolar ridges in complete denture wearers: A mixed longitudinal study covering 25 years. J Prosthet Dent 27:120, 1972.
31. Härle F: Visor osteotomy to increase the absolute height of the atrophied mandible. J Maxillofac Surg 3:257, 1975.
32. Härle F: Follow-up investigation of surgical correction of the atrophic alveolar ridge by visorosteotomy. J Maxillofac Surg 7:283–293, 1979.
33. Hopkins R: A sandwich mandibular osteotomy: A preliminary report. Br J Oral Surg 20:155–167, 1982.
34. Peterson LJ, and Slade EW: Mandibular ridge augmentation by a modified visor osteotomy: Preliminary report. J Oral Surg 35:999–1004, 1977.
35. Schettler D, and Holterman W: Clinical and experimental results of a sandwich technique for mandibular alveolar ridge augmentation. J Maxillofac Surg 5:199–202, 1977.
36. Lekkas K: Absolute augmentation of the mandible. Int J Oral Surg 6:147–152, 1977.
37. Stoelinga PJW, Tideman H, Berger JS, and deKoomen HA: Interpositional bonegraft augmentation of the atrophic mandible. J Oral Surg 36:30–32, 1978.
38. deKoomen HA, Stoelinga PJW, Tideman H, and Huybers TMJ: Interposed bonegraft augmentation of the atrophic mandible. J Maxillofac Surg 7:129–135, 1979.
39. Fitzpatrick BN: Visor/sandwich osteotomy progress report. Int J Oral Surg 10:87–92, 1981.
40. Frost DE, Gregg JM, Terry BC, and Fonseca RJ: Mandibular interpositional and onlay bonegrafting for treatment of mandibular bony deficiency in the edentulous patient. J Oral Maxillofac Surg 40:353–360, 1982.
41. Baker RD, Terry BC, Davis WH, and Connole PW: Long term results of alveolar ridge augmentation. J Oral Surg 37:486–489, 1979.
42. Maloney F, Stoelinga PJW, Tideman H, and deKoomen HA: Recent development with interposed bonegrafting of the atrophic mandible. In preparation.
43. Brown LJ: A surgical solution to a lower denture problem. Br Dent J 95:215–216, 1953.
44. Downton D: Mylohyoid ridge resection. Dent Rec 74:212–214, 1954.
45. Kelly JF, and Friedlaender GE: Preprosthetic bone graft augmentation with allogeneic bone: A preliminary report. J Oral Surg 35:268, 1977.
46. Marx RE, Kline SN, Johnson RP, Malinin TI, Matthews JG, 2nd, and Gambill V: The use of freeze-dried allogeneic bone in oral and maxillofacial surgery. J Oral Surg 39:264, 1981.

7

IMPLANTS USED IN PREPROSTHETIC RECONSTRUCTIVE SURGERY

*John Helfrick, D.D.S., M.S.,
P. I. Brånemark, M.D., Ph.D., D.M.D.,
T. Albrektsson, M.D., Ph.D.,
Hans Bosker, D.M.D.,
Lucas VanDijk, D.M.D.,
Charles A. Babbush, M.Sc.D., D.D.S.,
George J. Collings, D.M.D.,
Gerald A. Niznick, D.M.D., M.S.D.,*
and *Francis V. Howell, D.D.S.*

IMPLANTS USED IN RECONSTRUCTIVE SURGERY

The goals of restorative dentists are clearly the provision of excellent masticatory function, esthetics, and phonation. These should be provided permanently and without any deleterious side effects. Because these goals are utopian, it is unlikely that they will ever be completely attained. However, it appears that progress has been made and is continuing. With the loss of a few teeth, fixed prostheses often approach an ideal solution, but when many or all teeth are lost, the problem becomes much more complex and difficult. The removable prosthesis and surgical aids could usually provide an infection-free restorative milieu but with obvious deficiencies in stability, comfort, and masticatory efficiency.

It is thus not surprising that a resurgence of interest in fixed prostheses via dental implants began in the early 1950's. However, these early efforts with subperiosteal and blade-type implants were almost always plagued by the presence of a peri-implant fibrous capsule, which predisposed to infection and loss of adjacent bone.

With few exceptions, the long-term results of dental implants have been poorly reported. Because of the interest and controversy generated with dental implants, a conference was held at Harvard University in June, 1978.

The Harvard Conference was designed to assess the safety and efficacy of dental implants. The conference was convened primarily in an attempt to predict the survivability of the various dental implants. Considerable attention was devoted to data on efficacy, i.e., benefit versus risk. Although many "successes" had been reported by dentists, attending members at the conference were concerned about whether the patient had actually benefited from the implant, whether the implantable device served the purpose for which it was designed, and whether the implants performed at or above standards previously accepted by dental reconstructive procedures.

Four commonly used implants were evaluated: the subperiosteal, transosteal/staple, vitreous carbon, and blade implants. Unfortunately the work of Brånemark et al. was not addressed at the conference, although it had been published in 1977. The definition of success was that *"the dental implant provides functional service for five years in 75 per cent of the cases."* The subjective criteria included (1) adequate function, (2) absence of discomfort, (3) improved esthetics, and (4) improved emotional and psychological attitude.

Objective success was determined by the following criteria: (1) bone loss no greater than one third of the vertical height of the implant; (2) good occlusal balance and vertical dimension; (3) gingival inflammation amenable to treatment; (4) mobility of less than 1 mm in any direction; (5) absence of symptoms and infection; (5) absence of damage to adjacent teeth; (7) absence of paresthesia or violation of the mandibular canal, maxillary sinus, or floor of the nasal passage; and (8) healthy collagenous tissue.

As a result of the statistics, the conference attendees accepted the following:

1. Subperiosteal implants (supporting a full arch mandibular denture and opposing a removable denture), including the work of five investigators with a total of 200 implants, suggest the five-year survival rate may be as high as 90 per cent and the ten-year survival rate as high as 65 per cent. One investigator reported data on 44 patients with a five-year survival as low as 46 per cent and a ten-year survival as low as 39 per cent.

2. Mandibular staple bone plate implants (7-pin) had a 95 per cent survival rate for five years in 43 patients; however, these statistics were based on the work of a single investigator.

3. Vitreous carbon implants have about a 55 per cent survival rate (range of 50 to 60 per cent) for three years, based on the work of two investigators and a sample of 133 single interdental implants.

4. Blade implants used in free-end applications, which primarily involve bridges with one pontic and two or more natural abutments, have a five-year survival rate as high as 90 per cent. This statistic was based on the work of two investigators reporting on 200 implants. Two other investigators reported on 70 implants in which the five-year survival rate was as low as 65 per cent. Insufficient data prevented a vote on blade implants acting as distal support for three-unit bridges with one pontic and one natural abutment, or five-unit bridges with two pontics and two natural abutments. Blade implants used to support a full arch (no natural teeth) have a five-year survival rate of 75 per cent, based on the work of one investigator reporting on 89 implants.

Four categories were established into which the conference participants were asked to place the various implants. The categories were: A—unrestricted use, B—use with guidelines, C—clinical trials only, and D—human application contraindicated. None of the implants were placed in the A or D categories.

Subperiosteal and blade implants in free-end and interdental sites when used as partial support for a fixed bridge were placed in category B. Transosteal (other than the staple bone plate), full arch blade (with no natural teeth), and vitreous carbon implants were placed in category C.

Although the mandibular staple orthopedic bone plate was not endorsed for category B (reports on success were from a single investigator), the FDA, following a review of the Harvard deliberations and subsequent publications by other investigators, elevated the staple to Class II (category B) status in 1983. Helfrick et al. published a survey of 250 staple patients who had been followed for up to 7.5 years.[1] They found at the time of their paper that 242 of their patients were functioning well; 17 (6.6 per cent) had experienced reversible complications, and 223 (89.2 per cent) of their patients had experienced no postoperative problems. The types and nature of their complications are shown in Table 7–1.

The Harvard Congress evaluated the types and significance of various complications associated with implants and agreed upon the following criteria for their removal:

1. Chronic pain
2. Significant movement
3. Infection
4. Progressive loss of supportive bone
5. Intolerable paresthesias and/or anesthesias
6. Oro-antral or oro-nasal fistulae
7. Bone fracture
8. Significant medical or psychiatric illness
9. Irreversible implant breakdown
10. Irreversible damage to adjacent teeth
11. Cosmetic problems

If the Harvard Conference were held today, the criteria for success of dental implants would be considerably elevated. This elevation would be primarily related to the excellent research findings of Brånemark et al., as well as Small and Bosker.

The salient factors of the Brånemark system which contributed to the success rate appear to be (1) minimal trauma to the bone adjacent to the fixture during placement; (2) a biocompatible material that would allow integration with bone at the level of light microscopy; and (3) passivity of the implant until integration occurs. This is discussed more fully later in this chapter.

With the apparent importance of osseointegration in implantology, the staple systems of Small and Bosker are being observed to evaluate the degree of osseointegration of these modalities, as their success rate has

TABLE 7–1. COMPLICATIONS OF THE MANDIBULAR STAPLE BONE PLATE

Complications	No. of Patients	Etiology	Treatment
Stress loosening	10	Denture not tissue-borne (prosthetic overload).	Remake denture. 3 staples removed due to severe mobility and extrusion.
Fractured staple	5	All fractures occurred in staples that had 3/32-inch transosteal pins that are no longer being used. Pins are now 7/64-inch in diameter.	2 removed and replaced. 2 asymptomatic with conventional dentures. 1 functioning with one staple abutment and an overlay denture.
Infection	5	Poor patient resistance; possible contamination at time of surgery.	I&D and antibiotics. 2 staples removed due to mobility and uncontrollable infection.
Hyperplasia	3	Pins placed labial to ridge.	Excise hyperplasia around pins.
Psychological	1	Psychotic—poor patient selection.	Psychiatrist advised staple removal.

SUMMARY OF CASES

Cases	Cases with No Complications	Cases with Reversible Complications	Cases with Irreversible Complications (Removed)	Cases Functioning at This Time
250	226 (90.3%)	14 (5.7%)	10 (4.0%) (2 staples reinserted)	242 (96.0%)

From Helfrick JF, Topf JS, and Kaufman M: Mandibular staple bone plate: Long-term evaluation of 250 cases. J Am Dent Assoc 104:318–320, 1982.

---

been encouraging. Both of these systems have had good follow-up studies.

Other implant systems with variations from the work of Brånemark et al. are proliferating. Some of these systems are included in this chapter. However, there appear to be varying degrees of success with these other systems, and their ultimate usefulness has yet to be validated by good long-term studies.

Selection of the Implant Candidate

The judicious selection of a candidate for an elective procedure is the key to the success of that operation. Second to the appropriate candidate selection is the determination of a suitable treatment plan, correct selection of the indicated implant modality, and implementation of superior surgical and prosthetic care. These factors have been given only modest attention in the past[2-6] but recently have been given greater attention.[7,8]

Medical Evaluation

The implant candidate may reveal many important findings when a comprehensive health history is carried out. The American Dental Association's Health Questionnaire (long form) renders a very complete and uniform outline. If metabolic bone disease is suspected, additional evaluation may be appropriate as outlined in Tables 1–4 and 1–5. By using standardized forms such as these, a systematic review is easily carried out but a stereotyped form is not mandatory. Various conditions or pathologic entities may be identified which would contraindicate the use of dental implants. An adequate history not only provides information about an individual's known health problems but may also lead to the detection of previously undiagnosed general medical diseases.

A detailed discussion of the various diseases that may play a part in evaluation of a patient relative to dental implants is presented in Chapters 1 and 3.

Dental Evaluation

Dental History

The dental evaluation of the implant patient is just as important as the medical evaluation. Individuals may lose their teeth for a variety of reasons. Periodontal disease, caries, trauma, and tumor are the most prevalent forms of tooth loss. Periodontal disease and caries may be due to neglect on the part of the patient. If a patient was not interested and/or knowledgeable enough to care for his own natural dentition, he may not be motivated to maintain dental implants properly.

Evaluation of the Oral Cavity

One of the factors contributing to a favorable prognosis for dental implants is whether or not the oral cavity is in a good state of health to accept and maintain implants. In creating a treatment plan for a candidate, the implant placement and reconstruction should be the last stage of the plan.

For the partially edentulous patient all oral surgery, periodontal therapy, and endodontic therapy should be completed. Carious lesions should be eliminated and individual dental units temporized (Fig. 7–1). The individual who has a poor state of dental health should be placed into a controlled program of oral hygiene for a 6- to 12-month period. Some patients will require the fabrication of a transitional prosthesis for purposes of function and esthetics during this phase. The clinician is able to assess the patient's ability to learn and willingness to cooperate during this period, which will give some

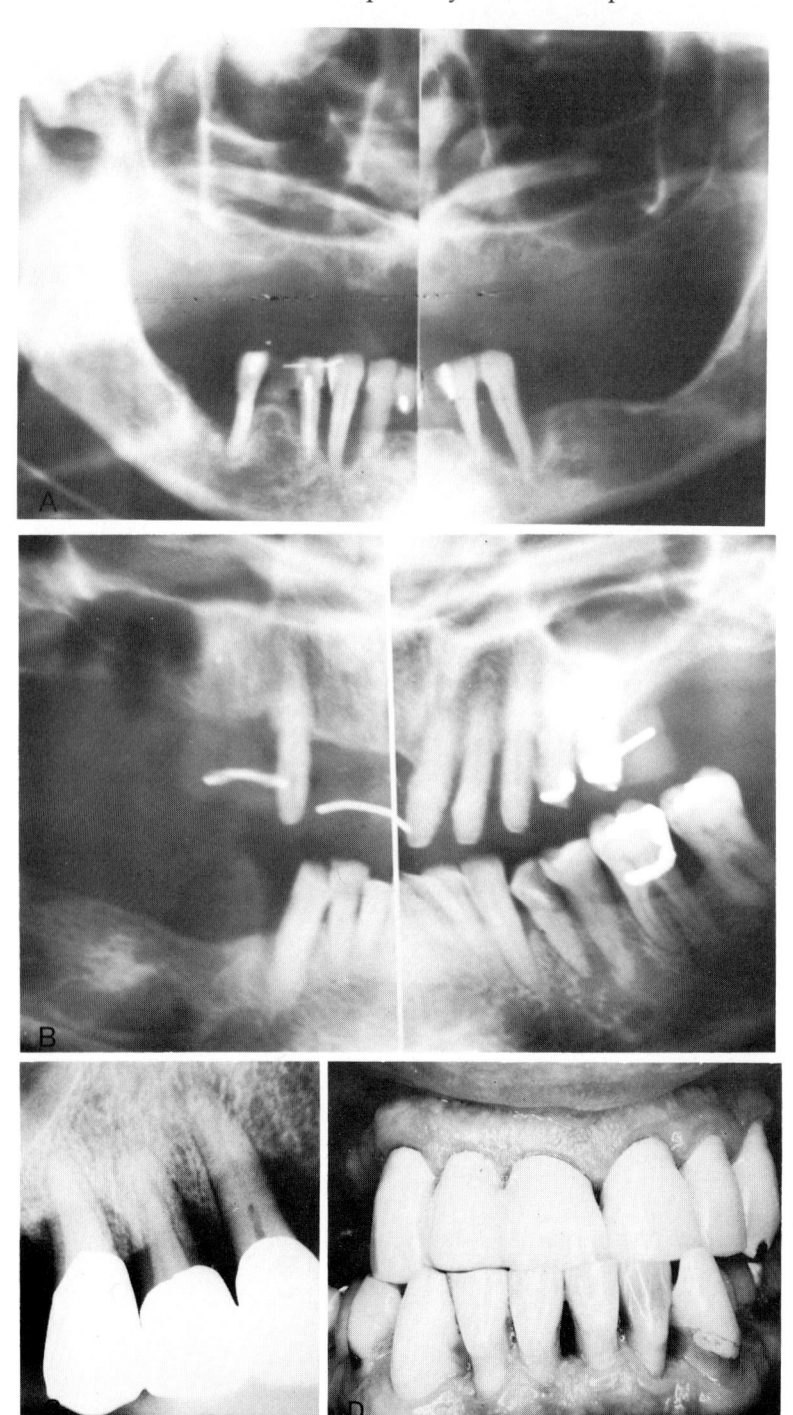

Figure 7–1. All necessary endodontic, periodontal, oral surgical, and restorative procedures must be carried out prior to final treatment planning for the implant restoration. The patient with poor history of cooperation and maintenance in dental care should be placed into a control program for 6 to 12 months.

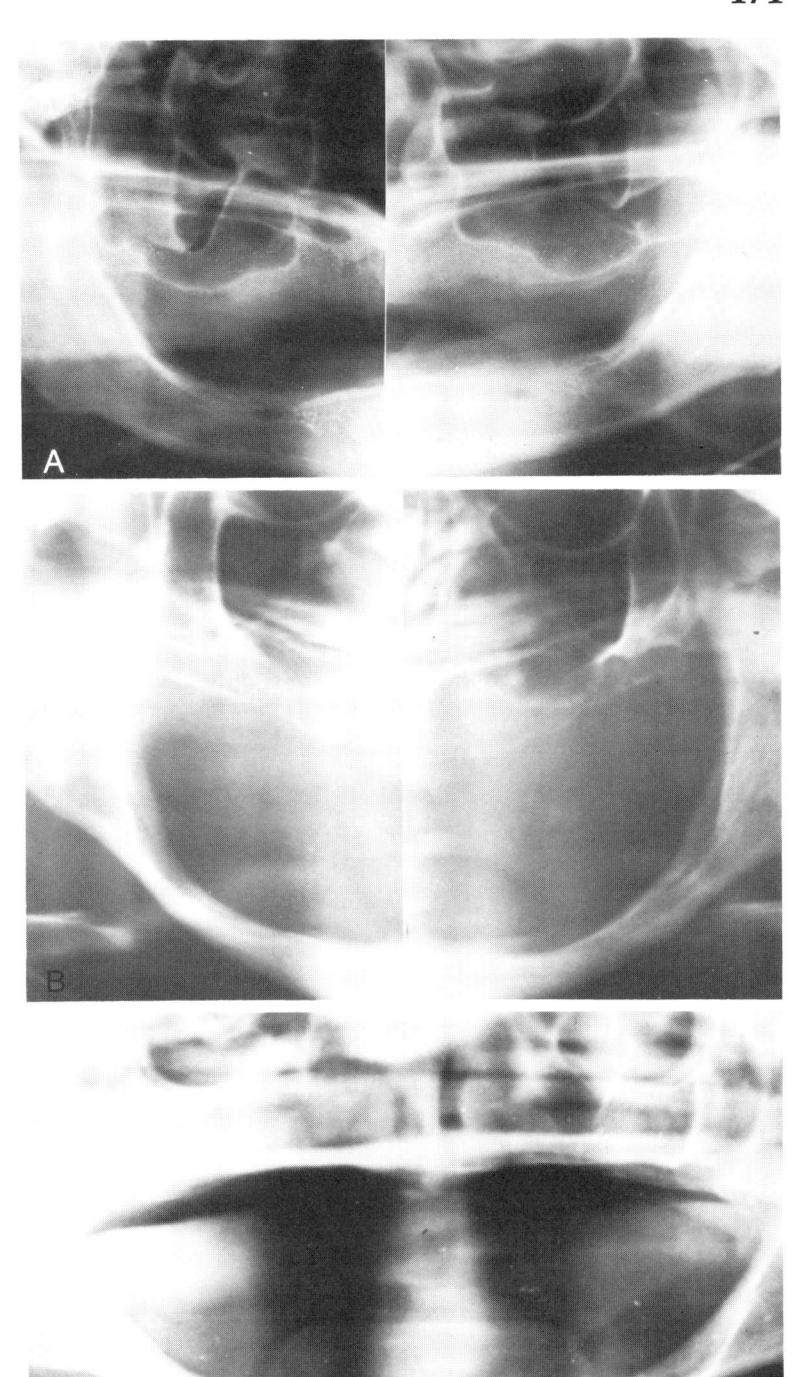

IMPLANTS USED IN PREPROSTHETIC RECONSTRUCTIVE SURGERY / **171**

Figure 7–2. *A,* Radiograph displaying rather advanced atrophy of the maxilla. The mandible has a minimal amount of resorption, and most endosteal implants could be placed with a favorable prognosis. *B,* Panoramic radiograph displaying moderate degrees of both maxillary and mandibular atrophy, indicating the use of a mandibular subperiosteal implant. *C,* Panoramic radiograph demonstrating severe advanced atrophy of both jaws. No implant could be used in this case. Bone grafting procedures are indicated.

guidelines as to the long-range prognosis for implants. If the pretreatment evaluation period is favorable, the treatment plan, which includes implant reconstruction, can be initiated.

Radiographs

The radiograph is a valuable diagnostic aid for implant planning. The appropriate radiographs will allow visualization of the anticipated area of implantation. The surrounding and adjacent structures such as the floor and walls of the maxillary sinus, the floor of the nasal cavity, the inferior alveolar canal, the mental foramina, and the height of the alveolar ridges must be visualized (Fig. 7–2). The presence of pathologic lesions may also be determined. A combination of periapical and panoramic radiographs allows for visualization of the above outlined entities (Fig. 7–3). Additional radiographs such as a lateral cephalometric radiograph may be desirable to determine more precisely the height of the symphysis for anterior implants. This is

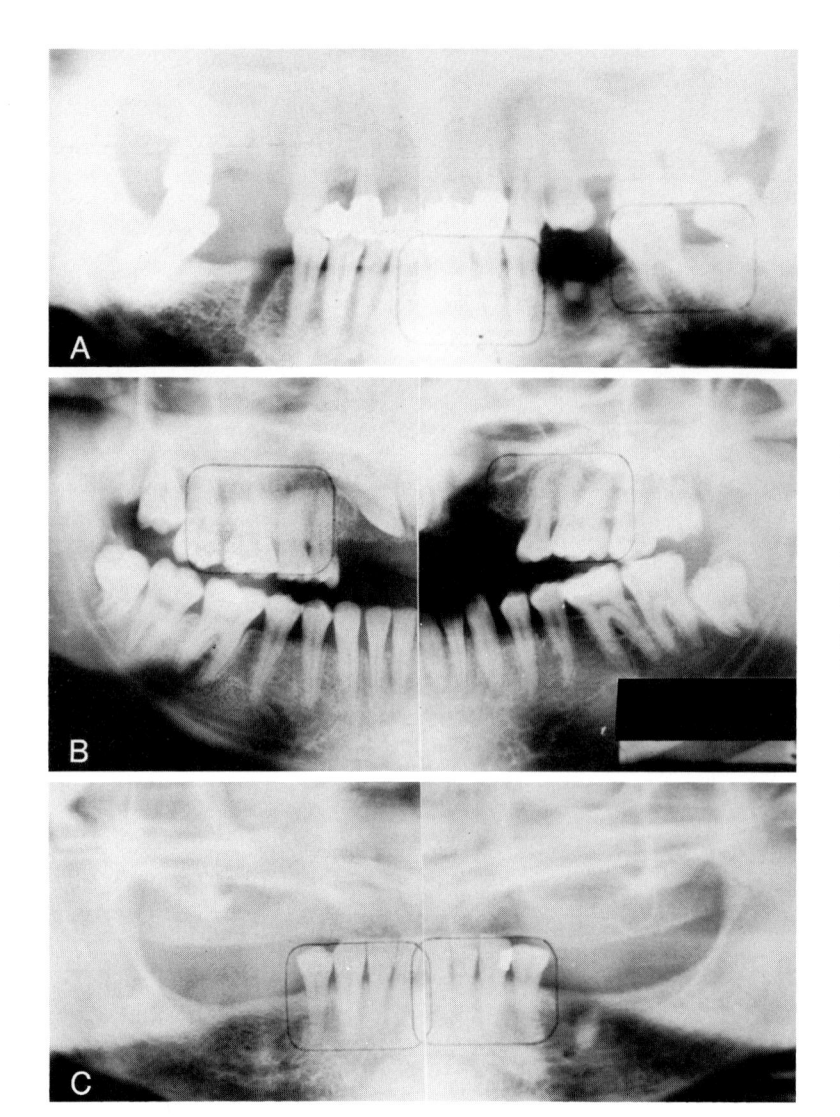

172 / IMPLANTS USED IN PREPROSTHETIC RECONSTRUCTIVE SURGERY

Figure 7–3. *A,* A retained root tip in the mandibular bicuspid region and an incompletely healed postextraction defect were not revealed in this patient's periapical radiographs sent by the referring doctor. A maxillary third molar was demonstrated in the panoramic radiograph. *B,* The maxillary impacted cuspid was in the line of insertion of an endosteal implant. *C,* The mandibular retained root tip was in the line of insertion of an endosteal implant.

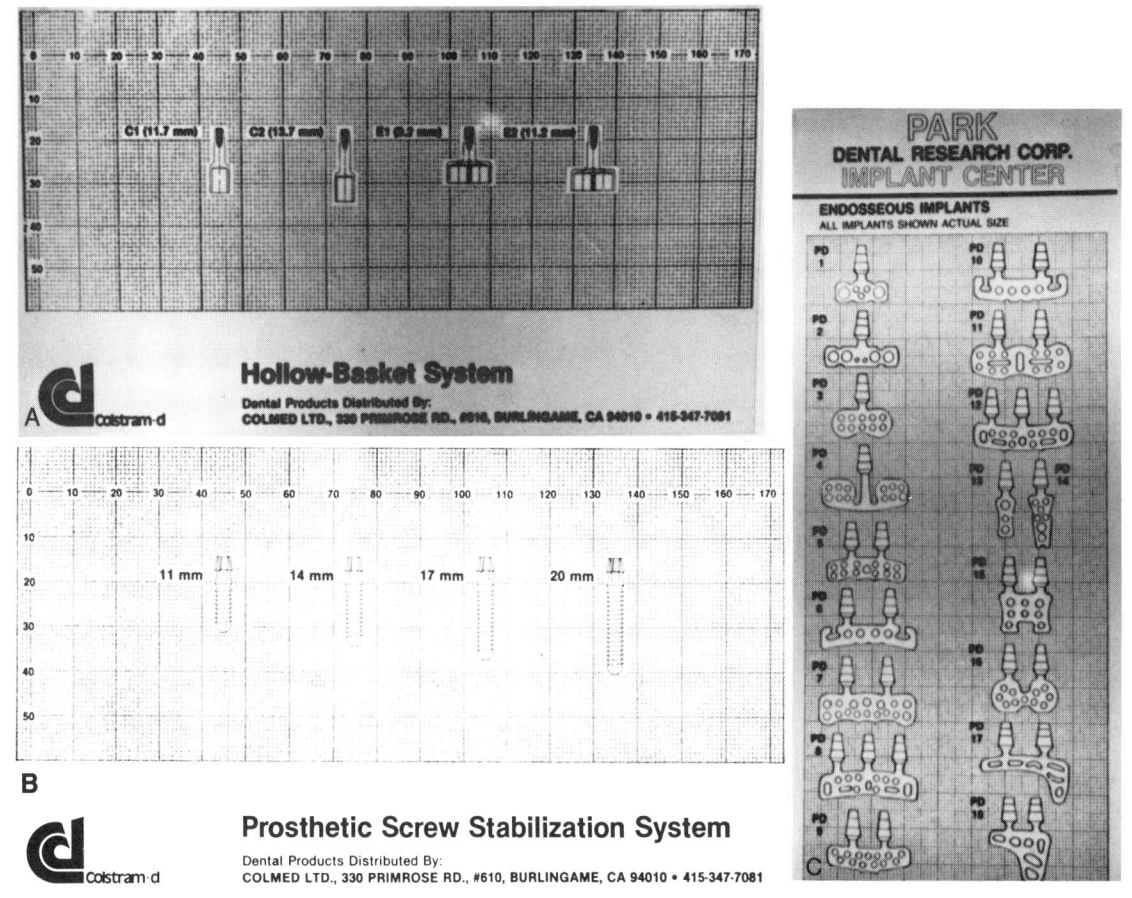

Figure 7–4. Plastic templates are available with most endosteal implant systems: *A*, Endosteal Hollow-Basket System. *B*, Titanium Plasma Spray Screw Implant System. *C*, Endosteal Blade-Vent Implants.

particularly applicable for the Brånemark type restoration of the edentulous mandible.

When endosteal implants are required in the posterior region of the mandible, the relationship to the inferior alveolar canal becomes critical. The proximity to the antrum may not be as critical as once thought. Titanium implants, as reported by Brånemark et al., have penetrated the antrum without a deleterious result, although this is a preliminary observation.

A clear plastic overlay template is available with some endosteal implant modalities (Fig. 7–4). The template is superimposed over the panoramic radiograph to aid in the selection of the appropriate size and shape of implant (Fig. 7–5). The largest implant that will be accepted in a given area without impinging

Figure 7–5. The clear plastic template is superimposed over the radiograph to aid in the selection of the appropriate size TPS Screw Implant.

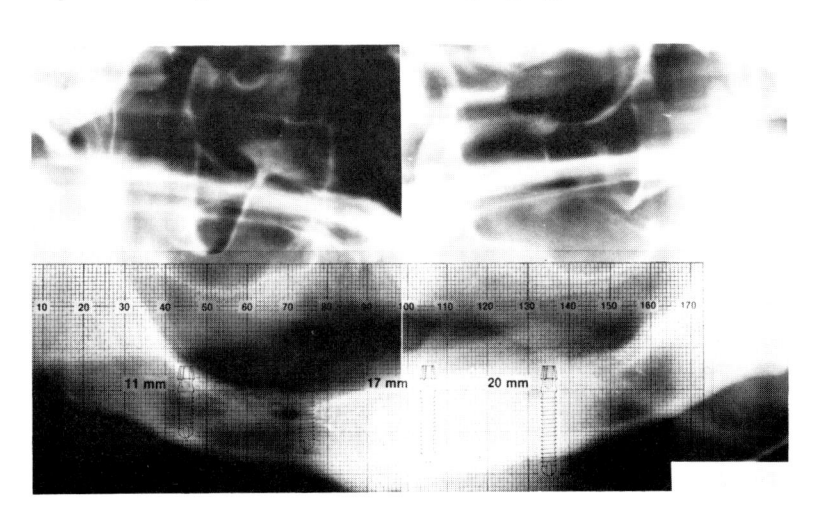

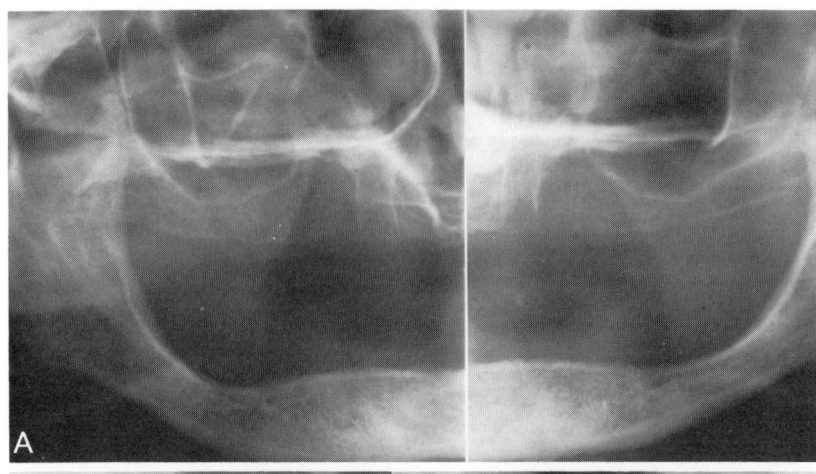

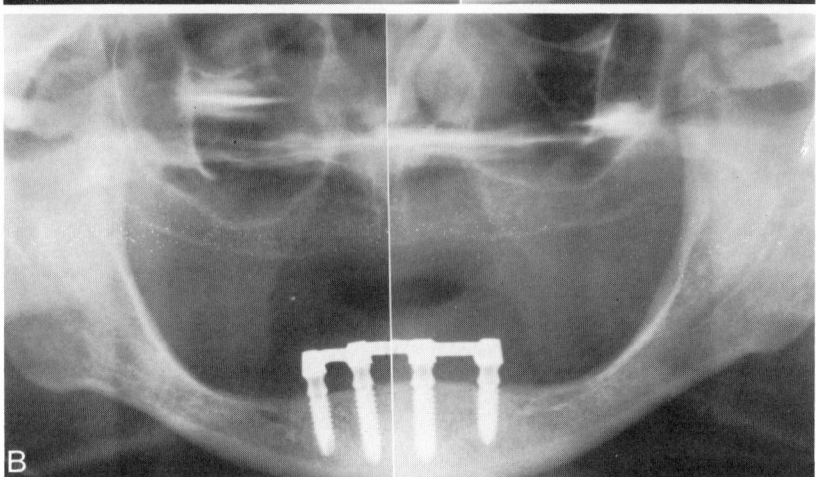

174 / IMPLANTS USED IN PREPROSTHETIC RECONSTRUCTIVE SURGERY

Figure 7–6. *A*, Preoperative radiograph reveals sufficient vertical height of bone in the mandibular symphysis for placement of a TPS Screw System. *B*, The postoperative radiograph demonstrates implants in position without perforation of the inferior cortex.

upon vital structures should be used in order to obtain the most favorable bone-to-implant ratio. Some ultra-short or shallow design implants are of insufficient size. This does not allow for a satisfactory bone-to-implant ratio for achieving good long-range success; these implants should not be used. Various types of implants are depicted in Figures 7–6 to 7–9. Additional types of implants to treat similar anatomic situations will be found later in the chapter, especially the Brånemark system.

Any pathologic abnormalities should be excised prior to implant placement (Fig. 7–10). If these areas involve the receptor site for an implant, a postsurgical waiting period of 6 to 12 months is necessary, or at least until there is no radiographic evidence of a de-

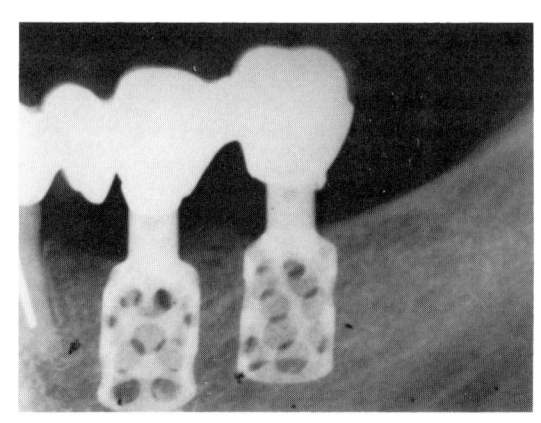

Figure 7–7. Postoperative radiograph revealing sufficient vertical bone to accommodate Endosteal Hollow-Basket Implants without encroachment on the inferior alveolar canal.

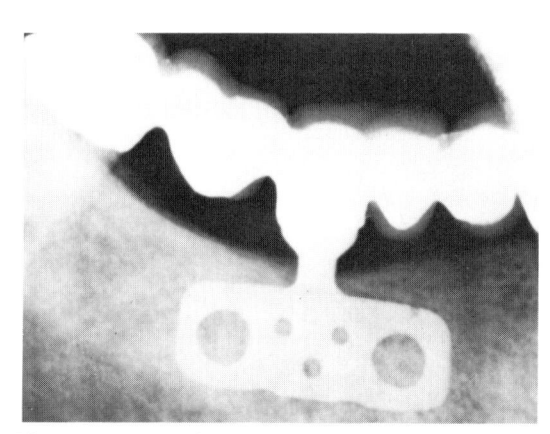

Figure 7–8. Radiograph demonstrating the presence of an Endosteal Blade-Vent Implant with no encroachment on the inferior alveolar canal.

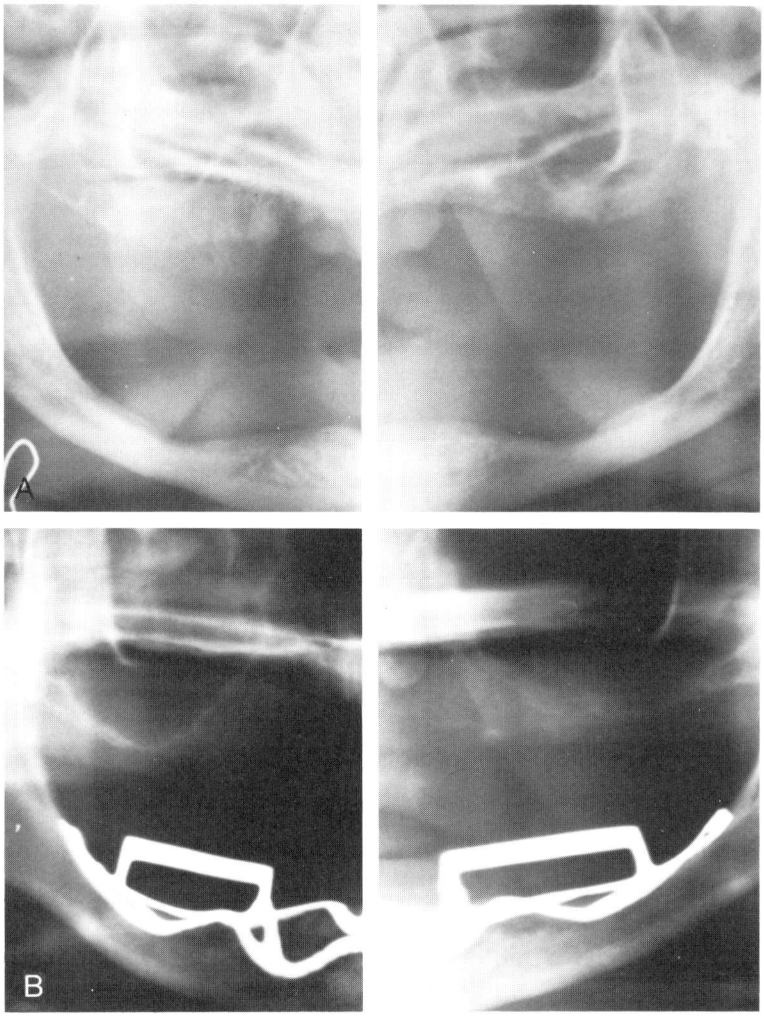

Figure 7-9. *A,* Preoperative radiograph demonstrating rather advanced mandibular atrophy. *B,* Postoperative radiograph demonstrating the successful placement of a subperiosteal implant.

fect. The same waiting period is required following extraction.

Study Casts

Mounted, articulated study casts are desirable and occasionally essential for preoperative study and evaluation. The various concepts involving centric relationships, interarch occlusal clearance, and occlusal discrepancies can be more carefully evaluated in this manner.

Photographs

Pretreatment facial and intra-oral photographs are desirable to record the patient's facial appearance and dental condition (Fig. 7-11). Often the restoration of either good or normal function, i.e., the ability to masticate food, to speak, and to retain a prosthesis with security, is the issue that the patient discusses preoperatively. Postoperatively, the patient's needs are more esthetically oriented. If the cosmetic improvement does not match the patient's underlying expectations, a functional success may be negated. Sometimes, showing the patient the preoperative photographic record to compare with a mirror view of the present result will help overcome postoperative concerns.

If the mental/dental evaluation is carried out in a systemic fashion, and the clinician's past clinical experience and judgment are utilized, successful implant restoration can be accomplished (Fig. 7-12).

TRANSOSTEAL IMPLANTS

THE MANDIBULAR STAPLE

John Helfrich

In 1964, Small conceived the idea of an orthopedic bone plate that could be used to reconstruct the edentulous mandible. To es-

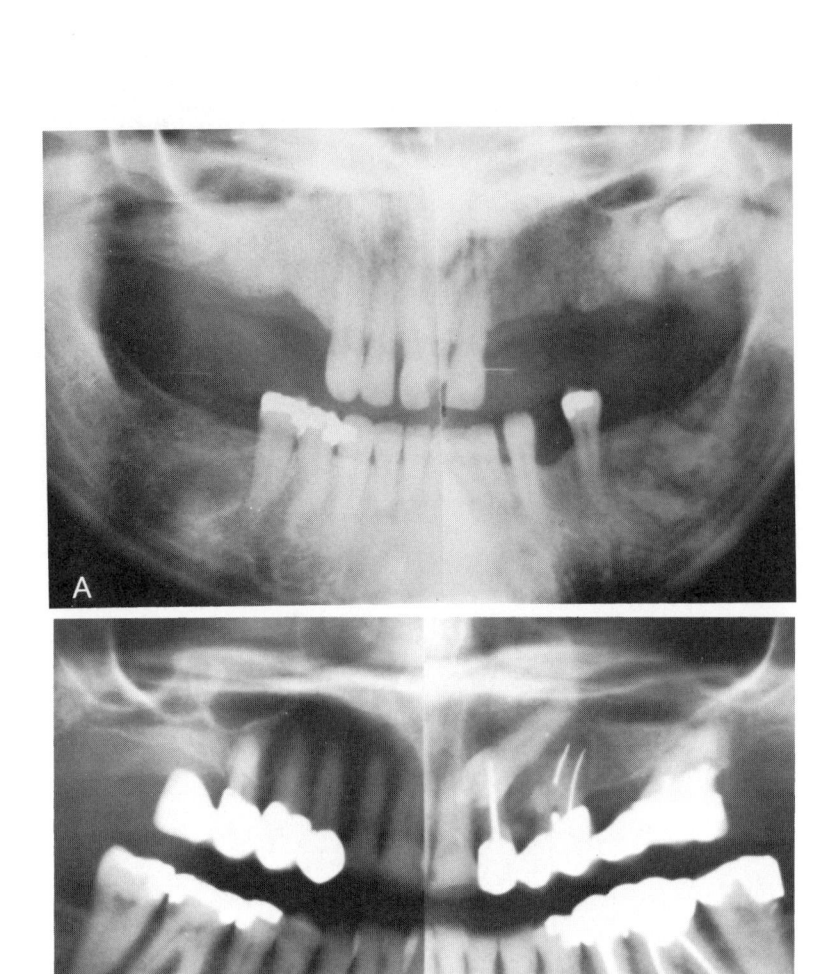

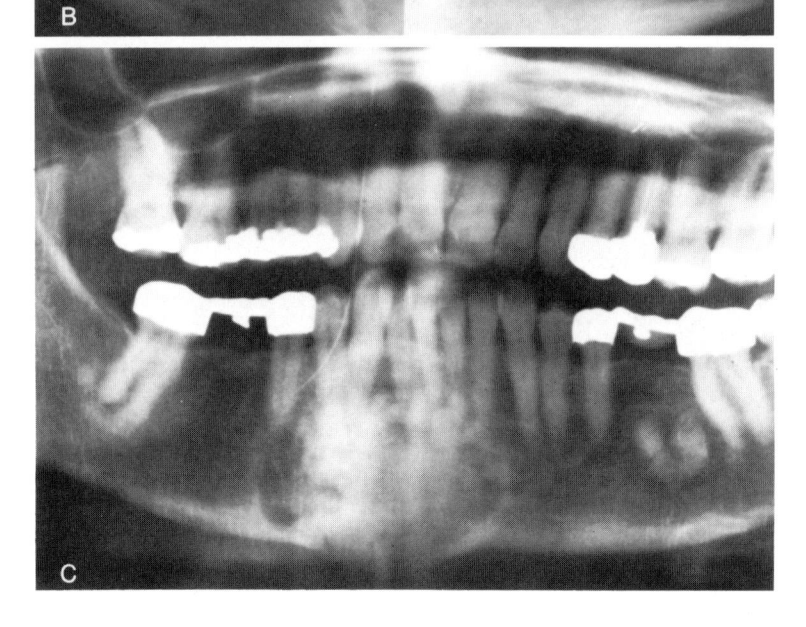

176 / IMPLANTS USED IN PREPROSTHETIC RECONSTRUCTIVE SURGERY

Figure 7–10. *A*, An impacted molar is present in the right maxillary tuberosity region along with an area of fibrous dysplasia in the right posterior mandible. *B*, An impacted cuspid is present in the anterior maxilla. *C*, A large ossifying fibroma occupies the mandibular symphysis completely.

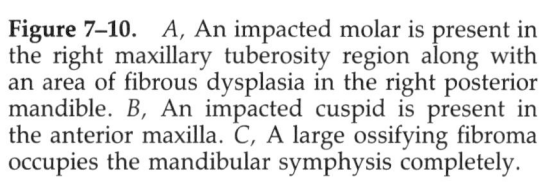

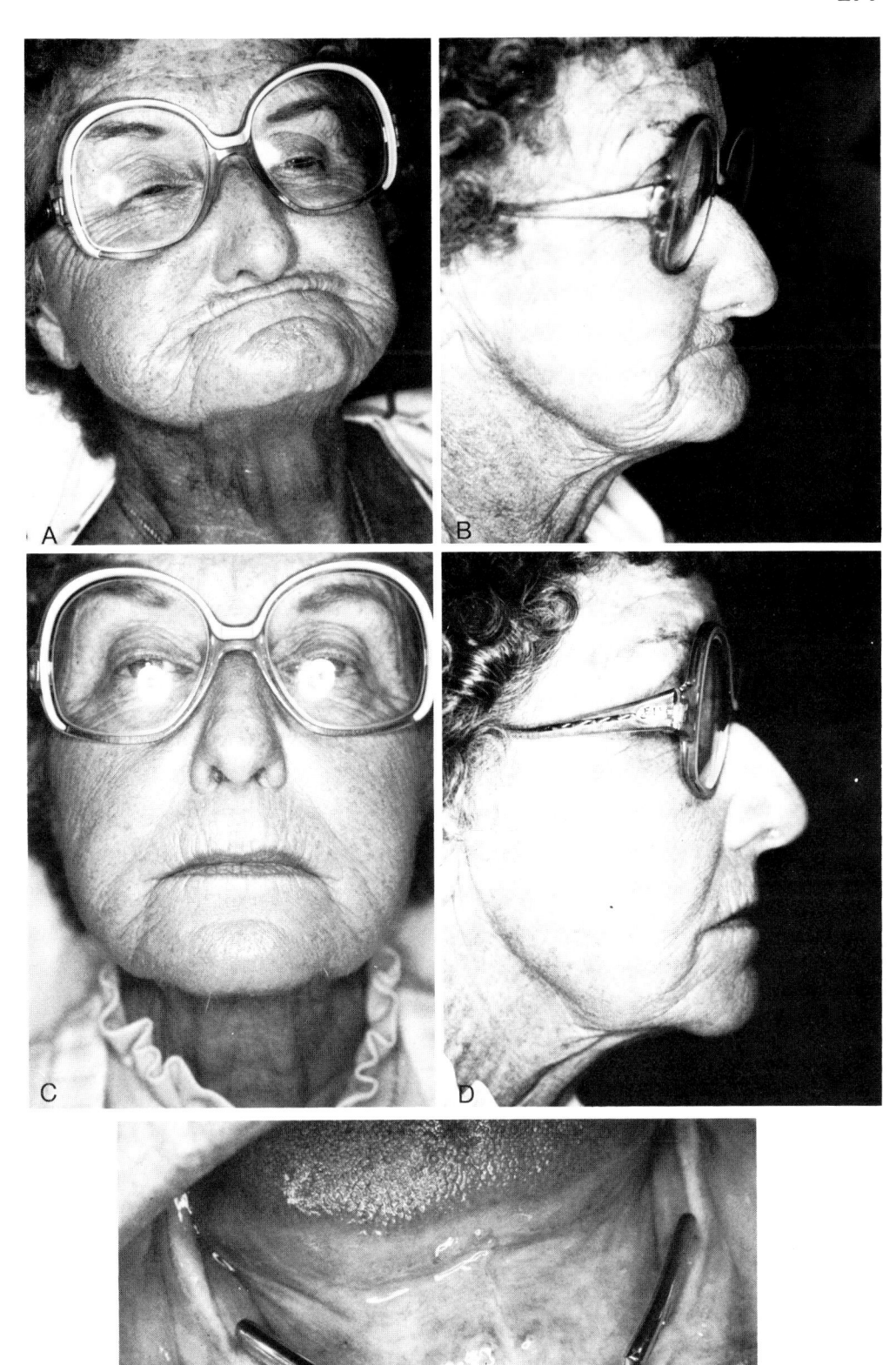

Figure 7–11. *A–D*, Pre- and postoperative full and lateral facial views of a mandibular subperiosteal implant patient. *E*, Postoperative intraoral view of the mandibular subperiosteal implant.

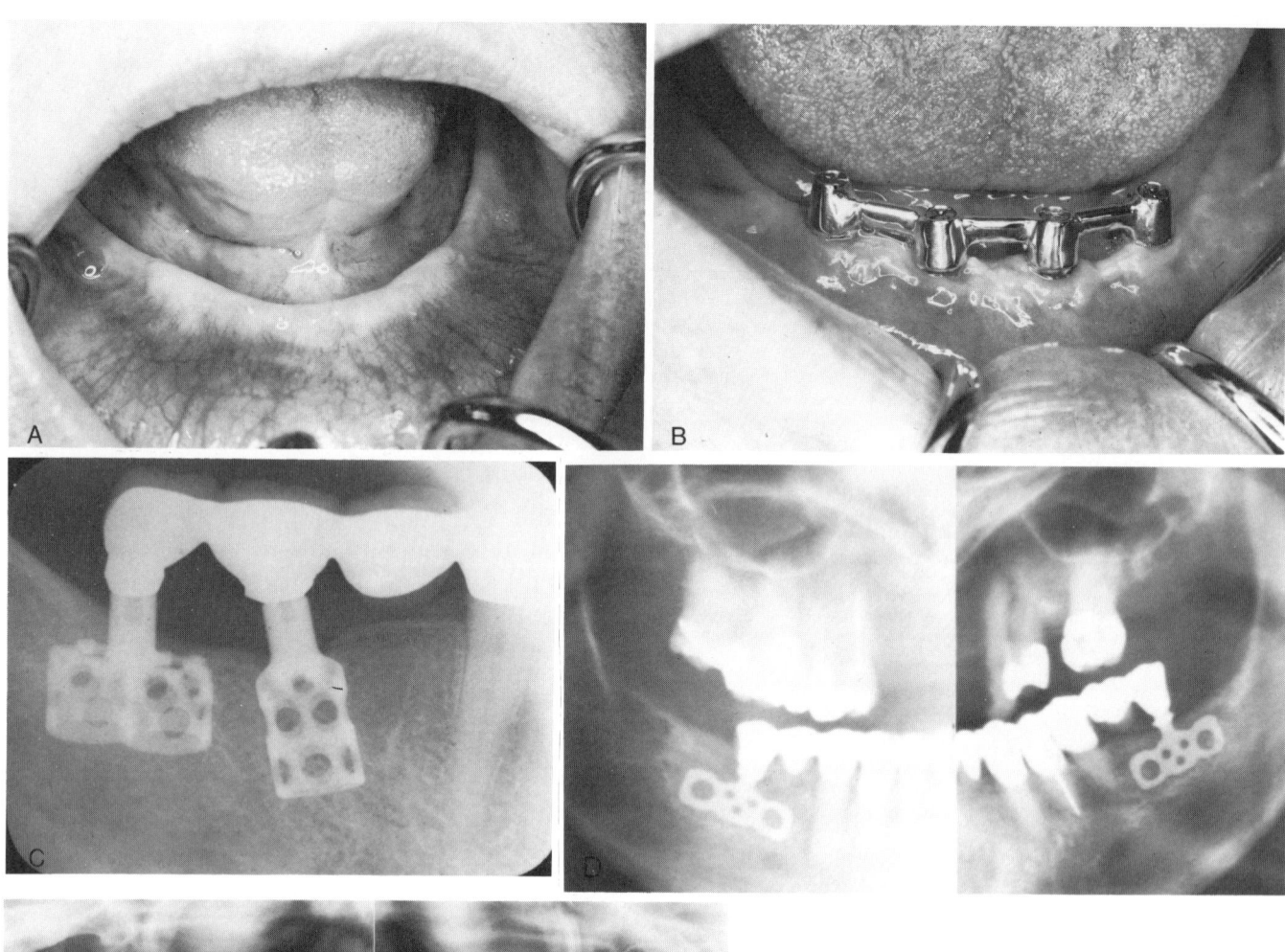

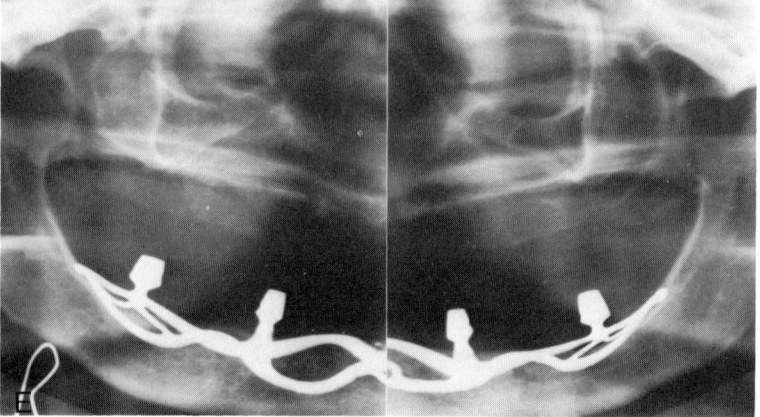

Figure 7–12. *A,* Preoperative intra-oral view of a moderately atrophic mandible. *B,* Clinical view of TPS Screw Implant restoration at 2.6 years. *C,* Endosteal Hollow-Basket Implant restoration at 2.6 years. *D,* Endosteal Blade-Vent Implant restoration. *E,* Mandibular subperiosteal implant restoration at 11 years.

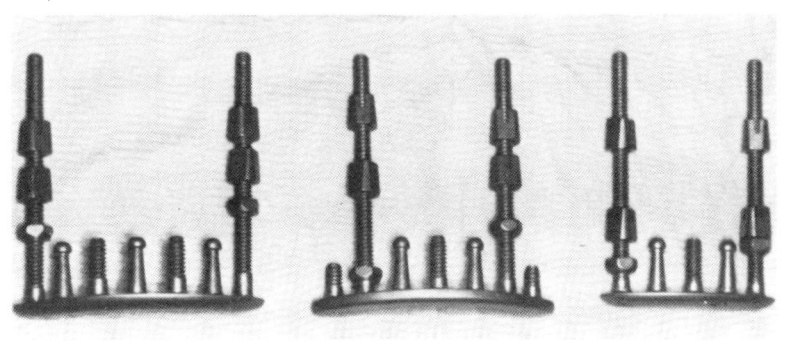

Figure 7–14. Three configurations of the mandibular staple are available: 7-pin, modified 7-pin, and 5-pin.

tablish a scientific basis for this device, he conducted a two-year laboratory research project on dogs (Fig. 7–13).[9]

In 1968, when the laboratory project was successfully completed, a five-year clinical trial was begun on 35 patients. The mandibular staple bone plate was used in this group of patients to reconstruct their severely atrophic mandibles. Upon completion of the project in 1974, this initial group of patients was evaluated by members of the Section of Oral and Maxillofacial Surgery at Sinai Hospital of Detroit. Stringent clinical and radiographic criteria were used in their evaluation.[10] As a result of this peer review process and an evaluation of the laboratory and clinical project by the Sinai Research Committee, the staple was approved for routine clinical use. Small and others have continued to publish results of successful staple bone plate implants.[2, 11-14]

The staple is constructed of a titanium alloy consisting of 90 per cent titanium, 5 per cent aluminum, and 4 per cent vanadium. The strength and resistance to fracture of this alloy, combined with its biocompatibility, are important factors in the success of the implant. The staple is manufactured in three configurations: 7-pin, 5-pin, and a modified 7-pin (Fig. 7-14). The choice of staple depends on the size and shape of the mandible to be reconstructed. The majority of cases require the 5-pin implant; when possible, however, the modified 7-pin staple is utilized, as it results in 30 per cent more retention. The 7-pin staple is rarely used, as the transosteal pins enter the oral cavity in a prosthetically unfavorable (posterior) position on the alveolar ridge.

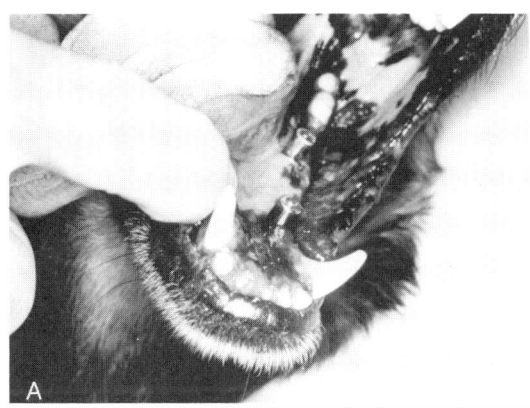

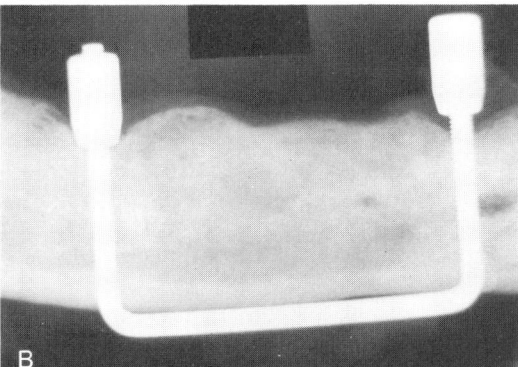

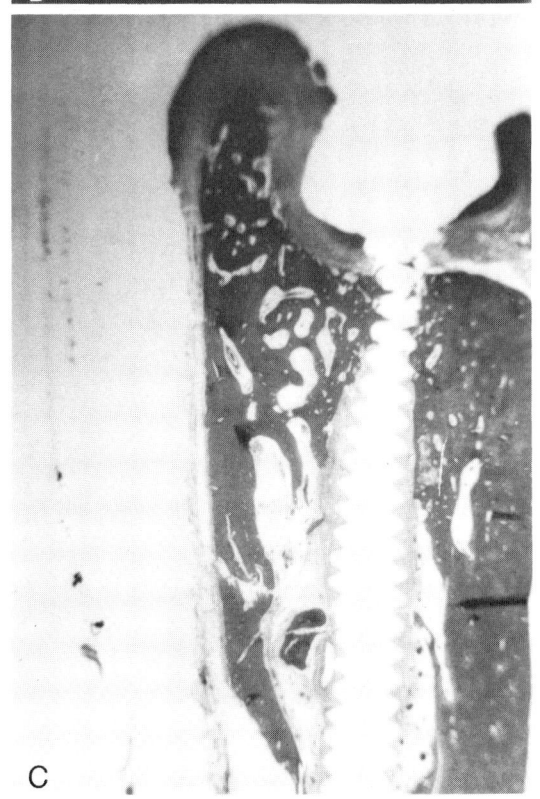

Figure 7–13. Dr. Irwin Small completed a two-year laboratory project on dogs to determine the efficacy of transosteal implants. The potential success of this type of device was assessed by evaluating the implant in the animals (A) clinically, (B) radiographically, and (C) histologically. The positive findings resulted in a five-year clinical project.

Patient Selection

Proper patient selection based on structured clinical criteria is critical in determining the long-term success of any dental implant; the staple is no different. The *indications* for mandibular reconstruction with the staple bone plate are as follows:

1. Severe or moderate EBL of the mandible of not less than 9 mm of vertical mandibular height. The intermediate pins of the mandibular staple bone plate measure 9 mm in vertical height; therefore, the inferior border–to–alveolar ridge crestal height must be at least 9 mm.
2. Mandibular bone loss as a result of trauma or tumor surgery.
3. Insertion as a means of limiting edentulous bone loss following dental extractions or in cases of congenital absence of dentition. The staple bone plate stabilizes the mandibular prosthesis and therefore equalizes the pressures and forces applied to the alveolar ridge and slows the resultant bone resorption.

The *contraindications* to the insertion of the mandibular staple bone plate are as follows:

1. Bone height of less than 9 mm between the mental foramina.
2. ASA Class III patients—those who have significant and potentially life-threatening medical problems.
3. Evidence of infection in the area of staple insertion.
4. Diabetes. This is a relative contraindication, and a significant amount of clinical judgment must be exercised in patient selection. Insulin-dependent diabetics have a higher incidence of morbidity associated with implants than do adult-onset, diet-controlled diabetics.
5. Osteoporosis, blood dyscrasias, psychiatric disease, and the presence of natural maxillary dentition are all relative contraindications.
6. Prior to staple insertion, the patient's mouth must be evaluated for the presence of neoplasia, hyperplastic tissues, and gross alveolar irregularities. Since it is highly desirable to have attached oral mucous membrane labial to the transosteal pin, it may be necessary to perform a mucosal or skin graft vestibuloplasty prior to staple insertion. If it is probable that the transosteal pins will enter the oral cavity anterior to the alveolar attached mucosa in the unattached labial sulcus tissue, a vestibuloplasty is indicated to provide for additional attached alveolar soft tissue. The movement of unattached labial mucosa against the threads of the transosteal pins may create hyperplastic tissue that must be periodically excised. The placement of a skin or mucosal graft prior to staple insertion provides an area of attached tissue through which the staple pins enter the oral cavity. The procedure decreases the potential for mucosal hyperplasia.

Preoperative Preparation

Measurement of the vertical height of the mandible in the symphysis region can best be achieved by correlating a panoramic x-ray with a lateral jaw radiograph taken of the mandibular symphysis. An occlusal dental film can be utilized to obtain the lateral jaw x-ray. In this latter technique, the cone of the x-ray machine is placed in a horizontal position on the opposite side of the patient's jaw, to allow the x-ray beam to enter at a right angle to the film, which is held extraorally by the patient.

Prior to surgery, an impression is taken of the patient's mandibular alveolar ridge and a plaster study model is constructed. On this model, a clear acrylic template can be fashioned and used as a guide at the time of surgery. This template should not exceed 1/4 inch in vertical height and should be overextended in the lingual and buccal sulcus areas to ensure stability. The crest of the alveolar ridge and mandibular midline can be marked on the study model with a marking pencil. The acrylic splint is then placed on the study model and the marking guide is used to drill two holes in the acrylic splint. This will correspond to the position of the pins on the drill guide (Fig. 7–15).

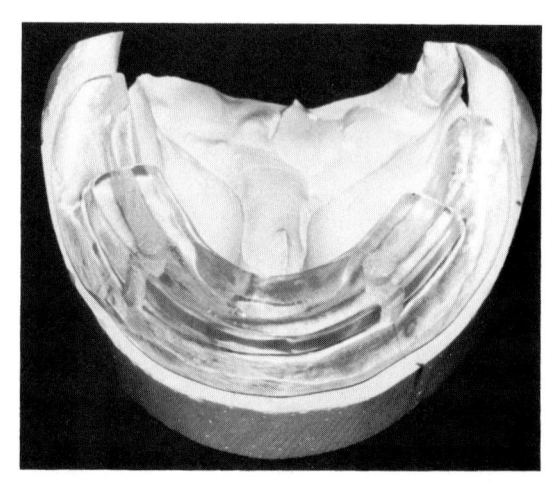

Figure 7–15. An acrylic splint is fabricated which is utilized at the time of surgery as a template. Two holes placed through the occlusal rim portion of the splint will correspond to the entry point on the ridge of a 7-pin staple. The guide used in drilling these holes is displayed in Figure 7–18*i*. The center pin of this device is placed at the mandibular (splint) midline and the two lateral pins, which correspond to the actual width of the transosteal pins on a 7-pin staple, dictate the points at which the holes should be placed.

If there is any question as to the proper location of the hole in relationship to the alveolar ridge, it is best to place them slightly to the lingual. This will ensure that the transosteal pins, particularly in a 5-pin staple or modified 7-pin staple, will enter the oral cavity with attached alveolar mucosa present on the labial aspect of the pins (Fig. 7–16). If the pins enter the oral cavity anterior (labial) to the attached alveolar mucosa, the potential for the development of hyperplasia around the pins is enhanced. By ensuring the presence of attached mucosa labial to the pins, this potential is minimized.

Because of the natural shape of the mandible, the smaller the jaw, the more V-shaped (from an inferior border perspective) it becomes. This V rather than U shape results in the transosteal pins in a 5-pin staple entering the oral cavity on the labial aspect of the ridge. This occurs even though the drill guide (which has been designed for a 7- and modified 7-pin staple) has been placed in an ideal position on the inferior border of the mandible. The more V-shaped the inferior border, the more anterior to the ridge the pins will enter, unless this factor is considered and appropriate adjustments are made when the guide holes are drilled in the template.

Although the acrylic splint is helpful, some surgeons prefer to replace the drill guide director pins, which fit into the template with the stabilizing "claws," and perform the surgery without using the acrylic splint. However, in cases in which there is a very tall and spinous alveolar ridge or a significant height disparity between the left and right alveolar ridges, the use of the drill guide "claws" will not provide for proper stability. For these reasons, it is the authors' opinion that it is preferable to have the acrylic splint available for all procedures in case the claws do not provide for adequate stability.

Prior to surgery, it is extremely important to educate the patient. Preferably, this education will include preoperative instructions with a model of the mandible into which a staple bone plate has been implanted. The patient should also be informed prior to surgery of his obligations regarding diet and postoperative hygiene. An example of a mandibular staple consent form is shown in Figure 7–17.

Proper instrumentation is imperative in the successful placement of a mandibular staple bone plate. The success of this implant has been due in great part to the instrumentation developed by Small. The minimum set of instruments is depicted in Figure 7–18.

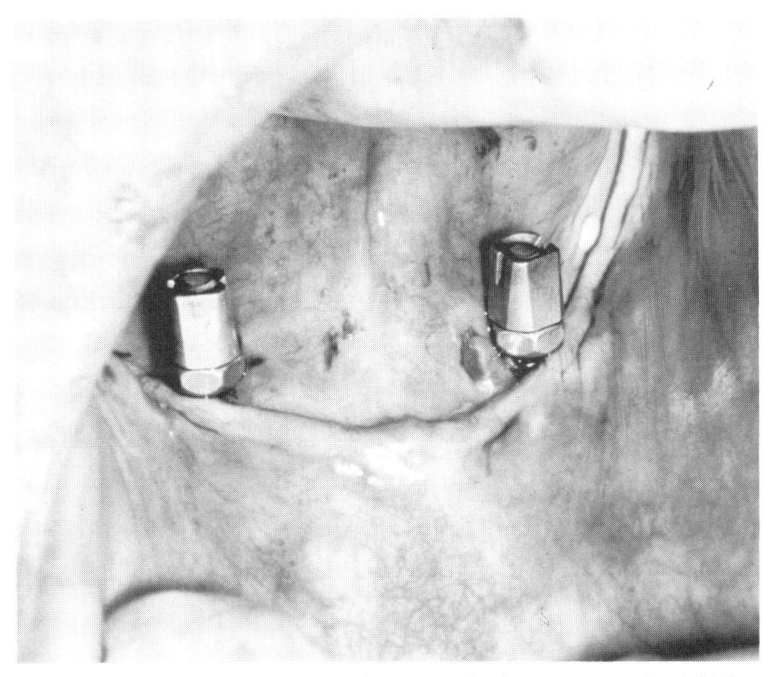

Figure 7–16. It is important to have attached mucosa on the labial aspect of the transosteal pins. If an inadequate amount of attached mucosa is present, a skin or mucosal graft vestibuloplasty should be performed prior to staple placement.

UNDERSTANDING THE MANDIBULAR STAPLE OPERATION

The Mandibular Staple is an implantable titaniuim device used to reconstruct the atrophic lower jaw in cases of severe bone loss. It permits attachment of a lower denture so that the denture is firm and stable. The denture can be removed for cleansing and the staple is kept clean by means of a toothbrush and a Water Pik.

The staple is inserted through an incision beneath the chin and is placed in the jaw by drilling from five to seven parallel holes. The holes are placed so that injury to the nerve of the jaw is avoided in most cases. The old lower denture can be worn a few days after surgery. Your dentist will drill holes in the old denture and reline it temporarily until the new denture can be made.

The staple and new denture should provide stability and improved chewing efficiency. The possible complications are (1) a rare metal reaction which might result in an allergic-like swelling; (2) loosening of the staple because of infection—this should be controllable with antibiotics in most instances; (3) fracture of the metal or jaw due to stress concentration or a blow; and (4) some numbness of an area of the lip or chin.

The staple should last for many years but cannot be guaranteed to last for any specific amount of time. Should it have to be removed, the patient should be able to wear a conventional denture or could possibly have a second staple inserted.

- -

I hereby consent to the insertion of a Mandibular Staple in my lower jaw with the understanding that no guarantees have been made or implied.

Signed:＿＿＿＿＿＿＿＿＿＿

Date:＿＿＿＿＿＿＿＿＿＿

Figure 7–17. Patient orientation form.

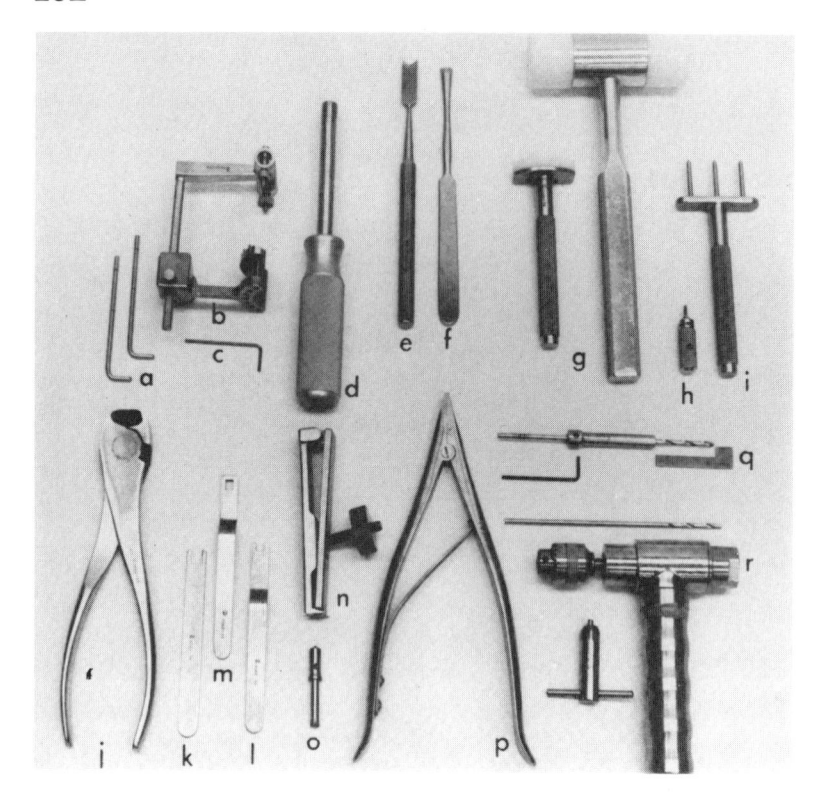

182 / IMPLANTS USED IN PREPROSTHETIC RECONSTRUCTIVE SURGERY

Figure 7–18. The instruments necessary for the successful placement of a mandibular staple bone plate are as follows: *a*, stabilizing pins; *b*, drill guide; *c*, Allen wrench; *d*, lock-nut wrench; *e*, digastric elevator; *f*, metatarsal elevator; *g*, mallet and staple driver; *h*, beveling device; *i*, drill hole measuring guide; *j*, pin cutter; *k*, lock-nut wrench; *l*, fastener-nut wrench; *m*, fastener-nut wrench; *n*, staple distractor; *o*, staple pin trephine; *p*, staple distractor pliers; *q*, drill bit with stop; *r*, drill.

Surgical Technique

At the time of surgery, the patient is intubated by a nasoendotracheal route. The patient is placed in the thyroid position and the chin is elevated. The patient is then prepared and draped so that the submental area and the oral cavity are isolated from each other. Although iodophor has been used for surgical preparation of the mouth, most surgeons have switched to hexachlorophene. Several patients complained of loss of smell (anosmia) following the staple surgery. It is likely that the iodophor prep solution cauterized the olfactory nerve endings in the nasal pharynx and resulted in anosmia.

The patient's chin is elevated and the submental skin crease is marked with a marking pencil. The drill guide is placed onto the anticipated incision line to determine the proper length of the incision, and the incision is then marked (Fig. 7–19). Several milliliters of 0.5 per cent lidocaine with epinephrine 1:200,000 are infiltrated into the surgical incision (Fig. 7–20). The incision is made through skin, subcutaneous tissues, and platysma muscle to the inferior border of the mandible (Fig. 7–21). Utilizing a periosteal elevator, the periosteum is stripped from the inferior border of the mandible. A minimal amount of stripping should be performed on the lingual aspect of the mandible; extensive stripping results in postoperative sublingual edema and ecchymosis. However, it is helpful to strip the periosteum on the anterior aspect of the inferior border extending toward the labial sulcus (Fig. 7–22). This allows for adequate anterior retraction of the soft tissues when the drill guide is in place. Care should be taken to remove soft tissue debris from the inferior border, and all bleeding should be controlled (Fig. 7–23).

One of the assistants enters the mouth and places the acrylic splint on the alveolar ridge. The drill guide director rods are then inserted into the previously drilled acrylic splint holes and the portion of the guide

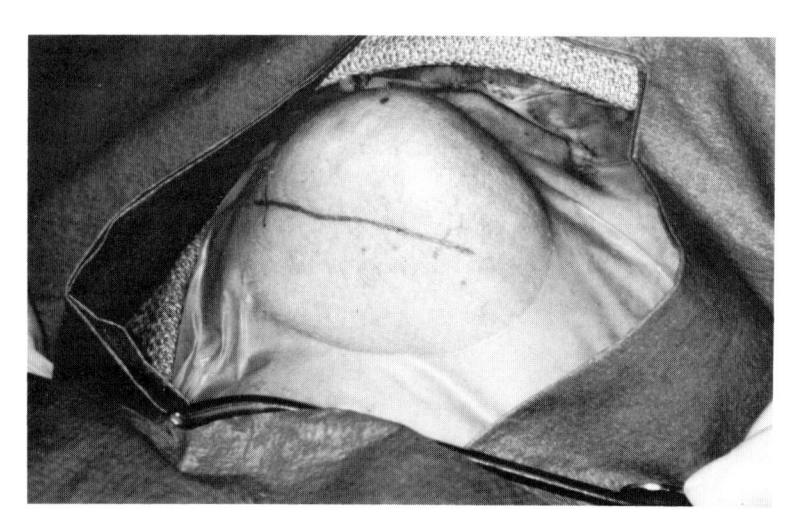

Figure 7–19. The incision line is placed and marked in the area of the submental crease. The portion of the drill guide that fits on the inferior border of the mandible is used as a guide in determining the length of the incision.

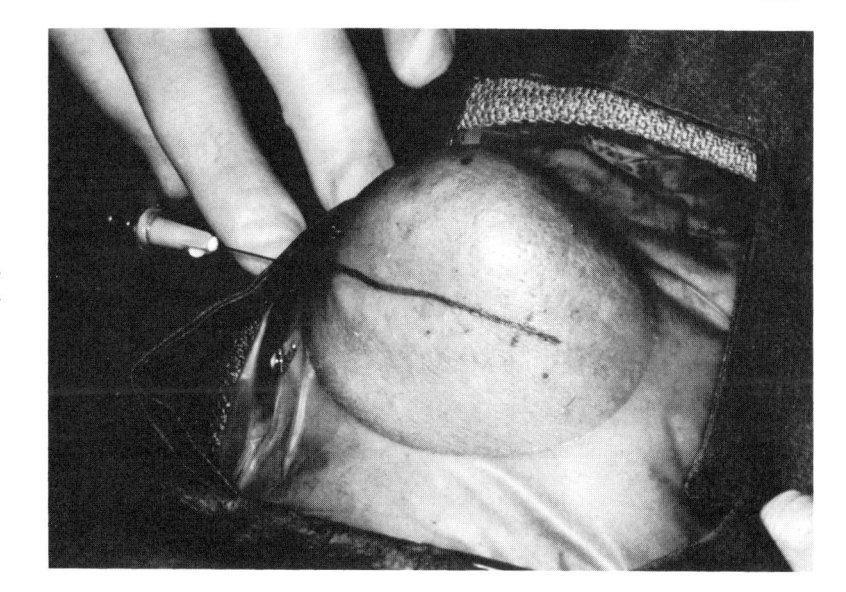

Figure 7–20. Local anesthesia with a vasopressor is infiltrated in the area of the skin incision.

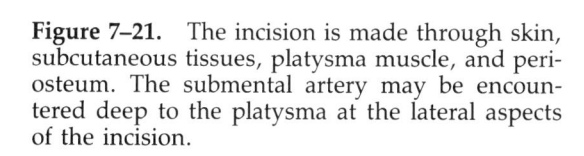

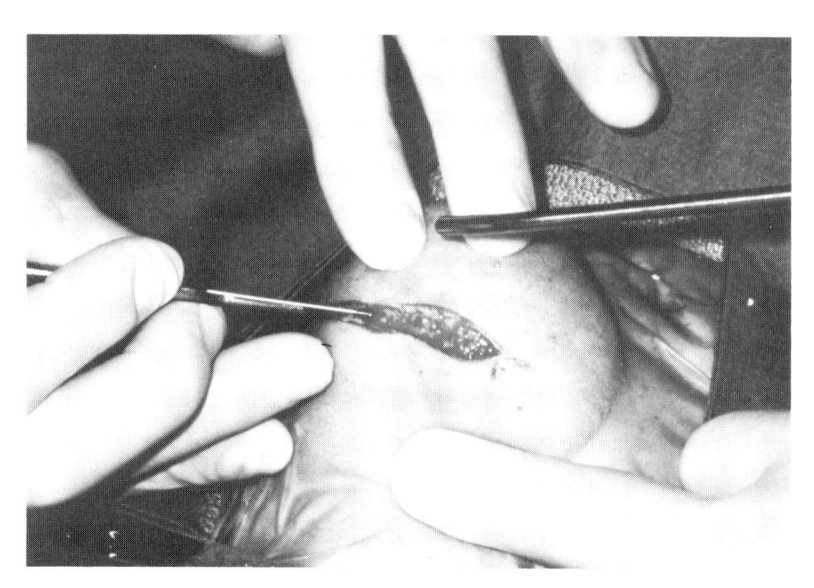

Figure 7–21. The incision is made through skin, subcutaneous tissues, platysma muscle, and periosteum. The submental artery may be encountered deep to the platysma at the lateral aspects of the incision.

Figure 7–22. Minimal stripping is performed on the lingual aspect of the mandible; however, it is helpful to strip tissues on the labial aspect of the inferior border. In cases of severe atrophy, care must be taken not to enter the oral cavity or injure the mental nerve during the reflection procedure.

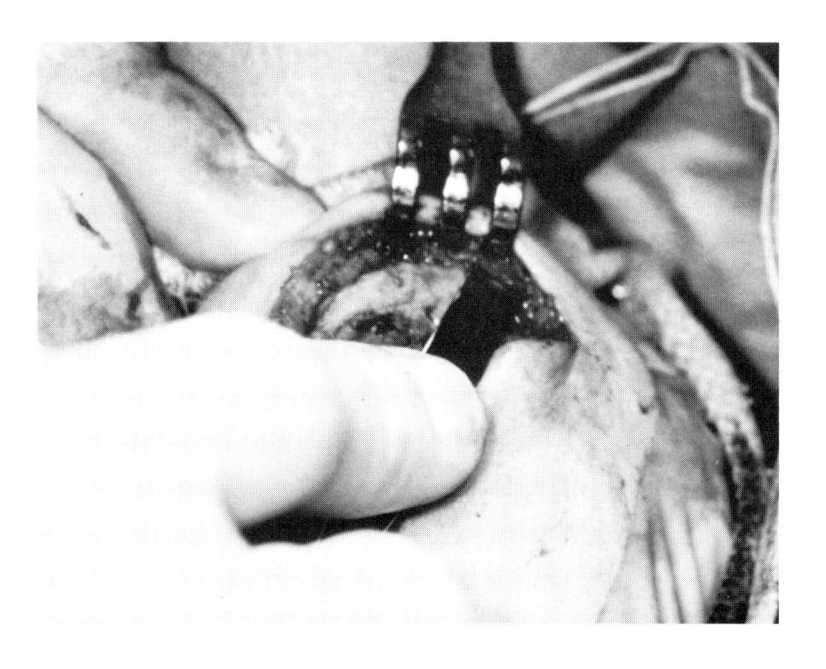

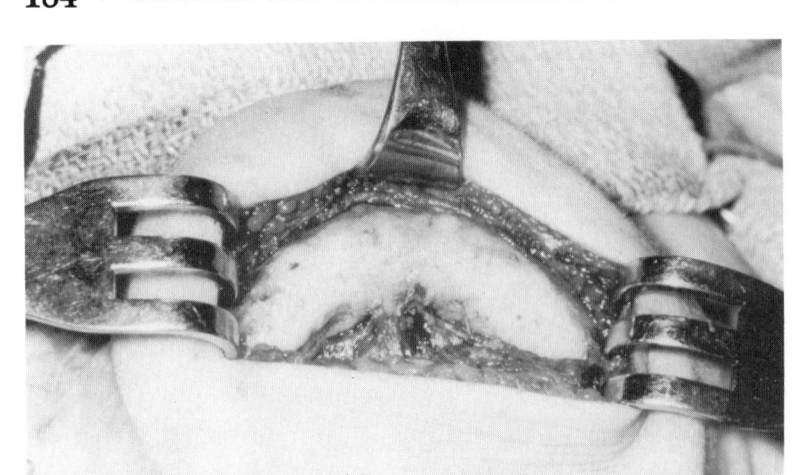

184 / IMPLANTS USED IN PREPROSTHETIC RECONSTRUCTIVE SURGERY

Figure 7–23. The inferior border must be totally devoid of soft tissue.

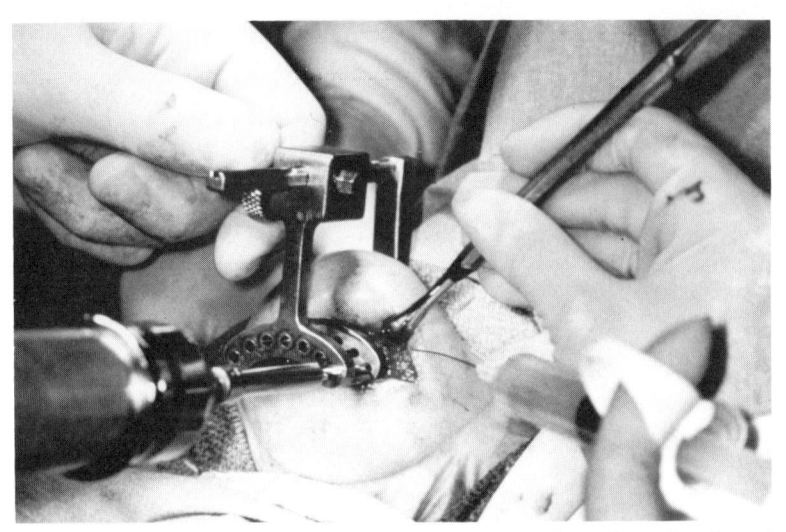

Figure 7–24. The drill guide must be flush with the inferior border of the mandible. Any gross irregularities should be removed with a reduction bur so that the drill guide is stable throughout the drilling process.

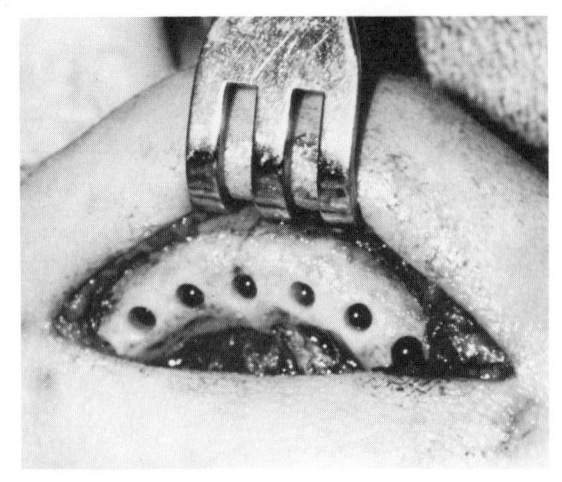

Figure 7–25. The holes should be placed at the midpoint of the inferior border. If the mandible is distorted, it is preferable to have the transosteal holes placed more toward the lingual aspect of the inferior border. All debris must be thoroughly irrigated from the holes.

from the bit so that the transosteal holes, which enter the mouth, can be completed.

The surgeon who is stabilizing the acrylic template must view the oral mucous membrane during the drilling of the transosteal holes. Once the drill bit begins to perforate the oral mucous membrane, he must notify the surgeon drilling the holes that the holes are complete and that the drilling should be stopped. The drill guide and the template are then removed. The inferior border is cleaned of all debris and the holes are thoroughly irrigated (Fig. 7–25). Because of flash at the junction of the staple pins and horizontal plate, a small beveling device is used to countersink all of the previously drilled holes (Fig. 7–26).

containing the drill holes is placed along the inferior border of the mandible. Any irregularities along the inferior border that do not allow for proper placement and stability of the drill guide should be removed with a reduction bur (Fig. 7–24).

The lateral holes are then placed with the "drill stop" attached to the drill bit. The drill stop is placed onto the bit utilizing an L-shaped marking gauge. This stop allows the holes to be drilled 1 mm longer than the length of the retention pins. Drilling is done with the Orthairtome II or an equivalent low-speed, high-torque drill. Copious irrigation is used during the placement of the pins.

Once the lateral holes have been drilled, the stabilizing pins are placed to secure the drill guide. The intermediate holes are then drilled and the stabilizing pins are moved from their previous positions into these intermediate holes. The drill stop is removed

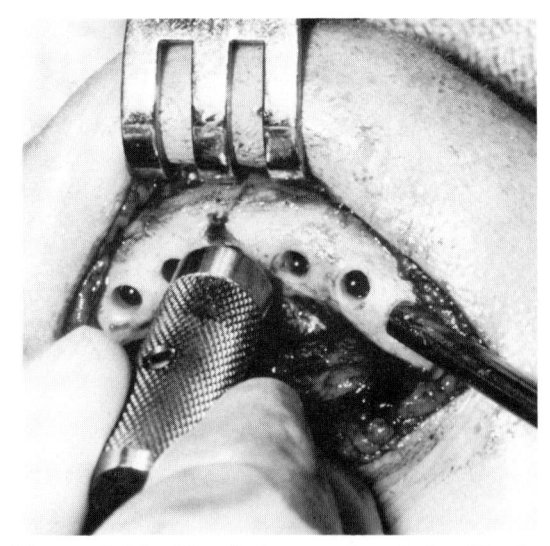

Figure 7–26. The holes are beveled with the bevelling device. This assures the complete seating of the staple bone plate.

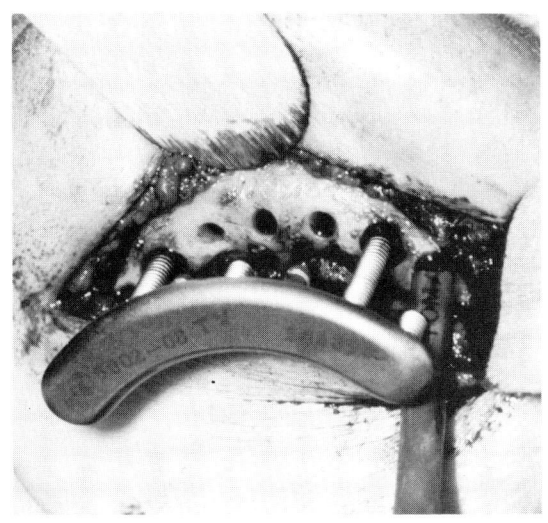

Figure 7–27. The staple can usually be inserted with hand pressure until the intermediate pins begin to contact their corresponding holes. Care must be taken to assure that no soft tissue is carried by the pins into the holes.

The fasteners are removed from the staple and it is inserted through the hole to a point just short of the oral mucous membrane. The surgeon who is responsible for the oral cavity then places a small incision in the alveolar ridge mucosa with a No. 15 blade. This allows for the penetration of the transosteal pin into the oral cavity without tenting of, or damage to, the oral mucosa. The staple can usually be inserted with hand pressure until the intermediate pins reach the osseous holes (Fig. 7–27). At this point, it is generally necessary to mallet the staple into place (Fig. 7–28).

Once the staple has contacted the inferior border of the mandible, tapping must be terminated (Fig. 7–29). No attempt should be

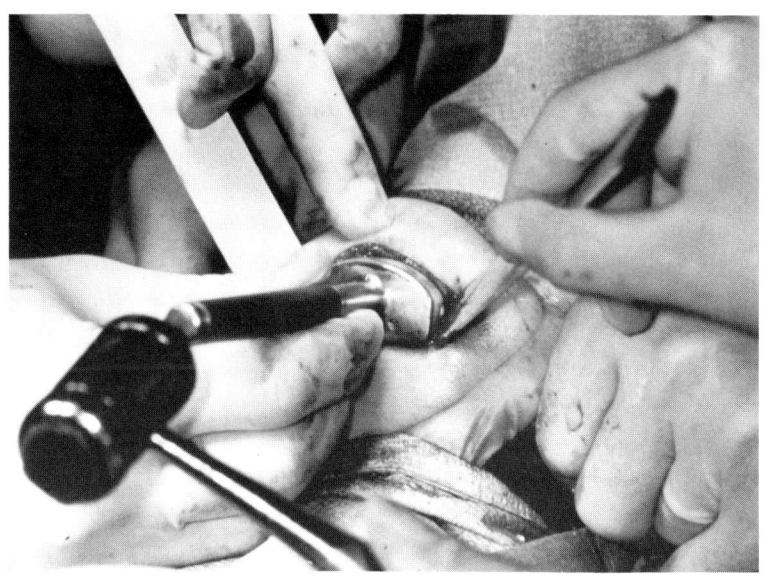

Figure 7–28. The staple must be gently malletted into place. Once any portion of the staple plate makes point contact with the inferior border, the staple is down and malleting should be discontinued.

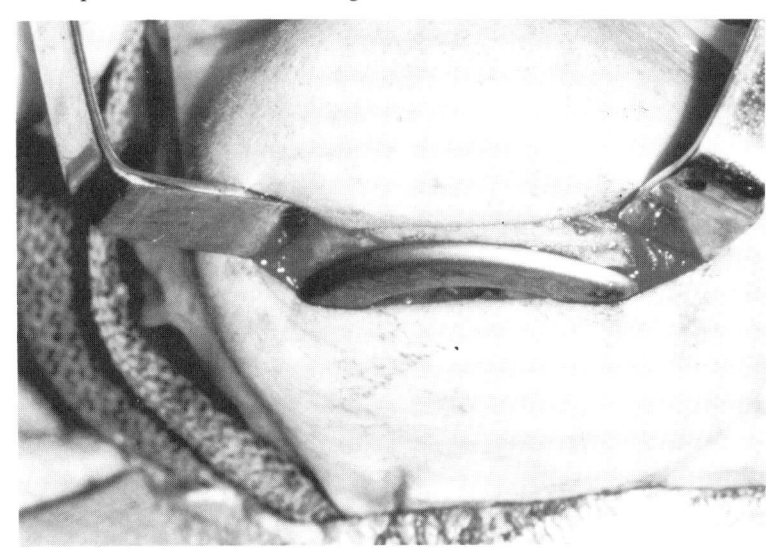

Figure 7–29. Although it is preferable to have the staple plate flush with the inferior border of the mandible, it is not uncommon for the plate to be 1 to 2 mm off the bone surface.

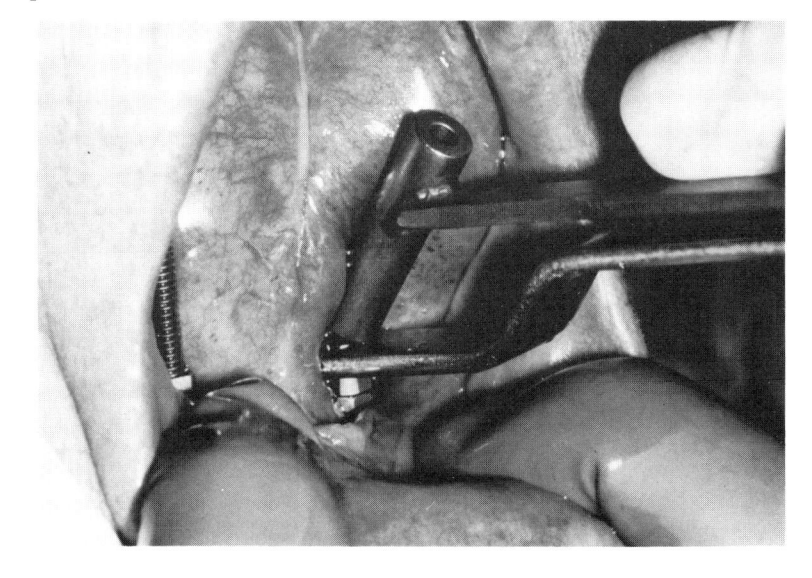

Figure 7–30. The excess pin is removed with a pin cutter or the specially designed pin breaker, which is included in the staple set.

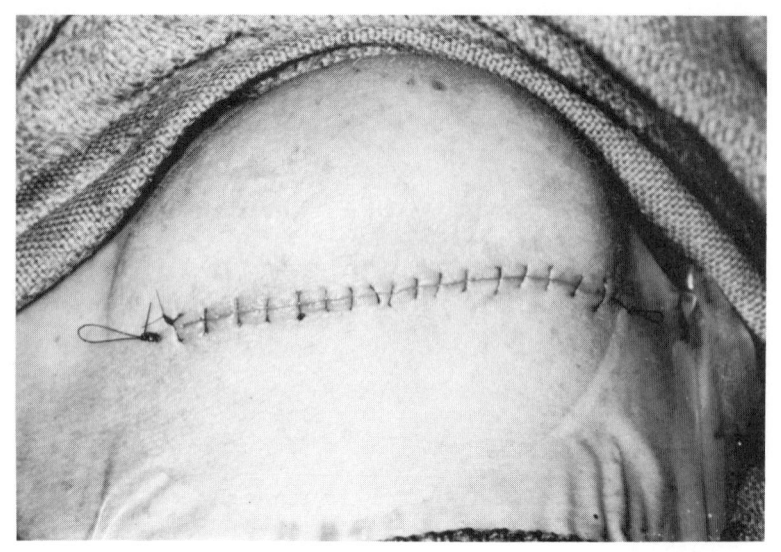

186 / IMPLANTS USED IN PREPROSTHETIC RECONSTRUCTIVE SURGERY

Figure 7–31. The wound should be thoroughly irrigated and closed in a layered fashion.

made to improve the relationship of the plate with the inferior border by additional vigorous tapping. The surgeon who has been working in the mouth applies the fasteners and cuts off the excess portion of the pin (Fig. 7–30). The extraoral wound is irrigated and closed in a layered fashion (Fig. 7–31). Steroids are generally used at the time of surgery to limit the swelling, and the patient is placed on antibiotics for one week.

Postoperative Management

The patient's denture can be adjusted to accept the fasteners and relined the following morning. Final denture construction can begin six weeks following surgery (Fig. 7–32). The patient should remain on a soft, edentulous diet until the final prosthesis has been completed. Proper postoperative diet and hygiene instructions must be given to the patients at the time of discharge.

Although postsurgical complications are unusual, 6 to 7 per cent of staple patients will experience a postoperative problem. By far the most common problem relates to a transosteal pin entering the oral cavity through unattached labial mucosa. This positioning, which is often unavoidable because of mandibular anatomy, may result in the development of hyperplastic tissue adjacent to the pin. This can be best managed by excision of the hyperplastic tissue and meticulous oral hygiene. The placement of a mucosal graft anterior to the pin may be necessary in cases of chronic mucosal hyperplasia.

Early postoperative infections can be effectively managed with the aggressive use of antibiotics and standard measures of surgical intervention, even when the staple has been exposed to purulence. Late infections can also be eradicated; however, the prognosis in these cases is guarded if the staple is mobile. Stability of the staple appears to be very critical in determining the long-term prognosis in these cases. For this reason, it is highly desirable to save natural mandibular teeth and include them as fixed restorative components of the prosthetic reconstruction. In the authors' experience, this approach has a mutually beneficial effect on the teeth and the staple. Stress loosening of the staple can occur if the denture is not tissue-borne. Prosthetic overload must be avoided and, if the staple becomes mobile, the denture should be remade, relined, or removed until the implant stabilizes.

Prosthetic Reconstruction

Proper prosthetic reconstruction is imperative following mandibular staple implant surgery. The denture must be tissue-borne and fastened to the superstructure by a stress-broken precision attachment. The most frequently used attachments are the Dalbo and Ceka.

The Dalbo is used in cases in which the mandibular height is greater than 10 mm and in those in which there are no natural opposing teeth. These attachments are long-lasting, require little maintenance, and provide good retention and lateral stability. However, they provide minimal stress-breaking capability, and some patients have complained of difficulty in inserting and removing the denture because of the preciseness of these attachments.

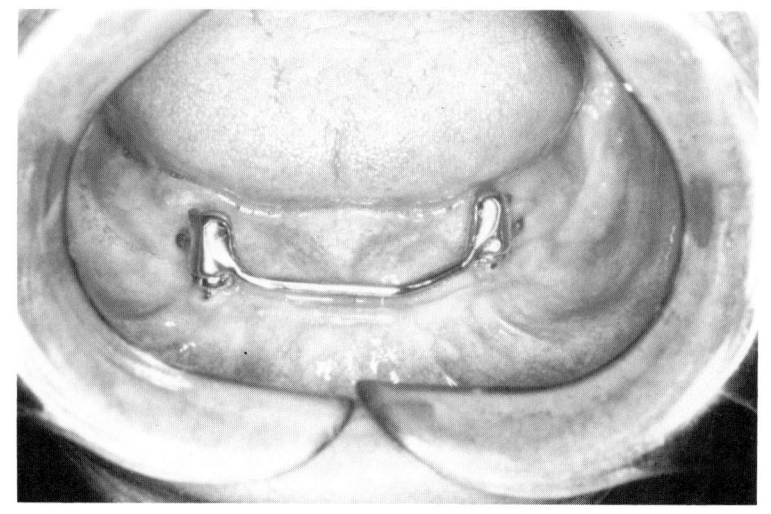

Figure 7–32. The final precision appliance is completed six to eight weeks following staple placement. The denture is fastened to the superstructure by means of a stress-broken attachment.

The Ceka attachments can be used in various ways: in very atrophic mandibles, in cases in which the denture is opposing maxillary natural dentition, in bruxers, and in cases in which a patient has had a hemimandibulectomy and the remaining mandible is being reconstructed with a staple bone plate. The Ceka has 360 degree stress-breaking capabilities, is easy to insert and remove, and is responsible for a minimal amount of stress to the staple. Because of the stress-breaking capabilities, some patients do complain that food becomes entrapped beneath the denture and that the attachments have to be periodically replaced. Although prosthodontists have devised alternative attachment methods, the greatest long-term experience and documentable staple survival rates have been with the Dalbo and Ceka attachments.

In summary, the surgical and prosthetic principles of the staple implant are to (1) insert the staple in a sterile (operating room) environment; (2) place the intermediate retention pins in the dense cortical plate at the inferior border of the mandible; (3) place the transosteal pins between the mental foramina; (4) place the transosteal pins through attached mucosa on the crest of the alveolus; (5) join the transosteal pins with a bar so that a rigid box configuration is formed; (6) construct a prosthesis that is tissue-borne and fastened to the superstructure by a stress-broken precision attachment.

The Versatility of the Mandibular Staple Bone Plate

The mandibular staple bone plate can be utilized to reconstruct mandibles that have been deformed as a result of various etiologic factors. The staple has been used routinely in reconstruction following maxillofacial trauma, tumor surgery, congenital deformities, and severe bone loss due to osteomalacia and osteoporosis. The following cases illustrate the various uses of the staple in mandibular reconstruction.

Severe mandibular atrophy, as a result of osteoporosis or osteomalacia, results in a significant functional and esthetic deformity. Figure 7–33 depicts the severely atrophic mandible of a 66-year-old female. Because of the extensive atrophy, which exceeded the 9 mm minimum for staple placement, the decision was made to reconstruct the mandible with an iliac crest bone graft. A block iliac crest bone graft was utilized, and Figure 7–34 depicts the adjustment and placement of the bone graft on a dental model at the time of surgery.

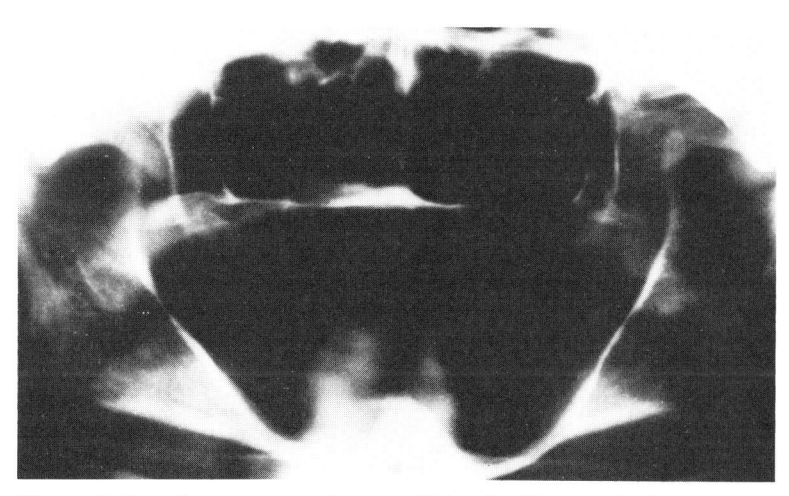

Figure 7–33. Severely atrophic mandible of a 66-year-old female.

The block bone graft is then placed on the crest of the mandibular ridge and wired into position with circummandibular wires (Fig. 7–35). Figure 7–36 is a panoramic x-ray taken immediately postoperatively. It shows the iliac crest bone graft in position and wired securely with circummandibular wires. Figures 7–37 and 7–38 display the patient's mandible six months postoperatively. The x-ray shows a bone graft that has been totally incorporated into the patient's mandible and one that, because of the extent of the healing, is physiologically prepared to accept the staple bone plate. Figure 7–37, a panoramic x-ray taken immediately postoperatively, shows the staple bone plate in position.

The final two x-rays (Fig. 7–39) disclose the patient's mandible at five years and nine years. It is important to note that there has

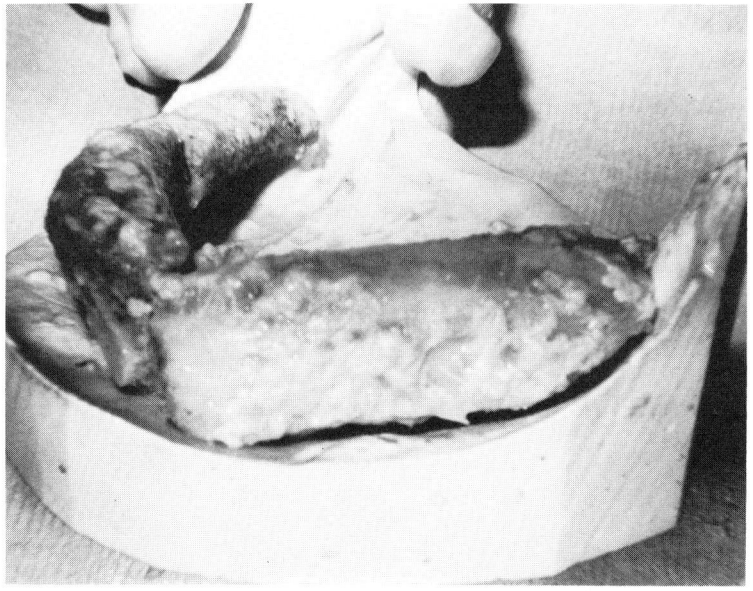

Figure 7–34. Adjustment and placement of a bone graft on a dental model at the time of surgery.

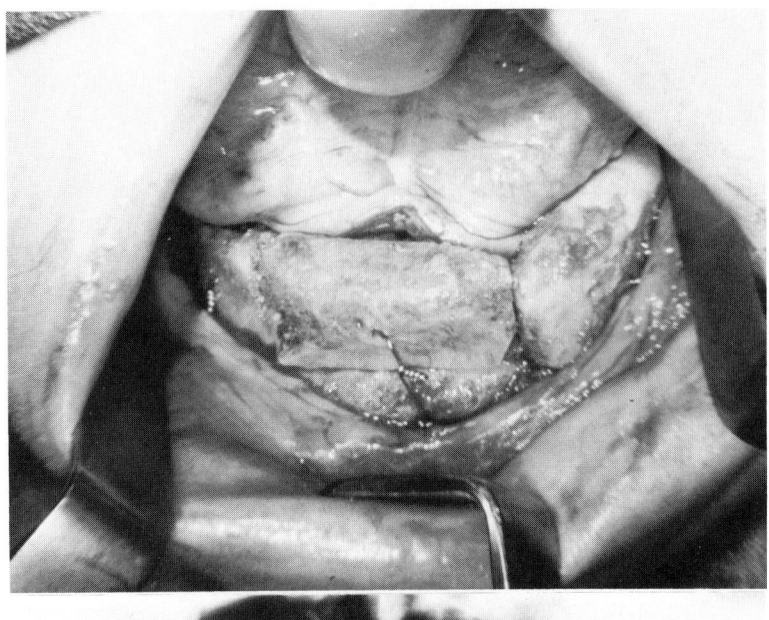

Figure 7–35. Block bone graft on the crest of the mandibular ridge wired into position with circummandibular wires.

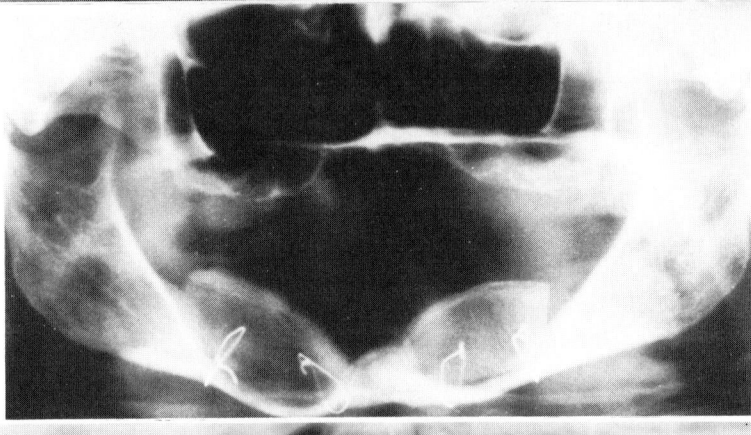

Figure 7–36. Panoramic x-ray taken immediately postoperatively.

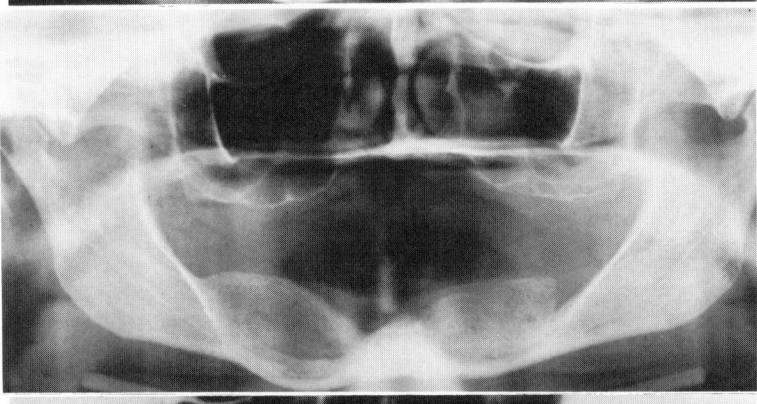

Figure 7–37. Panoramic x-ray taken immediately postoperatively.

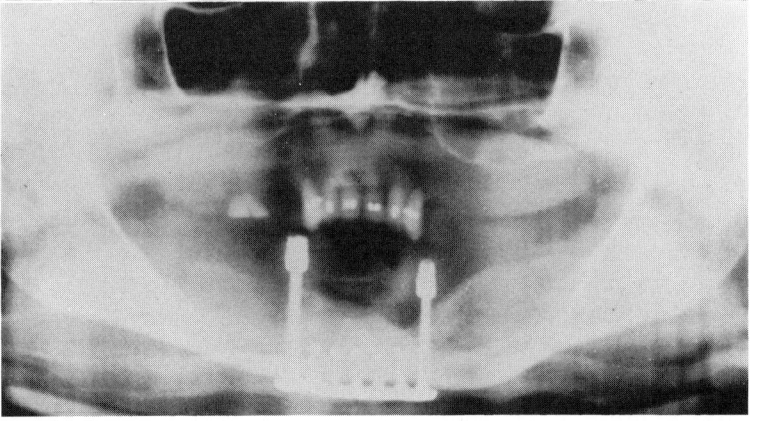

Figure 7–38. Patient's mandible six months postoperatively.

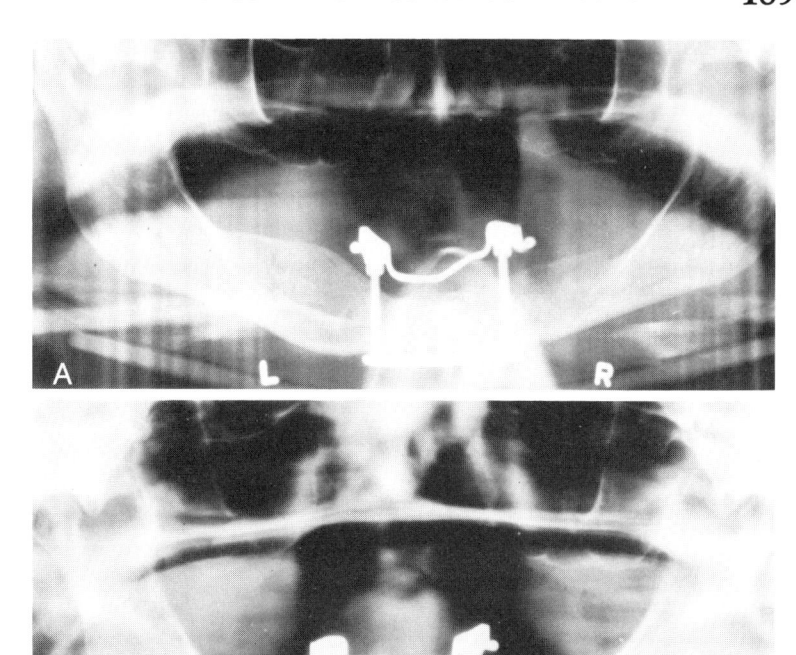

Figure 7–39. Patient's mandible at (A) five and (B) nine years postoperatively.

been minimal loss of mandibular bone height, most likely as a result of stabilization of the mandibular prosthesis by the staple bone plate. It is also interesting to note the maturation of the bone, as evidenced by the trabecular pattern, which has occurred between the fifth and ninth years.

Although iliac crestal bone is the graft material of choice, the mandible can be augmented in height with autogenous rib. Figure 7–40A and B presents pre- and postoperative photos of a patient in whom a rib graft was utilized to augment the mandibular alveolar height. The patient was an avid jogger, and it was felt that the risks involved with an iliac crest bone graft did not warrant the use of this graft material in the augmentation procedure. In addition, the patient required augmentation of the maxillary alveolus and for these reasons rib was chosen as the graft material of choice.

The panoramic x-ray discloses the rib graft, which has been fenestrated and cured to fit the configuration of the alveolar ridge. The graft was then wired into position with circummandibular wires. These wires were removed six weeks prior to the insertion of the mandibular staple bone plate.

As with iliac crest bone graft augmentation procedures, the staple is placed six months following the insertion of the augmentation rib graft. Figure 7–40C shows a panoramic x-ray of the patient's mandible immediately following the insertion of the staple bone plate. The final x-ray, Figure 7–40D, shows the patient's mandible five years following the staple insertion and demonstrates a well-consolidated rib graft. It is once again important to note the alveolar height that has been maintained as a result of the stabilization of the mandibular denture by the staple bone plate.

The staple has also been used to reconstruct the mandible following tumor resections. Figure 7–41A is a panoramic x-ray of a 27-year-old physician who had a mandibular resection for the management of odontogenic myxoma. An iliac crest bone graft was utilized to reconstruct the symphysis of the mandible at the time of tumor resection. Figure 7–41B shows the well-healed and consolidated iliac crest bone graft and a removable partial denture in position. The patient found the removable appliance unsatisfactory and strongly requested further reconstruction.

As a result of her request, an iliac crest bone graft was utilized to augment the initial graft (Fig. 7–41C). A mandibular staple bone plate (Fig. 7–41D) was then placed, and the prosthodontists reconstructed the dentition with a fixed bridge that extended from second molar to second molar. It was supported in the symphysis region by the staple bone plate.

The staple has been utilized in many cases of mandibular reconstruction in which natural dentition remains in the mandibular arch. The success rate of the staple in these patients, 100 per cent in the authors' experience, is due to several factors. First, the natural dentition, if supporting a fixed bridge

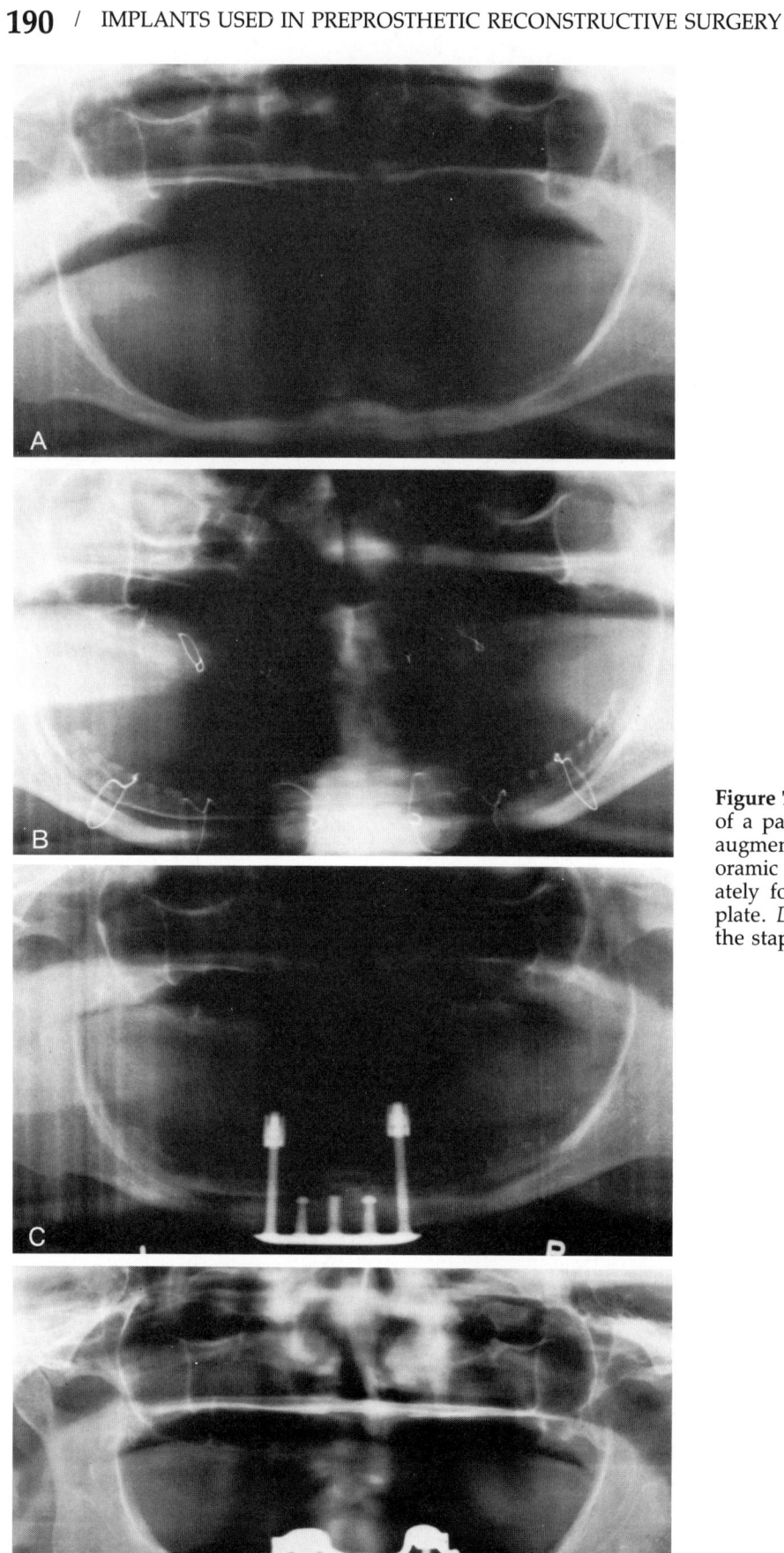

190 / IMPLANTS USED IN PREPROSTHETIC RECONSTRUCTIVE SURGERY

Figure 7–40. *A,* Pre- and *(B)* postoperative views of a patient in whom a rib graft was utilized to augment the mandibular alveolar height. *C,* Panoramic x-ray of the patient's mandible immediately following the insertion of the staple bone plate. *D,* Patient's mandible five years following the staple insertion.

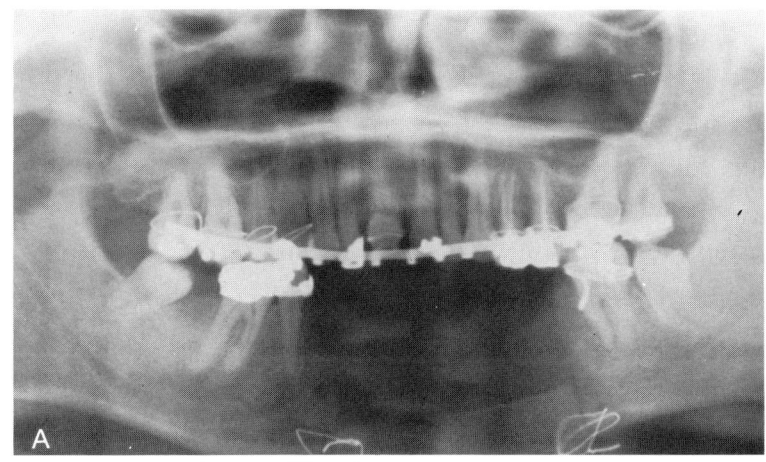

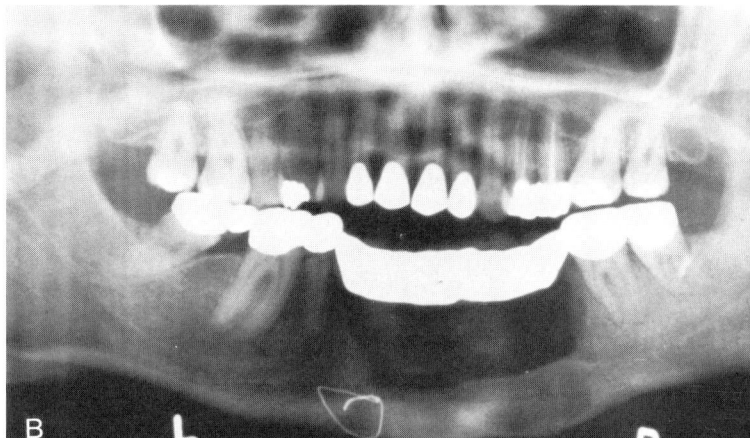

Figure 7–41. *A*, Mandibular resection for the management of odontogenic myxoma. *B*, Well-healed and consolidated iliac crest bone graft and a removable partial denture in position. *C*, Iliac crest bone graft utilized to augment the patient's original bone graft. *D*, Mandibular staple bone plate.

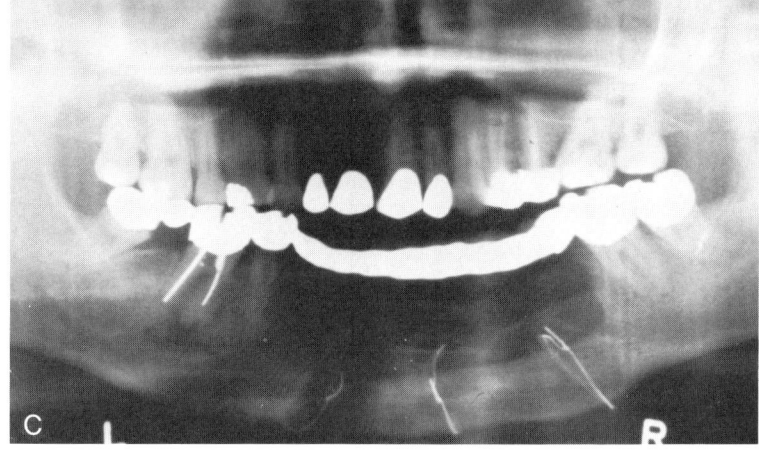

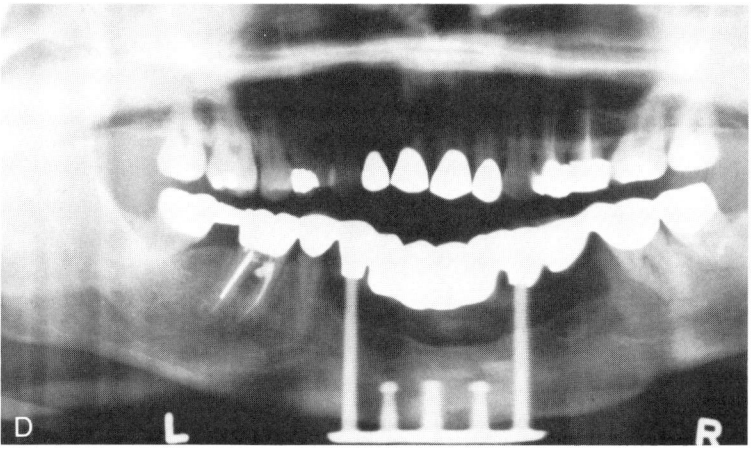

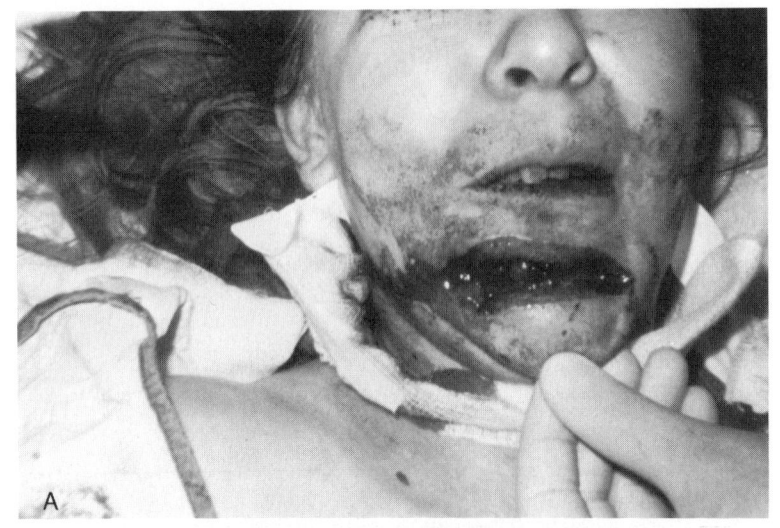

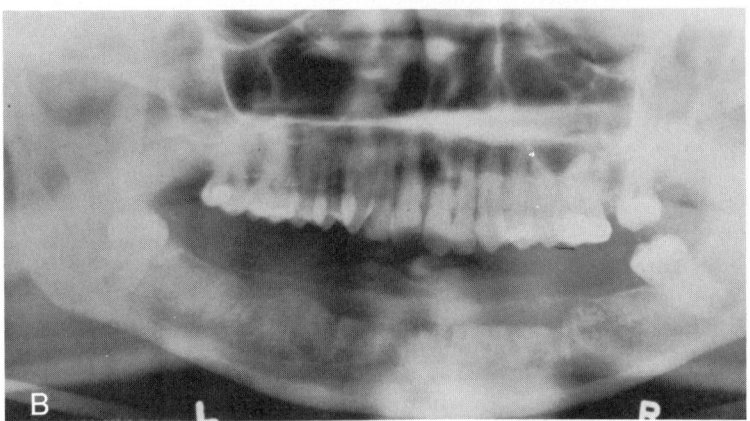

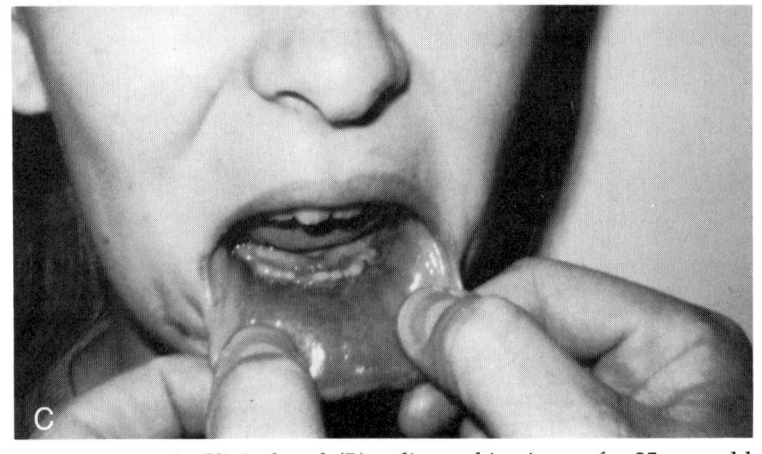

Figure 7–42. *A,* Clinical and *(B)* radiographic views of a 25-year-old female who received severe chin and mandibular alveolar injury as a result of an automobile accident. *C,* Ridge deformity resulting from the injury.

that incorporates the staple, supports the implant during the first three critical months of healing. Once the mandible has become osseointegrated about the intermediate staple pins, the staple then becomes a "periodontal support" for the remaining natural dentition. Secondly, in those cases in which a lone standing molar is utilized for additional support of a complete mandibular denture, that remaining molar provides significant stability to the mandibular prosthesis against the tremendous vertical forces generated during mastication. Finally, the greatest threat to staple longevity involves infection associated with a mobile staple. If the staple bone plate can be incorporated into a framework that is supported by natural dentition, any ensuing infection can be managed with antibiotics. However, if an infectious process is complicated by staple mobility, the prognosis for salvaging the implant is extremely poor. Therefore, when feasible, natural mandibular dentition should be maintained and utilized to assist in the stabilization of the mandibular prosthesis or should be incorporated into the mandibular staple superstructure. The following cases illustrate the use of the mandibular staple bone plate in these various clinical situations.

Figure 7–42A and B illustrates a 25-year-old female who received a severe chin and mandibular alveolar injury in an automobile accident. The through and through laceration of the chin caused loss of the patient's alveolus and dentition. The ridge deformity that resulted from the injury is shown in Figure 7–42C. The impacted left mandibular third molar was surgically removed and an alveoloplasty was performed. It was the recommendation of the prosthodontist that the mandibular right second molar be retained and utilized in the reconstructive procedure. Figure 7–43 shows the staple reconstructive procedure, the final superstructure, and the postoperative panoramic x-ray. Instead of using the remaining molar for retention, the prosthodontist chose to place a thimble crown on this tooth and utilize it as a vertical stop in an attempt to minimize the downward vertical forces of mastication. Because the patient had natural dentition, there was some concern about the potential for extrusion of the staple bone plate during the first three months of function following staple insertion. The presence of this molar provided significant stabilization of the mandibular prosthesis and limited the amount of vertical stress on the staple.

Figure 7–44A–D shows the final prosthetic reconstruction of the patient. Because of the patient's natural maxillary dentition, the prosthodontist chose to place gold occlusals posteriorly to assure proper occlusion and to limit the wear through attrition of the mandibular prosthetic teeth. The final photograph (Fig. 7–44E) shows the patient following reconstruction.

The next case involves a 25-year-old model who was injured in an automobile accident. This injury resulted in a chin laceration and

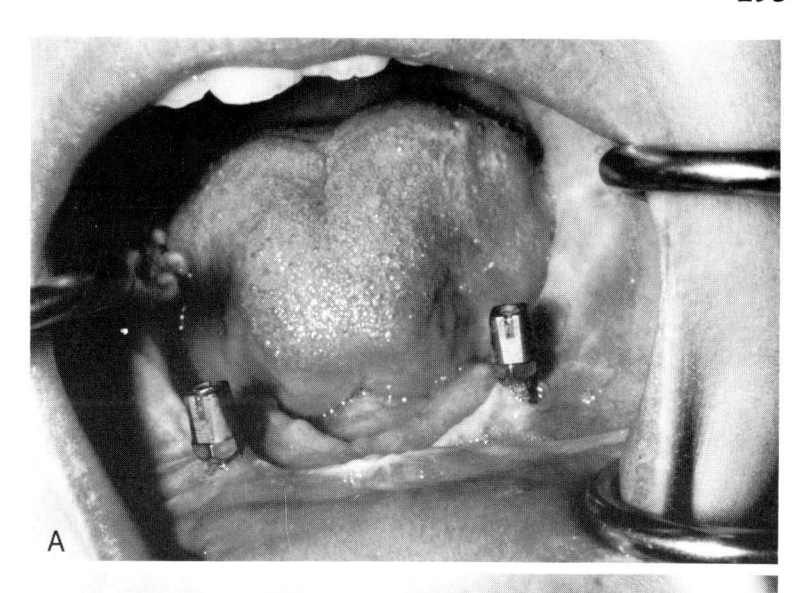

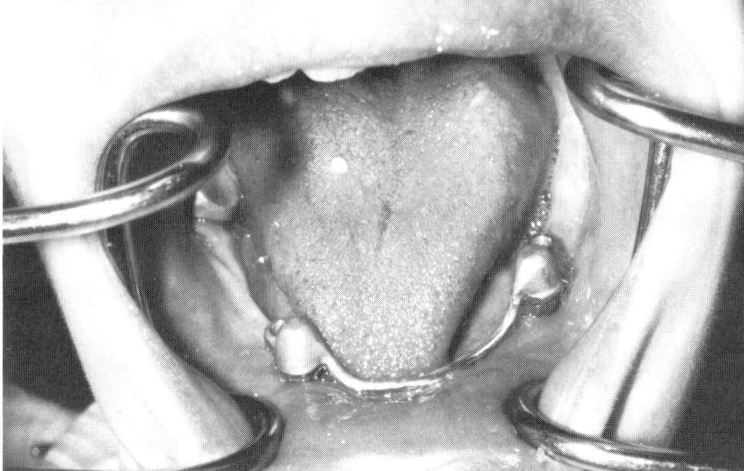

Figure 7–43. Repair of injury to mandible shown in Figure 7–42. *A*, Staple reconstructive procedure. *B*, Final superstructure. *C*, Postoperative panoramic x-ray.

the loss of mandibular alveolar supporting bone and anterior mandibular dentition. Figure 7–45 shows the patient at the time of injury and the alveolar deformity that resulted from the trauma.

The patient was very desirous of fixed prosthetic reconstruction, and it was the prosthodontist's opinion that anterior stabilization would be necessary because of the length of the edentulous span. The decision was made to utilize the staple in the reconstructive procedure. Figure 7–45C is a postoperative panoramic x-ray showing the staple implant and final bridge. The use of a

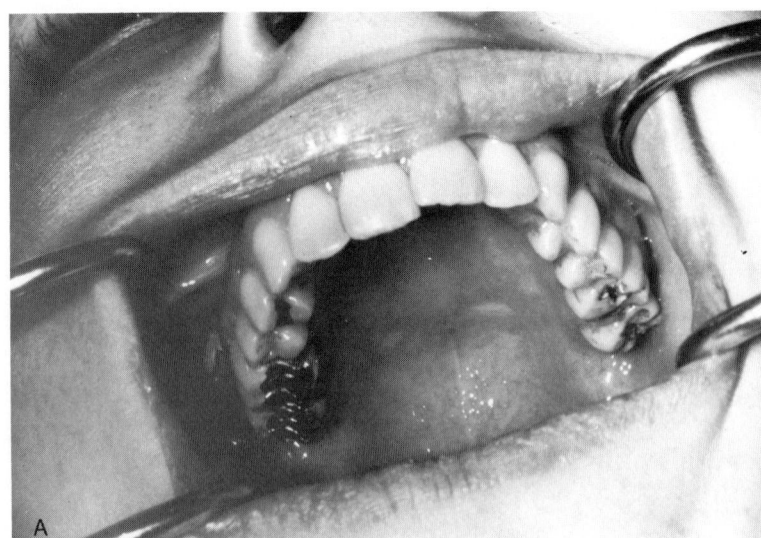

194 / IMPLANTS USED IN PREPROSTHETIC RECONSTRUCTIVE SURGERY

Figure 7–44. Final prosthetic reconstruction of the patient shown in Figures 7–42 and 7–43.

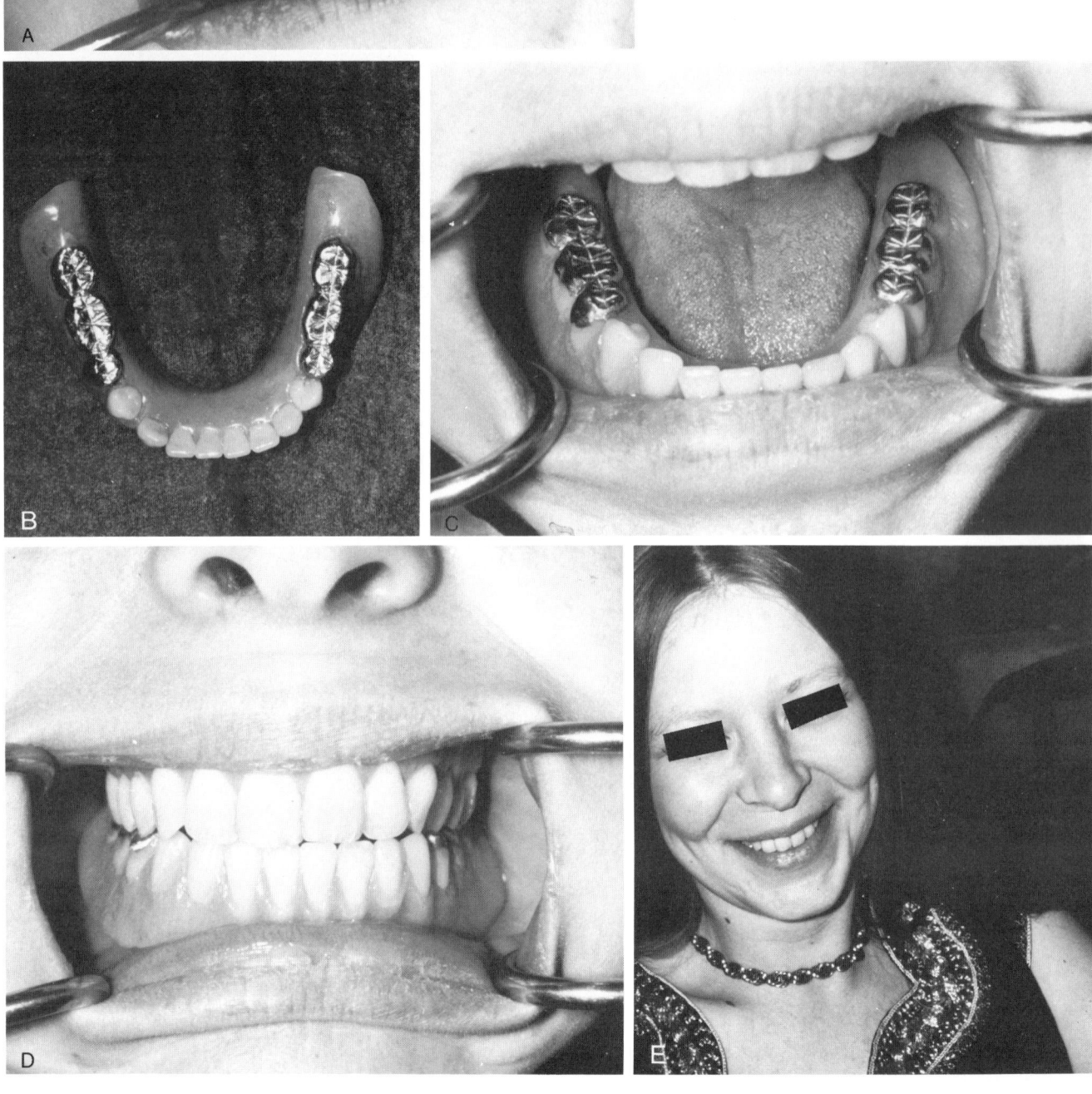

IMPLANTS USED IN PREPROSTHETIC RECONSTRUCTIVE SURGERY / **195**

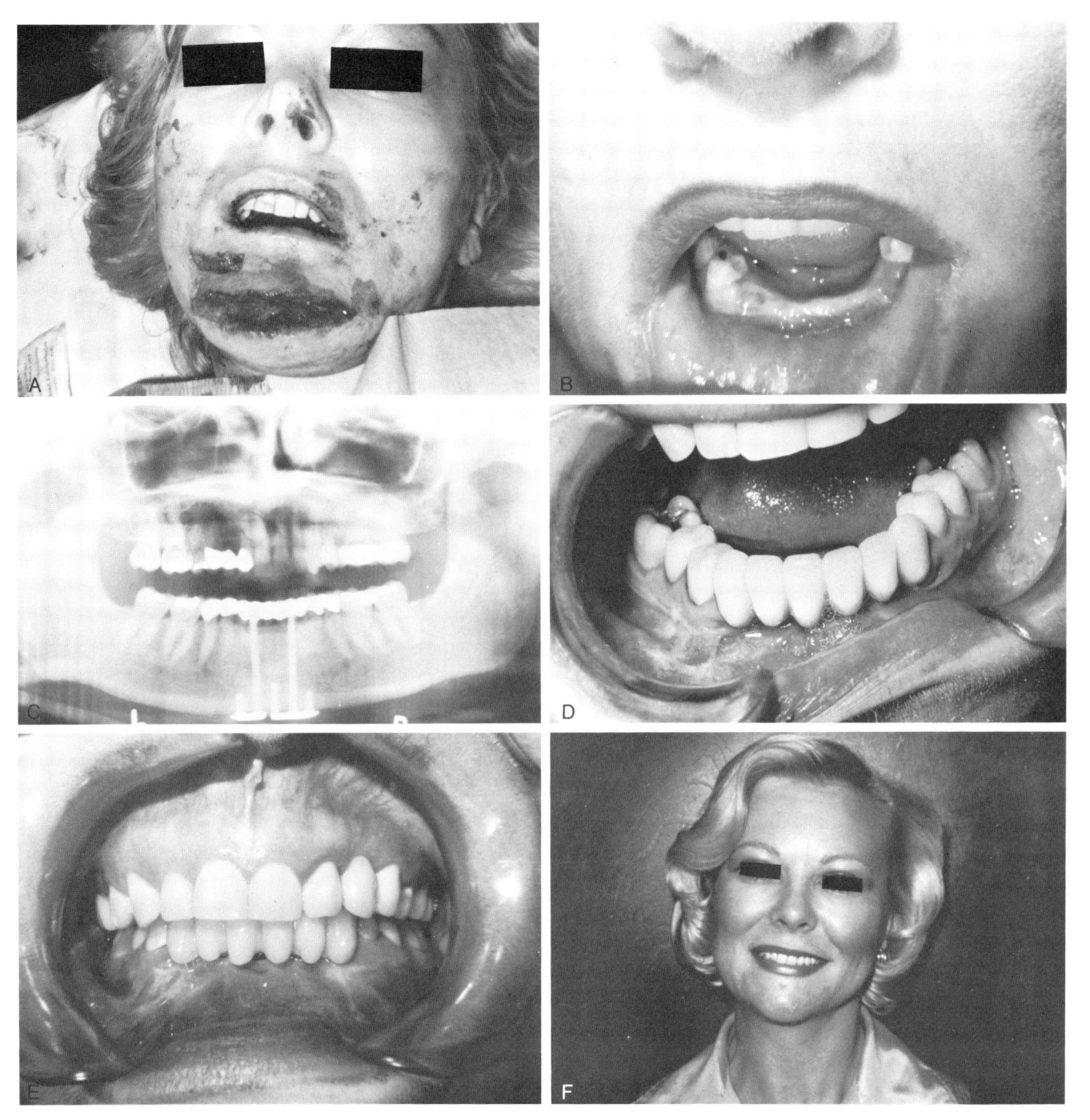

Figure 7–45. *A*, Patient at the time of injury. *B*, Alveolar deformity, that resulted from the trauma. *C*, Postoperative panoramic x-ray of the patient in Figure 7–46, showing the staple implant and final bridge. Final bridge *(D)*, occlusion *(E)*, and esthetic results *(F)*.

196 / IMPLANTS USED IN PREPROSTHETIC RECONSTRUCTIVE SURGERY

standard 5-pin staple would have placed the transosteal pins in direct opposition to the natural bicuspid teeth. Therefore, it was decided at the time of surgery to section a modified 7-pin staple and place two implants that would locate the transosteal pins in a more anterior and favorable position. The final ridge, occlusion, and esthetic results are shown in Figure 7–45D–F.

The panoramic x-ray in Figure 7–46A shows a mandibular alveolar ridge injury that resulted in the loss of six mandibular teeth and an alveolar arch fracture involving the mandibular right central and lateral incisors. Fortunately, the alveolar arch fracture healed and the mandibular incisors were salvaged. Figure 7–46B is a photo of the patient following crown and bridge reconstruction.

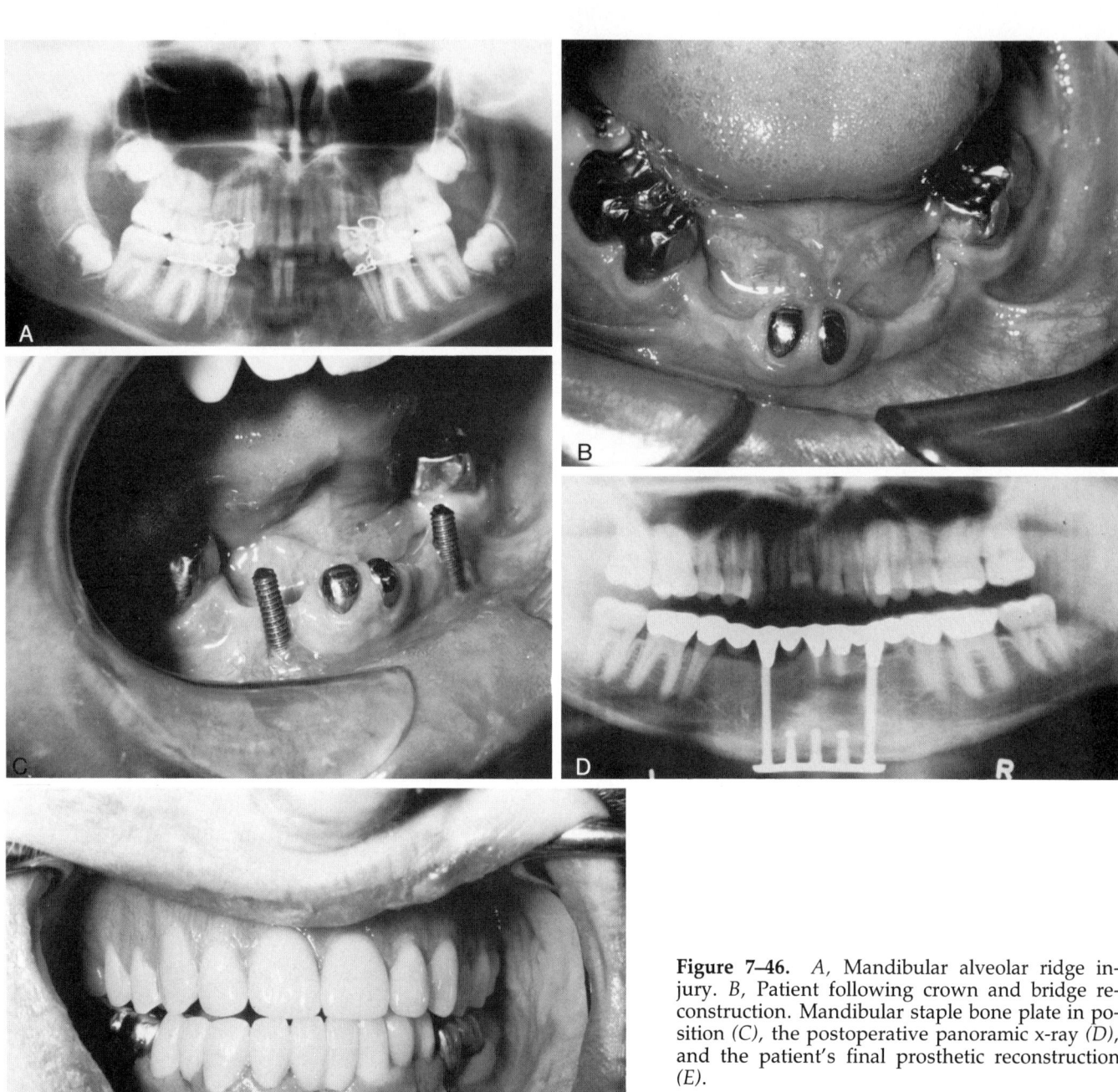

Figure 7–46. *A,* Mandibular alveolar ridge injury. *B,* Patient following crown and bridge reconstruction. Mandibular staple bone plate in position *(C),* the postoperative panoramic x-ray *(D),* and the patient's final prosthetic reconstruction *(E).*

A removable partial denture was constructed at that time and the patient functioned with that appliance for one year.

The patient returned to our office one year following the automobile accident and asked if it were possible for the mandibular arch to be reconstructed with a fixed appliance. Appropriate measurements were taken, and it was our opinion that a 5-pin staple could be utilized to straddle the remaining mandibular incisors. Figure 7–46C–E shows the mandibular staple bone plate in position, the postoperative panoramic x-ray, and the patient's final prosthetic reconstruction.

Future of Staple Implant Surgery

The goal in reconstructive implant surgery is to restore efficient masticatory function in the edentulous or partially edentulous patient. Ideally, this is accomplished by the replacement of missing teeth in a manner that will provide long-term comfort and masticatory efficiency while limiting morbidity to that expected in the dentulous patient. It now appears, as a result of research efforts and carefully documented clinical trials, that the dental profession is nearing this goal. With the development of new instruments, techniques, and materials, and as a result of a more clearly defined cost-benefit ratio, the gap between gadgetry and scientifically sophisticated implantable devices has been narrowed.

The ideal implant would have a firm, direct, and lasting connection with vital bone. Most implants to date have been associated with the existence of a connective tissue layer between the bone and the implant. The presence of this "pseudo-periodonteum" has resulted in inadequate long-term resistance of the implant to mechanical, chemical, and microbial trauma. The development of osseointegrated implants (devices fused to bone) would eliminate this undesirable connective implant-bone interface.

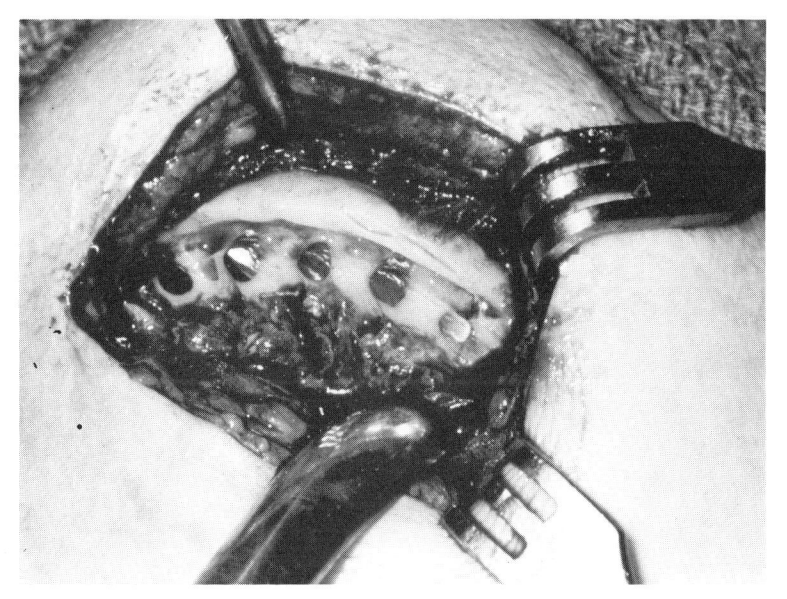

Figure 7–47 shows the inferior border of the mandible of a patient who requested removal of her mandibular staple bone plate. The patient's request was based upon her psychiatric illness. The photograph shows osseous integration involving the intermediate pins of the staple bone plate. At the time of removal, there was no soft tissue between the bone and pins and removal of the appliance was extremely difficult. This case illustrates one implant that lends itself to osseous integration and is one of the primary reasons that the mandibular staple bone plate has been successful.

Figure 7–47. Inferior border of the mandible of a patient who requested removal of her mandibular staple bone plate.

THE TRANSMANDIBULAR IMPLANT

Hans Bosker and Lucas VanDijk

Approximately ten years ago the transmandibular implant was developed by Dr. Hans Bosker in the Netherlands. Through a careful protocol with rigorous follow-up, over 472 patients have been treated by this technique with only ten failures. The implant is a functional one designed to withstand the direct forces of mastication. The implant is constructed of a gold alloy that is to be biocompatible. This development allows construction of a functional prosthesis without augmenting the mandibular body with bone and without stimulating further resorption or injury to the nerve (Fig. 7–48).

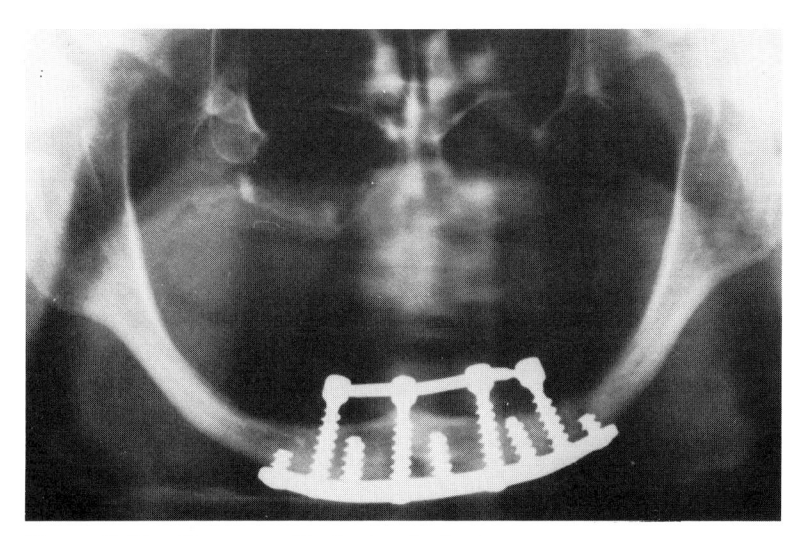

Figure 7–48. Transmandibular implant.

Anatomic Aspects

During the development of the implant, the form of the inferior border of the mandibular body of 95 jaws was measured. The mandibles came from human cadavers of varying age, race, and sex. This investigation showed that the ventrocaudal contour of the mandibular body had an identical centerline in all these jaws. In addition, at the level of the attachment of the digastric muscles, the protuberances were curved to various degrees. Little variation was noted in the measured distance from mental foramen to mental foramen when projected on the inferior border of the mandibular body and measured along its curvature. The measurement was never less than 37 mm. This occurred in all jaws, even those with deciduous teeth and those that were edentulous. The difference in the distance between the mental foramina thus measured derives principally from a difference in resorption on the lateral side of the mandibular body. This commonality can also be explained embryologically.

Embryologic Aspects

The bones of the skeleton and the skull are derived from the mesoderm. Meckel's cartilage and the membranous bone of the mandible, maxilla, and zygoma are exceptions, being derived from the ectomesenchyme of the neural crest.[16-19] In humans, cartilage plays no direct part in the composition of the mandible but is intimately involved in its formation. On the lateral side of Meckel's cartilage, during the sixth week of embryologic development, a condensation of ectomesenchyme occurs in the corner, being formed by the splitting of the inferior alveolar and mental nerves. From this corner, the intramembranous bone formation takes place. The formation of the bone goes through to the ventral part, closely following the outside of Meckel's cartilage.

The left and the right segments remain separate in the midline until shortly after birth. Both growing centers located in the symphysis disappear in the first year of life.[20] The change of shape of the ventral part of the mandibular body now takes place only through periosteal bone formation and resorption. Any further increase in mandibular length originates in the growing centers of the mandibular condyles.

Development of the New Implant

In highly atrophic mandibles, the roof of the mandibular canal is often resorbed to the point that the mental nerve lies on the crest of the residual ridge. Even minimal denture forces and forces of mastication on or directly over the nerve can cause pain. Implants for patients with atrophic mandibles should adequately support the denture and be able to withstand these masticatory forces.

The supporting structure of such a device must be situated between the mental foramina in order to spare the nervous innervation of the chin and the lower lip. To regain the chewing capacity of the posterior teeth, construction of a denture supported by an implant is a possible solution.

Implant Design

Owing to the previously determined equality in measurements of the ventrocaudal part of the mandibular symphysis, a uniform base plate could be developed, enabling fixation of the threaded posts in the centerline of the inferior border of the mandible (Fig. 7–49) of each patient. The base plate is fastened to the inferior border by means of five cortical screws, supports for the four threaded posts. With the help of a drill and an adjustable drill guide, drill holes can be made in such a way that each threaded post comes out at the highest point of the mandibular ridge. The threaded posts are fixed to the base plate by means of locking screws. The threaded posts, which perforate the oral mucosa, have a diameter of 1.7 mm and are intra-orally connected with

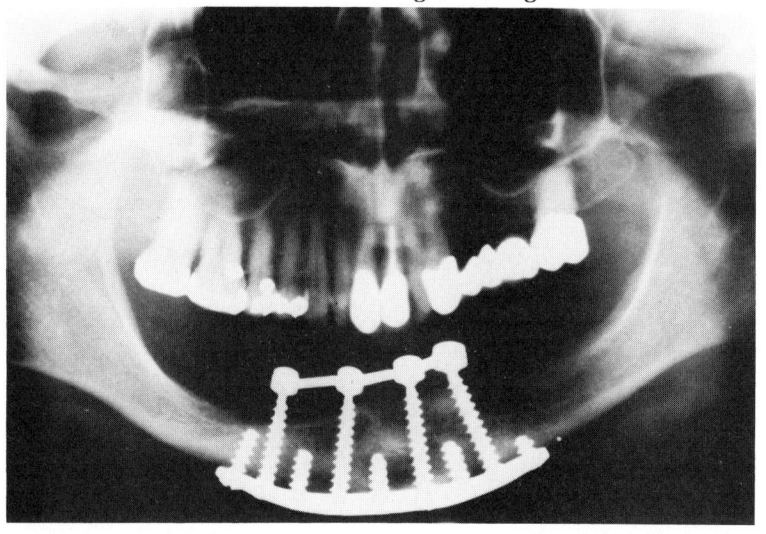

Figure 7–49. A uniform base plate could be developed, enabling fixation of the threaded posts in the centerline of the inferior border of the mandible.

each other by means of a bar construction. In the denture, the matrix, which is the retention sleeve of the Dolder bar, has been fixed so that the implant supports the prosthesis. Cortical screws are located on either side of the threaded posts (Fig. 7–50), connecting the base plate with the mandible. The most lateral ones lie well beneath the mandibular canal and penetrate the bone to the depth of 4.7 mm. The three remaining cortical screws are fixed into the cortex with either 4.7 or 9.0 mm screws, depending on the height of the symphysis. The intraosseous portion of the implant material has a pore size of 1.68 to 2.10 mm so that the surface area of the bone-implant interface can be increased.

Implant Principles

Dental implants can be divided into three categories: (1) cosmetic, (2) semifunctional, and (3) fully functional.

A cosmetic implant can replace one or more teeth but cannot withstand masticatory force. Crowns on such implants have to be left out of occlusion. An example of a cosmetic implant is the Tübinger implant.

A semifunctional implant can stabilize a denture, but the masticatory force has to be guided to the mucoperiosteum. An example of a semifunctional implant is the mandibular staple bone implant.

A fully functional implant can replace one or more teeth or support a denture and is loaded with masticatory force. Functional implants are the T.M. implants and the Brånemark implant.

Cosmetic and semifunctional implants have a limited use. The conditions that determine the clinical success of an implant are the biocompatibility, the mechanical dynamic properties of the implant material, the bearing and damping capacity, and the pretension in the implant design.

The mechanical properties of implant materials concern mainly the strength and the elasticity of the material. To resist many years of masticatory force, the implant has to be made of a material with high mechanical values, especially with reference to fatigue strength. The type of bond that exists between implant and bone is dependent on the material used: bioactive materials (e.g., glass ceramics, hydroxyapatite ceramics, and bioglass) cause bonding osteogenesis, whereas bioinert materials (e.g., aluminum oxide [Al_2O_3], carbon materials, precious metals, titanium, and tantalum) cause contact osteogenesis. Strength, biocompatibility, and elasticity are discussed more fully on pages 199 to 202.

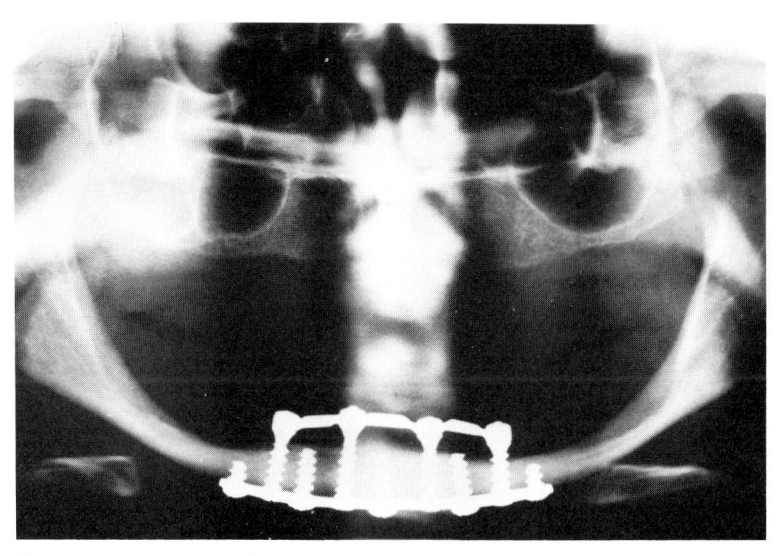

Figure 7–50. Cortical screws are located on either side of the threaded posts.

Implant Materials

Many materials have been investigated for use in general surgical and dental implant applications. These materials include ceramics, polymers, composites, and metals. The choice of the material for an implant depends on several factors, including strength, biocompatibility, elasticity, and implant design. Taken together, these factors act like a chain in which the weakest link determines the strength of the whole chain.

Oral implants are in contact with saliva, mucoperiosteum, bone, and tissue fluid. This is a highly complex environment in which all surfaces are continuously moist and are subjected to periodic temperature changes. The saliva is known to vary between pH4 and pH8 but commonly has a pH of 6.5 to 7.0.[21, 22] Localized changes may also arise from the deposition and accumulation of plaque and calculus. The oral cavity contains some 1100 ppm of chloride, 44 ppm of fluoride,[21, 23, 24] and many types of microorganisms that can vary widely with changes in systemic and intra-oral environment.

Strength

Clearly any material used in oral implantology must have sufficient strength to withstand masticatory stresses. The measured maximum masticatory force in the molar area with rigidly fixed implants is 40 to 75 kgf.[25] On simultaneous measurement in all three directions the maximum components are 20 kgf in the vertical direction, 11 kgf in the transverse direction, and 5 kgf in the sagittal direction. An implant may be required to resist these forces for 50 years if it is placed in a young person. To withstand such stress the implant has to be made of a material with high mechanical values, especially in reference to fatigue strength.

Ceramics. Ceramics are mechanically weak and brittle, having little flexural strength and no ductility. Furthermore, they have minimal impact resistance, and fabrication into complex shapes is difficult. In general, the strength of a ceramic material will decrease with increasing pore size.[26, 27] Bony ingrowth occurs when the pores exceed 150 to 200 μm.[28-33] The compressive strength for dense calcium phosphate ceramics without pores is around 410 ± 75 MPa. The tensile strength is 39 ± 4 MPa.[34] Calcium phosphate ceramics that are subjected to torque tend to fail mechanically *in vivo* because of their susceptibility to fatigue failure.[35]

Polymers. The mechanical properties of polymers can be altered by various additives or by variation of the polymer chain lengths. Since polymers are generally of low strength, any further decrease will adversely affect the mechanical usefulness of the polymer. Loss of strength and embrittlement can occur from hydrolytic leaching of components from implanted polymers. Polymers have poor abrasion resistance.[21]

Polymers may be susceptible to metabolization and disintegration by the biosystem.[36] This breakdown of polymers, which can involve both oxidation and hydrolytic degradation, would influence both the mechanical efficiency and the tissue tolerance of implanted polymers.

Polymers are polyethylene, Teflon, silicone rubber, polypropylene, and polymethylmethacrylate (PMMA). The compressive strength (e.g., for dense porous PMMA) is 500 to 600 kg/cm^2, and with a porosity of 50 per cent, 100 to 250 kg/cm^2. Owing to the porosity, the mechanical strength of the cement is impaired, indicating that the material should be used as a bone substitute only in low-stress situations.[37]

Polytetrafluoroethylene (Teflon) has low resistance to abrasion. It has been shown that particles of polymers loosened by abrasion will cause inflammation in the surrounding tissues.[38] Teflon used in combination with a titanium joint prosthesis will cause fretting of the titanium, because polytetrafluoroethylene contains 100 ppm of fluorides.

Metals. As the mechanical and/or physical properties of pure metals are generally inadequate for implants, alloys are used. The alloys and metals used for implants are wrought stainless steel, cast cobalt chromium, wrought cobalt chromium, wrought titanium alloy (Ti-6al-4V), gold alloy 18 carat 5 per cent (Au.Pt.Cu.Ag), and tantalum (Table 7–2). All these metals have sufficient strength to withstand masticatory stresses, but the design of the implant imposes severe restrictions on the type of metal that can be used.

Biocompatibility

An implant material is biocompatible if it is not toxic, allergenic, carcinogenic, mutagenic, harmful to the surrounding tissues, or disruptive to the healing of the tissues.

Ceramics. The best ceramics seem to be the dense form of hydroxyapatite with the formula $Ca_{10}(PO_4)_6(OH)_2$.[35, 39] This ceramic has been investigated in toxicologic studies in the soft tissues of rats and rabbits, in millipore chamber experiments in dogs, and in repair of femoral defects in dogs.[40, 41] The $Ca_{10}(PO_4)_6(OH)_2$ ceramic causes no adverse host reaction and no evident resorption. In this way hydroxyapatite is a biocompatible material. Implantation of hydroxyapatite can lead to a bone-implant interface within three to six months[41] when the implant material has adequate stabilization. Inadequate stabilization leads to the growth of fibrous tissue around the hydroxyapatite.

Polymers. Polymers corrode but do not form chemically insoluble passive films as some alloys do. Polymers are built up from molecules having a range of molecular weights, so that they contain low molecular weight components and, in some cases, residual monomers. In addition, stabilizers and antioxidants, together with other additives such as plasticizers and miscellaneous impurities, are present in the polymers.

TABLE 7–2. MECHANICAL PROPERTIES OF METAL IMPLANTS

Metal or Alloy	Tensile Strength (N/mm^2 MPa)	Yield Strength (0.2% N/mm^2 MPa)	Elongation at Fracture(%)	Hardness (HV)
Wrought stainless steel	500–1480	200–1450	12–40	160
Cast cobalt chromium	650–700	450–560	4–12	250
Wrought cobalt chromium	860–1700	300–1275	10–50	440
Wrought titanium	450	275	22	180
Ti-Al-V	930	870	10	310
Au.Pt.Cu.Ag.	880	840	3.5	250

These additives and low molecular weight compounds may be leached from the polymers and elicit adverse tissue reactions ranging from mild inflammatory response to osteomyelitis and other serious conditions.[42-46]

Metals. Almost every alloy, with the exception of certain precious metal alloys, corrodes in the mouth. The consequence of corrosion is diffusion of metal ions throughout the organism.[47, 48] In the short term certain metals can have toxic and allergenic effects. In the long term certain metals can present major health risks, such as mutagenic and carcinogenic effects.[49, 50] For this reason, nickel, cadmium, and chromium cobalt alloys are prohibited by the Swedish National Health Agency for use as implant materials.[51] The local or systemic effects of an alloy that corrodes in the mouth are those of its ingredients.

Some metals, however, form a stable oxide spontaneously, subject to certain conditions. This oxide has the very special property of developing a continuous, passivating film on the surface of its metal, protecting the latter from corrosion by the ambient medium. However, this shield is fallible and can be destroyed by wear and by ions in the saliva. For example, the oxide of chromium will be destroyed by Cl⁻ ions, and the oxide of titanium will be destroyed by F⁻ ions.[52, 53] Only 20 ppm of fluoride will cause fretting of titanium.[54] Human plaque normally contains 44 ppm of fluoride. This explains the high concentrations of titanium found in tissue in the vicinity of implants and the tendency toward accumulation of the metal ions in spleen and lung.[55-57] As far as we know titanium in low concentrations is not toxic. This fretting also explains the epithelial downgrowth that occurs by plaque accumulation along the implant.

The corrosion of titanium also takes place when titanium is used in a total hip replacement: of 667 patients treated, Scales[46] observed that 62.6 per cent of the stainless steel, 21.7 per cent of the vitallium, and 22.6 per cent of the titanium total hips were corroded. By the use of different alloys, phenomena of corrosion induce galvanic currents and cause diffusion of metallic ions from the alloy metal having the lowest corrosion potential.

To avoid local and general disorders, polymetallism is undesirable and highly electropositive metals should be favored (Table 7-3).

The following metals are present in the organism: constitutional origin (oligo-elements) Mg, Mn, Fe, Ca, Co, Cu, Zn, Mo. However, two of these oligo-elements, Co and Cu, can also be cytotoxic, depending on

TABLE 7-3. ELECTRODE POTENTIAL OF METALS

METAL	ELECTRODE POTENTIAL AGAINST "HYDROGEN" (VOLTS)
Au+	+1.50
Au+++	+1.36
Pt++	+0.86
Ag+	+0.80
Cu+	+0.47
Ni++	-0.25
Co	-0.28
Cd++	-0.40
Cr++	-0.56
Ti++++	-1.63
Al+++	-1.60

the concentration in the alloy used and means of entry into the tissues. For this reason, Co and Cu may be used only in an alloy metal that does not corrode. Gold and platinum do not corrode in the mouth. When an alloy of gold and platinum with copper or palladium has been fabricated, corrosion will take place when the nonprecious ions are dotted in the alloy. However, when a homogeneous crystal has been formed and the gold-platinum composition is 75 per cent or more, the alloy will not corrode.[58, 59] Such an alloy should not be caset afterward, because heating will change the crystal form and cause dotting of the nonprecious ions, which will then be available for diffusion throughout the organism.

The bone-metal interface of a 70 per cent gold–5 per cent platinum alloy is formed by osteocementum in close relationship to the alloy (Fig. 7–51). Epithelial downgrowth is not apparent with implants of such an alloy.

Tantalum has also been used as an implant material. However, fluoride attacks tantalum at room temperature, and hydrofluoric acid (aqueous or anhydrous), gasseous hydrogen fluoride, and acid solutions containing more than 2 or 3 ppm of fluoride ions all corrode and embrittle tantalum.[60]

In conclusion, precious alloys with a composition of at least 75 per cent gold and platinum are, if the metal alloy is treated in the right way, safe and biocompatible implant materials.

Elasticity

The type of bond that exists between implant and bone is dependent on the material used. The clinical success of an implant depends on its maintaining the bone-implant interface during long-term functional stresses. Failure of implants is caused by de-

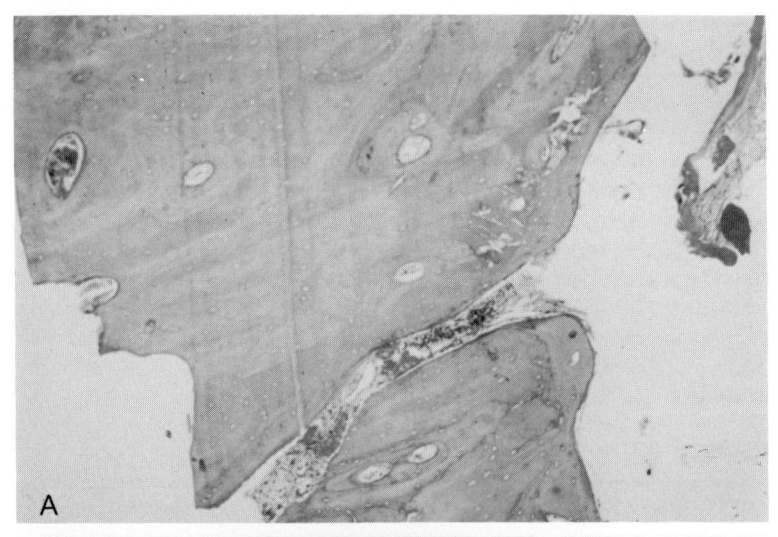

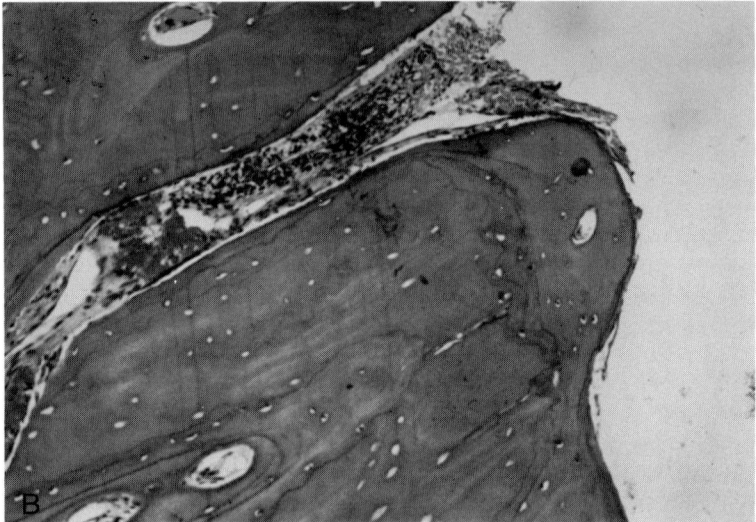

Figure 7–51. The bone-metal interface of a 70 per cent gold–5 per cent platinum alloy is formed by osteocementum in close relationship to the alloy.

struction of the interface between bone and implant by an intervening layer of connective tissue, which will interfere with the bond between the implant and the bony bed.[61] From this point of view the results will be the same for a bioactive and a bioinert implant: namely, a loose implant.

The mechanical dynamic properties of implant materials differ considerably from natural bone. The differences in the elasticity moduli that are specific to the materials involved exert a disrupting effect in the region of contact between implant and bone. The elasticity modulus of calcium hydroxyapatite, for example, is around 15 times that of bone, titanium and tantalum around 4 times that of bone, and 18/5 carat precious alloy metal 3 times that of bone. This means that if an implant is loaded with masticatory force, the deformation of the implant material exceeds that of the adjacent bone, which may result in a fracture through the osteocementum in the case of a bioactive implant material or a fracture of the osteocementum on the implant side in the case of a bioinert implant material. This difference in elasticity has to be diminished by the damping capacity of the implant system. The more the elasticity modulus of the implant material differs from that of the bone, the greater the damping capacity that must be built into the implant design.

The shearing strength of adjacent bone to the implant is also an important factor in maintaining the bone-implant interface. The shearing strength of the bone is, dependent on the time after operation, 0.7 to 0.74 MPa. The tensile strength is between 1.1 and 2.2 MPa.[62]

The masticatory force in the case of stable implants is around 65 kgf. In order to avoid fracture of the composite layer or osteocementum adjacent to the implant, the masticatory force has to be distributed over the bearing area of the implant in such a way that the tolerable shearing strength of the bone is not exceeded. This is called the "bearing capacity" of the implant. Increasing bearing capacity decreases the elasticity problem.

Choice of Material

The choice of material to be used is influenced by the demands ultimately made upon the implant and by reaction of the tissues in which the material is fixed. The transmandibular implant makes contact with the oral mucoperiosteum, saliva, the mandibular symphysis, and the submental periosteum and muscles.

When the vast body of alloy research is reviewed, very few metals can be found that do not react with human tissue. All alloys show corrosion while in contact with tissues of the human body, but those of precious metals do so the least.

Since the transmandibular implant supports the dental prosthesis, the alloy used for the implant should be the same as that of the retentive parts in the dental prosthesis. This prevents galvanic currents. Precious metals such as gold and platinum are thermodynamically stable and are not subject to corrosion. The optimum combination of biologic and mechanical qualities is an 18 carat, 5 per cent alloy. This alloy consists of 70 per cent gold, 5 per cent platinum, 12.8 per cent silver, and 12.2 copper. The ratio of 70 per cent gold to 12.2 per cent copper seems to offer the best resistance to corrosion.

An allergic potential has, however, been attributed to copper, and it may be an etiologic factor in lichen planus.[63] Patients being considered for transmandibular implants are therefore questioned about possible reactions to gold rings and chains and are examined for the presence of lesions on the mucous membrane near gold fillings or crowns.

If a positive history is elicited, allergy tests can be carried out. True allergy will contraindicate the placement of a transmandibular implant.

The mechanical values of the 18 carat, 5 per cent alloy are determined according to the DIN method 50-145*: yield point 0.2 per cent elasticity—840 N/mm^2; tensile strength—880 N/mm^2; breaking strength over 100 mm—15 per cent; hardness according to Vickers—230.

Instrumentation

The relation between the inferior symphyseal border and the crest of the alveolar ridge differs both in height and in direction.

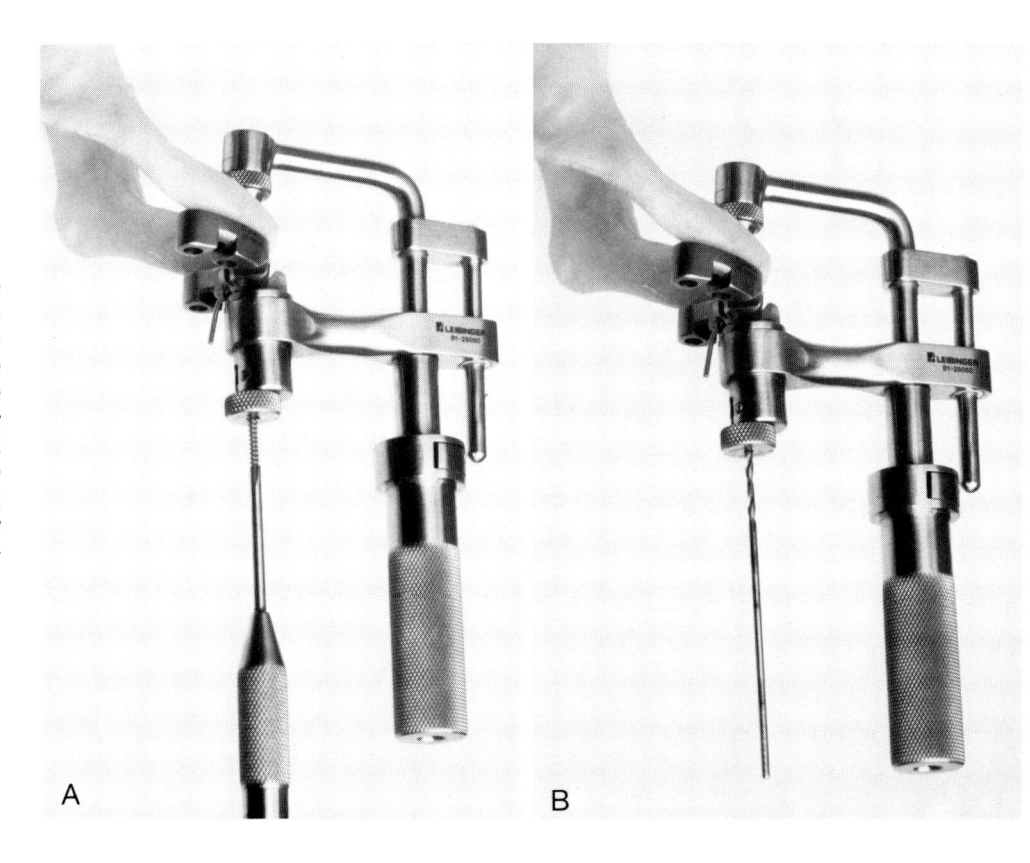

*According to a report of H. Drijfhout and Zoon's Edelmetaalbedrijven B.V., Amsterdam.

The difference in the direction is caused by the extent of resorption and by the position of the alveolar process in relation to the symphyseal basal bone. To place the threaded post in the inferior surface of the mandibular symphysis, a drill guide and an adjustable drill guide (Fig. 7–52A) are needed, so that the threaded post to the highest point of the ridge crest can be directed while passing through the proper location in the base plate. The holes for the threaded posts are drilled and tapped. The height of the symphysis can be read off the adjustable drill guide.

The holes for the cortical screws are drilled via the superstructure on the drill guide and are tapped through the drill guide after removal of the drill guide superstructure (Fig. 7–52B). By means of the drill guide, superstructure, and adjustable drill guide, the implants can be placed without injury to the mental or inferior alveolar nerves.

Further instruments used are a template to detect unevenness at the attachment of the digastric muscle; forceps to place the superstructure on the threaded posts; drills with diameter of 2 mm: (a) drills with a length of 10 mm for placing the threaded posts; and (b) drills with a stop for drilling holes for cortical screws beneath the mandibular canal; and taps with a diameter of 3.5 mm.

Figure 7–52. *A,* To place the threaded post on the inferior surface of the mandibular symphysis, a drill guide and an adjustable drill guide are needed. *B,* The holes for the cortical screws are drilled via the superstructure on the drill guide and are tapped through the drill guide after removal of the drill guide superstructure.

Indications and Contraindications

Indications

For the reconstructive surgery, patients were referred to the oral and maxillofacial surgeon. Patient complaints were the principal reason for considering surgical correction. These complaints were mainly pain, poorly functioning dentures, and appearance. The oral and maxillofacial surgeon's examination consisted of a thorough inspection of the supporting tissues. Attention was paid to sharp crests, bony undercuts, exostoses, flabby ridges, and areas of chronic irritation. Panoramic, lateral, and oblique mandibular radiographs determined the resorption and abnormalities in the cortical bone. Patients who might require symphyseal or ridge augmentation[64] were considered for implants as an alternative. Transmandibular implants are also useful for patients with a dentulous maxilla and an edentulous mandible; players of wind instruments, both to prevent resorption and to make blowing possible; patients with mandibular bone loss for any reason, such as trauma or tumor surgery; and youthful edentulous patients, such as those having ectodermal dysplasia or cleidocranial dysostosis.

Contraindications

Any contraindications to general anesthesia also contraindicate placement of the implant. The implant is also contraindicated in the following situations: uncontrolled endocrine diseases and the metabolic disorders[65]; immunodeficient states[65]; presence of metallic foreign bodies in the mandible[65]; psychologic instability; and allergy to the 18 carat, 5 per cent alloy.

Surgical Technique

Any needed intra-oral reconstructive surgery is performed four to six weeks before implant surgery. These corrections may consist of removal of any sharp bony crests, knife-edged ridges, or undercuts, and excision of epithelial hyperplasia or areas of chronic irritation. Following this surgery, the

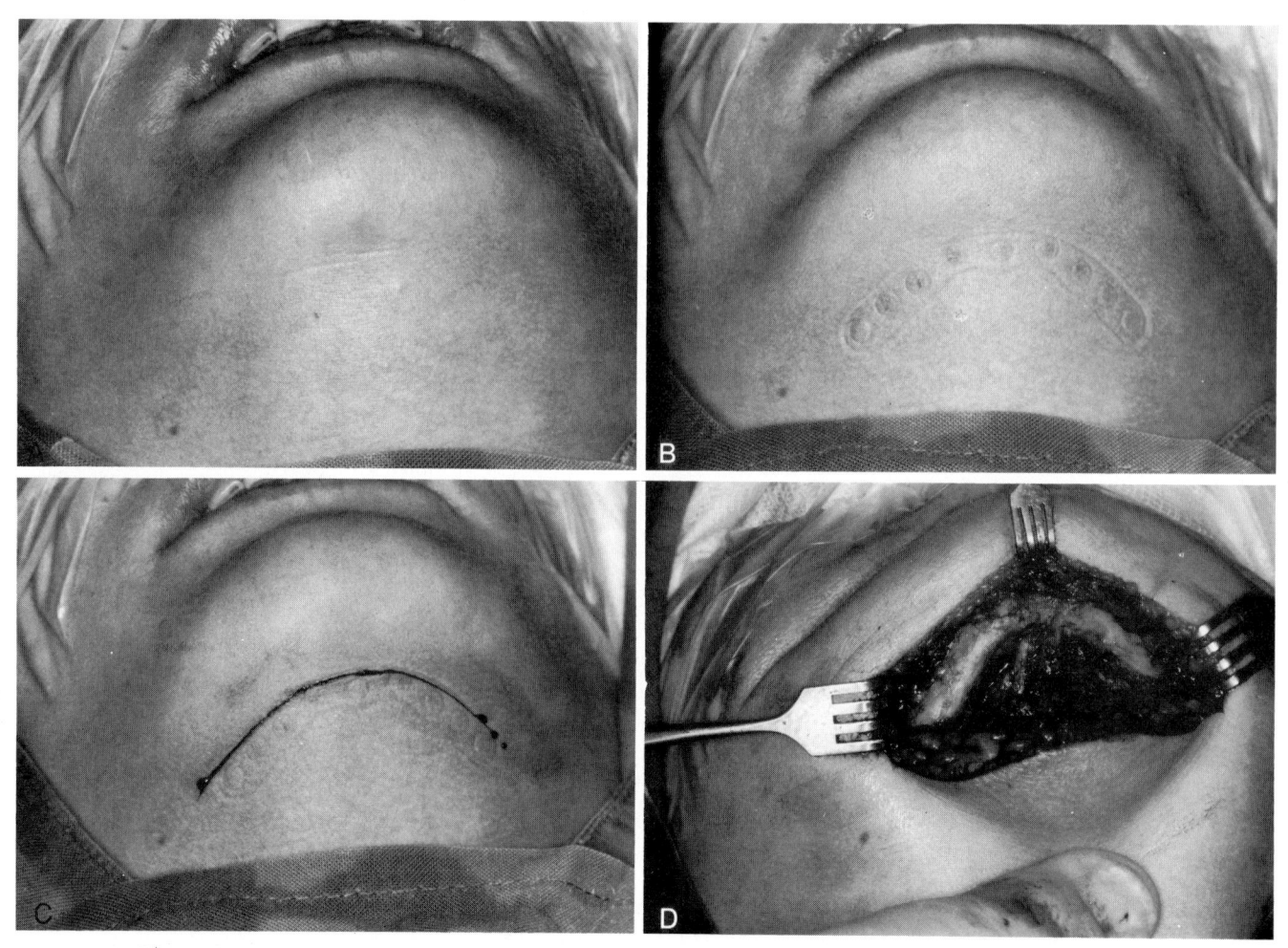

Figure 7–53. The length of the incision is determined by the length of the base plate plus 5 mm.

IMPLANTS USED IN PREPROSTHETIC RECONSTRUCTIVE SURGERY / **205**

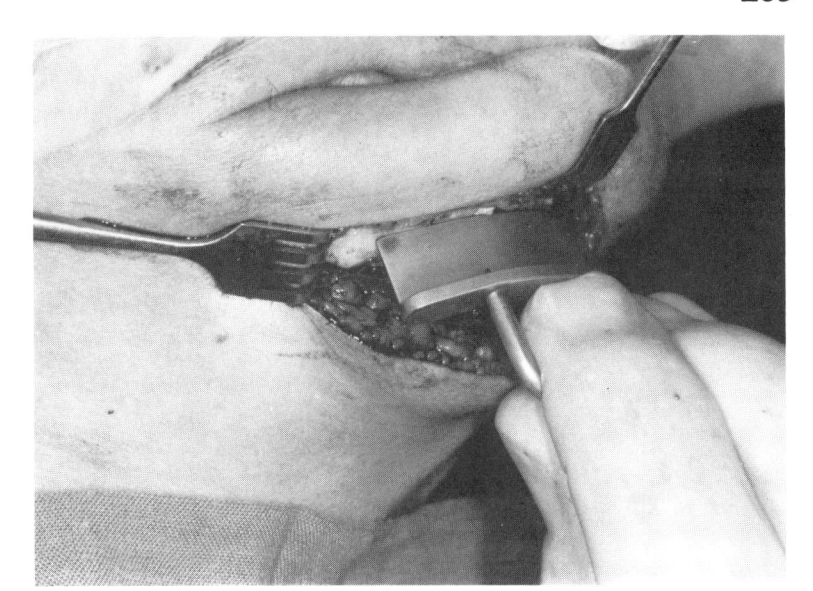

Figure 7–54. Using the template, correction is made of any bone protuberances at the site of the attachment of the digastric muscle.

denture can be relined temporarily with any tissue conditioner. The insertion of the transmandibular implant takes place under general anesthesia with appropriate prophylactic antibiotics.

The inferior border of the mandibular symphysis is exposed by means of curvilinear incision over the submental region of the mandible. The length of the incision is determined by the length of the base plate plus 5 mm (Fig. 7–53). Using the template, any bone protuberances at the site of the attachment of the digastric muscle are removed (Fig. 7–54). The drill guide is then placed (Fig. 7–55) and the drill holes for the cortical screws are drilled with the drill guide superstructure *in situ* (Fig. 7–56). The drill guide is locked with three cortical screws into the

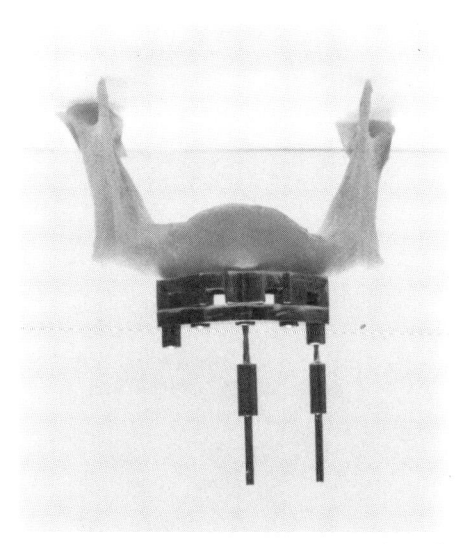

Figure 7–55. The drill guide is placed as shown on this model.

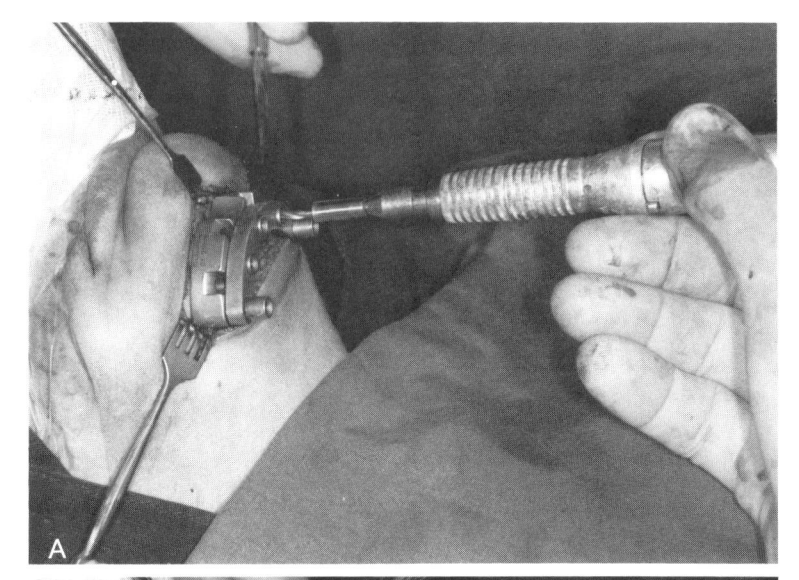

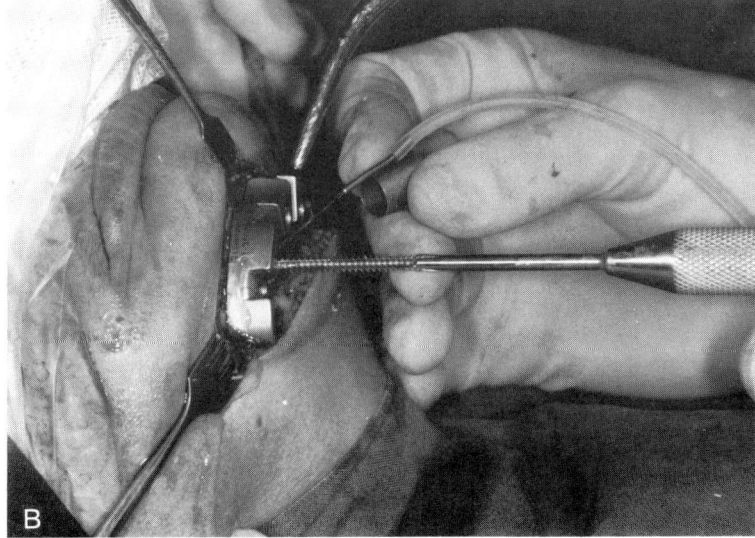

Figure 7–56. The drill holes for the cortical screws are drilled with the drill guide superstructure *in situ*.

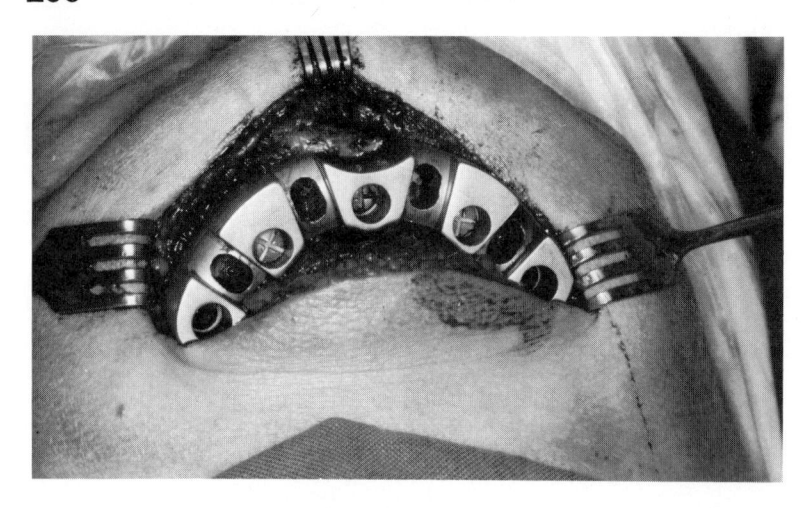

206 / IMPLANTS USED IN PREPROSTHETIC RECONSTRUCTIVE SURGERY

Figure 7–57. The drill guide is locked with three cortical screws into the symphysis.

symphysis (Fig. 7–57). The remaining two holes for the cortical screws are then drilled and tapped.

With the adjustable drill on the drill guide, the direction of each individual threaded post is determined. Through the adjustable drill guide, the holes for the threaded posts are drilled and tapped while being cooled with sterile water (Fig. 7–58). After removal of the drill guide, the threaded posts are placed (Fig. 7–59A) and the base plate is fastened to the threaded posts with lock screws (Fig. 7–59B). The incision is closed in layers (Fig. 7–59C) after the placement of the cortical screws.

At the crest of the ridge, the four long threaded pins should now be visible. The base plate of the superstructure and the fastener nuts for determining the position of the Dolder bars (Fig. 7–60A) are fixed on these pins. With the fastener nuts *in situ* an impression is taken. One day following the surgery, the bar construction is placed on the base plate and fixed with lock nuts. This re-establishes the function of the alveolar process (Fig. 7–60B). Four weeks after the in-

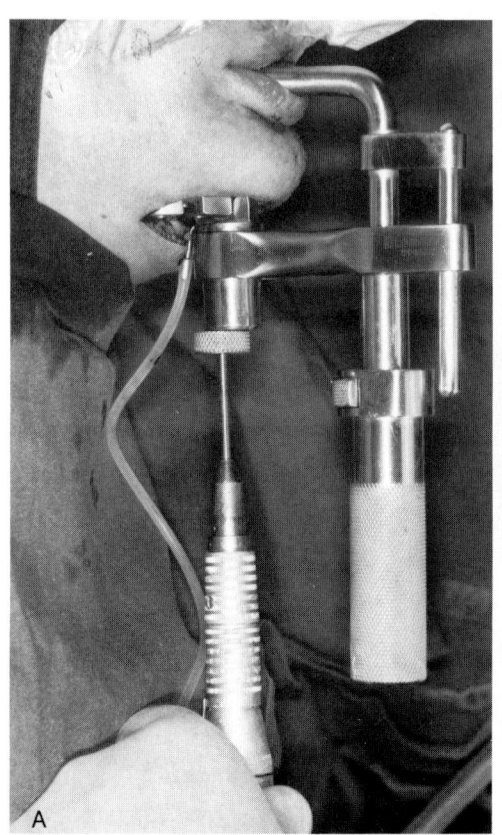

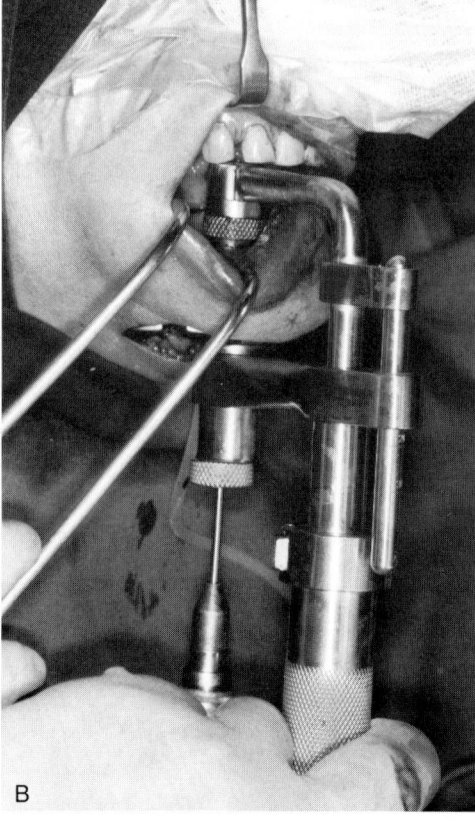

Figure 7–58. Through the adjustable drill guide, the holes for the threaded posts are drilled and tapped while being cooled with sterile water.

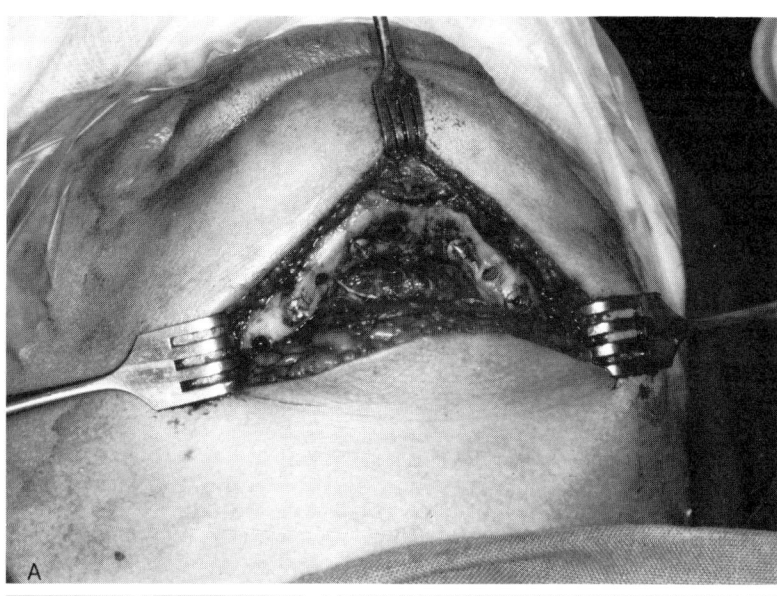

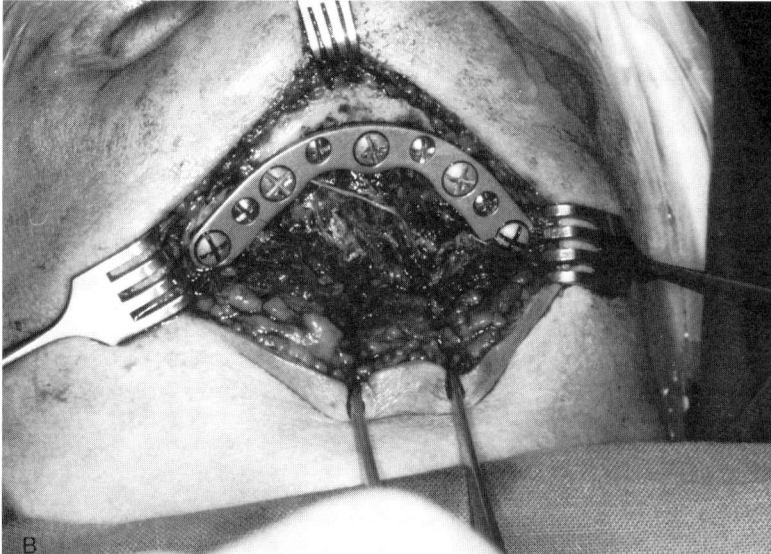

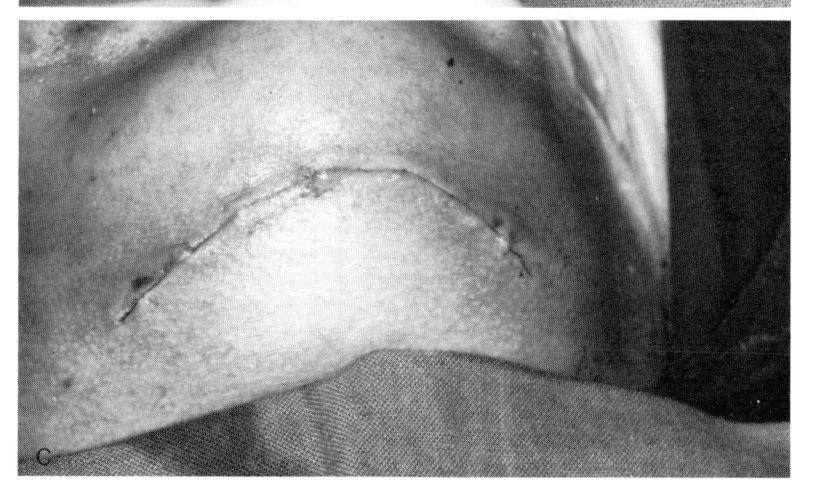

Figure 7-59. *A*, After removal of the drill guide, the threaded posts are placed. *B*, The base plate is fastened to the threaded posts with lock screws. *C*, The incision is closed in layers after the placement of the cortical screws.

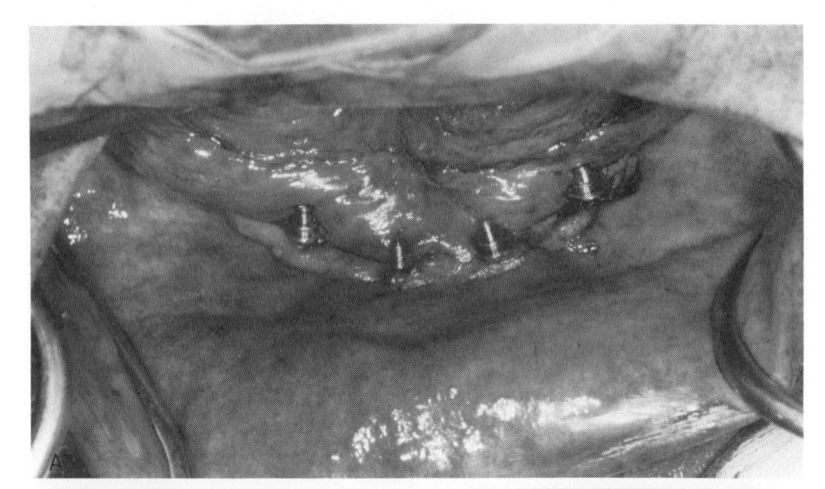

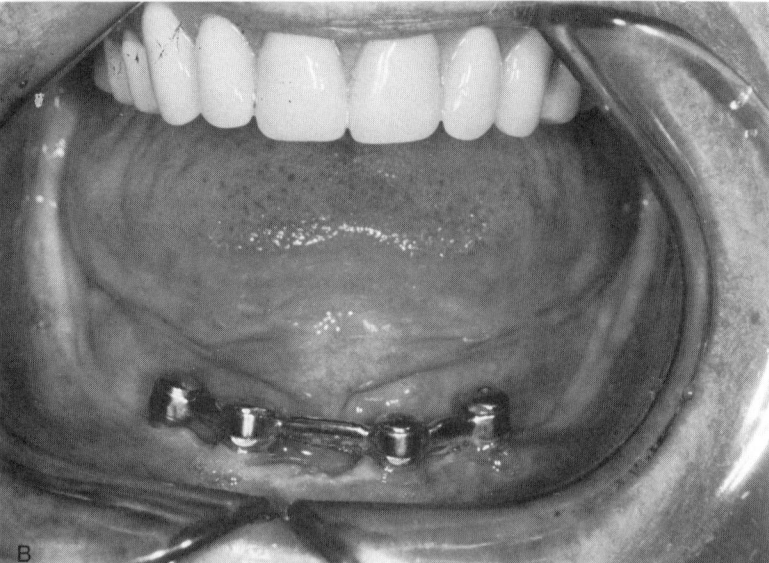

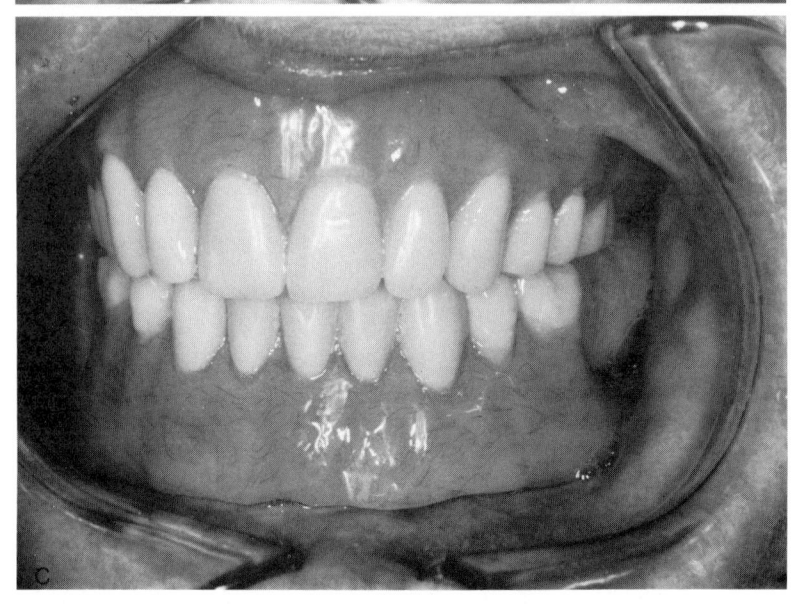

208 / IMPLANTS USED IN PREPROSTHETIC RECONSTRUCTIVE SURGERY

Figure 7–60. *A*, The base plate of the superstructure and the fastener nuts for determining the position of the Dolder bars are fixed on the pins. *B*, The bar construction is placed and fixed with lock nuts. *C*, Finished denture in place.

sertion of the implant, denture construction can begin (Fig. 7–60C).

The Construction of the Denture

The portion of the denture between the mental foramina is supported by the implant, because the matrices resting on the bars are fastened without degrees of freedom. The implant receives most of the forces of mastication. The chewing force to the implant can be increased by shortening the tooth-bearing portion of the area. As already stated, a highly resorbed mandibular alveolar process is an indication for the insertion of the transmandibular implant. In these cases, the mylohyoid ridge is frequently situated near the denture-bearing surface. This part of the mandible is formed by a cortical bony ridge and therefore receives no pressure from the denture. Since the denture has no need for lingual flanges because of the presence of the implant, the mylohyoid ridge can also be used as a supporting part of the dental prosthesis. The course of a superficial inferior alveolar and/or mental nerve can be relieved from the undersurface of the prosthesis if necessary.

To prevent tipping of the denture during biting, the lower anterior teeth must be set directly above the most anterior bar. While they are wearing a conventional denture, the chewing force of most patients is restricted by the pain threshold of their compressed mucosa. As the supporting surface of the edentulous mandible is smaller than that of the maxilla, the chewing force exerted in these cases may be diminished. If this threshold is increased by insertion of a transmandibular implant, limitation of chewing force may be the pain threshold of the mucosa of the maxilla. Thus, the total exerted chewing force can increase. To prevent rapid resorption of the maxillary alveolar process as a result of the increased chewing force, the arrangement of the teeth in the upper denture is crucial.

Like the mylohyoid ridge, the hard palate consists of dense cortical bone that resists loading forces. Thus, the posterior denture teeth should be placed just palatal to the crest of the alveolar process. This technique can lead to a cross-bite posteriorly but presents no obstacle to a good occlusion and balanced articulation. Sagittal contact between lower and upper anterior teeth and cuspid occlusion should be avoided. If the articulation curve is determined with the help of gypsum carborundum walls, molars without cusps can be used. If an average curve is utilized for the arrangement of the teeth, the use of teeth with cusps is preferable. Correction through selective grinding of the cusps makes it possible to achieve a balanced occlusion.

Research Goals

Clinical Experience

The original surgical procedures were performed by two oral and maxillofacial surgeons in the Diakonessenhuis Hospital in Groningen.

The dentures of 45 patients were fabricated by one dentist, and 52 other patients had their dentures constructed by various dentists. The entire study spans eight years and examines a total of 97 patients who received implants inserted in the aforementioned manner (Fig. 7-59). More recently, the transmandibular implant has also been placed in over 350 patients in other surgical clinics in the Netherlands. These patients form a selected group, all exhibiting extreme resorption of the mandible. They all experienced varying difficulties in wearing a lower denture, and all appeared motivated to undergo the operation.

The original 97 patients who received the implant consisted of 60 females and 37 males. In five cases, a vestibuloplasty was performed at the same surgical session. In three cases, a chin reduction[66] was also performed. The ages varied from 28 to 73; the average age of all patients was 47 years. The length of the hospitalization was five to six days. After a healing period of four weeks, denture construction was begun. The dentures were seated seven to eight weeks after surgery, and all patients have had yearly follow-up.

Follow-up examinations monitored the surgical results and the functioning of both implant and denture. Concurrently, possible unfavorable results were also monitored. All examinations were carried out by an oral and maxillofacial surgeon and a dentist at one and five years after insertion of the implant.

Ninety-two patients had no complications in the postoperative phase. Their response to the surgical treatment, the postoperative healing process, and their hospital stay was that the entire procedure exceeded their expectations. In particular, patients who had undergone a prior preprosthetic surgical correction were surprised at the absence of pain and sensibility disturbances. There was minimal to moderate submental swelling. Postoperatively, these patients did not request analgesic medication.

Complications

In three patients, postoperative inflammation appeared subcutaneously in the submental regions. No pathogenic micro-organisms could be cultured in these cases. Drainage and irrigation of the wound produced a rapid recovery in two of the patients within one and two weeks, respectively. In the third patient, pathogenic gram-positive cocci were cultured from the purulent drainage. These turned out to be penicillin-resistant. This sequela appeared following discharge from the hospital, about six days after the operation. In addition to the submental inflammation, a maxillary sinusitis had also developed. As the micro-organisms appeared to be sensitive to tetracycline, doxycycline was prescribed. Twelve days after surgery, the patient was again asymptomatic. The scar under the chin, however, had remained clearly visible.

In one patient (date of operation: June, 1977), ten weeks postoperatively and two weeks after the seating of the dentures, a submental fistula developed. Pathogenic micro-organisms could not be cultured. On x-ray, it appears that there was bone resorption around the threaded posts. In September, 1977, the extremely mobile implant was removed. In January, 1978, another implant was placed in this patient. The dentures were again seated after 14 weeks. Since that time the implant has functioned adequately.

In one patient (date of operation: October, 1977), the implant was removed in May, 1981. The patient was an undiagnosed alcoholic and blamed all her pain on the implant, although clinically it functioned well and radiographically did not show any breakdown. At surgery, it appeared that the base plate was covered with bone. The screws could only be removed by trephination of the bone that had grown over them. In one patient, a sequestrum developed between the lateral cortical screw and the threaded post. X-rays showed good bone ingrowth three months after removal of the fragment.

With two implants it appeared that the threaded posts became loose as a result of a defect in the manufacturing of the lock-screws. After replacement of the lock-screws, the function of the implant appeared to be restored again.

One patient complained about pain in both upper and lower jaws. The origin of the pain could not be related to either the implant or the denture.

The Functioning of the Dental Prosthesis

The function of the dental prosthesis was related to the extent of satisfaction of the patient, the chewing ability, the resorption of the maxillary and mandibular alveolar processes, and the stability of the prosthesis. Five years after the operation, 95 patients appear to be very satisfied with the function of the dental prosthesis. This satisfaction was expressed by the enthusiasm with which they compared their present situation to the functioning of their denture before the implant was inserted. There was a decided absence of complaints of pain and denture sores. They were pleased with the fact that they were again able to chew tough foods. The chewing force was said by many to be comparable to that of their natural dentition.

One patient who complained about numerous pains in the mandible and maxilla was not satisfied with the result. Allergy tests with 18 carat, 5 per cent alloy were negative. Clinically and radiographically no abnormalities were demonstrable.

In none of the 96 patients with a dental prosthesis supported by an implant was there any evidence of further resorption of the symphysis. The extent to which resorption takes place can be measured by using the cortical screws as points of reference and also by standardized radiographs taken with a panoramic x-ray machine. By means of a removable superstructure substituted for the denture on the implant, the mandibular position can be reproducibly fixed in the apparatus of the panoramic x-ray machine.

The resorption of the maxillary alveolar process appeared to be less than we initially expected. Because of the absence of a standardized measuring technique, maxillary resorption cannot be quantified in units.

The function of the retentive sleeves or matrix on the dental prosthesis appears to have remained unchanged over the intervening years. Reactivation seldom is necessary. The reason appears to be that there is no space between the interlocking parts, and the only forces on these parts are those elastic forces occurring during insertion and removal. When loaded by the chewing forces, the matrix rests in a nonactivated position on the implant superstructure.

Unfavorable Side Effects

At present we have not observed any side effects. No toxic or allergic reactions have occurred. It appears that, as a result of inadequate cleaning of the superstructure in a number of cases, calculus deposition occurs around the posts and bar parts. Although this deposition does not lead to bone resorption around the posts, hyperplasia of the mucosa can result. Excision of the hyperplasia and improvement of the oral hygiene are then required.

Summary

The transmandibular implant is designed as an alternative to augmentation of the mandible. The aim is to restore the function of the resorbed body by means of the dental prosthesis and to prevent further resorption of the mandibular symphysis without causing injury to the inferior alveolar and mental nerves.

ENDOSTEAL DENTAL IMPLANTS IN THE TREATMENT OF THE EDENTULOUS JAW

THE BRÅNEMARK IMPLANT

P. I. Brånemark and T. Albrektsson

One of the most controversial fields in the medical sciences is that of dental implants. Since the 1950's, practitioners have inserted dental implants, many times without sound scientific analysis and acceptable control of the clinical outcome. The clinical results have shown, over short follow-up periods, that less than 50 per cent have been successful.[67–69] Because of the poor success rate, most universities would vote against the routine use of dental implants in clinical practice. According to Schnitman and Shulman[70] there has been no scientifically controlled and successful dental implant system with a sufficiently long follow-up period to justify routine use of implants.

At the Laboratory of Experimental Biology in the Department of Anatomy and later at the dental faculty at the University of Gothenburg, Sweden, a scientifically controlled program using dental implants was initiated with experimental studies in the early 1960's. The clinical insertion of osseointegrated dental implants started in 1965. By June 30, 1983, 3510 osseointegrated implants had been inserted in Gothenburg in 585 jaws, the majority of which (94 per cent) were totally edentulous. All patients were monitored annually, and there were no patient drop-outs, permitting complete and accurate statistics on each inserted implant.[71] This was the first time it had been possible to analyze scientifically the results of a large, consecutive, and complete clinical dental implant program over a long period of time.

The initial experimental studies demonstrated the importance of controlling implant material, surgical trauma, and loading conditions if a favorable outcome with the implantation was to be expected.[72–74] There were, however, some aspects of these and other important background factors that were not experimentally verified as early as the 1960's. Therefore, while continuing the controlled clinical program, several Ph.D. theses on hard tissue biology were published at the Laboratory of Experimental Biology at Gothenburg University.[75-83] The close connection between the Research Laboratory and the clinical specialties at Gothenburg University was an important factor in achieving good clinical results.

An ordinary tooth is attached to the jaw bone via a highly differentiated periodontal ligament; theoretically the re-establishment of the ligament would constitute the ideal anchorage for a dental implant. The periodontal ligament, of course, is histologically quite different from the relatively undifferentiated fibrous tissue membrane. This has been demonstrated in the boundary zone around most currently used dental implants. A lasting, proper periodontal ligament around a dental implant has never been re-established.

Our titanium implants are osseointegrated. Osseointegration is defined as a direct contact between living Haversian bone and implant without any intervening fibrous tissue layers.[84] In the following evaluation, possible advantages of osseointegrated implants in comparison to implants anchored in fibrous tissue will be discussed with regard to clinical results in a complete patient program that was followed up over an adequate period of time. Ledermann et al.,[85] who worked with the Straumann system of dental implants that have been followed over a one- to three-year period, claimed this "adequate time" to be at least ten years. We will present here five- and ten-year results of osseointegrated dental implants.

The first part of this overview is a survey of the experimental studies that constitute the biologic background to the system of osseointegrated dental implants. Thereafter, the method of osseointegration is described and the clinical results are presented. The discussion ends with a review of dental implants in general and with an outline of other clinical applications of the osseointegrated system.

Experimental Analyses

The Use of Titanium as Implant Material

Experiments with canine dental implants of either titanium, tantalum, or vitallium resulted in the preference for pure titanium as implant material.[86] It was demonstrated that dental implants of titanium could be inserted in the jaw bone of dog or man without becoming encapsulated in fibrous tissue.[84] The experimental plastic plug technique (Fig. 7–61) for ultrastructural analyses of the bone-implant interface[87] showed titanium to have a more natural boundary zone than any other tested material. In fact, the tissue

POLYCARBONATE PLUG FOR INTERFACE ANALYSIS

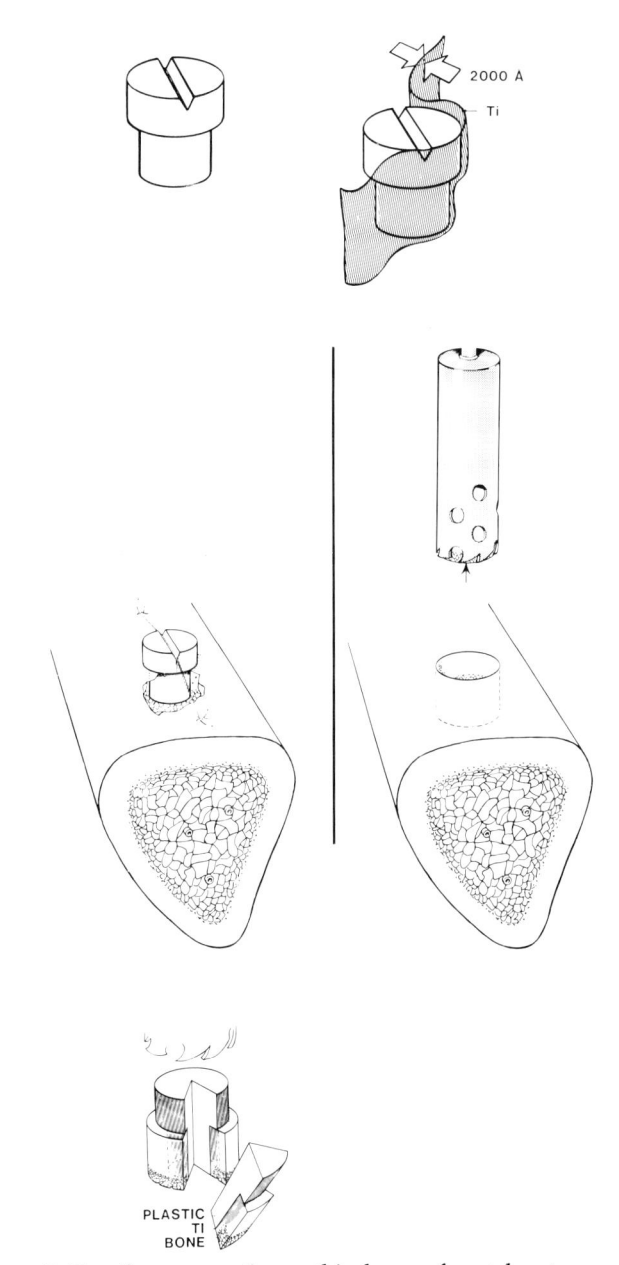

Figure 7–61. By evaporating a thin layer of metal onto a soft core of plastic it is possible to obtain sections for ultrastructural investigations of the intact interface between bone and metal. The implants are inserted in the rabbit tibia and removed with a trephine three to six months later. With this technique there are other possibilities, such as measuring the width of the proteoglycan layer that always surrounds an implant.

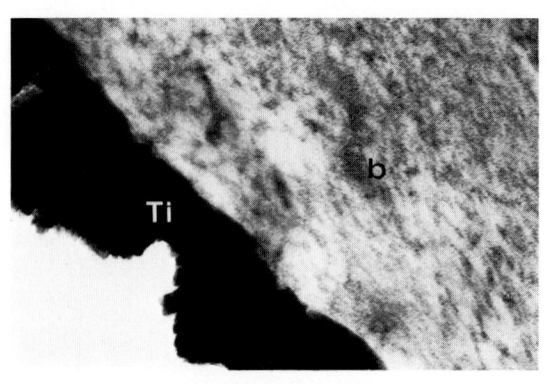

Figure 7-62. Intact interface between bone tissue and titanium (magnification × 100,000). The titanium (Ti) is in apparent direct continuity with the bone (b). In a narrow zone of 20 to 30 nm adjacent to the implant there is slightly reduced calcification and a positive staining reaction to proteoglycans.

characteristics around a bone-integrated titanium implant resembled those found between individual cells where no implants had been inserted. A partly calcified ground substance with an interface layer of only 20 to 30 nm was found around titanium bone implants.[87, 88] Gold,[87] stainless steel,[89] and zirconium[90] demonstrated much wider proteoglycan layers with clearly reduced calcification in the boundary zone. The high degree of biocompatibility of pure titanium is further documented in recent review papers.[91, 92] Figure 7-62 shows the bone interface of an experimental titanium plug implant inserted in a rabbit tibia. Figure 7-63 shows the interface between bone and titanium in a clinical case seven years after implantation in the mandible. There are no studies known to the present authors that demonstrate a similar bone tissue acceptance at the ultrastructural level of frequently used *non-metallic* implant materials such as carbon, glass ceramics, and Al_2O_3. Furthermore, carbon and glass ceramics are brittle, and a similar potential hazard exists with aluminum oxides after longer periods of implantation.

Implant Macro- and Microstructure

The screw form is an advantageous design compared to a smooth, nonporous implant as described by Skalak.[93] A screw can carry shear stresses even in the absence of bonding by compression onto the inclined faces of the threads, assuming, of course, a close apposition between bone and screw as in the case of the osseointegrated implant.[94] In comparison, a smooth, porous implant is subjected to potentially dangerous stresses, particularly in the early phases after implant insertion when bone growth into the pores has not yet occurred. Micromovements of an implant in this early phase after insertion may prove deleterious to implant fixation and may lead to a fibrous tissue encapsulation, as demonstrated by Uhthoff[95] and Schatzker et al.[96]

The microstructure of the implant is of a considerable importance for osseointegration. The small irregularities of the surface interlock can aid in transfer of shear stresses to the threads of the screw, as discussed above.[94] The microroughness of the implant surface is an aid in carrying stresses while fostering intimate contact between bone and implant surfaces. An example would be the osseointegrated dental implant inserted in the canine or the human jaw. Furthermore, cellular processes have been shown to adhere more readily to rough implant surfaces than to polished ones (Fig. 7-64).[89]

Surface energy, protein binding, and the exact nature of the titanium oxide are other important factors in the long-term outcome of the implantation.[92] A minor alteration of the surface conditions may cause implant failure in the long run because of unwanted side effects that become apparent only after some time. In such cases, implant loss may occur several years after implantation, although its fate was determined at insertion. A seemingly well-functioning dental implant may thus prove later to be a failure. This is one important reason why short follow-up

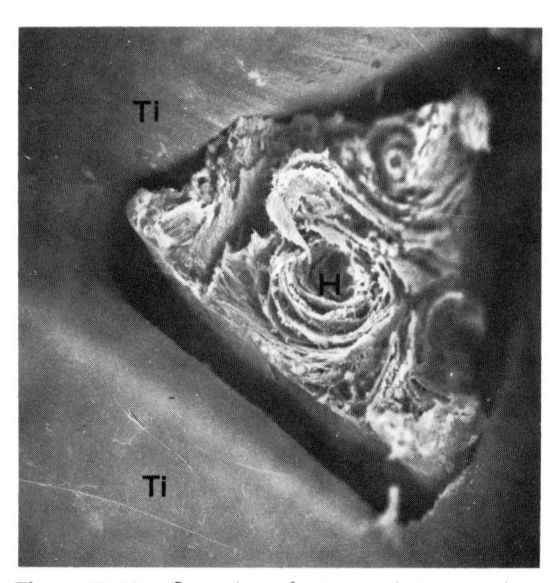

Figure 7-63. Scanning electron microscope image of bone tissue with Haversian systems (H) in a thread of a titanium (Ti) implant from a clinical case after seven years of function. The bone is partially detached from the titanium owing to the decalcification procedure.

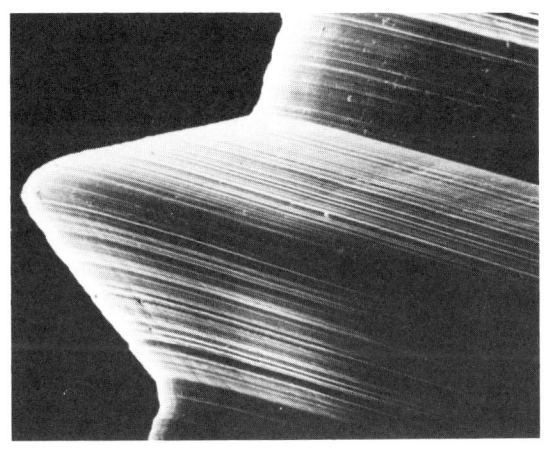

Figure 7–64. Scanning electron microscope image of implant surface, showing minor irregularities that have proved important for cellular attachment.

times (less than five to ten years) of a dental implant are of limited interest to the clinician. The clinician wants to evaluate the true success level of a dental implant system in relation to the patient's need for several decades of undisturbed function.

To avoid minor, but later potentially hazardous, surface alterations, there is a need to strictly control the manufacturing of a dental implant as well as the handling of it afterwards. Ultrasonic cleaning in poorly defined solutions, uncontrolled autoclaving, or metallic pollution from surgical instruments may alter the surface conditions from favorable to less favorable.[97] Titanium implants should, for instance, be handled only with titanium instruments.

The Importance of the Implant Bed

Much of the basic and applied research at the Laboratory of Experimental Biology has been devoted to various morphologic analyses of bone tissue and bone tissue reactions to an implant. It was early established that osteoporosis was no contraindication to the insertion of dental implants.[84] Neither was advanced resorption of the mandible accompanied by less clinical success. Brånemark et al.[84] and Adell et al.[71] found no indications for bone grafting in the anterior area. There is almost always enough bone for anchorage between the mental foramina. However, in cases of severe resorption with extremely thin remaining mandibular bone in the molar area, a bone graft may be in order to increase the mechanical strength of the corpus. The anterior part of the mandible, even if extremely thin, has in our experience never suffered a fracture or failure of bone strength after insertion of osseointegrated implants. In the upper jaw, on the other hand, about 10 per cent of the cases show such resorption that there is not enough bone left to carry the osseointegrated implant. In such cases, augmentation of the alveolar ridge with preformed bone grafts containing integrated fixtures gave better clinical results than did the use of conventional bone grafts (Breine and Brånemark, 1980). Preformation of a bone graft is a two-step procedure: the first being the insertion of a mold in the donor site, usually the upper tibial metaphysis or the iliac crest, and the second being the actual grafting. Advantages of preformation are that the graft can remodel according to the demands at the host site before removal from the donor bone, that fixtures may be incorporated in

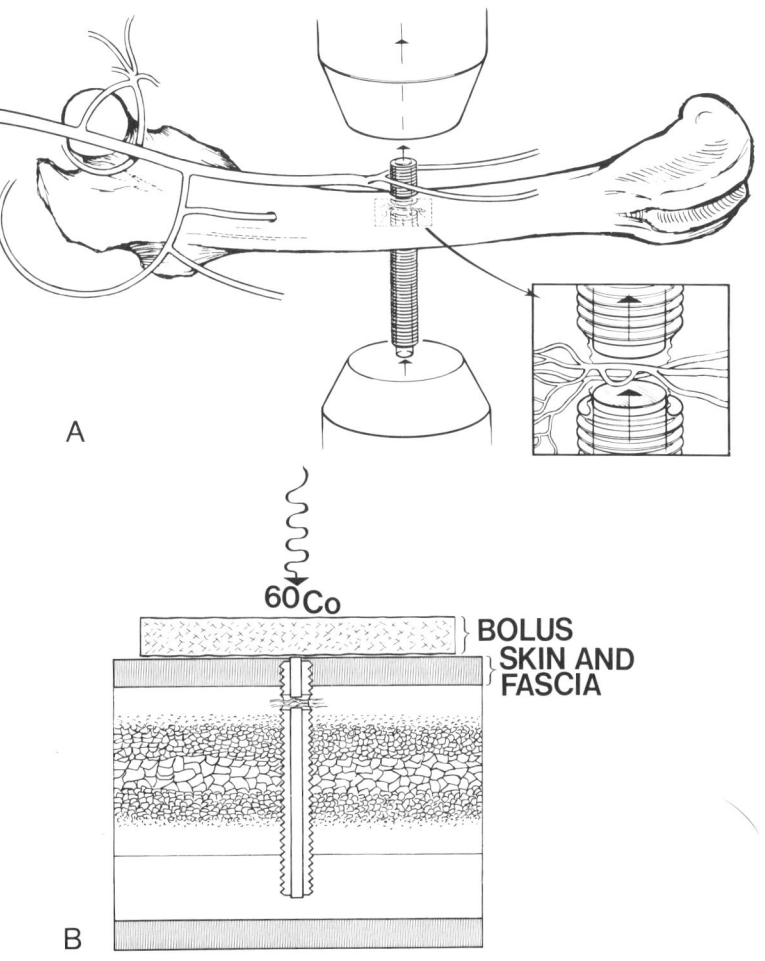

Figure 7–65. *A,* The optical chamber is a hollow titanium implant into which two glass rods are glued in such a manner as to leave a space of 100 microns in between. If the chamber is inserted in the bone with a very gentle surgical technique, bone and vessels will grow through this space between the rods. It is then possible, in the living animal, to transilluminate the ingrown bone tissue and register the tissue on cine film or slides at periodic follow-up. *B,* The chamber may be used, for example, in studies of irradiation effects on bone tissue. In such a case the bone is primarily inspected and photographed before irradiation. Thereafter, vital microscopic registrations are performed weekly, thus recording the dynamics of the establishment of an irradiation injury.

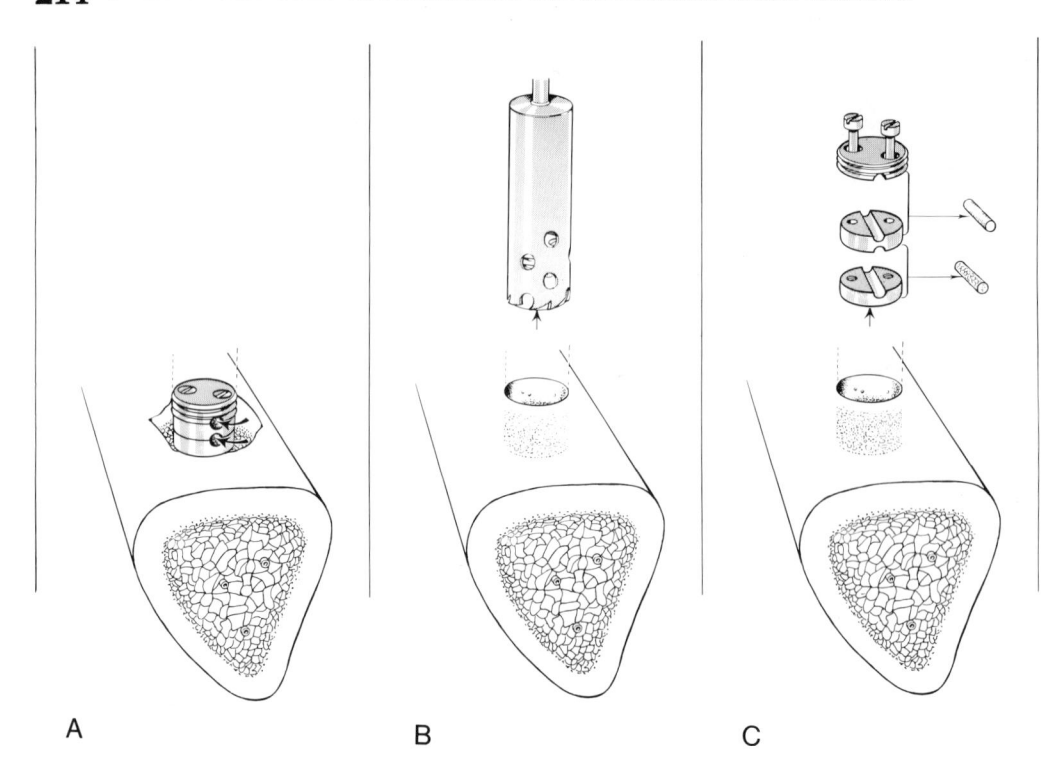

Figure 7–66. The Bone Growth Chamber is a dividable titanium implant that is inserted in each tibia of the animal with a strictly controlled surgical technique (A). The bone that invades the canals of the implants may be obtained after animal sacrifice (B, C). The amount of bone is assessed by microradiography followed by a computer analysis. In such a way it is possible to compare the bone formation rate under controlled circumstances, after irradiation or heat trauma, for example.

the donor bone to provide improved stability at host sites at a later time, and that actual grafting can be performed with a minimally traumatizing surgical technique.[98–100]

While everyone would agree that an infected bone bed is unsuitable as the anchor site for a bone implant, controversy prevails concerning whether an implant should be inserted in an irradiated bed. Jacobsson et al.,[101] have used such methods as the optical bone chamber (Fig. 7–65) and the Bone Growth Chamber (Fig. 7–66), developed at the Laboratory of Experimental Biology,[72, 102] to analyze the healing capacity of irradiated bone. A single irradiation dose of 1500 to 2500 rads to the rabbit tibia resulted in bone necrosis. If an implant was inserted in a bed that had received only 500 rads, a significantly reduced osteogenesis prevented osseointegration. However, preliminary data indicate that one year after irradiation the bone regains its capacity for healing and a seemingly normal osseointegration may occur in spite of previous irradiation. This also seems to be true with doses higher than 500 rads.[103]

The Surgical Trauma at Implant Insertion

One important factor that governs the outcome of an implantation procedure is the control of surgical trauma.[84] When the implant site is prepared and the implant inserted, a necrotic border zone is inevitably established around the foreign device owing to the frictional energy generated by drilling or sawing. This border zone must heal with new bone instead of with fibrous tissue if osseointegration is to occur. It was not known until recently at what critical temperature bone tissue necrosis occurs. Eriksson and Albrektsson[104] used the heat chamber, a modification of the original optical chamber (Fig. 7–67), and were able to demonstrate that lamellarized rabbit tibial bone showed signs of necrosis at a temperature of 47° C applied over one minute. Furthermore, if a modified Bone Growth Chamber was inserted in a bone bed that was simultaneously heated to 47° C for one minute, there was a significant reduction in the amount of ingrowing bone.[105] Not only is the early bone healing disturbed by a traumatizing surgical technique,[105] but also later bone repair is unlikely.[106] Lindström et al.[100] summarized several parameters to be controlled in a surgical procedure with a minimally traumatizing technique. Important precautions involve the use of well-sharpened drills, careful cooling during drilling, and the avoidance of excessive drill speeds. With the use of the drill machine developed by Brånemark and Stefech,[107] which can be run with adequate torque at low rotatory speeds of 10 to 15 rpm (drill diameter: 3.5 mm), drilling temperatures do not exceed 40° C, provided that adequate cooling and an intermittent drilling technique are used.[108] This temperature elevation is in contrast to what has been clinically demonstrated during the insertion

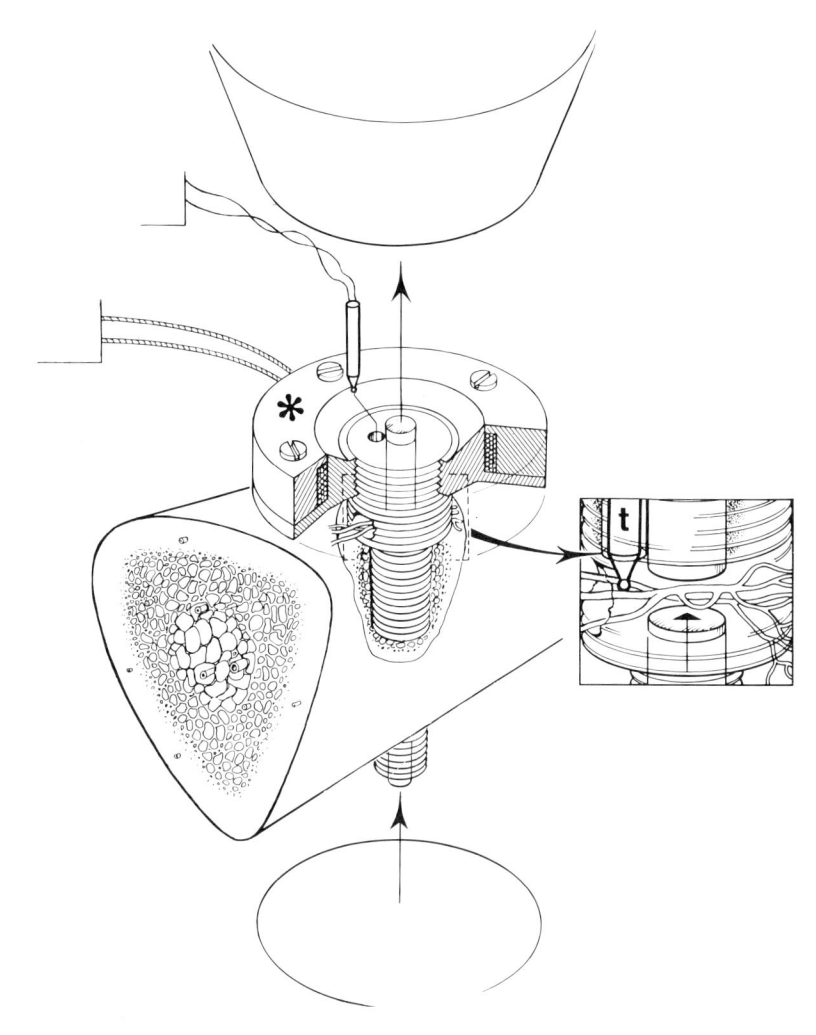

Figure 7–67. The heat chamber is a modified optical chamber in which a thermocouple (t) can be inserted in contact with the ingrown bone. An electrically regulated heating device (*) is attached on top of the chamber. In this way it is possible simultaneously to heat up the tissue to the desired temperature for the desired length of time and to study the effects acutely and over a long follow-up period.

of a Richards plate in the human femur, when temperatures around 89° C were registered.[109]

Loading the Implant

In the canine experimental series[73] and during the first years of clinical trial with osseointegrated implants,[84] loading was sometimes allowed as early as two to three weeks after implant insertion. Osseointegration occurred in many of such early-loaded cases. However, with longer (>three months) times of unloaded healing,[84] Albrektsson[110] found that the optical bone chamber demonstrated a much improved bone regeneration in the rabbit tibia. Over a follow-up period of one year, it was found that if the early osseointegration of the implant was disturbed, there were no signs of a subsequent bone incorporation of the titanium chamber even if the loading conditions were later controlled.[110] From these investigations, it can be concluded that early loading of the implant should be avoided to ensure optimal implant integration.

In the clinical situation, once the first months of bone healing have occurred uneventfully, the entire masticatory load can be carried by the osseointegrated implants. This is why osseointegrated implants are always inserted in the bone in a first surgical session. They are then connected to the dental bridge in a second surgical procedure at least three months after the first one. Haraldson[82] compared the masticatory loads of patients with osseointegrated dental implants with those of patients having the same extension of dentition but with teeth of their own. There were no significant differences between the groups in chewing efficiency or maximal bite load. In the osseointegrated group, the maximal bite force level measured was 412 N. In fact, since the great majority of clinically inserted osseointegrated dental implants have been installed into completely edentulous jaws,[71, 84, 86] we know that the implants are load-bearing. Most controlled clinical programs of dental implants are single replacements of individual teeth, in which cases the actual loading of the implant is uncertain. In the case of a single implant, the major masticatory load may well be carried by the adjacent functioning teeth.

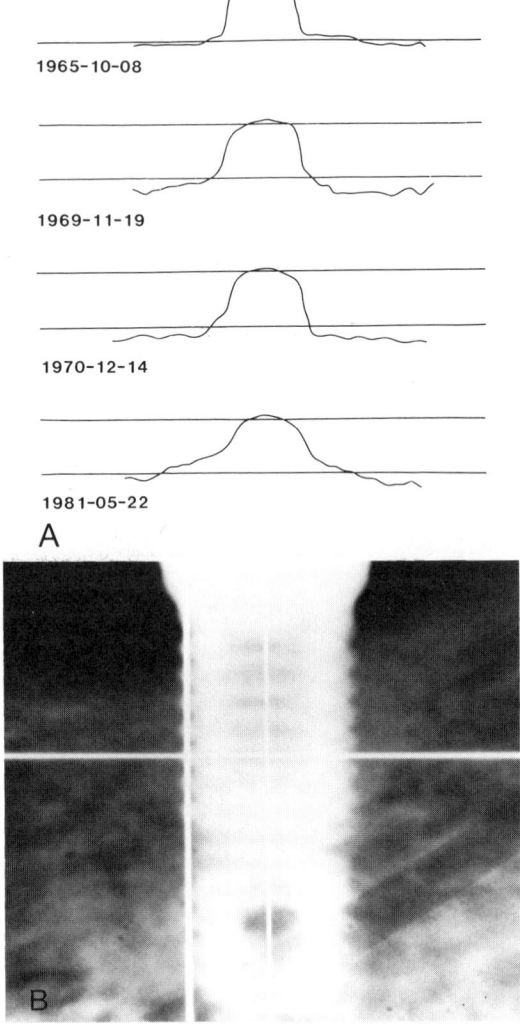

Figure 7–68. Repeated density analyses *(A)* obtained from radiographs *(B)* of the bone tissue around the same mandibular implant from the time within one year after insertion to 15 years afterward. Note the gradual increase in density adjacent to the implant, evidence of bone corticalization because of load adaptation.

With increasing time of osseointegration, there is bone condensation around the implant noticed in radiograms. Figure 7–68 shows a density analysis, performed with an IBAS I + II computer, of a typical osseointegrated dental implant that had been functioning for ten years in the lower jaw of a patient. We regard this bone condensation as a clear indication of a structural adaptation of the bone to the load-bearing implant.

Summary of Experimental Data

The experimental analyses have demonstrated that pure titanium is the most suitable material for dental implants. The use of a threaded design with microgrooves on the implant surface is beneficial for implant incorporation. Implants may be inserted with an extremely gentle surgical technique in irradiated beds if a defined time lapse has occurred since the irradiation.

Osseointegrated implants can be inserted in the mandible without bone grafting, even in the most severe cases of bone resorption. Utmost care to avoid excessive surgical trauma is imperative for proper osseointegration. Before direct loading, the implants should be primarily incorporated; the process will require at least three months.

Osseointegrated implants are capable of carrying the entire masticatory load over long periods of implant function and have been demonstrated to function over followup periods of up to 18 years. The experimental data point to some clinical conditions for proper long-term implant function. The superstructure that is mechanically connected to the implant must fit perfectly to avoid stress concentrations and material/bone fatigue. It is equally important to control occlusal forces by a careful adaptation of the dental bridge.

Methodologic Aspects of Osseointegrated Dental Implants

The Implant

The implant is a screw of pure (99.75 per cent) titanium (Fig. 7–69) with an outer di-

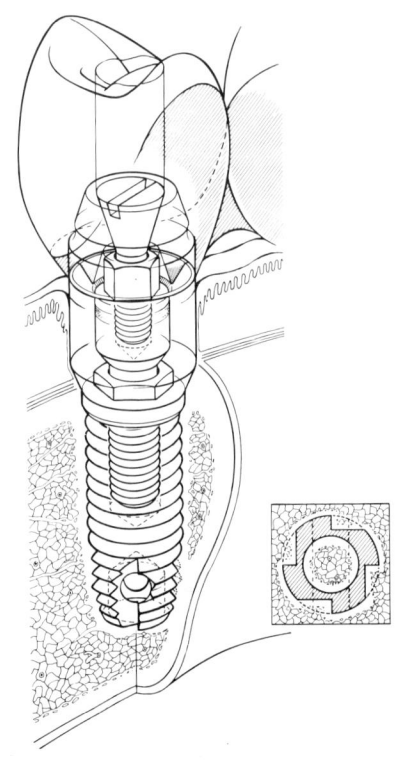

Figure 7–69. The titanium implant is a screw with a diameter of 3.75 mm. It has a controlled surface on the microscale.

ameter of 3.75 mm and a length of either 7, 10, 13, or 15 mm. At manufacturing, a precise engineering method is used that ensures a standardized surface. The outer edges of the threads are rounded according to Skalak.[93] The implant is supplied with a cover screw and has an inner threading and hexagonal top that fits the abutment, i.e., the piece that after the primary bone healing period is used to penetrate the mucous membrane.

Handling of the Implant

Once the implant is manufactured, utmost care is taken to avoid any accidental alterations of the surface.[97] The titanium implants are handled only with instruments of pure titanium to avoid metallic contamination. They are ultrasonically cleaned in defined solutions and autoclaved. These various procedures result in a structurally well-defined titanium implant that, at the time of surgery, is covered with an 8-nm oxide layer.

Implant Insertion (Fig. 7–70)

All surgery is performed under aseptic conditions and usually under local anesthesia. First, the buccal mucoperiosteum is incised in a horizontal line at about half the height of the residual alveolar process. Thereafter, a lingually or palatally pedicled mucoperiosteal flap is raised by sharp dissection close to the bone surface (Fig. 7–71). The dissection is continued until, in the mandible, the neurovascular bundles from the mental foramen are reached or, in the maxilla, the osseous covering of the anterior parts of the sinus is defined. Generally, six implant sites are prepared in the mandible and four to six in the maxilla.

In order to keep a relative parallelism between the implant sites, preparation is generally started close to the midline. The first implant site is carefully oriented with regard to the residual bone volume, the opposite jaw, and the planned direction of the bridge teeth. A direction indicator is installed in the first site and the remaining implant sites are prepared accordingly. Specially designed spiral drills of successively increasing dimensions, to reduce the surgical trauma, are used at a speed of about 1500 rpm. Final adjustments to the entrances of the sites are made by a countersink procedure that gives them a proper topography with regard to the implant, implant holders, cover screws, and abutments. The most crucial part of the preparation is the threading of the implant

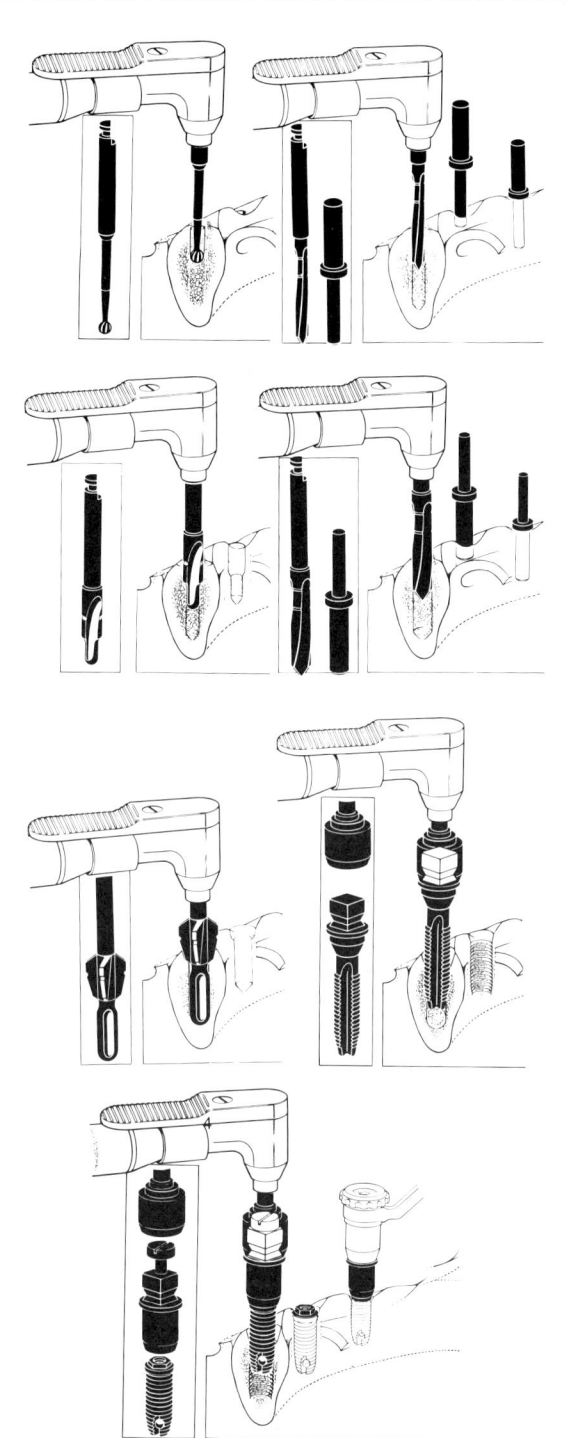

Figure 7–70. A strictly controlled insertion technique is used with osseointegrated dental implants. In this example of insertion of a mandibular implant, the technique of using gradually larger drills to minimize the surgical trauma is demonstrated. The tap is run at a speed of 10 to 15 rpm. The implants are gently inserted and allowed to heal *in situ*, without loading, for about three months.

sites and the installation of the implant. Both procedures are performed at a speed of 10 to 15 rpm. The implants are partly self-tapping and have a vertical and horizontal canal for

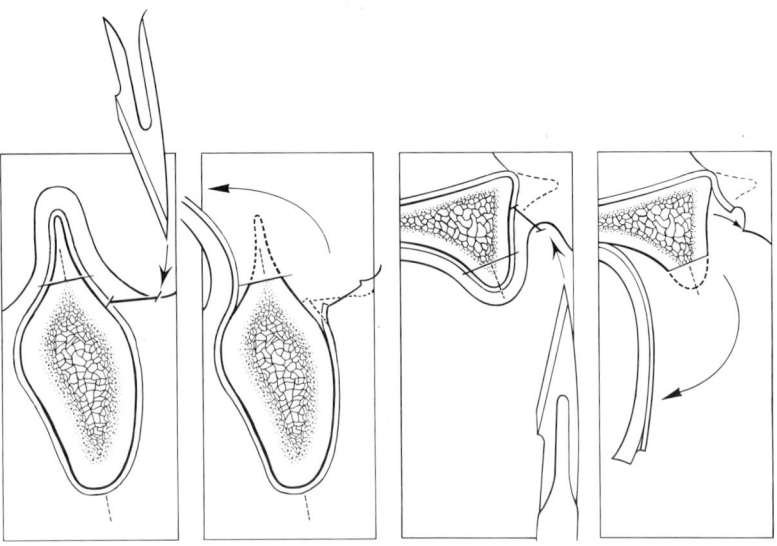

Figure 7–71. Mucoperiosteal flap procedure in the mandible and maxilla. Sharp dissection is performed through the muscle fibers under tight stretching of the lip. The muscle fibers are successfully loosened. The periosteum is cut between the canine regions. With the help of a dissector, a very careful subperiosteal dissection is performed as close to the bone surface as possible. The top of the crest is laid bare with a dissector, and any fibrous adhesions are removed. The very thin periosteal layer on the lingual side of the jaw must not be perforated.

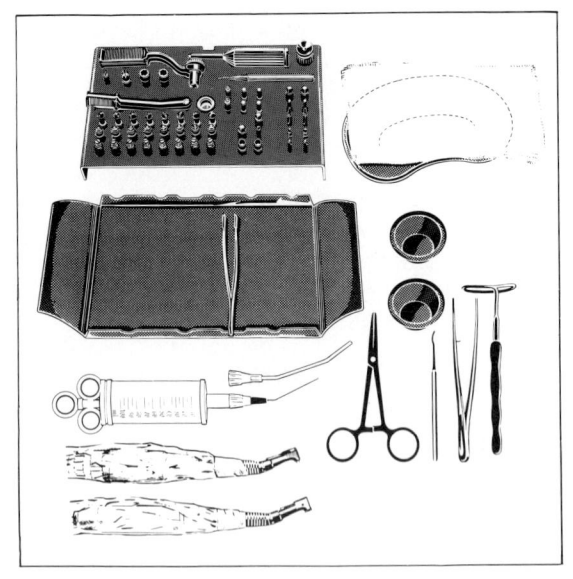

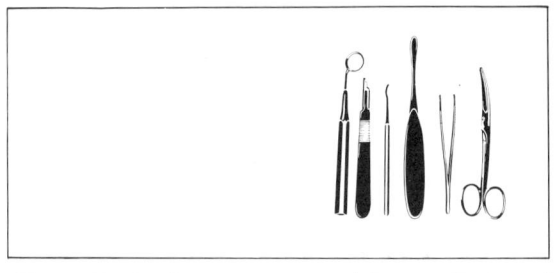

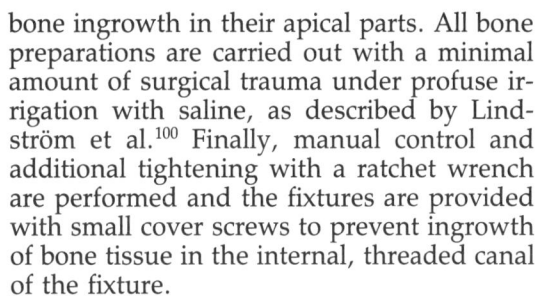

Figure 7–72. Instruments used for installation of osseointegrated dental implants.

bone ingrowth in their apical parts. All bone preparations are carried out with a minimal amount of surgical trauma under profuse irrigation with saline, as described by Lindström et al.[100] Finally, manual control and additional tightening with a ratchet wrench are performed and the fixtures are provided with small cover screws to prevent ingrowth of bone tissue in the internal, threaded canal of the fixture.

The operation is finished with careful readaptation of the flap by means of interrupted polyamid 4-0 mattress sutures, attempting full periosteal covering of the entire anchorage region. Postoperatively, the patients are asked to bite on gauze rolls for a few hours in order to prevent or reduce hematoma and edema formation. The instruments used for installation of an osseointegrated implant are shown in Figure 7–72.

Healing-in of Implants

The implants are left to become incorporated in the bone for at least three months. In some cases of severely resorbed maxillary bone, an incorporation time of more than six months without direct implant loading is required. After the first postoperative week, when only liquid and semisolid food is recommended, patients may wear ordinary dentures. Penicillin V is given prophylactically during the first five postoperative days.

Abutment Operation

An incision is made at the top of the crest over each implant, and the covering gingiva is removed with a punch. Then the cover screws are removed and the abutments are attached to the implant. The height of the abutment is chosen to fit the thickness of the mucoperiosteum, extending about 1 mm. The abutment is preferably penetrating an attached part of the mucosa. The gingiva is sutured around the abutment.

Prosthetic Treatment

The prosthetic treatment starts two weeks after the abutment operation. Impressions, either in hydrocolloid or in a plaster material, are taken with the aid of special copings. Stone casts are made (Fig. 7–73). A conventional recording of jaw relations is made. An occlusion rim is made of wax with an acrylic base plate with notches and holes for guides or fastening screws. It is thus possible to screw the template onto the abutments. The color and shape of the future

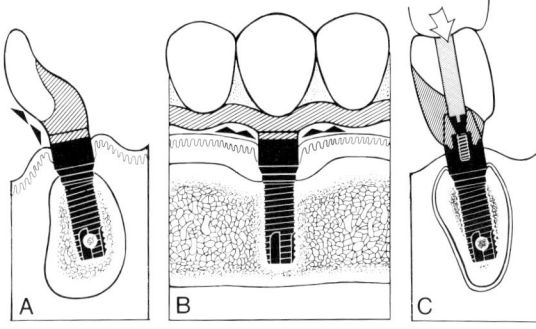

IMPLANTS USED IN PREPROSTHETIC RECONSTRUCTIVE SURGERY / **219**

Figure 7-74. The bridge should be studied carefully so that there are no buccal or palatinal overhangs, as these inevitably produce retention places for plaque *(A)*. All surfaces against the abutment connection must be convex *(B)*. The screw holes can be temporarily covered by pushing white gutta percha into them *(C)*.

bridge are determined in cooperation with the patient according to the usual methods and rules. A bar is made of gold alloy and the set of teeth is made of acrylic resin. It is important that the bridge lie passively against all abutments and that plastic work be checked for porosity and discoloration. Selective grinding is performed to achieve balanced occlusion and articulation. The bridge is made so that there are no buccal or palatinal overhangs, as these inevitably produce retention places for plaque and are inaccessible to hygienic measures (Fig. 7-74). The patient is informed not to bite too hard on the bridge at the beginning. A list of aids to oral hygiene is given to the patient. At re-examination one week later, the occlusion and articulation of the bridge are again checked and adjusted if necessary. Further postoperative check-ups are performed one, three, and seven months later and thereafter at least once annually.

Overview of the Clinical Studies

Number of Treated Patients

The first osseointegrated dental implant was inserted in man in 1965, and a total of 6100 implants had been inserted in 991 jaws through June 30, 1982. Until 1978, no implants were used outside the University of Gothenburg, Sweden. Since 1978, several other universities have joined the clinical program. By the end of 1983, 58 university teams, from all five populated continents, had been trained in the method of osseointegration. In the United States there are currently twelve universities with clinically established osseointegration programs and several others are to start in the near future.

All treated patients have been included in careful follow-up. As there have been no pa-

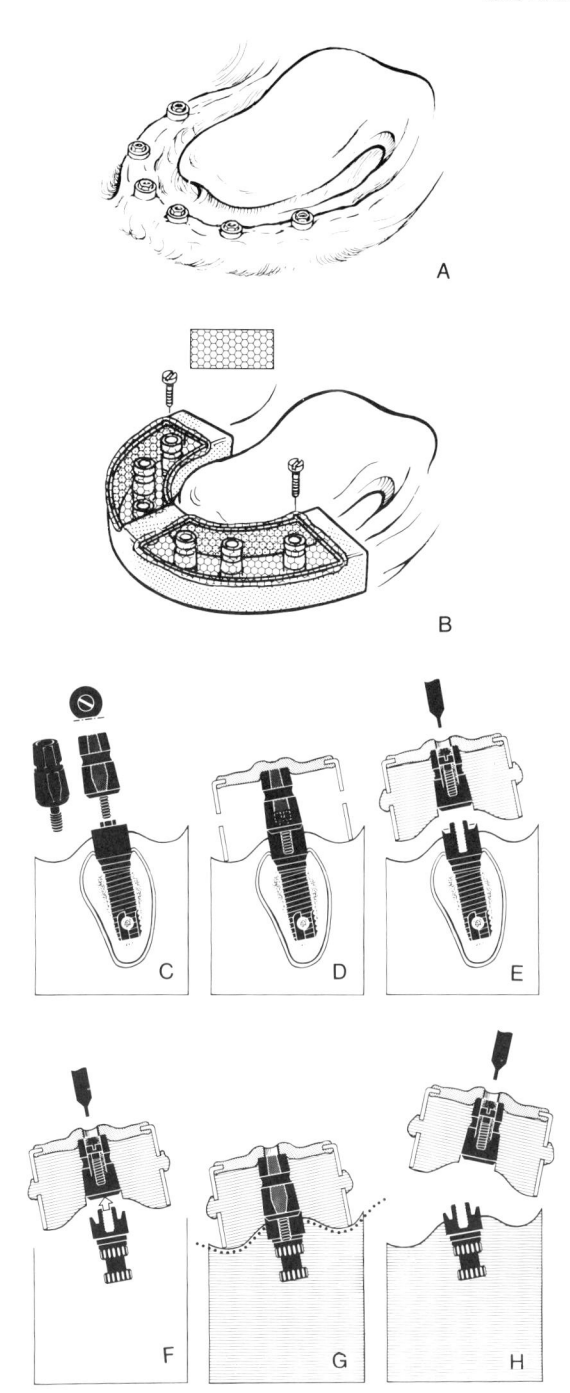

Figure 7-73. At the beginning of prosthetic treatment, special impression copings are tried on the replicas. They are then mounted on the abutments to check that the components fit tightly *(A,B)*. The screw holes are sealed with blue wax and the perforated impression tray without a cover is tested and any necessary adjustments made *(C)*. Tenax wax is applied as a cover. When the impression tray is finally tried in the mouth, impressions are made in the wax cover by the impression copings *(D)*. After setting, the wax is scraped off the screw holes of the impression copings and the impression is unscrewed. The replicas are mounted on the impression copings set in plaster, and the plaster impression is coated with separation varnish, after which the impression is filled with plaster as soon as possible *(E-H)*.

tient drop-outs in the entire program of the Gothenburg clinic, we have a unique opportunity to assess the success rates and to identify possible mechanical and histologic complications of a comparatively large, consecutive clinical program of dental implants that have been followed up for as long as 18 years. Preliminary results from other teams indicate even better success rates than have been observed in Gothenburg.[111]

Adell et al.,[71] in a review of the patients treated in Gothenburg through September 30, 1980, found the mean age of the patients at the time of surgery to be 53 years (sd = 11), with a range of 20 to 77 years. Females comprised 62 per cent of patients. Eighty-one per cent had osseointegrated bridges in both jaws, while the remaining patients had either natural teeth or dentures in one jaw. The majority of the patients (93 per cent) were totally edentulous in the treated jaw.

Selection of Patients

As described by Adell et al.,[71] the following *indications* have been observed for treatment with osseointegrated dental implants: (1) insufficient retention of a denture, generally due to extreme resorption of the alveolar process; (2) mental inability to accept a denture in cases with technically adequate or inadequate denture retention; (3) functional disturbances, e.g., severe nausea and vomiting reflexes caused by a denture.

Relative *contraindications* to treatment have been (1) presence of the edentulous state for less than one year (necessary for a proper judgment of the indications listed above); (2) psychotic disorders; (3) severe bone resorption of the maxilla (about 10 per cent of all maxillary cases) necessitating a bone grafting procedure; (4) jaw bone irradiation (e.g., in tumor cases) less than one year before treatment.

Except in the 10 per cent of maxillary cases in which bone grafting was necessary, the extent of alveolar ridge atrophy was not a problem or contraindication.

Control of the Patients

All patients were carefully examined at least twice prior to surgery and then at one-week and at three-month intervals during the first year after surgery. Thereafter, annual check-ups have been performed. At these visits, occlusion, implant and bridge stability, stress distribution, and the state of the marginal periabutment tissues were examined. Roentgenographic studies were performed at each check-up after the first three postoperative months, when roentgenography was avoided because of the potential risk of disturbing the early phases of osseointegration. The marginal bone height level could be accurately established by comparison with the implant threads.

In a series of 17 consecutive cases with 101 implants, a careful scoring of plaque and gingival indices, defined as a percentage of affected periabutment quadrants, was registered. In the same patient samples, the clinical pocket depth and proximal marginal bone height were assessed.[71]

Summary of Methodologic Aspects and Clinical Material

In this clinical study we have used only pure titanium implants of a defined surface finish and geometry. They have been inserted in the jaw bone of edentulous patients by means of a delicate surgical technique. Direct, immediate loading of the implants has been avoided. The manufacturing of the implants and the handling of them afterwards, prior to insertion, have been meticulously controlled to avoid possible contamination or alteration of the surface conditions. The Gothenburg study comprises 3510 implants inserted into 585 jaws. There have been no patient drop-outs over the entire follow-up period of 18 years. The long-term patients have been examined at least once a year. The following material describes clinical results from 100 consecutively inserted upper jaw and 100 lower jaw implants followed for ten years and another 100 upper jaw and 100 lower jaw implants followed for five years. In early publications,[71, 84] the entire clinical program was evaluated.

Results of Treatment with Osseointegrated Dental Implants

Percentage of Persisting Maxillary Implants After Ten and Five Years of Function

The outcome of 100 consecutively inserted upper jaw implants, inserted during 1971 and 1972, showed a ten-year success rate of 84 per cent. Most of the implant losses occurred during the first year after implantation and depended on primary failure to achieve osseointegration. Discounting the losses during the first year after implantation, the ten-year success figures for the upper jaw were 97 per cent. From the study by Adell et al.,[71] we know that continuous long-term bridge stability was achieved in about 90 per cent of maxillary cases.

The outcome of 100 consecutively inserted upper jaw implants installed during 1976 and 1977, and thus followed for five years, showed a clinical success of 91 per cent. Again, nearly all losses occurred during the first year after implantation, after which a 98 per cent five-year success rate is found. Therefore, the better results in the five-year group compared to the ten-year group reflect an improvement of the implantation. It is likely that the ten-year results of bridge stability will reach more than a 90 per cent success level. In other words, the edentulous maxilla can be restored to long-term clinical function with osseointegrated implants without the need for additional implants in 90 per cent of the cases. The long-term results of Adell et al.[71] indicate that continuous bridge stability in the future may be expected in more than 96 per cent of all maxillary cases.

Based on the above figures, it seems reasonable to conclude that a most reliable prognosis can be given for the outcome of an osseointegrated maxillary dental implant after the first year. In the 10 per cent of the maxillary cases in which a bone graft has been used, or in the instances in which an implant penetrates the bone wall of the sinus or nasal cavity, there was a slightly less favorable five-year prognosis reported by Brånemark et al.,[86] who found success rates around 80 per cent in sinus-penetrating implants. Maxillary implants in general show less favorable results than do mandibular ones: in the upper jaw there is often less and weaker bone to anchor the osseointegrated implant than is the case in the lower jaw.

Percentage of Persisting Mandibular Implants After Ten and Five Years

The outcome of 100 consecutively inserted lower jaw implants installed during 1971 and 1972 showed a ten-year success of 91 per cent. All implant losses occurred during the first year after implantation. After discounting these primary losses, the ten-year success rate of mandibular osseointegrated implants was 100 per cent. A continuous bridge stability was achieved in 100 per cent of treated mandibles, as demonstrated by Adell et al.[71]

The outcome of 100 consecutively inserted lower jaw implants installed during 1976 and 1977 and thus followed for five years showed a clinical success rate of more than 96 per cent. All losses occurred during the first year after implantation. This high level of success with mandibular osseointegrated implants indicates that a reliable long-term prognosis for the outcome may be given in almost every individual case, regardless of the degree of alveolar ridge resorption. However, this favorable outcome is achieved only with the use of strictly controlled surgery, prosthodontics, and the precautions mentioned in the methodologic sections of this chapter.

Indications of Implant Failure

There are different reasons for failure to achieve osseointegration: (1) poor control of the surgical trauma, leading to impairment of bone healing; (2) perforation through the covering mucoperiosteum during bone healing; (3) repeated overloading with microfractures in the surrounding bone; (4) persisting gingivitis that leads to progressive marginal bone loss.

After a defined healing period had occurred, implants that failed to achieve osseointegration were removed and, in many cases, replaced with new ones. Adell et al.[71] presented a diagrammatic representation of the percentage of failures and replacements with osseointegrated implants. Implants that are not stable at a manual test at the first evaluation, three to six months after insertion, will not become osseointegrated and should be removed. If a loose implant is not diagnosed by the surgeon, it will soon be indicated by the radiographic demonstration of a radiolucent zone around it. It must be stressed that the loss of a single fixture does not necessarily imply loss of the dental bridge. In several cases it may successfully be carried by four or five instead of six fixtures. The necessity for replacement depends on the location of the lost implant.

The most severe complication is the loss of all fixtures in a treated jaw. This has occurred in about 1 per cent of all operated maxillary cases. In such cases, reoperation with new fixtures has been possible after tissue healing, and there have been no cases of destructive osteitis reported.

Fracture of the implant occurred in 3.5 per cent of inserted implants in the study by Adell et al.[71] Most of these fractures occurred in maxillary implants within five years after surgery. It should be noted that the largest number of implant fractures was encountered in those patients in whom the prosthetic construction was based exclusively upon fixed prosthodontic technology. This resulted in rather heavy gold frameworks that were difficult to cast accurately. Consequently, adverse stresses were imposed upon the supporting implants, leading to their fracture. This prosthetic design, with the subsequent loading problem, has been remedied by introducing different laboratory technologies, e.g., combined complete and removable partial dentures. Since this change was implemented, implant fractures have decreased to less than 1 per cent.

Marginal Bone Height Measurements

After the first year has passed and the osseointegration of the implant has been established, the annual bone loss has been less than 0.1 mm on the average. This very minute amount of bone resorption is valid for follow-up periods of ten years or more. There have been no significant differences between mandibular and maxillary implants in this respect. It is possible to achieve a very good reliability in the evaluation of the marginal bone height in the radiograms. The implant threads can be used as a reference.

Status of the Soft Tissues

Evaluation of gingivitis and plaque indices have given values of 7.6 per cent and 13.7 per cent, respectively. This result was regarded as satisfactory by Adell et al.,[71] as there had been a six-month interval since the oral hygiene instructions were given to the tested group. Plaque at the abutment-gingival junction was found to cause gingivitis in 6.7 per cent of the periabutment quadrants. Albrektsson et al.,[108] in an ultrastructural investigation of the interface between soft tissue and abutment, demonstrated normal epithelial cells glued to the titanium oxide surface by a thin layer of proteoglycans. Hansson et al.[112] observed hemidesmosome-like formations between epithelial cells and the titanium implant. These findings probably explain the relative absence of pathogenic bacteria and the absence of chronic inflammatory cells around osseointegrated dental implants.[113] Mean pocket depth around osseointegrated dental implants was found to be 2.6 mm, a value that Adell et al.[71] regarded as indicating a healthy situation.

Results of Psychiatric Evaluation

Blomberg and Lindqvist[114] performed a study of 26 randomly chosen patients with osseointegrated implants. They were matched against 26 control patients with regard to sex, age (±5 years), and the degree of resorption of the alveolar crest in the lower jaw. All patients were completely edentulous and most of them had been using dentures for more than ten years. The psychiatric evaluation included a semistructural clinical examination of about 30 minutes duration, Eysenck's Personality Inventory (EPI), and a questionnaire regarding dentures vs. a jawbone-anchored bridge. The control group had, prior to the study, been supplied with complete new dentures. The experimental group was treated with osseointegrated implants. They were tested at examinations three months and two years after treatment.

Retention problems improved significantly in the osseointegrated group. The patients regarded the jawbone-anchored bridge as part of their body, in contrast to the denture, which was regarded as a foreign body. The postoperative improvement in the experimental group was still seen two years after surgery. The differences between test and control group were significant at the $p < 0.01$ level. It was concluded that treatment with an osseointegrated dental bridge means an odontologic and psychosocial restitution *ad integrum*.

Comments on Results

Individual implants of the long-term follow-up study showed a ten-year success level of 84 per cent in the maxilla and 91 per cent in the mandible. Corresponding five-year success rate figures were 91 per cent and 96 per cent, respectively. The implant losses occurred almost exclusively during the first two years after implant installation. After ten years, the results will probably be comparable to the five-year success rate. Marginal bone height evaluations, implant-surrounding soft tissue examinations, and the conclusions of a controlled psychiatric investigation have all demonstrated the benefits of osseointegrated dental implants. Indications for treatment have been limited to patients who have severe problems in wearing ordinary dentures. Good long-term results in treated patients lead us to assume that indications for implants will be widened in the future. Edentulousness can be treated with osseointegrated implants in a controlled manner, from both functional and cosmetic points of view, in almost all observed cases. This is verified by a continuous bridge stability in the upper jaw of 90 per cent and in the lower jaw of 100 per cent.

Dental Implants, General Aspects

Anchorage in fibrous tissue of a bone implant is an indication of failure.[84] However, it does not mean that less biocompatible implant materials will always become surrounded by a poorly differentiated soft tissue layer, nor does it imply that a biocompatible material such as titanium will become anchored in Haversian bone. Control of the surgical trauma, the tissue bed, and the loading conditions are equally important in achieving solid bone anchorage of dental implants, with predictable long-term results. The multidimensional problem of ensuring a firm bone integration of an extracorporal substitute can be successfully met[84, 89] with a meticulous clinical approach and control of these several parameters.

A fibrous tissue–anchored implant, evidenced by mobility or by radiography, should be removed to avoid further damage to the bone. Even if a soft tissue–anchored implant remains *in situ* and is part of the "ceramic smile" for some time, it has an inferior capacity to carry load and would best be replaced with a new, properly integrated implant. Until the osseointegrated implant is no longer considered experimental, it is essential to establish a reliable, preferably computer-based, evaluation program. The clinician is responsible for a standardized technique of implant insertion and can estimate the clinical success of the insertion. The procedure of evaluation must be strictly standardized. The human organism is indeed multifactorial, and solitary favorable long-term results may be achieved with most currently used dental implants. Therefore, to provide a scientific basis for evaluating the outcome of dental implants, it is imperative that single inserted implants be registered and followed up and that the patient be examined regularly on a yearly basis. It is important to note that patient drop-outs must be regarded as failures.

In order to evaluate a dental implant system, the results of the five- and ten-year studies must be considered using the criteria of the Harvard consensus (see below), which represents a complete patient study of adequate size. Suggestions on criteria and evaluation for a successful dental implant system were presented at the Harvard Consensus Meeting. The objective criteria for implant success are bone loss that is not greater than a third of the vertical height and mobility of less than 1 mm in any direction. We would remove an implant long before these two criteria have been reached, as they represent to us clear signs of failure and the risk of progressing local tissue damage and loss. There is a great need for a reliable basis to evaluate the outcome of various dental implants. The Harvard Consensus, although liberal in its criteria, was important in its standardization of subjective and objective criteria for evaluating the success of implants.

Other Clinical Applications of Osseointegrated Implants

The principles of osseointegration are also applicable in other clinical situations. Principally, titanium implants similar to those described here have been inserted in the retroauricular region of man in certain cases of auditory dysfunction in which the need for a bone conduction hearing aid exists. In such cases, the titanium screws were anchored in the temporal bone and allowed to permanently penetrate the skin. This provided a direct bone attachment to the hearing aid. The result has been improved hearing.[115, 116] When loss of the pinna, eye, or nose has occurred, especially after trauma or cancer surgery, three or four skin-penetrating titanium implants have been used as anchorage for a facial prosthesis. This has resulted in a much improved cosmetic and psychological outcome.[117, 118] To date, 198 such skin-penetrating bone-anchored implants have been inserted in man. The osseointegration failed in two cases, and one implant was removed by request of the patient. The remaining 195 implants are still *in situ* and function for their purpose. Eighteen of those implants have been followed clinically for more than five years. They represent the first consecutive series of functioning skin-penetrating implants ever published in the literature.

Osseointegrated screws have demonstrated that they function as stable anchorage for metacarpophalangeal joint replacements,[119, 120] although the clinical results have been followed for only three years. Other areas of application include various types of bone grafts[98, 102] and different amputee cases. The most challenging field today for scientific studies of osseointegrated titanium screws is that of joint reconstruction using osseointegrated implants.

Conclusion

The outcome of any implantation procedure is determined by the regenerative capacity of the tissues. The principles behind the osseointegration of a dental implant are based on biologic analyses of healing tissue. We believe it is important to recognize the cellular contribution to implant success rather than to focus only on the possible technical details and refinements. This principle makes it possible to present a valid prognosis for the outcome of treatment with osseointegrated dental implants in the individual edentulous patient. Nevertheless, in any implantation procedure it is imperative to strictly control the manufacturing and later handling of the implant to avoid possible surface contamination of the foreign devices. Such contamination may become the cause of many "unexplainable" late failures. EDITOR'S NOTE: The work of Brånemark et al. has demonstrated a breakthrough in the provision of fixed restorations for edentulous patients. Other osseointegrated systems may prove as efficacious as that of Brånemark et al.; however, the research of Brånemark et al. should not be applied to support other systems, since no other system as yet produced exactly duplicates that of Brånemark in material, design, and method of placement.

THE CORE-VENT™ SYSTEM FOR IMPLANT PROSTHODONTICS*

Gerald A. Niznick

Implant prosthodontics has, from a clinical standpoint, two basic components: the surgical operation and the restorative technique. They can be separated procedurally, but each must still be done with the same degree of skill if consistent success is to be achieved. The Core-Vent Implant System[121-123] encourages the division of responsibilities between these two disciplines while incorporating the features in the osseointegrated implant. This encourages success of a cylindrical, submergible titanium alloy basket (Fig. 7–75).

---

*Core-Vent Corporation, 14724 Ventura Boulevard #502, Sherman Oaks, CA 91403

The Core-Vent Implant System achieves versatility and adaptability by using a two-component implant:

1. An endosseous hollow, vented screw that is available in three diameters (5.5, 4.5, and 3.5 mm), each modifiable to eight lengths, thus allowing for maximum use of available bone.
2. Four different abutment inserts that facilitate a spectrum of prosthetic appliances.

Diagnosis and Treatment Plan

After confirming that there are no medical problems that would contraindicate or compromise routine oral surgery procedures, the edentulous area is evaluated. By means of a panoramic radiograph and intra-oral examination, the initial determination is made as to the prosthetic objectives and proposed implant sites. Where the amount of available bone is marginal, an alternate treatment plan should also be considered. The buccal-lingual width of the proposed implant site cannot be confirmed until the time of surgery.

Surgical Phase

The Core-Vent Implant System is biomechanically designed to absorb and distribute

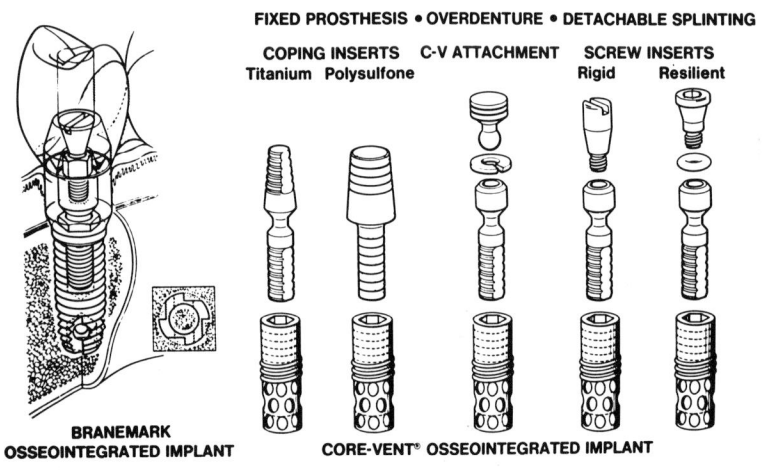

Figure 7–75. Drawing of the Brånemark Implant and the Core-Vent Implant. The Core-Vent Implant is available in three diameters (5.5 mm, 4.5 mm, 3.5 mm) and the system offers a selection of four inserts (left to right: Titanium Coping Insert [TCI], Polysulfone Coping Insert [PCI], Core-Vent Attachment [C-VA], Titanium Screw Insert [TSI]). A fifth insert option is achieved by selecting an alternate titanium screw for nonresilient support of a detachable fixed prosthesis or by shortening the titanium screw and deleting the O-ring for rigid splinting with a cast tissue bar for overdenture support and retention.

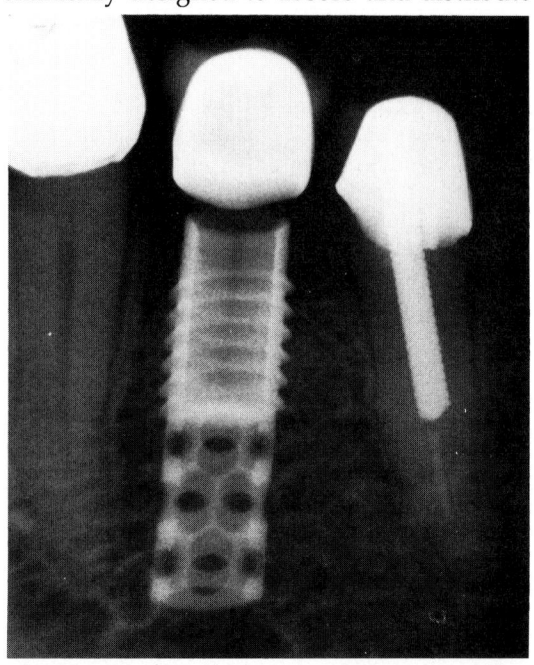

Figure 7–76. Single tooth replacements. Panoramic radiograph of 3.5-mm Core-Vent Implants (left, Mod. 6; right, Mod. 4) with Titanium Coping Inserts bent approximately 45 degrees owing to the fact that implants must be placed toward the palate to avoid devitalizing buccal cortical bone.

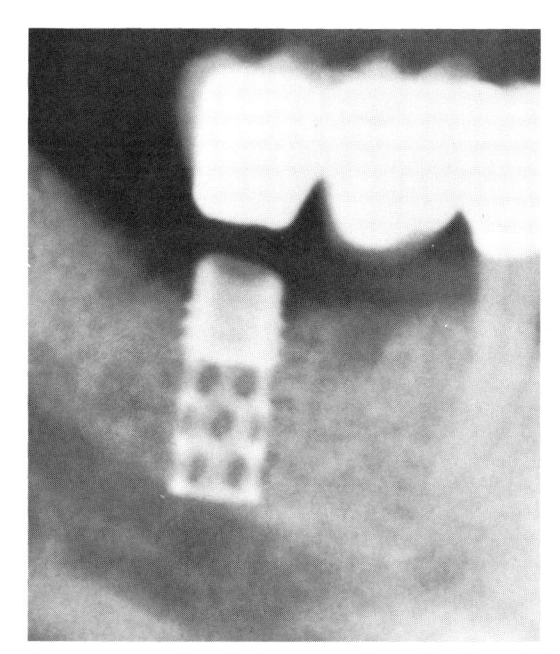

IMPLANTS USED IN PREPROSTHETIC RECONSTRUCTIVE SURGERY / **225**

Figure 7–77. Distal abutment for a fixed partial prosthesis. Periapical radiograph of 5.5-mm Core-Vent Implant (Mod. 4) with a Polysulfone Coping Insert (1 year postoperatively).

masticatory forces. It is capable of functioning as a free-standing device for single-tooth replacement (Fig. 7–76), as an abutment (Fig 7–77), and as a free-standing device for overdenture retention (Fig. 7–78). The endosseous portion of the Core-Vent Implant is a titanium cylinder (titanium alloy—6Al/4Va) modifiable to 8 lengths—16 mm to 7 mm (Fig. 7–79A). It has a self-tapping, threaded neck that uses flat-based threads for better loading while keeping the differ-

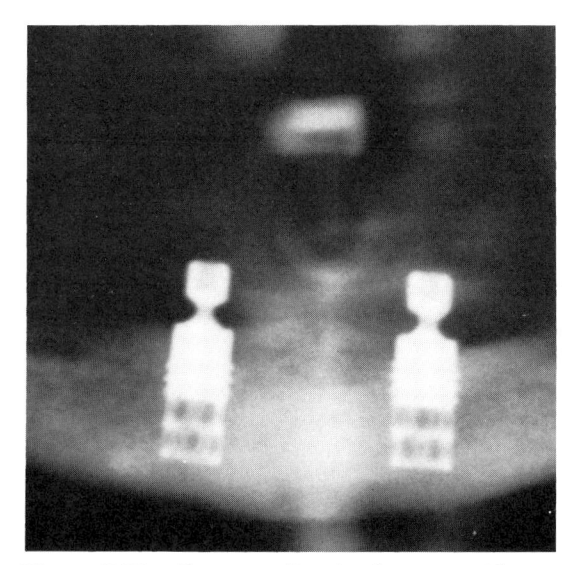

Figure 7–78. Free-standing implants provide retention and lateral stability to a tissue-supported removable prosthesis. Panoramic radiograph of 4.5-mm Core-Vent Implants (Mod 6) with Core-Vent Attachment Inserts.

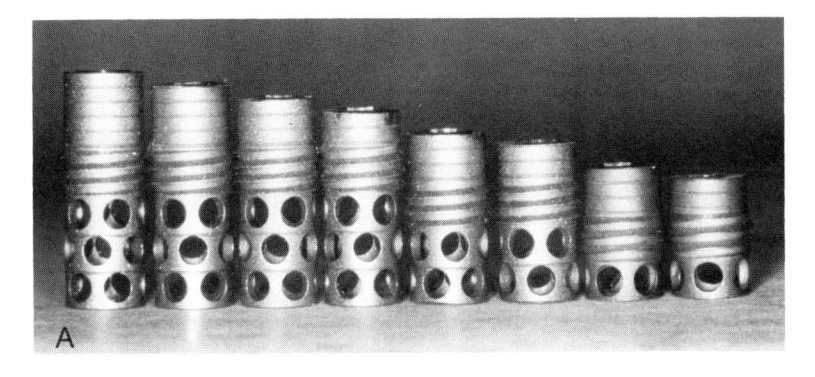

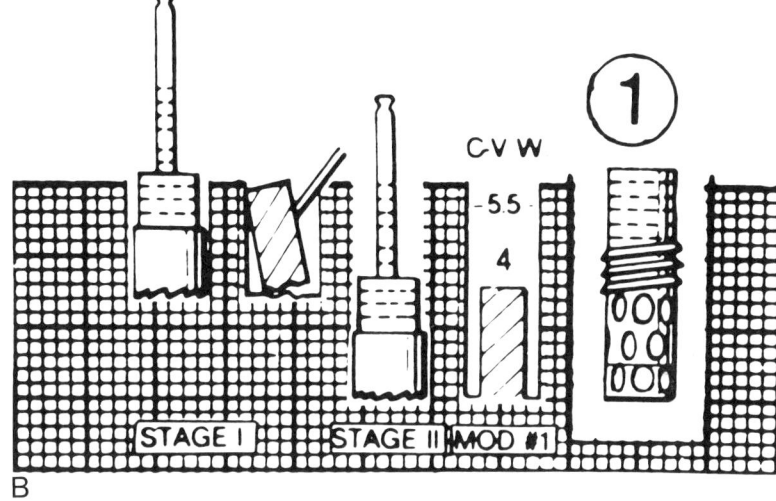

SELECT, PLACE AND MODIFY FOR MAXIMUM USE OF AVAILABLE BONE
— PLACE NECK 1mm ABOVE CREST — PREPARE PER CHART
— ELIMINATE EXPOSED PORTION OF THREADS — EACH 1mm APART

THREE DIAMETERS — C-V N: CORE = 3.5mm D   THREADS = 4.3mm OSD • 6.5mmL
C-V M: CORE = 4.5mm D   THREADS = 5.3mm OSD • 6.5mmL
C-V W: CORE = 5.5mm D   THREADS = 6.3mm OSD • 3.5mmL

EIGHT LENGTHS — MAXIMUM = 16mm (8.5mm NECK/THREADS + 7½mm CORE)

MODIFI-CATION #	AVAILABLE BONE	SHORTEN NECK	REMOVE ROW OF VENTS	PREPARE IMPLANT SITE WITH 7½mm CORE DRILL STAGE I CORE LINES	STAGE II SHANK LINES
1	15 mm+	0	0	TOP LINE	TOP LINE
2	14 mm	−1 mm	0	2nd LINE	2nd LINE
3	13 mm	−2 mm	0	3rd LINE	3rd LINE
4	12 mm	−3 mm	0	DIAM CHANGE	4th LINE
5	10½ mm	−2 mm	−2½ mm	3rd LINE	5th LINE
6	9½ mm	−3 mm	−2½ mm	DIAM CHANGE	6th LINE
7	8 mm	−2 mm	−5 mm	3rd LINE	TOP CL + ½mm
8	7 mm	−3 mm	−5 mm	DIAM CHANGE	2nd CL + ½mm

Figure 7–79. A, The Core-Vent Implant can be modified to eight lengths (16 mm to 7 mm). B, Schematic drawing showing depth of penetration for stage I and II preparation for Modification 1 (full length 15 mm in bone and 1 mm above crest. C, The chart specifying how to achieve the corresponding implant length and receptor site for Modifications 1 to 8.

ence between the outside and inside diameter of the threads only 0.4 mm to avoid compression necrosis of the bone. The lower half consists of a hollow vented core opening downward.

The Core-Vent Implant is made with a hexagonal shaped hole (hex-hole) extending down, but not through, the upper half. This facilitates ratcheting of the implant into a preparation site that is precision machined to match (±0.004 inch) the preselected diameter and length modification. Preparation is accomplished with a minimum of trauma using a fairly slow-speed, 10-1 reduction contra-angle handpiece. The handpiece prepares the bone, allowing internal irrigation through the hollow shaft and permitting precise depth control using gauge lines marked on the drill. The correct length modification is selected by the use of a 25 per cent magnified schematic printed on a transparency (Fig. 7–79B). A corresponding chart specifies how to modify the implant and which guide lines on the trephine instrument should be followed to limit bone penetration. This is important to reach the precise depth for each of the two stages of bone preparation (Fig. 7–79C). Following the chart has many advantages: (1) The results will be in 1 mm of the implant above the crest of the ridge for ease of future location when the implant is to be exposed (three to six months). (2) An area of epithelium attachment will not be disturbed during the uncovering procedure. (3) The part of the implant that passes through the crest of the bone will be rigid, even if flexible inserts are later cemented into the hex-hole. In the full length of the implant (modification 1), 15 mm will be endosseous: 7.5 mm of threaded neck and 7.5 mm of vented core. The implant can be placed even with the crest of the bone in cases of immediate replacement of an extracted tooth. It can also be placed where more than 1 mm of bone loss can be anticipated, by modifying the implant for one modification number but preparing the bone for the preceding modification number. For example, select Modification 3 but prepare the bone according to the lines specified in Modification 2 (Fig. 7–79C).

The trephine instrument, which is self-limiting at 7.5 mm, prepares the receptor site in two stages, as follows.

Preparatory. A guide pin is placed into a starting hole prepared to the exact diameter and length of the cutting surface of a No. 557 carbide bur (high speed), or the diameter of a No. 0.012 twist drill (low speed, penetrates 4 mm). This helps align the direction of the bone preparation, select the appropriate diameter of implant, and start the cut without the peripherally cutting trephine instrument running across the bone.

Stage I. This stage provides a cylindrical chamber for the threaded neck portion of the implant. The bone core is removed and the bottom of the chamber is flattened with an end-cutting rotary instrument (depth gauge drill) with lines corresponding to the trephine drill. A depth gauge is further provided to verify the correct depth and the creation of a flat bottom to the Stage I chamber. (Any bone spicules left after the bone core is fractured off would impede the penetration of the trephine drill during Stage II.) Both the depth gauge and the guide pins are used to aid parallelism between adjacent implants, available bone permitting.

Stage II. This stage leaves a central core of bone that ultimately becomes encompassed by the vented lower half of the implant. The bone core inside the circumference of the implant is separated from the bone that is in intimate contact with the external surface of the implant by only 0.75 mm.

Submerging. A polysulfone rod is placed into the hex-hole protruding 0.5 to 1.0 mm beyond the implant and then covered by the mucoperiosteal flap (submerged). The rod allows the bone to reunite through the vents and vital bone to reorganize at the implant-bone interface in a sterile, isolated environment, removed from any detrimental, external forces. After a suitable healing period of three to six months (depending on the quality and quantity of bone and the stress to be placed on the implant), the hex-hole on the superior aspect of the implant is exposed by creating a 2- to 3-mm opening in the tissue with a diamond rotary instrument. Each polysulfone rod is removed simply by engaging it with a No. 34 or No. 557 carbide bur.

Verification that each implant is firmly anchored to the bone (osseointegrated) is done by using radiography, clinical mobility, and percussion tests. A longer polysulfone surgical rod should be cemented in the hex-hole with a 50 per cent mix of temporary cement and vaseline to maintain the tissue opening. The abutment insert is later permanently attached by cementation into the hex-hole in the superior aspect of the implant using a composite cement (see Fig. 7–90).

Restorative Phase

For *fixed prosthetics*, the Titanium Coping Insert (TCI) provides a tapered abutment head (Fig. 7–80) that can be modified from the base to achieve proper tissue relationship. It should be shortened from the top for occlusal clearance and bent up to 35 degrees for parallelism. Alternatively, a flexible Polysulfone Coping Insert (PCI) can be prepared for parallelism, and used as a distal abutment for a short-span fixed prosthesis in the lower jaw where the natural abutment has a +1 or greater mobility. It can also be used as a middle abutment in a long-span fixed bridge. The PCI is potentially more susceptible to fracture than the rigid TCI and, there-

Figure 7–80. Modify the Titanium Coping Insert (TCI) for fixed prosthetics: shorten the shaft (smaller diameter is for 3.5-mm implant) to achieve the desired gingival relationship with the head of the insert. If the top of the implant becomes exposed, esthetic requirements or the desire for a longer clinical crown may necessitate additional shortening of the shaft so that the narrow neck will end up inside the hex hole. Shorten and/or modify the head for occlusal clearance and bend up to 35 degrees for parallelism. A flexible Polysulfone Coping Insert (PCI) is available that can be prepared for parallelism. Use it only as a distal abutment for a short-span tower fixed bridge under controlled loading conditions.

fore, should not be used unless the direction of the occlusal forces is ideal and the magnitude is well-controlled by proper occlusal design.

For *overdenture* support and/or retention, two titanium inserts are available that can be bent for better head alignment. Core-Vent Attachments (C-VA) (Fig. 7–81) are used in conjunction with two implants in the symphysis for a tissue-supported overdenture. Titanium Screw Inserts (TSI) (see Figs. 7–86 and 7–90) are used with four or more Core-Vent Implants in either the upper or lower edentulous jaw for a totally implant-supported overdenture. This system may be used in both arches to increase functional capabilities. The implant-supported overdenture can be retained by a variety of methods such as Hader nylon and Dolder or round bar metal clips. A choice of modifiable screws is available for use with the TSI depending on whether the tissue bar is to be stress-broken by interposing O-rings between the bar and the head of the insert or rigidly connected to the threaded inserts. Evaluation of the need for a resilient tissue bar depends on opposing occlusion, extent of cantilevering, and the total implant-bone interface area achieved. This is indicated for all cases in which the implants have been shortened to Modification 7 or 8 (two rows of vents have been removed). Remaining natural teeth can be used in combination with Core-Vent Implants for overdenture retention and/or support by cementing the C-VA into endodontically treated roots or by splinting copings or crowns with cast tissue bars to TSI in Core-Vent Implants.

1. The Core-Vent Attachment (C-VA), a snap-socket with a constricted opening in the superior aspect of the titanium insert through which an ultra high molecular weight polyethylene ball can pass, provides 5 lb of retention (see Fig. 7–80). The ball is attached to the tissue side of the acrylic denture base, with the use of

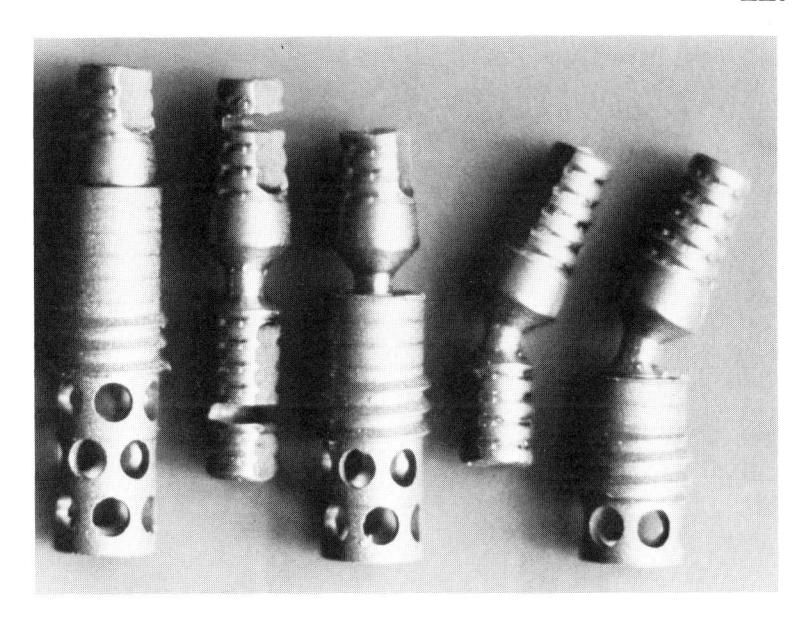

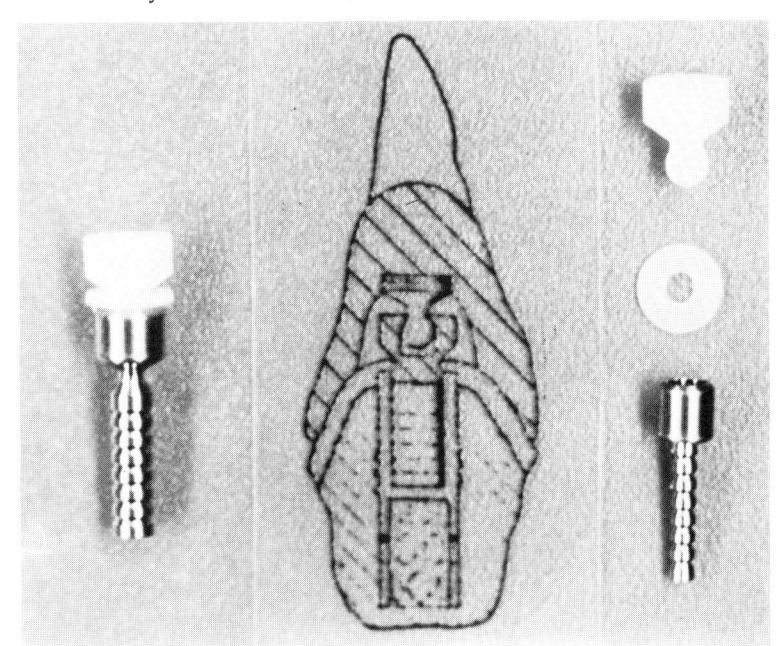

Figure 7–81. The Core-Vent Overdenture Attachment is designed for use with the Core-Vent Implant (left) as well as with endodontically treated roots (center). The Core-Vent Attachment combines a durable utra high molecular weight polyethylene male and a titanium female to minimize wear and breakage (right). Prior to cementation into the Core-Vent Implant, shorten the shaft to establish tissue contact with the head and bend the head for approximate parallelism. Eliminate any undercuts in the denture flanges that can deflect the denture on insertion, preventing proper seating of the male component. Either attach the male component to the denture with cold-cure acrylic directly in the mouth (block out any undercuts if the neck is exposed), or place a second pair of inserts into the final or relined impression to facilitate attachment during laboratory processing. After attachment of the plastic male to the denture, remove the spacer and generously clear the denture acrylic from any contact with the head of the insert.

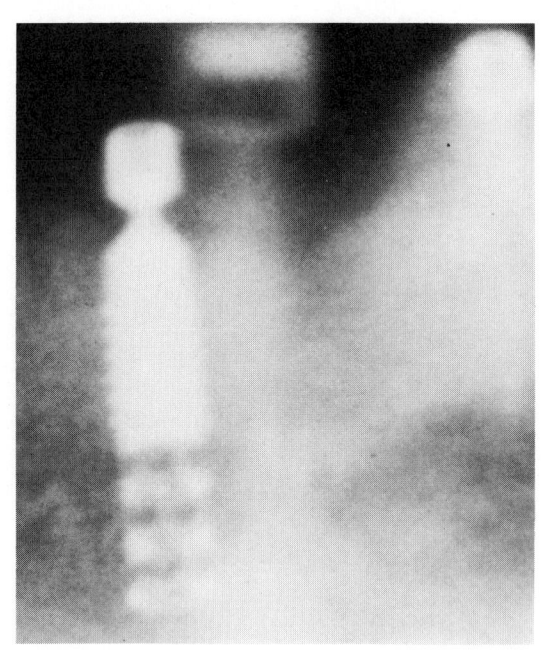

228 / IMPLANTS USED IN PREPROSTHETIC RECONSTRUCTIVE SURGERY

Figure 7–82. Panoramic radiograph of Core-Vent Attachment cemented into both the implant and the endodontically treated root. This system provides a simple, economic method of retaining an overdenture using natural teeth (without the need for impressions and expensive laboratory procedures) and free-standing Core-Vent Implants.

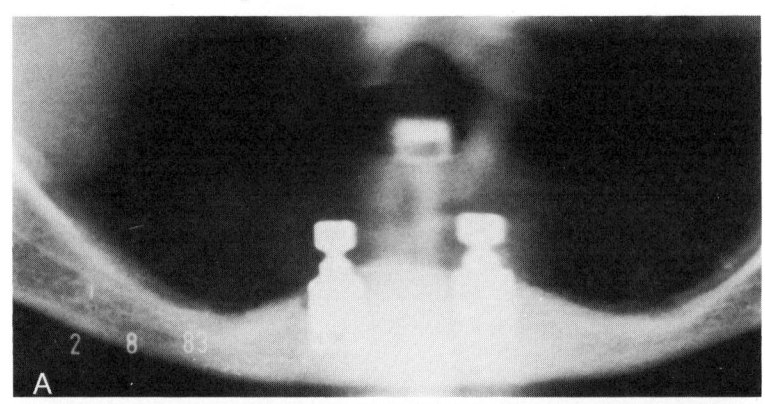

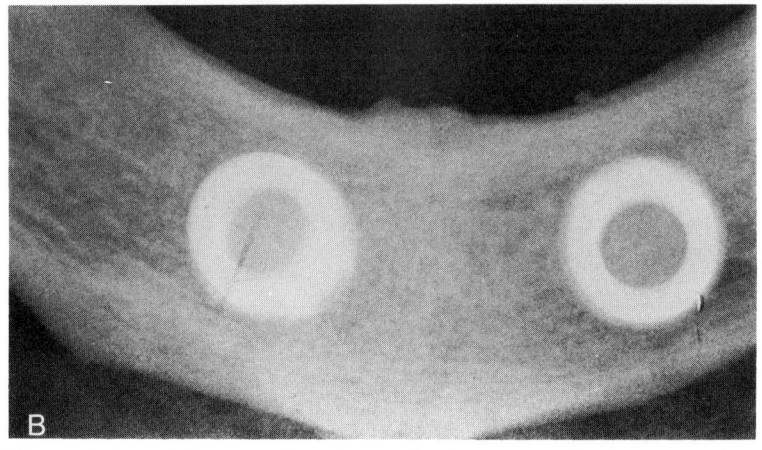

Figure 7–83. *A*, Panoramic radiograph of a 5.5-mm Core-Vent Implant (Mod. 8). The genial tubercle is higher than the 7-mm endosseous portion of the implant. *B*, Occlusal radiograph of a 5.5-mm Core-Vent Implant (Mod. 8).

a spacer to ensure that the ball is situated just inside the constricted opening of the socket, in the absence of occlusal forces. In function, the male of the overdenture attachment flexes, rotates freely, and moves 0.5 mm deeper in the socket, minimizing the stress on the free-standing Core-Vent Implant. This allows the prosthesis to be tissue-supported while providing lateral stability and retention. The C-VA is available in a smaller diameter head and a 1.5-mm diameter shaft (with a corresponding pair of drills) for use in endodontically treated roots (Fig. 7–81). This facilitates the combination of natural teeth and Core-Vent Implants for overdenture retention with a conformity of retention and stress-breaking features (Fig. 7–82). The osseointegrated Core-Vent Implant, in combination with the stress-reducing features of the C-VA, distributes stress to such an extent that even in cases where the implant is used in Modification 8 (5.5-mm diameter), the implants may be able to function free-standing to retain an overdenture (Figs. 7–83 and 7–84).

2. The Titanium Screw Insert (TSI) allows fixed/detachable splinting for overdenture retention and support as well as a detachable fixed prosthesis (Figs. 7–83 to 7–89). A choice of screws is available that attach vertically into the superior threaded aspect of a titanium insert cemented into the Core-Vent Implant.
   a. For overdentures, the screw (TS/O) (see Fig. 7–86) is designed with a 3-

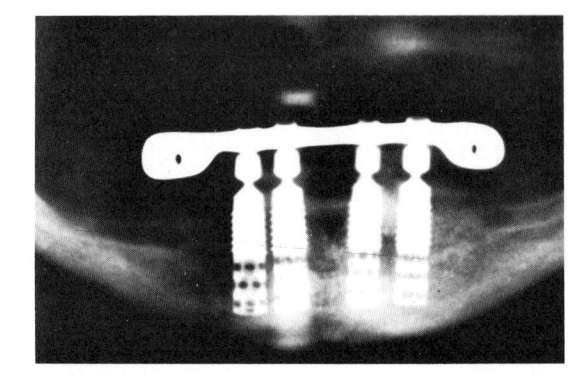

Figure 7–84. Restoration of the atrophic mandible with an implant-supported overdenture on fixed/detachable splinting. Panoramic radiograph shows that four Modification 1 Core-Vent Implants (4.5 mm diameter) have made maximum use of available bone in the symphysis. The 2-mm tapered section of the TSI accommodates 0.080-inch acrylic base plate material (Omnivac) for fabricating the pattern for casting the chrome cobalt superstructure. The holes are for Lew Passive Attachments (LA).

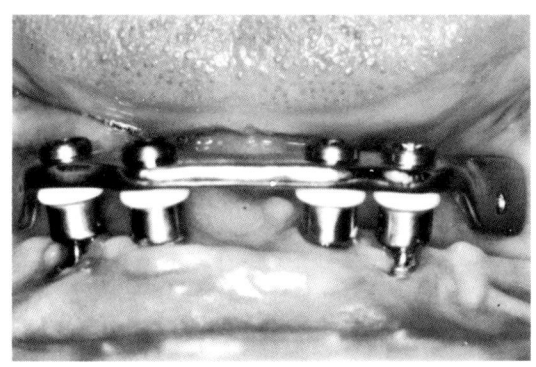

Figure 7–85. Four Core-Vent Implants in the symphysis with Titanium Screw Inserts (TSI). A cast superstructure that cantilevers distally and rests on resilient O-rings connects the implants and provides a fixed/detachable support for an overdenture. The tapered neck of the Titanium Screw (TS) allows for vertical and lateral movement of the bar as occlusal forceps compress the resilient O-rings.

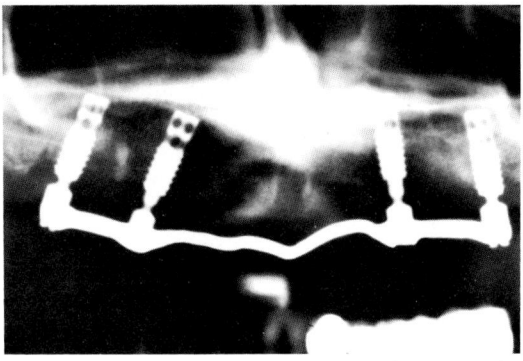

Figure 7–87. Four Core-Vent Implants in the maxilla splinted together with cast tissue bars (Hader and 13-gauge round plastic patterns available with gold and nylon clips [BS]). Keep the insertion of the implants angled to the lingual for maximum bone maintenance on the buccal. Perforation of the sinus should be avoided if possible but does not necessarily result in a failure. For nonresilient support (as in this case) the 4-mm head of the Titanium Screw can be modified to 2 mm by cutting off halfway down the tapered portion with a carborundum disc and then cutting a slot to facilitate screwing into the TSI. The TSI is bendable in order to avoid having to overcontour the prosthesis. Parallelism is not a factor, since the bar is attached by screws that are independently placed into the head of the TSI.

mm shaft, with a straight 1-mm section next to the top of the insert (just above the threaded portion) to accommodate a 1-mm Titanium Washer (TW) during the laboratory construction of a connecting bar. It ultimately accommodates a 1.3-mm resilient O-ring. A 2-mm tapered portion located between the straight section and the 1-mm flat head of the screw passes through a cast metal bar. The cast bar compresses the O-rings under function as it sep-

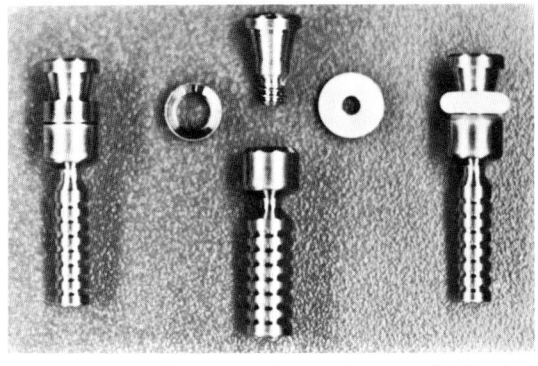

Figure 7–86. Titanium Screw Inserts (TSI) plus components for constructing and attaching a resilient tissue bar. The 2-mm tapered section of the 4-mm long Titanium Screw/Overdenture (TS/O) is the same thickness as 0.080-inch acrylic base plate material (Omnivac). Use this for fabricating the pattern for casting the superstructure (chrome cobalt, gold, or nonprecious alloy). The 1-mm Titanium Washer (TW) is used for the laboratory phase to create the space for the resilient O-ring. The overdenture can be retained by Lew Passive Attachments engaging a hole in the cantilevered part of the metal casting.

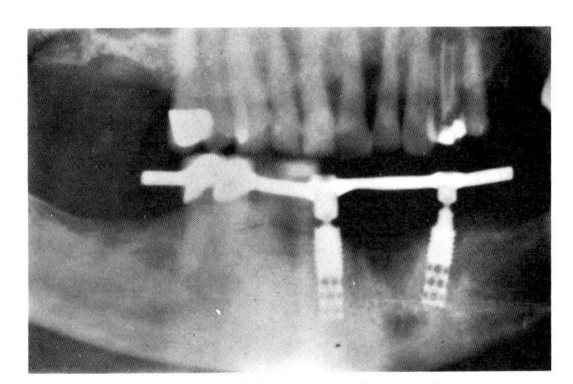

Figure 7–88. The Titanium Screw Insert provides nonparallel, nonresilient splinting to two ankylosed natural teeth with cast bars and nylon Hader clips. The TSI in the midline Core-Vent Implant was used with the Titanium washer for rigid splinting and in order to obtain a relatively horizontal bar. The left Core-Vent Implant was inserted at approximately a 30-degree angle to avoid the bone defect left by the extraction of tooth No. 22 (implant placed same appointment as extraction) and to avoid the mental foramen. The TSI was used in the left implant with a modified Titanium Screw (shortened by 2 mm) to obtain vertical clearance and nonresilient splinting. Although parallelism is not essential when using TSI's, the head was bent to facilitate construction of the bar.

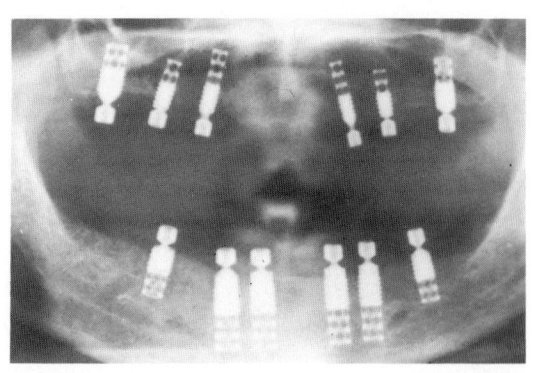

Figure 7–89. Total rehabilitation of the edentulous mouth is now feasible using Core-Vent Implants and Titanium Screw Inserts after Osseoventegration™ is verified clinically by the absolute rigidity of the implant in the bone and radiographically by the congruency of implant and bone. The heads of the upper TSI's were bent to allow construction of a prosthesis within the confines of the dental arch. The following restoration options are available using the versatile Titanium Screw Insert: Overdentures on a fixed/detachable tissue bar using the Titanium Screw (TS/O) with the neck designed for the resilient O-rings; Detachable Fixed Prosthesis (acrylic and metal) using the Titanium Screw (TS/F) with a narrow, 6-mm long neck: the occlusal 3-mm section has a diameter of 3 mm while the apical half tapers down evenly to the threaded section. This allows shortening (and recutting of the slot) depending on the height of the pontic it must pass through.

arates slightly from the tapered portion of the shaft of the screw. It buffers the effect of both vertical and lateral occlusal forces. The TSI allows a number of Core-Vent Implants to be splinted together, regardless of parallelism, by a cast bar that can cantilever distally in order to provide support for an overdenture even in the areas of a dehiscent mental foramen. Where resilience is not required (connecting to ankylosed natural teeth or splinting of multiple implants without cantilevered extensions), the titanium washer can be used instead of the O-ring or the screw can be modified (Fig. 7–91). This is particularly true in cases in which vertical clearance is inadequate and can be done by removing the 1-mm flat head and 1 mm of the tapered portion with a carborundum disc and subsequently cutting a slot in the top to facilitate tightening of the screw. The head of the TSI can be bent to facilitate the proper contours in the overdenture or fixed detachable prosthesis.

b. For a detachable fixed prosthesis, a titanium screw (TS/F) (Fig. 7–91) is available that tapers down evenly to the threaded portion. This allows the screw to be modified occlusally and the slot recut depending on the length needed to allow the screw to pass through the pontic. Fixed reconstruction of the totally edentulous mouth is possible using four to six Core-Vent Implants and titanium screw inserts to provide implant-supported fixed bridges. Usually these can be removed by the dentist to mitigate future possible implant or prosthetic complications and to reduce the risks and improve the prognosis of extensive rehabilitation with implant prosthodontics.

c. The laboratory procedures for constructing fixed/detachable splinting of either resilient or nonresilient tissue bars, as well as detachable fixed reconstruction, are simplified by the fact that, after the TSI's are cemented in the implants, regardless of modifications or bending, a sec-

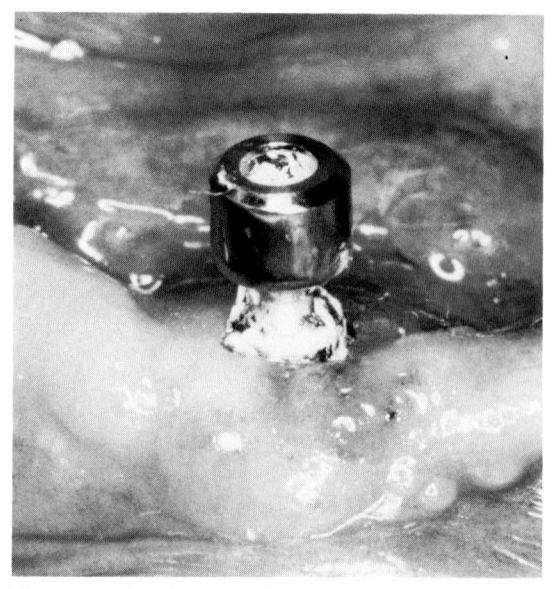

Figure 7–90. Cement the appropriate insert into the implant after completing all modifications. Before cementation, lubricate the narrow neck with vaseline unless it is to be cemented into the hex-hole. Use a Centrix syringe to inject Den-Mat composite cement into the hex-hole. Immediately after seating the insert, make an impression and place a second set of inserts into it prior to pouring the stone working model. Likewise, a second TCI can be used as a metal transfer die. Since only the position of the heads is important to the laboratory procedure, it is irrelevant whether the necks of the cemented inserts have been bent or the shafts shortened.

ond set of TSI's can be placed in the impression as transfers and become incorporated in the working stone cast. The final prosthesis can then be fabricated using accepted prosthetic principles (Fig. 7–92).

Summary

Because of design features of the Core-Vent Implant System that result in the achievement and maintenance of osseointegration, the dental profession now has an alloplastic tooth substitute that can function free-standing to replace a single tooth or to stabilize a removable prosthesis. The method of fixed/detachable splinting using Core-Vent Implants and titanium screw inserts is similar to that of the Brånemark system in that it allows for the removal or treatment of individual implants without affecting other implants or the continuous stability of the prosthesis. This is an essential factor in the long-term considerations when advocating intervention with dental implants for extensive reconstruction. The built-in precision and simplicity of the system reduce operator error and minimize the cost and risk to a level that justifies the intervention. This makes it possible for the Core-Vent Implant System to serve as a viable alternative to conventional dentistry.

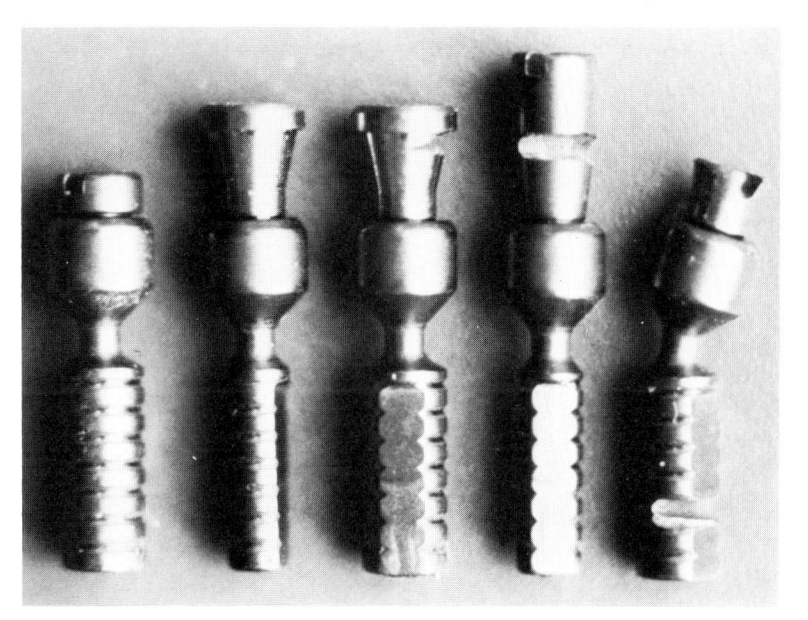

Figure 7–91. Three screws are available for the TSI insert. Left to right, A short screw (TS/H, for hygiene) is used to keep the threaded end of the TSI clean during the time between cementing the TSI and completion of the prosthesis. For nonresilient fixed/detachable splinting with a tissue bar, the 4-mm head of the TS/O can be modified by 2 mm by sectioning it just under the 1-mm lip with a carborundum disc and then cutting a slot. A longer (6 mm), narrower (3 mm) screw (TS/F) can similarly be shortened for retaining a fixed prosthesis or a metal-based overdenture that can be detached only by the dentist. The TSI is bendable in order to avoid having to overcontour the prosthesis, but absolute parallelism is not essential.

TITANIUM PLASMA SPRAY (TPS) SCREW IMPLANT SYSTEM FOR RECONSTRUCTION OF THE EDENTULOUS MANDIBLE*

Charles A. Babbush

Artificial metallic dental implants may be helpful to patients who can no longer tolerate or function with conventional removable dentures. Lack of tolerance or loss of function can have a psychological and/or a physical etiology. The mandibular symphyseal area provides the greatest quality and quantity of osseous components, devoid of vital structures in the maxillofacial complex. The TPS screw implants form the basis for a superstructure that will subsequently ensure retention of a mandibular prosthesis.

---

*I wish to thank Dr. Philippe Ledermann, Herzogenbuchsee, Switzerland, and Mr. Franz Sutter and Dr. Fritz Straumann, Institute Straumann, Waldenburg, Switzerland, for their advice and support as well as the technical and photographic information for this work. In addition, I wish to thank Mr. Bart Colucci, President, Colmed LTD, Half Moon Bay, California, for his cooperation in the clinical aspects of this work.

Engineering Considerations

In the development of the Association for Osteosynthesis (AO) and its philosophy of orthopedic internal fixation, the Institute Straumann was able to create a team concept. This close cooperative effort was established among clinicians, metallurgists, engineers, and other allied scientists. Because of the vast experience of this group over 20 years, the development of certain basic concepts in oral implantology was possible. These concepts were used in the Endosteal Hollow-Basket and TPS Screw Implant Systems.[124]

The choice of biocompatible materials is essential for a good prognosis in implant reconstruction. Of equal or perhaps greater importance is the bioengineering designs of the implant. The structural strength of the implant is of paramount consideration. It is most desirable to avoid high specific peak loads (peak pressure), as resorption may otherwise occur at the bone area adjacent to these impact points. The design must feature an anchoring surface of the greatest

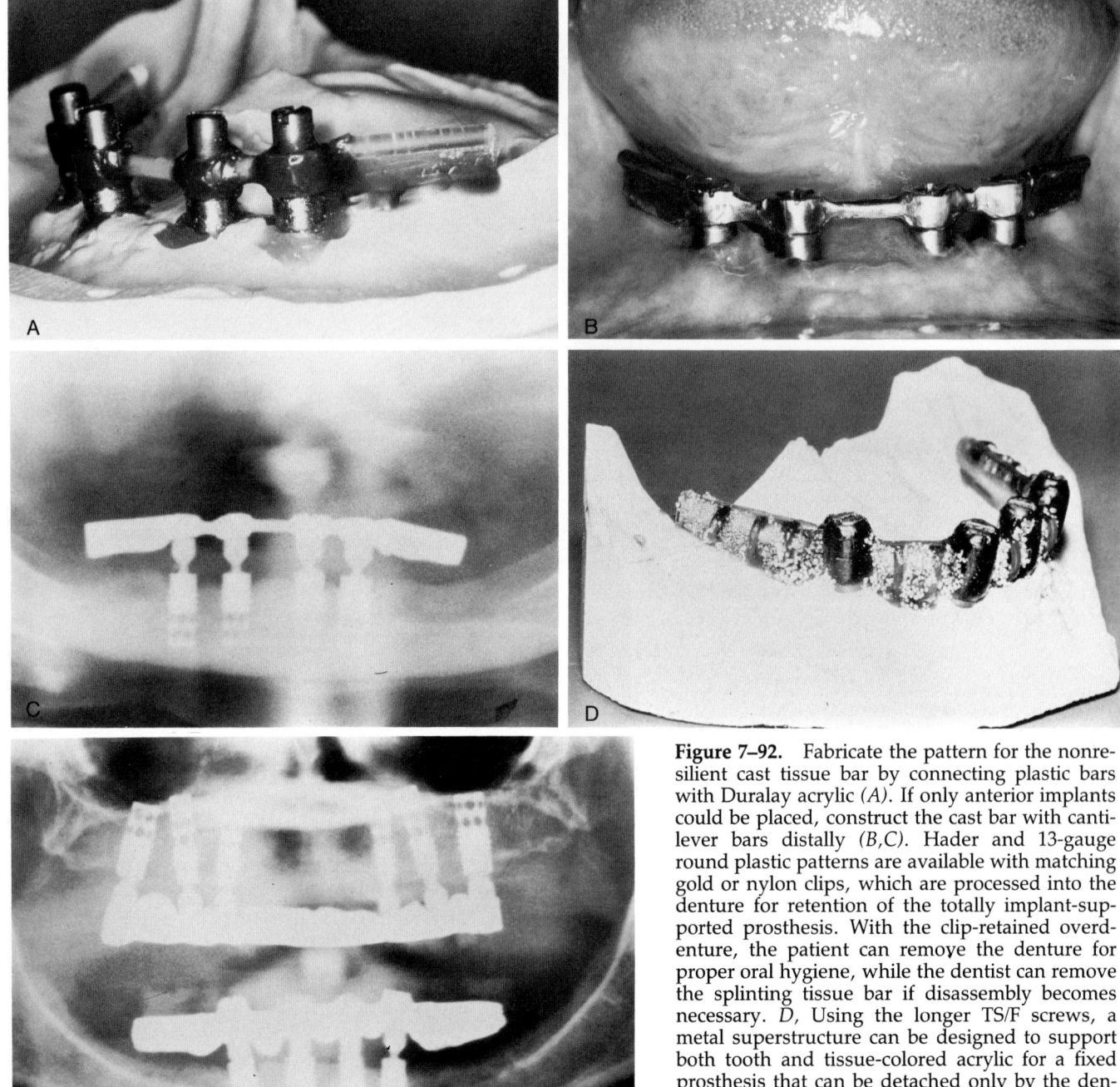

232 / IMPLANTS USED IN PREPROSTHETIC RECONSTRUCTIVE SURGERY

Figure 7–92. Fabricate the pattern for the nonresilient cast tissue bar by connecting plastic bars with Duralay acrylic (A). If only anterior implants could be placed, construct the cast bar with cantilever bars distally (B,C). Hader and 13-gauge round plastic patterns are available with matching gold or nylon clips, which are processed into the denture for retention of the totally implant-supported prosthesis. With the clip-retained overdenture, the patient can remove the denture for proper oral hygiene, while the dentist can remove the splinting tissue bar if disassembly becomes necessary. D, Using the longer TS/F screws, a metal superstructure can be designed to support both tooth and tissue-colored acrylic for a fixed prosthesis that can be detached only by the dentist. Wax up the entire length of the screw so that when the screw is shortened for form and occlusal clearance, it will be surrounded by metal. E, Full-mouth rehabilitation with fixed/detachable metal superstructure and Iviclar acrylic and composite denture teeth.

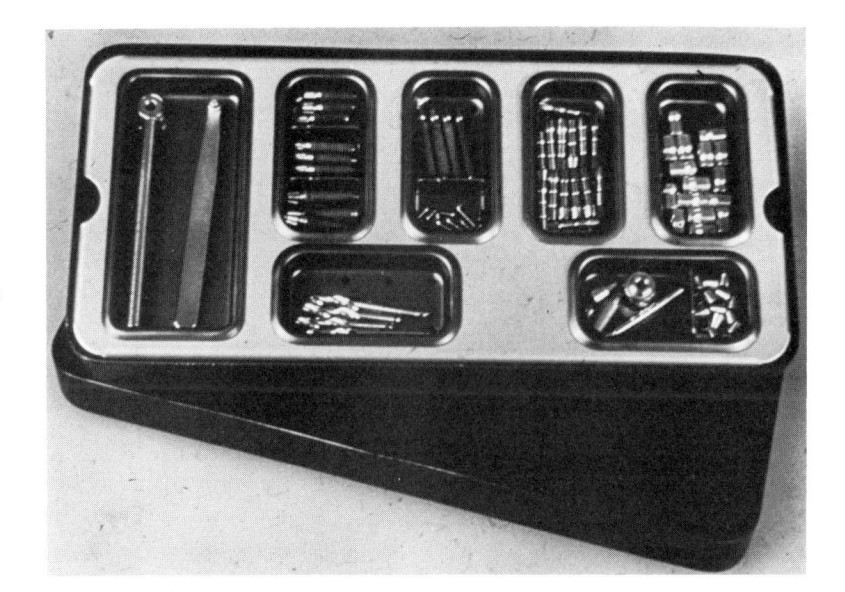

Figure 7–93. The autoclavable Eloxal cassette with all the system parts.

possible area in order to lower the specific pressure per unit area, since lower specific pressures will inevitably create better conditions for the integration of the implant into the bone tissue. The screw implant corresponds to the basic design of the AO cortical traction screw. The material used is technically pure titanium, ASTMB standard 265-58T, with a resistance of 80 kg/mm and a melting point of 1670° C. The screw prepared from this material is additionally coated with a titanium plasma–sprayed layer.

Titanium Plasma–Sprayed (TPS) Screw Implant System™

The Titanium Plasma–Spray System is easily sterilized in the autoclavable cassette container and tray. The entire sterile system can then be carried into the operative field (Fig. 7–93). The TPS screws are available in four lengths: 11 mm, 14 mm, 17 mm, and 20 mm (Fig. 7–94). The outer diameter of the implant body is 4 mm, wtih a 3.2-mm threaded core diameter. All implants have certain design concepts: the head, neck, and shoulder, and the thread with its self-tapping tip (Fig. 7–95). Four vertical slots are designed into the 3-mm cone-shaped head. These slots serve as a positive seat for the corresponding

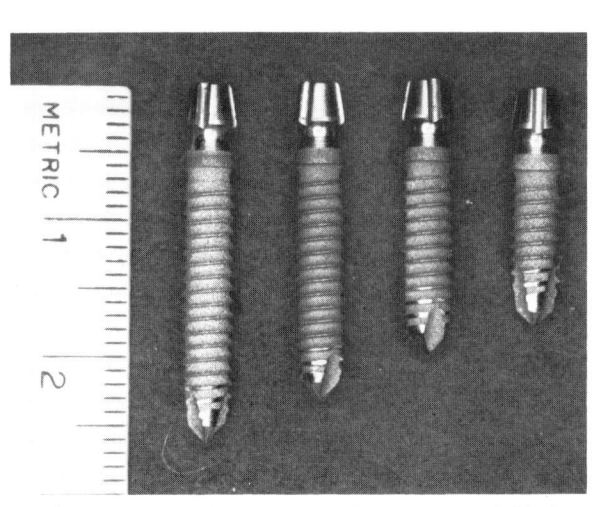

Figure 7–94. The screw implants are available in four lengths, 11 mm, 14 mm, 17 mm, and 20 mm.

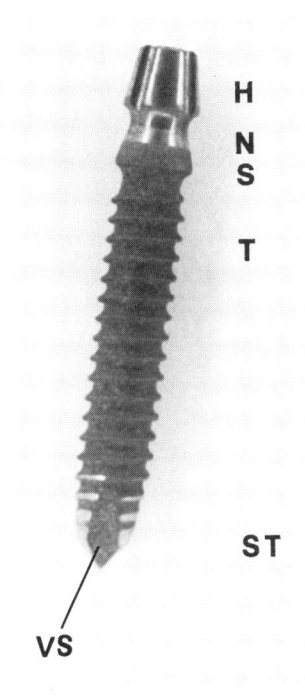

Figure 7–95. The implant has differently designed sections: head (H), neck (N), shoulder (S), thread (T), self-tapping tip (ST), and vertical slot (VS).

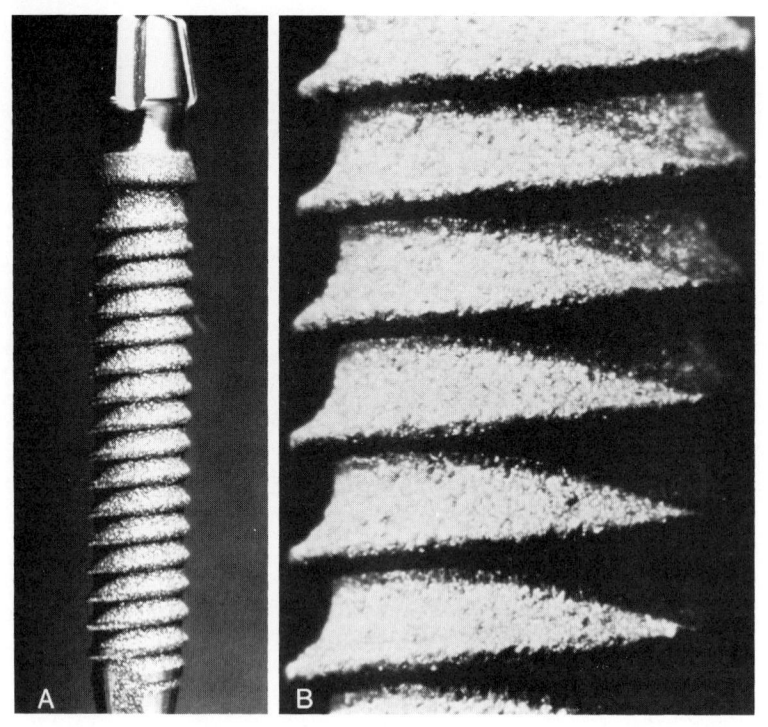

Figure 7–96. *A*, The threaded portion of the implant is coated with a titanium plasma spray. *B*, Magnified view of plasma-sprayed surface.

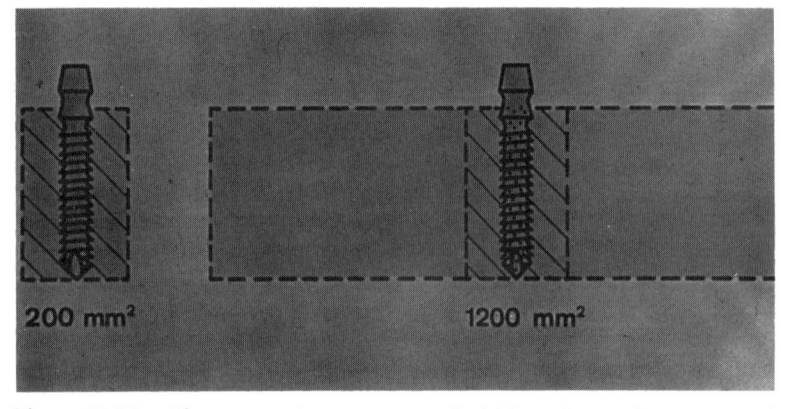

Figure 7–97. Plasma coating creates a six-fold surface enlargement of the anchored implant portion.

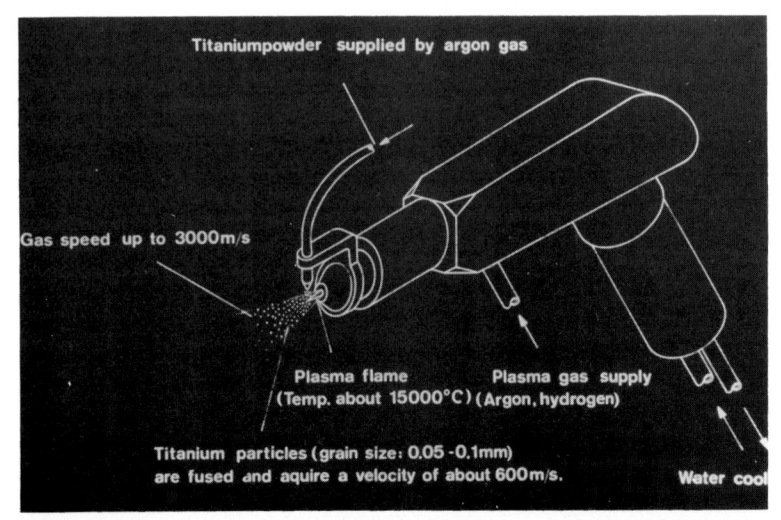

Figure 7–98. The process of plasma spraying is a complex one.

system parts, such as the impression caps, die pins, and gold telescopes. The socket wrench and the hand ratchet lock into these slots for accurate implant insertion. The head has an internally threaded area 5 mm deep and 2 mm in diameter. This accepts a 4-mm or 8-mm occlusal screw, which anchors the superstructures into a fixed position. The construction between the head and threaded body of the implant is referred to as the neck of the implant and is 3 mm in length. This area produces a favorable contour and the correct shape for attachment of the gingival tissues. The cylindrical shoulder is 1 mm long and 4 mm in diameter. It extends downward from the neck and should be level with the crest of the alveolar bone.

The implant body is threaded as a cortical bone screw with gently rounded outer threads. This design produces a consolidation and compression of the medullary bone at the rounded crest of the thread. It does not develop excessive specific loads at the bone points involved. Thread intervals are minimized in order to reduce as much as possible the potential of microfractures of the bone trabeculae. Sharp line angles and point angles on the implant surfaces are eliminated. This is the principal requirement for the achievement of bonding with bony material. The self-tapping aspect of the thread becomes anchored in the bone, producing an optimum degree of initial retention. The apical tip has 120-degree ground extensions. Because of this design concept, immediate stability and retention are achieved. This stability enables the placement of the connector bar superstructure immediately following implant placement, with restoration of the patient to function. The threaded portion of the implant surface is coated with a titanium plasma spray (Fig. 7–96). This process provides an irregular surface on the threaded area of the implant.[125] Hulbert demonstrated that porosity, such as with plasma-coated surfaces, led not only to a more rapid healing but also to a substantially lesser foreign body reaction.[125] Scanning electron microscope investigations show that bone is able to grow into these pores without a connective tissue membrane.[126,127] A six-fold surface enlargement of the anchored implant portion is achieved, which improves the microanchoring characteristics of the bone[124,126–128] (Fig. 7–97). Titanium plasma–sprayed coating is achieved by argon gas flame spraying where the base material is not heated above 220° C. This process results in a plasma layer 0.04 to 0.05 mm thick on the thread area of the implant (Fig. 7–98). A bond strength of c 0.5 kp/mm² plasma coating does not impair fatigue resistance.

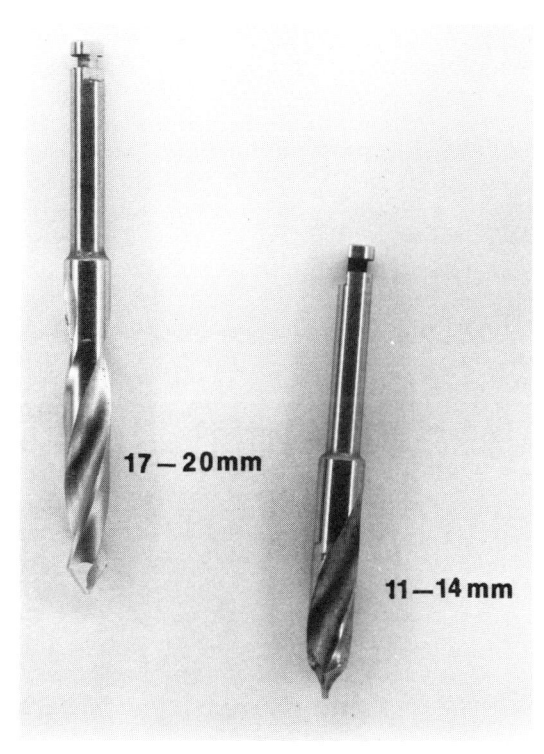

IMPLANTS USED IN PREPROSTHETIC RECONSTRUCTIVE SURGERY / **235**

Figure 7–99. Two twist drills are available, a short one for the 11-mm and 14-mm implants and a long one for the 17-mm and 20-mm ones.

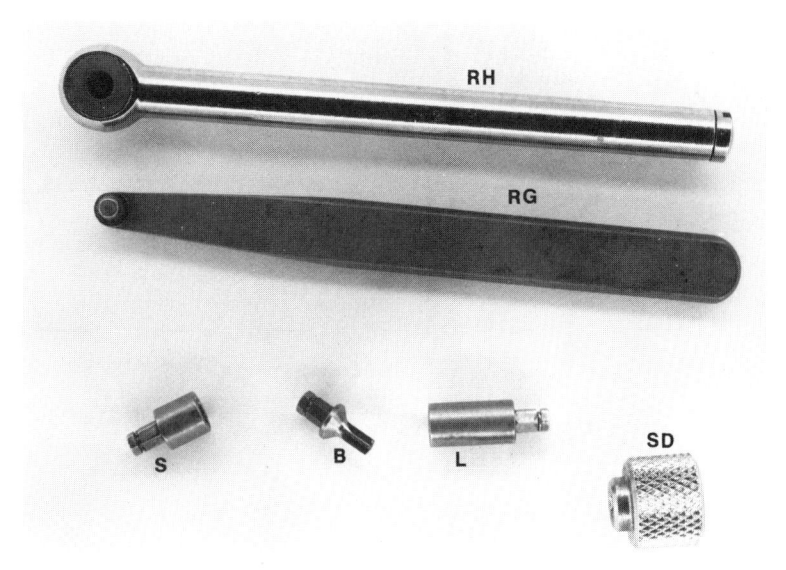

Figure 7–100. A ratchet handle (RH) with a short (S) and long (L) adaptable head is part of the inserting instruments. By turning the handle over, either a forward or reverse direction can be used. The ratchet head has four vertical ribs that engage the vertical slots on the implant head for optimum retention for the implant insertion. A ratchet guide (RG) is used with the inserter for improved implant alignment during insertion. A small, "fingertip" screwdriver handle (SD) with replaceable blades (B) is used for placement of the occlusal screws.

The most impressive feature of the TPS screw implant is its ability to utilize the full depth of the mandible down to its anchoring in the inferior cortex. Two lengths of twist drills, short and long, are used in a standard latch-type contra-angle with half-speed gear reduction handpieces (Fig. 7–99). A maximum speed of 600 to 800 rpm with copious irrigation by sterile saline for cooling is recommended. The burs are 3.2 mm in diameter, which is the core diameter of the implant. The short drill bit is used to prepare the osseous site for the 11-mm and 14-mm implants. The long drill bit is used to prepare the site for the 17-mm and 20-mm implants. The osseous preparation is considered adequate if the implant can be seated so that the shoulder is level with the alveolar crest.

The implant is inserted via the ratchet handle and either the long or short adaptable head. The ratchet head has four ribs projecting from its sides on the inner surface. These ribs engage the four vertical slots in the implant head to create a precision fit and optimum retention for implant insertion. The ratchet is two-directional, one side forward and the other reverse. This instrument will also accommodate the occlusal screwdriver blade for easy placement of the occlusal screw to secure the Dolder bar superstructure. The ratchet guide functions as a stabilizer arm for the ratchet and screwdriver blades. During placement of the implant or occlusal screw, the guide allows the clinician to keep the implant aligned and to apply slightly downward pressure. A small, round, knurled "fingertip" screwdriver handle can be used with interchangeable screwdriver blades (Fig. 7–100). This instrument is used for the insertion of the occlusal screws, for insertion or removal of the Dolder bar, and in the laboratory as well. In order to verify the depth of the osseous preparation, the depth gauge with 3-mm interval markings is tried in and out of the bone (Fig. 7–101). The gauge is marked at 11-mm, 14-mm, and 20-mm depths. It is a good idea to have three

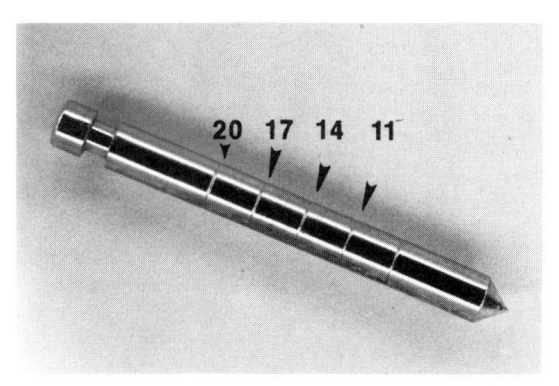

Figure 7–101. A depth gauge marked with 3-mm intervals, which correspond to the length of the implants, is used to check the depth of the osseous preparation site.

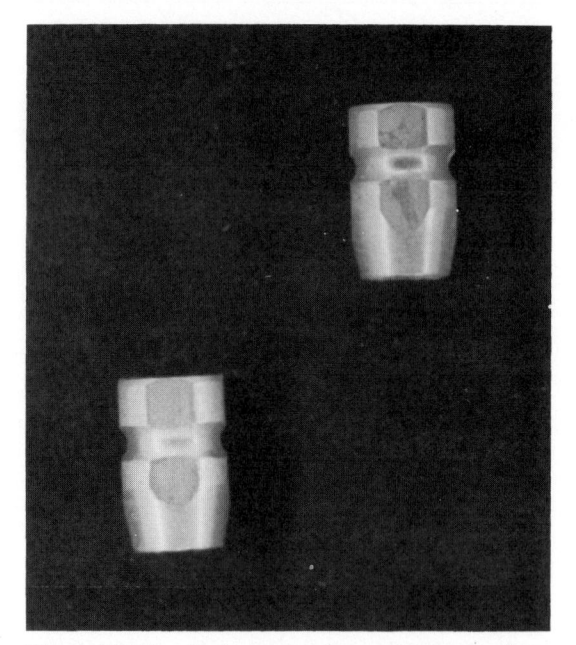

236 / IMPLANTS USED IN PREPROSTHETIC RECONSTRUCTIVE SURGERY

Figure 7–102. Impression caps with four projecting ribs are placed over the implant heads and into the vertical slots. The transfer copings are picked up with the impression material.

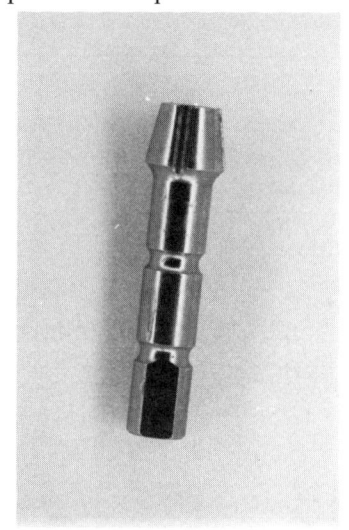

Figure 7–103. Transfer pins are placed into the impression caps.

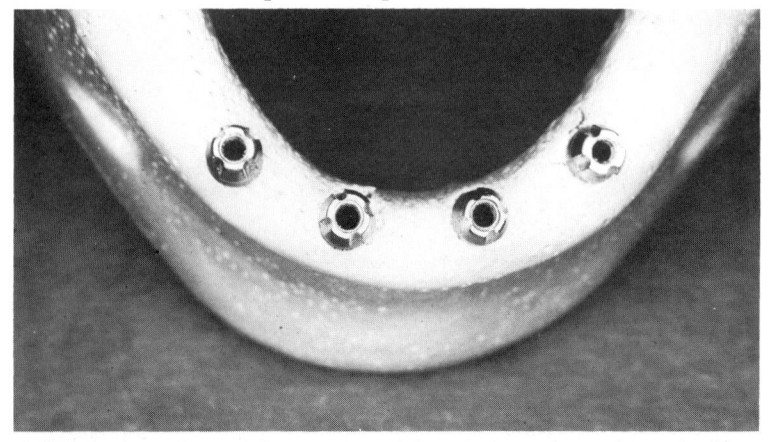

Figure 7–104. Stone laboratory model with die pins in place, duplicating the actual case.

of these gauges. Once the first site is completed, the depth gauge is left in position. This acts as a point of orientation and aids in controlling parallelism during the preparation of the second implant site. This is then repeated with the second and third depth gauges and the corresponding preparation sites.

Transfer copings are supplied with the system (Fig. 7–102). These impression caps are placed over the heads of the implants at the conclusion of the suturing of the mucoperiosteal flaps. A cold-cure occlusal matrix is placed over the impression caps to relate them to one another. The impression caps are picked up in the impression material when the impression is obtained. Precision-designed die pins are placed into the impression caps (Fig. 7–103), and a stone model is then poured to create a duplication of the implants *in situ* for the laboratory (Fig. 7–104). Prefabricated, precision-made telescopic gold copings are used to fabricate the Dolder bar superstructure (Fig. 7–105*A*). Occlusal screws of 4-mm and 8-mm lengths are used to secure the soldered Dolder bar structure to the implant heads (Fig. 7–105*B*).

Special Principles

All mucoperiosteal osseous surgical procedures should be carried out under sterile conditions using the standardized instrument set supplied with the system. The procedure must be carried out in an atraumatic

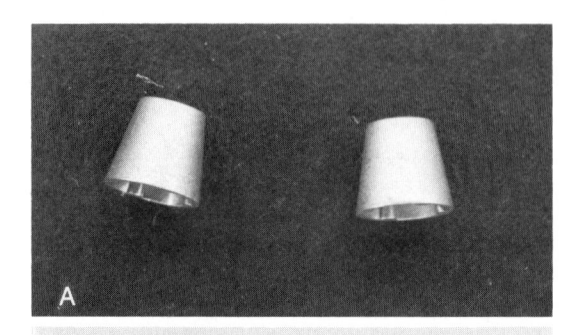

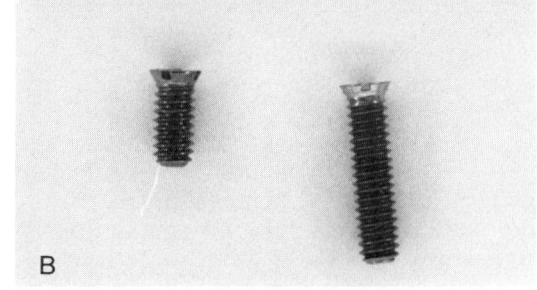

Figure 7–105. *A*, Prefabricated precision-made gold copings. *B*, Occlusal screws 4 mm and 8 mm in length are used in the superstructure fabrication.

fashion to obtain a favorable prognosis. It is recommended that the same length implant be used throughout the case unless variations in bony contours dictate a difference.[129] When the surgical placement of the implant(s) is complete, no mobility should be present. Initial primary anchorage is essential to good bone healing. The screw implants should be splinted within 48 to 72 hours postoperatively and thus placed into function immediately.[129] A new denture can be fabricated prior to the procedure. If the screws are splinted by the Dolder bar, they can be left indefinitely without the denture prosthesis. Alternately, the patient's existing denture can be hollowed out to fit over the implant abutments and Dolder bar. The denture can be relined with soft tissue conditioners to be worn as a temporary prosthesis until complete healing has occurred, and the final prosthesis can then be fabricated.

Preoperative Procedure

The instrument system should be checked to ensure that all equipment and parts of the armamentarium are available. Any missing instruments or an instrument demonstrating wear from previous procedures should be replaced. Normal sterilization for implantation requires autoclaving the entire system in the cassette available. The implants themselves are packaged clean but not sterile at this time. The transparent implant template (Fig. 7–106A) is superimposed over the panoramic and lateral radiograph (Fig. 7–106B) to aid in the selection of the appropriate length of implant. The approximate position is outlined and the proper implant size is chosen.

Anesthesia

The implants are designed to be placed in the mandibular symphysis anterior to the mental foramen and its neurovascular bundles. Local anesthesia of choice can be selected by the surgeon (Xylocaine 2 per cent with 1:100,000 epinephrine, Carbocaine 2 per cent with 1:20,000 Neo-Cobefrin, etc.). Vasoconstrictors should not be used in patients with known sensitivity or a medical history that contraindicates their use. Bilateral mental blocks with infiltration in the anterior mucobuccal vestibule as well as the anterior floor of the mouth should be sufficient to carry out this procedure. Premedication via the intravenous, intramuscular, or oral route is at the discretion of the surgeon.

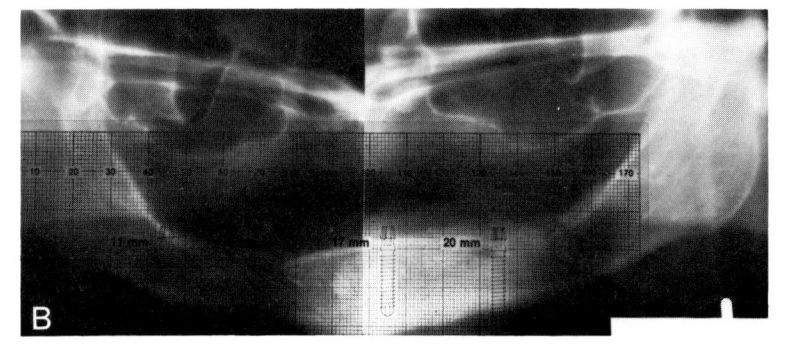

Implantation Procedures

A midcrestal incision is made with a No. 15 scalpel blade (Fig. 7–107) slightly distal to

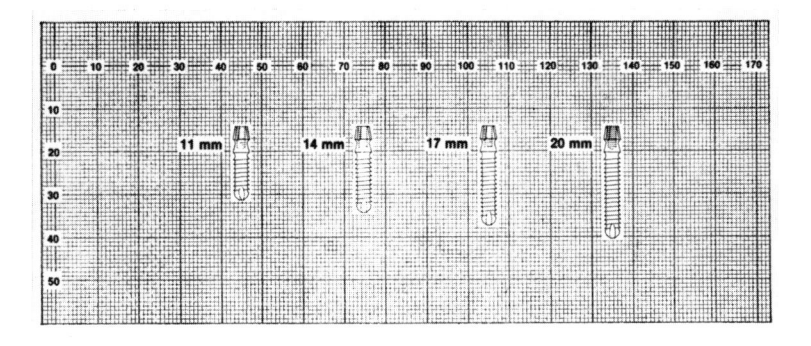

Figure 7–106. The transparent template (A) is superimposed over the radiographs (B) to determine proper implant length selection.

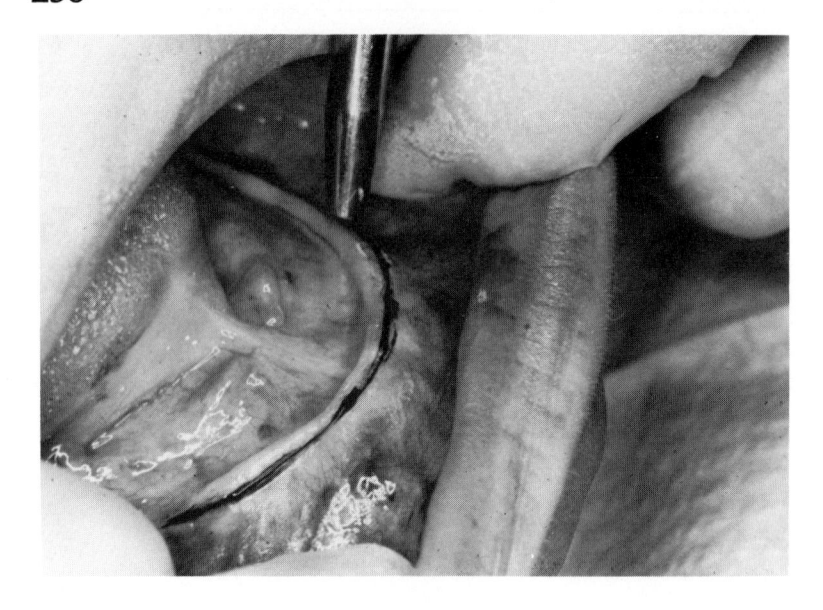

238 / IMPLANTS USED IN PREPROSTHETIC RECONSTRUCTIVE SURGERY

Figure 7–107. A midcrestal mucoperiosteal incision is made with a No. 15 scalpel blade. The incision extends from the second bicuspid region of one side around to the same region of the opposite side.

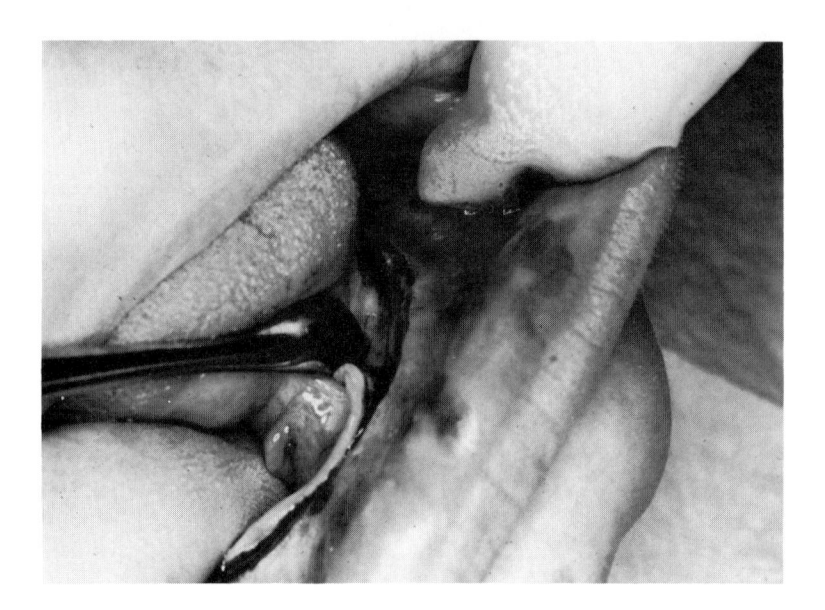

Figure 7–108. The lingual and labial mucoperiosteum is reflected to expose the full thickness of the alveolar ridge.

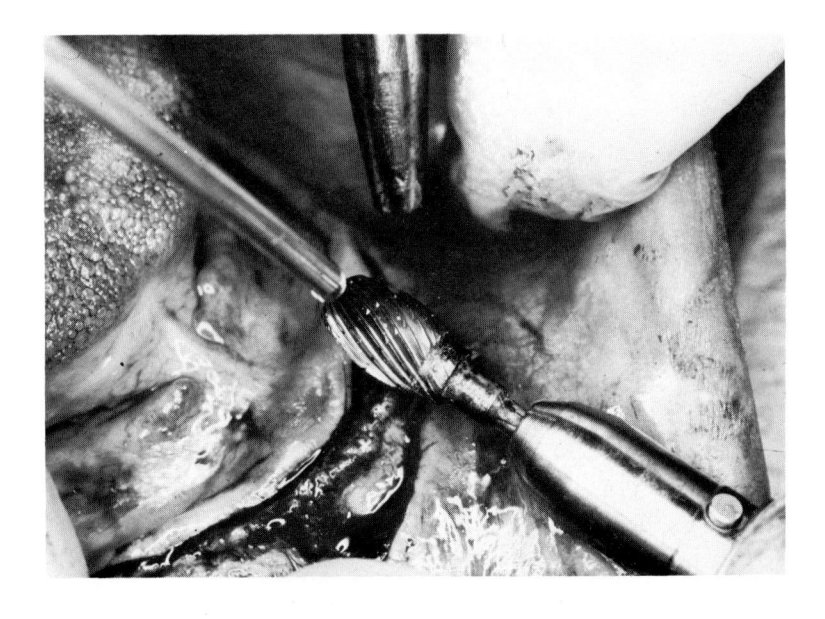

Figure 7–109. A large acrylic laboratory bur is used to plateau the alveolar crest.

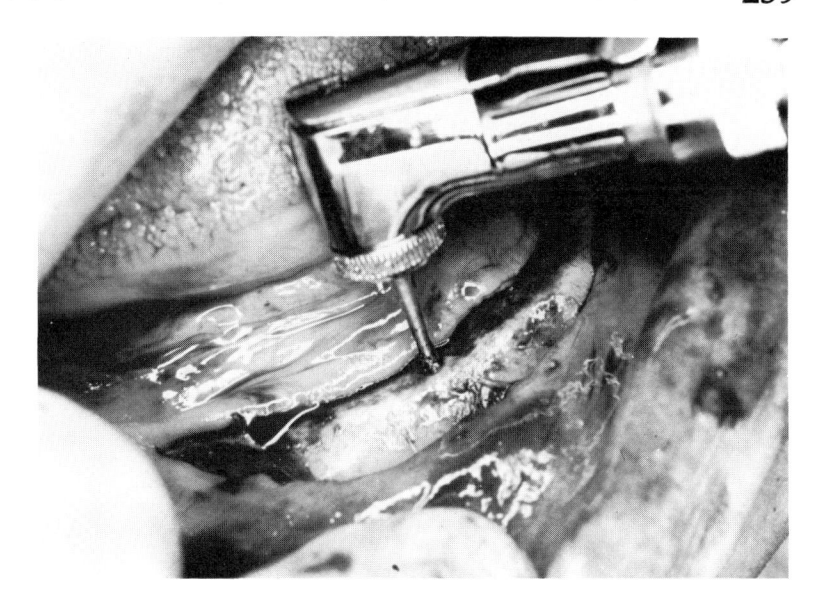

Figure 7–110. The purchase points are equally spaced anterior to the mental foramen and placed with a No. 4 or 6 round bur.

the mental foramen on one side and continued around to the opposite side. The incision should be carried through the mucoperiosteal tissues. The flap should be reflected in both a labial and a lingual direction to expose the width of the alveolar ridge (Fig. 7–108). Care must be exercised to not traumatize the mental neurovascular bundle. The extension of the incision beyond the mental nerve allows direct visualization of the neurovascular bundle when the mucoperiosteal flaps are reflected, greatly reducing potential trauma to this area.

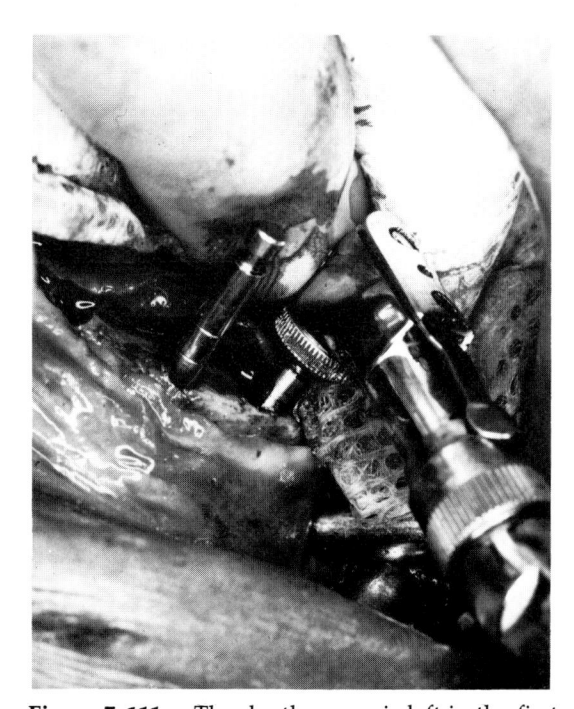

Figure 7–111. The depth gauge is left in the first site while the second site is prepared, allowing for good spacial relationships and parallelism.

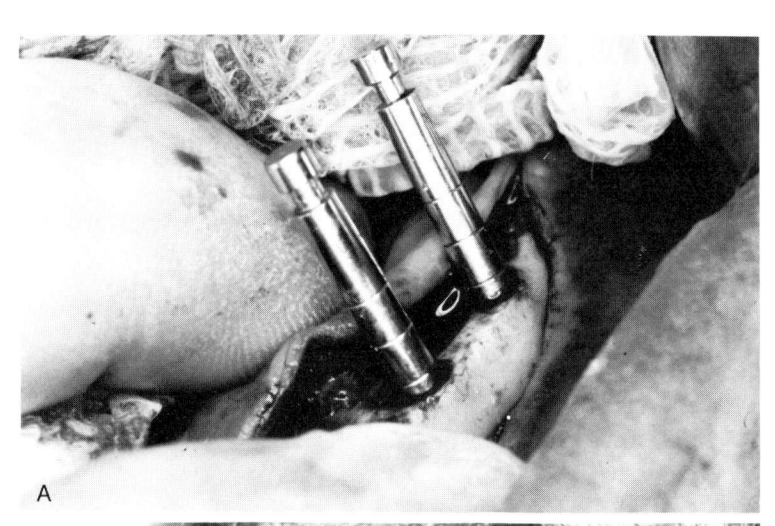

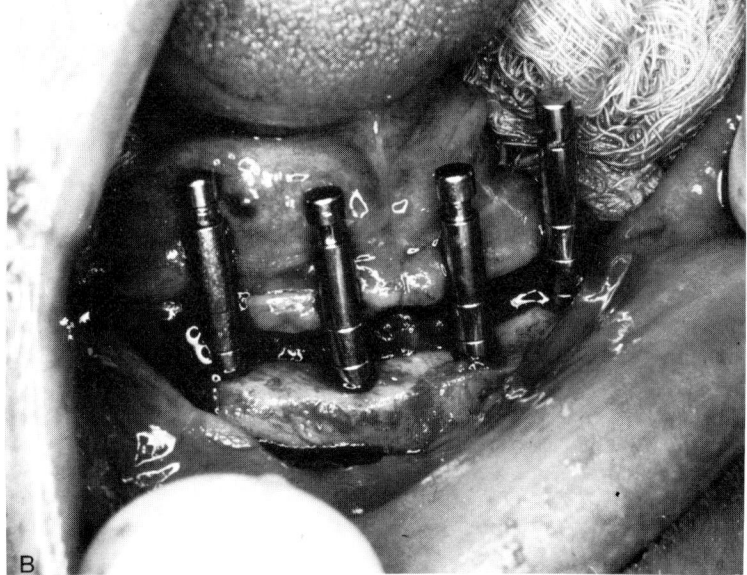

Figure 7–112. *A,* With each preparation a depth gauge is placed for improved parallelism. *B,* All four sites should be parallel to each other.

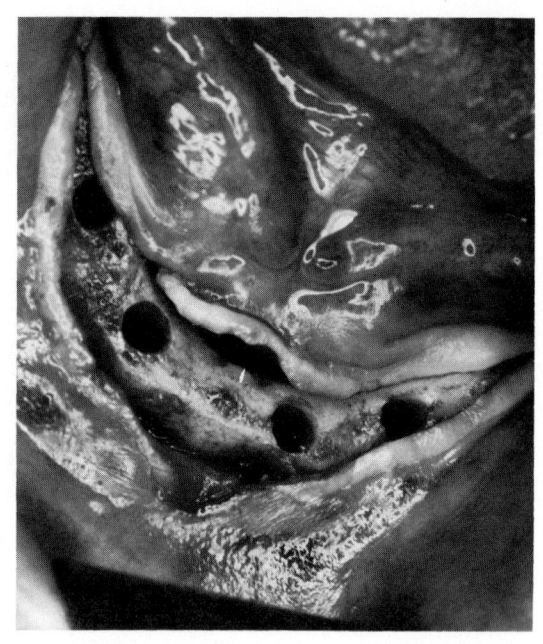

Figure 7–113. When the site preparation is completed, thoroughly clean out any bone splinters or debris with suction and rinse with sterile saline.

In numerous instances once the mucoperiosteal tissues are reflected, spinous processes or knife-edge ridge crests are revealed. These areas can be reduced by using a bone file to burnish or remove these projections. In addition, a large acrylic laboratory bur in a slow-speed handpiece can be used to recontour the alveolar crest until a plateau is created for the initiation of the implant placement (Fig. 7–109). Bilateral palpation, using the index finger on the lingual and the thumb on the labial area during all site preparations and implant placements, will detect any potential perforation of the bony cortices. As depth is increased while drilling, the thumb may be placed externally, under the chin, to detect the obvious "bite" of the drill into the lower cortex, indicating maximum drill depth required.

The distalmost implants are placed 2 mm mesial to the mental neurovascular bundles, with the mesial implants 4 to 6 mm mesial to that position. With this placement, a larger space is available in the midline. This method of placement allows for the inclusion of only one clip in the prosthesis. Subsequently, the prosthesis can rotate somewhat around the superstructure and thus reduce torque on the distalmost implants. A No. 4 or 6 round bur is used to initiate purchase points on the ridge crest (Fig. 7–110). This procedure allows for accurate introduction of the twist drill into the bone without slipping off the ridge crest.

The depth of the implant site is monitored with the system's depth gauge. The depth gauge is marked at 11 mm, 14 mm, 17 mm, and 20 mm to accurately relate the depth of the preparation site to the indicated implant. The second borehole is drilled, leaving the depth gauge in the first hole as an axis-direction aid for the second drilling (Fig. 7–111). All four implants should be set as closely as possible to the same spacial orientation (Fig. 7–112). After drilling, any bone splinters or debris should be thoroughly removed with suction and irrigation with a sterile saline solution (Fig. 7–113).

The appropriate implant length should be selected. The implant should be 1 to 2 mm shorter than the depth of the receptor site in order to avoid stripping the bone thread (i.e., if the depth gauge reads 20 mm, use the 17-mm implant). The screws are then introduced into the bored preparation sites. The hand ratchet is used to place the first screw (Fig. 7–114). A light pressure is exerted on the ratchet guide, preventing a tilting or sliding of the screw while it is being

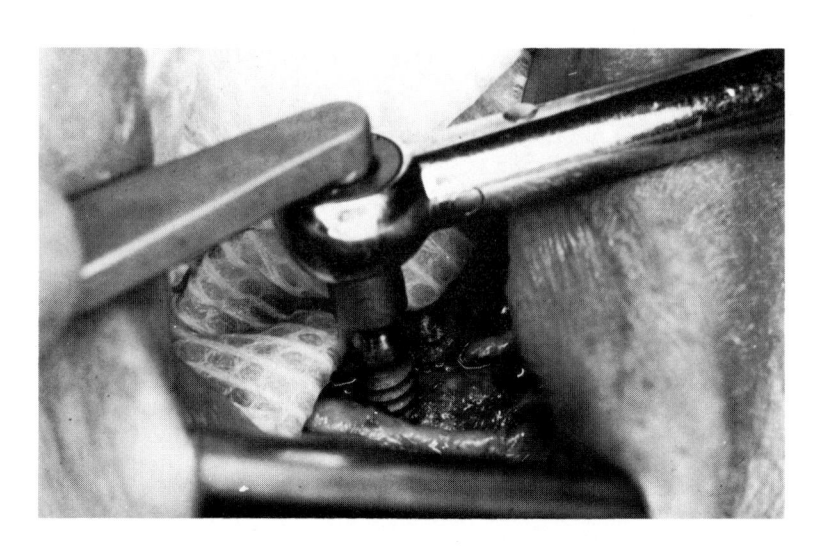

Figure 7–114. Using the hand ratchet, the first implant is placed. Continue insertion until the shoulder is in contact with the bony crest and/or you feel resistance.

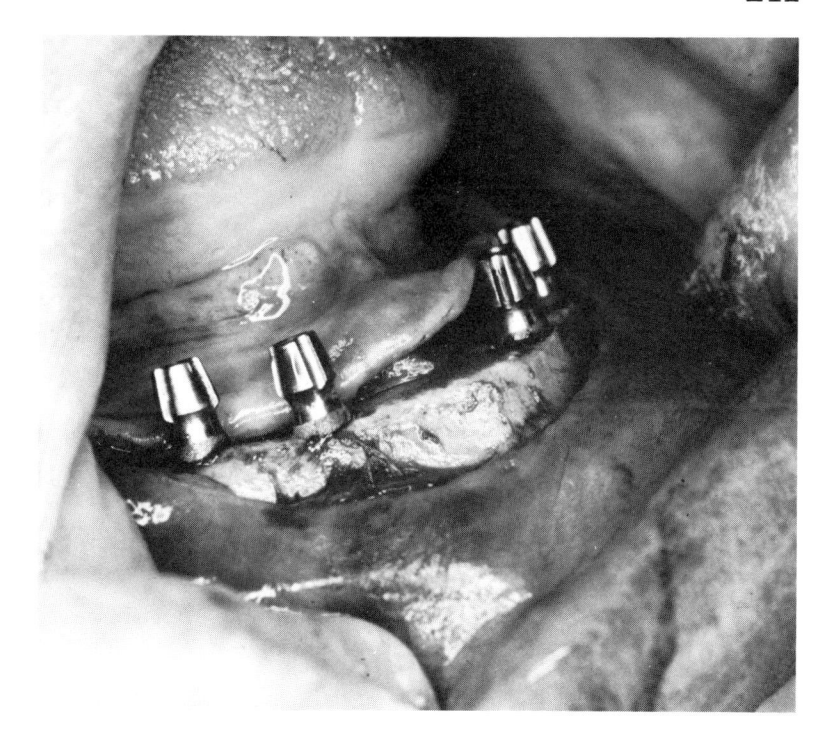

IMPLANTS USED IN PREPROSTHETIC RECONSTRUCTIVE SURGERY / **241**

Figure 7–115. All four implants are appropriately seated.

placed. The second, third, and fourth implants are placed in the same manner. No attempt should be made to overtighten the implants (Fig. 7–115). Tightening should stop at the first resistance. The surgical sites are irrigated and the mucoperiosteal flaps repositioned. Excess tissue is removed with a tissue punch and the flaps are sutured (Fig. 7–116). Immediately after implantation (i.e., at the same session), the impression is taken over the prefabricated impression caps in order to be able to insert the superstructure as quickly as possible. The impression caps are set on the implant heads (Fig. 7–117). They are examined to be sure that adjacent soft tissue and suture materials are not trapped between the cap and the implant, making removal difficult. A Duralay or cold-cure acrylic template is fabricated *in situ* over the impression caps prior to impression taking. This will aid in accurately transferring the registration to the laboratory model (Fig. 7–118). Using standard procedures, a rubber-base or silicone impression should be taken. The impression caps will be picked up when the impression is removed (Fig. 7–119). The die pins are positioned into the caps, which are embedded in the impression material (Fig. 7–120). A stone model is poured with the die pins in place to reproduce the exact relationship in a working model (Fig. 7–121).

The gold telescopic copings are placed on

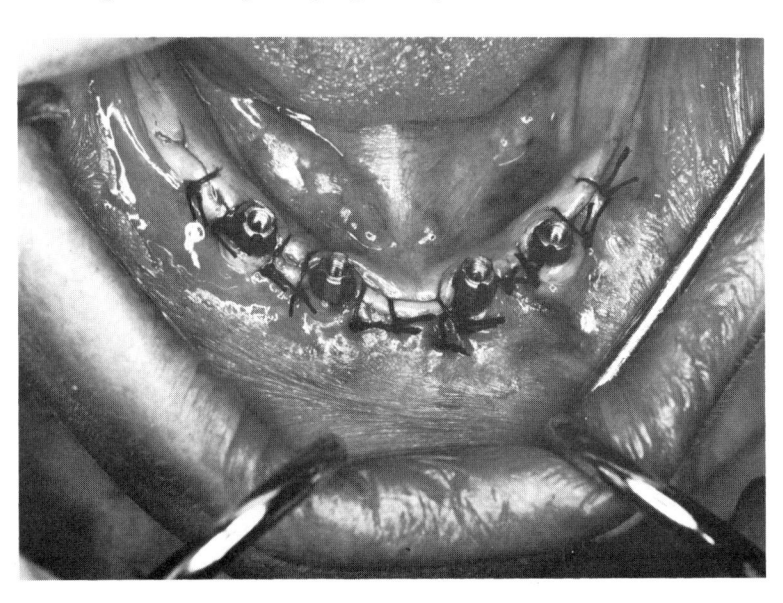

Figure 7–116. The mucoperiosteal flaps are repositioned and sutured with 3-0 black silk interrupted sutures.

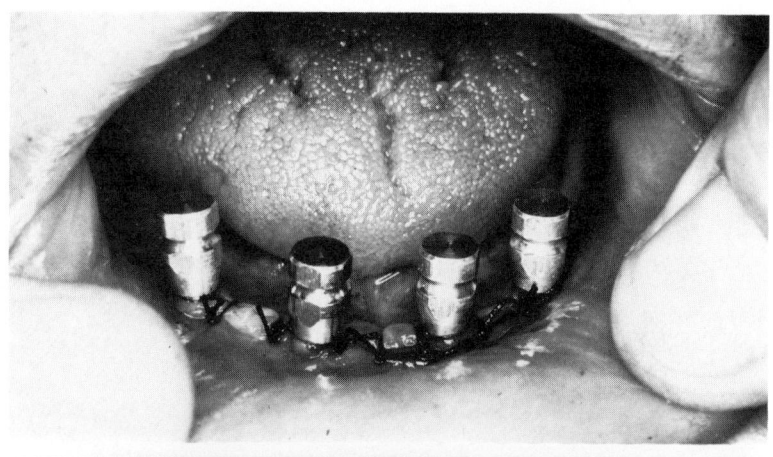

242 / IMPLANTS USED IN PREPROSTHETIC RECONSTRUCTIVE SURGERY

Figure 7–117. The impression caps are placed on each implant head, making sure that no soft tissue or suture material is trapped between them, which would make removal difficult.

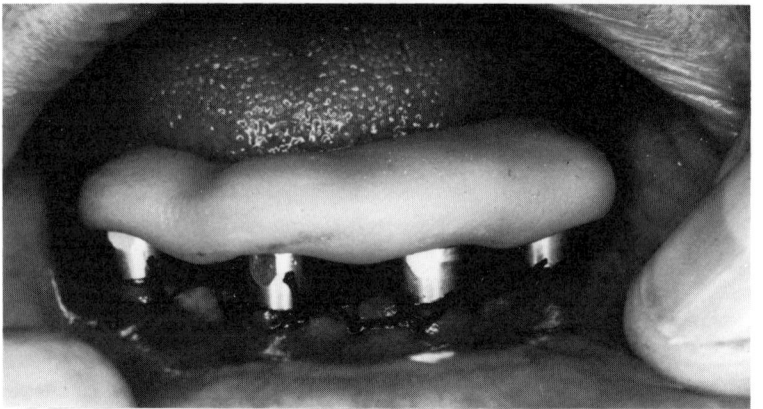

Figure 7–118. An acrylic matrix is fabricated intra-orally to aid in accurately transferring the registration to the laboratory model.

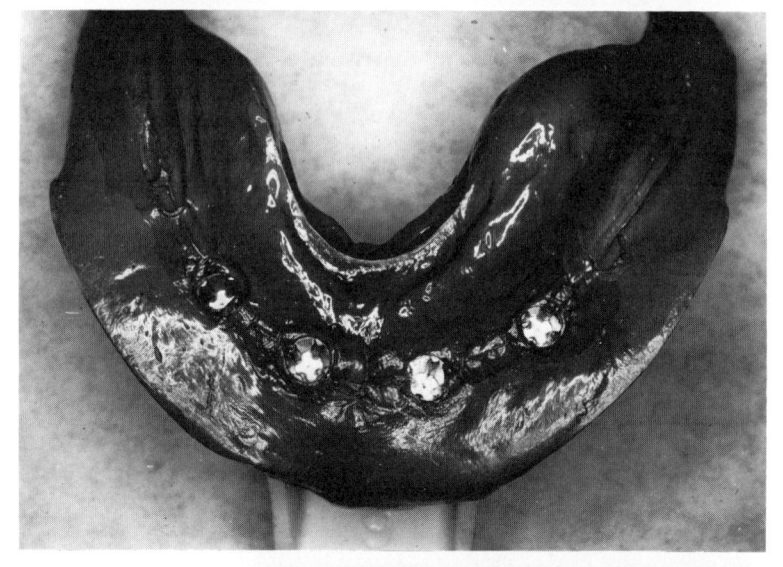

Figure 7–119. The impression caps and matrix are picked up in the impression.

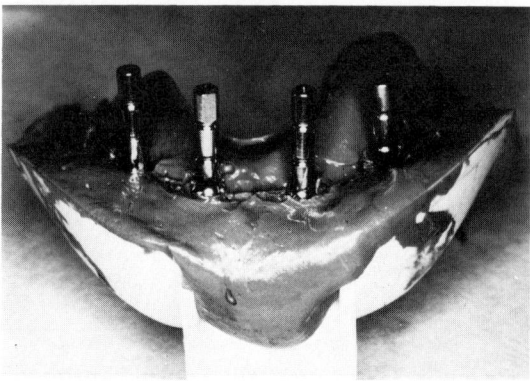

Figure 7–120. The die pins are placed into the impression caps in the impression.

IMPLANTS USED IN PREPROSTHETIC RECONSTRUCTIVE SURGERY / **243**

Figure 7–121. A stone model is poured with the die pins in place, reproducing the oral relationship in the laboratory.

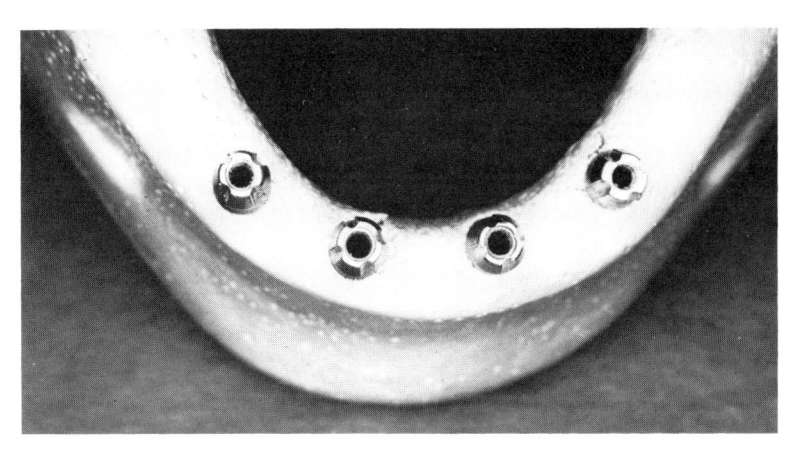

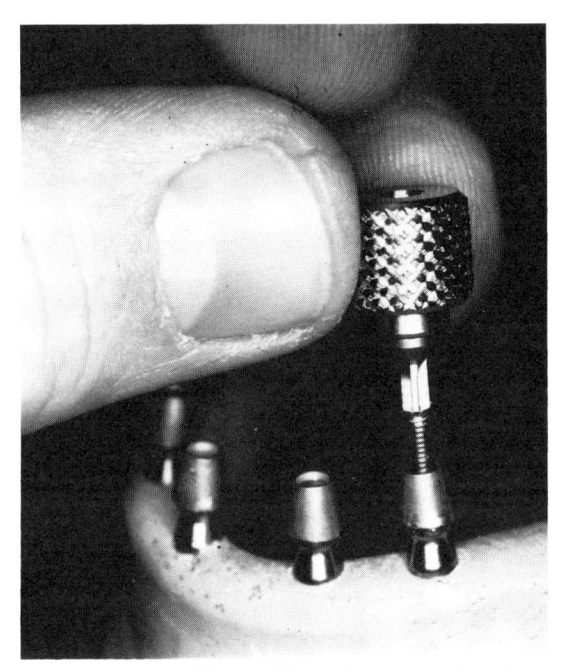

Figure 7–122. The gold copings are placed on the die pins and secured with the occlusal screws.

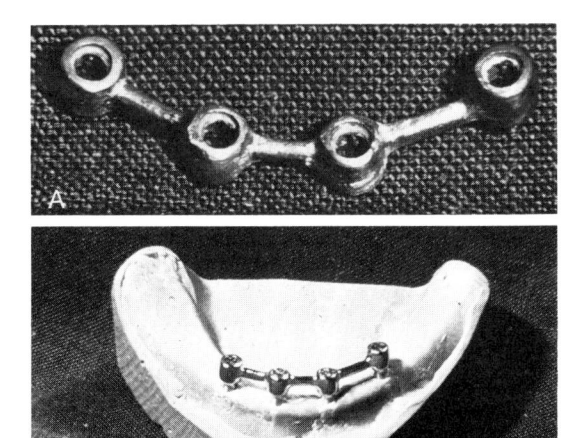

Figure 7–123. *A*, The Dolder bar fabrication is completed. *B*, The Dolder bar is replaced on the model and finished.

each die transfer in this model. The occlusal screws secure the copings in place (Fig. 7–122). The model is then ready for the laboratory technician to solder the prefabricated Dolder bar. The bar should be level with the occlusal surface and have a polished finish (Fig. 7–123).

The clinician then removes the completed Dolder bar from the model by removing the occlusal screws and places it on the implants in the mouth. Riders are applied to the bar. Both the occlusal openings of the gold copings and the areas of the bar lying below are waxed in (Fig. 7–124). The bar should be 1 to 2 mm above the gingival surface to allow for proper oral hygiene.

The denture should be finished by heat-cured laboratory denture construction, which is the preferable procedure. If cold polymerization is used, care must be taken to cool the denture during the curing phase. The bar is separated from the riders and mounted and secured by tightening the occlusal screws with the ratchet and guide

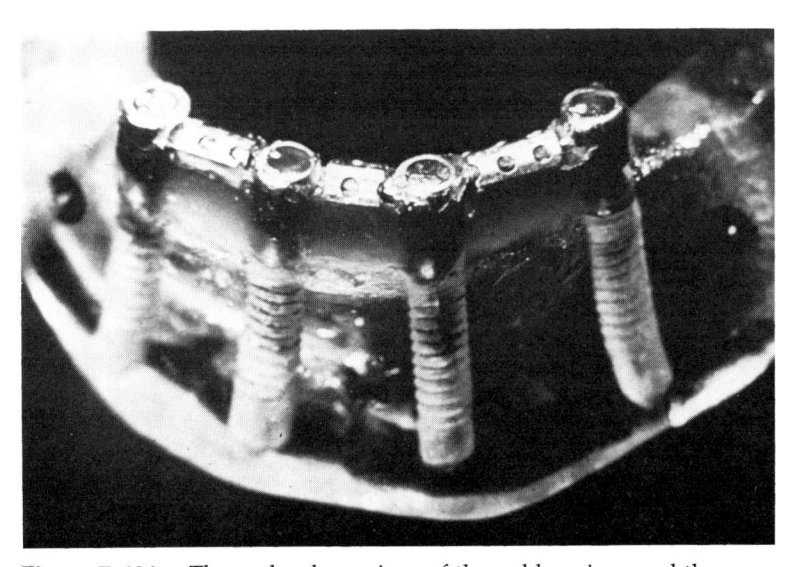

Figure 7–124. The occlusal openings of the gold copings and the areas of the bar lying below are waxed in, so that the clips may be picked up and fabricated into the denture.

244 / IMPLANTS USED IN PREPROSTHETIC RECONSTRUCTIVE SURGERY

Figure 7–125. The completed Dolder bar (*A*) is placed in the mouth and secured with the occlusal screws (*B*). *C*, The denture is completed.

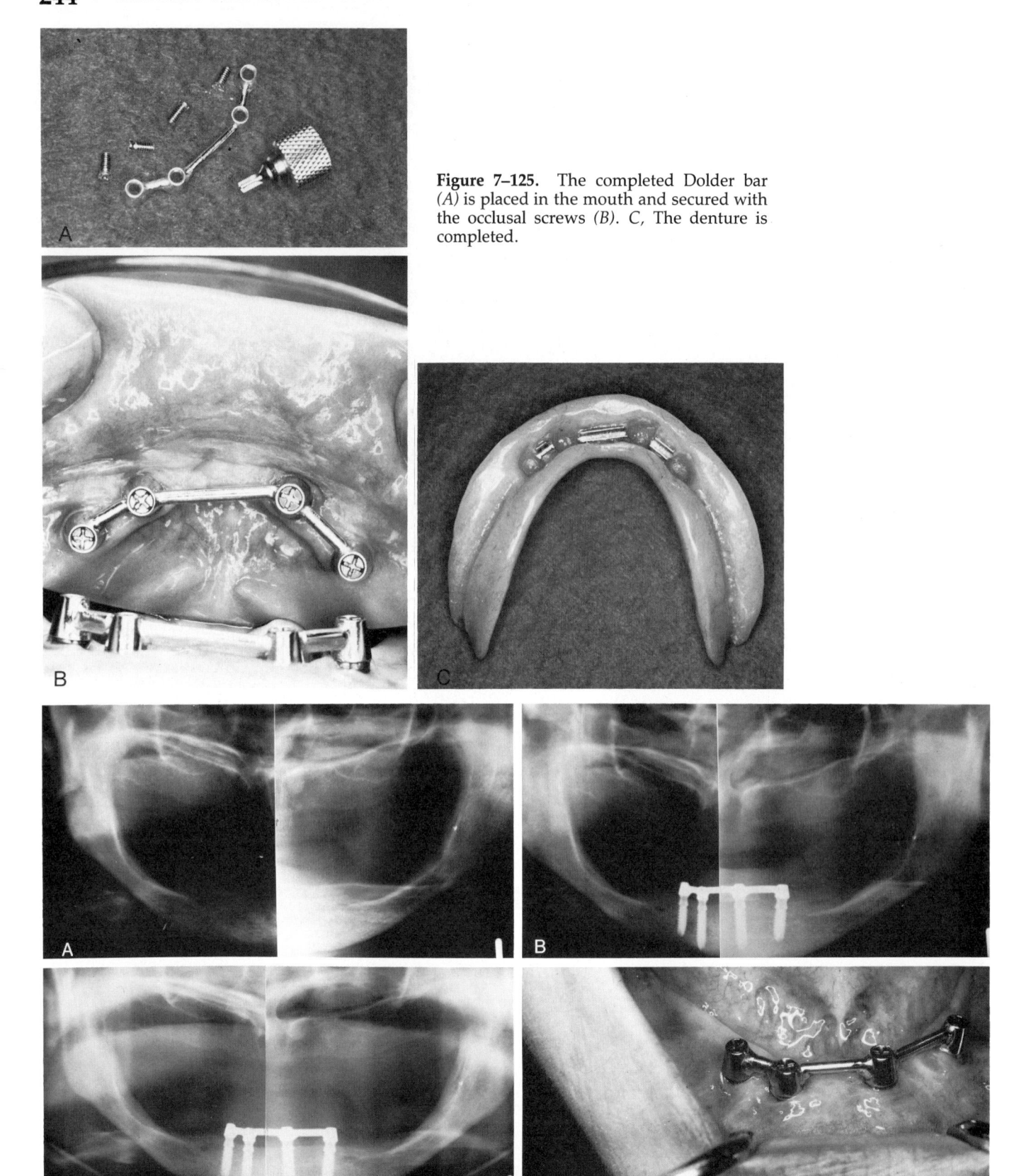

Figure 7–126. *A*, Preoperative panoramic radiograph. *B*, Postinsertion panoramic radiograph with TPS screws in position in the anterior mandible and Dolder bar inserted. *C*, The implants in the panoramic radiograph 24 months after insertion. *D*, Clinical view at 24 months.

(Fig. 7–125). The denture is positioned and the occlusion checked and equilibrated for optimum load bearing.

Summary

Historically, a variety of screw implants have been used in implant dentistry.[130–134] When the anatomy, quality, and quantity of bone in the symphysis of the completely edentulous mandible allows, the screw configuration seems to be best suited. Studies have confirmed several desirable characteristics that, coupled with the screw configuration, result in a superior endosteal implant.[126, 135]

The TPS Screw Implant System has been developed as an entirely standardized system that provides for minimal surgical trauma during preparation of the implant site and final insertion of the screws. The system has been designed to adhere to the guidelines of good surgical and prosthetic principles (Figs. 7–126 and 7–127).

Owing to the material characteristics of titanium, the TPS screw dimensions are optimal for load bearing. The thread design, coupled with the titanium plasma–sprayed coating, maximizes the implant-bone surface contact area. By chemical calculation the contact area increases at least six-fold, resulting in excellent primary stabilization and good force distribution. The highly polished neck allows for a connective tissue seal in the region of the mucogingival junction; the mucosa adheres closely to the new abutment.[128]

If complications should arise with the TPS screw implants, the superstructure can be removed atraumatically by unscrewing the occlusal screws and removing the offending unit. The superstructure can be replaced and, if there is no radiographic evidence of a bony defect at the end of a three- to four-month waiting period, a new TPS screw can be placed. The superstructure can then be cut and resoldered if necessary and replaced. The case is thus salvaged.

ENDOSTEAL BLADE-VENT IMPLANTS

Charles A. Babbush

The first endosseous blade-vent implant was introduced to the dental profession over 15 years ago.[136] The use of the blade-vent has increased steadily in frequency.[137–146]

As with the roots of natural teeth, the endosteal blade-vent implant is inserted into

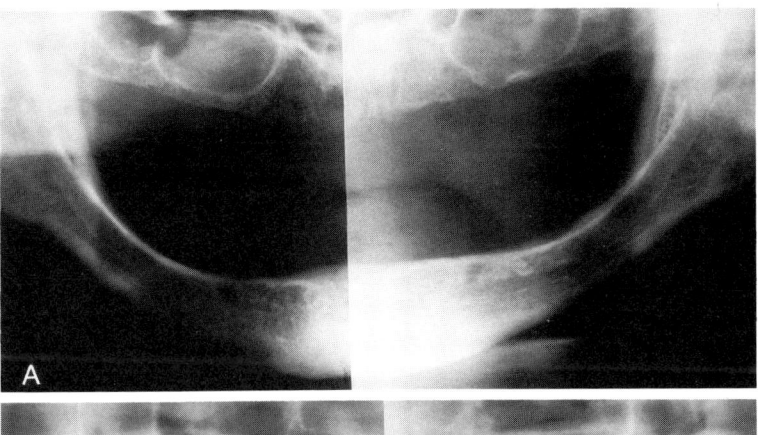

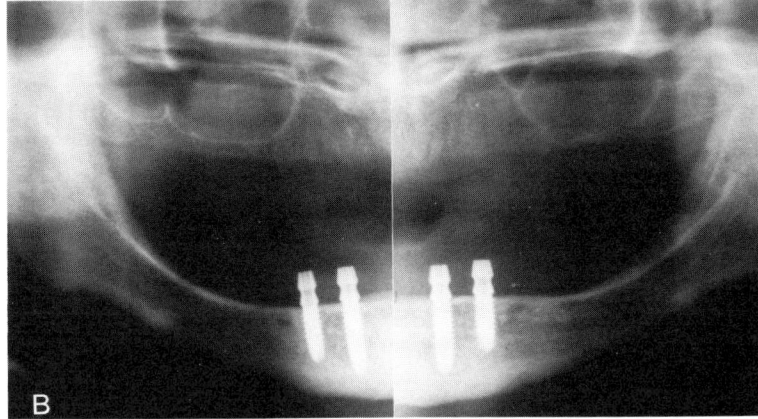

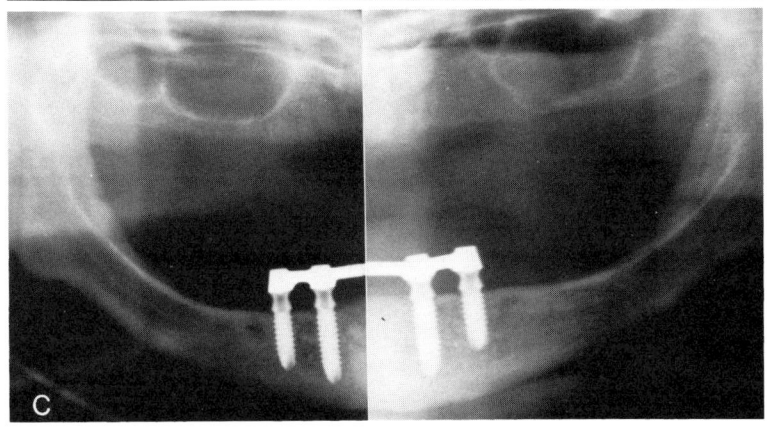

Figure 7–127. *A,* Preoperative panoramic radiograph. *B,* Immediate postinsertion panoramic radiograph with the TPS screws in position in the anterior mandible. *C,* The 12-month postinsertion radiograph demonstrates normal healing.

the residual alveolar ridge. The subperiosteal implant, however, is placed on the basal bone of the mandible and beneath the mucoperiosteal tissues.

Several changes have been made in the endosteal blade-vent implant since its origination. In recent years, design modifications have improved it to the level of use we have today.[138, 147, 148]

The blade-vent implant is not indicated for use as an unsupported replacement for a single tooth. Nor is it indicated as an abutment for a removable prosthesis or as a support unit for a cantilevered restoration. Classically, the blade-vent has been indicated and used as a distal abutment for distal free-end cases, or as an intratooth support for long-span fixed prosthetic appliances. It also requires a sufficient width and height of alveolar bone without violating the boundaries of the inferior alveolar canal and mental neurovascular bundle in the mandible, or the floor of the maxillary sinus or nasal cavity in the maxilla. An overdenture with internal clip fixation has been a successful means of restoring the alveolar ridge that is not atrophied. Additionally, four and as many as six endosseous blade-vent implants, in an edentulous arch with a Dolder-type connector bar, are used as mesostructures.

Implant Design

Each and every implant has a certain design concept basic to the implant. Basically, the endosteal blade-vent is made with an abutment head, a neck, and a body that contains various designs of vents and small recessed areas in the shoulder or superior aspects of the body (Fig. 7–128). All blades of recent vintage are made of titanium. Most blades are surface texture coated, which creates a more biologic environment and increases the implant-bone ratio.

The abutment head is usually etched or demarcated in a millimeter measurement to allow for adjustments related to the occlusal surface of the opposing dentition. The abutment head is usually designed to simulate the preparation of a natural abutment for full crown coverage. It is tapered to allow for appropriate parallelism of adjacent abutments and for adequate primary retention of the prosthesis. Tapering also allows for distribution of functional loading in a physiologic manner. The outer circumference of the vents is beveled to increase the implant-bone

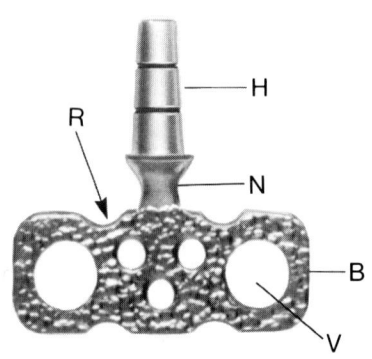

Figure 7–128. The basic structures of the endosteal blade-vent implant are head (H), neck (N), body (B), vents (V), and countersink recess (R).

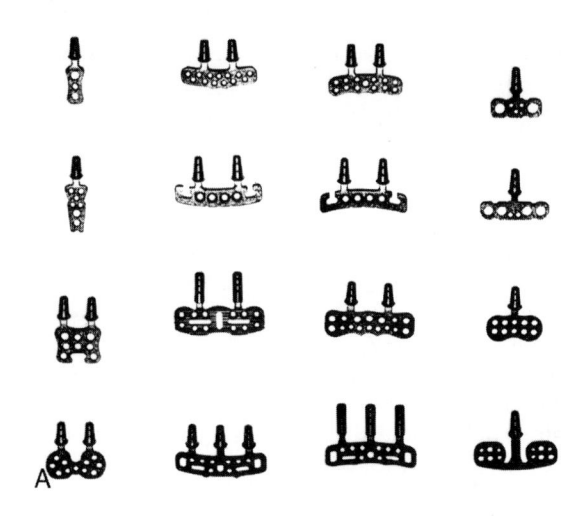

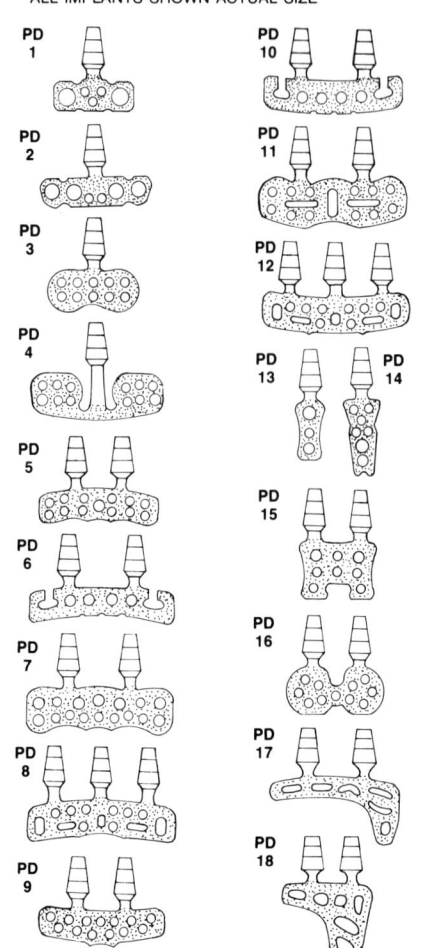

Figure 7–129. Numerous prefabricated designs are available to accommodate the various anatomic sites in both the maxillary and mandibular ridges.

ratio, thereby increasing retention. Numerous prefabricated designs are available to accommodate the various anatomic sites in both the maxillary and mandibular ridges (Fig. 7–129).

Armamentarium

When mucoperiosteal osseous surgical procedures are carried out, autoclaving of all instruments, materials, and implants is indicated. A variety of containers is available for storage and sterilization of the implants. The container and its contents are sterilized prior to each procedure. Some type of pick-up instrument should be included in the implant container so that a sterile field can be maintained throughout the procedure.

A series of instruments has been designed and fabricated with titanium tips. This instrument package has precision fittings for the implant and is biocompatible for a more favorable prognosis (Fig. 7–130). Additionally, standard surgical instruments are selected to carry out the mucoperiosteal and osseous preparations. The use of noncompatible material or design or inadequate instrumentation will cause trauma to the surrounding or adjacent tissues, damage to the implant itself, and/or improper placement of the implant.

Channel Burs. A special pair of carbide burs has been designed. The neck of the bur is tapered so that binding at the ridge crest does not occur and a sufficiently deep preparation can be made to accommodate the body plus the neck of the implant. The bur sizes are 700XL and 700XXL. The 700XL bur is used with all implant sizes for the initial entry at the ridge crest. The 700XXL is used to its complete depth for the osseous preparation in the longer implant designs. The thickest or widest portion of the implant buccolingually is 1.2 mm at the shoulder. The bur is matched to this dimension. Use of any other burs results in an improper osseous preparation. An undersized bur would prepare a channel of insufficient size to accommodate the implant. When attempting to insert the implant in the osseous preparation site, overcompression of the buccal and lingual walls of the osseous sites may occur. If resistance is encountered on insertion, the inserting mallet may be overused, causing fracture of a cortical plate. Overcompression could be responsible for an avascular necrosis of the surrounding bone with resultant failure. An excessively large bur would result in a mobile implant, which is completely contraindicated in endosteal implantation.

Both burs must be used with generous amounts of irrigation, both from the handpiece and from syringes held by the assistant. This irrigation will act as a lubricant and a coolant to prevent overheating of the osseous tissues, which creates the potential for sequestration.

Channel Depth Measure (Titanium-Tipped). The horizontal markings on the blade of the instrument are scaled at 1-mm intervals. In this manner, a comparison between channel depth and implant seating potentials can be accurately made.

Single-Headed Seating Instrument (Titanium-Tipped). The tip is hollow and telescopes over the implant abutment head in a precision fit. It is used with the surgical mallet. Several light taps are sufficient to seat the implant in its final position.

Double-Headed Seating Instrument (Titanium-Tipped). The tip of this instrument is wide enough to telescope over both heads of a double-headed implant. It is used with the surgical mallet. Several light taps are sufficient to seat the implant in its final position. It can be used in an eccentric position to seat either the mesial or distal portion of the implant when necessary.

Counterseating Instrument (Titanium-Tipped). This instrument is engaged in the final stage of implant insertion, more so with the single than with the double abutment. It is employed to prevent damage to the crestal bone, as the tip is narrower than the channel and the shoulder of the implant. It engages

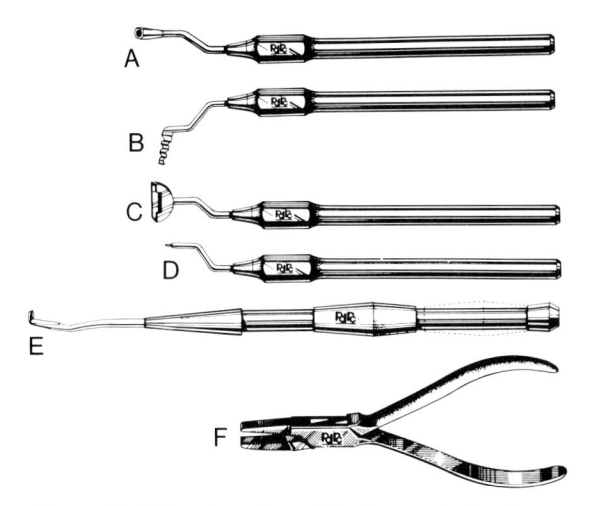

Figure 7–130. A series of instruments has been designed and fabricated with titanium tips. These instruments should be used during the insertion of the implant. They are *(A)* single-headed seating instrument, *(B)* channel depth measure/curette, *(C)* double-headed seating instrument, *(D)* counterseating instrument, *(E)* implant remover, and *(F)* a pair of contouring pliers.

the depression in the shoulder of the implant and is used for eccentric adjustments when the implant requires additional mesial-distal alignment.

Contouring Pliers (Titanium-Tipped). The pliers are used only in pairs. In some instances, especially in the cuspid and first bicuspid regions, a curvature of the arch is present. The pliers are used to contour the body of the implant to fit the contour of the arch and its subsequent channel preparation.

Tapping Mallet. The instrument should have Teflon tips to reduce trauma. It is used in conjunction with the single- and double-headed inserting instrument and the counter-seating instrument. No more than three to five gentle taps should be necessary for the final seating of an implant. If excessive tapping is necessary, remove the implant with the implant remover instrument and reevaluate the channel. Further bony preparation may be necessary.

Implant Remover (Titanium-Tipped). The prongs at the tip of the instrument are designed to fit around the implant next to and under the base of the abutment. It is a reverse tapping mallet. It is used to remove the implant when further preparation of the channel or contouring of the implant is necessary.

Semilunar Tissue Punch. In some instances when the mucoperiosteal flaps are repositioned, bunching and straining of the soft tissue occurs. The tissue punch is used to create a neat semilunar removal of gingival tissue at the buccal or lingual aspect of the neck. This technique should be used only if a sufficient amount of attached gingival tissue remains. Additionally, it is necessary to have available a needle holder, suture scissors, and suture material of choice.

Technique

The selection of the appropriate implant will mark the initiation of the procedure. Using the mounted study cast, the panoramic radiograph, and visual assessment of the oral cavity will produce the best results. The transparent template is superimposed over the radiograph in the area of intended implantation (Fig. 7–131). The size of implant should be the largest that will fit in the area without impinging on or violating vital adjacent structures. An appropriate margin of 2 to 3 mm from such vital anatomic areas as the inferior alveolar canal, mental foramen, floor of the maxillary sinus, and floor of the nasal cavity is recommended.

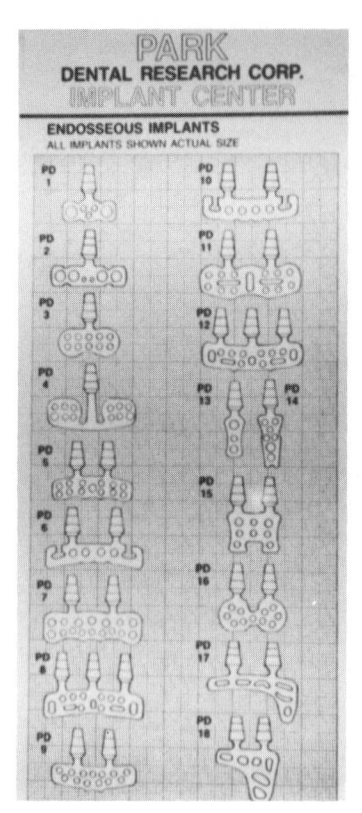

Figure 7–131. The transparent template is superimposed over the preoperative radiograph to aid in the appropriate implant selection.

The proper implant size should be obvious. Usually, neither periapical radiographs alone nor panoramic radiographs alone are sufficient to make this selection. Panoramic radiographs should be used in conjunction with periapical film.[149]

The adjacent natural abutments should have been prepared preoperatively for full crown coverage. Additionally, a temporary prosthesis that covers these preparations and extends over the area of implantations is fabricated. This prosthesis is now placed in the mouth. A mark with a sterile magic marker is made on the buccal mucosa opposite the crown. This provides a reference point for the placement of the implant (Fig. 7–132).

The incision should be made at the crest of the alveolar ridge and through the mucoperiosteum (Fig. 7–132). It should be 1.5 times longer than the mesial-distal length of the implant to allow for sufficient operating room. The mucoperiosteum is reflected in both a buccal and a lingual direction to expose the complete buccolingual width and direction of the bony ridge (Fig. 7–133).

A knife-edged or spiculated bony crest is frequently encountered, more so in the maxilla than in the mandible. The irregularities can be eliminated by using a large ovoid car-

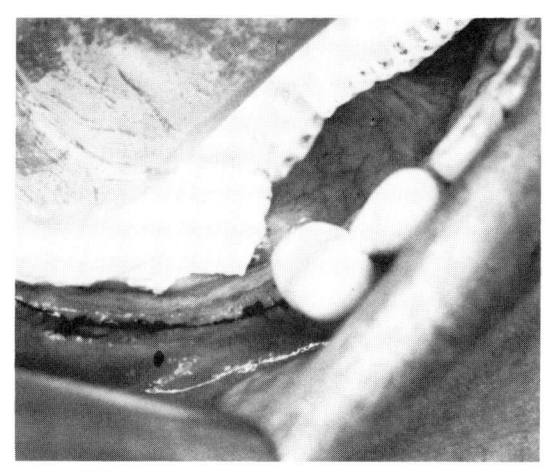

IMPLANTS USED IN PREPROSTHETIC RECONSTRUCTIVE SURGERY / **249**

Figure 7–132. A sterile magic marker is used to mark a point of reference on the buccal mucosa, as a guide in the placement of the implant. A full-thickness mucoperiosteal incision 1.5 times longer than the length of the implant is made over the midcrestal area.

bide acrylic laboratory bur in a straight handpiece to plateau the bone. This bone should be reduced until a buccolingual ledge of at least 2 mm is created. This dimension will then accommodate the 1.2-mm width of the implant. If soft-tissue tags or other bony spurs remain, they should be burnished with a bone file. The bony channel should be placed at the ridge crest, parallel to the buccal and lingual bony cortex. The implant should be held against the bony ridge to estimate the length of the preparation, which should be 1 to 2 mm longer than the implant to facilitate ease of insertion. The 700XL and 700XXL burs in a high-speed contra-angle handpiece, with copious amounts of water, are used for the osseous preparation (Fig. 7–134).

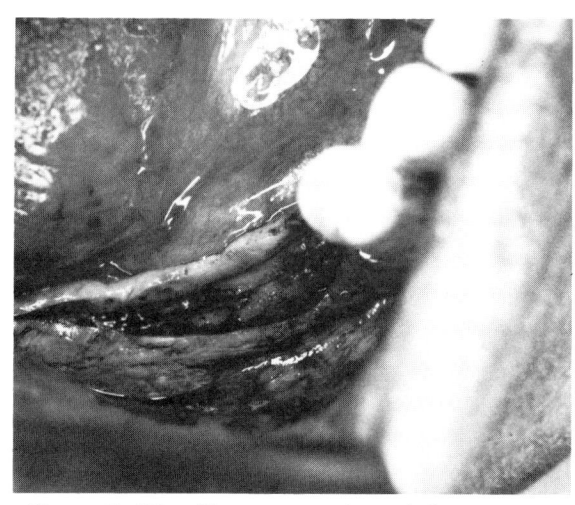

Figure 7–133. The mucoperiosteal flaps are reflected in both the buccal and lingual directions. The full buccolingual width and direction of the bony ridge must be exposed.

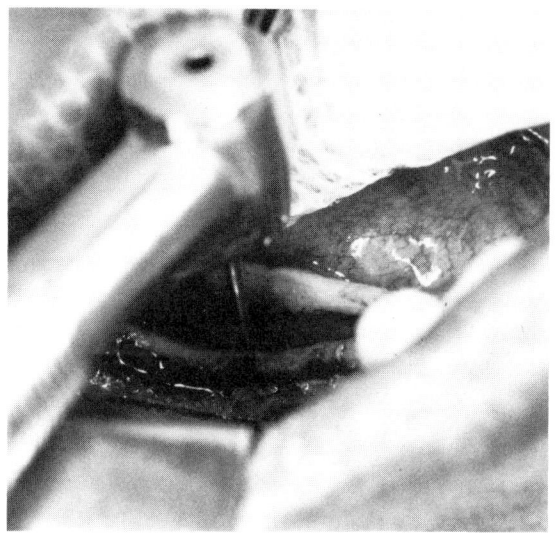

Figure 7–134. The 700XL and 700XXL burs in a high-speed contra-angle handpiece, with copious amounts of water, are used for the osseous preparation.

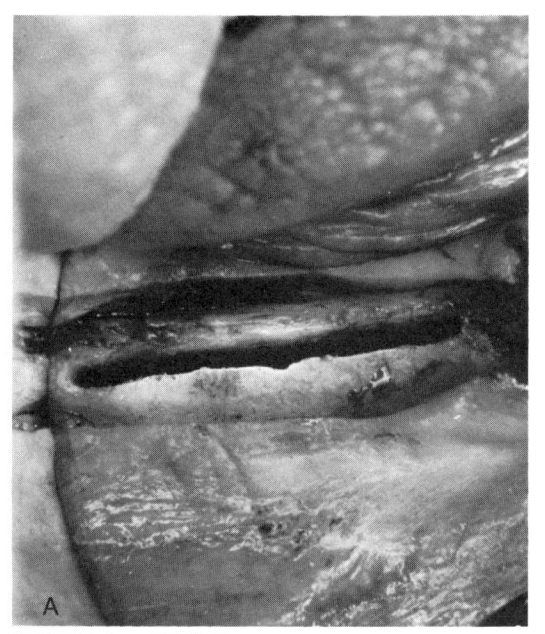

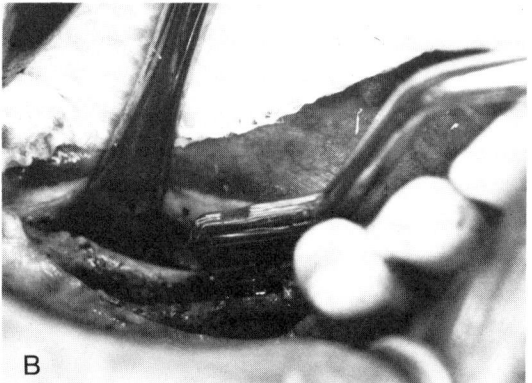

Figure 7–135. When the osseous preparation is complete, the area should be completely irrigated with saline (A) and the depth of the preparation verified with the channel curette/depth gauge (B).

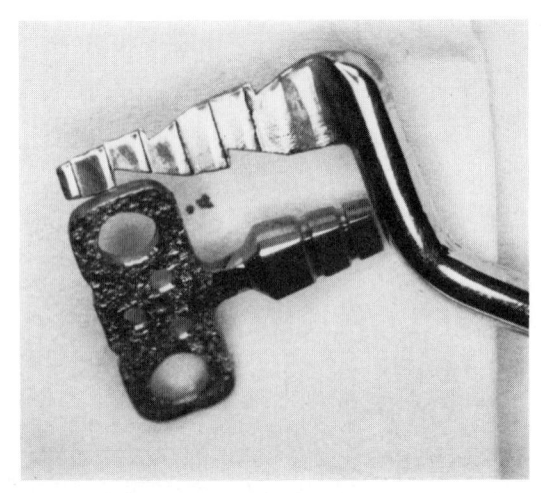

Figure 7–136. The implant is held alongside the depth gauge and an estimation of osseous depth, the body plus the neck, is obtained. This is transferred to the bone depth with the gauge.

One of two techniques can be used to initiate the bony preparation. Numerous puncture points can be made in the ridge crest along the length of the preparation. These are spaced at 3- to 5-mm intervals and then connected together with the drill. Alternatively, the bur can be used like a paint brush and stroked gently back and forth until the groove is initiated in the ridge crest. Regardless of technique, the drilling is carried to a depth that will accommodate the vertical measurement of the body plus the neck of the implant. When the base of the abutment head contacts the crest of the alveolar ridge, the implant is completely seated. When the osseous preparation is completed, the channel should be irrigated and cleansed with water and the channel curette (Fig. 7–135). In addition, as the channel curette/depth gauge is drawn from mesial to distal in the channel, the depth of the preparation is verified as the gauge rises and falls (Fig. 7–136). If further preparation is necessary, it should be carried out at this time.

The implant is then placed into the channel with finger pressure only. If the preparation is appropriate, the implant should easily be inserted until two thirds of the body is in the channel. The parallelism with the adjacent natural teeth, the alignment with the opposing arch, and the occlusal clearance for the prosthesis fabrication are checked at this time. If any alterations are necessary, the implant should be removed with the implant remover (Fig. 7–137). *Under no circumstances* should any adjustments be carried out with the implant in the channel. Damage to or fracture of the adjacent and surrounding osseous structures may result.

Angulation of the head is carried out with the contouring pliers, as a pair, to adjust for alignment with the opposing arch (Fig. 7–138A). The angle should not exceed 15 degrees, as functional forces will then be carried outside the long axis of the implant and will adversely affect the long-range prognosis (Fig. 7–138B). In many instances, the reduction of the height of the abutment head will be necessary. The use of a medium-grit diamond or a separating disc will be satisfactory. Once the reduction is carried out, with 1.5 to 2.5 mm clearance, the cut end should be repolished with a Burlew sulci disc. The implant should then be cleansed in an ultrasonic cleaner, rinsed in water, and sterilized in a bead sterilizer.

The implant is once again placed in the channel and checked for correct alignment and parallelism. The inserting instrument is placed over the abutment head and tapped into final position with the mallet (Fig. 7–139). Final position is achieved when the base of the abutment head is in contact with the crestal bone. If the alignment of the head is mesiodistally incorrect, the implant will require adjustment with the counterseating instrument (Fig. 7–140).

Final inspection should be carried out with special attention to mobility. As a general rule, all endosteal implants must be totally immobile upon final seating. If any mobility exists, the implant should be removed. In the case of the blade-vent, it is usually an excessively large channel that causes this problem. Once again, the implant should be removed with the implant remover. The body of the implant can be bowed with a pair of contouring pliers. If this is not sufficient, the mesial and distal ends of the body are bowed to the buccal or lingual to form an "S" shaped body. In addition, the buccal

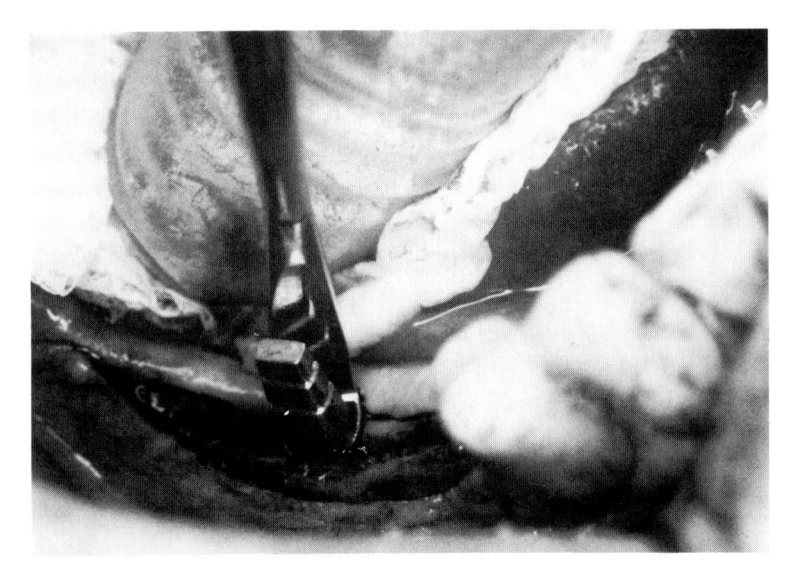

Figure 7–137. The implant can be removed with the implant remover when any modifications are necessary.

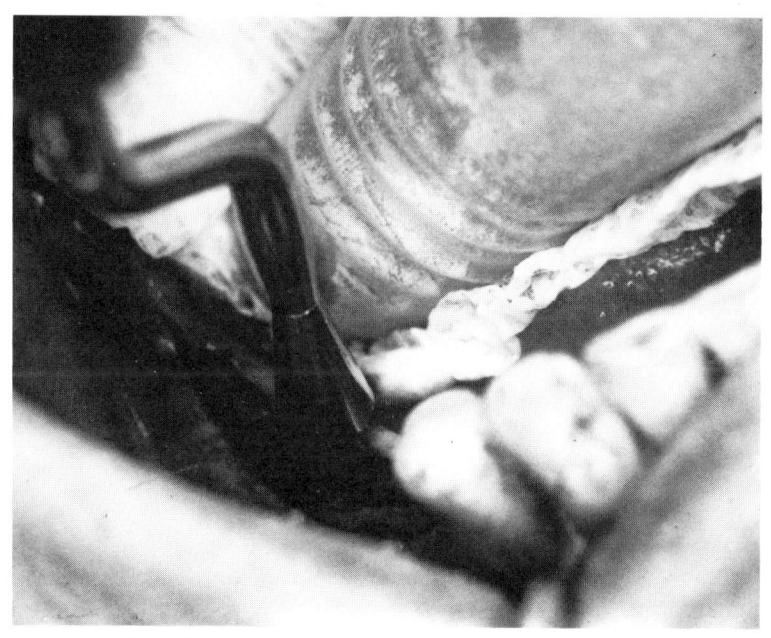

IMPLANTS USED IN PREPROSTHETIC RECONSTRUCTIVE SURGERY / 251

Figure 7–139. The inserting instrument is placed over the abutment head and tapped with the inserting mallet into final position. Four to six light taps should be sufficient for complete seating if the channel has been prepared properly.

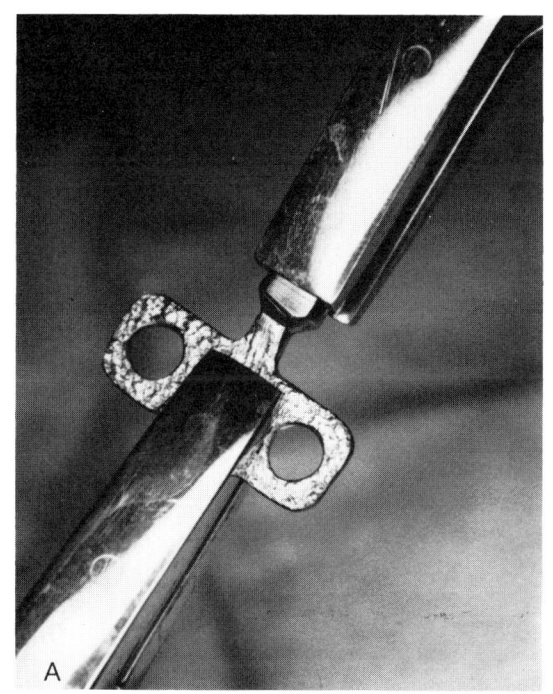

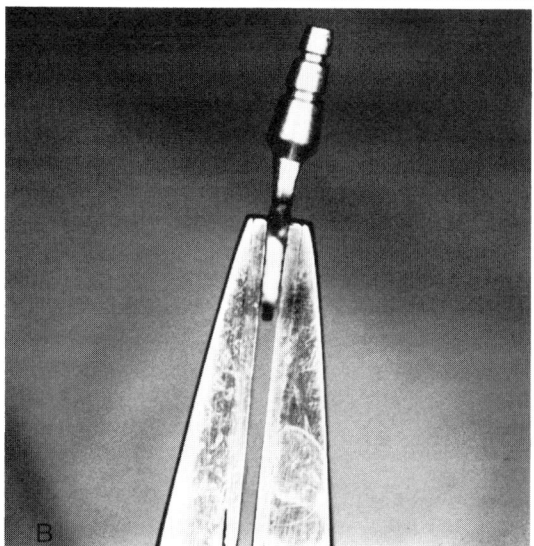

Figure 7–138. *A,* Angulation of the head is carried out with the contouring pliers, as a pair, to adjust for alignment with the opposing arch. *B,* The angle of adjustment should not exceed 15 degrees, as functional forces will then be outside the long axis of the implant.

stances, when an endosteal implant is seated, the base of the abutment will encounter the more superior lingual wall and prevent complete seating on the *buccal.* To correct this situation, it is necessary to *create* a countersunk area at the abutment on the lingual with the high-speed 700XL bur. The implant is once again seated and the shoulder is completely countersunk in both the buccal and lingual areas (Fig. 7–141).

The area is irrigated with copious amounts of saline, and the mucoperiosteal flaps are repositioned. The soft tissue in the area of the abutment head is inspected. Occasion-

and lingual cortices should be inspected for possible fracture. If a fracture is present, the implant must be removed and the soft tissues reapproximated and sutured. The patient should be informed of the problem. If he is still desirous of having an implant placed in this area, a six- to nine-month waiting period is advisable.

The natural resorption of the maxillary and mandibular alveolar ridges leaves the lingual aspect of the ridge in a more superior position than the buccal aspect. In *many* in-

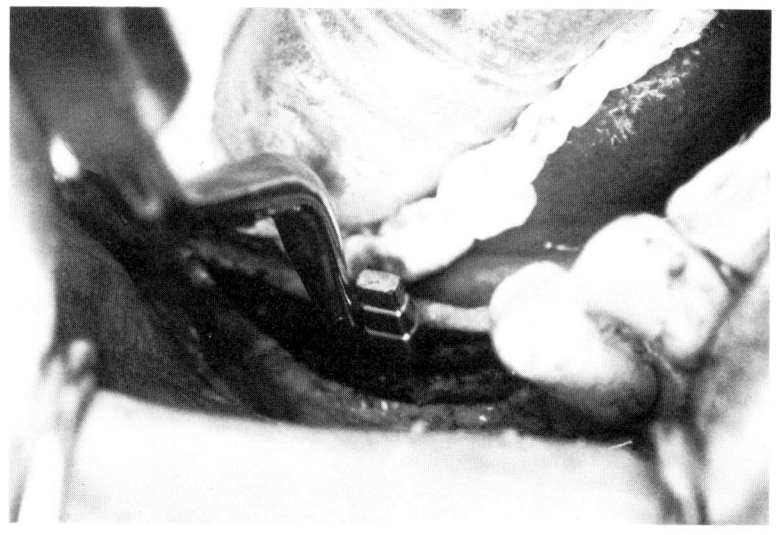

Figure 7–140. The counterseating instrument is used to improve the mesial-distal alignment of the implant without traumatizing the crestal bone.

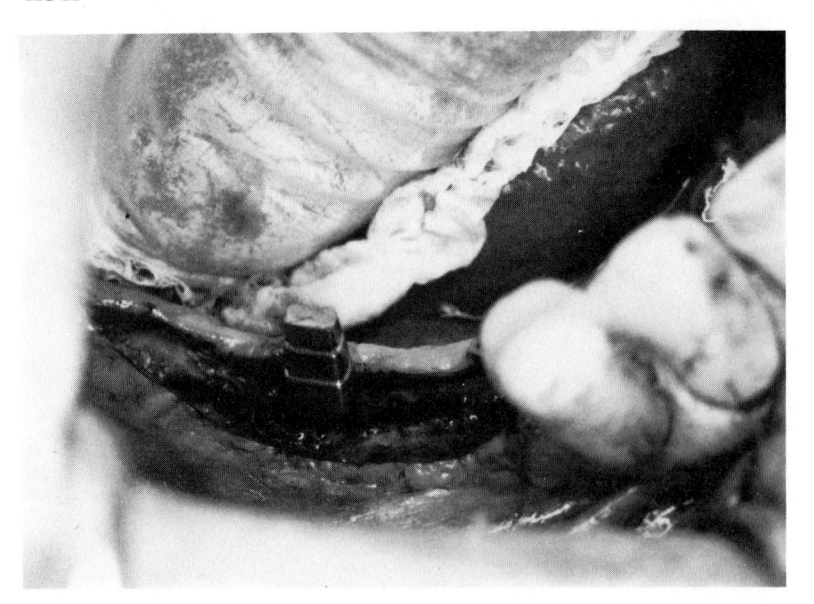

Figure 7–141. The implant is completely seated when the base of the abutment head is in contact with the crestal bone and the shoulder is more than 2 mm below this point.

ally, this area will have an excess bulk of gingival tissue, which can be removed with the semilunar tissue punch to create a more physiologic healing environment. One must be careful not to remove too much of the attached gingival tissues. The flaps are then approximated and sutured with 3-0 black silk interrupted sutures (Fig. 7–142). In most cases, an immediate postinsertion radiograph is advisable to check the position of the implant in relation to adjacent vital structures.

Temporization of the endosteal blade-vent implant has been a controversial issue. Temporization offers several advantages. The endosteal blade-vent implant is a two-dimensional implant, having height and width but no depth, the third dimension. It was never designed to be used as a self-standing un-

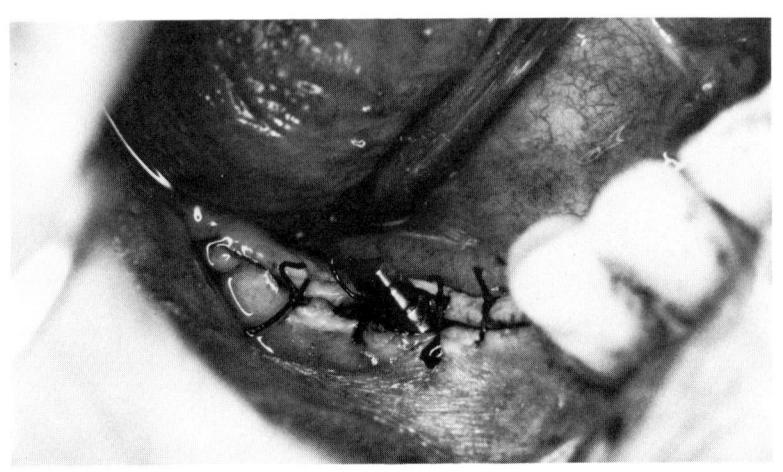

Figure 7–142. The mucoperiosteal flaps are re-approximated and sutured with 3-0 silk interrupted sutures.

splinted entity. Therefore, it should have support at the time when it is weakest, during the immediate postinsertion period. When bone is traumatized, as in the preparation of the osseous channel, the response of that bone is a catabolic one. During the 10- to 21-day postinsertion period, the implant may become slightly mobile and should be splinted. Psychologically, the temporary prosthesis serves as a confidence builder for the patient, as he can be discharged with an esthetically pleasing functional unit.

A prefabricated, heat-cured, temporary prosthesis should be supplied by the dental laboratory. The design should include coverage of the adjacent natural abutments and extend into the area of the anticipated implant abutment post. The pontic should be of a sanitary design so that there is no impingement on the crestal soft tissues. The occlusal table should be narrowed to reduce trauma. The finish line on the implant abutment should be supragingival to avoid tissue impingement and maintain a self-cleaning environment. If a small square of rubber dam is placed over the abutment head, ingress of cementing material around the neck of the implant and along the incision line will be prevented. When the prosthesis is seated, the rubber dam is pulled to the buccal and cut with scissors. It will then slide out from around the abutment neck and from under the bridge.

Routinely, the patient is given only a prescription for analgesics and is instructed about the proper oral hygiene techniques. He is told to resume a normal diet but is cautioned not to carry this to excess. Because he is wearing only a plastic prosthesis, it will not withstand the excessive trauma of such foods as candy apples, caramels, etc.

The sutures and temporary prosthesis are removed five to seven days later. The implant should be inspected for tenderness or mobility as well as the progress of the soft tissue healing. Usually by the end of two or three weeks, postsurgical edema has completely subsided so that the final impression can be obtained. The case is completed following good standards of fixed prosthesis reconstruction (Figs. 7–143 to 7–147).[150]

Five years have elapsed since the Consensus Development Conference at Harvard University and 15 years since the first clinical use of endosteal blade-vent implants.[151] The recommendation of "use with guidelines" is still in effect. Every procedure should have guidelines so that a clear set of indications and contraindications are available to the professional. The guidelines are an endorsement of and not a limitation to these proce-

IMPLANTS USED IN PREPROSTHETIC RECONSTRUCTIVE SURGERY / **253**

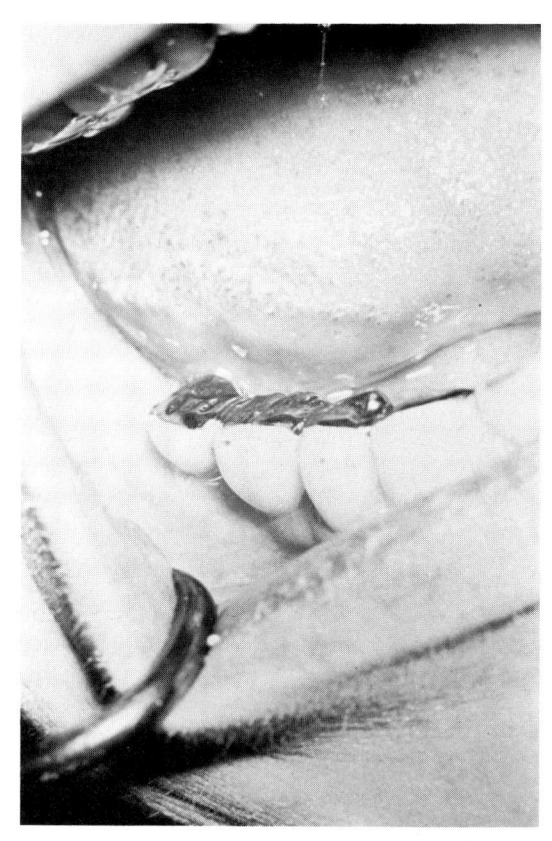

Figure 7–143. The case is completed after the soft tissue healing has reached the final phase.

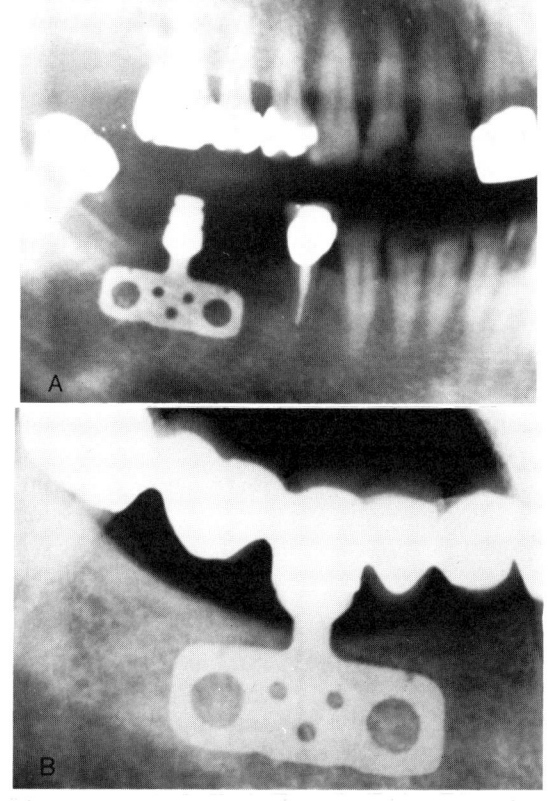

Figure 7–144. *A,* Immediate postinsertion radiograph of a blade-vent implant as an intermediary support for a long-span bridge. *B,* Three-year postinsertion radiograph.

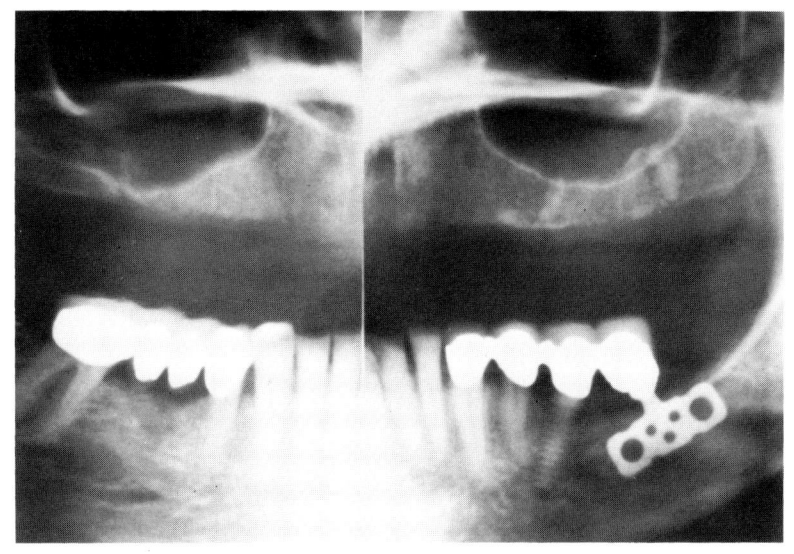

Figure 7–145. A five-year postinsertion radiograph of a distal abutment for a fixed prosthesis.

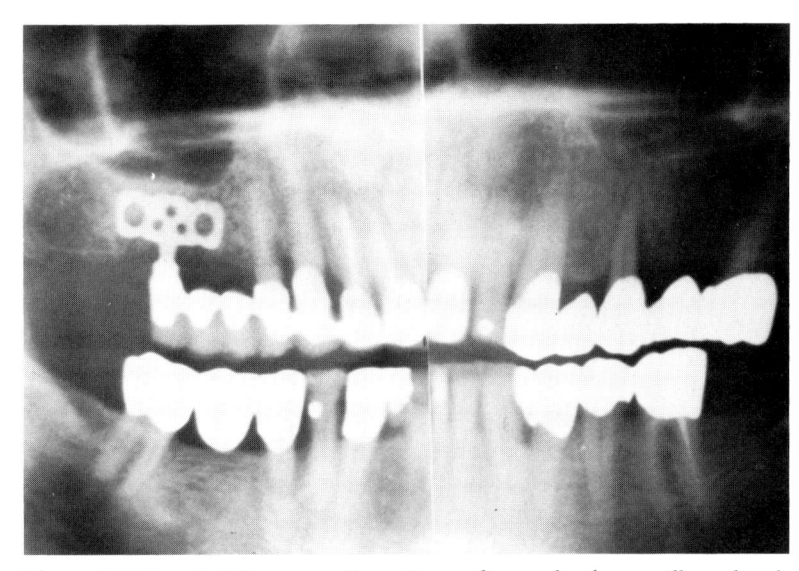

Figure 7–146. A 6.5-year postinsertion radiograph of a maxillary distal abutment for a fixed prosthesis.

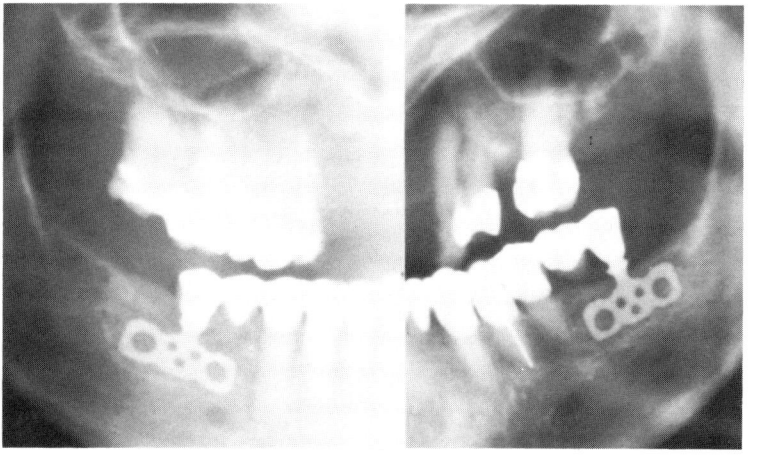

Figure 7–147. A six-year postinsertion radiograph of bilateral mandibular distal abutments for a fixed prosthesis.

dures. Endosteal implants can be used as an alternative to other conventional restorative procedures. A more favorable prognosis can be expected when there is adequate vertical bone height, with sufficient intermaxillary space, and when fixed prosthetics are indicated. The doctor must have an adequate training program on a continuing education basis. If the above criteria are met, a minimum of 75 per cent five-year survival of the implant can be expected. If a failure should develop, the patient should have no residual sequelae after removal of the implant or be left in a poorer state of function than before the procedure was carried out. The five-year survivals in my series have been at the 90 per cent level. The ten-year survivals have ranged between 70 and 80 per cent.

ITI Endosteal Hollow-Basket Implant Systems*

Charles A. Babbush

Since the advent of dental endosteal implant restoration with the placement of stainless steel screws by Stroch and Stroch, a variety of shapes, materials, and surgical techniques has been used. Most of these early implants had a very low percentage of success. Many failures were due to faulty stress-strength calculations. Incorrect mechanical designs cause bone resorption or compressive loading. As implants are designed, it is imperative that the biocompatibility of the implant material and the microstructure of the implant surface be considered.[152] (1) The implant configuration should guarantee high strength characteristics as well as maximum anchoring surface with a minimum loss of bone. (2) The micromorphologic surface quality should favor the healing process. (3) The implant must possess good biocompatibility and adequate mechanical strength.

Because of the differences in bone quality and quantity between the anterior and posterior aspects of the jaw and the maxilla and mandible, the development of an ideal implant configuration, suitable for all these anatomic sites, is most difficult and challenging. Therefore, a variety of configurations have been developed to meet these diverse requirements. The ITI Hollow-Basket design, with lateral fenestrations, was selected as the primary prototype (Fig. 7–148).* These systems are indicated primarily for use in the cuspid through molar region of the mandible, with modification for anterior mandibular reconstruction and for the maxilla.

The major design consideration related to the microscopic features of this implant is the open structure and the constricted area at the implant neck. The various perforations of the cylinder create conditions for good blood supply. In addition, growth of calcified tissue over the shoulder area takes place quickly and continuously until it reaches the neck area (Fig. 7–149). The most favorable implant shape would be one that could withstand functional loads in three dimensions; height, width, and depth. The Hollow-Basket designs meet these criteria. Additionally, the Hollow-Basket allows for a precision fit in the initial preparation site due to high quality technology of the entire system, which results in primary stability. The plasma spray surface promotes maximum implant-bone ratios with a resultant osseointegrated (ankylotic) relationship. Since placement of the system uses a trephined osseous preparation, minimal removal of bone is possible. Extensive laboratory and clinical evaluations of these implants have documented the efficacy of these systems.[153]

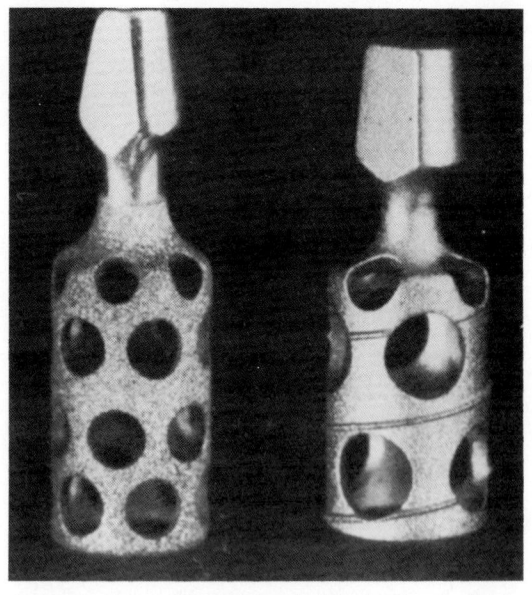

Figure 7–148. The original 1974 hollow cylinder and hollow screw implants with vented body and shoulder regions.

---

*I wish to thank the International Team for Implants (ITI), Professor Dr. Andre Schroeder, its President, Mr. Franz Sutter, and Dr. Fritz Straumann of the Institute Straumann, Waldenburg, Switzerland, for their advice and support as well as the technical and photographic information for this work. In addition, I wish to thank Mr. Bart Colucci, President, Colmed LTD, Half Moon Bay, California, for his cooperation in the clinical aspects of this work.

*Institute Straumann

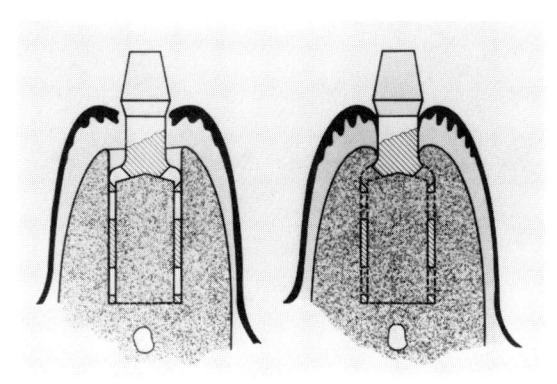

Figure 7–149. Hollow-Basket implant immediately after insertion (left): after eight weeks bone proliferates over the shoulder and through the vents (right).

The actual material and surface finish are the remaining essential factors necessary for a successful implant. Many researchers and authors have documented the importance of the biocompatibility of the material.[154-164] Long-term laboratory research, animal studies, and clinical evaluations have shown titanium to be the material of choice for the Hollow-Basket Systems. These implants are then coated with titanium plasma spray (TPS), which promotes direct bone opposition (ankylosis, osseointegration).[165, 166] TPS causes a six-fold increase in the surface area of the implant over the nonsprayed core. Thus the implant-bone ratio is greatly increased, for a more favorable long-range prognosis.

The question of fenestrations (vents) has long been a controversial one, dating back as far as the original Linkow Endosteal Blade-Vent Implant. The Hollow-Basket Systems were designed with a specific bioengineering concept in the use of these vents and their value has been substantiated by animal studies.[166] Once bone has proliferated over the shoulder and through the vents, postoperatively, a significant reduction in shear load along the bone-implant interface takes place. The Straumann Institute research staff has proven that this bone bridge, on models, supports at least 25 per cent of the axial load of any given Hollow-Basket Implant (Fig. 7–150).

Indication for Implant Placement According to Design

The osseous variations in the alveolar ridges are considerable. In order to accommodate the large numbers of anatomic variations, a variety of implant designs is needed. These designs must consider the mesiodistal, buccolingual, and inferior-superior measurements of available residual edentulous bone (Fig. 7–151). The adjacent vital structures, such as the inferior alveolar and mental neurovascular bundles, must be circumvented with at least a 2-mm margin of safety.[167]

The Hollow-Basket Implant Systems have been used since 1974 to restore the mandibular bicuspid and molar regions. Choice of implant designs "C," "E," "K," "H," and "F" depends on the available bone, for placement must be made without impinging on adjacent vital structures.

Owing to the extremely sophisticated bioengineering of the inserting mechanisms, these implants are easily placed for restoration of the oral apparatus. The design of the Hollow-Basket Implants, as compared to that of comparable solid implants, has several favorable characteristics. The vented hollow cylindrical design presents a tremendously increased bone-implant contact surface, with resultant reduced loading per unit area (Fig. 7–152).

In the "C" and "E" implants the anchoring surface is approximately one third greater. The "K" is 310 sq mm as compared to 240 sq mm. The "H" design represents 340 sq mm as compared to 230 sq mm. With a reduction in bone removal, owing to the trephining preparation of the osseous site, bone trauma is considerably reduced. The "C" implant is reduced by almost half and the "E," "K," and "H" greater than 50 per cent reduction. Likewise, the implant volume has been reduced in the Hollow-Basket as compared to solid configurations. The "C" implant is 75 per cent less, the "E" is two thirds less, the "K" is 2.5 times smaller, and the "H" is almost 50 per cent reduced in volume. The results, related to these factors are maximization of surface area for bone integration, reduction of bone loss at implant site preparation, and minimal implant volume.

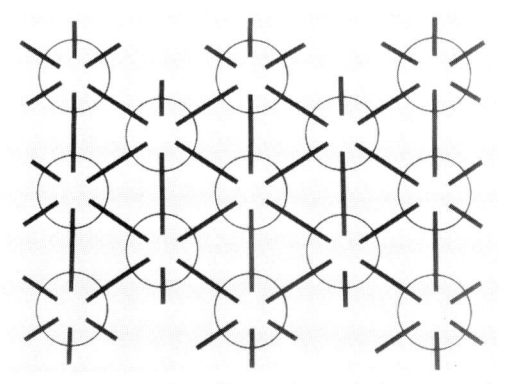

Figure 7–150. The illustration of the vent designs, by the Straumann Institute Research Staff, demonstrates the reduced shear forces between the bone and implant and allows bone bridges to the core.

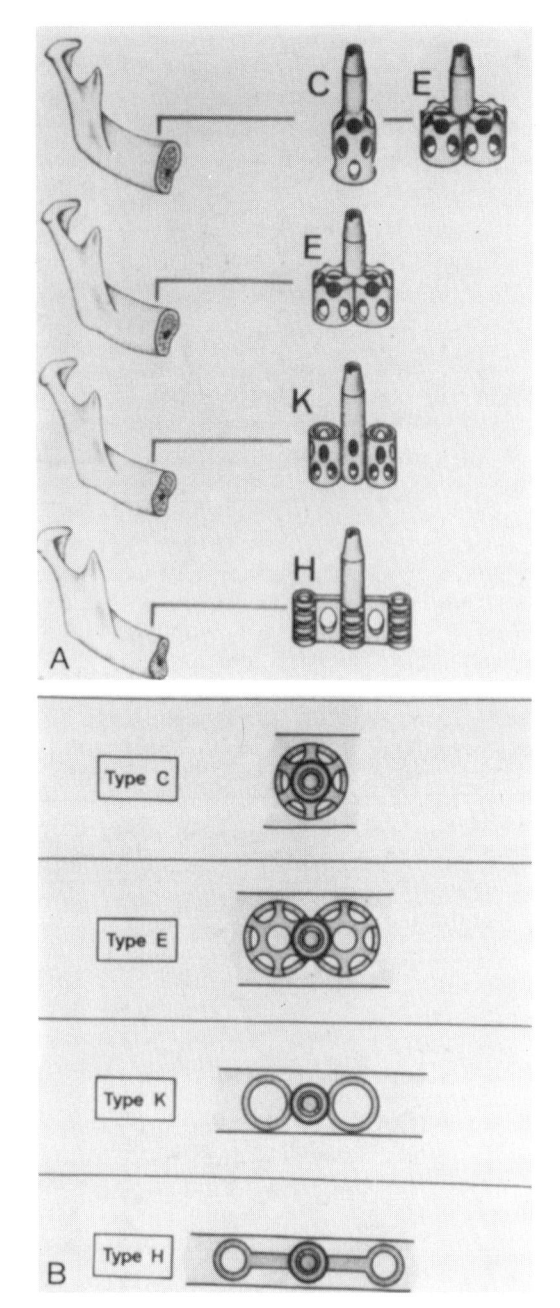

256 / IMPLANTS USED IN PREPROSTHETIC RECONSTRUCTIVE SURGERY

Figure 7–151. *A*, ITI implant system indications as to bone quantities. *B*, Occlusal views of these Hollow-Baskets clearly demonstrate the cylindrical concept in models C, E, K, and H.

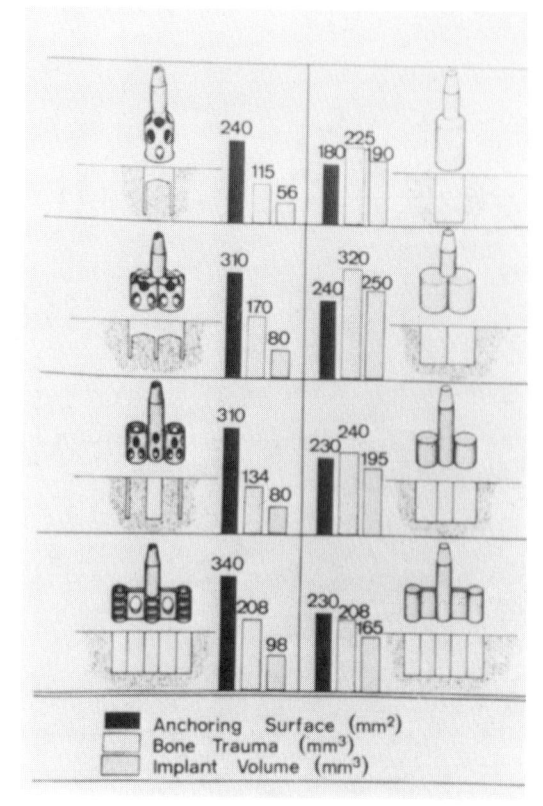

Figure 7–152. Hollow-Basket and Solid-Body implants are compared using anchoring surface, bone trauma, and implant volume.

"C" Endosteal Hollow-Basket Implant System

The type "C" is a single 5.5-mm diameter Hollow-Basket Implant (Fig. 7–153). The basket is 9.5 mm in length, and the neck is available in 4.2-mm and 6.2-mm lengths. Neck length is selected according to the vertical measurement of bone and/or the interocclusal space. A transparent plastic template is supplied with the system which can be superimposed on the radiograph to aid in proper implant selection. This design is used in the bicuspid and molar regions of the mandible.

The procedure is initiated via a midcrestal mucoperiosteal incision. If the ridge crest is irregular or knife-edged, a bevelling procedure can be carried out using a large oval

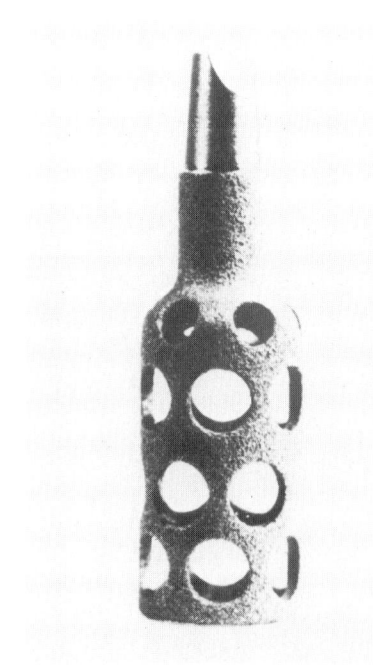

Figure 7–153. The "C" Single-Basket Implant.

Figure 7–154. *A,* The No. 1 trephine is used to make the initial entry into the bone. The try-in template is used to ascertain correct reduction of the core as well as preliminary depth of the osseous walls. *B,* The No. 2 trephine is used to deepen the walls of the osseous preparation site without further reducing the core. The implant can then be seated in the bone.

laboratory carbide bur. The implant site should be inspected to verify that the trephine is placed to obtain maximum parallelism with the adjacent abutments and proper alignment with the opposing arch.

The No. 1 trephine, single groove on the shaft, is used to make the initial entry into the bone. The bur is used in a low-speed, reduction, latch type contra-angle. A pumping motion with copious irrigation is suggested. The trephine will reduce the osseous core 3 mm below the ridge crest and prepare the walls to a depth of 5 mm. Therefore, the total depth is 8 mm (Fig. 7–154*A*). The trephine is then changed to No. 2, two grooves in the shaft. This trephine will not reduce the core any further but will deepen the preparation of the walls to 9.5 mm. The try-in template is inserted in the site to ascertain correct preparation. If the longer neck implant is to be used, each trephine will have to be used to a greater depth. The implant can then be inserted, usually with slight pressure, until the shoulder is 3 mm below the ridge crest (Fig. 7–154*B*).

The mucoperiosteal flaps are repositioned

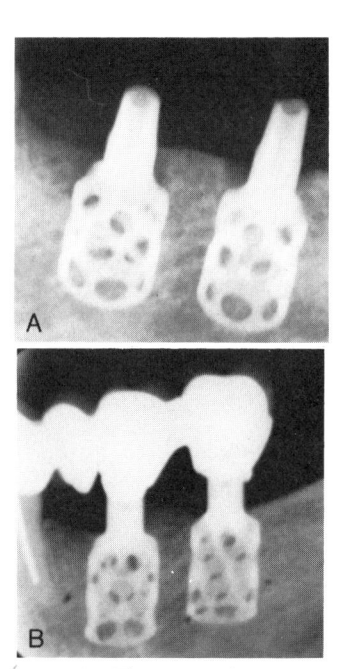

Figure 7–155. *A,* The immediate postinsertion radiograph of two "C" type implants to restore a distal free end case in the mandible. *B,* A 30-month follow-up radiograph.

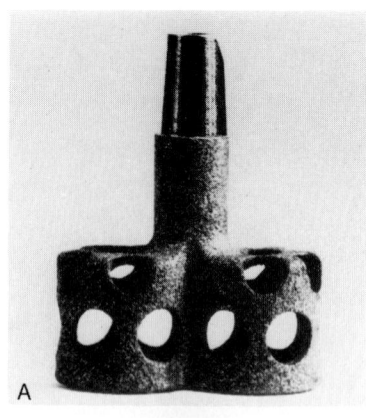

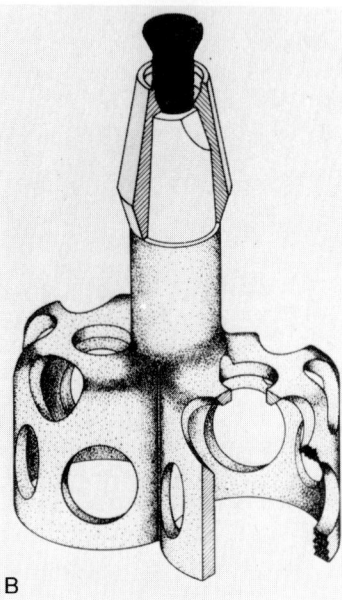

Figure 7–156. *A*, The "E" Double Hollow-Basket Implant. *B*, A cutaway diagram of the "E" implant, with the 4-mm occlusal screw securing the prefabricated gold telescope.

and sutured with interrupted 3-0 or 4-0 silk sutures. The patient is given routine postoperative instructions and analgesics. The sutures are removed five to seven days postop-

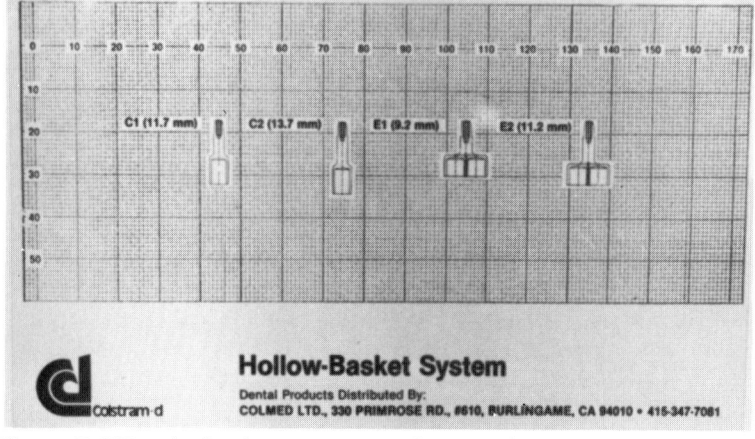

Figure 7–157. A plastic transparent plate can be superimposed over the preoperative radiograph to aid in appropriate implant selection.

eratively. The patient is seen every two weeks for the first two months. The final prosthetic reconstruction can then be completed (Fig. 7–155).

"E" Endosteal Hollow-Basket Implant System

The "E" implant is a double-basket design with a vertical basket height of 5 mm (Fig. 7–156). The diameter is 5.5 mm and the length 10.5 mm. This design is indicated for use in the mandibular molar region. The "E" implant is available with a long (6.2 mm) or a short (4.2 mm) neck. The appropriate size is chosen on the basis of the vertical height of the bone and the interocclusal distance. The minimum buccolingual width for placement of this system is 7.5 mm. A transparent plastic template is available (Fig. 7–157) for determination of an appropriate implant selection by superimposition on the preoperative radiographs.

A midcrestal mucoperiosteal incision, approximately twice the length of the implant, is required for this procedure. This length of exposure will allow for the placement of the drill guide. Since the abutment head is located in the middle of the implant body, appropriate determination of the exact location must be made prior to the osseous preparation. The adjacent and opposing natural abutments must be considered in this site selection in relation to the final prosthetic reconstruction.

The No. 1 trephine, single groove on the shaft, is used for this entire preparation. It is placed in a slow-speed, reduction, latch-type contra-angle. It is used with a pumping motion with copious irrigation. If the preparation is on the left side of the mandible, the most distal area is prepared first. The same drill guide is used on both the right and left sides of the mouth, as the handle can be adjusted for each side. A sleeve-type projection is located on one half of the guide, the other half having a perfectly aligned opening. The sleeve is located on the left of the distal and on the right of the mesial of the oral cavity. Therefore, proper alignment can be obtained only when the sleeve-type projection can be placed into mesial preparation on the right or distal preparation on the left.

The trephine is carried into the bone until the row of holes is level with the crestal bone (Fig. 7–158*A*). The preparation will then be countersunk 3 mm from the crest and 5 mm along the walls for a total depth of 8 mm. The single depth gauge is placed to check the preparation. The drill guide can then be positioned (Fig. 7–158*B*). The same is used

IMPLANTS USED IN PREPROSTHETIC RECONSTRUCTIVE SURGERY / 259

Figure 7–158. Insertion of the "E" Double Hollow-Basket Implant. *A,* The No. 1 trephine is used for the entry into the bone for the "E" implant preparation. *B,* The try-in is used to determine adequate reduction of the core and depth of the osseous walls. *C,* The drill guide is positioned into the first preparation site, thereby aligning the second site in a precision manner. The No. 1 trephine is used once again. The trephine is carried inferiorly, into the drill guide, until the top of the trephine is level with the superior aspect of the drill guide. *D,* The drill guide is removed and the double try-in is inserted to check the accuracy of the preparation. *E,* The implant is inserted into the osseous site; it should be countersunk 2 to 3 mm below the alveolar bone crest.

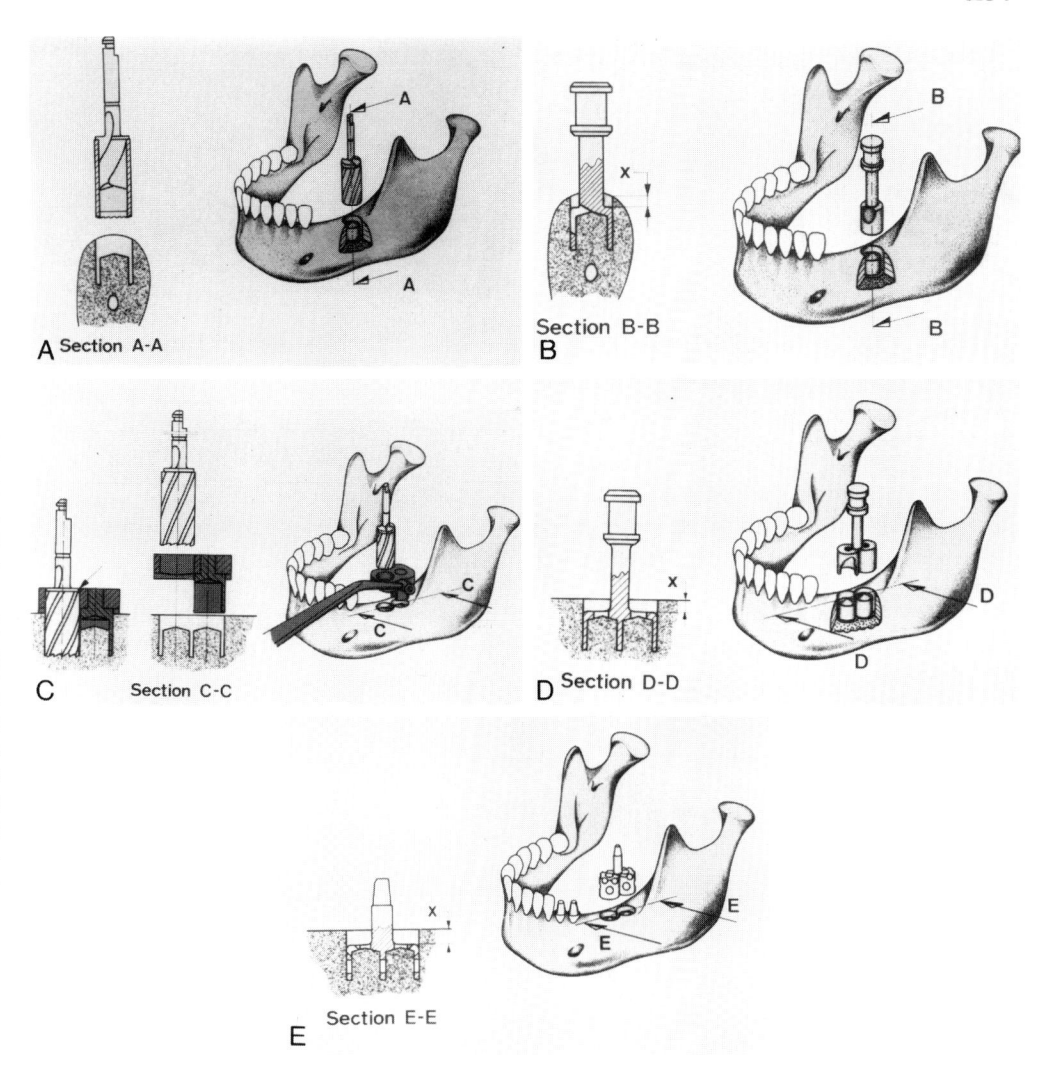

for the second chamber. The drill should be started prior to placement in the drill guide. Once again, a pumping motion with copious irrigation should be used. Sufficient depth has been achieved when the top of the trephine is level with the top of the drill guide (Fig. 7–158C). The guide is removed and the double depth gauge is placed to ascertain if the preparation is 3 mm below the crestal bone (Fig. 7–158D). The implant is then placed (Fig. 7–158E). If necessary, slight pressure can be exerted on the outer shoulder with the wrench. No malletting should be used, as distortion of the implant can occur.

The mucoperiosteal tissues are repositioned and sutured with 3-0 or 4-0 interrupted silk sutures. The patient is discharged with routine postoperative instructions and analgesics. The sutures are removed five to seven days postoperatively. The patient is seen every two weeks for the next eight weeks. At that time, the final prosthetic reconstruction is carried out (Fig. 7–159).

"H" Endosteal Hollow-Basket Implant System

The "H" implant incorporates the original endosteal blade-vent implant and the concepts of the endosteal hollow-basket systems (Fig. 7–160). It is intended for use in the posterior aspect of the oral cavity in the bicuspid and molar regions. Unlike other blade-vent implants, these cannot be modified by bending or contouring the body, neck, or abutment head. Therefore, the placement in the anterior alveolar ridge is almost impossible owing to the natural curvature of the arch. The implant may be used as a distal and/or intermediary abutment for fixed prosthesis reconstruction. It is not advisable to use it as an abutment for a removable prosthetic appliance.

The implant is fabricated with a mesiodistal length of 10.5 mm and a body height of 5 mm. The buccolingual width is 3 mm at the basket areas and 1.1 mm at the connecting arms. Therefore, the minimal vertical bone

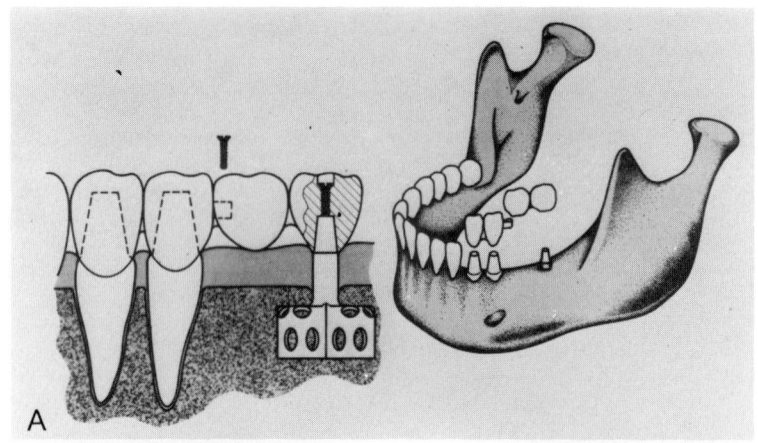

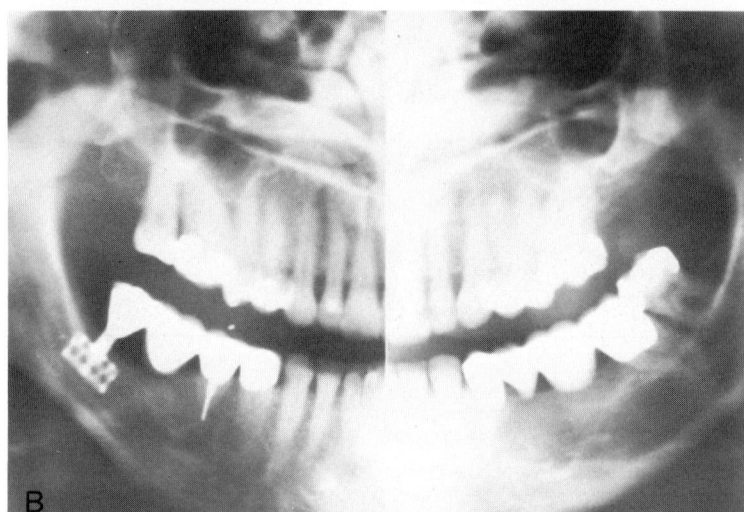

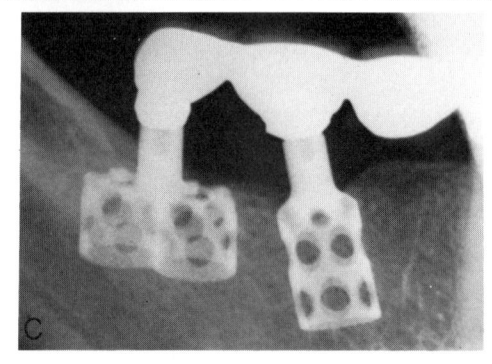

260 / IMPLANTS USED IN PREPROSTHETIC RECONSTRUCTIVE SURGERY

Figure 7–159. *A,* The area is allowed to heal for a period of 6 to 10 weeks, at which time the case is completed. *B,* This 28-month panoramic radiograph illustrates an "E" Hollow-Basket Implant as a distal abutment for a four-unit fixed prosthesis. *C,* This 36-month radiograph demonstrates a "C" and an "E" implant as distal and intermediary supports for a long-span fixed prosthesis.

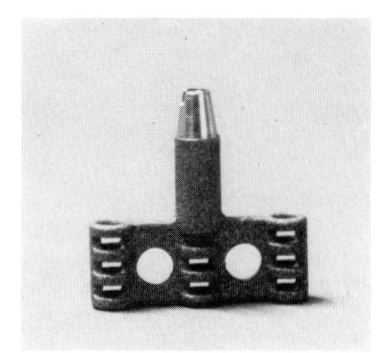

Figure 7–160. The "H" Hollow-Basket Implant.

be 1.5 to 2.0 times the length of the implant so that the drill guides will be able to be seated directly on the residual ridge. The center perforation in the No. 1 drill guide should be positioned opposite the opposing abutment both buccolingually and mesiodistally to obtain appropriate position of the abutment post.

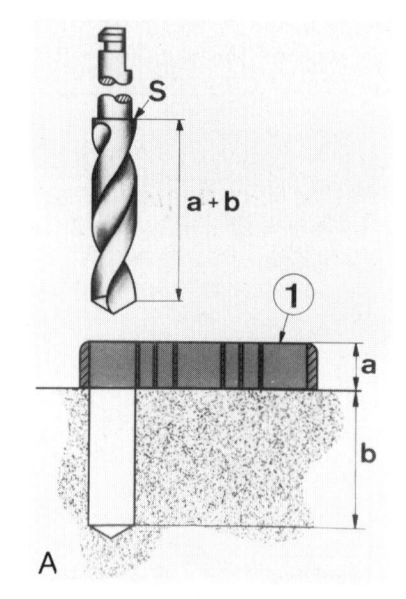

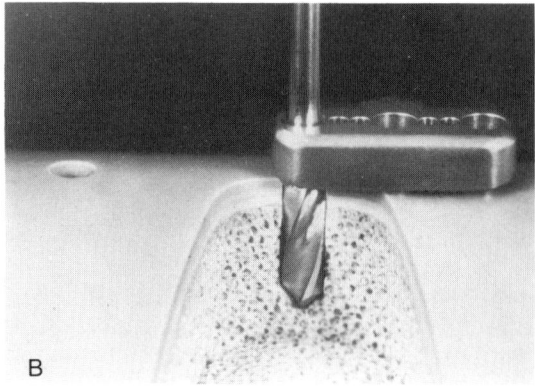

Figure 7–161. The 3-mm twist drill is used with the No. 1 drill guide to prepare the first of three osseous sites. The appropriate depth (a and b) is obtained when the shoulder of the twist drill is level with the top of the drill guide.

height necessary for placement is 9 mm above the inferior alveolar canal or below the maxillary sinus. The minimum buccolingual ridge width is 5 mm, thereby allowing 1 mm of bone on each side of the implant. The mesiodistal length, of course, is 10.5 mm, allowing for the appropriate length of implant.

The surgical procedure is initiated as with the other implant modalities. The anteroposterior mucoperiosteal incision length should

The osseous preparation is carried out with the 3-mm diameter twist drill (Fig. 7–161). A low-speed, latch-type, reduction contra-angle is used with all of these systems. The drill speed should not exceed 600 to 800 rpm, thereby ensuring that internal temperatures do not exceed 50° C and keeping bone trauma to a minimum. The drill should be started prior to placement in the drill guide to prevent binding and/or skidding of the bur. The handpiece should be used with a pumping motion, with copious amounts of sterile water or saline irrigation. The drilling should be continued until the top surface of the drill body is even with the top of the drill guide. This ensures adequate depth of preparation in the bone. The retaining pin is then placed through the hole in the drill guide and down into the preparation site. Either the mesial or distal site is prepared using the same technique (Fig. 7–162). The second retaining pin is then placed to lock the drill guide into position, thus preventing slippage or rotation. The third site is then prepared. The two retaining pins are then placed into the mesial and distal sites with the flat side facing the center of the drill guide (Fig. 7–163). This will allow sufficient room for the preparation of the small connection arm osseous sites with the 1.1-mm special single flute twist drill "C" (Fig. 7–164). The same techniques are used for this stage of the preparation. This drill guide is then removed.

The second drill guide, with projections extending from the mesial and distal aspects, is placed into the mesial and distal osseous preparation sites. The 1.3-mm special single flute twist drill is used to prepare each of the six sites through the guide surface (Fig. 7–165). The appropriate depth is achieved when the drill stop contacts the superior surface of the drill guide. When the drill guide is removed the preparation of the three basket areas and the connecting arm is complete. These six osseous penetrations are one-half diameter overlays of the original four preparations with the No. 1 drill guide. The area should be thoroughly irrigated and the try-in placed in the osseous site to check for adequate preparation (Fig. 7–166).

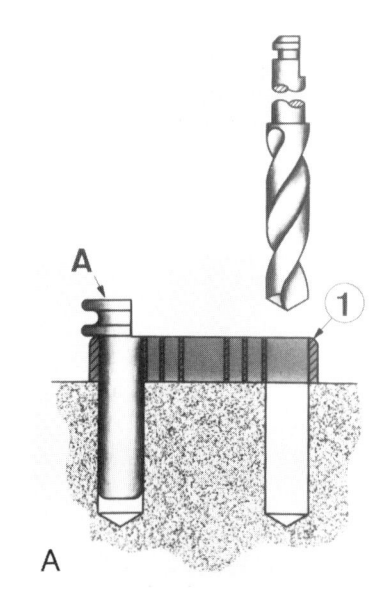

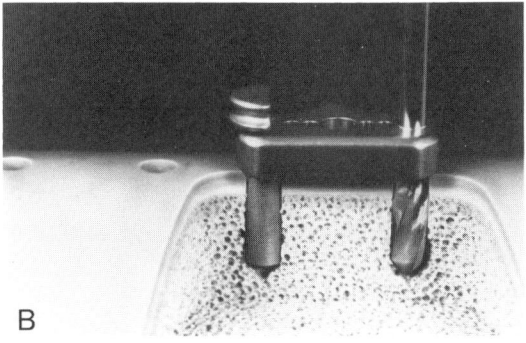

Figure 7–162. The stabilizing pin (A) is placed into the drill guide (1) and down into the osseous site, thus stabilizing the drill guide. The second osseous site is prepared.

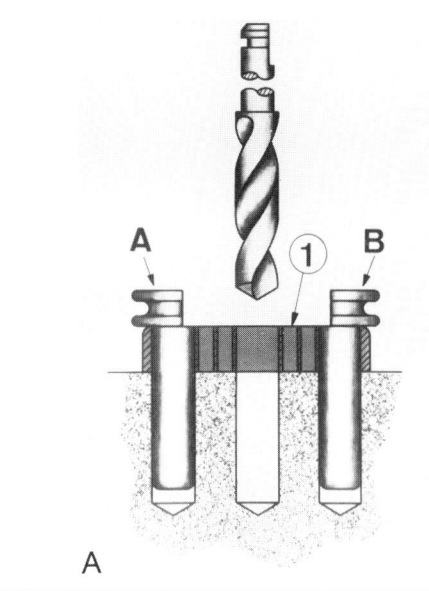

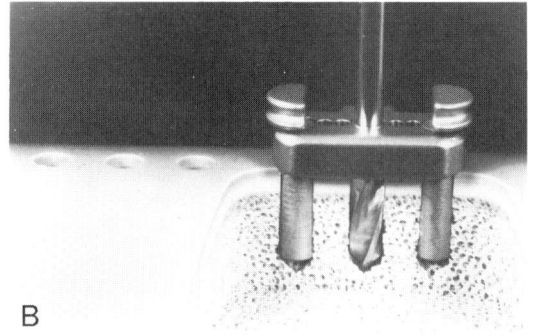

Figure 7–163. The second stabilizing pin (B) is placed into the drill guide (1) and osseous site. The third site is prepared.

The implant is now ready for final seating. Owing to the well-rounded edges and the highly precise osseous preparation, the implant will move easily into position. If any resistance is encountered, the wrench can be employed as a pusher over the mesial and distal basket areas. No tapping or hitting with a mallet is indicated. In its final position the shoulder of the implant should be 2 to 3 mm below the alveolar crest. There should be no mobility on the implant when it is finally seated (Fig. 7–167).

The mucoperiosteal tissues are repositioned. Usually no modification of the soft tissue is necessary. The neck of the implant is narrow enough to be accommodated without recontouring procedures. In order to maintain good oral hygiene and reduce trauma to the tongue and buccal mucosa, the prefabricated gold telescope is placed over the abutment and secured with the occlusal screw. The patient is instructed in *oral hygiene* techniques. Routine post-surgical instructions are reviewed. The patient is seen in five to seven days for suture removal, and

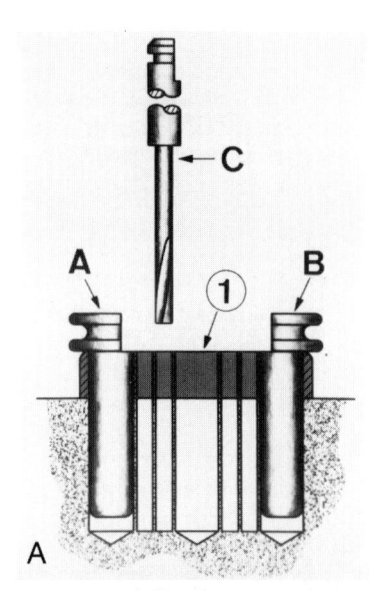

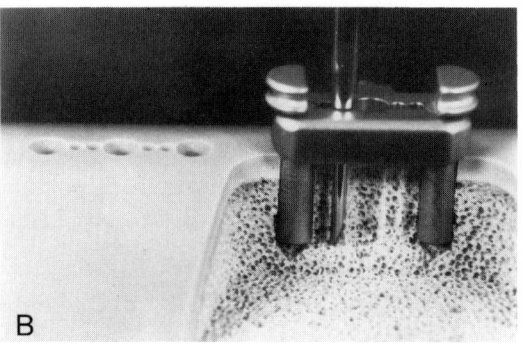

Figure 7–164. The stabilizing pins (A and B) are rotated until the flat side is facing inward. The 13-mm single flute twist drill (C) is used to prepare the first four connecting arm sites.

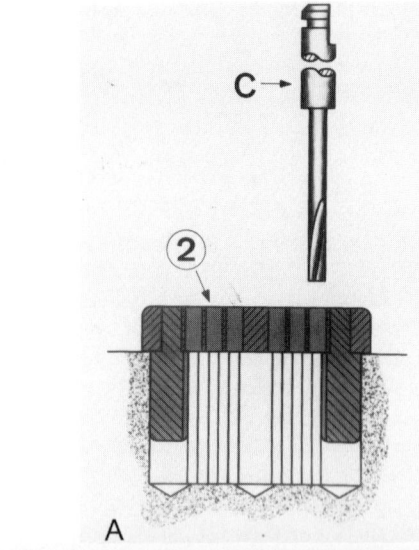

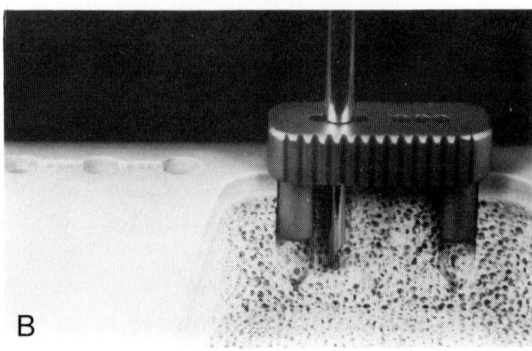

Figure 7–165. The first drill guide is removed and the second drill guide (2) is positioned into the prior osseous preparation sites. The remaining six 1.3-mm sites are prepared with the single flute drill (C).

the implant is checked for soft tissue healing, mobility, and sensitivity. The patient is checked in a similar manner over the next six to eight weeks. If at that time healing of the soft tissues is adequate, final prosthetic reconstruction is initiated (Figs. 7–168 and 7–169).

"K" Endosteal Hollow-Basket Implant System

The "K" implant is designed with an open shoulder (Fig. 7–170), which allows for reduced bone removal and the use of a trephine preparation. The implant has a 4-mm buccolingual dimension, allowing for a ride of 6 mm in width. The body is 5 mm high. The implant has three cylinders.

The 3-mm twist drill is used to initiate the first step, after the reflection of the mucoperiosteal tissues. The site of this drill entry will be the position of implant abutment. The drill is carried into the bone until the su-

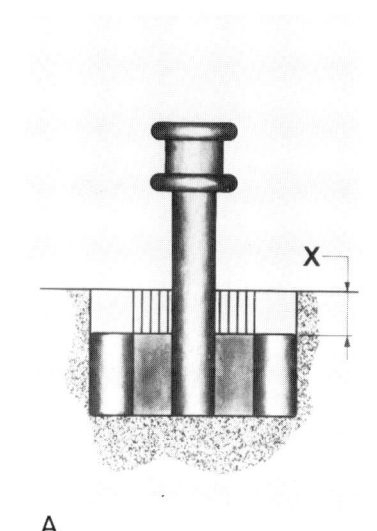

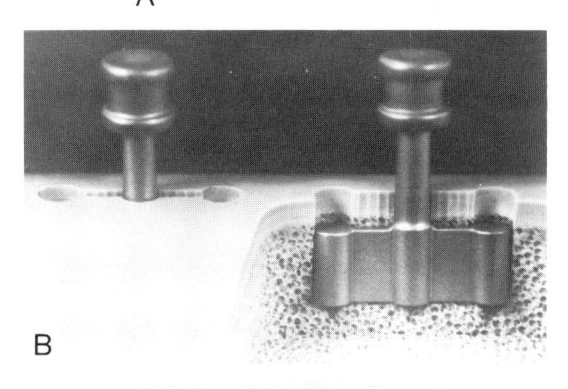

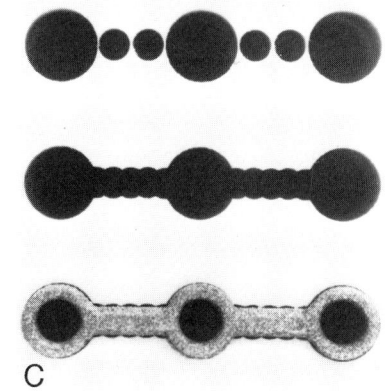

Figure 7–166. *A, B,* The depth gauge is positioned into the osseous site, ascertaining that it is countersunk 2 to 3 mm below the ridge crest (x). *C,* An occlusal view of the stages of preparation of the osseous implant sites.

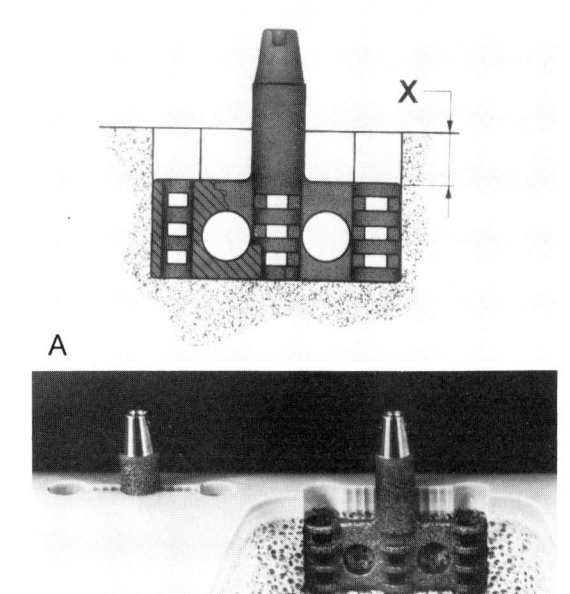

Figure 7–167. The "H" implant is inserted so that the shoulder is countersunk 2 to 3 mm below the ridge crest (x).

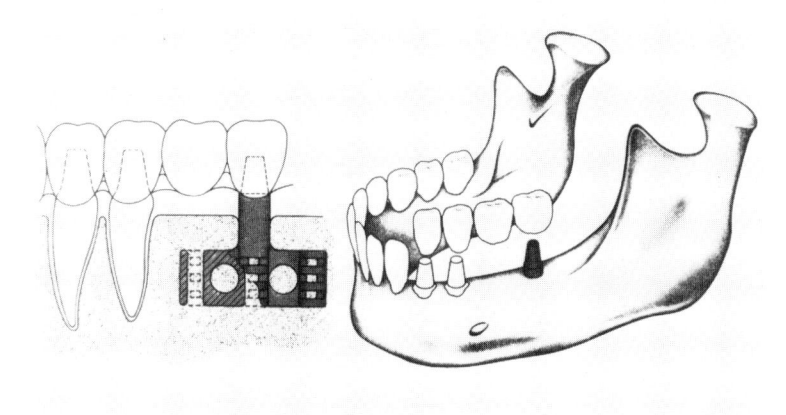

Figure 7–168. Six to ten weeks after insertion, the prosthesis is completed and inserted.

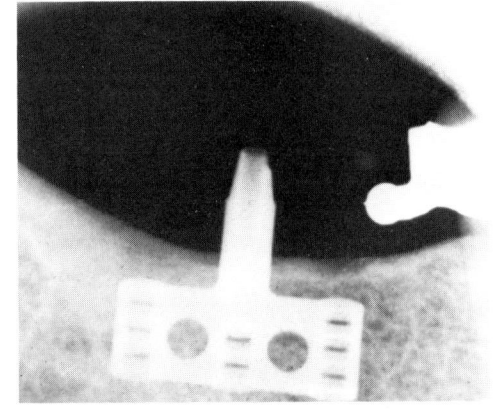

Figure 7–169. A 25-month postinsertion radiograph. The prosthesis has been removed for prophylaxis and follow-up examination.

perior edge of the shoulder is level with the alveolar crest (Fig. 7–171). Once again the reduction handpiece with copious irrigation is used.

The drill guide for the "K" implant has a center projection that telescopes into the first osseous preparation site. When the drill guide is seated in this position, the appropriate trephine drill is used to prepare the mesial and distal cylinders. The drill should be

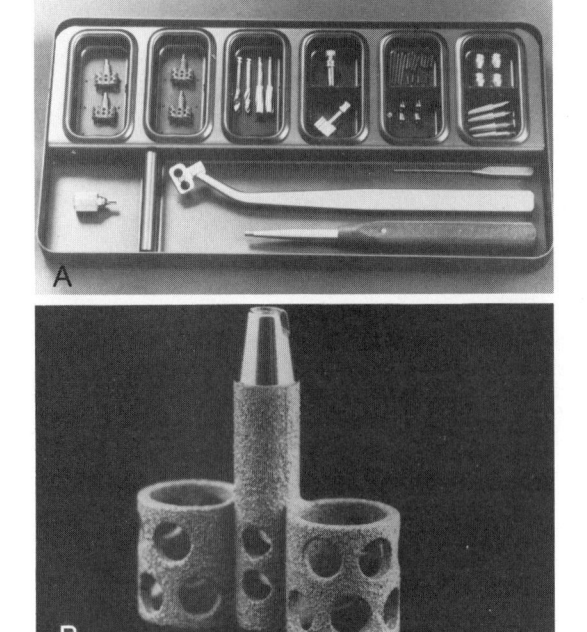

264 / IMPLANTS USED IN PREPROSTHETIC RECONSTRUCTIVE SURGERY

Figure 7–170. *A,* All ITI Hollow-Basket Implants are supplied in sterilizable containers. The system is composed of implants, transfer copings, die pins, occlusal screws, telescopes, drills and trephines, drill guides, depth gauges, and a screw driver. *B,* The "K" Hollow-Basket Implant.

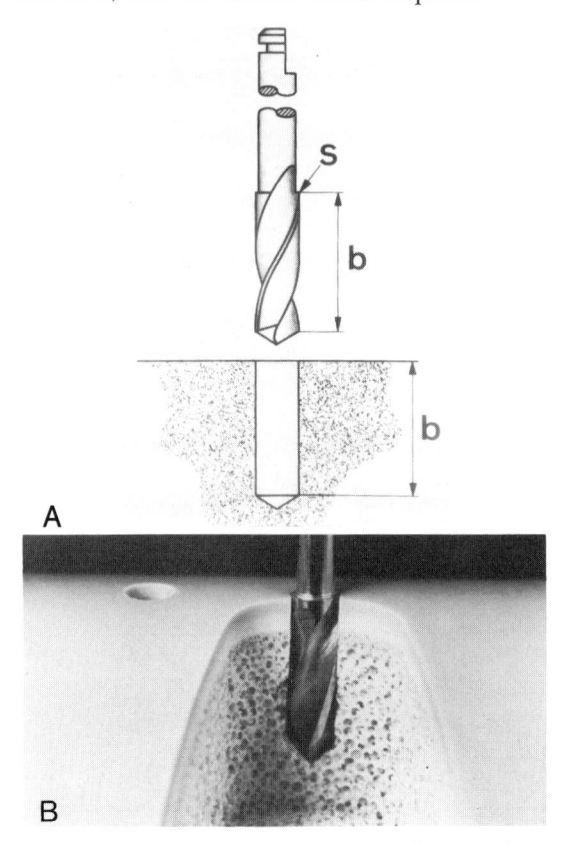

Figure 7–171. The 3-mm twist drill is used to prepare the central osseous site. The drill is inserted into the bone (b) until the shoulder (s) is even with the ridge crest.

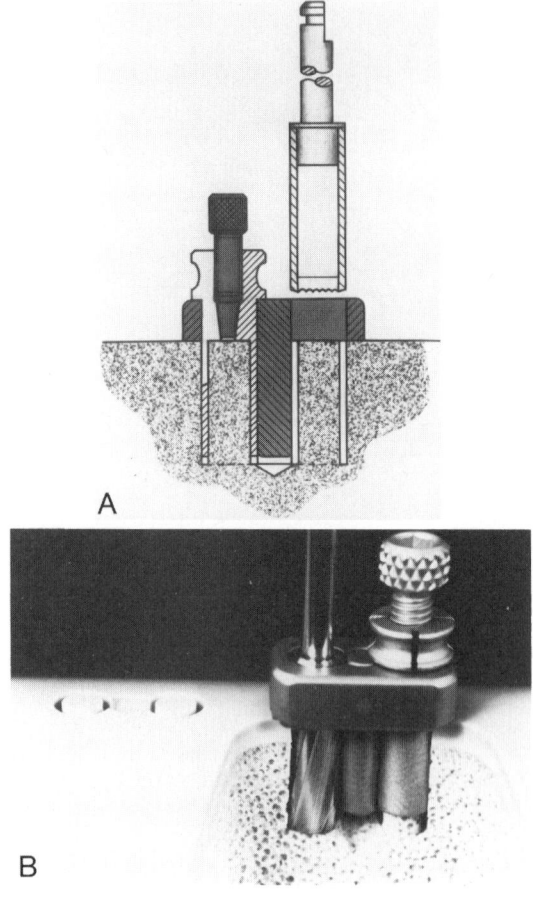

Figure 7–172. The drill guide is inserted into the first osseous preparation site. The 4-mm trephine is used to prepare the first core. The trephine is inserted until the shoulder is level with the superior aspect of the drill guide.

started prior to entry into the drill guide to prevent binding and reduce trauma to the sharp edges of the drill. The drill speed should be 600 to 800 rpm with a pumping motion and copious amounts of irrigation. The appropriate depth is achieved when the shoulder of the trephine is even with the superior surface of the drill guide platform (Fig. 7–172). When one cylinder is completed, the trephine drill is withdrawn, the site irrigated, and the adjustable stabilizing pin inserted. The set screw at the superior aspect of the stabilizing pin is tightened, thus locking it and the drill guide into position. Then the drill guide is stabilized for completion of the preparation of the second cylinder (Fig. 7–173). Once the cylinder is prepared, the set screw on the retention pin is loosened and removed and the drill guide is removed. The area is irrigated and the try-in is placed into the osseous preparation and fit and depth of position are evaluated (Fig. 7–174). The implant is placed into the osseous preparation (Fig. 7–175). Owing to the accuracy of the preparation and the rounded

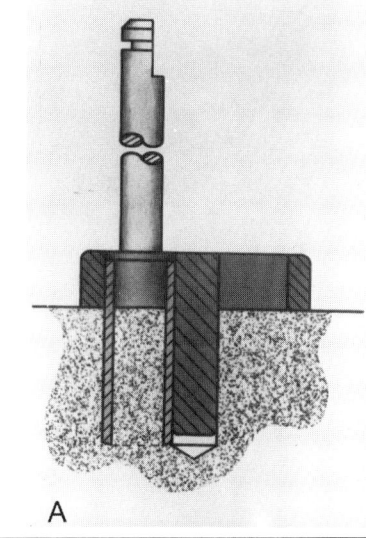

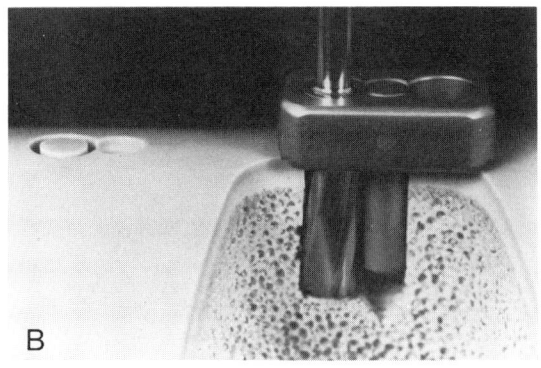

Figure 7–173. The stabilizing pin with the locking screw is inserted and tightened into position, thereby locking the drill guide into place. The second osseous core is prepared.

inferior edges as well as the slight taper toward the base of the implant, the implant should be able to be seated with finger pressure. If some binding should occur owing to uneven seating, the wrench may be used as a pushing instrument. The implant should not be tapped with a mallet, especially on the abutment head, as there is a good chance of stripping the internal thread, making use of the occlusal screw impossible. The implant should be countersunk 2 to 3 mm below the crest of the bone.

The mucoperiosteal tissues are repositioned and sutured with 3-0 or 4-0 silk interrupted sutures. Because the osseous defects are only 0.5 mm wide, a minimum amount

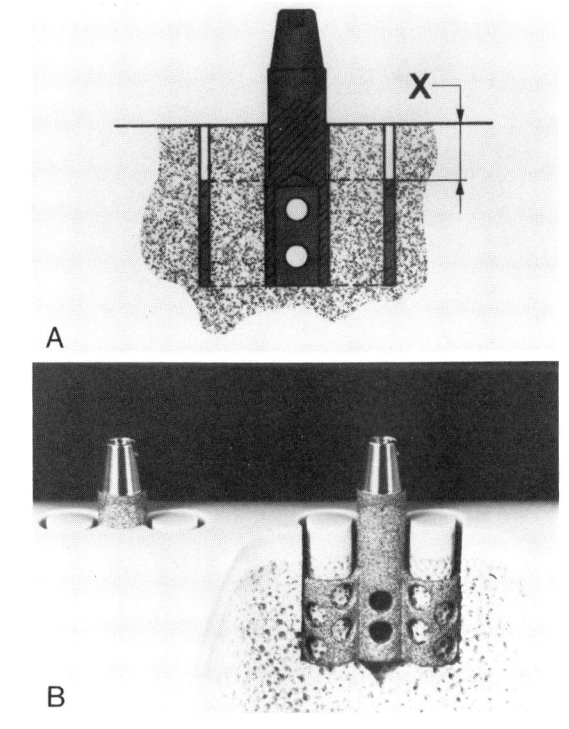

Figure 7–175. The "K" Hollow-Basket Implant in the final seated position (x).

Figure 7–174. *A, B,* The drill guide is removed. The depth gauge is inserted to check the osseous preparation site. The shoulder should be 2 to 3 mm inferior to the ridge crest (x). *C,* An occlusal view of the osseous preparation demonstrates the minimal amount of bone removal in this technique.

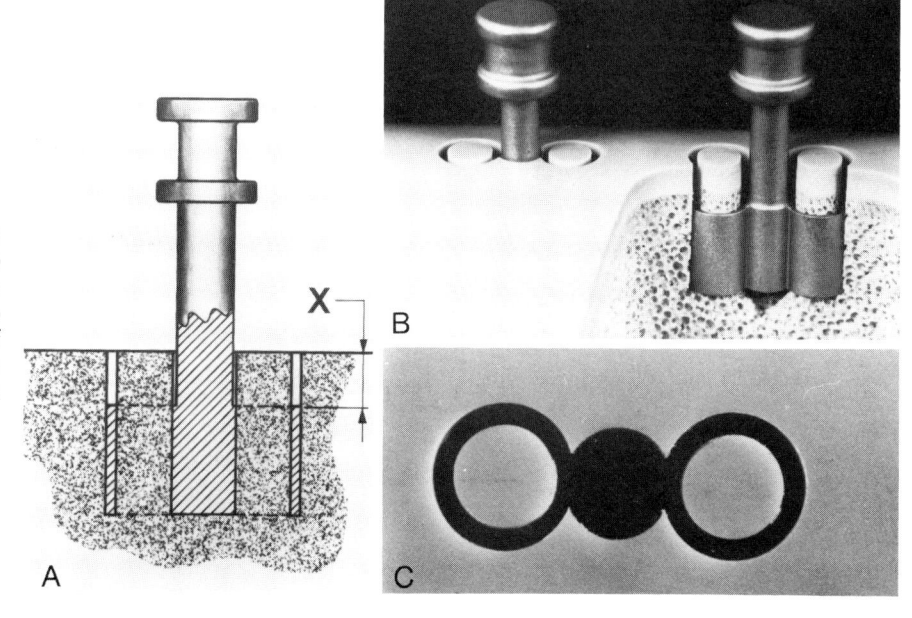

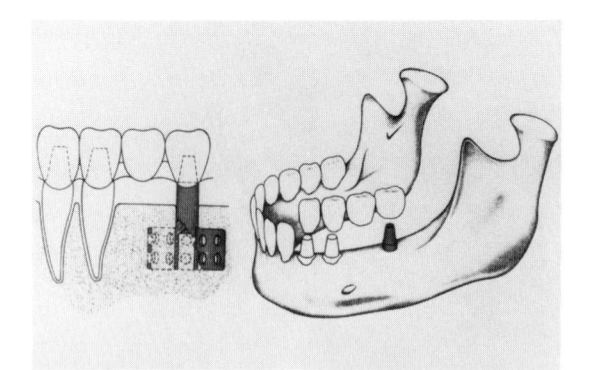

Figure 7–176. Reconstruction with a prosthesis can be done 8 to 10 weeks after insertion.

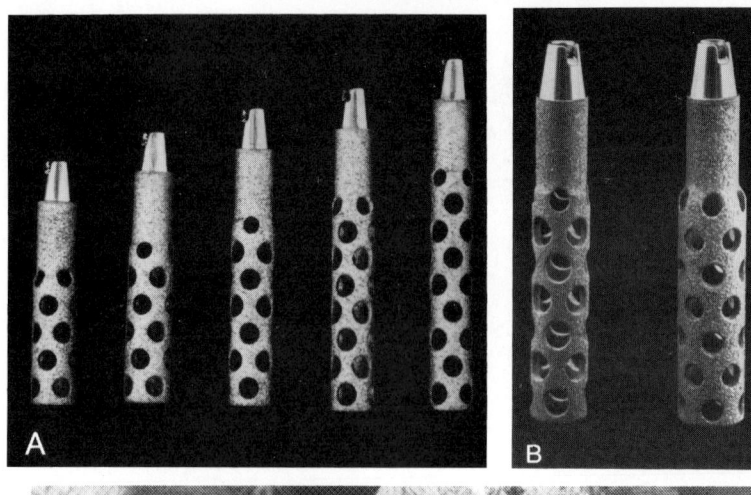

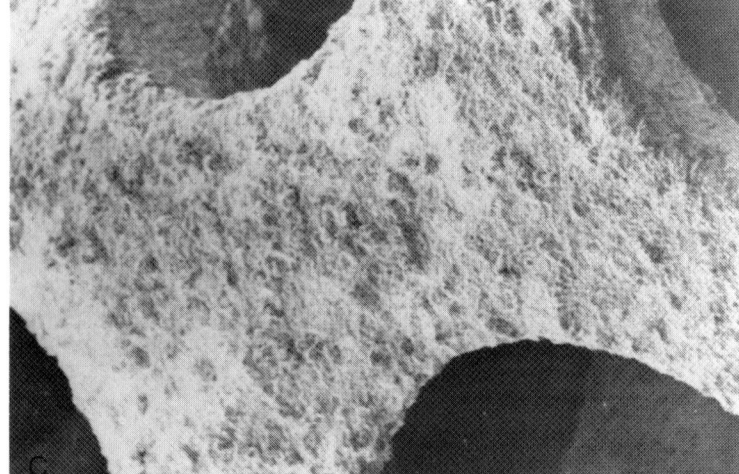

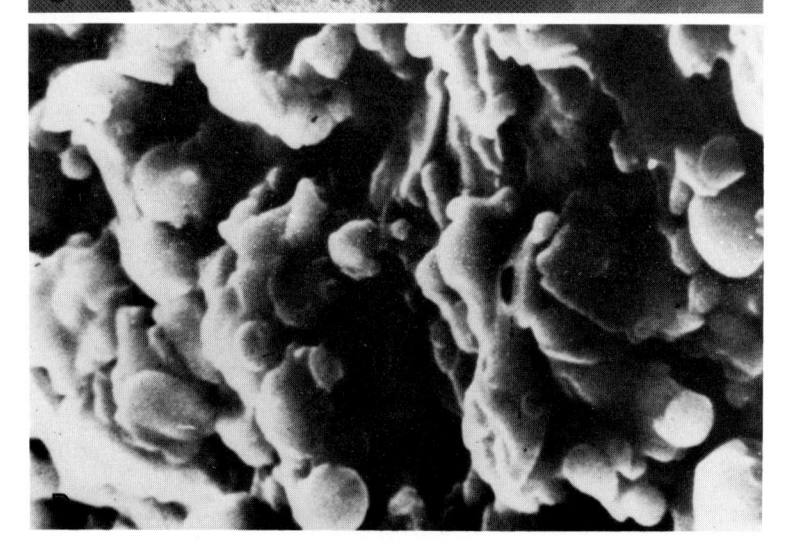

Figure 7–177. *A*, The "F" Hollow-Basket design is available in 9-, 11-, 13-, 15-, and 17-mm lengths. *B*, The "F" Hollow-Basket design is available in the 3.5- and 4.0-mm diameters. *C*, All Titanium Screw and Hollow-Basket Design Implants are coated with titanium plasma spray (TPS). *D*, Titanium plasma–sprayed implant surface (scanning electron micrograph ×5000).

of bone regeneration is required. This, combined with the extremely stable design of the implant, allows the implant to support large multidirectional loads, as they are distributed over a considerable area. The implant site is usually well-healed after six to eight weeks. Reconstruction with a fixed prosthesis can be carried out at that time according to guidelines previously described (Fig. 7–176).

"F" Endosteal Hollow-Basket Implant Systems

This Hollow-Basket design is intended to be used as a single tooth replacement or as support for a fixed prosthesis (Fig. 7–177). The "F" type may be used in both the maxilla and mandible. The design is basically a modification of the "C" single-basket, 5.5-mm diameter implant. It is available in five lengths, 9, 11, 13, 15, and 17 mm, and two diameters, 4.0 mm and 3.5 mm. The above-mentioned lengths are the body lengths, shoulder to inferior tip. A length of 2 to 3 mm must be added to this for the amount of available vertical height of bone so that the shoulder will be adequately countersunk below the ridge crest on final seating (Fig. 7–178). The neck is 3 mm in diameter and 6 mm in length. The abutment head is 3 mm long.

The "F" type implant is supplied in a metallic, autoclavable, compartmentalized container. A transfer coping (impression cap), die pin, prefabricated gold telescopic coping, and occlusal screw are part of this system. Also supplied are both a hollow-core trephine and hollow depth gauge or, alternatively, a twist drill and a solid pin depth gauge (Fig. 7–179). A countersinking bur is supplied with the system (Fig. 7–180).

The site selected must provide at least 6 mm of bone horizontally and sufficient vertical height to accommodate the length of the baskets. This is in addition to 2 to 3 mm of neck plus a 2-mm safety zone adjacent to any vital structures. Most of these procedures can be carried out under local anesthesia.

A full-thickness mucoperiosteal flap should be reflected over the proposed implant site. Bony spurs or irregularities can easily be removed with a bone file. Levelling of the alveolar ridge can be done with a large carbide laboratory bur. A No. 4 or 6 round bur can be used to make the initial entry into the ridge crest (Fig. 7–181A). The special 4-mm diameter starter bur is used to countersink a 4-mm area (Fig. 7–181B and C). The trephine, which comes in five lengths to

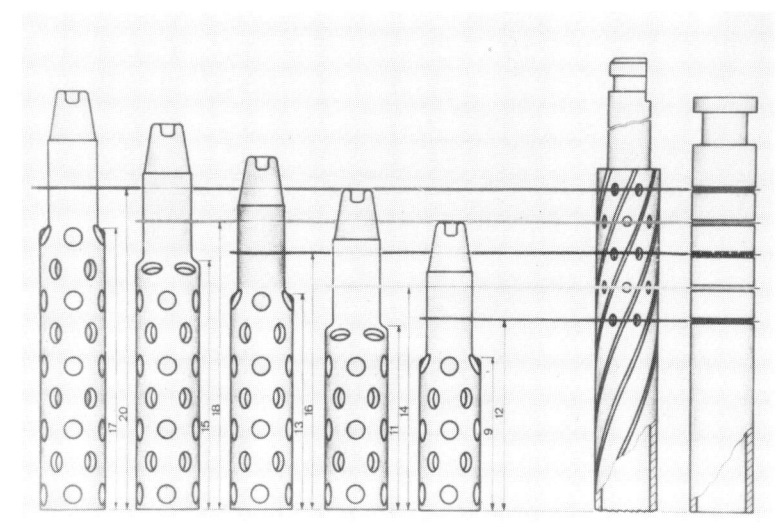

Figure 7–178. The lengths of the "F" implants are coordinated with the trephine and the depth gauge.

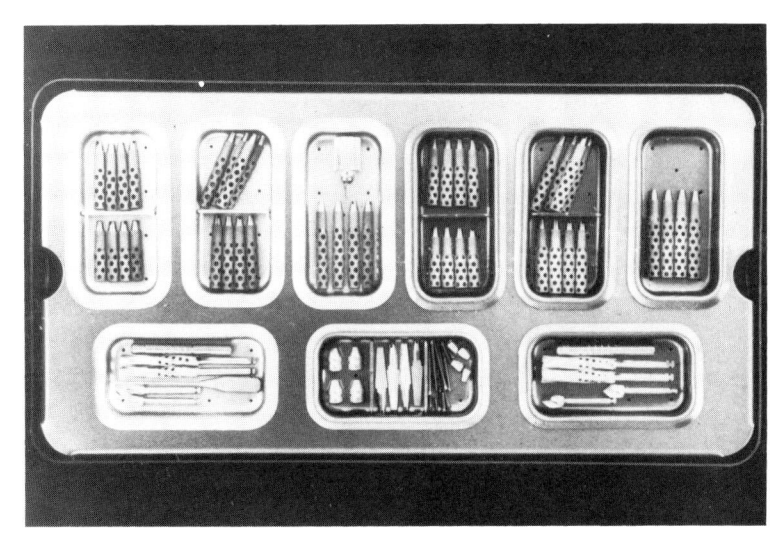

Figure 7–179. The system is supplied with the various lengths and widths of implants as well as transfer copings, die pins, gold telescopes, occlusal screws, trephines, depth gauges, and a screw driver.

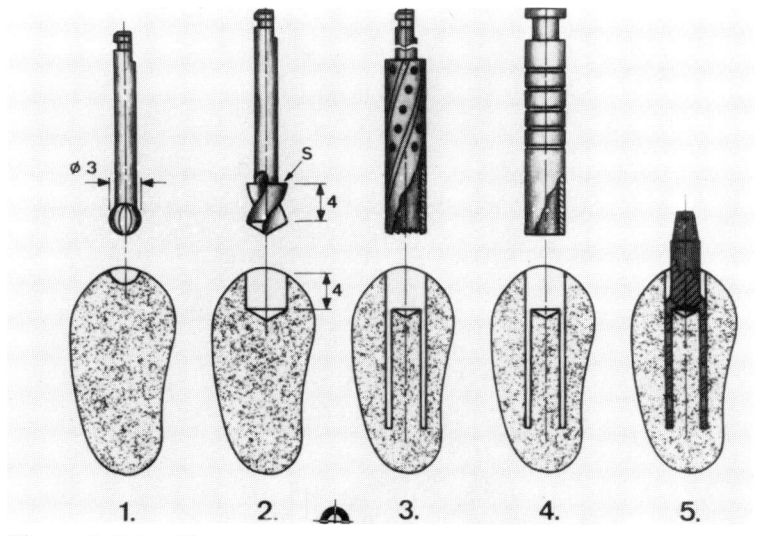

Figure 7–180. The preparation of the "F" implant site.

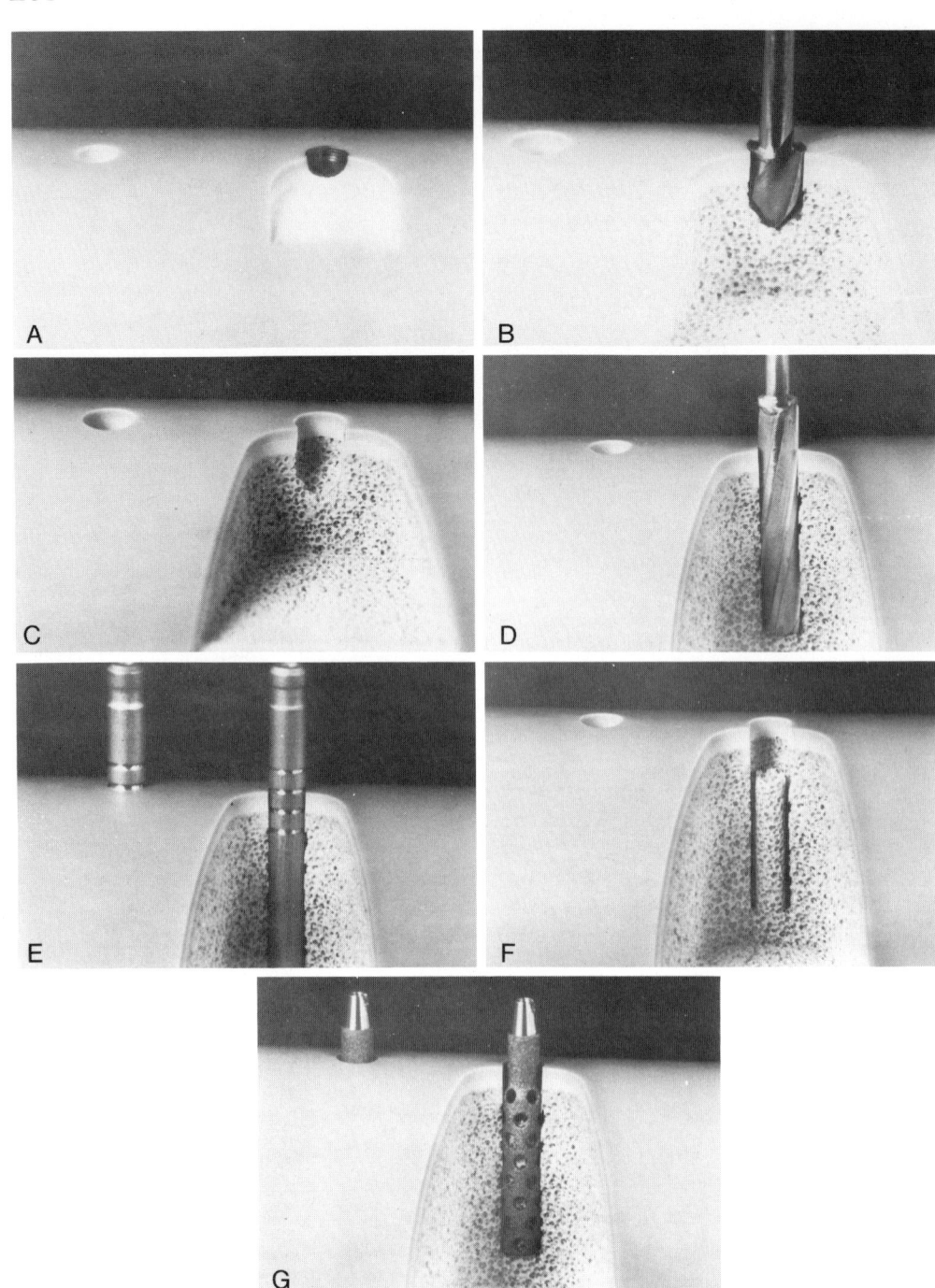

268 / IMPLANTS USED IN PREPROSTHETIC RECONSTRUCTIVE SURGERY

Figure 7–181. *A*, A No. 4 or 6 round bur is used to create a purchase point in the crest of the ridge. *B*, The 4-mm starter bur is used to countersink a 4-mm area (*C*). *D*, The trephine is used to prepare the site. *E*, The depth gauge is inserted over the core to verify the appropriate depth. *F*, The completed preparation. *G*, The "F" implant is inserted.

match those of the implants, is used to carry the core preparation to the appropriate depth, which is the length of the basket plus the 3-mm neck (Fig. 7–181*D*). The depth gauge is also matched to the depth of the implant and is color-coded with them (Fig. 7–181*E* and *F*).

Preparation may also be done with a solid drill, thus eliminating the bony core. With the loss of the core, osseous regeneration is prolonged; the trephine technique is therefore preferred. The inferior area of the basket is slightly tapered and the edges are rounded, making nontraumatic insertion easier (Fig. 7–181*G*).

The mucoperiosteal tissues are repositioned and sutured with 3-0 or 4-0 interrupted silk sutures. If the implant is placed in the anterior region of the oral cavity, it may be necessary to use temporization for esthetic reasons. The implant should not be loaded for six to eight weeks. A temporary shell crown can be adapted to the prefabricated gold telescope that has been fixed into position by the occlusal screw and bonded to the adjacent teeth as a splint. Final pros-

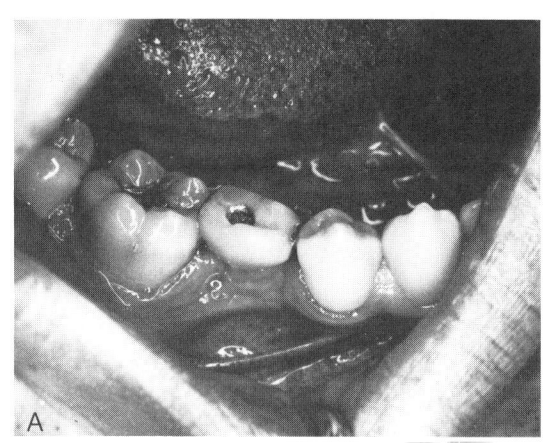

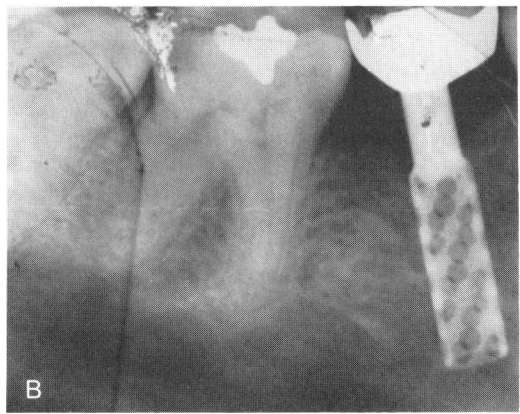

Figure 7–182. These 24-month clinical and radiographic pictures demonstrate the 4.0-mm "F" implant. It is a self-standing, unsplinted replacement for a congenitally missing mandibular second bicuspid.

thetic fabrication can be carried out 60 days after insertion of the implant (Fig. 7–182).

Summary

The ITI Endosteal Hollow-Basket Implant Systems are used in a variety of reconstructive situations, ranging from single-tooth unsupported units to complex dental rehabilitation of semiedentulous to totally edentulous arches. These systems have been documented over the past ten years by the ITI and have been used in the United States since 1981. The titanium implants with TPS coatings have successfully stimulated calcified tissue integration, which has been maintained over many years.

As with all implant systems, a predictable long-range favorable prognosis is dependent on several factors: bioengineering, biocompatibility, good surgical technique, adequate prosthetic design and fabrication, and good oral hygiene and maintenance by the patient. Controlled clinical evaluations from Switzerland, Sweden, and the United States document success in all these areas.

SUBPERIOSTEAL MANDIBULAR IMPLANT*

Charles A. Babbush

Goldberg and Gershkoff[168] carried out the first mandibular subperiosteal implant in the United States over 30 years ago (Fig. 7–183). Because of the efforts of various men in the field of dental implantology,[169–176] utilization of this technique has increased. With the refinement of surgical techniques, improvement of impression materials, developments in biomaterials, and modifications of laboratory procedures, the subperiosteal implant

---

*I wish to thank Mr. Jack Wimmer, CDT, President, Park Dental Research Corporation, NY, NY, for the models, the laboratory information, and his technical advice for this section.

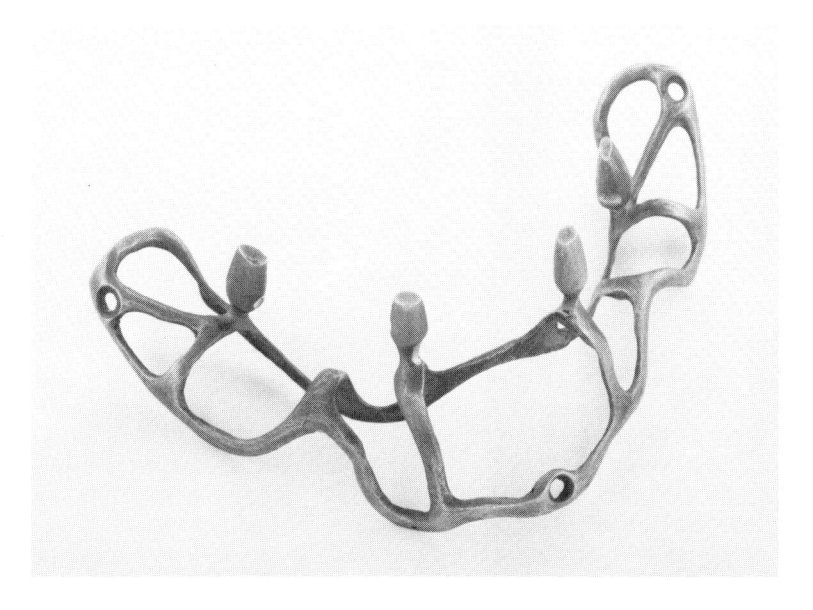

Figure 7–183. Early subperiosteal framework with four abutments. The distal portion of the casting extends up the ascending ramus. The secondary struts cross the ridge in several places.

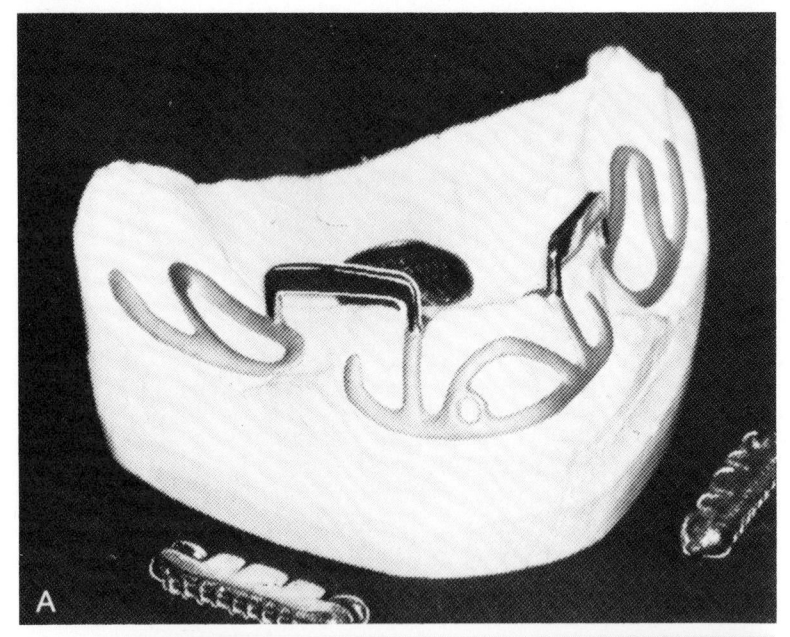

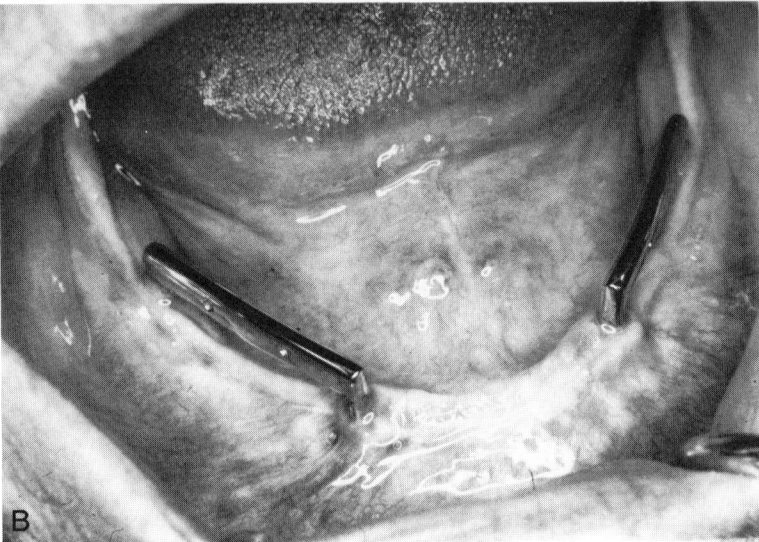

Figure 7–184. *A*, Framework of newest design modifications with simplified strut work, shortened distal coverage, and anterior-posterior connector bars. *B*, Clinical view of anterior-posterior connector bar design.

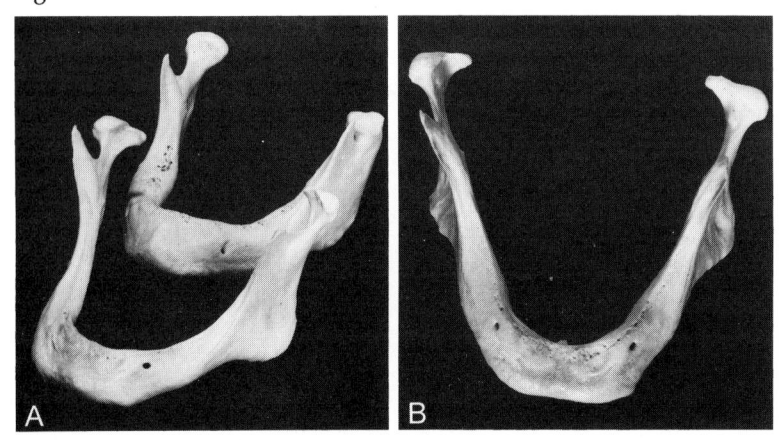

Figure 7–185. *A*, Postextraction mandibles with (below) and without (above) atrophic changes demonstrate the more superior position of the mental foramen. *B*, The genial tubercle is located in a relatively superior position.

has been used with some frequency for the atrophic mandible (Fig. 7–184). Recently the introduction of a preoperative model created from computerized tomography has reduced the surgical procedures needed for some subperiosteal implants.

Patient Selection

Potential candidates for this procedure, as with other restorative techniques, must be evaluated as outlined previously.[177] Painful episodes during function, the inability to function properly, to eat, and to speak, and a lack of confidence in their ability to retain a prosthesis are the factors that cause patients to seek a fixed restorative procedure. Historically, these patients will usually have had several other conventional prosthetic devices, none of which alleviates their problems. The problem of functional pain is related to mandibular atrophy and progressive impingement of a prosthesis on the mental neurovascular bundle, which is located in a more superior relationship to the crest of the residual alveolar ridge (Fig. 7–185A). When functional forces are applied to a conventional denture, pressure is exerted on the neurovascular bundle, eliciting pain. With this atrophy, the genial tubercle becomes situated in a more superior position than the ridge itself (Fig. 7–185B), and the conventional denture cannot be seated adequately without eliciting functional pain. Additionally, any movement of the tongue, because of the high muscle attachments of the genioglossus, will cause the denture to be dislodged. Many atrophic residual ridges will be severely knife-edged or will exhibit numerous spinous processes. An alveolectomy should be carried out to correct these problems, followed by a waiting period of six months prior to initiating the implant reconstruction.

Any type of metallic substance upon or within the mandible, such as bone plates, screws, wires, or amalgam tattoos, should be removed preoperatively to prevent potential reactions with the metal framework of the implant (Fig. 7–186). All odontogenic pathology must be corrected preoperatively. After the removal of these foreign bodies or pathologic conditions, a minimum six-month waiting period is required. If the atrophic area is more extensive, a 12-month wait would be desirable. If a natural opposing detention still exists in the maxillary arch, subperiosteal reconstruction is contraindicated (Fig. 7–187). Because the implant framework rests on residual bone, it is not able to withstand the functional forces of natural dentition and will eventually fail.

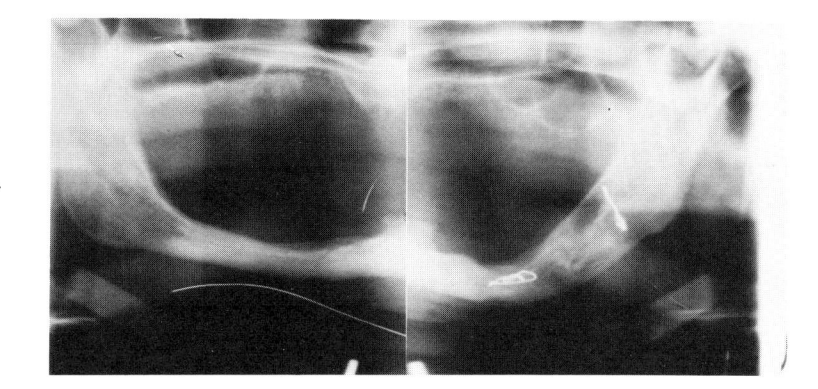

Figure 7–186. All foreign objects should be removed preoperatively.

As with any prosthetic device, the structure is composed of various parts, principally the framework, the superstructure, and the prosthesis. The framework rests directly on the mandibular residual bone beneath the mucoperiosteal tissues. The outer portions of the framework are referred to as the major connectors or peripheral struts. The portions of the framework that cross the alveolar crest and connect the labial with the lingual peripheral struts are called the minor connectors or secondary struts. These are usually located in the cuspid and first molar areas bilaterally. The abutment neck is that portion of the framework which connects the secondary struts to the abutment heads or mesobar (Fig. 7–188). The classic design consists of four abutment heads, whereas later designs may be fabricated with anteroposterior connector bars or a continuous monorail type of bar. The superstructure is embedded into the final denture and becomes an integral part of it. Only retentive clasps are not covered by acrylic. The denture fits over the abutments of the mesobar and can be removed for oral hygiene purposes. The denture is completely implant-borne, and there is no soft-tissue compression between the denture and underlying implant framework.

The denture should have shortened peripheral flanges to ensure that no soft-tissue impingement occurs. Only acrylic zero-degree teeth should be fabricated into the final denture in order to avoid undue lateral stresses and reduce functional loads that otherwise would surpass the physiologic limits of the underlying bone. Obtaining proper centric relation of the occlusion is of the utmost importance.

The procedure is divided into several phases:

Phase I Stage I—Surgical Procedure: Direct Bone Impression
Phase II Laboratory Procedure: Fabrication of the Implant Framework
Phase III Stage II—Surgical Procedure: Insertion of Framework
Phase IV Temporary Prosthesis
Phase V Final Prosthesis

The surgical procedures will be described first, followed by a discussion of laboratory considerations.

Stage I: Direct Bone Impression

The procedure is initiated by measuring and recording the thickness of the mucoperiosteal tissues in the first molar and cuspid areas bilaterally. The tissue thickness in these areas will determine the length of the

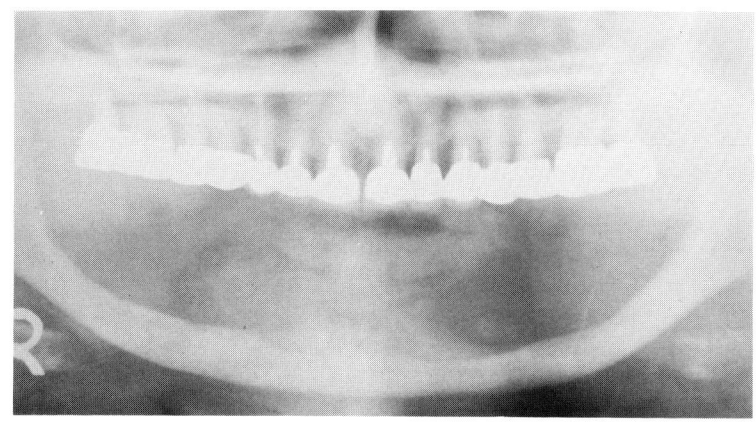

Figure 7–187. The subperiosteal mandibular bone plate is contraindicated when natural dentition remains in the maxilla.

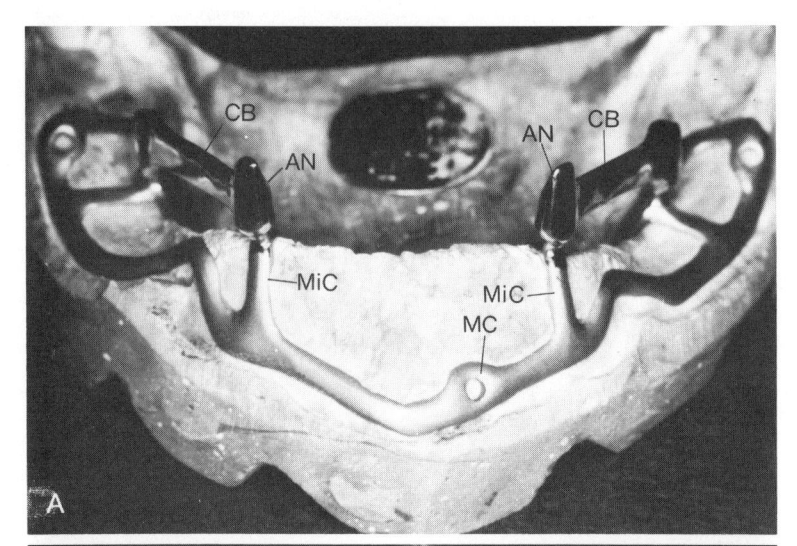

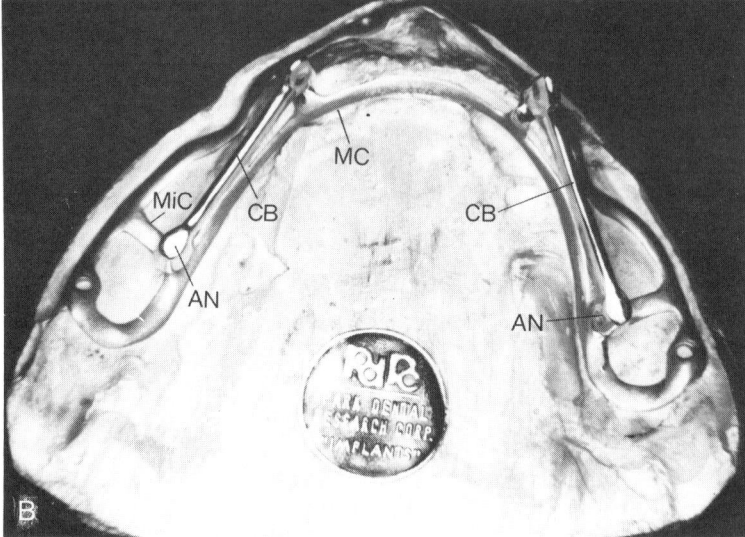

272 / IMPLANTS USED IN PREPROSTHETIC RECONSTRUCTIVE SURGERY

Figure 7–188. The subperiosteal framework is composed of several parts: major connectors (MC), minor connectors (MiC), abutment neck (AN), and connector bars (CB).

neck of the abutment. This can be accomplished with an explorer and a small square of rubber dam as a stop or a periodontal probe demarcated in millimeters (Fig. 7–189). The patient's centric relation is also recorded.

Anesthesia for these procedures can be either intravenous sedation or general anesthesia, depending on the medical history and the patient's and doctor's mutual choice. Intravenous infusion of Ringer's lactate with 5 per cent dextrose is usually maintained throughout the procedure. Lidocaine 2 per cent with 1:100,000 epinephrine, block and infiltration, is administered for its vasoconstrictive as well as anesthetic properties.

A straight-line incision is carried through the mucoperiosteal tissues at the midcrestal area of the residual alveolar ridge. The incision extends from one retromolar region to the other (Fig. 7–190). If radiographic review and clinical palpation show the mental foramen and its neurovascular bundle to be in a superior position or located near the ridge

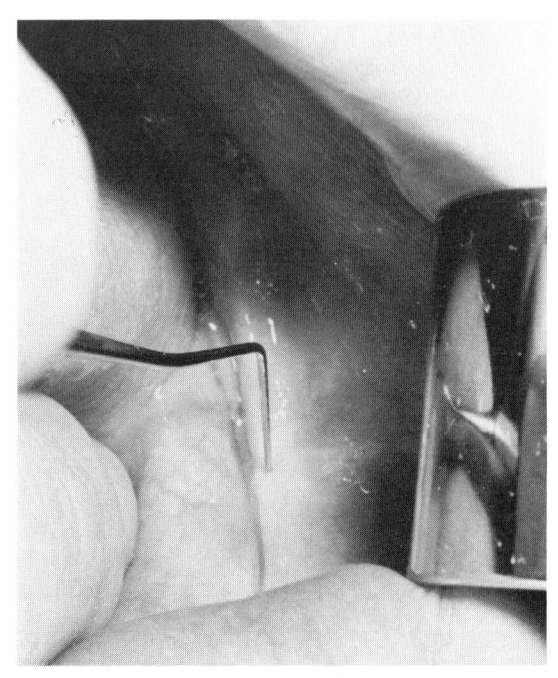

Figure 7–189. The tissue thickness measurement is obtained in the cuspid and first molar area bilaterally.

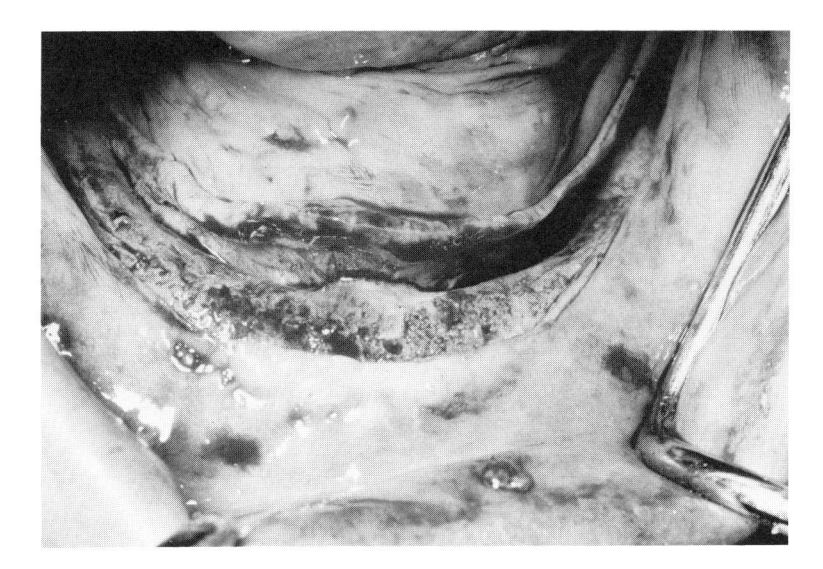

Figure 7–190. The incision extends from one retromolar region to the other.

crest, extra care must be taken in the placement of the incision, which should be carried off to the lingual aspect of the ridge crest. Likewise, if there is evidence of a dehiscent inferior alveolar canal, alternate sharp and blunt dissection will help prevent trauma to these vital structures. In each of these cases, the patient should be warned preoperatively of the potential of paresthesia. In 16 years we have encountered less than 10 per cent transient paresthesia apparently related to the surgical edema and trauma of the impression procedure.

Once the incision has been completed, the tissues are reflected in both the buccal and lingual directions with a periosteal elevator. Care must be exercised in the region of the mental neurovascular bundle to ensure its continued attachment to the buccal flap (Fig. 7–191). The dissection should not be carried inferior to the neurovascular bundle, as impression material will then flow around the bundle, causing increased trauma and entrapment of the impression, making removal very difficult.

In order to obtain an accurate impression of the mandible, the following anatomic landmarks must be exposed via reflection of the mucoperiosteal flaps: the external oblique ridges, the mental foramina and associated neurovascular bundles, the mylohyoid ridges, the mandibular symphysis, the genial tubercle, and the concavity on the lingual aspect of the mandible located between the genial tubercle and the beginning of the mylohyoid ridges (Fig. 7–192). The genioglossus and geniohyoid muscles should not be detached. The peripheral areas of the major connectors of the implant framework rest on these dense bony landmarks and the implant obtains its retention in this manner.

Once these anatomic areas are exposed, the lingual flaps are sutured from the anterior of the right to the posterior of the left, and the posterior of the right to the anterior of the left, with 3-0 black silk sutures. When these sutures are tied, they form an X across the floor of the mouth and retract the tongue posteriorly (Fig. 7–193). In this manner, the flaps are self-retaining for ease of insertion of the impression tray and material and accuracy of the impression. If the buccal flaps are to be sutured to the buccal mucosa, the sutures should be placed just distal to the mental nerve. This technique will create further exposure of the mandible with self-retaining flaps (Fig. 7–194). In those cases in which extreme atrophy has occurred or in small-boned individuals, a midline relieving inci-

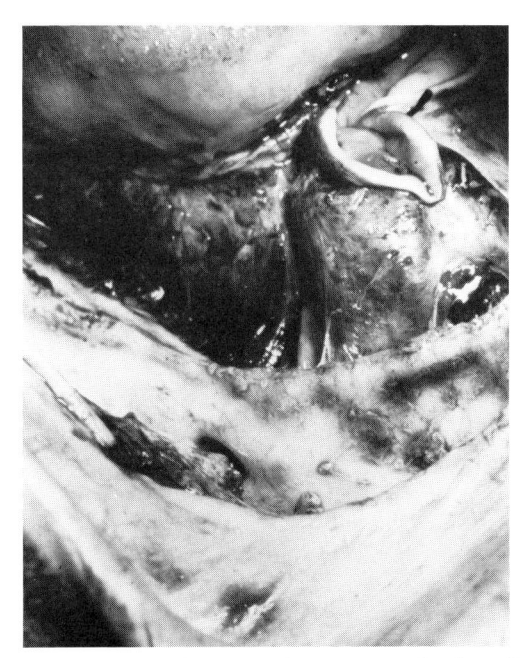

Figure 7–191. The mental neurovascular bundle will in many instances be located near the crest of the ridge.

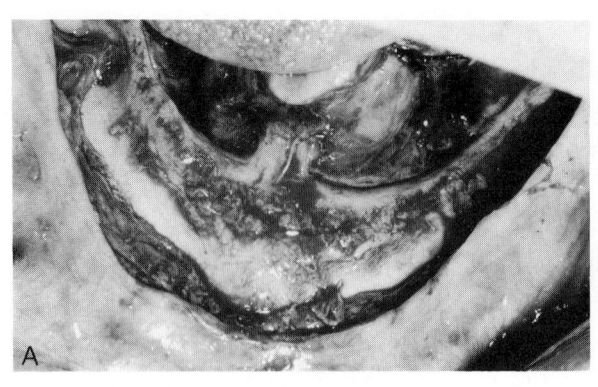

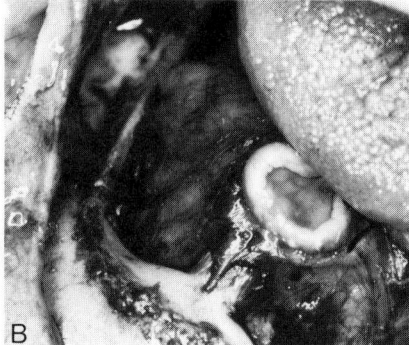

Figure 7–192. The reflection of full-thickness mucoperiosteal flaps should expose the mandibular symphysis, genial tubercle, mental neurovascular bundles, external oblique ridges, and mylohyoid ridge.

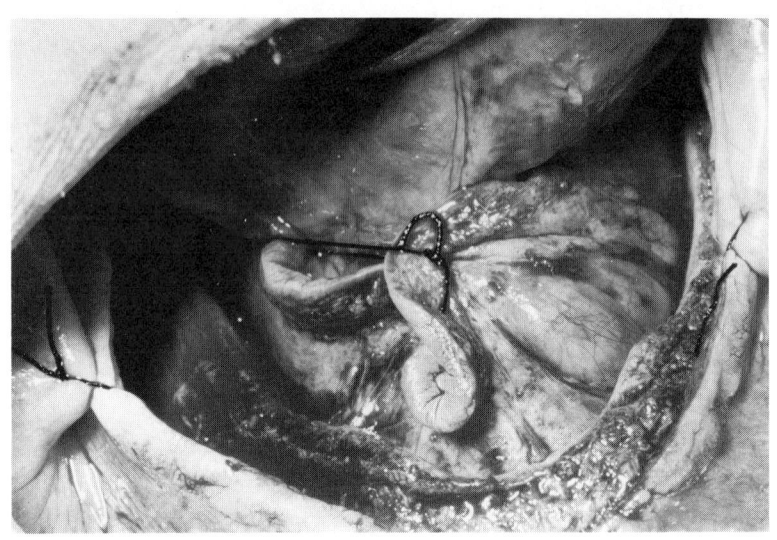

Figure 7–193. Retention sutures are placed in an "X" fashion between the lingual flaps in the floor of the mouth.

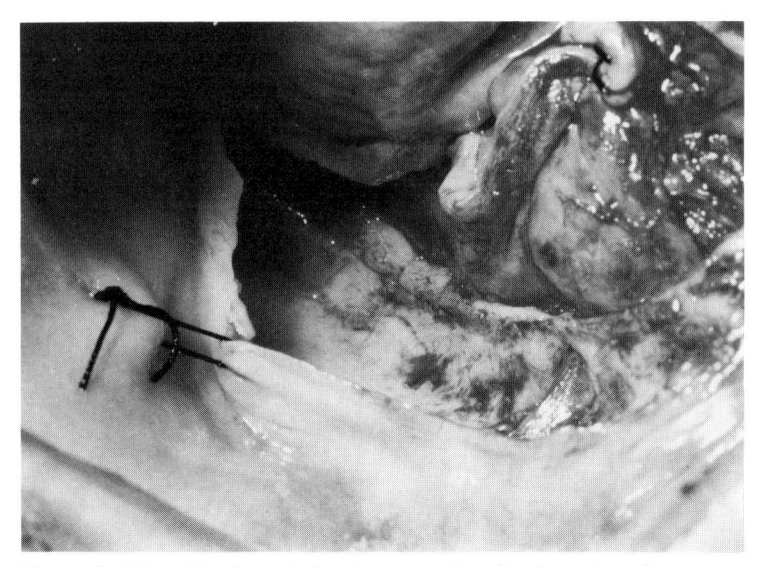

Figure 7–194. The buccal flap is sutured to the buccal mucosa.

sion is necessary to gain full access to the mandibular symphyseal area.

Prior to the surgical procedure, the prosthodontist obtains an overcompressed impression of the mandibular arch. From the subsequently poured models, two surgical impression trays with handles are fabricated and a surgical bite registration tray is prepared (Fig. 7–195).

The impression and bite registration trays are sterilized in glutaraldehyde (Cidex) and thoroughly rinsed in sterile saline. The trays are positioned to ensure ease of manipulation under the flaps and to check the relationship to the previously outlined anatomic landmarks. In many instances, adjustments will be necessary in the region of the mental neurovascular bundle and the mandibular symphysis.

The exposed bone is then packed with saline-moistened gauze sponges, and the trays are coated with adhesive to lock in the impression materials. A polyvinyl ether impression material, which is accurate and easy to handle, has been used in recent years.

The saline packs are removed from the exposed bony areas while simultaneously two impression syringes are loaded with the light-bodied material. The material is injected under the flaps and around the outer circumference of the dissection. The assistant must be sure that the periphery of the tray is located under the soft tissue flaps to obtain as accurate an impression as possible. The tray is held under pressure for five minutes while the material sets. The impression tray is then removed, usually with some difficulty, as considerable retention develops with this technique. Manipulation of the tray handle will usually loosen the impression.

If dissection has been carried below the mental neurovascular bundle, impression material may flow below it and become trapped. As the impression tray is removed, these areas should be carefully watched. If

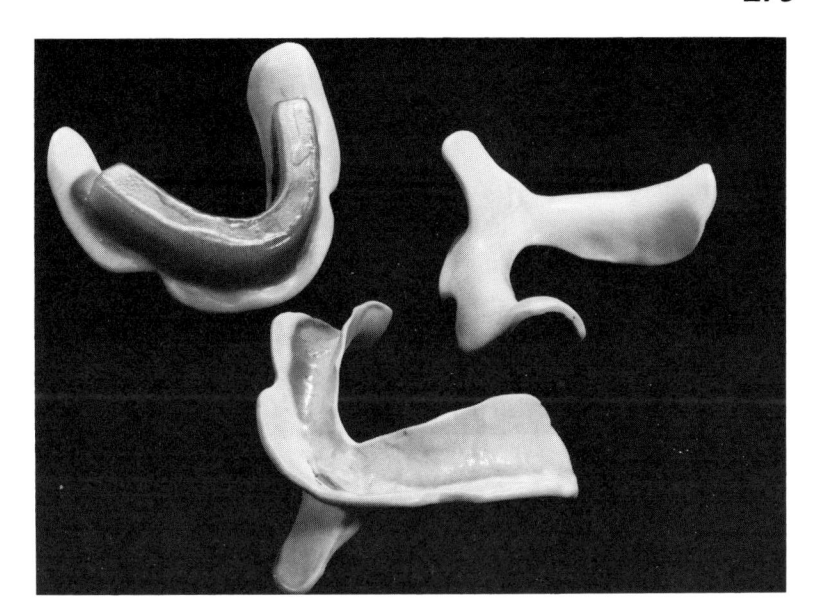

Figure 7–195. Surgical impression trays and a bite rim are fabricated preoperatively.

resistance is noted, the area should be inspected further. If impression material is present and encircles the bundle, the impression material can be cut with scissors at the inferoanterior aspect of the bundle. The impression should then be easily removed *without* trauma to this vital structure.

Once the tray is removed, the impression should be checked for the presence of defects and irregularities as well as registration of all anatomic landmarks, which should extend slightly beyond the external oblique ridges bilaterally, the mental neurovascular bundles bilaterally, the mylohyoid ridges bilaterally, the mandibular symphysis, the genial tubercles, and the concavity on the lingual aspect of the mandible (Fig. 7–196). The impression should then be washed, dried, and inspected once again. If the impression is not absolutely perfect, a second one should be made. The surgeon should irrigate under the flaps and inspect the areas for residual impression materials before making a second impression. The next step is placement of the surgical bite rim, in which the bony mandibular ridge is positioned and occluded with the patient's maxillary denture. The previously marked centric registration should be checked, as this relates the residual mandibular bony crest to the opposing occlusal table. This space will establish a guideline as to the height of the abutment head and the accompanying mesostructure. This technique also allows for the fabrication of the transitional denture. The surgical bite rim is filled with light-body impression material and seated on the ridge. Soft wax is then added to the impression and the mandible is occluded with the maxillary denture. The entire bite registration is removed and inspected.

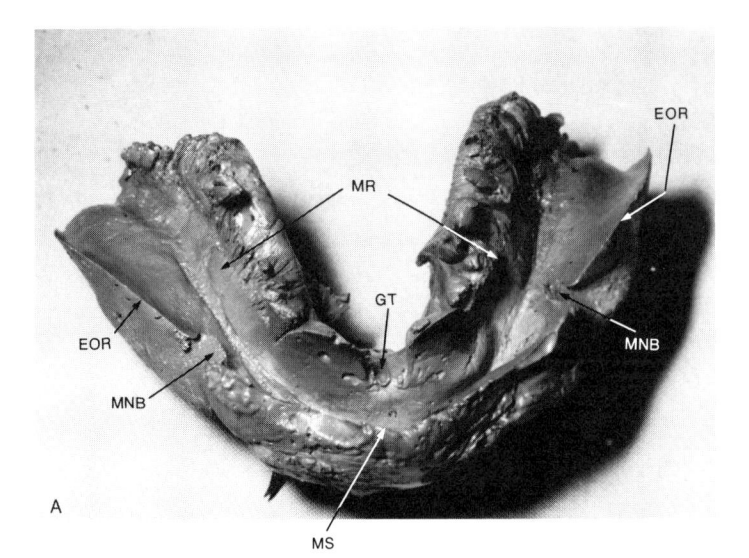

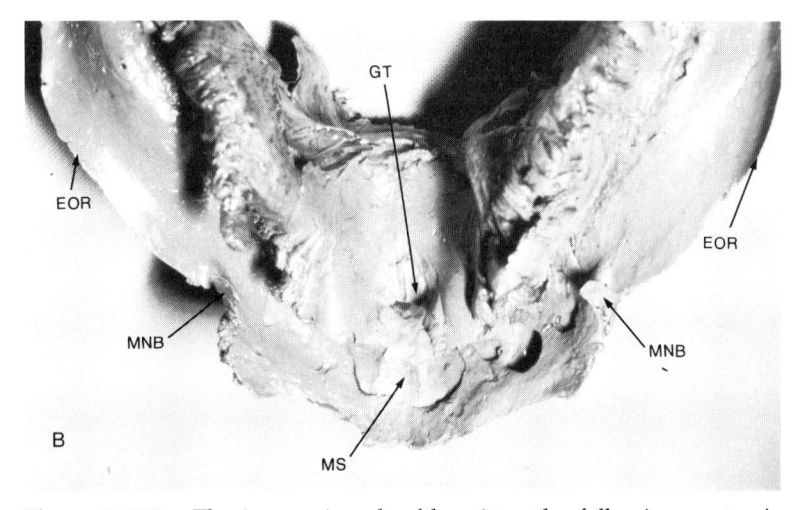

Figure 7–196. The impression should register the following anatomic landmarks: external oblique ridges bilaterally (EOR), mental neurovascular bundles bilaterally (MNB), mylohyoid ridges bilaterally (MR), mandibular symphysis (MS), genial tubercle (GT), and concavity on the lingual aspect of the mandible.

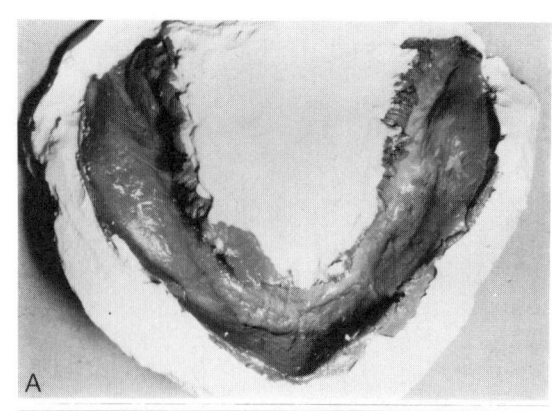

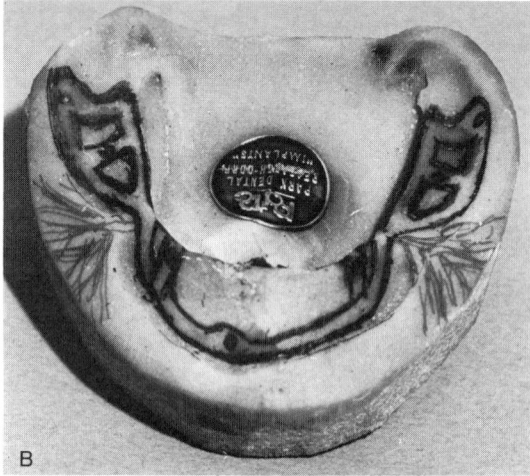

Figure 7–197. The impression must be boxed and poured so that no distortion of the impression occurs. *B,* The design for the casting is drawn on the master model and forwarded to the laboratory.

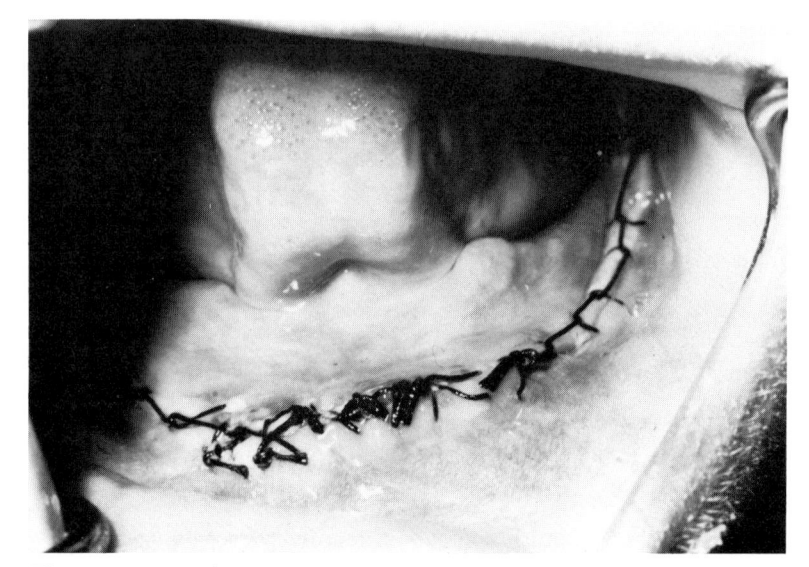

Figure 7–198. The mucoperiosteal flaps are repositioned and sutured using continuous sutures in the posterior area and mattress sutures in the anterior.

The best impression is selected and boxed in, and a master cast is poured (Fig. 7–197A). The framework is then designed on the master cast, the work authorization form is completed, and the entire case forwarded to the laboratory (Fig. 7–197B).

The sutures retaining the lingual and buccal flaps are removed, and these areas are once again irrigated and inspected for residual impression material. The mucoperiosteal flaps are repositioned and sutured with a combination of 3-0 silk continuous sutures in the posterior and 4-0 mattress sutures in the anterior region (Fig. 7–198).

Postoperatively the patient is maintained on continuous intravenous fluid infusion over the course of the hospital stay. Analgesics are prescribed and corticosteroids are used to reduce postoperative edema.

Stage II: Insertion of the Framework

When the subperiosteal procedure was first conceived, a six- to eight-week period of time elapsed between Stage I and Stage II, surgical insertion of the implant.[168–174] Recently, this time has been reduced to 10 to 14 days, the actual time being determined by the geographic proximity of the laboratory, which governs the shipping or mailing time, and the actual laboratory time required for fabrication of the implant.

The reduction in time between stages was initiated for two reasons. First, some atrophy of the bone will occur during the six- to eight-week waiting period. Second, the psychological impact of waiting for many weeks is traumatic to some patients. The shortened interval minimizes dimensional change in the bone, tissue shock, and delayed healing, and the patient is happier with the procedure.

The laboratory should return the original master cast and impression, the cast framework, the superstructure, the temporary prosthesis, screws when applicable, and a radiograph of the casting. The framework must be thoroughly examined for its fit on the master cast, for completeness of finish and polish, and for irregularities on the tissue-bearing surfaces (see Figs. 7–135 and 7–136). The radiograph must be viewed with variable-intensity illumination to detect internal defects (Fig. 7–199). The temporary prosthesis is composed of acrylic posterior bite blocks and six anterior teeth (Fig. 7–200). The tissue surface is fabricated to telescope in a passive fashion over the abutment posts or bar. The patient is given an appliance to wear and function with from the time the framework is inserted until the final prosthe-

IMPLANTS USED IN PREPROSTHETIC RECONSTRUCTIVE SURGERY / 277

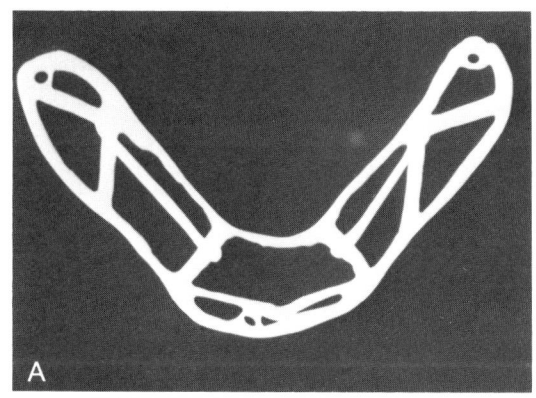

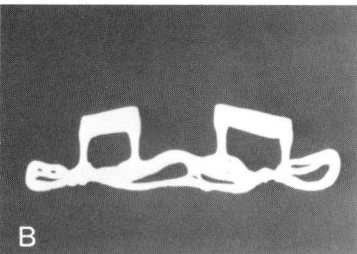

Figure 7–199. The radiographs of the casting must be viewed with variable-intensity illumination to detect the presence of any internal defects.

sis is completed. If adequate retention cannot be obtained with the prosthesis alone, the use of denture adhesive is helpful. The denture flanges must be totally clear of soft tissue, even allowing for post-surgical edema. The occlusion must be checked and spot ground until there is no evidence of premature contact or imbalance. Major deficiencies can be compensated for with the addition of cold-cure acrylics to the posterior bite blocks.

The implant framework is placed on the master cast, with the superstructure in place to prevent warping or trauma to the casting, and autoclaved, permitting the entire mechanism to be carried into the sterile operative field.

The anesthetic technique is the same as for Stage I surgery. The sutures are removed. Because of the brief interval between stages,

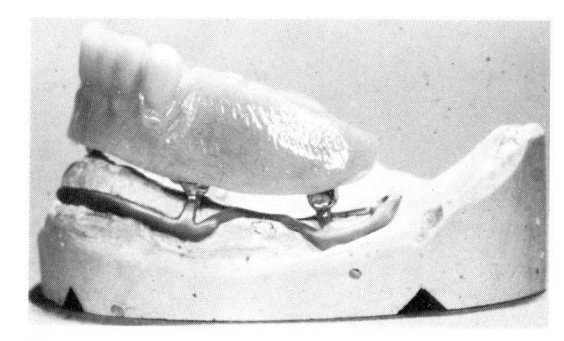

Figure 7–200. The temporary prosthesis is fabricated with six anterior teeth and posterior bite blocks and is totally implant-supported.

only a periosteal elevator is needed to reflect the mucoperiosteal flaps. The dissection can be less extensive than in Stage I, as it need not extend beyond the anatomic borders previously outlined.

The superstructure is placed on the implant and seated in place on the mandible. With this technique, the superstructure acts as a handle to ease manipulation and decrease the chance of deforming the casting. The framework should squeeze easily into position and should never be inserted or driven with a mallet. Once the framework is seated, the superstructure is removed. The major and minor connectors must be examined to ensure an accurate fit to the underlying bone. There should be no entrapment of the mucoperiosteal tissues (Fig. 7–201). Bone screws are usually not needed, but if the

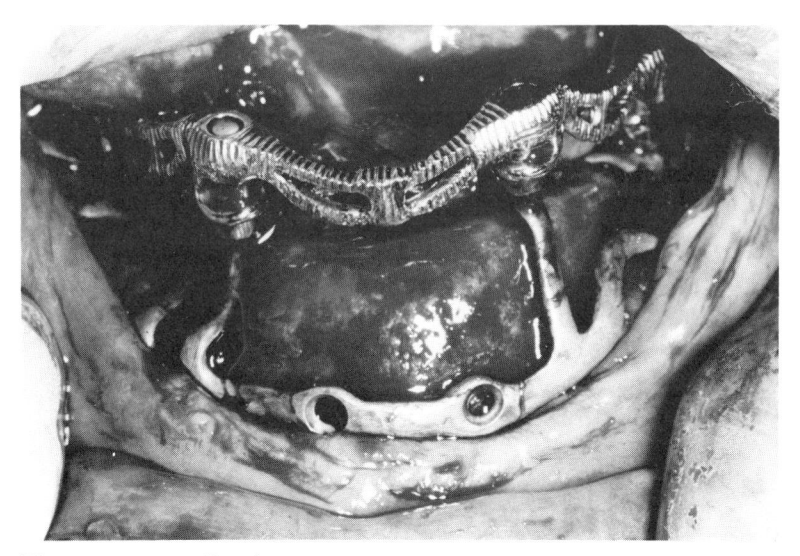

Figure 7–201. The framework is seated with the superstructure in place to prevent any deformation.

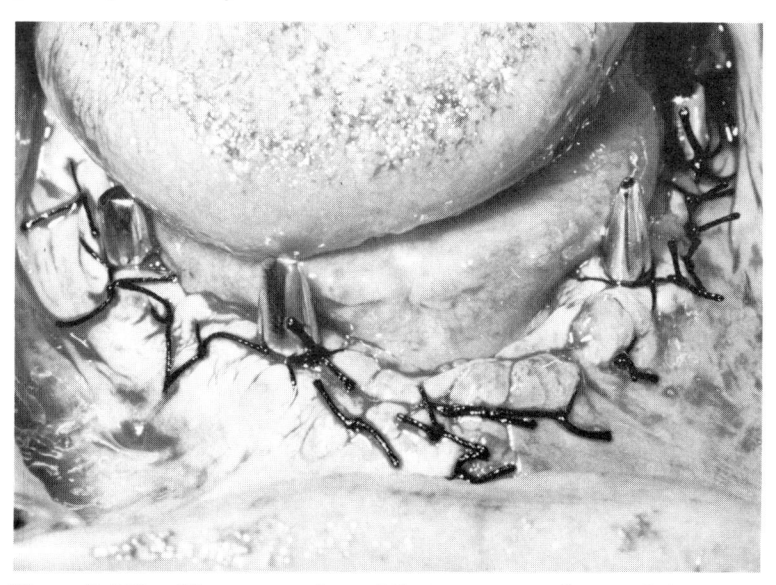

Figure 7–202. The mucoperiosteal flaps are sutured around the posts.

mandible is extremely flat, one screw placed into the symphyseal region may be useful. The mucoperiosteal flaps are sutured in the posterior region with 3-0 black silk sutures, using a combination of horizontal mattress and simple interrupted sutures (Fig. 7–202). In the anterior region, 4-0 silk horizontal mattress sutures are preferable. The transitional prosthesis is placed and checked for soft-tissue impingement and traumatic occlusion.

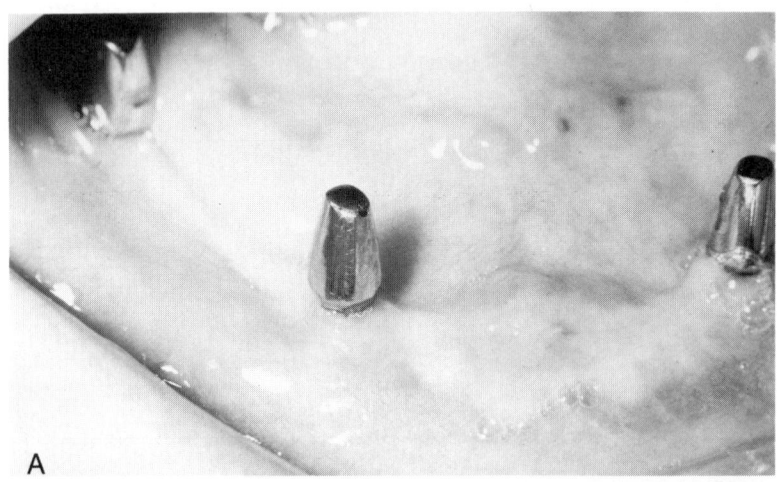

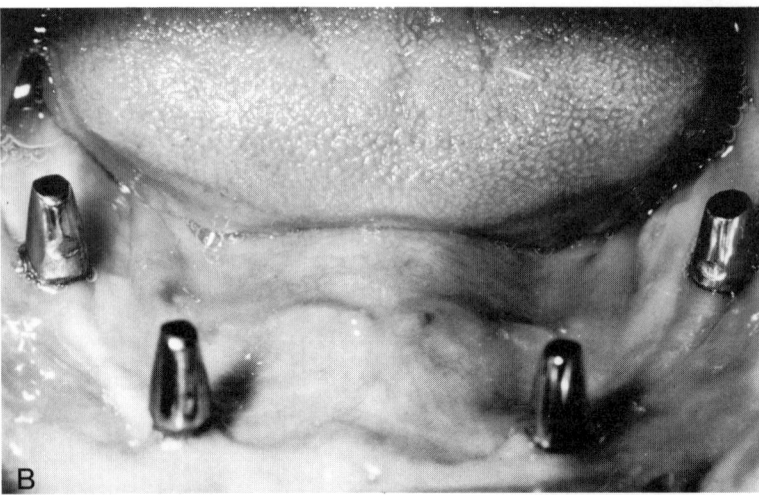

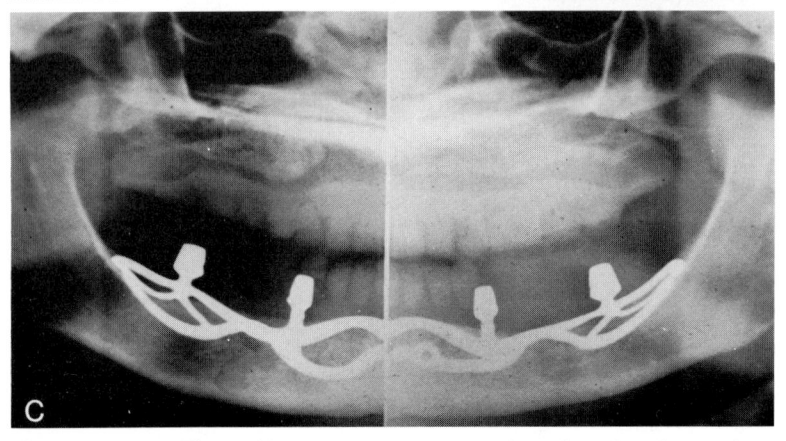

Figure 7–203. These 11-year postoperative clinical and radiographic pictures demonstrate excellent long-term results.

The same postoperative regimen is used for this period as for Stage I. The patient is usually discharged the next morning. The sutures are removed between the seventh and tenth postoperative day. During that time, the patient is maintained on a liquid to semisoft diet, followed by a semisoft to soft diet after two weeks. A regular diet may be resumed at three to four weeks. Initially, cleaning should be done with a soft toothbrush softened further with hot water, the gentle wiping away of debris, and manual irrigation and rinsing. After 10 to 14 days, a water-irrigation device at the lowest setting can be used. In addition, proper dental flossing techniques should be demonstrated to the patient.

The fabrication of the final prosthesis, with the superstructure incorporated into the tissue-bearing surface, is carried out four to six weeks postoperatively. The guidelines for the prosthetic fabrications are best outlined by Perel[176] (Fig. 7–203).

Laboratory Phase

Selection of the dental laboratory for the fabrication of this mechanism is of the utmost importance. Because this device is custom-made, its fabrication must be of the greatest accuracy and highest quality. The ordinary dental laboratory has neither the appropriately trained staff nor the sophisticated equipment to carry out these procedures properly. The clinician should visit the physical facility and discuss the needs and requirements for implant cases. Such a visit allows one to inspect other work in progress and judge the quality firsthand. It also affords the opportunity to clarify what the laboratory needs to fabricate an acceptable device for successful case completion.[178]

The first phase of the laboratory procedure involves the fabrication of the surgical bite rim and impression trays. These are constructed preoperatively from an overcompressed impression of the soft tissues of the lower arch, from which a study cast is poured. Stage I surgery is carried out using these trays (Fig. 7–204).

After the surgical impression is taken, the master cast is poured and the framework designed by the doctor. He then carefully writes out a prescription to the laboratory. In addition to general instructions, items that must be included are (1) the tissue thickness in the area of the implant post, (2) the number of screw holes and length of screws, (3) the height of the abutment heads or meseostructure, and (4) the design of the temporary denture and the color and type of teeth. The following items must be for-

IMPLANTS USED IN PREPROSTHETIC RECONSTRUCTIVE SURGERY / **279**

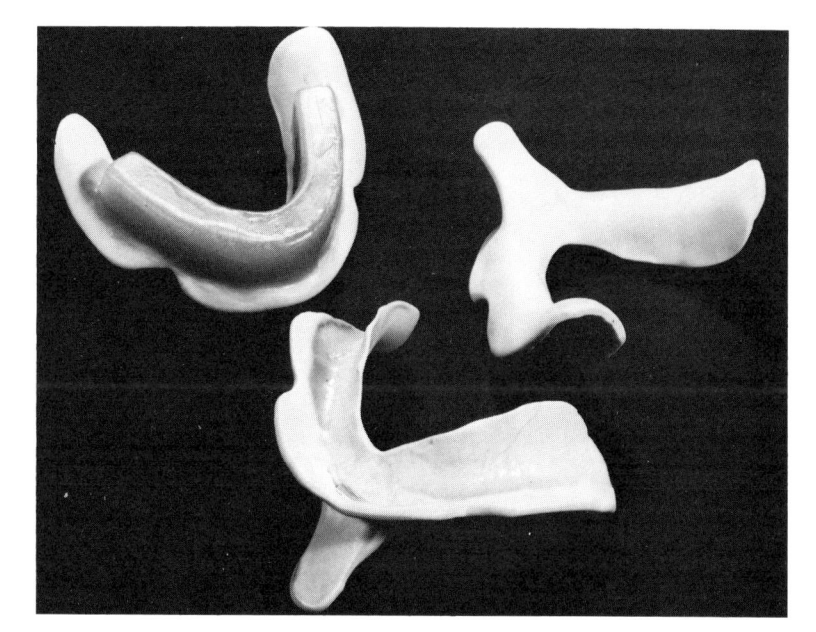

Figure 7–204. Surgical impression trays and bite rim are used to obtain accurate records for the laboratory during Stage I.

warded to the laboratory: (1) the final bone impression, (2) the master cast with the framework design, (3) the surgical bite with the bit rim in place, (4) the study cast of the maxillary denture or the denture itself, and (5) the written prescription for the fabrication of the frame.

Once the laboratory receives the case, a refractory or investment cast is made by duplicating the master cast (Fig. 7–205A). A very careful check of the accuracy of this step is essential, as fabrication of the framework will actually be carried out on this refractory model (Fig. 7–205B). The design, as outlined on the master model, is then duplicated (Fig. 7–205C).

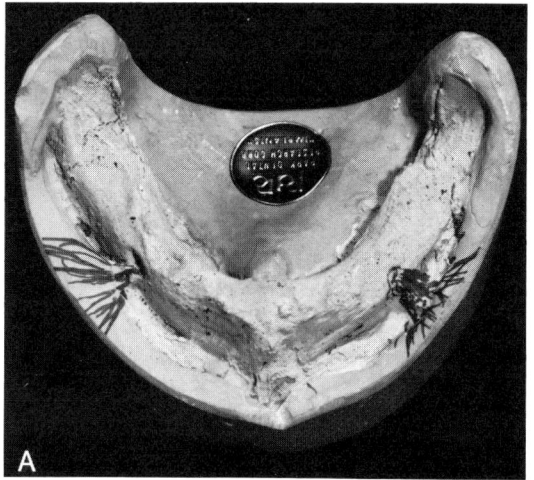

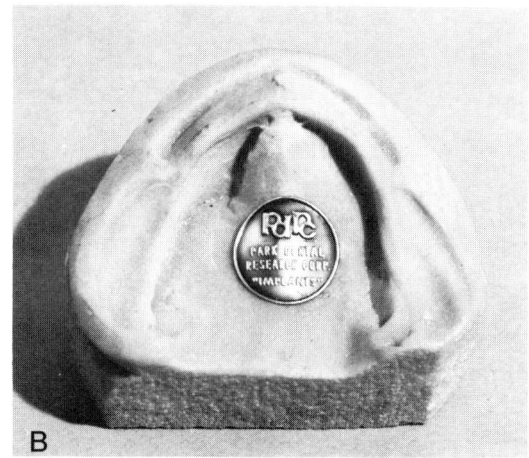

Figure 7–205. *A,* The master cast is duplicated. *B,* The investment cast is fabricated and used for the design and fabrication of the framework. *C,* The design is then duplicated on the investment cast.

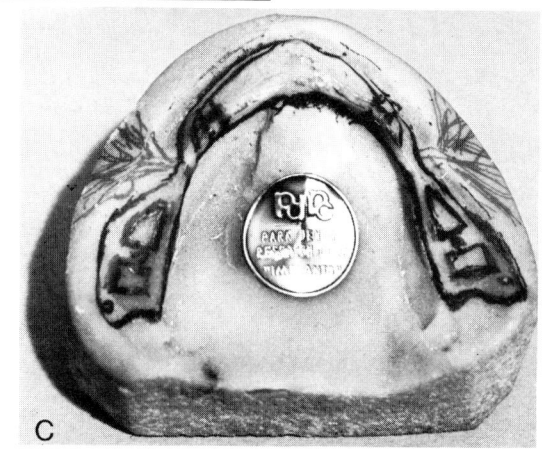

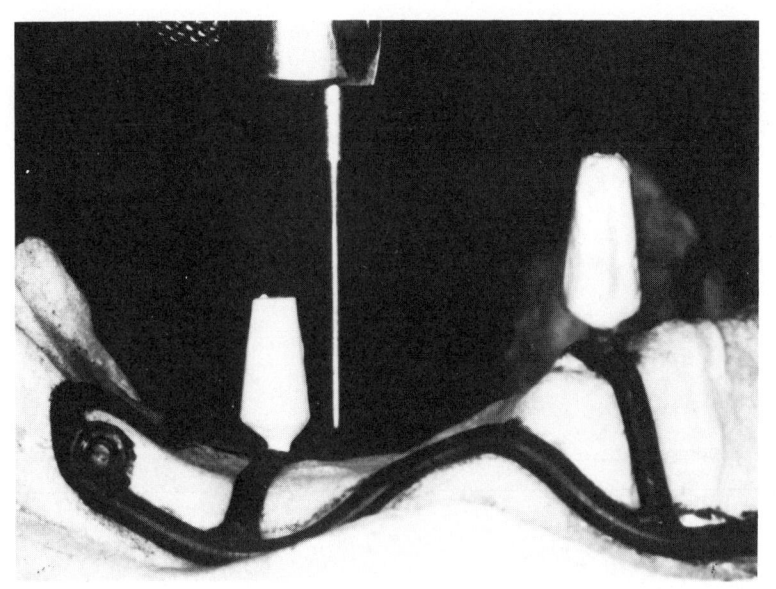

280 / IMPLANTS USED IN PREPROSTHETIC RECONSTRUCTIVE SURGERY

Figure 7–206. A surveyor is used to insure parallelism of the abutments.

In recent years, laboratory techniques and materials have greatly improved. Many of the wax portions are prefabricated, allowing for uniformity and accuracy of struts and abutments. When the abutment heads are positioned, they are paralleled with a surveyor (Fig. 7–206). The length of the abutment necks is based on the soft-tissue measurements. Once the framework has been waxed, the sprue is placed (Fig. 7–207). The model with the wax-up is examined, burned out, and cast in a centrifugal casting machine. Only virgin ingots of surgical grade vitallium should be used for the casting. Buttons from previous castings, flasking, or old framework should never be used in the new casting. This reduces the chance of contamination with impurities. Once the casting has been completed, it is cleaned and polished. The tissue-bearing surface should never be polished but only sandblasted. The abutment heads are polished.

At this point in the fabrication of the framework, further inspection is indicated. Industrial grade radiographic examination of the metallic framework has been used over the past decade. Several views must be made to allow evaluation of the casting from all angles (see Fig. 7–199). Interpretation of the radiographs must be done with a variable-intensity illuminating screen and a magnifier, and the cast framework should be available for comparison.

The temporary prosthesis, with six anterior teeth and posterior bite blocks, is fabricated in heat-cured acrylic. The tissue surface of this prosthesis is designed to passively telescope over the cast mesostructure. The prosthesis should be entirely implant-supported, with no soft-tissue contacts (Fig. 7–208).

The laboratory will then forward the following materials to the doctor, to be used in

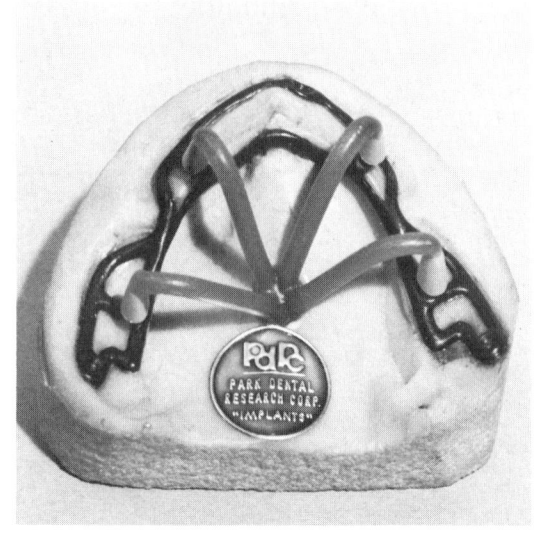

Figure 7–207. When the waxing is completed, the sprue is placed, the cast is invested, and the framework is fabricated.

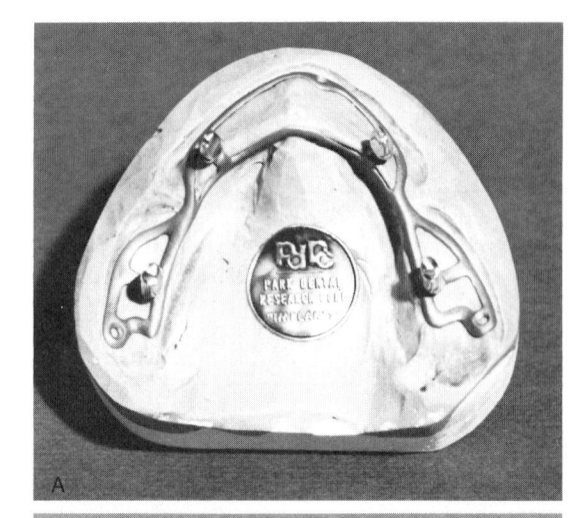

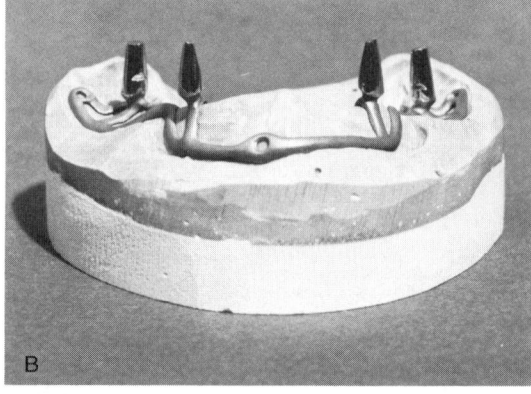

Figure 7–208. The completed cast is returned to the clinician for Stage II.

the completion of the case: (1) the master cast with the cast framework, (2) the superstructure in place on the implant framework, (3) the osseous screws, (4) the temporary prosthesis, (5) the laboratory radiograph, and (6) the surgical impressions and bite rims.

THE RAMUS FRAME

George J. Collings

The Basic Ramus Frame

Since the ramus frame was introduced by Harold Roberts, the mandibular ramus frame implant has been a part of the armamentarium of the implantologist, because it requires only a one-stage operation that patients often tolerate well.[180] It can be placed in a mandible with significant edentulous bone loss, and it may be placed by a versatile general dentist as well as by an oral surgeon or prosthodontist.

Advantages of a Ramus Frame Implant

1. It is a one-stage surgical procedure.
2. It can be utilized on a patient who cannot tolerate a two-stage surgical procedure.
3. The patient leaves the operatory wearing dentures.
4. It can be utilized when there is bony dehiscence of the inferior alveolar nerve from the molar region to the mental region.

Disadvantages of a Ramus Frame

1. There is a possibility of damaging the inferior alveolar nerve and blood vessels when the posterior crypt is made in the ascending ramus.
2. Portions of the frame may sink and impinge on the superior aspect of the mucoperiosteum, with attendant discomfort, infection, and bone loss.[181]
3. The anterior foot of the ramus frame may settle severely, necessitating removal of this portion through the inferior border of the mandible (see Failures of the Ramus Frame).

Patient Selection and Education

The patient should be fully acquainted with the benefits and risks involved in placing this implant and must be willing and able to undergo the physiologic and psychological trauma associated with it. Viewing a model of the implant, talking to another patient, and reading literature on the procedure may help allay anxieties.[182]

A thorough medical and dental examination should precede this operation, and the oral health and hygiene of the patient must be acceptable (see Chapter 3). The patient should have good health and nutrition and should not smoke or use alcohol to excess. A booklet may be given to the patient outlining a special diet.[183]

Preliminary Preparation

Articulated study models should be obtained. Before a clinical placement is at-

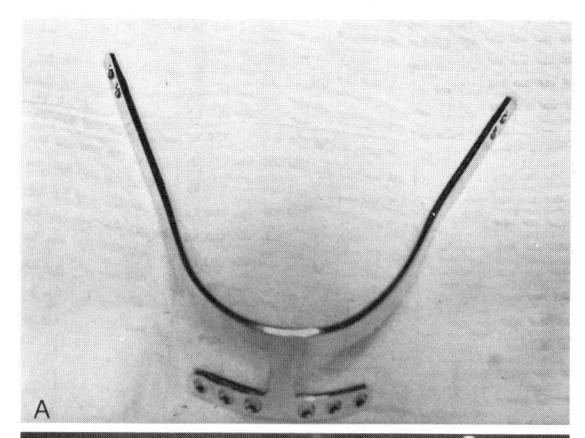

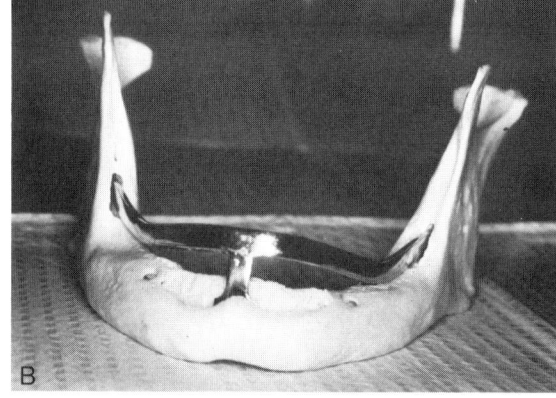

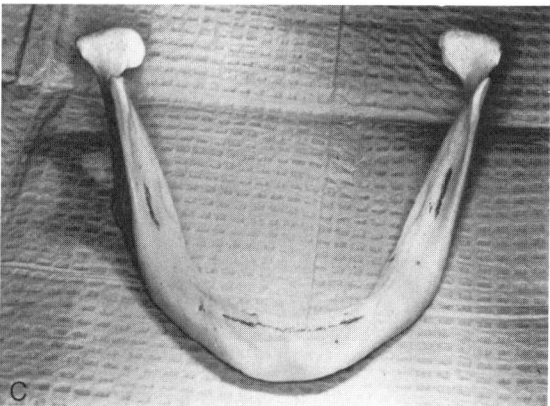

Figure 7–209. *A*, Basic ramus frame. *B*, Ramus frame in mandible. *C*, Bony incision areas.

tempted, a ramus frame (Fig. 7–209A) implant is placed on a dry mandible and retained for study and reference during the procedure (Fig. 7–209B), particularly as bone incisions are made (Fig. 2–209C). One can use the study model to practice the technique of bending and placing the frame; it also serves as a guide for the try-in during surgery. A panoramic radiograph is needed. The quantity and quality of bone and any pathology are evaluated.

Patient Preparation

Vertical measurements of the patient are taken with the existing dentures in place. It is imperative that up-to-date and accurate records be kept, including radiographs, photographs, and written records. The upper denture should be relined at this time if needed.

A duplicate set of dentures is made entirely of acrylic, which is easier to trim and insert. If the patient does not have a lower denture, a trimmed factory denture may be purchased (Fig. 7–210A) or the new lower plastic denture (Fig. 2–210B) may be trimmed to fit the laboratory model made prior to the operation (Fig. 2–210C). The duplicate denture will closely fit both the patient and the model, but the last molar in the duplicate denture may have to be removed if it interferes with the opposing occlusion.

The temporary denture will be utilized for approximately six months. As the frame for the implant adapts, equilibration of the dentures will be necessary. Equilibration is an important step in both the preparation and longevity of the implant and cannot be stressed enough.

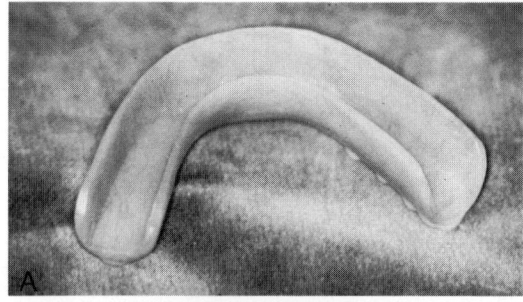

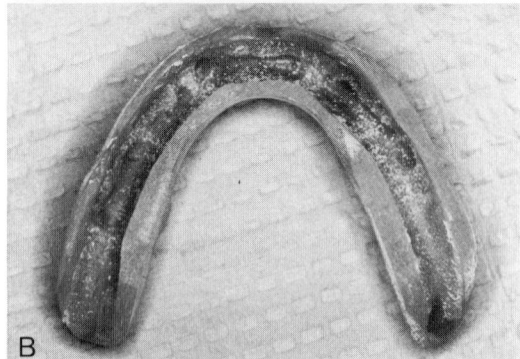

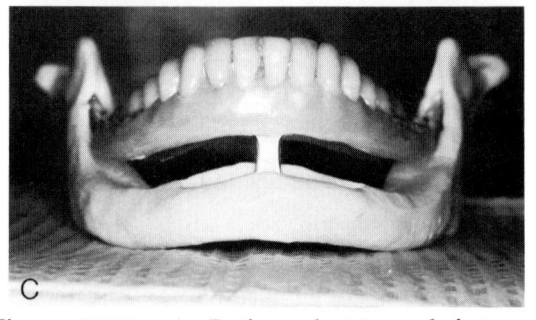

Figure 7–210. *A*, Preformed, trimmed factory denture. *B*, Patient's plastic denture. *C*, Trimmed dental on model.

Surgical Preparation

Several packaged sterile ramus implants of various sizes should always be available during surgery in case the bone structure is different than anticipated or an implant becomes contaminated. The basic frame is constructed of 316 surgical stainless steel. It can be easily bent and cut and has excellent strength and ability to resist the forces of mastication.[184, 185]

A good inventory of implants and instruments should include two 5 and 6 and one 7 implant (Fig. 7–211A); one try-in frame (Fig. 7–211B); two handpiece air rotors—one bayonet and one quiet-air right angle (Fig. 7–211A); necessary burs, including the No. 701 and No. 557 cross-cut fissure; tracing papers for checking occlusion; a set of 316 surgical stainless steel bending instruments (Fig. 2–209C). Standard surgical instruments for mucoperiosteal and osseous surgery should, of course, be available.

Dexamethasone (Decadron [5-12] pack) or equivalent and an appropriate antibiotic should be given just prior to surgery. A vitamin-mineral supplement should be considered if the patient's diet has been deficient.[186] Sedation and local anesthesia are usually appropriate,[187] along with corticosteroids to minimize swelling, if not contraindicated. A sterile technique is used.

Surgical Stage

The anterior surface of the ascending ramus is palpated to determine the width between the external and internal oblique ridges. An incision 14 mm long is made through the mucoperiosteum on the anterior surface of the ascending ramus and slightly buccally (Fig. 7–212), exposing the ascending ramus. The external and internal oblique ridges are then exposed and the tissue retracted. Using a Mid-West bayonet hand-

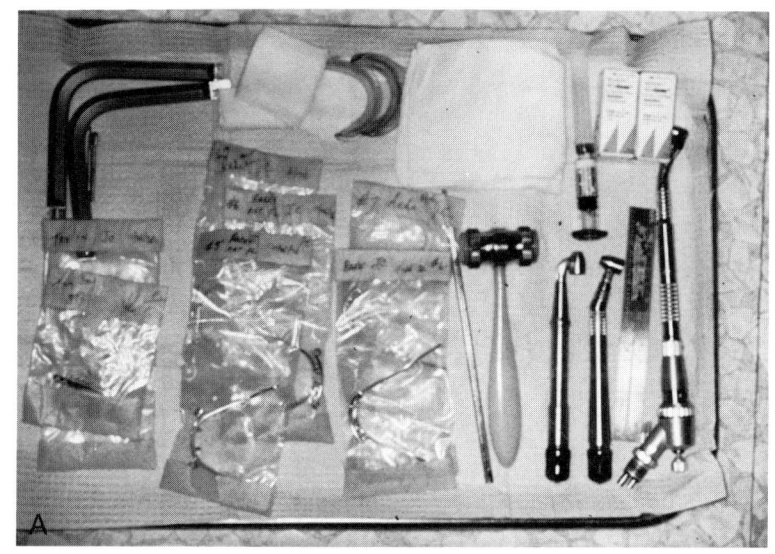

Figure 7–211. Surgical instruments for ramus frame implant. *A*, Ramus tray set-up. *B*, Three-piece try-in. *C*, Bending instruments.

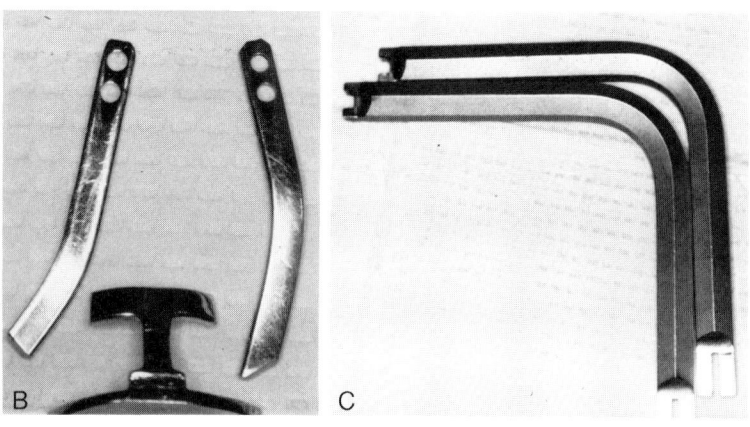

piece with a No. 557 cross-cut fissure bur that is 15 mm from tip to hub (Fig. 7–213), a bony channel 10 mm long and 15 mm deep is made under irrigation with copious amounts of sterile normal saline solution. Great care should be taken to keep the bur and handpiece parallel to the buccal surface of the ascending ramus (Fig. 7–214). The bur should be pointed slightly upward to ensure that the frame will have a correct occlusal line when inserted (Fig. 7–215).

A try-in, composed of the frame cut into three segments (see Fig. 7–211*B*), is inserted 15 mm deep. The posterior try-in has a notch made on the superior aspect 15 mm

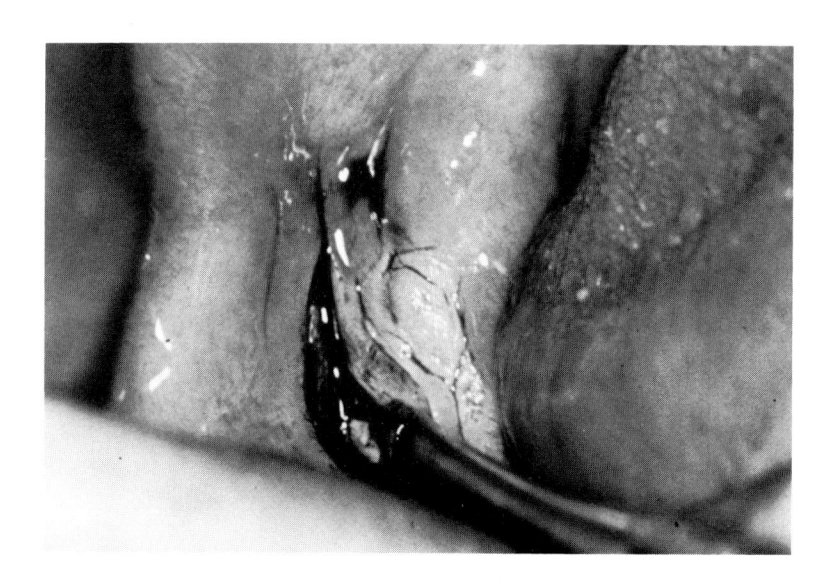

Figure 7–212. Incision on ascending ramus.

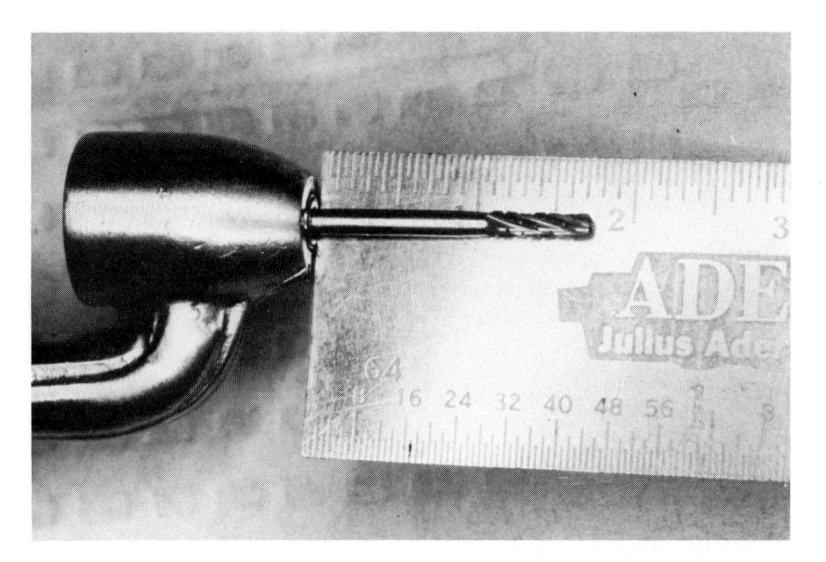

Figure 7–213. Measuring cross-cut fissure bur.

from the distal end (Fig. 7–216), and adjustments can be made at this time if necessary. This is repeated on the opposite side. When the final frame is seated in the symphysis it will shift anteriorly. If the distal portion extends less than 15 mm under bone in the ascending ramus, it will project only 11 to 12 mm into the ramus after the anterior portion is seated. A mark similar to the one on the try-in template is placed on the frame at the superior border 15 mm from its distal end so that the position of the frame in the ascending ramus can be determined.

An incision is made along the crest of the alveolar ridge from the area of the right first bicuspid to the area of the left first bicuspid (about 15 mm long). The lingual and labial mucoperiosteum is retracted just enough to allow the burs to make the anterior slot in the symphysis without traumatizing the tissue. It is of cardinal importance to avoid trauma to the mental neurovascular bundle. The crest of the alveolar process is scored with a No. 701 cross-cut fissure bur to obtain the length for the anterior try-in, which is established by placing the try-in on the crest of the exposed ridge. A No. 557 cross-cut fissure bur is used to cut the bone to its proper depth and width for insertion of the anterior try-in. Great care is taken to ensure proper width, depth, and length for a very close adaptation of the permanent anterior foot. To minimize heat damage, one should always use copious amounts of sterile normal saline solution when a bur is used on bone. *Be kind to your tissue.* The bony crypt should be approximately 6 mm deep and parallel to the anterior portion of the menton region of the mandible. This ensures approximately 1 mm of bone superior to the foot of the implant. The implant has a tendency to settle, so it should not be placed deeply into bone.

The anterior try-in is bent, using the bending instruments, to fit the bony crypt and is used as a template for the anterior foot of the implant (Fig. 7–217). The bony crypt should closely approximate the implant to minimize the invagination of epithelial tissue. If the bony incision is made too wide and epithelial tissue invagination occurs, pain results and the implant must be removed, the epithelial tissue curetted, and the bone allowed to heal for six months before the operation is repeated.

A frame of the proper size is selected and the ramus portions inserted into the two

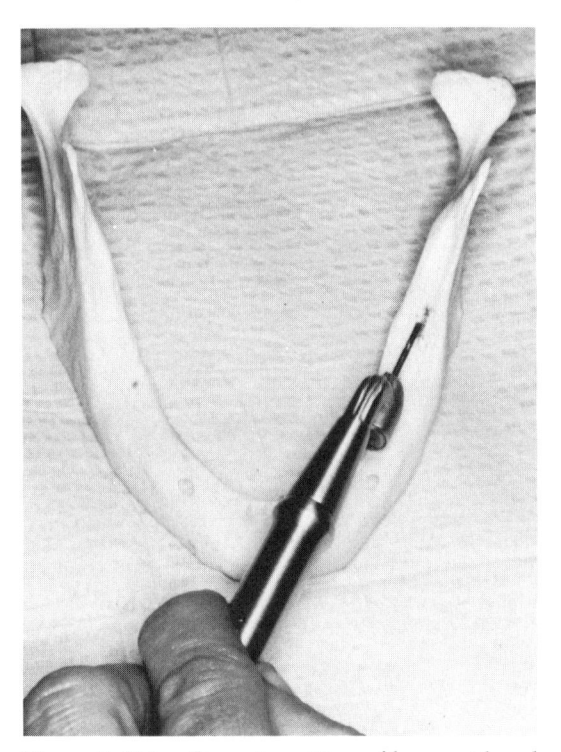

Figure 7–214. Correct position of bayonet handpiece.

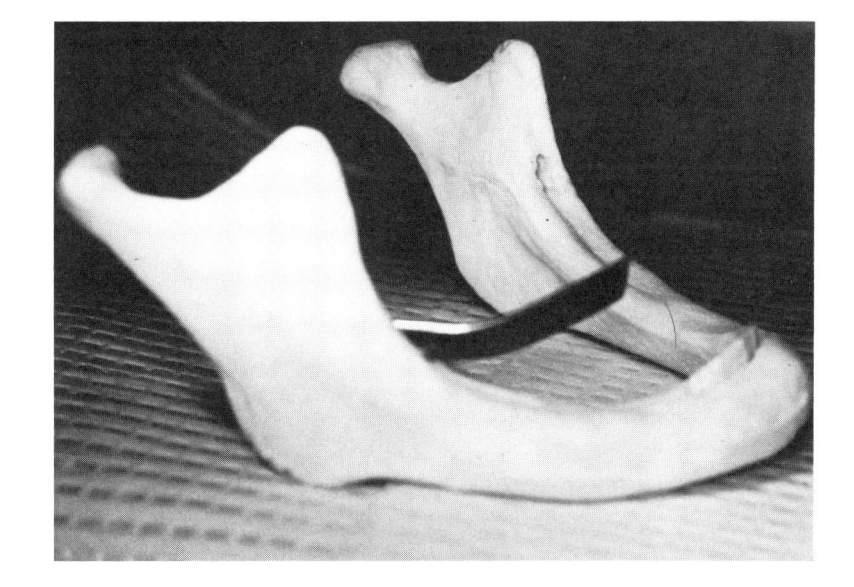

IMPLANTS USED IN PREPROSTHETIC RECONSTRUCTIVE SURGERY / **285**

Figure 7–215. Incorrect occlusal line.

Figure 7–216. Posterior try-in with notch.

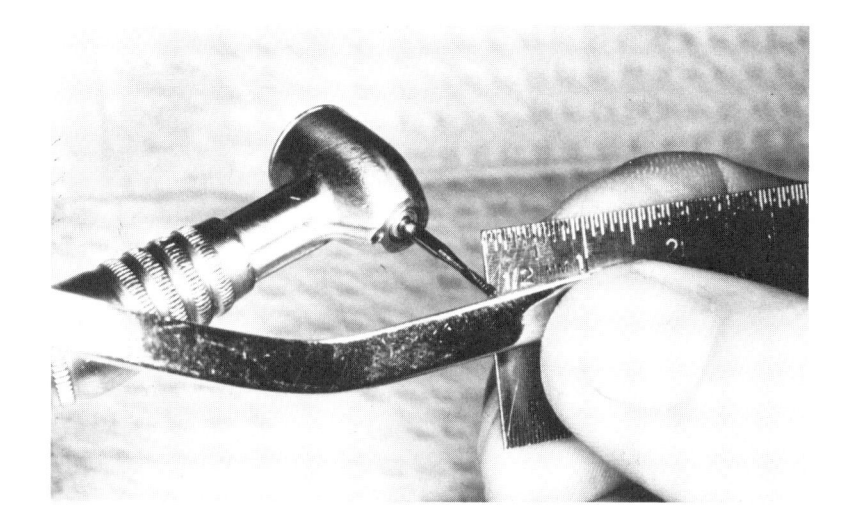

Figure 7–217. Transferring the try-in to the utilized frame.

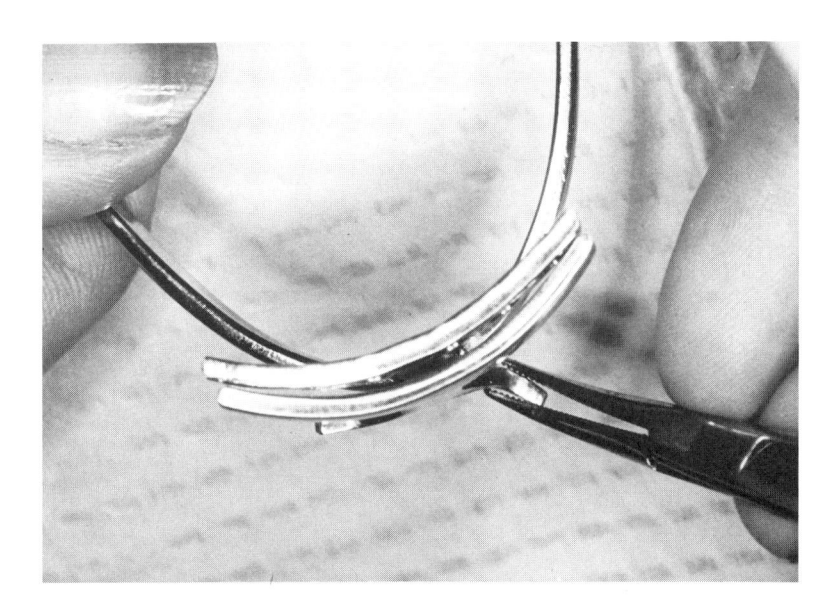

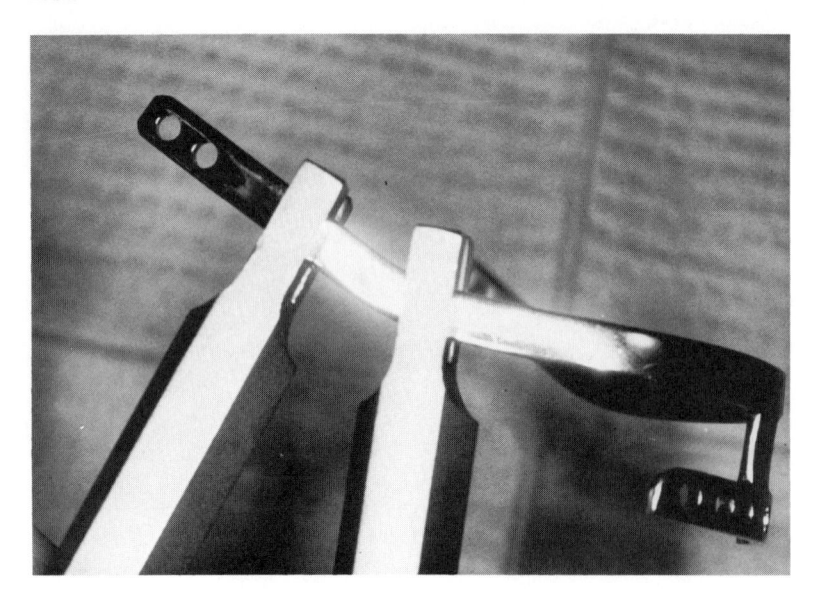

Figure 7–218. Bending the monorail correctly.

rami slots. The ramus portions may have to be bent with the special bending instruments (Fig. 7–218) until they have been inserted to their proper depth. The anterior portion should be lightly tapped into place. The center post should be in a midline position, and the frame solid and free from any movement or clicking. The frame may have to be bent and adjusted to eliminate any movement; this can be done with the bending pliers without removing the implant (Fig. 7–219). Both instruments are inserted on the monorail as far distally as possible, using minimum pressure, and one instrument is twisted to the left and the other to the right, care being taken not to fracture the internal or external plate of the ascending ramus. This should be done on both posterior portions of the monorail until no clicking or movement is noted. The implant is now solidly in place.

Suturing

A mattress suture of 2-0 nonresorbable material is placed around the anterior post with close adaptation. The mucoperiosteum is approximated with 3-0 sutures about 2 mm apart to counteract the tension from lip and tongue movement (Fig. 7–220A). The mucoperiosteum of the rami is approximated with two 3-0 sutures below the monorail and two above (Fig. 7–220B).

Temporization of the Dentures

The upper denture is inserted, and the trimmed, lower denture is placed on the frame and examined for midline, centric, and vertical occlusion. The cusps of both dentures and the internal surface of the lower denture can be reduced if necessary. Fine equilibration can be done once the lower denture is stabilized. The bite should not be

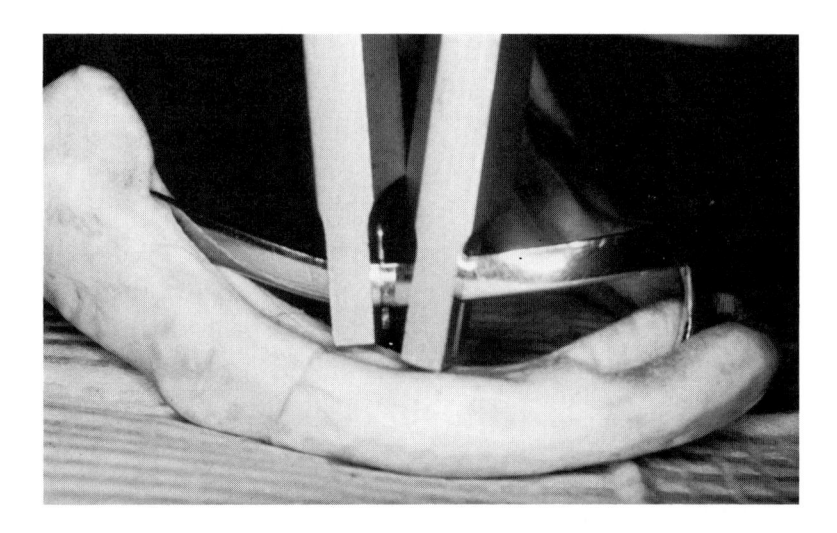

Figure 7–219. Demonstration of bending technique in the patient's mouth.

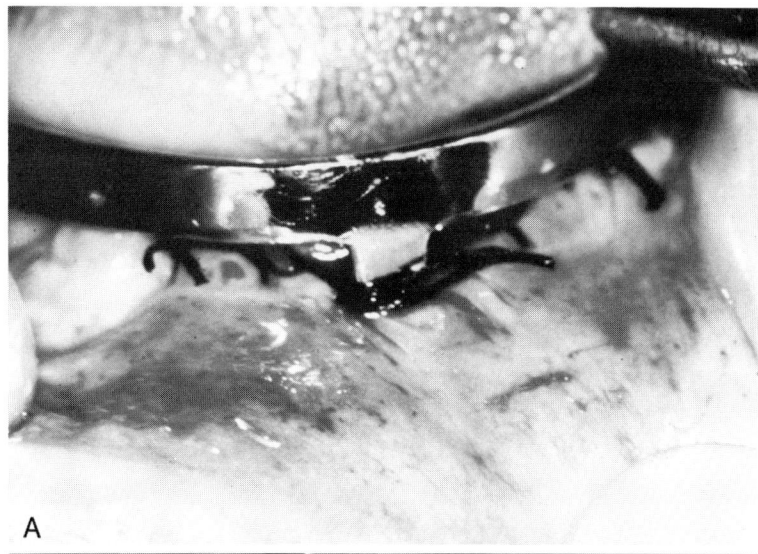

Figure 7–220. *A*, Anterior sutures in place. *B*, Posterior sutures in place.

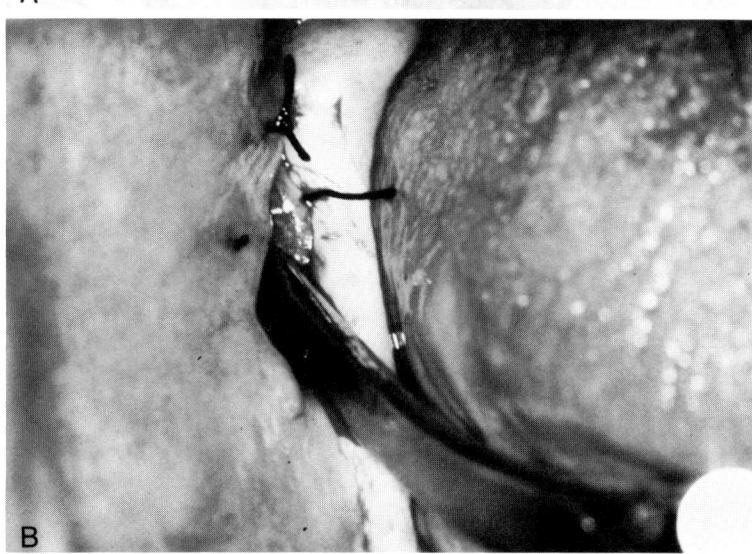

opened at this time. The lower denture is lined with quick-curing acrylic and placed in proper occlusal relationship with the upper denture after the monorail has been generously coated with petroleum jelly. Great care must be taken to prevent the acrylic from lodging under the frame, which would prevent removal of the lower denture. Just when the acrylic begins to set, the lower denture is removed and spurs and excesses are ground away (Fig. 7–221A). It may be necessary to repeat this procedure several times to stabilize the lower denture. Occlusal equilibration is repeated, as it is critical to the success of the implant.[188] The lower denture is then polished (Fig. 7–221B).

Postoperative Care and Medication

In addition to pain medication, an antibiotic should be continued for at least three days postoperatively. The patient should be instructed to load the denture minimally for at least three months.

The lower denture is left in place for 12 to 14 days before removal of the sutures. At this time, the patient is instructed on how to remove the lower denture to ensure proper cleaning of denture and frame. The patient is provided with a Butler brush (614 tip) to clean the inferior border of monorail and around the anterior post, a soft nylon pediatric brush to clean the monorail, and Q-tips soaked in equal parts of H_2O_2 and H_2O to clean and stimulate tissue around distal portions of the monorail. Patients are given a disclosing agent to make sure all plaque is removed, and periodic professional cleanings are done. The patient is also given strict home care instructions on diet and on what to expect. Occlusion must be carefully checked and radiographs taken every three months for the first nine months and yearly thereafter. At approximately six months,

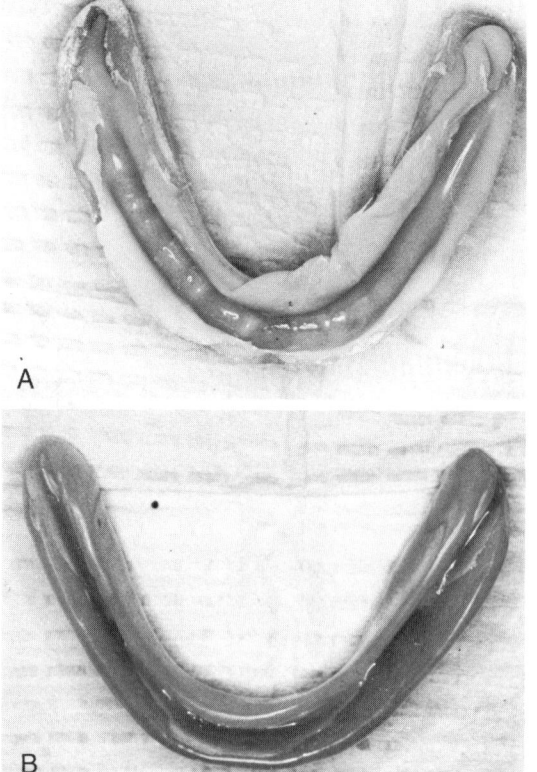

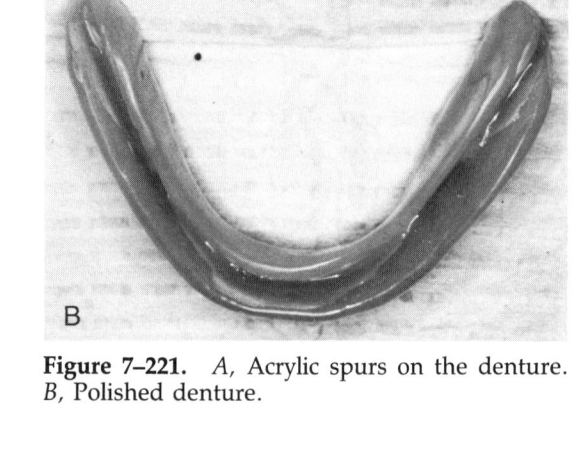

Figure 7–221. *A,* Acrylic spurs on the denture. *B,* Polished denture.

permanent dentures are made. The patient is then followed on a six-month or yearly basis.

Figure 7–222 shows a panoramic x-ray taken nine years postoperatively, revealing normal bone in the ramus, anterior foot, and post. Figure 7–223 shows no epithelial irritation around or adjacent to the anterior post or right and left ascending rami.

Permanent Fixation of Lower Denture

In the past friction against the monorail alone was used to stabilize the lower denture. This method has now been replaced by a combination of gold or stainless steel clips and Lew Locks.[189, 190]

Geltrate or a similar material is used to take the impression of the maxillary arch, and the same material may be used for the lower arch, but soft carding wax should be used under the monorail to help eliminate undercuts. The maxillary impression can be poured in the stone of choice, but the mandibular impression should be made with pink quick-curing acrylic, using a syringe technique to prevent bubbles. A wax model is then made for the clip-on portion, using the anterior portion of the monorail and right and left mandibular areas (Fig. 7–224). A Lew Lock pin is then inserted in the waxed-up lower denture and the tip of the Lew Lock is colored red (Fig. 7–225) so that when it is placed on the monorail, an exact hole may be drilled from this mark. Figure 7–226 shows clips in place with the Lew Lock, and Figure 7–227 shows a close-up of the Lew Lock in the finished denture. This method has decreased the need for periodic relining and is more stable and satisfactory.

The RA-2 Ramus Frame Implant

Many modifications of the basic ramus frame implant have been introduced to overcome the problem of the sinking or settling of these implants.

Ralph Roberts publicly introduced the RA-2 ramus frame implant in 1981 at the Alabama Implant Congress. According to his statistics, 675 RA-2 appliances (Fig. 7–228) have been placed, with 12 failures reported. Of these, 163 frames have been in place for two years or more. The author has placed approximately 15 since 1982, with one failure to date.

This type of frame is the most radical of all the modifications but the most practical approach to the settling problem. As stated in the discussion of basic ramus frames, the monorail is inserted 15 mm into the ascending ramus, which is porous. The pod or posterior portion of the RA-2 is 40 mm long (Fig.

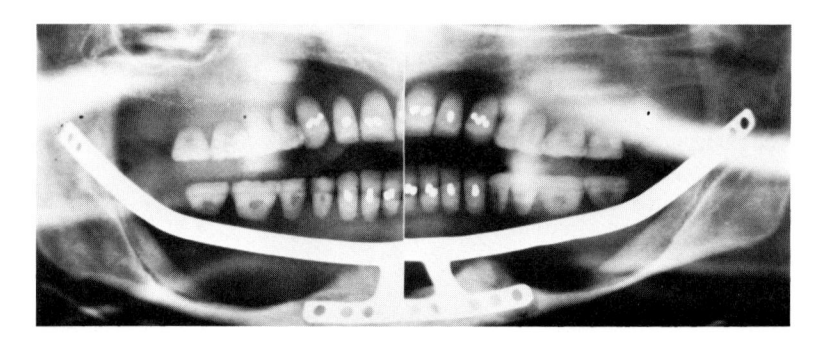

Figure 7–222. Nine-year postoperative panoramic radiograph.

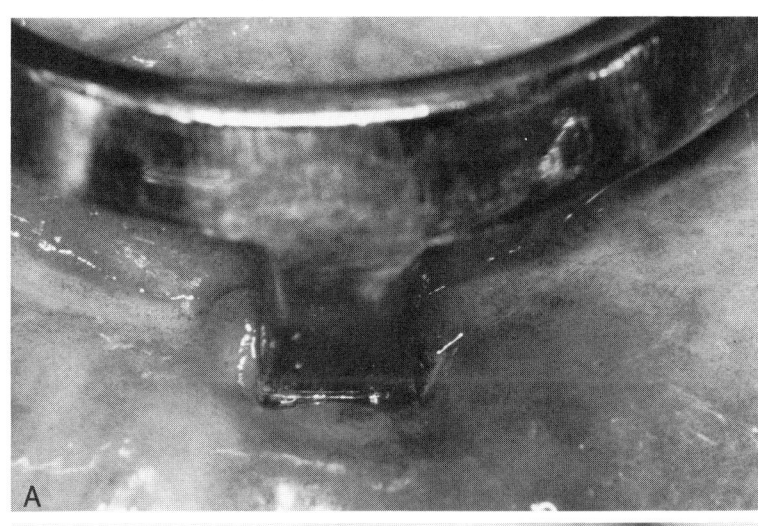

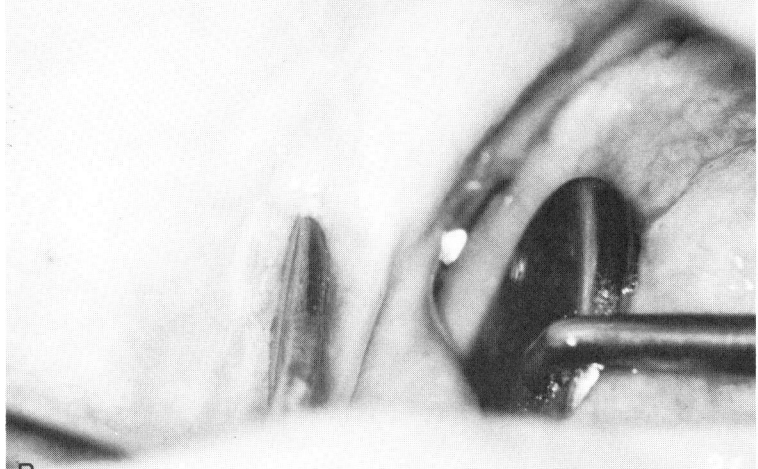

Figure 7–223. *A*, Anterior post with excellent healing. *B*, Right monorail with no epithelial irritation. *C*, Left monorail reveals normal epithelium.

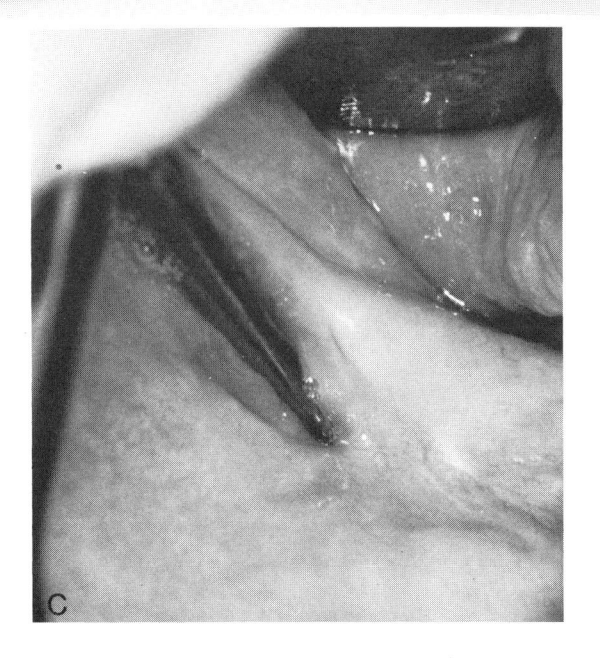

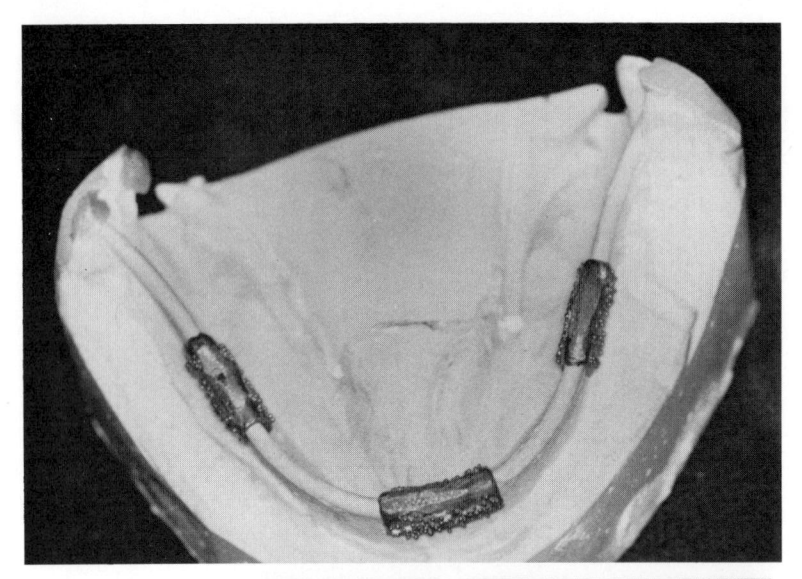

Figure 7–224. Three metal clip-ons in place.

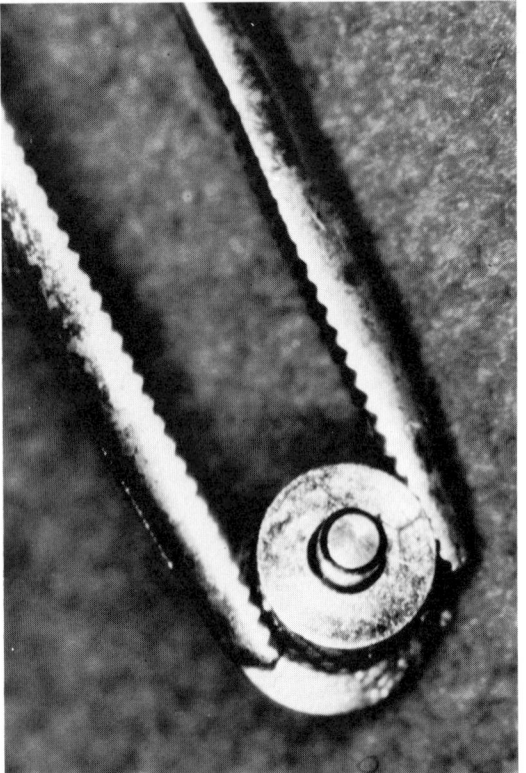

Figure 7–225. Lew Lock attachment with dot.

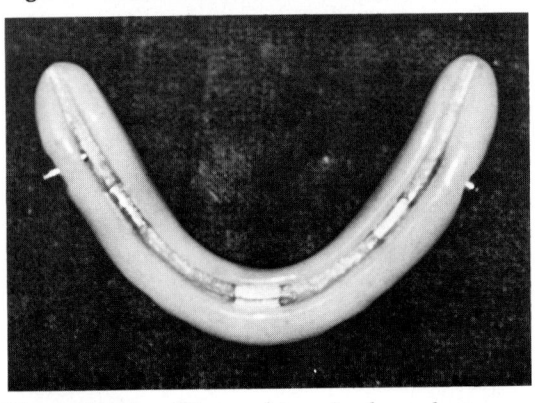

Figure 7–226. Clips and Lew Lock on denture.

7–229) and is inserted in the external oblique ridge, which is cortical bone. The posterior pod is also made with a buccal antisettling tab (see Fig. 7–228). The posterior pod is made either 5 or 10 mm from inferior aspect to superior border. The author's experience has been to utilize the 5-mm RA-2, as it is easier to insert and less bone has to be removed to insert it.

The sizes of the RA-2 implant are classified I, II, and III. It is made from 316 stainless steel or titanium.[191–193]

Advantages of the RA-2 Implant over the Basic Ramus Frame

1. The posterior border of the distal pod is 40 mm long, allowing greater resistance to occlusal stress. In addition, the device has antisettling tabs (Fig. 7–230).
2. The posterior pod is inserted in the external oblique ridge, thus eliminating the danger of severing the inferior bundle as it enters the ascending ramus.
3. The antisettling tabs adhere to the hard cortical plate of the external oblique ridge, which lessens settling.
4. The antisettling tabs on the anterior foot closely adhere to the cortical plate in the menton region, thus decreasing the settling in that area.

Disadvantages of the RA-2 Implant

1. It is more difficult to insert than the basic ramus frame.
2. Bending of the implant using the bending gig is very critical.
3. It is more time-consuming to insert than the basic ramus frame.

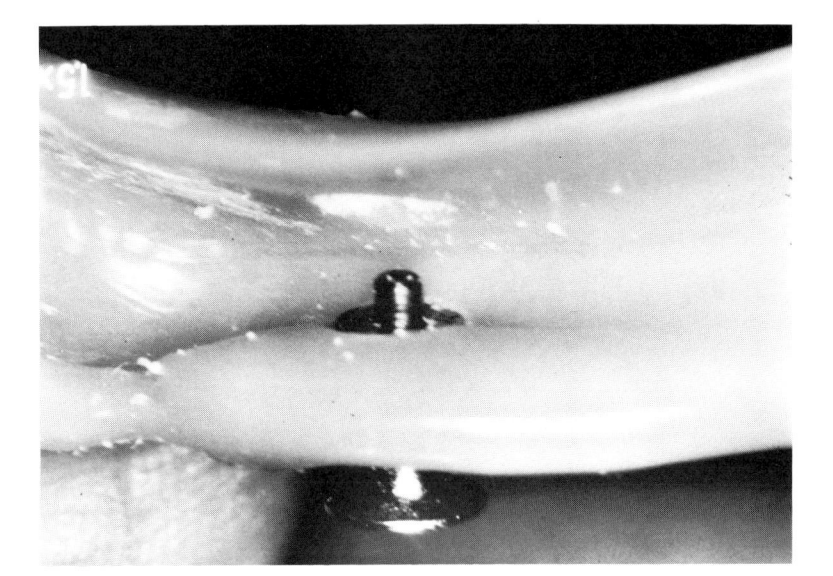

IMPLANTS USED IN PREPROSTHETIC RECONSTRUCTIVE SURGERY / **291**

Figure 7–227. Close-up of the Lew Lock in place.

4. Not enough time has elapsed to properly evaluate its merits.

Owing to the complexity of insertion of the RA-2 implant the following guidelines are suggested to reduce the possibility of operative failures.

1. If the posterior pod is not seated to the proper and desired depth before the anterior foot is seated, tension will be placed on the implant bar when seating of the anterior foot is attempted. The net result will be a loose anterior foot and a failing implant.
2. When the implant is seated, if the posterior osteotomies are not extended far enough anteriorly, the pods will make contact with the anterior portion of the trenches and prevent proper seating.
3. Improper depth of the osteotomies promotes failure.
4. Improper bending of the appliance promotes failure. Bending of the device is done with great caution and only as a last resort.
5. Overcutting of the osteotomies results in a loose implant.

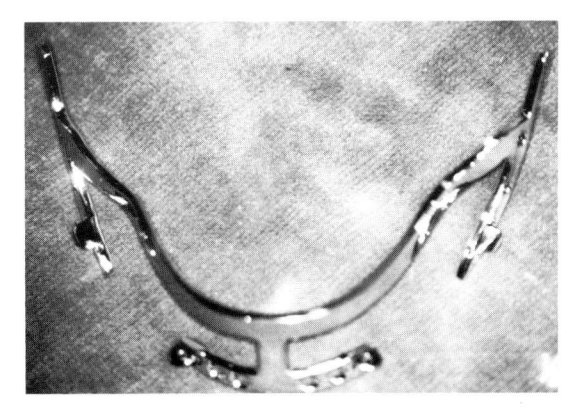

Figure 7–228. RA-2 ramus frame with antisettling tabs.

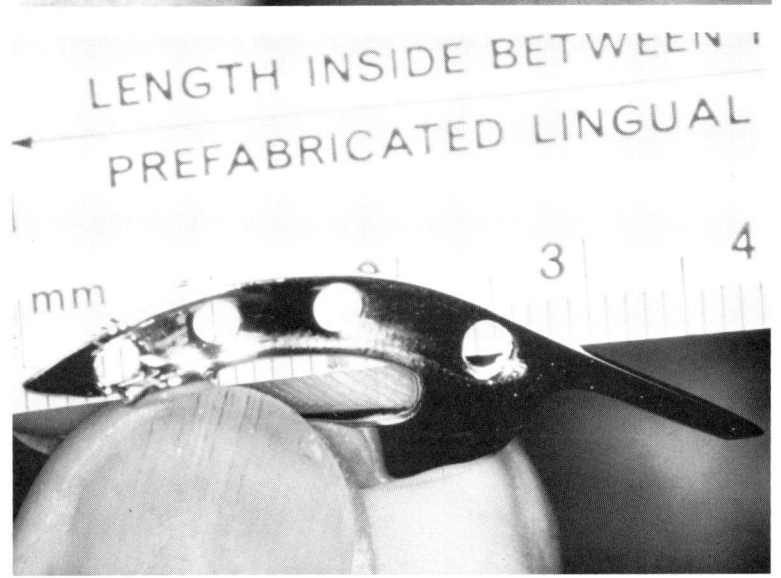

Figure 7–229. Measuring posterior try-in (40 mm long).

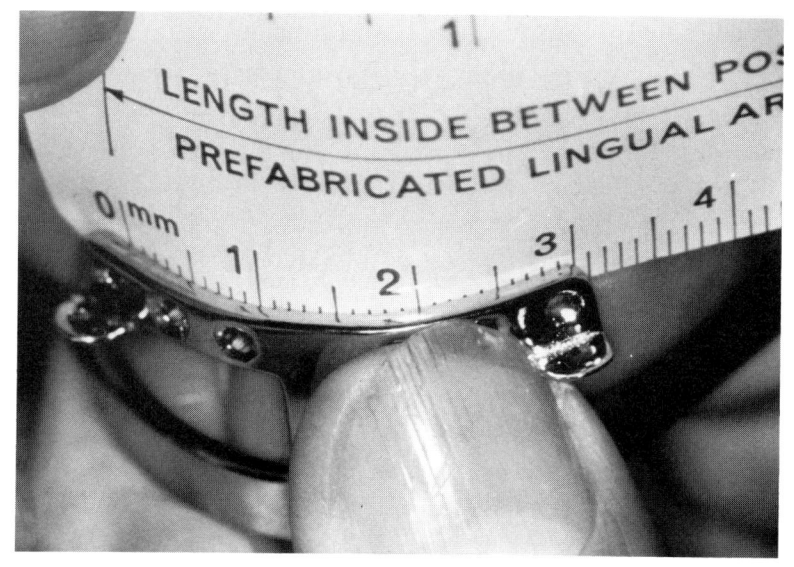

Figure 7–230. Measuring length of anterior foot (30 mm).

6. Trauma to soft tissues can result in soft-tissue invagination and bone destruction.

7. Proper patient selection is an important consideration.

8. Improperly applying the seating chisel, denting the implant, or fracturing into one of the holes of the implant foot leads to failure.

9. Incomplete seating of the foot (or pods) of the implant promotes failure.

Preliminary Preparation

Preliminary preparation is the same as for the basic ramus frame implant, with the exception that the operator should place three or more RA-2 implants in a dry mandible to familiarize himself with the complexities of bending and seating the RA-2 (Fig. 7–231A) in the patient's mandible (Fig. 7–231B). Radiographic analysis is utilized as in the basic ramus frame implant.

Surgical Preparation

Again, the surgical set-up is the same as for the basic ramus frame except that a divider (Fig. 7–232A) with two sharply pointed ends is added (Fig. 7–232B). This may be purchased from a mechanical drawing equipment dealer. It must be made of stainless steel for autoclaving. A spring-driven mallet may be used with a 316 stainless steel tip (Fig. 7–233) and a try-in consisting of a ramus portion (Fig. 7–234A) and an anterior try-in (Fig. 7–234B). All parts that come in contact with each other must be of the same metal.

Surgical Stage

This stage is the reverse of that for the basic ramus frame. An incision is made through the mucoperiosteum high and slightly buccal to the midline in the ascending ramus. As the incision line proceeds anteriorly, it is directed to the midline on the crest of the alveolar process. It terminates in a like fashion on the opposite side.

The mucoperiosteum is retracted approximately 4 mm labially and lingually in the anterior region from mental neurovascular bundle to mental neurovascular bundle, with great care taken not to traumatize this structure. A No. 557 cross-cut fissure bur is

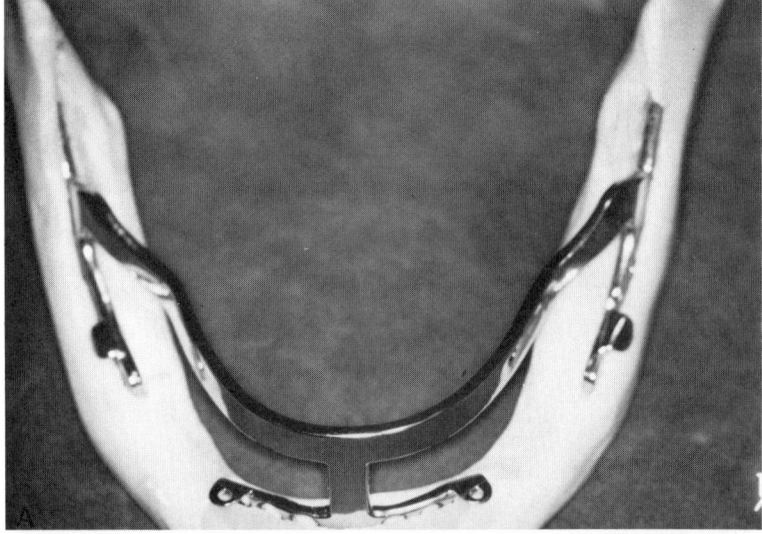

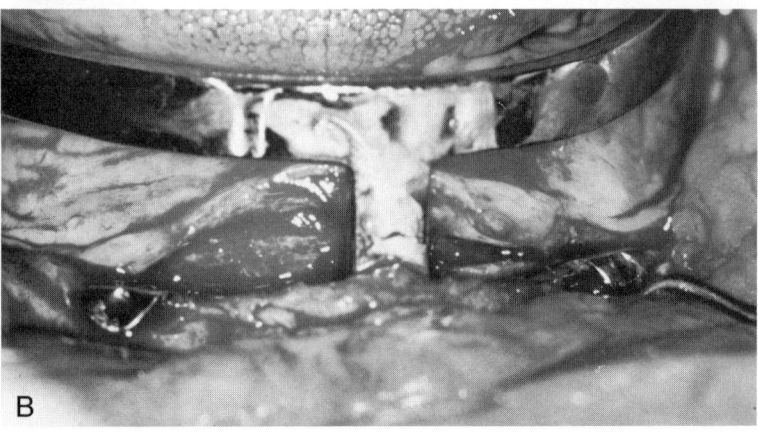

Figure 7–231. *A,* RA-2 frame in dry mandible. *B,* RA-2 frame in patient.

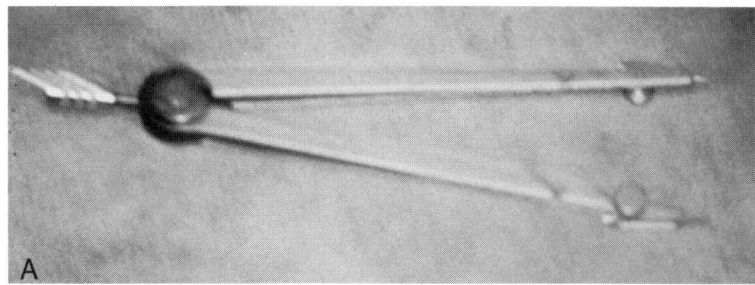

IMPLANTS USED IN PREPROSTHETIC RECONSTRUCTIVE SURGERY / **293**

Figure 7–232. *A*, Stainless steel dividers. *B*, Close-up of stainless steel points.

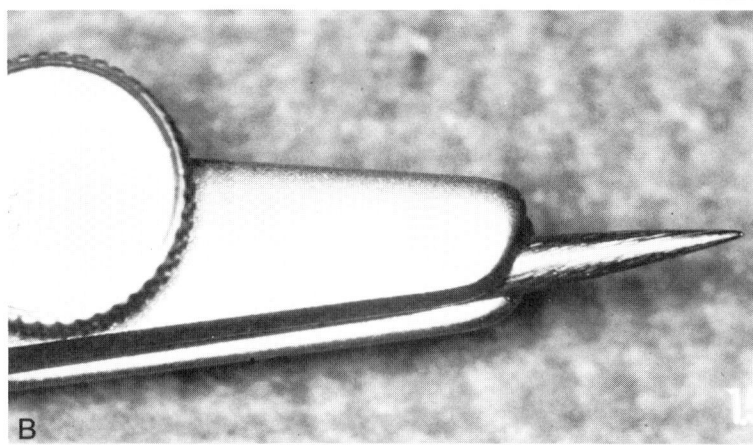

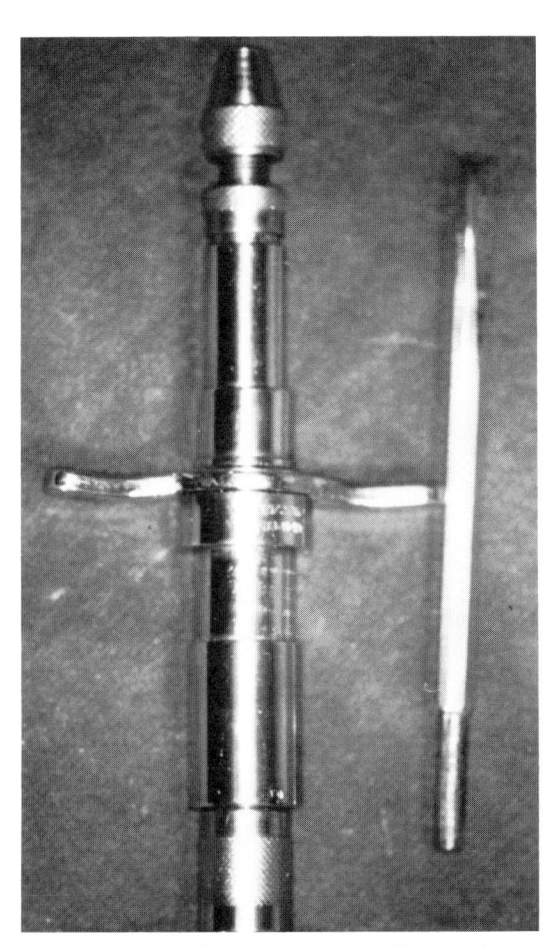

Figure 7–233. Spring-driven mallet with 316 stainless steel tip.

utilized to make a half-moon incision just wide enough and deep enough to accommodate the foot of the anterior try-in (Fig. 7–235*A*). This contour is then transferred to the implant to be inserted (Fig. 7–235*B*).

The mucoperiosteum is now retracted on the body and ascending ramus both lingually and buccally. The dividers are separated 18 to 20 mm from point to point. The

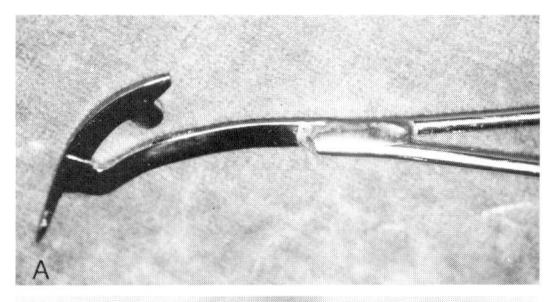

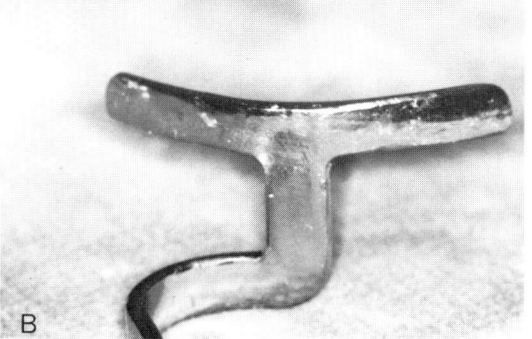

Figure 7–234. *A*, RA-2 try-in. *B*, Anterior try-in.

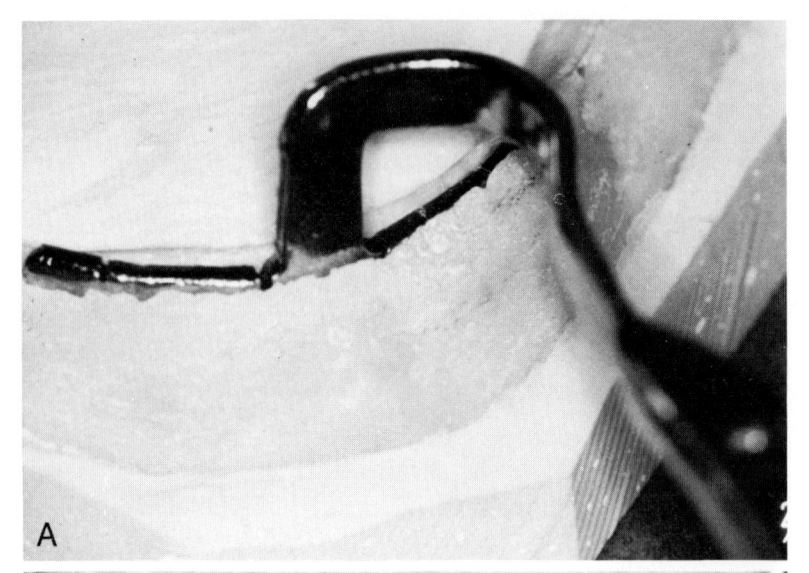

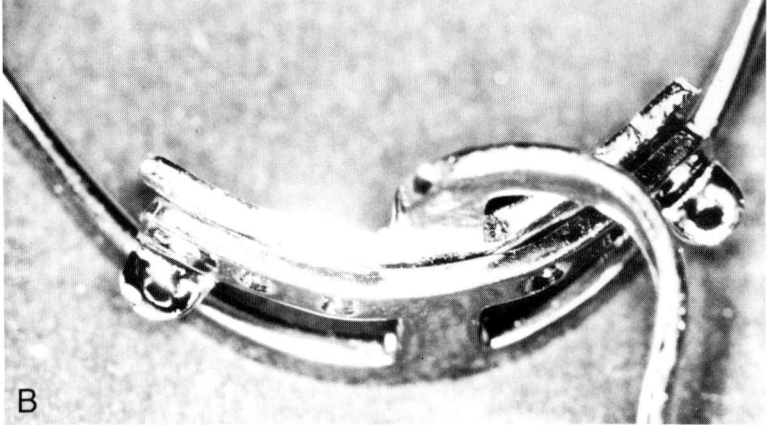

Figure 7–235. *A*, Anterior try-in placed in dry mandible. *B*, Transferring the contour to the implant for insertion.

anterior point is placed on the distal aspect of the anterior bony crypt and the distal end on the crest of the ridge, and a dot is made as a reference point (Fig. 7–236*A*). The dividers are then separated 30 mm and a mark is made on the distal point (Fig. 7–236*B*). These two marks are lined up with a series of dots (Fig. 7–236*C*), using a No. 4 round bur for a guide between the mesial and distal dots. The dots are now connected using a No. 557 cross-cut fissure bur to accommodate the posterior pod of the implant. A 10-mm crypt is then made with a No. 557 cross-cut fissure bur, using a bayonet handpiece (Fig. 7–236*D*) on the distal end of this slot under the cortical plate where the pointed end of the implant try-in will be inserted. The bayonet handpiece should be directed superiorly and distally. The posterior try-in is now ready for insertion (Fig. 7–237) utilizing the hand mallet (see Fig. 7–233). This portion, like the anterior portion, *must* adhere to the bony crypts (Fig. 7–235*A* and 7–237). It may be necessary to use the special bending gigs (Fig. 7–238) to achieve the correct occlusal plane.

This procedure is repeated on the opposite side, and the RA-2 frame is inserted using the spring mallet, the bending instruments used in the basic ramus frame, and the RA-2 bending gig (Fig. 7–238). Surgical sites should be thoroughly debrided before the mucoperiosteum is approximated and sutured. This procedure differs from that for the basic frame in that more sutures are required owing to the length of the incision.

Failures of the Ramus Frame

In addition to the inherent problems of implants that penetrate the mucosa, failure of ramus frame implants can occur owing to (1) the ramus crypt being too wide, too low, or too shallow; (2) the anterior bony crypt being too deep or too wide; (3) incorrect length of the ramus frame; (4) damage to the inferior alveolar or mental nerves; (5) inappropriate loading, such as excessive vertical dimension of dentures or faulty occlusion or patient bruxism.[194] It is probably best to provide three or more months with very light loading; (6) failure to note systemic conditions that might predispose to poor load re-

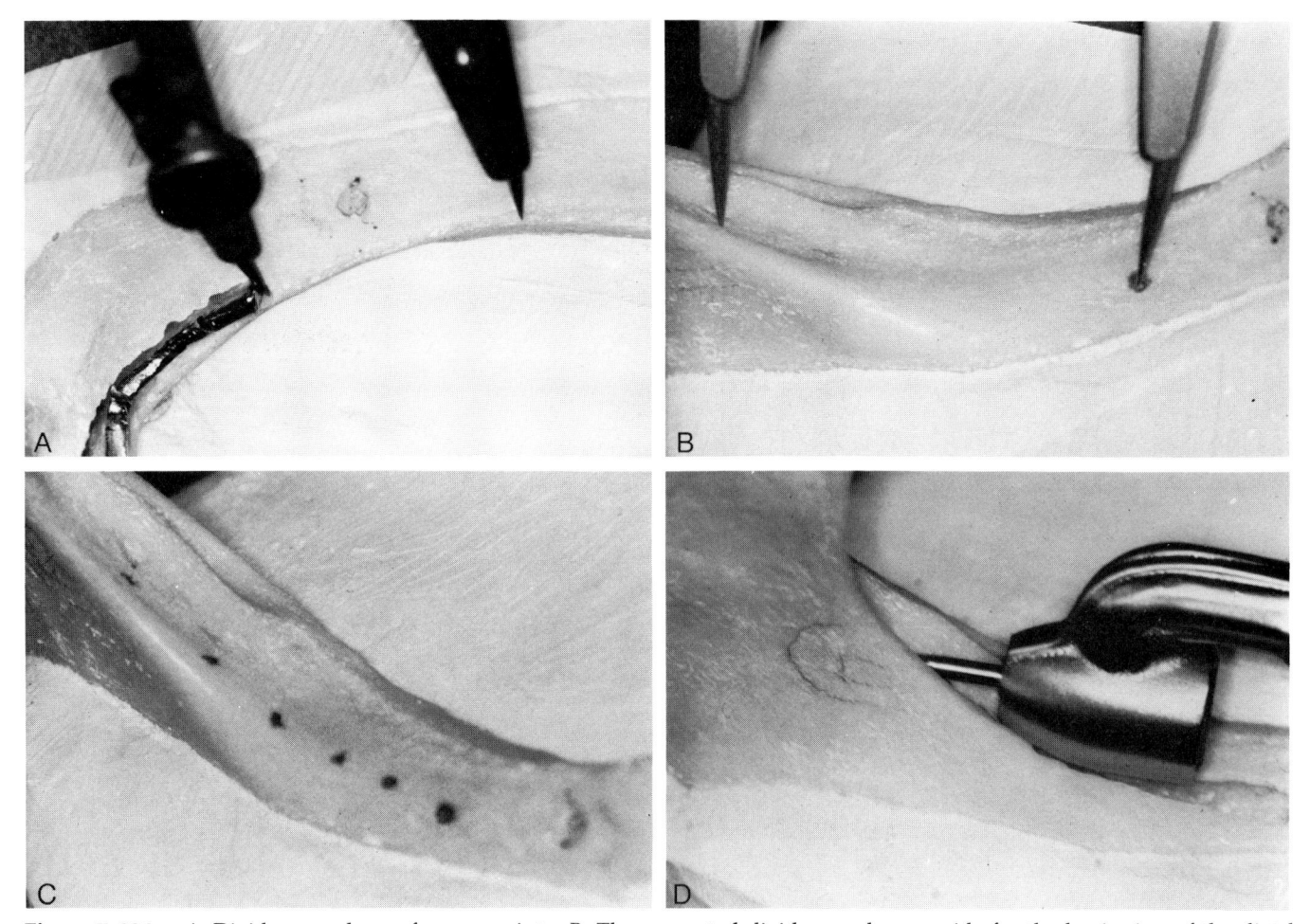

Figure 7–236. *A*, Dividers used as reference points. *B*, The separated divider used as a guide for the beginning of the distal crypt. *C*, Dots placed as guides for a No. 4 bur to make a crypt on the dry mandible. *D*, Bayonet handpiece at the correct angle to make a 10-mm crypt under the cortical plate.

sistance of bone, such as osteopenia; (7) poor patient cooperation in areas such as hygiene,[191] recall, and maintenance of general health.

Removing a Ramus Frame

When dysesthesia, infection, pain, or bone loss is significant the implant usually requires removal. In removing a ramus

Figure 7–237. Posterior try-in in the correct position in a dry mandible.

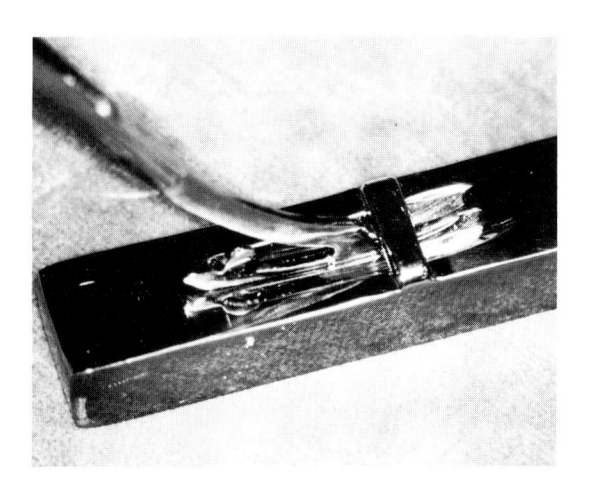

Figure 7–238. Special bending gig being utilized.

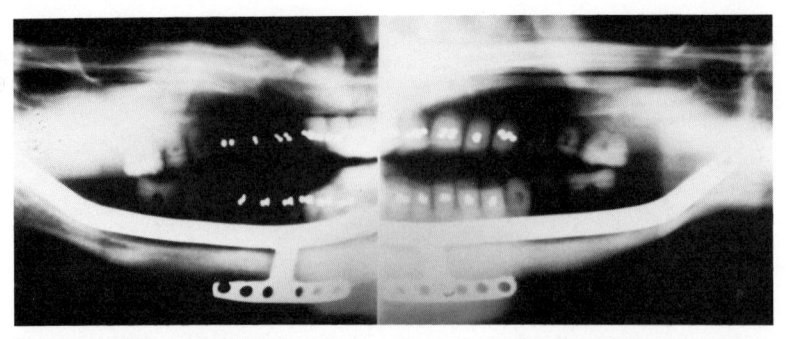

296 / IMPLANTS USED IN PREPROSTHETIC RECONSTRUCTIVE SURGERY

Figure 7–239. Anterior foot below the inferior border of the mandible.

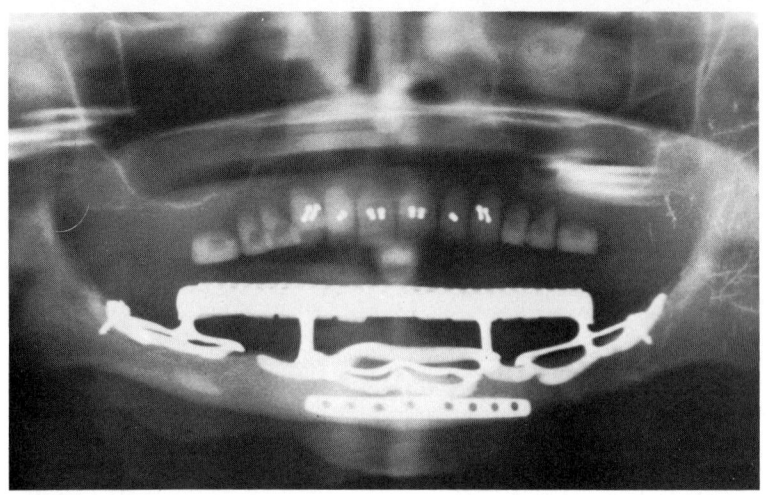

Figure 7–240. Subperiosteal segment in place with no bone pathology in the retained foot.

frame, the monorail is cut on each side of the anterior segment and the posterior arms are removed. The anterior segment may have penetrated the inferior border of the mandible, requiring that it be removed via a percutaneous approach (Fig. 7–239). In special circumstances, the bar of the anterior segment may be left in place (Fig. 7–240).

Conclusions

It is most rewarding to see the patient's increased confidence, improved appearance and ability to masticate and enjoy food, and definitely improved speech and smile. Since 1971, the author has performed 225 to 250 of the basic and modified ramus frame implants. After 13 years, most of the author's patients' implants are still functional.

SINGLE CRYSTAL SAPPHIRE: A NEW MATERIAL FOR ENDOSSEOUS IMPLANT

Francis V. Howell

Many different materials have been used for endosseous dental implants. Most of these have been metallic, a feature that gives the implant considerable strength and varying degrees of biocompatibility and crevicular adherence. Polycrystalline ceramic materials have also been investigated, but these possess a high degree of fragility and have surfaces that do not provide good epithelial contact. One of the most promising materials now available is the single crystal sapphire (alpha alumina oxide).[194] This material is biocompatible and has a hardness equal to that of a gem sapphire. Calcified and soft tissue adaptability produces excellent gingival and bone response, which has been demonstrated experimentally and in human subjects.[195–200]

In September of 1980, the material was approved for dental implants by the U.S. Food and Drug Administration. This approval was granted after animal and human experiments confirmed previous studies performed in Japan. The material is now available in the United States, and at the present time it is estimated that more than 300 dentists have placed these implants in approximately 2500 clinical cases.

The parent material was developed as a byproduct of the ceramic processes of the Kyocera Ceramic Company of Kyoto, Japan. The developmental dental program was initiated by Professor H. Kawahara at the Osaka Dental School in 1972. Initial human clinical applications began in 1975, and at the present time there have been more than 60,000 clinical cases reported, with a success rate of approximately 92 per cent over a five-year period. The studies, both animal and clinical trials, have demonstrated the biocompatibility and relative practicality of the use of the synthetic sapphire as an endosseous implant.

At Scripps Clinic and Research Foundation in La Jolla, California, human studies began in October of 1981. There have been nearly 300 implants, but "success rates" are difficult to interpret, as many implants have been placed in unusual sites and clinical situations. Development of two new devices using the material has resulted from the studies. Two types of implants are now in production and are available. One is basically a single crystal core with a polycrystalline shaft that incorporates a female receptacle for a Zest attachment. This Bioceram Zestplant* allows the use of the implant in edentulous areas for anchorage of dentures. The second adaptation of the material incorporates use as an intraosseous stimulator of

---

*Zest Anchors, Inc., San Diego, California.

IMPLANTS USED IN PREPROSTHETIC RECONSTRUCTIVE SURGERY / **297**

Figure 7–241. Depiction of the various forms of the single crystal synthetic sapphires. As noted, some contain polycrystalline shafts (A-type). This figure is from a plastic form that can be used over panoramic x-rays and compensates for the magnification of these films.

bone in cases of recent or impending loss of teeth due to periodontal and periapical inflammatory disease or trauma. Use of the specially shortened, single crystal sapphires (super short) as bone stimulators has led to a rapidly expanding study of the use of this material to stimulate bone. The buried implants can later be removed and the stimulated bone serves as an anchor for a conventional endosseous implant. In some cases, these sapphires can be retained in the bone to maintain adequate contour. The short sapphires can also be used in edentulous posterior ridges as "stops" for partial and full dentures.

At the present time, no patient in the Scripps studies has had an untoward reac-

Figure 7–242. *A,* Conventional E-type post and a "super-short" E-type. *B,* Bioceram Zestplant which combines a single crystal shaft with a polycrystalline sheath into which a Zest attachment can be placed.

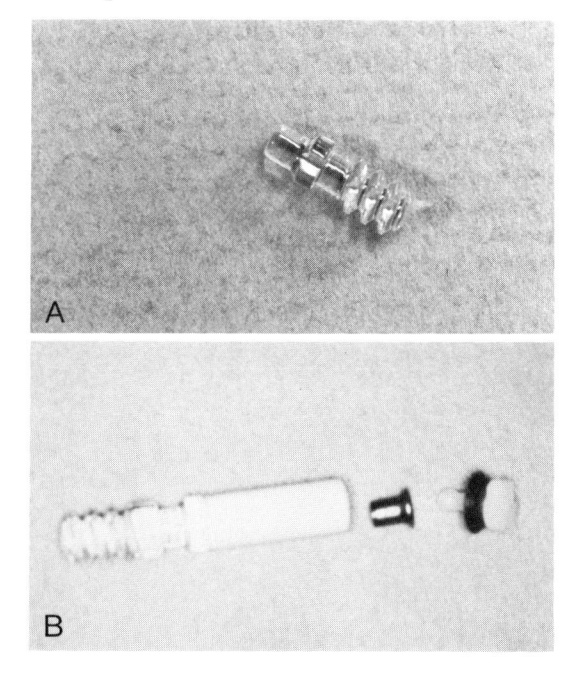

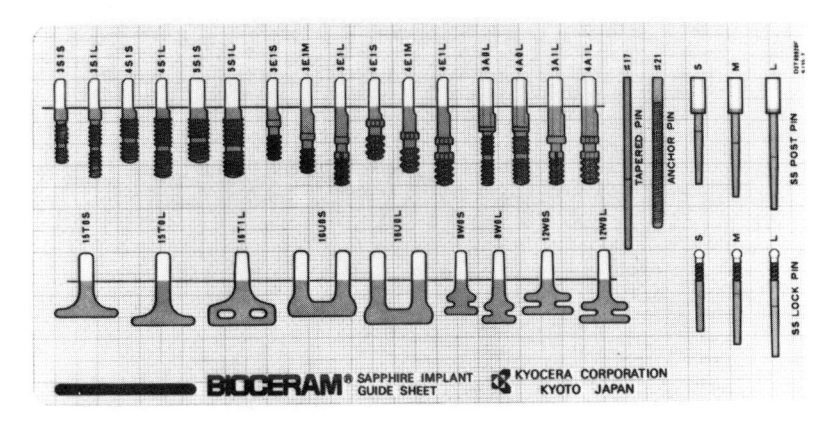

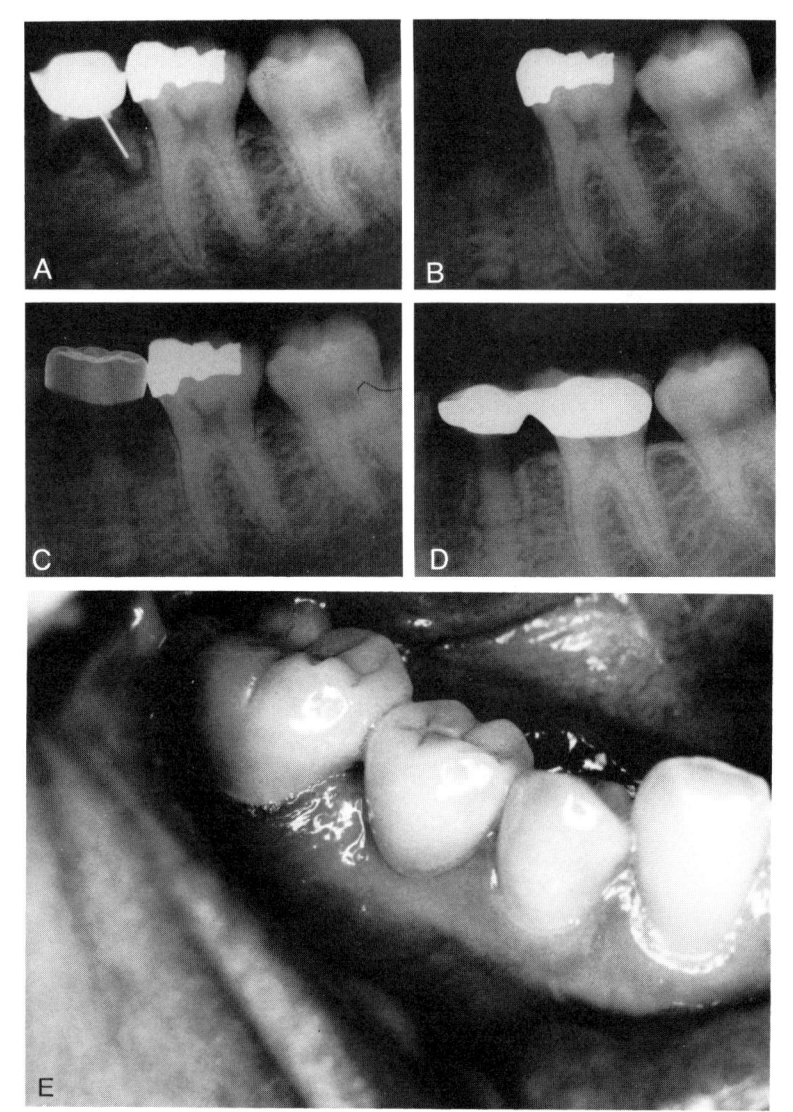

Figure 7–243. Thirty-three-year-old female with failing deciduous molar. *A,* Just prior to extraction. *B,* Immediate placement of E-type, medium length. *C,* Temporary stabilization, temporary crown. *D,* Restored sapphire and first molar tooth taken two years after placement. Note growth of bone around sleeve and shaft of sapphire. *E,* Clinical photograph of the patient. Restoration of the single crystal sapphire is stabilized with a crown on first molar. This produces a well-adapted biologic replacement.

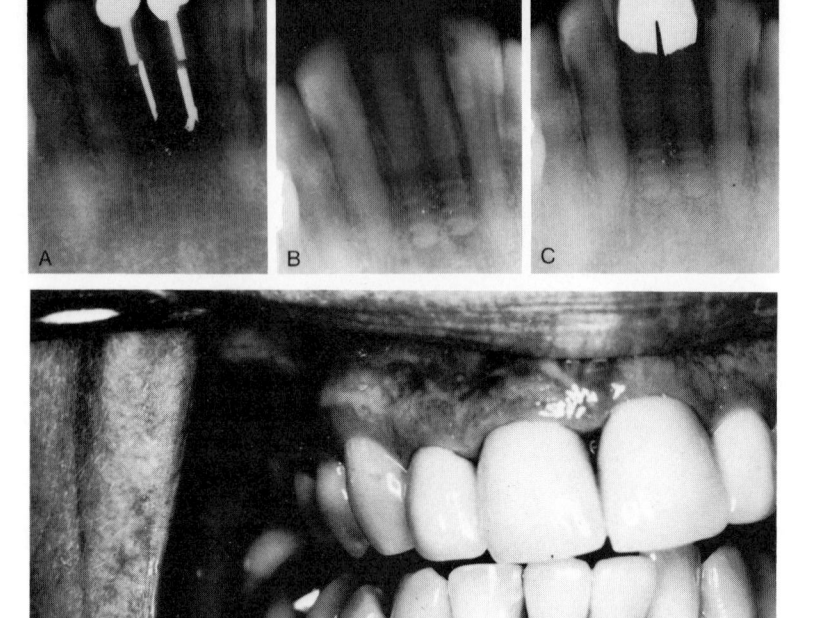

298 / IMPLANTS USED IN PREPROSTHETIC RECONSTRUCTIVE SURGERY

Figure 7–244. *A*, Preoperative radiograph of two mandibular central incisor teeth in a 44-year-old female patient. These were endodontic failures. *B*, Immediate postextraction insertion of three sapphires. *C*, Adaptation of bone to implants following stabilization by permanent dual crowns 16 months after insertion of implants. *D*, Clinical photograph taken 16 months following insertion of two sapphires replacing central incisor teeth.

tion to the material, and in the majority of "failures" the biocompatibility of the material is not a factor. As noted by many clinicians, in many implant "failures," adequacy of restoration is the determining factor in the actual success or failure of the case.

In Figure 7–241 the various forms of the implant material for endosseous purposes are illustrated. In the studies at this institution, the E-type implant has been used almost exclusively for "screw post" applications. Blades of U-type have also been used successfully. The two principal modifications are shown in Figure 7–242. *A* shows an E-type post that has an extremely short shaft and is utilized as a bone stimulator or as a solitary mucosal implant. The Bioceram Zestplant combines a single crystal–polycrystalline implant *(B)* with a polycrystalline shaft and is designed for edentulous areas. It is placed almost entirely within bone and mucosa except for the entrance into the concavity in the superior surface. The Bioceram Zestplant female attachment can be cemented into the opening.

There are many indications for the use of these endosseous implants. They are primarily designed for single tooth replacement and in most cases must be stabilized by direct connection to an existing tooth. They are not designed to be "free-standing" tooth replacements.

A patient missing a permanent bicuspid presented with a failing deciduous molar (Fig. 7–243). The preoperative radiograph *(A)* demonstrates the presence of adequate bone, *B* is the immediate postinsertion radiograph with temporary stabilization, *C* shows the temporary stabilizing crown, and *D* is a radiograph of the restored implant. Two years after placement, bone continues to form around the implant. This is considered successful, based on the established criteria.[199] *E* is a clinical photograph of the restored implant demonstrating the tissue compatibility. The implant produced a bone-stimulating anchor that eliminates the need for a three-unit bridge.

In Figure 7–244, *A* is a preoperative radiograph of two mandibular central incisor teeth that were endodontically treated with subsequent retrofill procedures that were unsuccessful. It was determined that both teeth were split. *B* is the immediate post-extraction film showing insertion of two 3-E sapphires. *C* demonstrates the adaptation of the bone to the implants and stabilization by

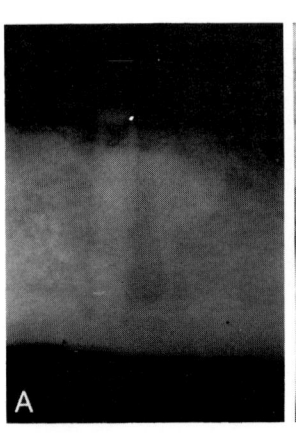

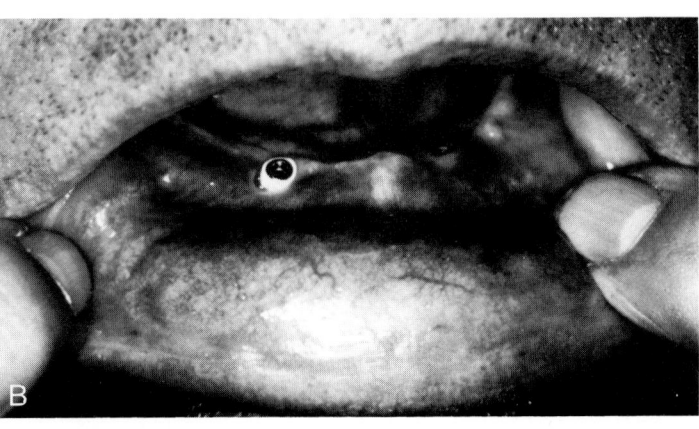

Figure 7–245. *A*, Insertion site of Zest combined E-type single crystal with polycrystalline shaft. *B*, Position in the mandible. The mucosa is well-adapted to the shaft.

permanent dual crowns. *D* is a clinical photograph of the restored teeth, showing their stability despite the lack of anchoring to adjoining natural teeth.

Figure 7–245*A* is a radiograph of the insertion site of a Zest combined E-type single crystal with a polycrystalline shaft. This is placed in an edentulous jaw, and *B* illustrates its position in the bone. The placement of the female Zest attachment makes it possible for the denture to be retained in much the same way as any other type of "overdenture."

A 57-year-old male patient involved in an automobile accident suffered complete luxation of mandibular central incisors and fracture of lateral incisors below the alveolar crest (Fig. 7–246*A*). *B* shows super-short, 3-E sapphires immediately inserted into the alveoli of the central incisors. The lateral incisors were not endodontically treated, as good blood clots had formed over the pulps. *C* is a clinical photograph of the patient three months following placement of super-short sapphires. There has been complete healing of the edentulous ridge, and the temporary bridge has been satisfactory. *D* was taken the same day as *C* after insertion of 3-E medium sapphires through small openings in the edentulous ridge. The openings allowed removal of "buried" sapphires. The patient is now wearing a fixed bridge from right cuspid to left cuspid with anchorage on endosseous implants.

The biocompatibility of the single crystal sapphire with both soft tissue and bone has been well established. The materials are acceptable to the patient, as natural healing is provided as well as physiologic replacement of diseased teeth and stimulation of bone where there has been damage by dental infection or injury.

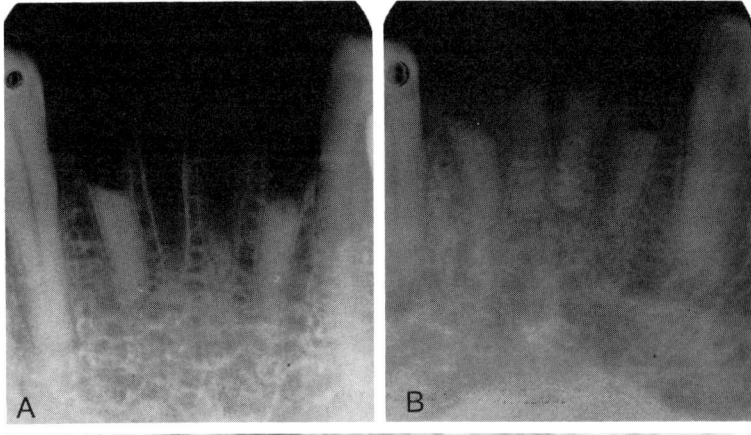

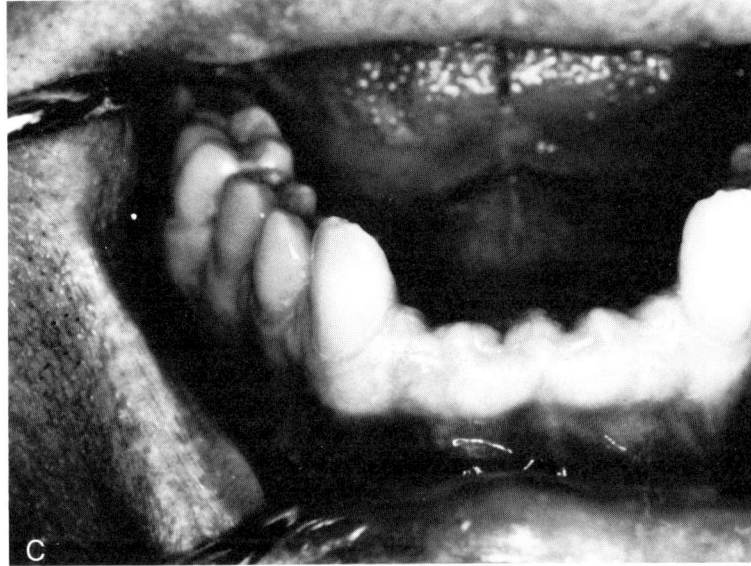

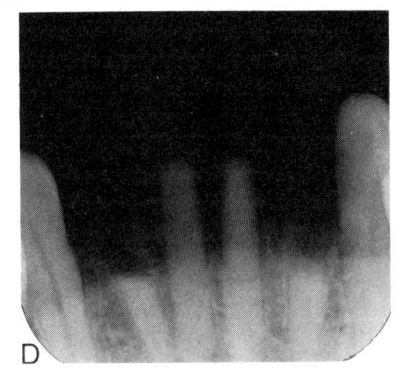

Figure 7–246. *A*, Luxation of mandibular central incisors and fracture of lateral incisors in a 57-year-old male. *B*, Super-short 3-E sapphires placed in alveoli of central incisors. *C*, Healing of the edentulous ridge three months following placement of the super-short sapphires. *D*, 3-E medium sapphires in the edentulous ridge.

BIBLIOGRAPHY

1. Helfrick JF, Topf JS, and Kaufman M: Mandibular staple bone plate: Long-term evaluation of 250 cases. J Am Dent Assoc 104:318–320, 1982.
2. American Academy of Implant Dentistry: Implant Criteria Workshop. Dearborn, Michigan, June, 1976.
3. American Dental Association, Council on Dental Materials and Devices and Dental Research: Workshop on Dental Implants. Chicago, Illinois, December, 1975.
4. Babbush CA: Medical contraindications and the implant candidate. Annual Meeting, American Academy of Implant Dentistry, Washington, DC, November, 1974.
5. Babbush CA: Selection of the implant candidate. Lecture, University of Southern California, July, 1975.
6. Bicol NA: Preparation, the keyword for implant dentistry. J Oral Implants 3:354, 1973.
7. Babbush CA: Selection of the Implant Candidate. Hagerstown, MD, Harper & Row, Publishers, Inc., 1979.
8. Babbush CA: Surgical Atlas of Dental Implant Techniques. Philadelphia, WB Saunders Co., 1980.
9. Small IA, and Kobernick SD: Implantation of threaded stainless steel pins in dog mandibles. J Oral Surg 27:99–109, 1969.

10. Small IA: Chalmers J. Lyons Memorial Lecture: Metal implants and the mandibular staple bone plate. J Oral Surg 33:571–585, 1975.
11. Small IA: Survey of experiences with the mandibular staple bone plate. J Oral Surg 36:604–605, 1978.
12. Small IA: Use of the mandibular bone plate in the deformed mandible. J Oral Surg 37:26–30, 1979.
13. Small IA: The mandibular staple bone plate for the atrophic mandible. CDS Review 73(7):27–30, 1980.
14. Small IA: The mandibular staple bone plate for the atrophic mandible. Dent Clin North Am 24:565–570, 1980.
15. Adell R, Lekholm U, Rockler B, and Brånemark P-I: A 15-year study of osseointegrated implants in the treatment of the edentulous jaw. J Oral Surg 10:387–416, 1981.
16. LeLievre C: Participation of neural crest derived cells in the genesis of the skull in birds. J Embryol Exp Morph 47:17, 1978.
17. Noden DM: The control of avian cephalic neural crest cyto-differentiation. I. Skeletal and connective tissues. Devl Biol 67:296, 1978.
18. Johnston MC, Noden DM, Hazelton RD, Coulombre JL, and Coulombre AJ: Origins of avian ocular and periocular tissues. Expl Eye Res 29:27, 1979.
19. Hall BK: Specificity in the differentiation and morphogenesis of neural crest–derived scleral ossicles and of epithelial scleral papillae in the eye of the embryonic chick. J Embryol Exp Morph 66:175, 1981.
20. Ten Cate AR: In Oral Histology. Toronto, The CV Mosby Co., 1980.
21. Fraunhofer JA: Oral implants. In Scientific Aspects of Dental Materials. London, Butterworths, 1975.
22. Harper HA: Physiological Chemistry. Los Altos, CA, Lange Med Publishers, 1963.
23. Ahrens G, Bramstedt F, and Naujoks R: Zur Standardisierung einzelner Bezugsgrossen fur biochemische Untersuchungen an Plaquematerial. In Advances in Fluorine Research and Dental Caries Prevention, Vol 2. London, Pergamon Press, 1964, p. 167.
24. Gulzow HJ, and Mardaus DW: Vegleichende Untersuchungen uber organische Plaquebestandteile. Dtsch Zahnarztl Z 28:351, 1973.
25. Spiessl B: The dynamic compression implant (DCJ) as a basis for allenthetic prosthetics. In New Concepts in Maxillofacial Bone Surgery. Berlin, Springer Verlag, 1976.
26. Young FA: Ceramic tooth implants. J Biomed Mater Res, Symp No. 2:281, 1972.
27. Denissen HW, and Groot K de: The response of the apatite ceramic surface to a simulated physiological environment. In Dental Implants. Munich, Carl Hanser Verlag, 1980.
28. Hulbert JE, Klawitter JH, Talbert CD, and Fitts CT: Materials of construction for artificial bone segments. In Research in Dental and Medical Materials. New York, Plenum Press, 1969.
29. Hammer JE, and Reed OM: The complex factors in tooth implantations. J Biomed Mater Res, Symp No. 2:297, 1972.
30. Hammer JE, and Reed OM: Implantable ceramic teeth. J Biomed Mater Res, Symp No. 4:217,
31. Busing CM, Schulte W, Hoedt B, and Heimke G: Histological results with biomechanically shaped implants with A1203 Ceramic. In Dental Implants. Munich, Carl Hanser Verlag, 1980.
32. Topazian RG, Hammer WB, Boucher LJ, and Hulbert SF: Use of alloplastics for ridge augmentation. J Oral Surg 29:792, 1971.
33. Topazian RG, Talbert CD, and Hulbert SF: The use of ceramics in augmentation and replacement of the mandible. J Biomed Mater Res, Symp No. 2:311, 1972.
34. Denissen HW, Veldhuis AAH, and Rejda BV: Het tandwortelimplantaat als pijler voor kroon- en brugwerk en de Dolder-prosthese. Ned Tijdschr Tandheelkd 90:89, 1983.
35. Groot K de: Ceramics based on calcium phosphates. Amsterdam, Elsevier, 1983.
36. Williams DF: The properties and medical uses of materials. Part 3: The reactions of tissues to materials. Biomed Eng 6:152, 1971.
37. Wijn JR de: Poreus polymethylmethacrylaat als botvervangend materiaal. Ned Tijdschr Tandheelkd 88:429, 1981.
38. Patha P, Slingerland ACH, Velzen D van, and Groot K de: Slijtage van een kop-halsprothese van de heup. Ned Tijdschr Geneeskd 127:152, 1983.
39. Kent JN, Quinn JH, Zide MF, Finger JM, Jarcho M, and Rothstein SS: Correction of alveolar ridge deficiencies with non-resorbable hydroxyapatite. J Am Dent Assoc 105:993, 1982.
40. Groot K de: Degradable ceramics. In Biocompatibility of Clinical Implant Materials, Vol. I. Boca Raton, FL, CRC Press, 1981, p. 199.
41. Chang CS, Matukas VJ, and Lemons JE: Histologic study of hydroxylapatite as an implant material for mandibular augmentation. J Oral Max Surg 41:729, 1983.
42. Autian J: Toxicologic aspects of implants. J Biomed Mater Res 1:433, 1967.
43. Guess WL, and Haberman S: Toxicity profiles of vinyl and polyolefinic plastic and their additives. J Biomed Mater Res 2:313, 1968.
44. Hornsey CA, Kent J, and Hinds EC: Materials for oral implantation—biological and functional criteria. J Am Dent Assoc 86:817, 1973.
45. Zwart JGN: Bone replacement of the maxillofacial area. Amsterdam, Acad Proefschrift, 1984.
46. Scales JT: Examination of implants removed from patients. J Bone Joint Surg 53B:344, 1971.
47. Dobbs HS, and Minsky MJ: Metal ion release after total hip replacement. Biomaterials 1:193, 1980.
48. Driessens FCM, and Hage MD: Overgevoeligheid voor nikkel, chroom en cobalt. Ned Tandartsenblad 704, 1983.
49. Hildebrand HP, and Herlant-Peers MC: Les metaux cancerogenese. Nat Med Travail 29, 1983.
50. Herlant-Peers MC, Hildebrand HF, and Kerckaert JP: In vitro and in vivo incorporation of 63 N1(11) into lung and liver subcellular fractions of BALB/C mice. Carcinogenesis 4:387, 1983.
51. Bergman M, Bergman B, and Scremark R: Tissue accumulation of nickle released due to electrochemical corrosion of non-precious dental casting alloys. J Oral Rehab 7:325, 1980.
52. Rudinger K: Korrosionsschutz durch die Werkstoffe Titan, Zirkonium und Tantal. Thyssen Edelst Techner 82:172, 1982.
53. Rudinger K: Titan und Titan-Legierungen. In Ullmann's Encyklopadie der Technischen Chemie. 23rd ed. 1983.
54. Bitter HG: Continent, Thyssen Edelstahlwerke AG. Personal communication. 1984.
55. Ferguson AB, Akahoshi Y, Laing PG, and Hodge ES: Characteristics of trace ions released from imbedded metal implants in the rabbit. J Bone Joint Surg 323, 1962.
56. Meachim G, and Williams DF: Changes in nonosseous tissue adjacent to titanium implants. J Biomed Mater Res 555, 1973.
57. Gettleman L: The problem of corrosion and tarnish of dental restorative and implant metals. Biomaterials 7, 1979.
58. Gasser K, Kunzi HU, and Henning G: Metalle im Mund. Berlin, Quintessenz, 1984.

59. Kato J: Influence of surface condition on the cytotoxicity of copper-gold alloy. Shiha Rikogahuzarshi 17(88):63, 1976.
60. Hampel CA: Tantalum. In Rare Metals Handbook. New York, Krieger Publishing Company, Inc., 1967.
61. Osborn JF, and Newesely H: Dynamic aspects of the implant-bone interface. In Dental Implants. Munchen, Carl Hamer Verlag, 1980.
62. Bunte M, Strunz V, Gross UM, and Bromer H: Deutscherk. Vergleichende Untersuchungen uber die Haftung verscheidene Implantatmateriale im knochen. Dtsch Zahnarztl Z 32:825, 1977.
63. Frykholm KO, Frithiof L, Fernstrom AJB, Moberger G, Blohm SG, and Bjorn E: Allergy to copper derived from dental alloys as a possible cause of oral lesions of lichen planus. Acta Derm Venereol 49:268, 1969.
64. Koomen HA de: De verhoging van de geresorbeerde mandibula. Nijmegen, Acad Proefschrift, 1982.
65. Babbush CA: Surgical Atlas of Dental Implant Techniques. Philadelphia, WB Saunders Co., 1980.
66. Bosker H, and Kijk L van. De heksenkin. Ned Tijdschr Tandheelkd 89:186, 1982.
67. Cranin NA, Rabkin MF, and Garfinkel L: A statistical evaluation of 952 endosteal implants in humans. J Am Dent Assoc 94:315–320, 1977.
68. Zarb GA, Smith DC, Levant HC, Graham BS, and Zingg GW: The effects of cemented and uncemented endosseous implants. J Prosth Dent 42:202–210, 1979.
69. Hench LL: Biomaterials. Science 208:826–831, 1980.
70. Schnitman PA, and Shulman LB: Recommendations of the consensus development conference on dental implants. J Am Dent Assoc 98:373–377, 1979.
71. Adell R, Lekholm U, Rockler B, and Brånemark P-I: A 15-year study of osseointegrated implants in the treatment of the edentulous jaw. Int J Oral Surg 10:387–416, 1981.
72. Brånemark P-I, Breine U, Johansson B, Roylance PJ, Rockert H, and Yoffey JM: Regeneration of bone marrow. A clinical and experimental study following removal of bone marrow by curettage. Acta Anat 59:1–46, 1964.
73. Brånemark P-I, Breine U, Lindstrom J, Adell R, Hansson B-O, and Ohlsson, A: Intra-osseous anchorage of dental prosthesis. I. Experimental Studies. Scand J Plast Reconstr Surg 3:81–100, 1969.
74. Brånemark P-I, Breine U, Hallen O, Hansson B, and Lindstrom J: Repair of defects in mandible. Scand J Plast Reconstr Surg 4:100–108, 1970.
75. Albrektsson B: Repair of Diaphyseal Defects. Thesis, University of Gothenburg, 1971.
76. Lundskog J: Heat and Bone Tissue. Thesis, University of Gothenburg. Scand J Plast Reconstr Surg (Suppl 9), 1972.
77. Adell R: Regeneration of the periodontium. An experimental study on dogs. Scand J Plast Reconstr Surg 8 (Suppl 11), 1974.
78. Linder L: Bone Cement Monomere. Thesis, University of Gothenburg, 1976.
79. Tjellstrom A: Tympanoplasty with preformed, autologous ossicles. Thesis, University of Gothenburg, 1977.
80. Hansson E-O: Success and Failure of Osseointegrated Implants in the Jaw. Thesis, Univ of Gothenburg. Swed Dent J (Suppl 1), 1977.
81. Albrektsson T: Healing of Bone Grafts. Thesis, Univeristy of Gothenburg, 1979.
82. Haraldson T: Functional evaluation of bridges on osseointegrated implants in the edentulous jaw. Thesis, University of Gothenburg, 1979.
83. Eriksson RA, Albrektsson T, and Albrektsson B: Heat caused by drilling cortical bone. Temperature measured in vivo in patients and animals. Acta Orthop Scand 55: 629–631, 1984.
84. Brånemark P-I, Lindstrom J, Hallen O, Breine U, Jeppsson P-H, and Ohman A: Osseointegrated implants in the treatment of the edentulous jaw. Experience from a ten-year period. Scand J Plast Reconstr Surg (Suppl 16), 1–132, 1977.
85. Ledermann P, Schroeder A, and Sutter F: Der Einzelzahnersatz mit Hilfe des ITI-Hohlzylinderimplantates Typ F (Spatimplantat), 1982.
86. Brånemark P-I, Adell R, Albrektsson T, Lekholm U, Lundvist S, and Rockler B: Osseointegrated titanium fixtures in the treatment of edentulousness. Biomaterials 4:25–28, 1983.
87. Albrektsson T, Brånemark P-I, Hansson H-A, Ivarsson B, and Jonsson U: Ultrastructural analysis of the interface zone of titanium and gold implants. In Lee AJC, Albrektsson T, and Brånemark P-I (eds): Clinical Application of Biomaterials. Advances in Biomaterials 4:167–177, 1982.
88. Linder L, Albrektsson T, Brånemark P-I, Hansson H-A, Ivarsson B, Jonsson U, and Lundstrom I: Electron microscopic analysis of bone-titanium interface. Acta Orthop Scand 54:45–52, 1983.
89. Albrektsson T: Response of bone tissue to surgical preparation and non-biological material. IRL press, 1985 (in press).
90. Albrektsson T, Hansson H-A, and Ivarsson B: Interface analysis of titanium and zirconium bone implants. Biomaterials 6:97–101, 1985.
91. Williams DF: Titanium and titanium alloys. In Williams DF (ed): Biocompatibility of Clinical Implant Materials. CRC Series in Biocompatibility 1:9–44, 1981.
92. Albrektsson T, Brånemark P-I, Hansson H-A, Kasemo B, Larsson K, Lundstrom I, McQueen D, and Skalak B: The interface zone of inorganic implants in vivo: Titanium implants in bone. Ann Biomed Eng 11:1–27, 1983.
93. Skalak B: Biomechanical considerations in osseointegrated prostheses. J Prosthet Dent 49:843, 1983.
94. Albrektsson T: Direct bone anchorage of dental implants. A review of biological aspects on the technique of osseointegration. J Prosthet Dent 50:255–261, 1983.
95. Uhthoff HK: Mechanical factors influencing the holding power of screws in compact bone. J Bone Joint Surg 55B:633–641, 1973.
96. Schatzker JG, Horne JG, and Sumner-Smith G: The effect of movement on the holding power of screws in bone. Clin Orthop 111:257–262, 1975.
97. Kasemo B: Biocompatibility of titanium implants. Surface Science Aspects. J Prosthet Dent 49:832, 1983.
98. Breine U, and Brånemark P-I: Reconstruction of alveolar jaw bone. An experimental and clinical study of immediate and preformed autologous bone grafts in combination with osseointegrated implants. Scand J Plast Reconstr Surg 14:23–48, 1980.
99. Albrektsson T, Brånemark P-I, Eriksson A, and Lindstrom J: The preformed, autologous bone graft. An experimental study in rabbits. Scand J Plast Reconstr Surg 12:215–223, 1978.
100. Lindström J, Brånemark P-I, and Albrektsson T: Mandibular reconstruction using the preformed autologous bone graft. Scand J Plast Reconstr Surg 15:29–38, 1981.
101. Jacobsson M, Albrektsson T, and Turesson I: Dynamics of irradiation injury to bone tissue. A vital microscopic study. Acta Radiol, in press.
102. Albrektsson T, Brånemark P-I, Hansson H-A, and Lindstrom J: Osseointegrated titanium im-

plants. Requirements for ensuring a long-lasting, direct bone anchorage in man. Acta Orthop Scand 52:155–170, 1981.
103. Jacobsson M, Albrektsson T, Jonsson A, and Turesson I: The effect of irradiation on bone regeneration at different dose levels. A quantitative study. Int J Radiol Oncol Biol Phys, accepted for publication.
104. Eriksson RA, and Albrektsson T: Temperature threshold levels for heat-induced bone tissue injury. J Prosthet Dent 50:101–107, 1983.
105. Albrektsson T: The healing of autologous bone grafts after varying degrees of surgical trauma. J Bone Joint Surg 62B:403–410, 1980.
106. Albrektsson T, and Linder L: Intravital, long-term follow-up of autologous, experimental bone grafts. Arch Orthop Traumat Surg 98:189–193, 1981.
107. Brånemark P-I, and Stefech V: A new-developed drill-machine for bone preparation. Unpublished report, Department of Anatomy, University of Gothenburg, Sweden, 1981.
108. Eriksson RA, and Albrektsson T: The effect of heat on bone regeneration. J Oral Maxillofac Surg 42:701–711, 1984.
109. Eriksson AR: Heat-induced Bone Tissue Injury. Thesis, University of Gothenburg, 1983.
110. Albrektsson T: The response of bone to titanium implants. CRC Critical Reviews in Biocompatibility, submitted for publication 1983.
111. Brånemark P-I, Albrektsson T, Skalak R, Symington J, and Zarb G: Osseointegrated dental implants. Transactions Eighth and Fourteenth International Biomaterials Symposium 5:132, 1982.
112. Hansson H-A, Albrektsson T, and Brånemark P-I: Structural aspects on the interface between tissue and titanium implants. J Prosth Dent 50:108–113, 1983.
113. Lekholm U, Brånemark P-I, Adell R, Rockler B, Lindhe J, Lindvall AM, and Yoneyama T: Marginal barrier tissue reactions at osseointegrated dental implants—a cross-sectional study. Int J Oral Surg, 1985, in press.
114. Blomberg S, and Lindqvist L: Psychological reactions to edentulousness and treatment with jawbone-anchored bridges. Acta Psych Scand 68:251–262, 1983.
115. Tjellström A, Lindström J, Hallén O, Albrektsson T, and Brånemark P-I: Osseointegrated titanium implants in the temporal bone. A clinical study on bone-anchored hearing aids. Am J Otology 2:304–310, 1981.
116. Tjellstrom A, Lindstrom J, Hallen O, Albrektsson T, and Brånemark P-I: Direct bone anchorage of external hearing aids. J Biomed Eng 5:59-63, 1983.
117. Tjellstrom A, Lindstrom J, Nyhlen O, Albrektsson T, Brånemark P-I, Birgersson B, Nero H, and Sylven C: The bone-anchored auricular episthesis. Laryngoscope 91:811–815, 1981.
118. Tjellstrom A, Lindstrom J, Nyhlen O, Albrektsson T, and Brånemark P-I: Directly bone-anchored implants for fixation of aural episheses. Biomaterials 4:55–57, 1983.
119. Hagert C-G, Sollerman C, Brånemark P-I, and Albrektsson T: Directly bone-anchored metacarpophalangeal joint implants. Transactions Eighth and Fourteenth International Biomaterials Symposium 5:33, 1982.
120. Hagert C-G, Albrektsson T, Strid K-G, Irsfam L, and Brånemark P-I: Osseointegrated implants for metacarpophalangeal joint prostheses. Scand J Plast Reconstr Surg, accepted for publication, 1985.
121. Niznick G: The Core-Vent Implant System. Oral Implantol 10(3):1982.
122. Niznick G: The Core-Vent Implant System. Implantologist 4(1): 1983.
123. Niznick G: Evolution of the osseointegrated implant. Oral Health (Can) 1983.
124. Sutter F, Schroeder A, and Straumann F: Engineering and Design Aspects of the ITI Hollow-Basket Implants, Sonderdruck aus ZWR/Zahnarztliche Welg/Rundschau 90 Jahrgang. Dr. A. Hiithig Verbag. Heidelberg. NY 50–59, 1981.
125. Hulbert F, et al: Attachment of prosthesis to the musculoskeletal system by tissue ingrowth and mechanical interlocking. J Biomed Mater Res, Symp No. 4:1–23, 1973.
126. Schroeder A, Ponler O, and Sutter F: Tissue reaction to a titanium hollow cylinder implant with titanium sprayed layer surface. Schweig Mschr Zahnheilkd 86:713–727, 1976.
127. Schroeder A, Stich H, Straumann F, and Sutter F: Deposition of osteocementum at the surface of a load-bearing implant. Schweig Mschr Zahnheilkd 88:1051–1058, 1978.
128. Claes LP, Hutzs Chenreuther P, and Pohler O: Losemomente von Corticaliszugsschrauben in Abhangigkeit von Implantationszeit und Oberflachenbeschaffenheit. Arch Orthop Unfall-chir 85:155, 1976.
129. Ledermann PD: Titanium-coated screw implants as alloplastic endosteal retention element in the edentulous problematic mandible (1+11). Quent Inter 12:484–491, 1981.
130. Stroch AE: Experimental work on direct implantation in the alveolus, anier. J Ortho Oral Surg 25:5, 1936.
131. Stroch AE, and Stroch MS: Further studies on inert mental implantations for replacement.
132. Traimonte S: A further report on intra-osseous implants with improved drive screws. J Oral Implant Transplant Surg 11:35, 1965.
133. Skinner PR, and Robinson RA: Intra-osseous metal implants for denture stabilization. Dent Digest 52:427, 485, 1946.
134. Linkow LJ: Clinical evaluation of various designed endosseous implants. J Oral Implant Transplant Surg 12:35–46, 1966.
135. Hahn H, and Palich W: Preliminary evaluation of porous metal surfaced titanium for orthopedic implants. J Biomed Mat Res 4:571, 1970.
136. Linkow LI: The blade-vent: A new dimension in endosseous implantology. Dent Concepts, Spring 1968.
137. Babbush CA: Endosseous blade-vent implants: A research review. J Oral Surg 30:168, 1972.
138. Babbush CA: Endosteal blade-vent implants: A clinical review. J Hyg Med 31:1499, 1973.
139. Babbush CA: Endosteal blade-vent implants. In Perel M (ed): Dental Implantology and Prostheses. Philadelphia, JB Lippincott, 1976.
140. Babbush CA, and Staikoff LS: The scanning electron microscope and the endosteal blade-vent implant. J Oral Implants 4:373–385, 1974.
141. Cranin AN: Oral Implantology. Springfield IL, Charles C Thomas, 1970.
142. Fagan MJ: New Concepts in Implant Dentistry-Implantodontics. Atlanta Dental Practice Plan, Inc., 1971.
143. James RA: The support system and the perigingival defense mechanism of oral implants. J Oral Implants 6:270–285, 1975.
144. Linkow LI: Histopathologic and radiologic studies on endosseous implants. Dental Concepts, Fall-Winter 1968.
145. Linkow LI: Statistical analysis of 173 implant pa-

8

RECONSTRUCTION OF THE ALVEOLAR RIDGE WITH HYDROXYLAPATITE*

*John N. Kent, D.D.S.,
and Michael Jarcho, Ph.D.*

THE EDENTULOUS ALVEOLAR RIDGE

Alveolar ridge resorption or deficiency occurs in a variety of forms such as undercuts, knife-edge appearance, concave ridge form rather than convex, and severe resorption patterns such as the very flat, pencil-thin mandible. The ability of a patient to wear a denture satisfactorily depends on a proper convex ridge form, adequate height, and an adequate surface area on a nonmobile keratinized mucosal base.

Each year many patients present in the dental office with deficiencies in ridge height and form and inadequate fixed soft tissue. A new denture would be unsatisfactory or only a temporary solution. Lack of retention and stability with varying degrees of discomfort are common complaints.

As the resorption process continues under pressure of denture function, denture bulk increases, mastication and speech worsen, and esthetic complaints increase. In addition, extensive resorption often produces a vertical and horizontal disharmony between the maxillary and mandibular alveolar ridges, resulting in further impaired function.

HISTORY OF ATROPHIC RIDGE MANAGEMENT

A variety of procedures can be used to reconstruct the alveolar ridge. Their indications for surgery are based on remaining ridge height and contour and the adequacy of fixed soft-tissue base and sulcus depth (Fig. 8–1). Also important in the mandible is the resistance to fracture (see Chap. 3).

Selection of a corrective procedure should not be determined by any specific ridge height measurement but rather by the degree and type of anatomic deficiency. Vestibuloplasty procedures such as the buccal and labial sulcus extensions, as well as lowering of the floor of the mouth, are helpful only if there is adequate alveolar ridge height and convex ridge form. A variety of procedures with or without soft-tissue grafts to improve sulcus depth and establish a fixed soft tissue base are available, as described in Chapter 5. Complete resorption of the soft alveolar bone to dense basilar bone would contraindicate soft-tissue vestibuloplasty and indicate hard-tissue augmentation. Methods to increase alveolar ridge height and retention of dentures in the past included onlay bone grafting and inlay or interpositional bone grafting, as well as the use of metallic dental implants.

Onlay bone grafts in the form of rib and iliac crest grafts can produce a tremendous increase in ridge height but have serious drawbacks.[1] Grafted bone may not produce a uniformly level ridge because its form is poor and resorption is unpredictable.[2] At least 40 to 60 per cent of grafted bone may be resorbed during the first one to two years and 60 to 100 per cent by the end of three to

*This material is referred to elsewhere as hydroxyapatite.

Figure 8–1. Reconstruction of the alveolar ridge.

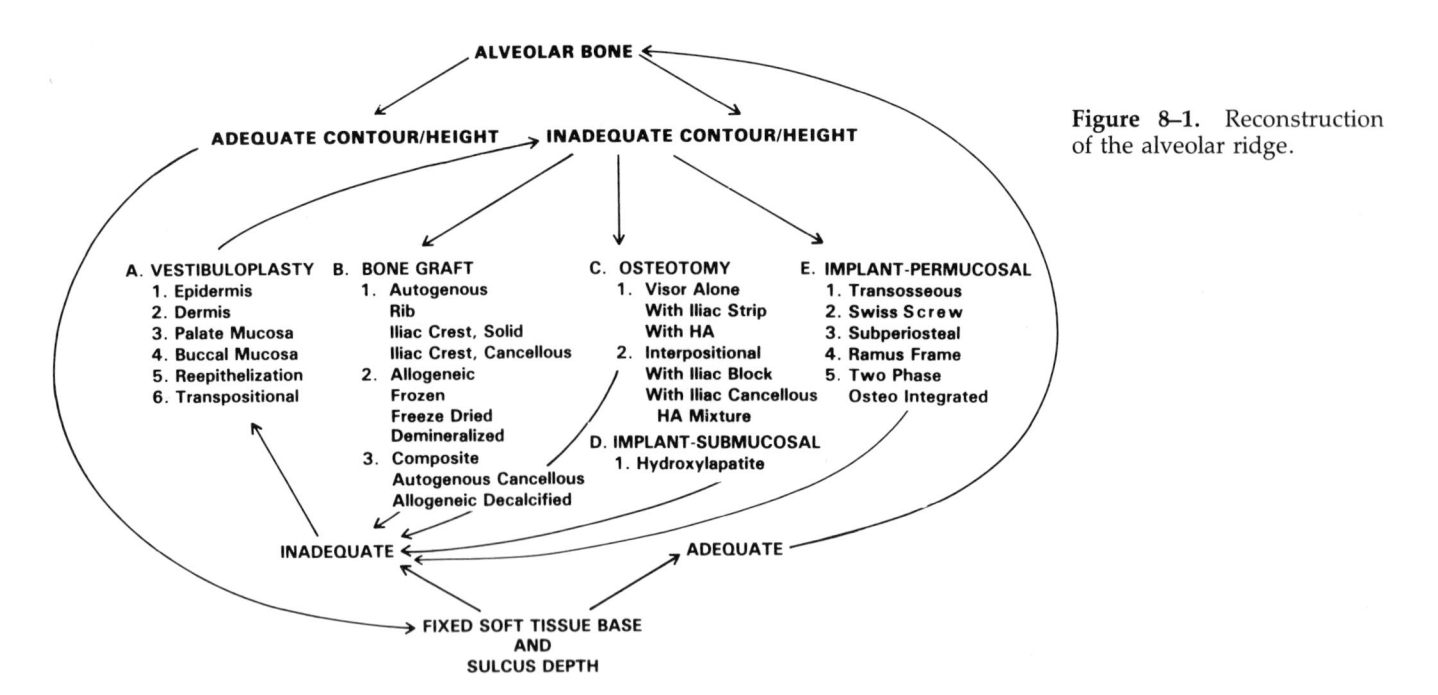

five years.[3-5] The success of these grafts lies in adding basal bulk or horizontal width to a thin mandible or maxilla. Resorption of onlay bone grafts is such a serious problem that patients are faced with a series of multiple denture relines, many weeks or months without dentures, an increased expense over other techniques, and possible donor site complications such as pneumothorax and prolonged hip pain. Allogeneic bone and demineralized bone eliminate the problem of donor site complications, but problems such as infection from dehiscence, varying degrees of resorption, and multiple denture problems such as numerous relines, discomfort, and time without dentures are similar to those of autogenous grafts.[6] Vestibuloplasties, usually necessary to provide a firm fixed soft-tissue covering over grafted bone, are generally not possible for four to six months until revascularization of the bone graft and formation of a viable periosteum occurs.

Visor and interpositional osteotomy techniques with grafts are an improvement over onlay bone grafting, with less postoperative resorption and loss of ridge height and contour.[7,8] However, donor site morbidity, limited vertical height, lateral resorption/deficiency (visor), frequent relines, and prolonged periods of inability to wear a denture are still significant disadvantages. These procedures are discussed in Chapter 6.

Most submucosal implants have had limited success as synthetic ridge augmentation materials. The methylmethacrylates are not completely inert and promote excessive encapsulation with fibrous connective tissue. This results in displacement and finally extrusion and infection. Silicone rubber, although more favorably bioinert, does not directly attach to bone, which can lead to slippage and extrusion. Proplast, a porous composite of vitreous carbon fiber and Teflon, showed early promising results with stability on bone by connective tissue ingrowth.[9] However, voids were often left when tissue failed to completely infiltrate the material. Infection liability was significant, particularly as compression under denture function reduced pore size and incited tissue necrosis. Many patients are not candidates for permucosal implant devices because of expense, lack of bone height, and concerns about failure of these devices. The latter problem, however, is significantly improved with newer modalities, as discussed in Chapter 7.

The search for a synthetic submucosal material capable of stimulating a direct biologic bone attachment unfolds with the physical characteristics and biologic profile of calcium phosphate materials, described below.

HISTORY OF CALCIUM PHOSPHATES

In the past, biomaterials research in the field of hard-tissue repair and replacement has traditionally concentrated on the development of new materials with improved mechanical (e.g., strength, flexibility) and toxicologic properties (inertness) to better withstand the rigors of the skeletal system. During the past decade, however, considerable effort has been directed toward the discovery, development, understanding, and exploitation of new concept hard-tissue prosthetic materials that interact with and may ultimately become an integral part of living bone tissue. What sets these new materials apart from the traditional surgical alloys is that they are composed of calcium and phosphate ions. These are the same ions that make up natural bone mineral, hydroxylapatite [$Ca_{10}(PO_4)_6(OH)_2$].

Hydroxylapatite (HA) and related calcium phosphates are very common substances that are found geologically in impure form and mined by the hundreds of millions of tons each year as the principal source of phosphate ion for the chemical industry.[10] In refined powder form, HA is used as a tableting agent in pharmaceuticals, as a calcium food supplement, and as an anticaking agent in baked goods and table salt. Because HA has long been recognized as the mineral component of vertebrate hard tissues, much research on this substance has been done by biologic scientists. Innovations that have emerged include preventive fluoridation and the development of the diphosphonates used in the treatment of Paget's disease.[11]

Early studies on the use of calcium phosphates as hard-tissue implants involved the use of fine powders. Some investigators reported accelerated healing,[12] while others observed little or no increase in bone healing rates.[13, 14] Present calcium phosphate implant materials began with the development of methods to produce strong macroforms of these substances. About ten years ago, successful methods of preparing ceramic forms of HA and other calcium phosphates began appearing in the literature.[15-23] Acceleration of animal and then human implant studies soon followed.[24-26]

PREPARATION AND PROPERTIES OF CALCIUM PHOSPHATE BIOMATERIALS

Virtually all current calcium phosphate bio-materials can be classified as polycrystalline ceramics. Their material structure is derived from individual crystals that have been fused together at the crystal grain boundaries by a high temperature process called sintering (Fig. 8–2). HA and TCP [$(Ca_3(PO_4)_2)$], the latter usually having a ß-Whitlockite (BW) crystal structure, have been the most widely investigated. The most widely used method of preparing these ceramics involves compacting calcium phosphate powders under high pressure into a given shape, which is then sintered at temperatures in the range of 1100° to 1300° C to produce the ceramic materials.[20, 22] Depending on processing conditions, both dense and porous structures can be produced.

Although HA and TCP have similar crystal structures and chemical composition, they differ significantly with regard to bioresorption. Numerous investigators indicate that HA ceramics in dense form can serve as permanent bone implants, showing virtually no tendency to bioresorb *in vivo*, while porous TCP and HA ceramics have a tendency to bioresorb in a more or less unpredictable fashion when implanted in hard tissues.[24, 25, 27, 28] The unpredictable bioresorption of porous TCP and HA may limit their use, since these porous implants *in vivo* frequently cannot be distinguished radiographically from surrounding bone. If significant amounts of these materials remain unresorbed or partially resorbed, they may be biomechanically detrimental to the restoration in the long term if it is a stress-bearing area. This is attributed to their lack of strength, as discussed below.

The main limitation of calcium phosphate implant materials is their mechanical properties. Like most ceramics, these materials are quite brittle and have low impact resistance and relatively low tensile strength. The mechanical properties of calcium phosphate ceramics versus currently used metallic mate-

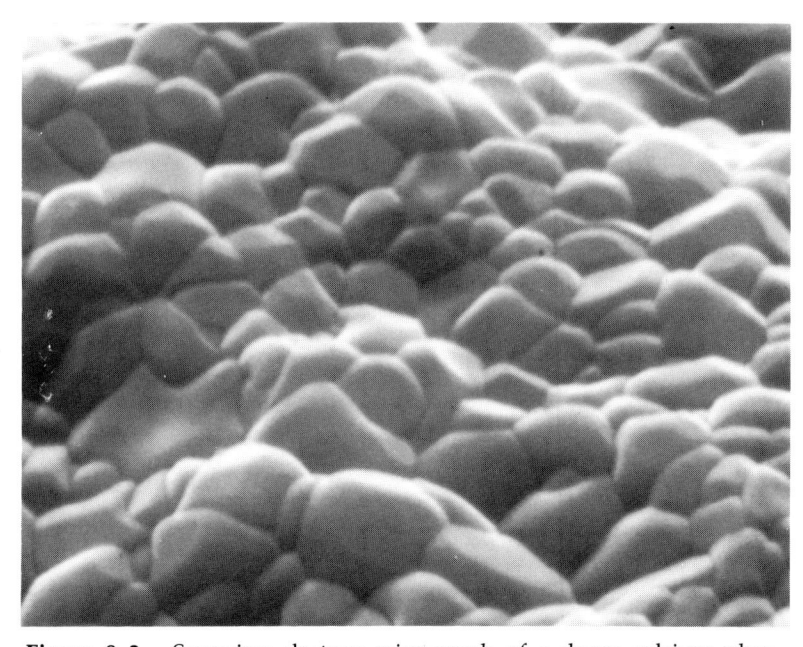

Figure 8–2. Scanning electron micrograph of a dense calcium phosphate ceramic showing individual crystals of approximately 0.5 to 3 μm fused together at the grain boundaries.

TABLE 8–1. THE MECHANICAL PROPERTIES OF BONE AND METALLIC AND CALCIUM PHOSPHATE IMPLANT MATERIALS[25]

Material	Compressive Strength (10^3 psi)	Tensile Strength (10^3 psi)	Modulus (10^6 psi)
Bone			
Cortical bone	20	10.0	2
Cancellous bone	6–9	0.5	—
Metals			
316 L Stainless	—	80–145	30–40
Cor-Cr alloy	—	97	30
Titanium	—	50	16
Calcium phosphates			
Dense	30–130	10–28	5–15
Porous	1–10	0.4	—

rials and bone are detailed in Table 8–1. Porous calcium phosphates have properties similar to cancellous bone, while the dense materials are significantly stronger than bone. However, because dense calcium phosphate ceramics are much less compliant than bone (elastic modulus of a 1×10^7 psi versus 2×10^6 psi for bone), they cannot withstand the rigors of implant sites that would be expected to endure significant bending, torsional, or impact forces. Metallic implants, on the other hand, because of their high strength, can withstand such forces.

Calcium phosphates, despite their lack of great strength, can be used as bone graft substitutes in a variety of situations that are currently not served by metals. For example, dense HA particles have been found to easily withstand the forces of mastication under denture function when used for alveolar ridge augmentation. Dense HA submerged root forms, when used to prevent postextraction alveolar ridge resorption, show no tendency to fracture under denture function after prolonged implantation in humans.[29] Dense HA block forms, when used as spacers in conjunction with orthognathic procedures, can readily withstand the associated forces, since they are mainly compressive in nature. As mentioned earlier, porous HA or TCP cannot be considered useful bioresorbable materials because of their lack of predictability. However, it is quite likely that implant materials with much more reliable resorption characteristics will emerge out of the exploitation of the calcium phosphate system. These materials will probably have approximately the same strength as autogenous cancellous bone and will serve as only a temporary scaffolding, being rapidly and fully replaced by normal bone. Therefore, the mechanical properties of these resorbable materials will not be a significant factor in their use. The judicious use of dense, permanent HA implant materials and porous bioresorbable calcium phosphates (when they become available), with full cognizance of their mechanical limitations, still offers the promise of generating many useful, new hard-tissue prosthetics.

BASIC BIOLOGIC PROFILE OF CALCIUM PHOSPHATE IMPLANT MATERIALS

These "new concept" calcium phosphate biomaterials are distinguished from previous hard-tissue implant materials by their basic biologic profile, which suggests that they are the most biocompatible hard-tissue implant materials known. Key features of this profile include the lack of local or systemic toxicity, inflammatory or foreign body response, and the absence of intervening fibrous tissue between implant and bone. They have an apparent ability to become directly bonded to bone by what may prove to be natural bone-cementing mechanisms. Since this profile has been observed with implant materials of varying chemical composition and material structure, it appears that this highly attractive profile is generic to all calcium phosphate implant materials.

The histology associated with the implantation of nonporous calcium phosphate materials in bone represents normal bone healing processes on and around the implant. At the interface of these materials, bone is usually found to be deposited directly on the surfaces without the presence of a fibrous tissue capsule (Fig. 8–3). Normal calcification also takes place at the implant sites. In one study of dense HA implants placed in artificially created defects in dog femurs, the implant sites were examined for calcium and phosphorus content and Ca/P ratios with the electron microprobe, using point counts, line ratemeter scans, and pulse images. Calcification processes were observed to occur at normal rates immediately adjacent to the implants (Fig. 8–4). After six months, mineralization within the implant sites was comparable to that of surrounding bone.[30] Similar observations have been made by others using microradiography and energy dispersive analysis.[31,32] This general pattern of healing and mineralization also takes place on the outer surfaces and pores of porous calcium phosphate implants. In the inner pores of these materials, however, the rate of tissue infiltration and maturation becomes significantly retarded.

Calcium phosphate implant materials also display a complete lack of local and systemic toxicity. This is due to the fact that they can release only calcium and phosphate ions.

Several studies have been conducted to determine the fate of these ions, particularly with regard to bioresorbable implants. Analysis of serum and urine calcium and phosphate levels and/or SMA 12 parameters carried out in conjunction with implant studies of a bioresorbable TCP material implanted in puppies (palate)[33] and dogs (orbital, iliac, mandible[34]; SC, IM, femur[35]; spine[36]) and with HA in dogs (alveolus[37, 38]) produced normal results. Tissue studies of major organs have been performed, including fine-detail kidney radiography, and no abnormalities or pathologic calcification was noted.[33, 35]

A study in rabbits (calvaria) used radiolabeled (Ca^{45}) TCP implant materials. Various areas (tibia, liver, skin, brain, heart, kidney, intestine, and lung) were examined for accumulation of labeled calcium six months following implantation. Measurable quantities of labeled calcium were found only in the tibia, indicating that implant-derived calcium was accumulated only in the relatively nonexchangeable pool of bone calcium.[39] These studies indicate that calcium and phosphate derived from these implants enter the body pool and are utilized (or removed) in a normal fashion.

Probably the most remarkable feature of calcium phosphate implants is their ability to become directly bonded to bone without benefit of a mechanical interlock. Numerous investigations have observed this bone-bonding phenomenon, which is manifested by the inability to remove even dense HA implants from surrounding bone.[30, 32–42] Rigorous attempts to remove these implants usually result in breaking of either the implant or the surrounding bone; separation rarely occurs at the interface.

Several investigators have attempted to reveal the structure of the bonding zone between bone and HA ceramics using electron

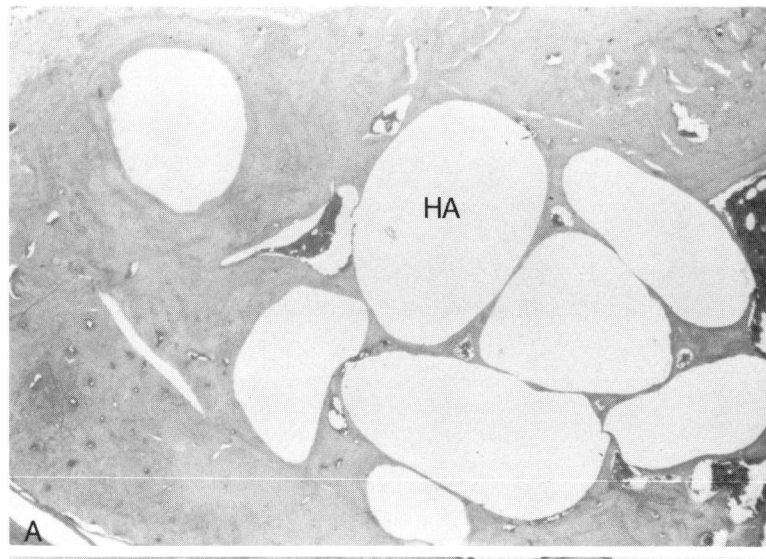

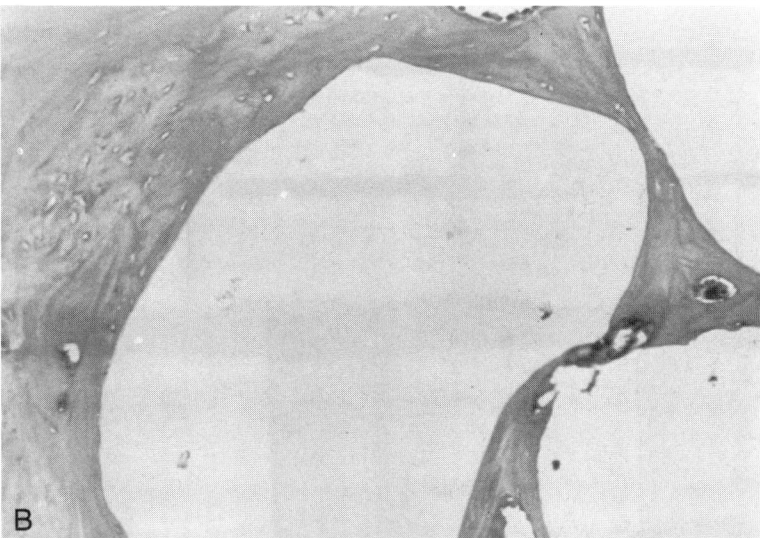

Figure 8–3. *A*, Low power micrograph of bone infiltrating HA particles in the proximal tibia of a rat two months after implantation. *B*, Higher-power micrograph of the same section, showing bone directly deposited on the surface of the implants (void area) without intervening fibrous tissue. (Courtesy of R. M. Meffert.)

Figure 8–4. EDAX pulse image of calcium density (left) and corresponding back-scattered electron micrograph (right) of a dense HA particle (P) embedded in new bone (N) near the old bone (O) interface.[42]

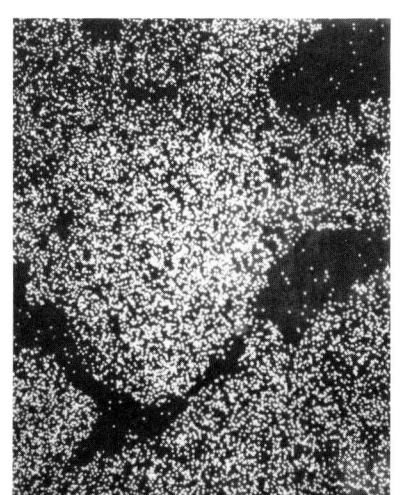

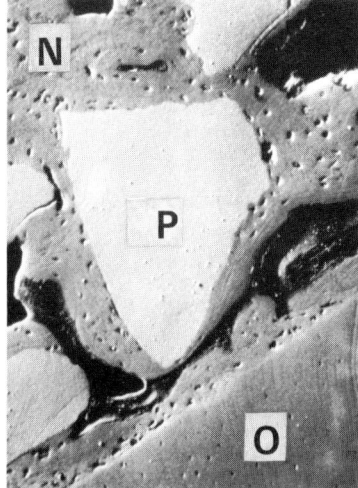

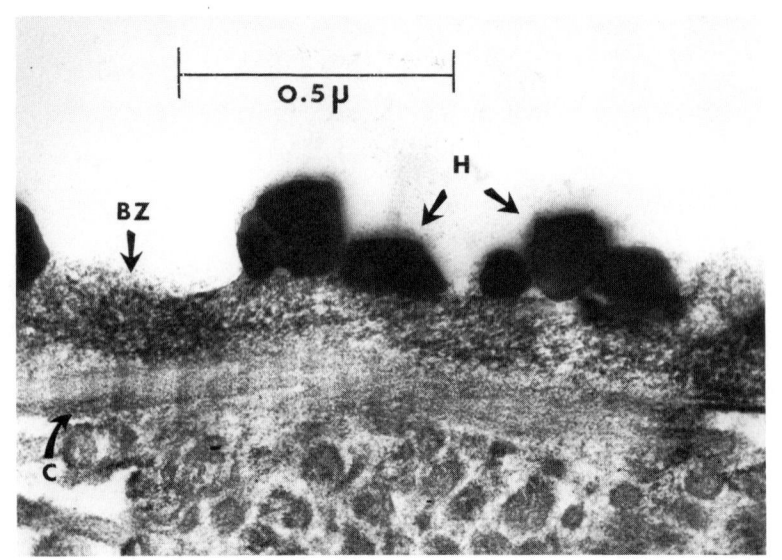

Figure 8–5. Electron micrograph of a decalcified bone-HA interface showing remnants of HA implant crystals (H) still attached to the amorphous bonding zone (BZ). A collagen fibril (C) is readily seen running parallel to the bonding zone and implant surface.[43, 44]

microscopy and other electron optical techniques. These studies have revealed the zone to be confined to a narrow band (50 to 200 nm wide) devoid of collagen fibers but containing an amorphous organic ground substance (Fig. 8–5).[43, 44] Crystals of biologic apatite were found to be embedded in this ground substance,[45] arranged in an orderly perpendicular palisade array directly on the surface of the HA implant (Fig. 8–6).[30, 42] The bone immediately adjacent to the bonding zone is normal in appearance and contains its usual complement of ground substance, collagen fibrils, and bone mineral.[30, 42–46] The characteristics of the bonding zone are very similar to those of natural bone cementing substance, which also has an amorphous ground substance that becomes mineralized.[47]

Calcium phosphate implants, composed of the same chemical substance of natural bone mineral, not only "fool" living bone cells into reacting as if they were natural autogenous materials, but also "fool" the intercellular matrix into bonding these materials to living bone. Therefore, it naturally follows that the factors that govern the "take" of a conventional bone graft also play a role in the success or failure of calcium phosphate implants. A prime factor is initial stabilization, with many investigators noting the need for tight fixation of the implant to adjacent bone as a prerequisite for effective healing.[30, 33, 35] Migration of the implant from a bony site into adjacent soft tissue, while undesirable, does not usually produce inflammatory responses. These materials are well-tolerated by soft tissues and are sequestered by a quiescent fibrous tissue capsule (Fig. 8–7). In fact, the infiltration of an HA particle mass by fibrous tissue yields a very tough, almost bonelike structure that plays a role in the successful use of HA for alveolar ridge augmentation.

The osteogenicity of calcium phosphate implants has also been the subject of some investigation. Although it is frequently asserted that these materials may stimulate osteogenesis,[48, 49] there is no real evidence to support this contention. To the contrary, experiments involving millipore chambers[50] or implantation into nonbony tissues suggest that these materials do not induce bone formation but instead serve as highly suitable substrates for hard-tissue growth. For example, subcutaneous implantation of a porous

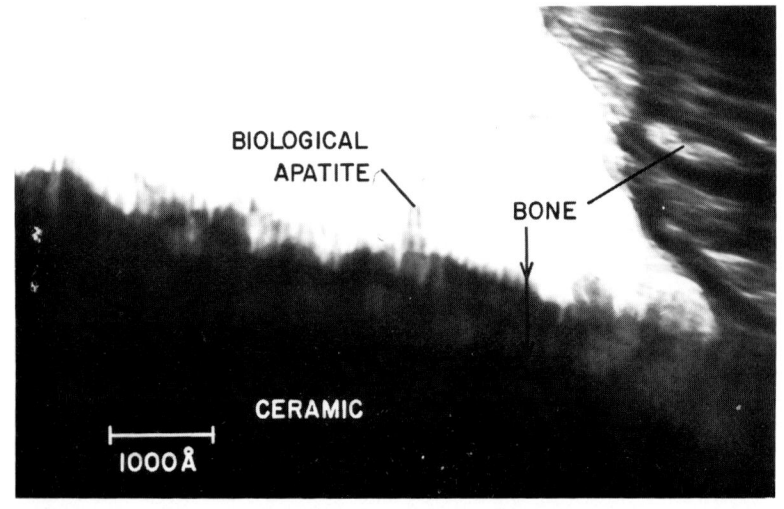

Figure 8–6. Direct transmission electron micrograph of an undecalcified ultrathin section of a bone-HA implant interface, prepared by ion beam micromilling.[30, 42] Biologic apatite is deposited directly on the surface of the implant in a perpendicular palisade fashion. The white space represents the area perforated by the ion beam.

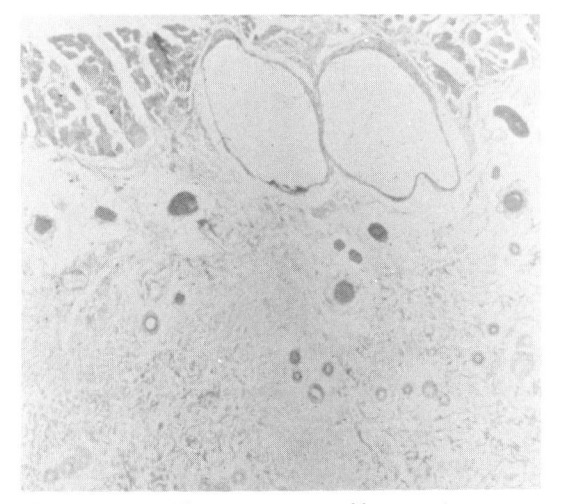

Figure 8–7. Thin quiescent fibrous tissue capsule surrounding HA particles two months after subcutaneous implantation in a rat. (Courtesy of R. M. Meffert.)

TCP material in rats, as opposed to the same material coated with calcitonin or viable autogenous marrow, revealed that bone formation took place only in the marrow-coated implants. This indicated that the material, either alone or coated with calcitonin, had no osteogenetic effect; it was noted, however, that the material was an excellent vehicle for osteogenetic marrow.[51]

Viable autogenous cancellous bone consistently has outperformed calcium phosphate implants in histologically determined healing rates of periodontal lesions (dogs),[52] spinal fusions (dogs),[36] and segmental replacements (rabbits).[53] In a study designed to determine the time required to effect bony bridging of rabbit tibia lesions, a porous TCP material in granular form was compared with autogenous cancellous bone and mixtures of the two. The autograft effected bridging at four to six weeks, the ceramic at 14 to 16 weeks, and a 50/50 mixture of the two at six weeks.[53] While this study revealed the superiority of the autogenous material, the results clearly point to using the material as an autograft extender.

As mentioned earlier, the healing rates of implant sites containing porous calcium phosphates are somewhat retarded relative to unimplanted control defects. For example, in one study evaluating a porous nonresorbable HA implant material in surgically created periodontal defects in dogs, empty control defects were completely filled with new bone after 16 weeks. The porous blocks of HA in the experimental sites still contained significant amounts of proliferating fibrovascular tissue.[38] Similar results were obtained by others using porous TCP particulate implants in essentially the same model.[52, 54] In contrast, surgically created periodontal defect implant sites containing dense HA implants in particulate form appear to allow for healing rates that are comparable to those observed in empty controls.[55] Similar findings of comparable healing rates with empty and implanted (dense HA particles) sites have also been reported for femur defect models.[30]

A possible explanation for this difference in histologically observed healing rates between dense and porous calcium phosphate implant materials lies in the nature of these porous materials (Fig. 8–8). All of them impose upon infiltrating tissue an unnatural pathway that must be followed if the porous implant is to become fully invested with bone. Since bone is a tissue that is notorious for proliferating and remodeling according to its own overall biomechanical dictates, it is expected to travel these unnatural pore pathways with some reluctance. Most bony structures also require some degree of mechanical stimulation to maintain vitality. One must question the long-term fate of bone residing deep within the pores of a rigid ceramic structure, an environment virtually devoid of mechanical stress. Additionally, the vascular system that supplies precursor fibrous tissue, and eventually bone, must follow the same tortuous pathway to get deep within such blocks. It would be expected that such a vascular system would be inefficient, both in its support of cell function and in its ability to serve as a conduit for systemic antibiotics, if infections arise at the implant site.

This theory is supported by a study wherein the calvaria of rabbits were implanted with porous blocks of a bioresorbable TCP material. Twenty-four hours prior to sacrifice (at three months), the animals were injected with radiolabeled calcium. Radioisotope analysis revealed that the uptake deep within the porous implant was approximately one tenth that of surrounding bone; at the periphery of the implant, however, the rates of uptake were about one half that of surrounding bone.[56] In one dog study, using a porous block form of HA derived from marine coral as an interpositional "sandwich graft" for alveolar ridge augmen-

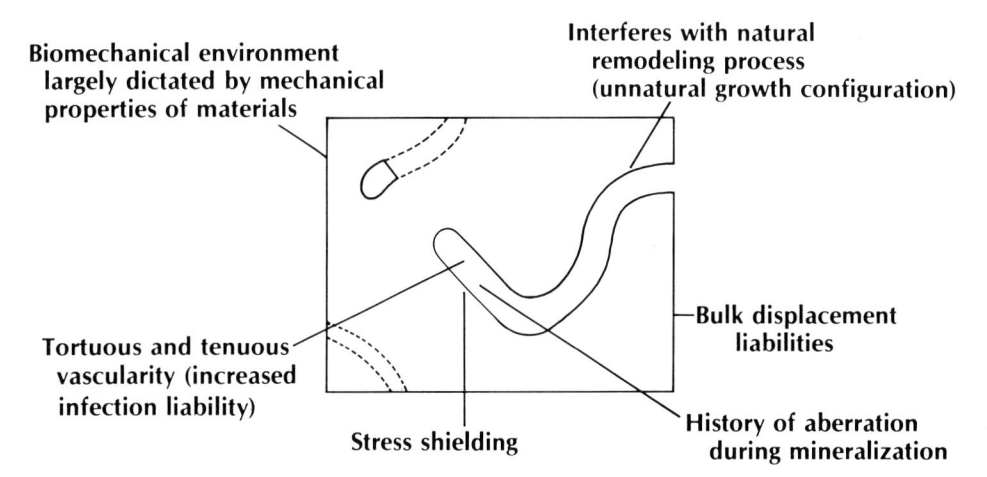

Figure 8–8. Problems with permanent porous implant materials.

- Biomechanical environment largely dictated by mechanical properties of materials
- Interferes with natural remodeling process (unnatural growth configuration)
- Tortuous and tenuous vascularity (increased infection liability)
- Bulk displacement liabilities
- Stress shielding
- History of aberration during mineralization

tation, the longest-term sample evaluated (40 weeks) still contained large areas within the porous implant that were devoid of osseous or soft tissue.[57] In another dog study using this same porous HA material in block form as an onlay graft for alveolar ridge augmentation, the authors noted both that bone ingrowth was slow and that the noninfiltrated ceramic crushed when the animals (initially on a soft diet) were returned to a solid diet 1.5 years after implantation.[58]

The above discussion on the perceived and verified limitations to the use of porous block forms of calcium phosphates (Fig. 8–8) clearly raises questions about their long-term suitability for use in man. The ideal porous calcium phosphate implant material would appear to be one that is bioresorbable, with resorption rates closely matching hard-tissue infiltration and replacement rates. While no such material has yet been reported in the literature, numerous laboratories are undoubtedly working to achieve this goal.

In contrast to porous implants, implant sites filled with dense, impervious calcium phosphate particles are far less restrictive to investing tissues, which can grow over and around the particles according to their own dictates.[30, 59] Since each discrete particle is capable of undergoing a certain degree of motion within the developing bone matrix, dictated by surrounding tissue, far less interference with normal bone remodeling patterns would be expected. Conceptually, this ability of dense calcium phosphate particles to move within the implant site should pose problems of gross migration or extrusion from the site. However, in practice the initial blood clot appears to be sufficiently adhesive to maintain the particles within the defect at early periods following implantation. At later periods, the restored site appears to function as a composite unit with no evidence of particle movement. The strength of such composite units can exceed that of normal bone.[60]

ALVEOLAR RIDGE RECONSTRUCTION

Clinical trials using particulate forms of HA for ridge augmentation were initiated at Louisiana State University in 1978. After evaluating atrophic ridge types and a variety of surgical techniques, an alveolar ridge classification based on severity of the deficient mandibular and maxillary alveolar ridges was developed by Kent to standardize and determine surgical approaches, material usage, and clinical performance of HA under denture function.[61, 62] Since actual ridge height and form vary considerably between and within sexes, an anatomic basis was selected to classify alveolar ridges (Table 8–2). The material was placed alone or in combination with finely crushed autogenous cancellous bone, through a subperiosteal tunneling technique, to obtain improvement in alveolar ridge height and form.[61, 62] Results in over 300 patients during the past six years have shown the material to be a simple, effective bone substitute to improve ridge height and form for denture function.[61–63] These early and more recent experiences are the bases for this chapter, since an estimated 20,000 patients in the United States have received HA ridge augmentation in 1982 through 1984.[64–66]

PREOPERATIVE PATIENT MANAGEMENT AND INSTRUCTIONS

Dentures are removed a few days preoperatively, if necessary, to allow for improve-

TABLE 8–2. CLASSIFICATION AND TREATMENT OF ALVEOLAR RIDGE DEFICIENCY

Class I
　　Alveolar ridge is adequate in height but inadequate in width, usually with lateral deficiencies or undercut areas. Patients received HA alone—2 to 4 grams for each anterior/posterior area and 6 to 8 grams for total ridge.

Class II
　　Alveolar ridge is deficient in both height and width and presents a knife-edge appearance. Patients received HA alone—3 to 5 grams for each anterior/posterior area and 8 to 10 grams for total ridge.

Class III
　　Alveolar ridge has been resorbed to the level of the basilar bone, producing a concave form in the posterior areas of the mandible and a sharp bony ridge form with bulbous mobile soft tissue in the maxilla. Patients received HA alone—8 to 12 grams or combined with autogenous iliac cancellous bone (1 gram HA: 1 cc bone).

Class IV
　　There is resorption of the basilar bone, producing pencil-thin, flat mandible or maxilla. Patients received HA—10 to 15 grams mixed with autogenous bone in a 1:1 ratio. Patient unable to permit harvesting of iliac bone may have HA alone to increase ridge heights modestly. HA combined with bone is recommended for larger augmentation and to strengthen the mandible.

ment of inflamed soft tissues. Patients with Class I and II lateral deficiencies or undercut areas augmented with HA may have their dentures modified so that they may be worn immediately after surgery (Table 8–2). Patients requiring a significant increase in ridge height (Class III and IV) should have their dentures modified or preferably a splint made from a cast with a wax-up that simulates the ridge augmentation (Fig. 8–9). In Class III and IV patients the splint is secured to the maxilla (palatal screws) or mandible (circumferential sutures/wires) for one to three weeks (Fig. 8–10). Vestibular depth is most likely maintained if splints are used for three weeks. Careful soft-tissue release to form a tunnel and control particles without a splint is also possible. New denture construction cannot begin until the fourth to sixth postoperative week or until the augmented ridge is rigid. Patients are also advised of a potential manipulation of or injury to the mental nerve that may result in varying degrees of lip anesthesia postoperatively. Postoperative pain and swelling vary but may be considerable in older patients whose loose tissues permit extensive edema and discomfort. In severe ridge deficiency, postoperative skin graft vestibuloplasty may be necessary to establish a sulcus, remove displaced particles, or provide a more fixed soft-tissue base. Antibiotics such as penicillin or a broad-spectrum antibiotic are routinely used. Oral penicillin (500 mg), for example, is administered to outpatients at the beginning of surgery, and 2 million units of aqueous penicillin intravenously is given to inpatients undergoing general anesthesia. Outpatients continue to receive penicillin, 250 to 500 mg q6h, or the appropriate antibiotic and equivalent dosage if they are allergic to penicillin. With inpatients, intravenous penicillin, 1 to 2 million units q4h, is given until the patient is able to receive oral peni-

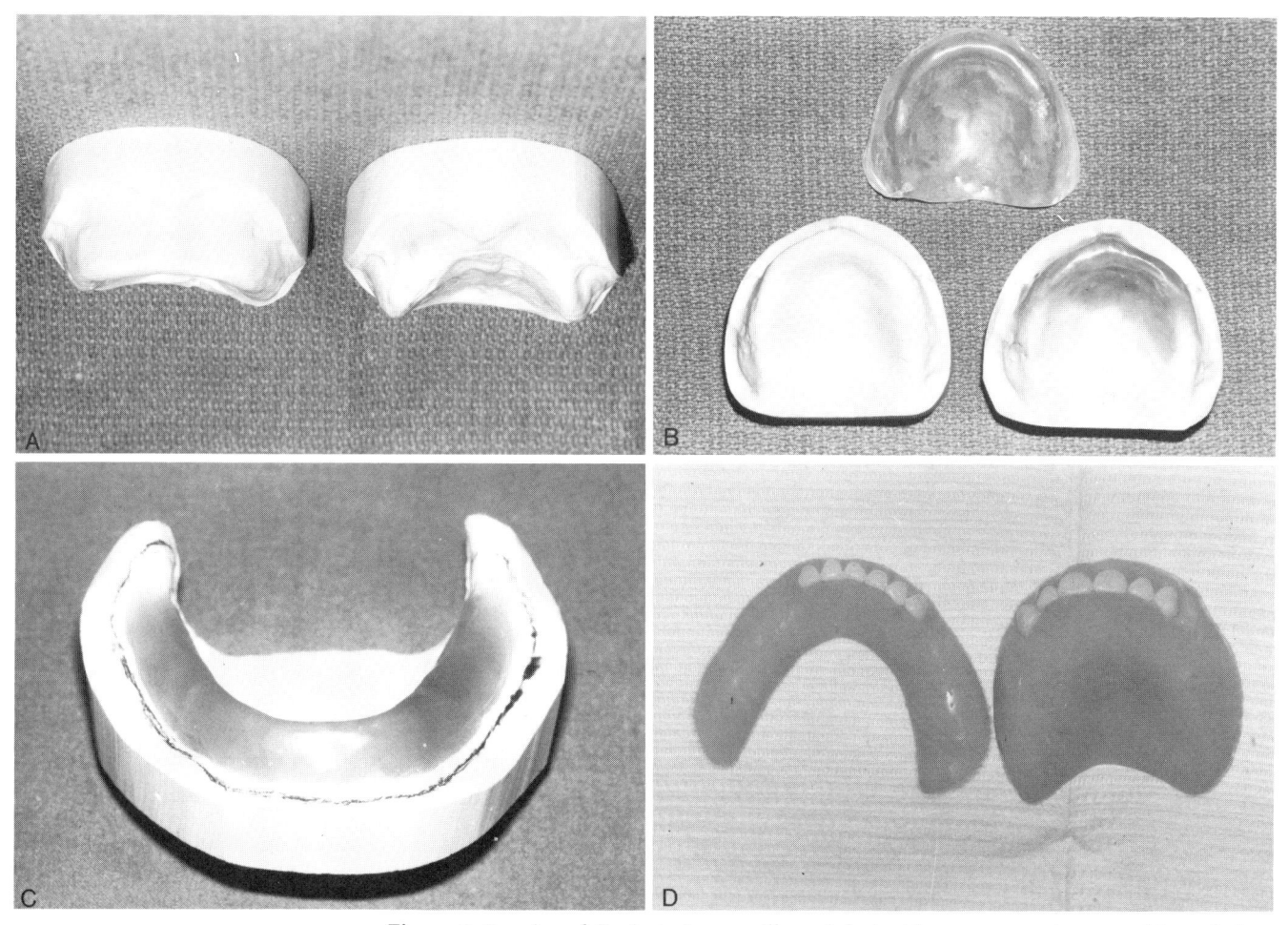

Figure 8–9. *A* and *B,* Anterior maxillary defect, ridge wax-up, stone model, and clear acrylic splint. *C,* Mandibular ridge wax-up does not include the retromolar pad but finishes along the external oblique ridge. The splint is constructed to the pencil line. *D,* Ideal maxillary and mandibular splints designed for control of particles, sulcus maintenance, and esthetics, but not function.

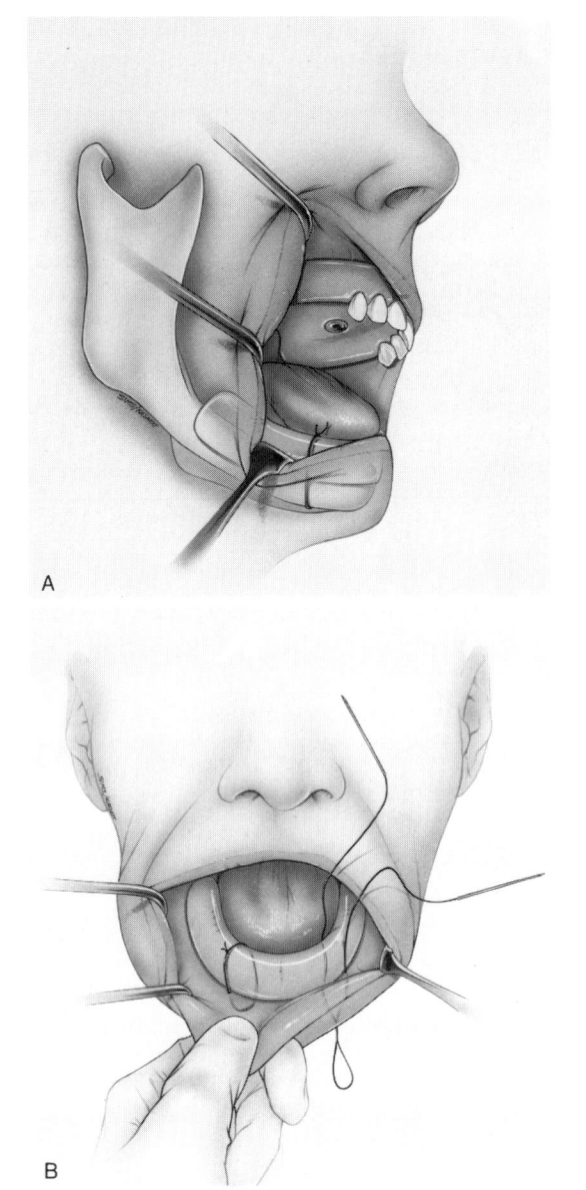

Figure 8–10. *A,* Maxillary and mandibular splints are secured in Class III and IV patients where vertical HA build-up requires control of particles. *B,* Circumferential sutures or wires are placed atraumatically with straight needles before HA is injected over the ridge crest.

cillin. A steroid regimen similar to that recommended for orthognathic surgery patients is helpful.

Construction of a Splint

The use of splints, dentures, tubes, etc., may be necessary to control HA particles and maintain the sulcus. If the denture is inadequate (most common) in height or width to permit augmentation or the flanges are insufficient in length, a splint with anterior teeth for esthetics is constructed on a wax model (Fig. 8–9D).

A well-extended modeling composition impression, which extends the vestibules, should be taken to identify bony outline on the stone model. For the complete alveolar ridge augmentation patient, the posterior limit is outlined just anterior to the retromolar pad in the mandible. This pencilled outline continues anteriorly along the external oblique ridge, swinging slightly medially in the region of the mental foramen. The width of the augmentation outline in the symphyseal area should be conservative. Lingually, the outline should be at the most superior lingual aspect of the alveolar crest of the mandible (Fig. 8–9C). In the maxilla, the outlines are placed on the palatal and buccal-labial surfaces. The posterior limit may be either at the tuberosity crest or in the hamular notch. The alveolar ridge is waxed-up to the desired height and width using the pencil outline as a guide (Fig. 8–9C). The patient's denture is then hollowed out to fit over the waxed-up ridge, or, more commonly, a splint is constructed (Fig. 8–10). Clear acrylic splints permit visualization of the underlying HA augmentation but may not satisfy esthetic requirements. A mandibular splint whose flanges extend beyond the external oblique ridge is preferred to avoid displacement "wings" of HA. Confinement of HA particles and sulcus maintenance can be accomplished with Silastic tubes, nasogastric tubes sutured to red rubber catheter, mattress sutures, or an equivalent (Fig. 8–11).

Surgical Technique for Minor Deficiencies (Class I and II Patients)

Minor deficiencies are easily augmented with HA under local anesthesia and, if necessary, sedation in the office. One of two types of incisions is used: a ridge crest incision or a vertical incision with subperiosteal tunneling.[61] Patients requiring complete augmentation of the anterior maxillary or mandibular area will require only a ridge crest or a single midline vertical incision from the crest of the alveolus to the vestibule, approximately 12 to 15 mm in length. If only the posterior aspects of the maxillary or mandibular alveolar ridge are to be augmented, ridge crest or bilateral vertical incisions in the cuspid areas are used. These same incisions may also be used for total ridge augmentation. The incision is carried continuously through mucosa, submucosa, and periosteum. The periosteum is elevated *only* in the area of desired augmentation. Traction sutures placed through both edges of the incision will facilitate the insertion of a small custom syringe and delivery of the HA particles (Fig. 8–12). A beveled syringe facili-

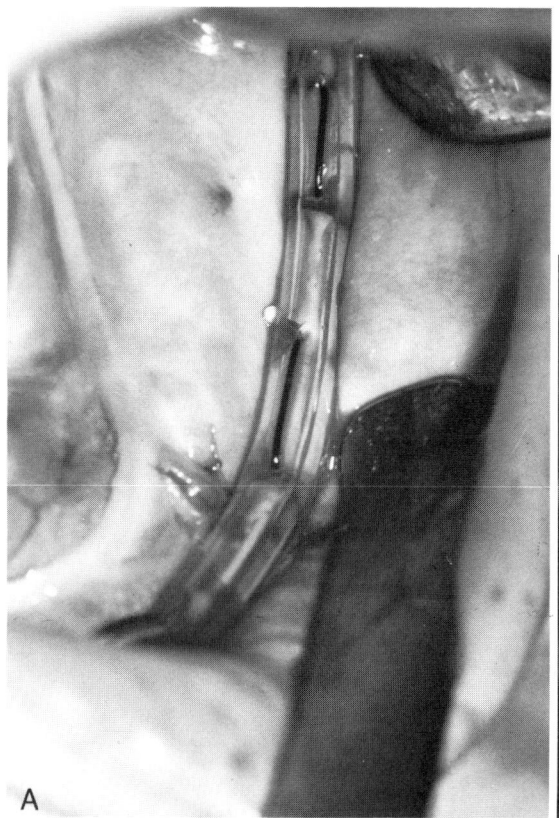

Figure 8–11. Nasogastric tube secured to a red rubber catheter maintains buccal and labial sulcus and controls HA particles.

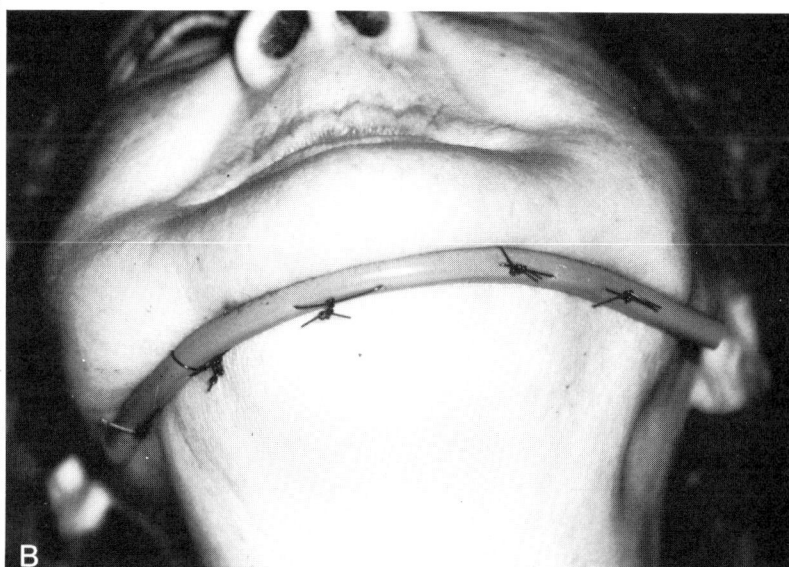

tates insertion and delivery by inserting the syringe with the point against the bone and rotating the syringe to deposit the particles (Fig. 8–12E,F). Supraperiosteal injection is avoided. In patients with a single midline incision, the subperiosteal pockets are filled from the posterior ends moving anteriorly toward the incision. In patients with bilateral vertical incisions in the cuspid area the filling extends from the posterior ends bilaterally to these incisions. One incision is closed, and the remaining anterior pocket is filled from the closed cuspid incision toward the opposite side. If the patient's denture or a previously prepared splint has been modified to accommodate the areas of augmentation, then the denture or splint can be worn immediately postoperatively. Securing the splint or denture with wires or screws is not necessary. Patients are placed on a nonchewing diet. Generally patients with high muscle attachments and inadequate sulcus depth are Class III and Class IV patients, and the surgery is modified as described below.

Surgical Technique for Major Deficiencies (Class III and IV Patients)

A larger subperiosteal pocket, dissection or avoidance of the mental nerve, excision of high muscle attachments, and maintenance of the sulcus areas are necessary in Class III and IV patients.[62] Augmentation may be accomplished in the office under local anesthesia and sedation or in the hospital under general anesthesia for patients augmented with HA alone or HA mixed with autogenous iliac cancellous bone.

Maxillary Augmentation. Class III and IV atrophic ridge patients require maintenance of the labial and buccal sulcus and a larger augmentation. The subperiosteal tissue elevation is frequently combined with a modified submucosal dissection.[64] A single vertical midline incision is made from the depth of the vestibule to the ridge crest through nonkeratinized mucosa only. Bilateral vertical incisions in the cuspid region may be necessary for an unusually broad maxilla. A submucosal dissection back to the tuberosity is accomplished over the facial side of the alveolar ridge. The initial vertical incision is then continued through the submucosal and periosteal layers and is extended to bone over the ridge onto the palate. A subperiosteal reflection is accomplished over the labial, buccal (limited in height), crestal, and palatal aspects of the alveolar ridge to the horizontal palatal surface. Two pockets are thus formed (Fig. 8–13A). With curved scissors the periosteal layer is incised at its attachment to the crestal mucosa to allow the periosteum to swing laterally (Fig. 8–13B). This produces a single large pocket lined by

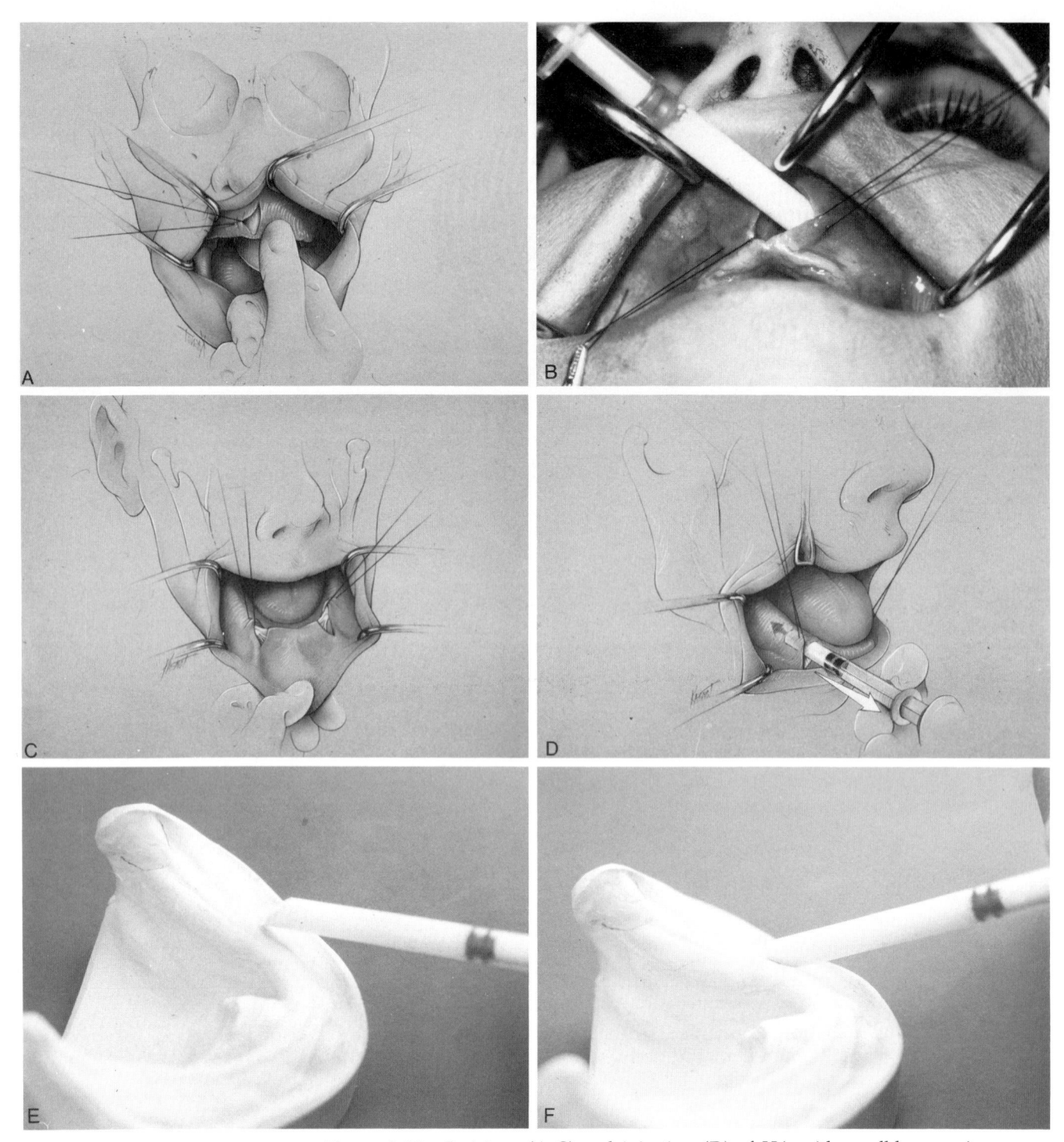

Figure 8–12. Incisions *(A–C)* and injection *(D)* of HA with small-bore syringe commonly used for injection of HA on minor ridge deficiencies. *E, F,* Beveled syringe facilitates HA injection.

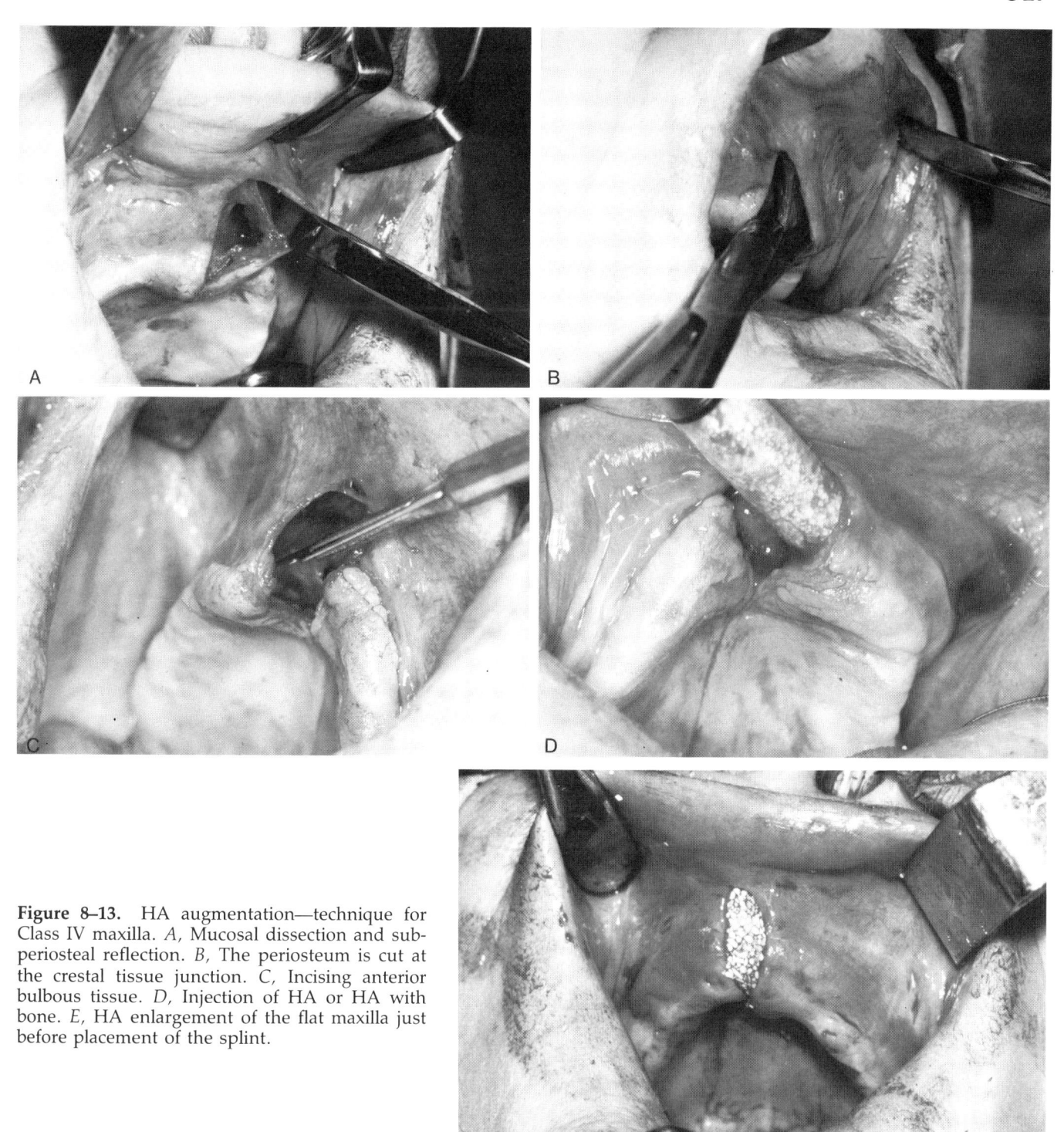

Figure 8–13. HA augmentation—technique for Class IV maxilla. *A*, Mucosal dissection and subperiosteal reflection. *B*, The periosteum is cut at the crestal tissue junction. *C*, Incising anterior bulbous tissue. *D*, Injection of HA or HA with bone. *E*, HA enlargement of the flat maxilla just before placement of the splint.

periosteum laterally and palatally and by mucosa over the crest (Fig. 8–13C). Incising anterior bulbous fibrous tissues from within the pocket provides additional tunnel space. Either a small-bore syringe for delivery of HA alone or a large-bore syringe for delivery of HA alone or a mixture of HA and autogenous cancellous bone is possible (Fig. 8–13D, E). Once the material is placed, contour is established by inserting the patient's splint. It is secured with one or two palatal screws into the nasal maxillary crest. Careful placement of the splint will prevent particles from being displaced. Manipulation of the soft tissues with the finger will remove particles that may be displaced high in the maxillary sulcus.

Mandibular Augmentation. In Class III or IV deficiencies it may be desirable to perform a modified submucosal dissection with the subperiosteal elevation to develop a large pocket, maintain an adequate buccal and labial vestibule, and excise high anterior muscle attachments[62] (Fig. 8–14A,B). The technique from 1978 to 1983 used bilateral vertical incisions immediately anterior to the mental nerve through mucosa only to allow for submucosal dissection with scissors back to the retromolar pad and over the symphysis. The vertical incisions are extended through the submucosal tissues and periosteum. Elevation of periosteum over the entire alveolar ridge is performed. The periosteal layer is then incised with scissors from its soft tissue crestal attachment along the most superior-lingual aspect of the alveolar ridge (Fig. 8–14A). Detachment of the periosteum beyond the external oblique ridge and on the lingual surface of the mandible is usually contraindicated. The mental nerve is easily dissected, if necessary, to avoid injury and ensure its placement to the lateral aspect of the augmentation material (Fig. 8–14B). Excision or inferior repositioning of a small portion of the mentalis muscle may be necessary in some cases. Bilateral circummandibular sutures or wires for the splint are placed *before* delivering the particles. Using a small- or large-bore syringe for HA alone or the large-bore syringe for HA mixed with cancellous bone, the ridge is augmented as previously described, injecting from the most posterior aspect of the pocket as the syringe is withdrawn (Fig. 8–14C). One vertical incision is closed with interrupted horizontal mattress sutures before the symphyseal area is augmented. Manipulation of the material with fingers on the buccal and lingual sulcus will permit even distribution of the material after the incisions are closed. The splint is then secured with circummandibular sutures. Quinn suggests placing the vertical incisions slightly posterior to the mental nerve for posterior tunneling. A midline incision is used to tunnel anteriorly to the nerve area[64] (Fig. 8–14D). The mental nerve is therefore not appreciably involved, since the periosteal reflection and HA augmentation are restricted in this area to minimize nerve damage.

Since 1983 a modification of our mucosal dissection and subperiosteal tunneling has reduced mental neuropathy, sulcus obliteration, and particle migration. A midline vertical incision is made from the crestal soft tissue to the vestibular depth through mucosa only (Fig. 8–14E). A submucosal dissection of the nonkeratinized or unattached mucosa with curved scissors is performed back to the retromolar pad bilaterally (Fig. 8–14F–H). The initial midline vertical incision and bilateral posterior ridge crest incision (beginning at the mental foramen region) are made through periosteum to bone (Fig. 8–14I). The posterior incision may be slightly medial to the submucosal dissection. In this case the lateral edge of the posterior incision is incised to open into the submucosal pocket dissection. The periosteum is then elevated over the ridge crest to the external obique ridge posteriorly and the mentalis muscle anteriorly through both incisions (Fig. 8–14J, K). Generally, the periosteum is *not* elevated on the lingual surface of the mandible, beyond the external oblique ridge, or beneath the retromolar pad. If the mental nerve is high or central over the ridge, periosteal elevation stops anterior to the nerve and begins again through the posterior incision (Fig. 8–14L). When the nerve is below or lateral to the ridge crest, a small amount of periosteum is elevated connecting the anterior and posterior incisions. The periosteum is then incised with scissors along its attachment to the fixed dense crestal tissues the entire length of the mandible (Fig. 8–14M, N). A large pocket is thus formed. Reflection or excision of the superior aspect of the mentalis muscle may be indicated. The posterior ridge crest incisions are used to deposit HA particles first from the mental nerve area to the retromolar pad. The posterior incisions are closed and the augmentation completed through the midline incision (Fig. 8–14O). If a splint has been prepared, circummandibular sutures or wires should have been placed outside the pockets *before* injection of the HA (see Fig. 8–10). The HA augmentation in severe ridge deficiency may be segmental or "sausage-linked" in contour, since dissection and periosteal involvement around the mental nerve are minimal (Fig. 8–14P, Q).

An open technique using a horizontal ridge crest incision, as in alveolectomy, along with horizontal releasing of the periosteum, can also be used. In this technique

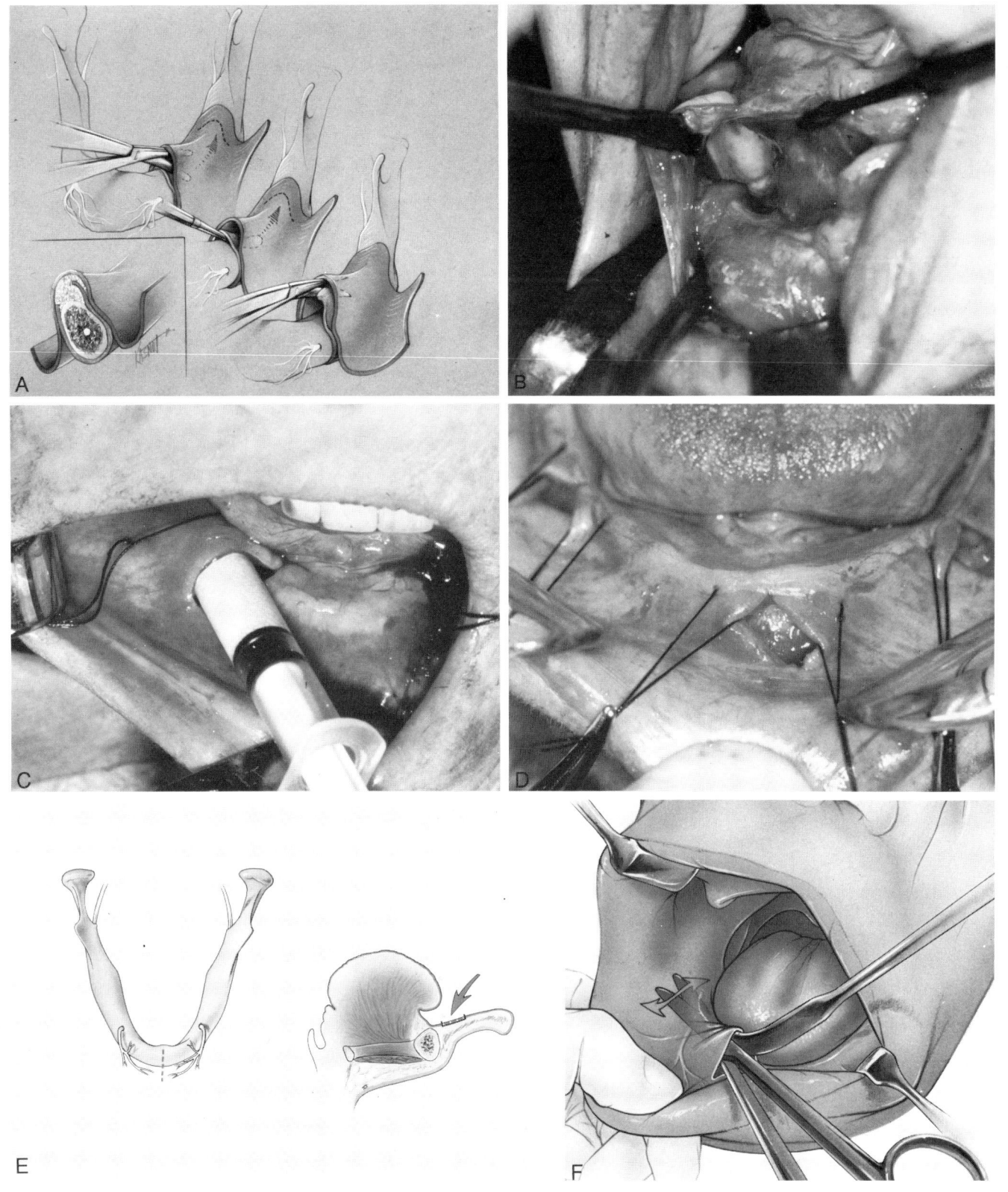

Figure 8–14. *A*, Combined mandibular mucosal dissection with periosteal reflection and detachment to develop a large pocket. *B*, Note the position of the mental nerve arising from the crest of the severely resorbed Class IV mandible. *C*, Delivery of HA particles on Class IV mandible after circummandibular sutures are placed. *D*, Incisions recommended by Quinn to minimize mental nerve involvement. *E–Q*, Technique recommended by Kent for Class III and IV deficient mandibles. *E*, The midline vertical incision begins at the crestal fixed tissue and extends to the vestibule.

Illustration continues on following page.

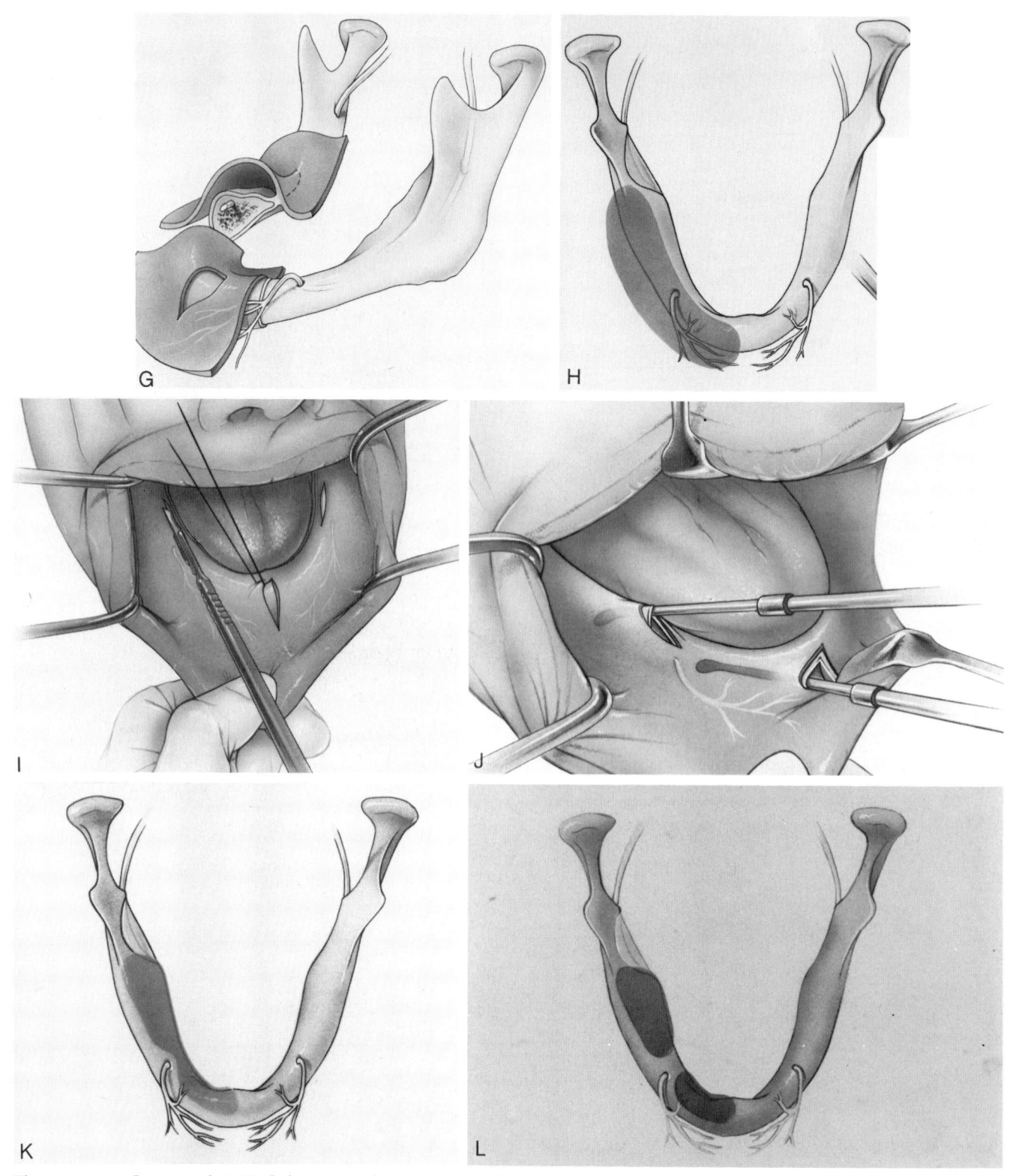

320 / RECONSTRUCTION OF THE ALVEOLAR RIDGE WITH HYDROXYLAPATITE

Figure 8–14. Continued. *F–H,* Submucosal dissection extends to the retromolar pad. *I,* Midline and posterior crestal incisions are carried to the bone. *J, K, L,* Elevation of the periosteum over ridge crest, between the external oblique ridge and the lingual surface of the mandible. The retromolar pad is usually not elevated. The periosteum is elevated marginally, or not at all, in the area of the mental nerve.

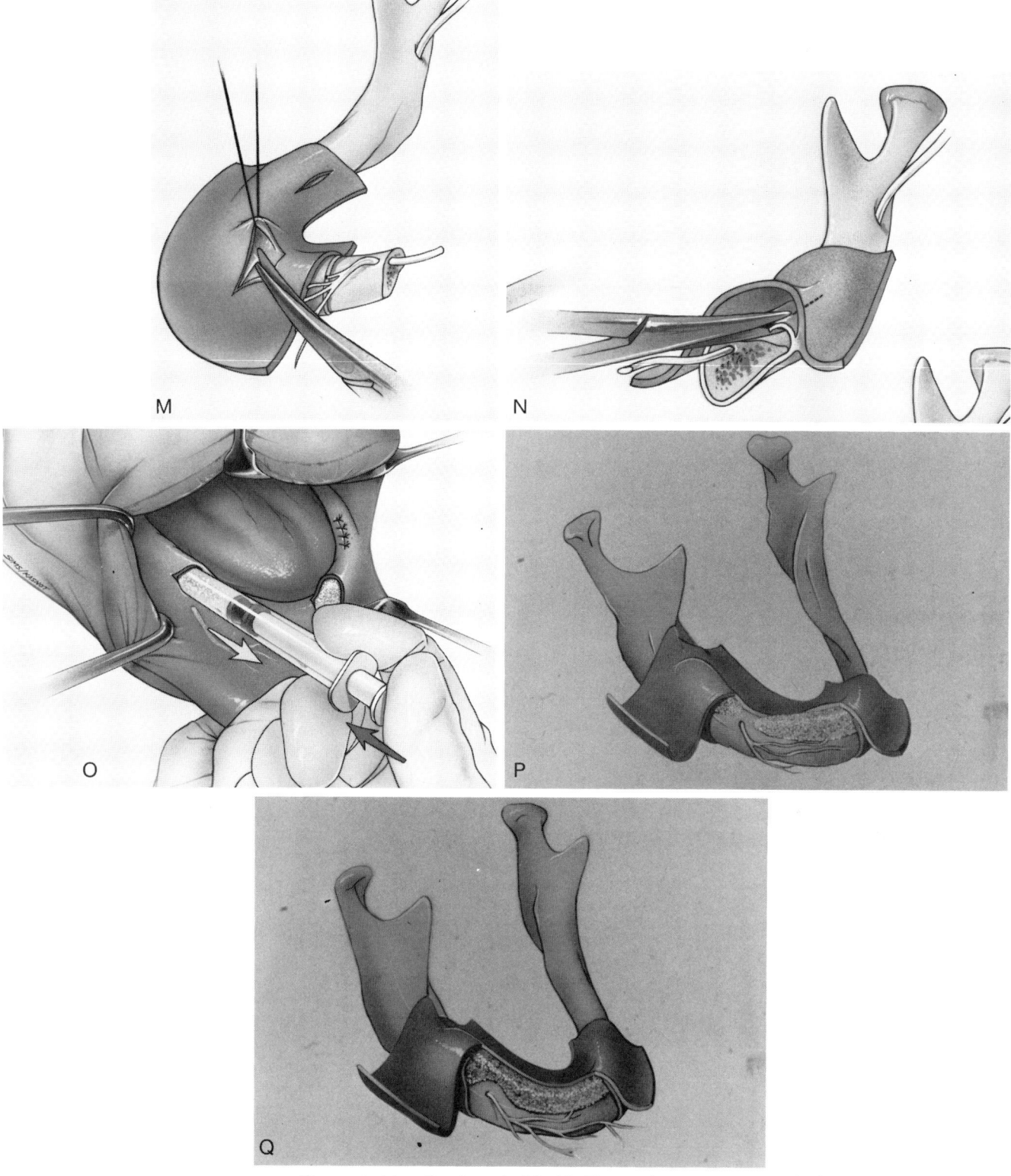

RECONSTRUCTION OF THE ALVEOLAR RIDGE WITH HYDROXYLAPATITE / **321**

Figure 8–14. Continued. *M, N,* The periosteum is incised along the junction with keratinized crestal tissue. *O,* Injection of HA beneath the periosteum begins at the posterior incision. Note that particles interface completely with bone but may not be completely covered with periosteum. *P, Q,* HA augmentation may be segmental or sausage-linked, depending on the position of the mental nerve in Class IV cases.

and the following lip switch procedure, HA is injected and the incision closed together, one alternating with the other until completed. Barsan and Kent described a lip switch technique in which a mucosal flap is developed just inside the lip and cheek and a periosteal flap is transposed to the facial side of the ridge to create a large mucosal pocket (Fig. 8–15). This technique minimizes lateral displacement of particles, maintains

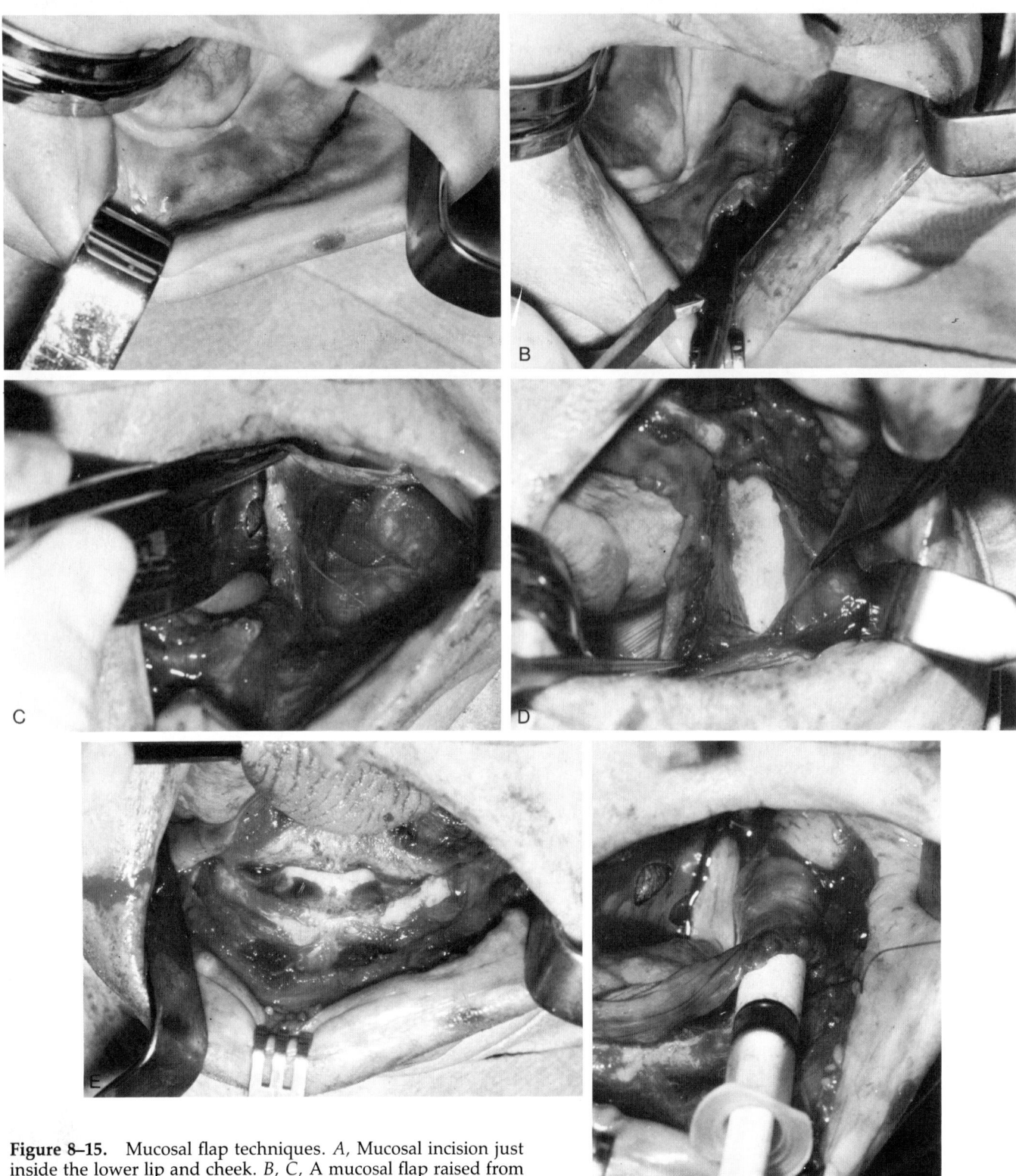

Figure 8–15. Mucosal flap techniques. *A,* Mucosal incision just inside the lower lip and cheek. *B, C,* A mucosal flap raised from retromolar to retromolar area to the lingual aspect of crest. *D,* The periosteum incised at the lingual crest and reflected laterally. *E,* In the anterior area the periosteum may be reflected lingually with the mucosal flap. *F, G,* Closure with injection of HA.

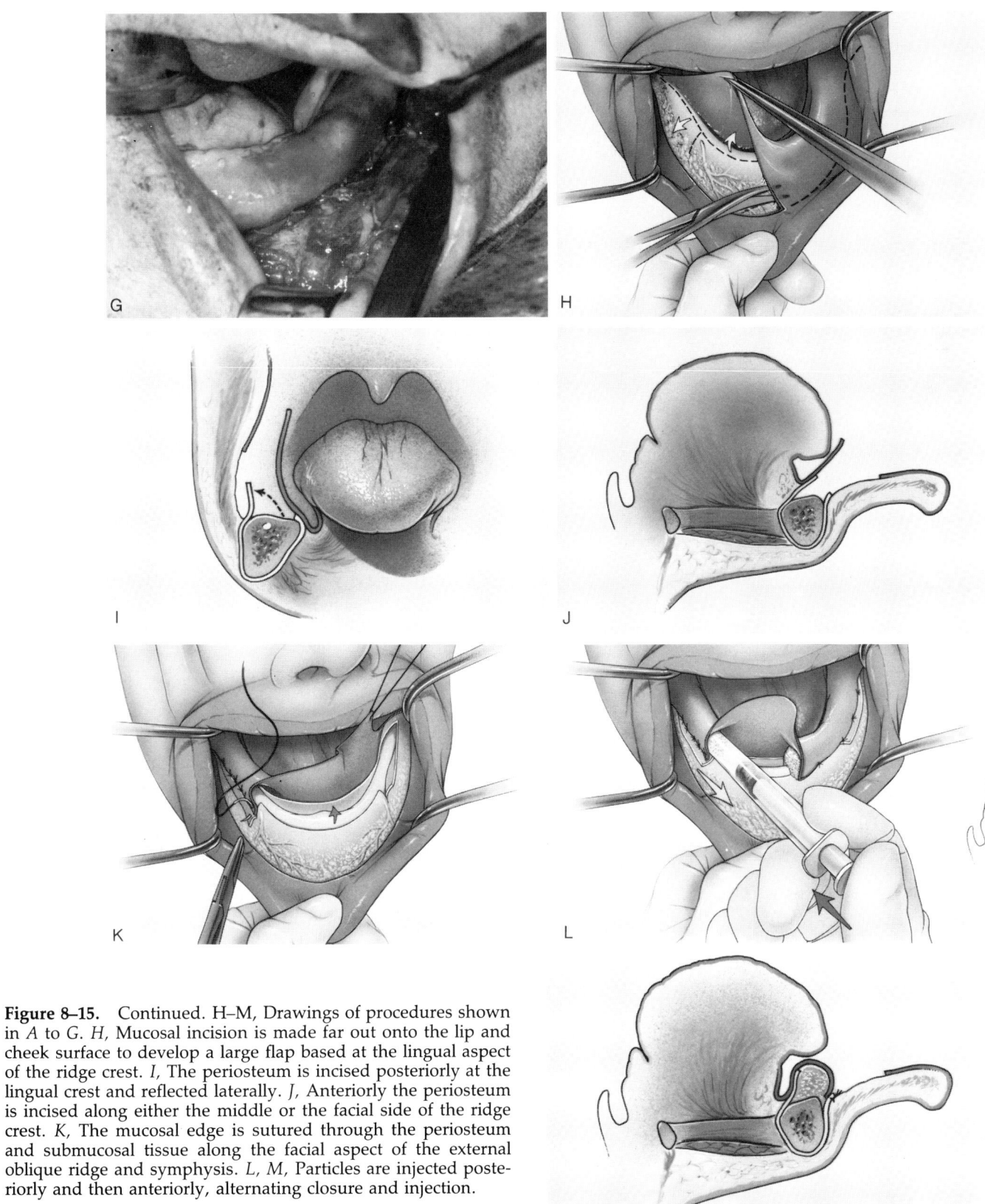

RECONSTRUCTION OF THE ALVEOLAR RIDGE WITH HYDROXYLAPATITE / **323**

Figure 8–15. Continued. H–M, Drawings of procedures shown in *A* to *G*. *H*, Mucosal incision is made far out onto the lip and cheek surface to develop a large flap based at the lingual aspect of the ridge crest. *I*, The periosteum is incised posteriorly at the lingual crest and reflected laterally. *J*, Anteriorly the periosteum is incised along either the middle or the facial side of the ridge crest. *K*, The mucosal edge is sutured through the periosteum and submucosal tissue along the facial aspect of the external oblique ridge and symphysis. *L, M*, Particles are injected posteriorly and then anteriorly, alternating closure and injection.

existing sulcus depth, and permits easy exposure with less damage to the mental nerve. A splint is not recommended or needed for the mandible. Splints are necessary and recommended for the maxilla with this technique. Disadvantages are increased surgical time, knife-edged sulcus, and possible lip inversion and mobile soft tissue.[65] Early results have been encouraging, and the procedure is useful for partially edentulous patients with esthetic ridge defects that need to be restored with a fixed or removable prosthesis (Figs. 8–16 and 8–17).

HA/Autogenous Bone. Close proximity of HA particles "cemented" together with thin fibrous connective tissue produces a firm convex ridge that mimics onlay bone grafting. Class IV deficient ridges such as the "pencil-thin" mandible may be dangerously thin in height and width. Augmentation with HA alone may not appreciably increase strength, since little bone growth occurs beyond the anatomic shape of the existing ridge. Biopsy may show occasional islands of calcified interparticular tissue. However, complete interparticular bone growth

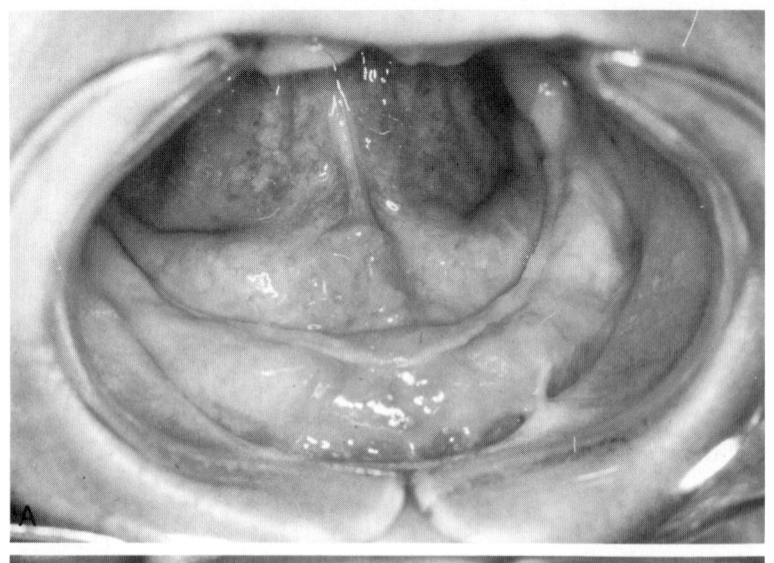

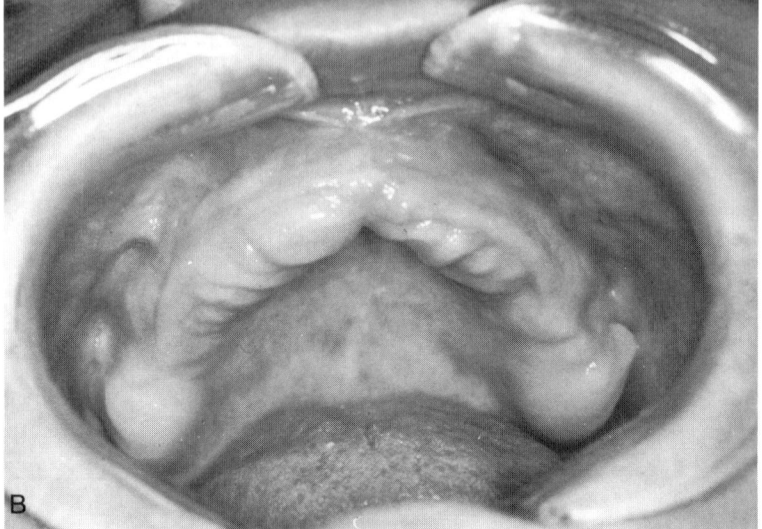

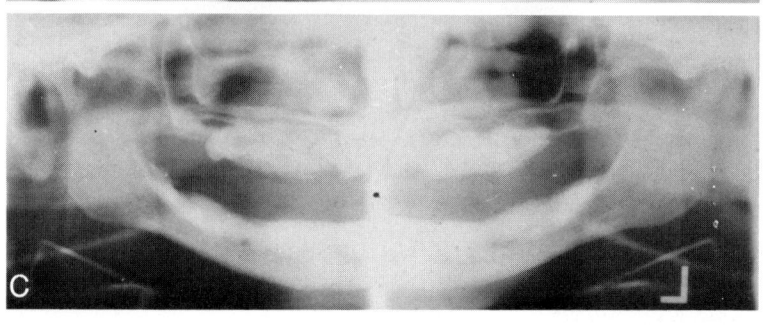

Figure 8–16. Result of HA augmentation using (A) open mucosal flap techniques (mandible) and (B) mucosal dissection/subperiosteal tunneling (maxilla).

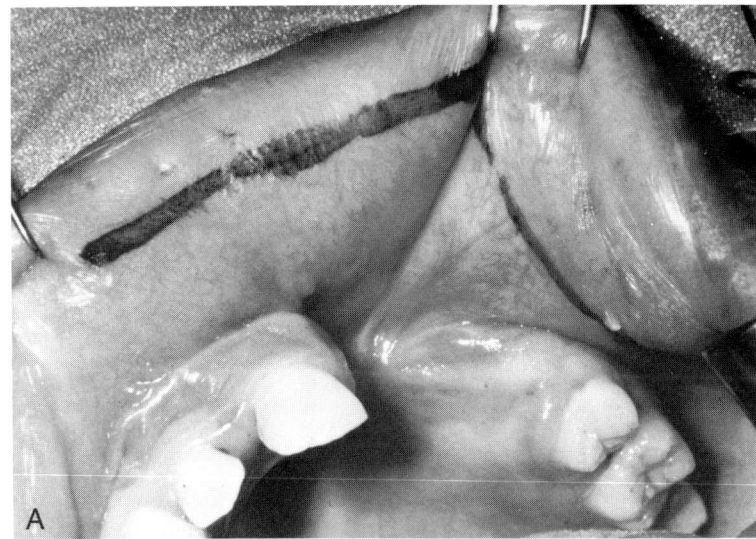

Figure 8–17. Lip incision (A) is also used for maxillary defects to improve ridge contour and esthetics for fixed or removal prostheses. B, Postoperative result.

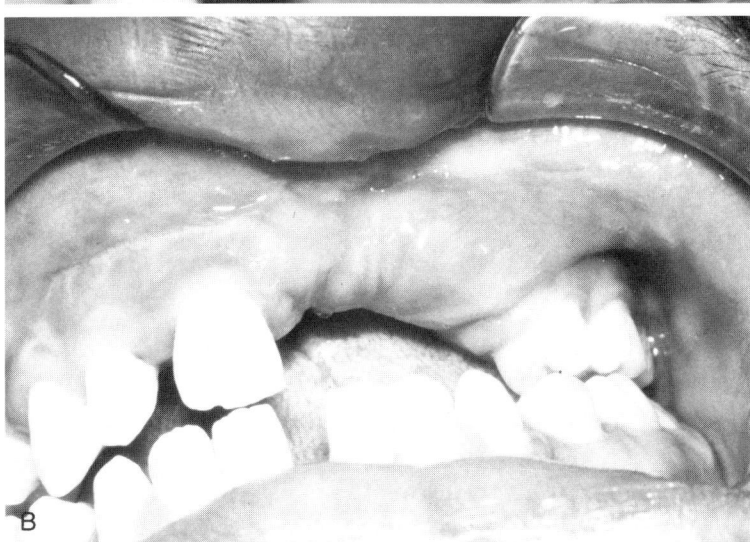

can be achieved only with a mixture of finely crushed autogenous cancellous bone and marrow with HA. The exact ratio of HA to bone is speculative, but experience by Kent et al. suggests a ratio of 1:1 (grams HA:cc bone).[62] Fine bone particles are necessary to achieve a uniform homogeneous mixture. Rongeurs and chisels may be inadequate. A bone grinder that produces small particles of similar size to the HA particle is preferred (Fig. 8–18). Since elderly patients, particularly postmenopausal women, may be deficient in iliac cancellous bone, ratios of 2:1 or perhaps 3:1 may result unless cortical bone is also used. Class IV patients unable to permit harvesting of iliac bone will, of course, benefit from HA alone. Class IV patients with wide mandibles may have significant increase in augmentation height. Class IV patients deficient in width as well are more difficult to provide large increases in height, since the HA surface area interfacing with the mandible is reduced. Stability of a large augmentation of HA alone may be compromised, resulting in postoperative HA movement. HA-bone mixtures are strongly recommended in this situation (Figs. 8–19 to 8–21).

POSTOPERATIVE MANAGEMENT OF THE PATIENT

Patients are maintained on antibiotics for at least one week (250 to 500 mg of penicillin q6h or an appropriate substitute). Meticulous oral hygiene is instituted with use of an effective anesthetic-germicidal mouthwash after meals and at bedtime and including brushing of the tongue. Sutures are removed after one week. Splints, when used, are maintained on both the maxilla and mandible for two to three weeks. Generally, control of particles is accomplished if the splint is removed at two weeks. However, sulcus maintenance usually requires wearing the splint for three weeks. Earlier removal of splints may allow the sulcus to rise. Impressions for construction of new dentures are

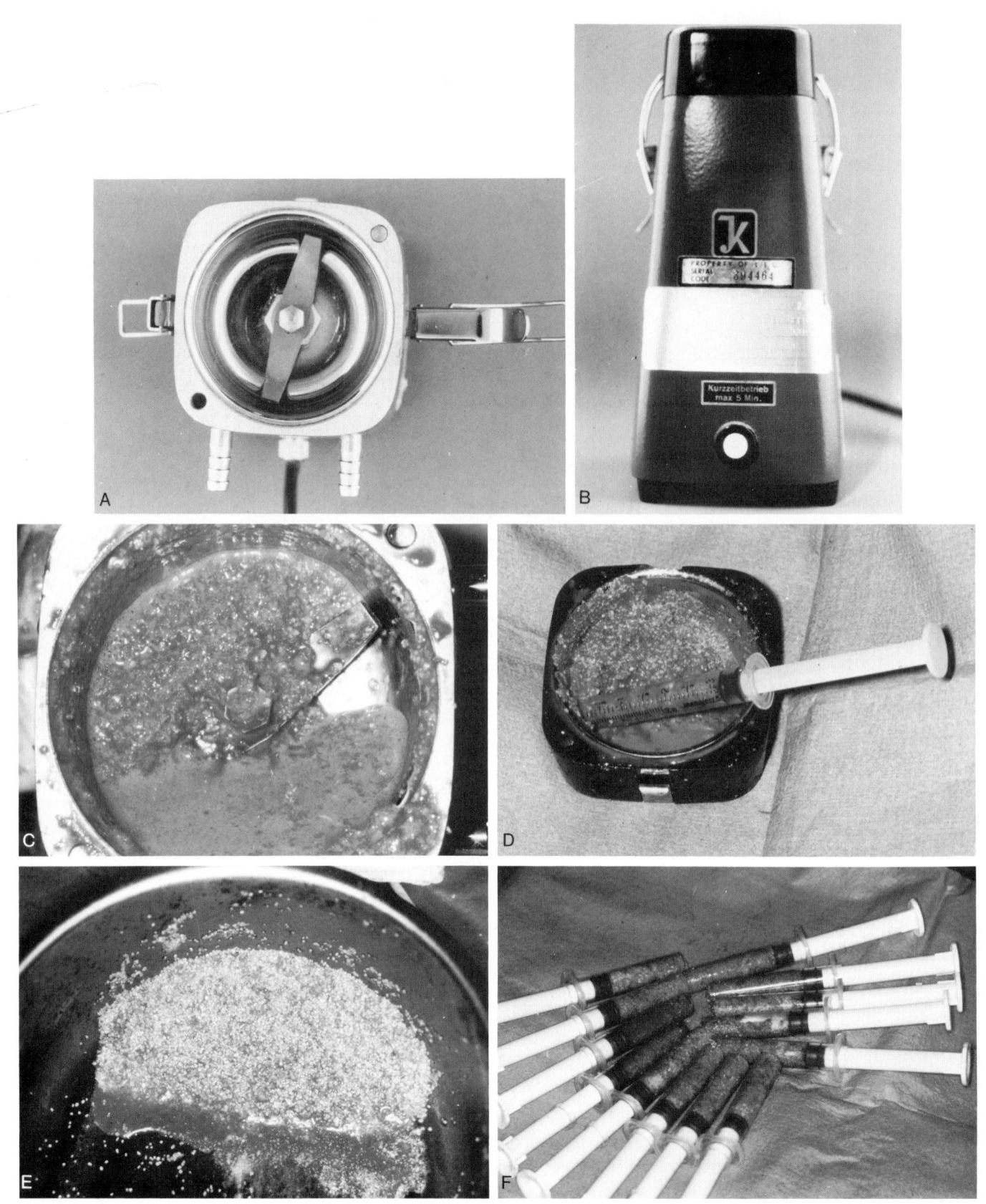

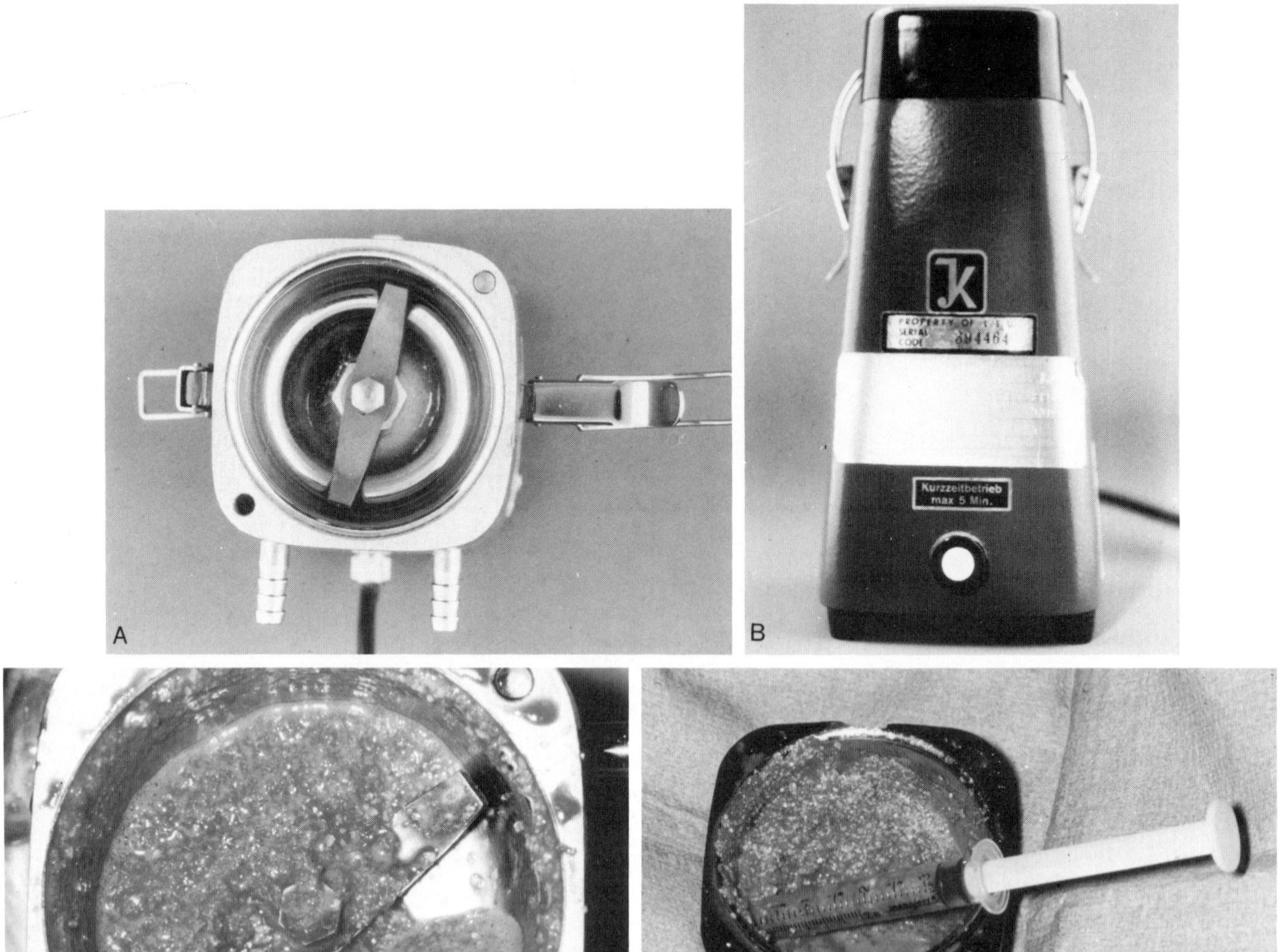

Figure 8–18. *A–C*, Bone mill (Tekmar Inc., Cincinnati, Ohio) used to grind cancellous bone from the patient's iliac crest. *D*, mixing bone and HA particles (1 gram HA to 1 cc bone) is done separately *after* bone is finely ground with the electric bone mill. If the patient is deficient in cancellous bone, a 2:1 or 3:1 ratio may be necessary *(E)* to obtain sufficient material for complete maxillary and mandibular augmentation *(F)*.

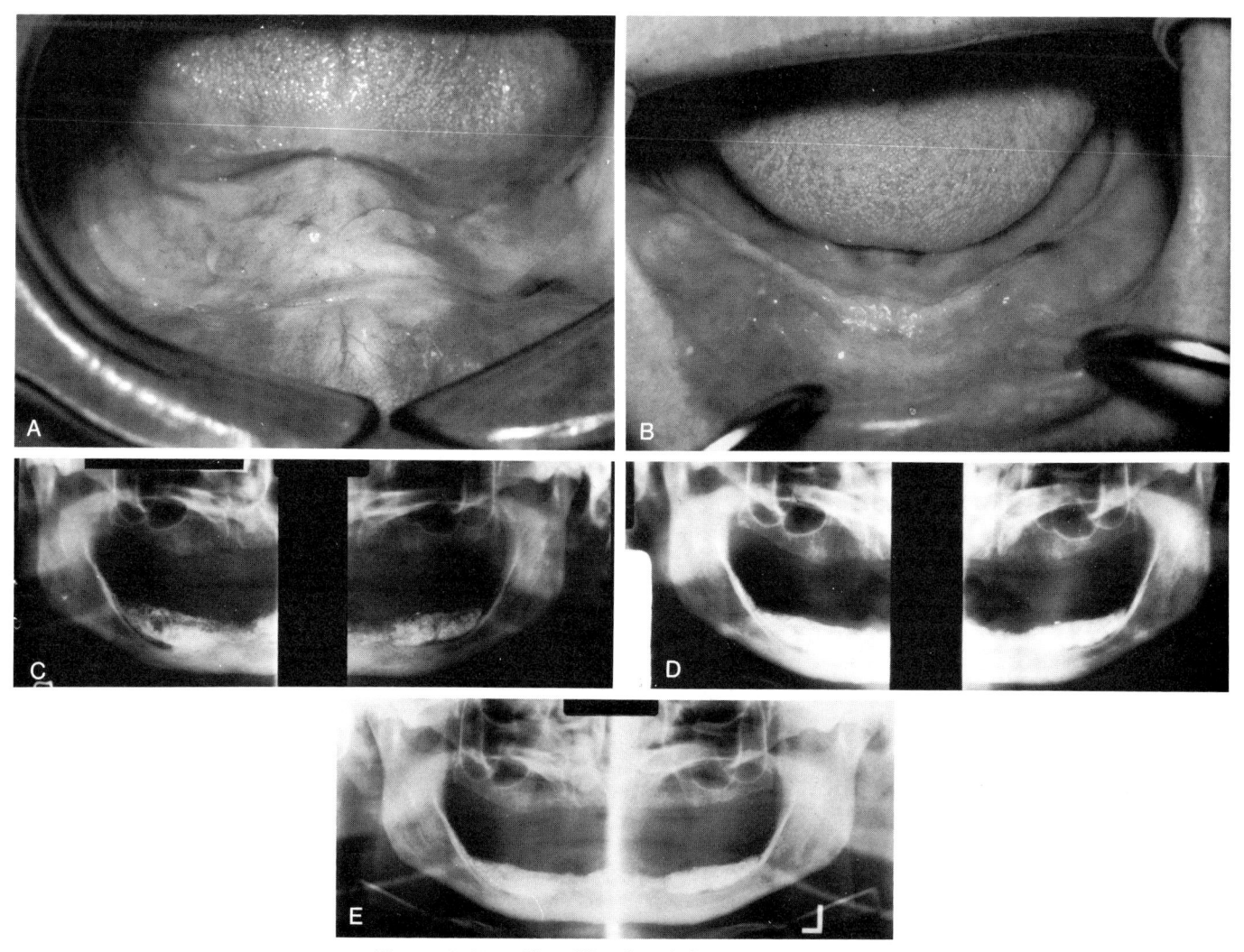

Figure 8–19. Class III ridge deficiency corrected with 1:1 HA and autogenous cancellous iliac bone using tunneling technique. *A,* Preoperative ridge; *B,* 24-month postoperative ridge; *C,* 12-month radiograph; *D,* 24-month radiograph; *E,* 48-month radiograph.

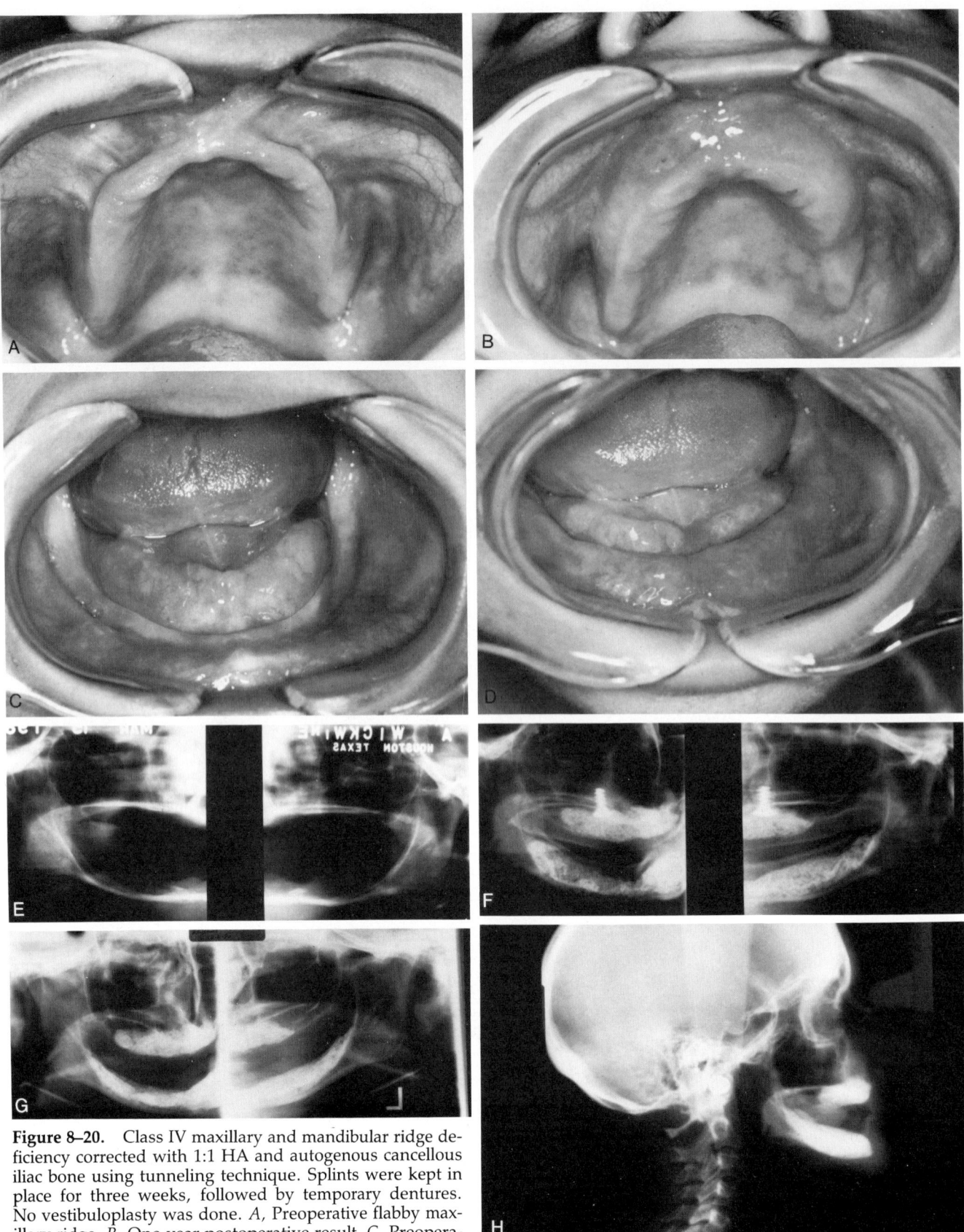

Figure 8–20. Class IV maxillary and mandibular ridge deficiency corrected with 1:1 HA and autogenous cancellous iliac bone using tunneling technique. Splints were kept in place for three weeks, followed by temporary dentures. No vestibuloplasty was done. *A*, Preoperative flabby maxillary ridge. *B*, One-year postoperative result. *C*, Preoperative concave ridge with complete bone resorption over the mandibular canal. *D*, One-year postoperative result. *E*, Preoperative radiograph. *F*, Immediate postoperative radiograph. *G, H*, One-year postoperative radiographs.

taken at the fourth to sixth postoperative week. If the augmented ridge is not firm at this time, final impressions are delayed and a nonfunctional splint or temporary denture is worn to maintain sulcus depth and ridge form.

Results of LSU Clinical Trials (1978 to 1983)

Deficient maxillary and mandibular ridges were classified according to the degree of deficiency. They were augmented with approximately 4 to 16 grams of 18-40 mesh irregular-shaped* or 20-40 mesh rounded† HA particles (Table 8–2). In some of the Class III and Class IV ridge deficiency patients, 12 to 20 grams of HA mixed with finely crushed autogenous cancellous iliac bone (1 gram to 1 cc) was used to provide increased strength and stability of the large amount of material added to the severely atrophic alveolar ridges. Surgical technique usually involved subperiosteal pocket tunneling through vertical mucoperiosteal incisions with or without a blind submucosal vestibuloplasty. Injection of HA into these pockets was done with a variety of modified plastic syringes. Maxillary and mandibular splints were used infrequently from 1978 to 1981. After that they were used to control the particles, maintain sulcus depth, and minimize the need for postaugmentation vestibuloplasty. Solidification of HA generally occurred by the fourth to sixth postoperative week, permitting impressions for denture construction. Skin and mucosal graft vestibuloplasty, if needed to increase sulcus depth after HA augmentation, was usually possible after two months because of the intense fibrous tissue infiltration between and over HA particles.

Up to five years (1978–1983) of follow-up has been done on 228 ridges in 208 patients of age 25–75, average 58 years, with a 2-to-1 female-to-male ratio.[66] Fifty-five ridges were augmented with irregular-shaped HA and 173 ridges with rounded particulate HA. Patients had worn dentures from 1 to 40 years, with an average of 18 years. The numbers of preoperative dentures for each patient ranged from one to ten with an average of three. The number of mandibular augmentations was over three times the number of maxillary augmentations. Class III ridge deficiencies were the most common augmentation in either arch. Tables 8–2 to 8–5 demonstrate the ridges reconstructed, demographic data, and mandibular and maxillary augmentation with respect to the ridge deficiency classification. Radiographic and clinical follow-up evaluations have been very satisfactory (Figs. 8–19 to 8–22).

Complications (Table 8–6) include various anesthesia, paresthesia, and hyperesthesia of the mental nerve, a need for postoperative vestibuloplasty, incision dehiscence, erosion of the mucosa from the use of splints, displacement of the material secondary to inadequate surgical technique, hematoma formation, and loose HA. In nearly all cases mental nerve dysesthesias improved, with normal sensation returning to the lower lip by the sixth postoperative month unless trauma to the nerve had occurred at surgery. No permanent complete lip anesthesias were observed; however, hyperesthesia in four patients necessitated re-entry to excise an enveloping fibrous cuff and remove adjacent HA particles. Vestibuloplasties may be necessary, particularly in Class IV patients, since a rise of the sulcus mucosa toward the ridge crest is inevitable when large augmentations are performed, particularly if the splint was removed before three weeks. This is usually predictable and as such is not necessarily a complication. As a complication, however, vestibuloplasties were performed to excise aggregates of particles displaced laterally. The etiology of this problem (the most common complaint of all complications) is overfill, excessive subperiosteal reflection, and manipulation of tissues for circummandibular sutures/wires placed after instead of before HA injection (Fig. 8–23). Displacement of material is also a problem related to the severity of the atrophic ridge (Class IV) and deficiencies in surgical technique. Incision dehiscence or erosion of mucosa within the first few postoperative weeks may result in a loss of particles in the immediate mucosal breakdown area. In all instances granulation tissue from the periphery and interparticulate fibrous tissue growth resulted in secondary closure without jeopardy to the augmentation material as a whole. Hematomas and seromas were common in Class III and IV ridge deficiencies prior to use of splints. The rare occurrence of a "loose" augmentation means failure of HA particles to attach directly to bone. Failure to elevate periosteum, hematoma, or excessive movement of particles from mastication during the first month permits formation of thickened intervening fibrous connective tissue at the bone-implant interface. A mobile mass should be removed if stability is not achieved by the third to fourth postoperative month. An open technique with a crest incision permits removal and immediate refill of material.

---

*Durapatite (Alveograph™), Sterling Winthrop Lab., Inc., Albany, NY.
†Calcitite™, RM, Calcitek, Inc., San Diego, CA.

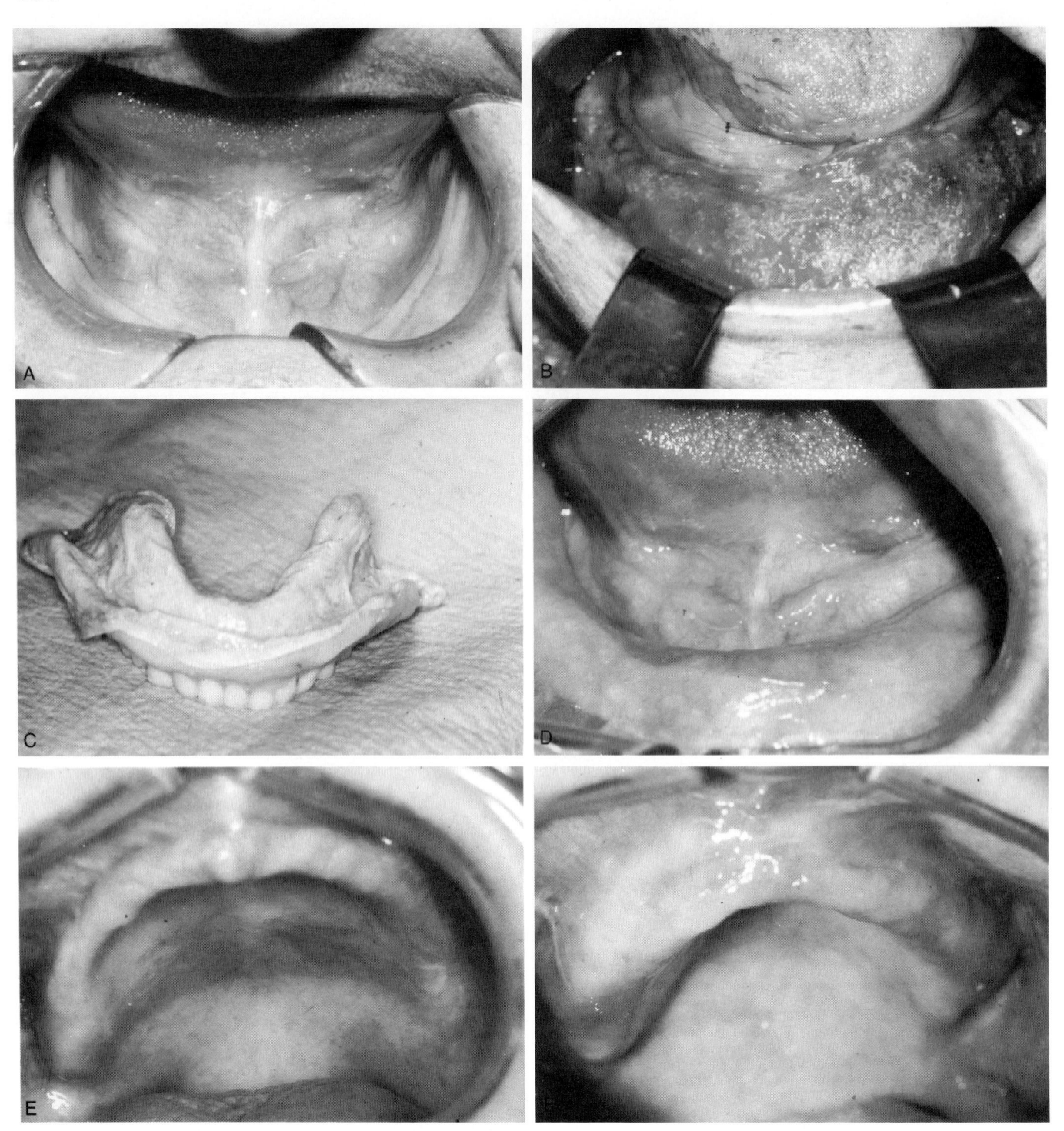

330 / RECONSTRUCTION OF THE ALVEOLAR RIDGE WITH HYDROXYLAPATITE

Figure 8–21. Class IV maxillary and mandibular ridge deficiency corrected with 3:1 HA-bone mixture. Splints were removed at one week. No temporary dentures were worn until four weeks postoperatively. Vestibuloplasties (maxillary re-epithelialization and dermis graft to the mandible) were performed at three months. *A*, Preoperative mandible. *B*, Vestibuloplasty. HA-bone ridge exposed for dermis graft at three months. *C*, Dermis graft lining temporary denture. *D*, 24-month result. *E*, Preoperative flabby maxillary ridge. *F*, Three-month result with HA particles in vestibule. *G*, Ridge and sulcus exposed to excise excess particles. The mucosa was sutured high in the sulcus and the augmentation healed by re-epithelialization. *H*, 24-month result. *I*, Preoperative radiograph. *J*, Immediate postoperative radiograph before vestibuloplasty. *K*, 24-month radiograph.

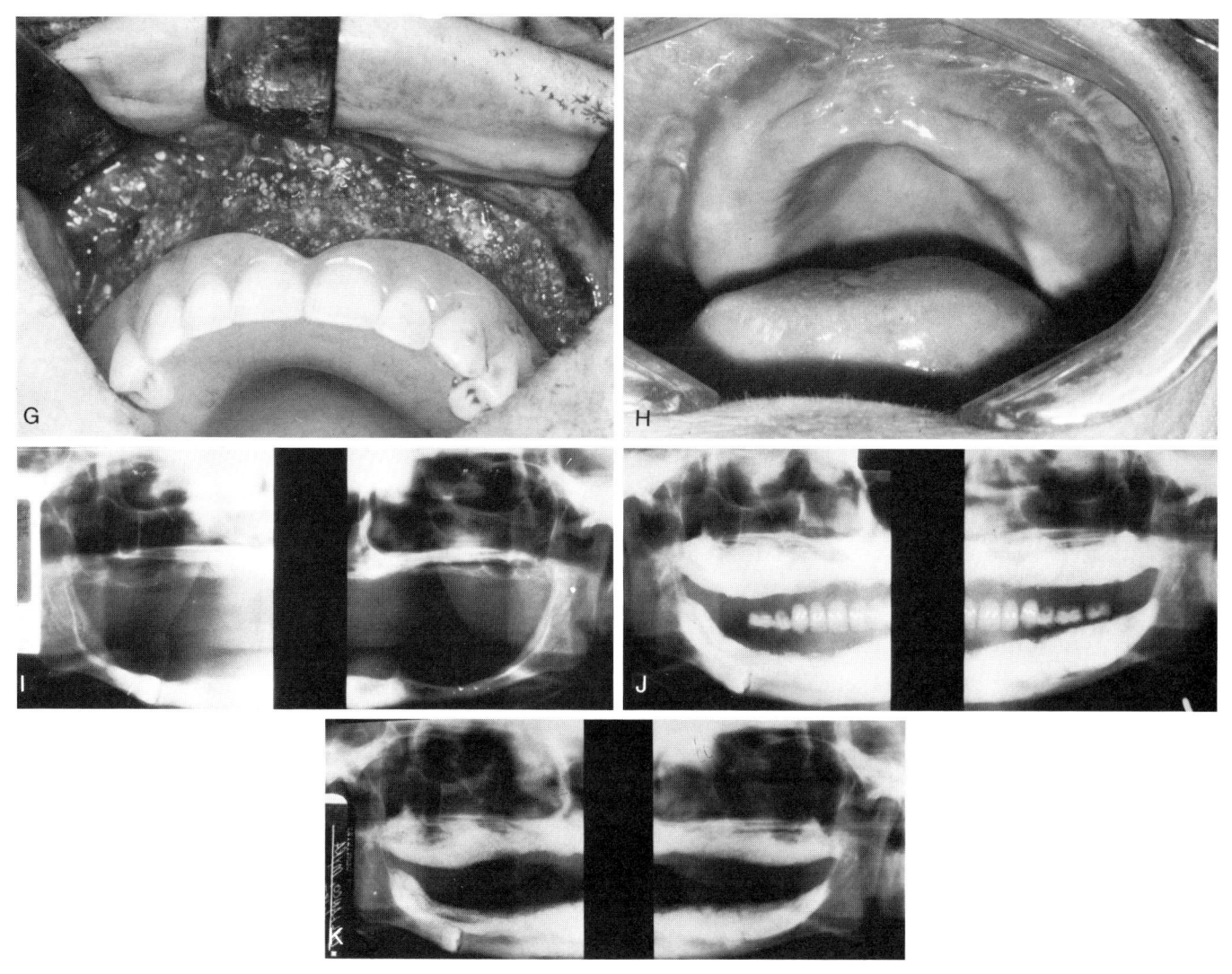

Figure 8–21 Continued.

TABLE 8–3. SUMMARY OF RIDGE RECONSTRUCTION

	Mandible	Maxilla
Ridges Reconstructed: 228		
HA alone	133	43
Durapatite 55		
Calcitite 173		
HA-Bone	40	12
Class I-II: 40%		
Class III-IV: 60%		
Totals	173 (76%)	55 (24%)

TABLE 8–4. DEMOGRAPHIC DATA ON RIDGE RECONSTRUCTION

Patients	Male	Female
208	64	144 (70%)

Ages: 27 to 74 years, average age 58
Number of dentures: 1 to 10, average 3
Years of edentulousness: 1 to 40, average 18

TABLE 8–5. MANDIBULAR AND MAXILLARY AUGMENTATION

MANDIBLE				
Class	I	II	III	IV
HA alone 115	20	34	47	14
HA-bone 33		3	17	13
Staple 13			8	5
Other dental implant 6		2	2	2
Visor 6		2	2	2
Total 173	20	41	76	36

MAXILLA				
Class	I	II	III	IV
HA alone 43	5	23	13	2
HA-bone 12		1	5	6
Total 55	5	24	18	8

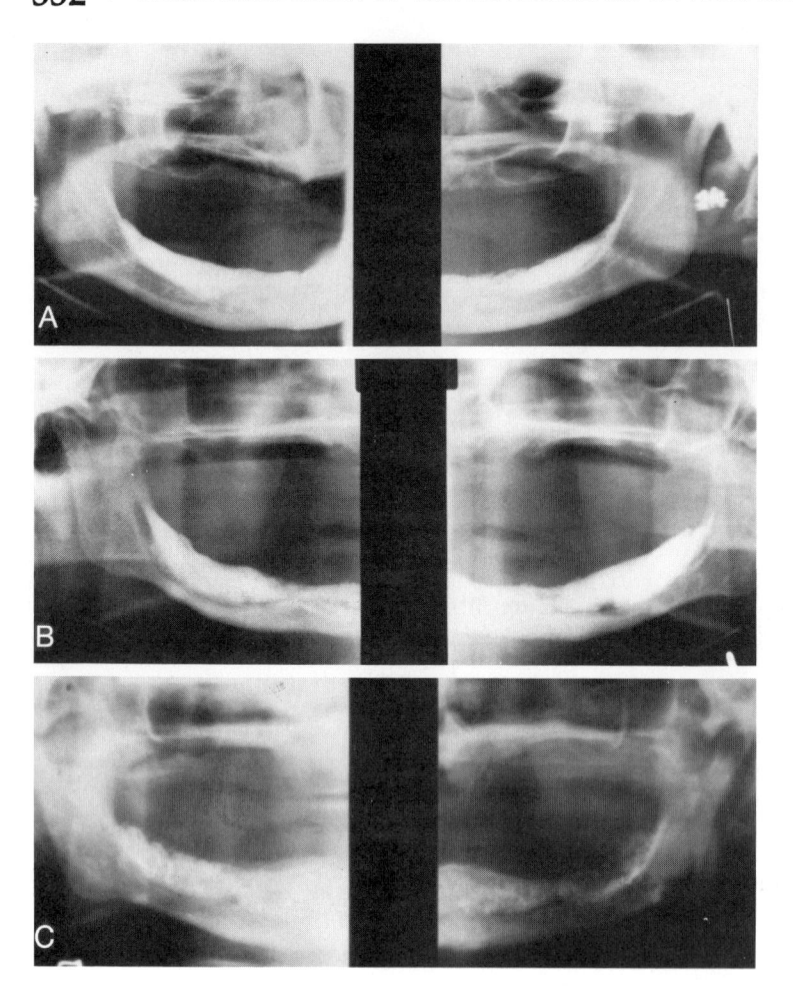

Figure 8–22. *A, B,* Three-year radiographs on Class III and IV ridge deficiencies corrected with HA alone. *C,* HA combined with visor osteotomy to avoid knife-edge ridge.

ADDITIONAL STUDIES

Radiographic studies by Kent et al.[67, 68] and Block and Kent[69] on 72 patients have analyzed the postoperative maintenance of ridge height augmentation of HA alone and HA combined with autogenous bone. Those reports of patients followed up to 48 months indicate a ridge height maintenance that is 90 per cent of the original augmentation height. There was no apparent statistically significant difference between HA alone and HA with bone augmentation (Fig. 8–24). Clinically this is an important observation. The decrease in ridge height following onlay autogenous bone grafts is approximately 40 to 60 per cent through two years of follow-up, with increasing resorption through longer-term follow-up.

TABLE 8–6. COMPLICATIONS OF RIDGE RECONSTRUCTION

Mental nerve impairment	37
Vestibuloplasty	32
Incision/mucosa breakdown	20
Displacement	17
Hematoma	10
Loose HA	3

Block and Kent have described the healing response in dogs of mandibular alveolar ridge augmentation with HA alone and with the addition of autogenous bone.[70] The augmented ridge at four weeks showed no bony ingrowth in either group. In both groups, HA particles were "cemented" by a thin, fibrous connective tissue with a mild inflammatory response. In the HA-bone specimens, small pieces of nonviable bone graft were seen with osteoclasts at their periphery. The 8-week and 16-week specimens contrasted with the 4-week specimens. HA-bone specimens demonstrated a definitive osteogenic ingrowth with bone interspersed among the HA particles throughout the ridge. (Figs. 8–25*A–E*). Dogs receiving HA alone, however, did not demonstrate bone ingrowth into the augmented ridge even at 16 weeks (Fig. 8–25*F*). Oxytetracycline fluorescent labeling in 8-week HA-bone specimens demonstrated diffuse mineralization and bone apposition. The HA-bone ridge in the 16-week specimens was lamellar in character, with haversian systems demonstrating maturation (Fig. 8–25 *E*). A sharp oxytetracycline pattern was isolated to the haversian system (Fig. 8–25*C*). The exact mechanism of

Figure 8–23. *A,* Immediate postoperative radiograph of *B,* HA particle displacement (overfill). *C,* Removal at four weeks. *D,* Fibrous encapsulation of excised implant particles (I). *E,* Preoperative radiograph. *F,* Postoperative radiograph after excision of displaced particles. Note how particles wrap around the thin inferior border.

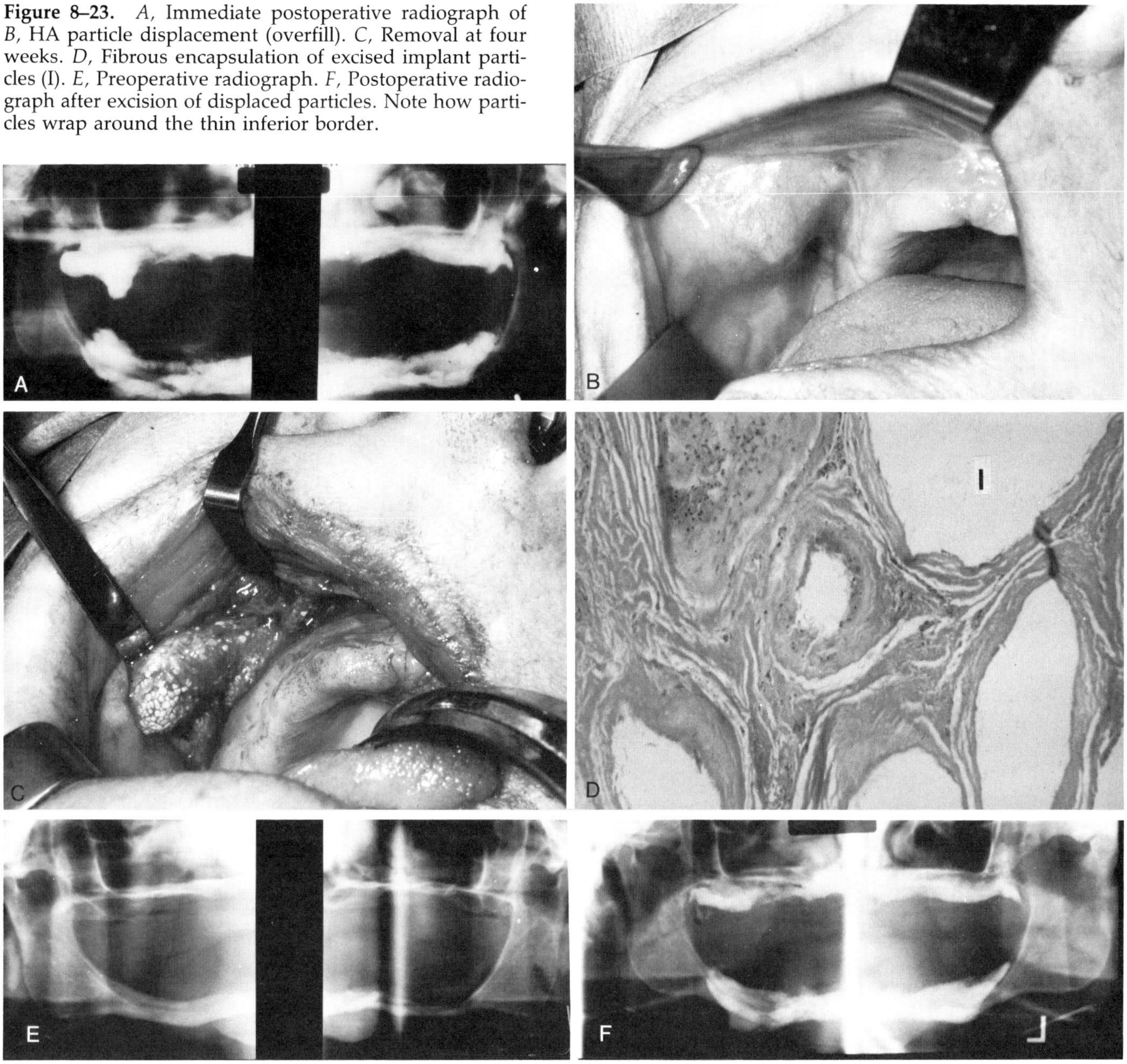

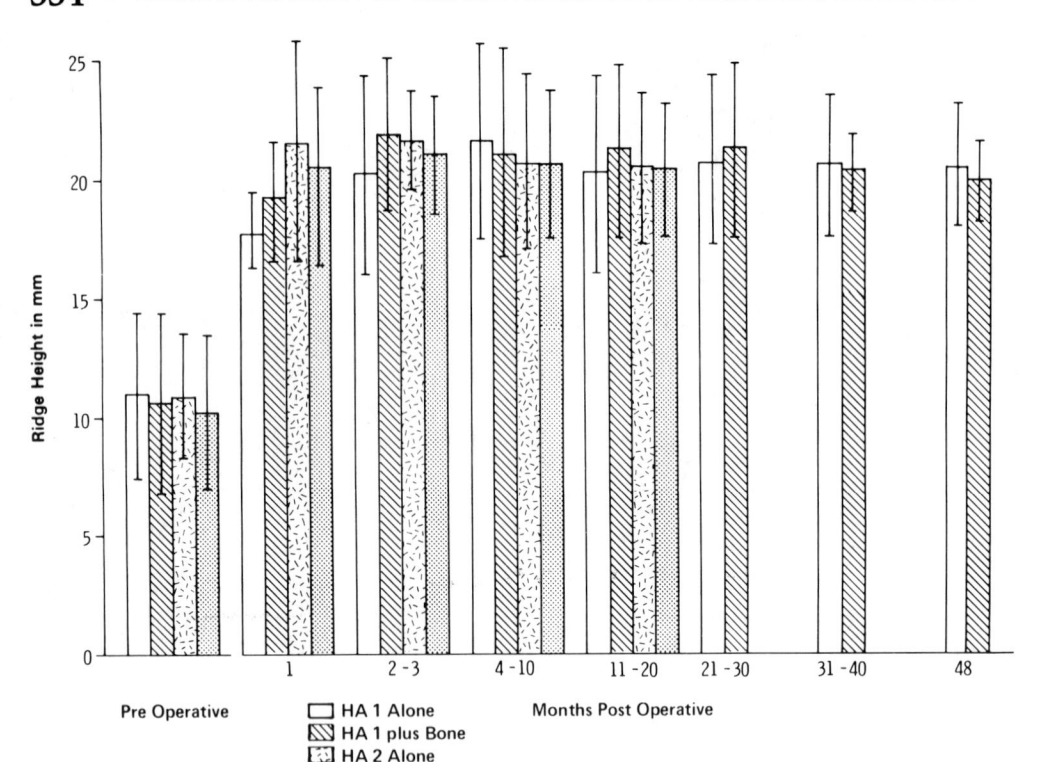

Figure 8–24. Graph of postoperative vertical height measurements for HA alone and HA-bone augmented patients.

bone induction did not appear to be a creeping substitution but rather was induced from bone morphogenic protein contained in the bone particles.

Chang et al. evaluated augmentation with HA alone on the dog inferior border up to nine months.[71] Each dog received HA placed supraperiosteally, subperiosteally, and subperiosteally with decortication. Poor mechanical stabilization, no bone formation, and dense collagenous fibers characterized the HA supraperiosteal group. In both subperiosteal groups, bone formation occurred from the bone base to the central implant particles by nine months. Bone formation in the decorticated bone group was slightly faster than in the nondecorticated ridge. Although HA is not osteogenetic in the traditional sense, both dog studies show bone formation, increasing in time, without the benefit of autogenous bone mixed with HA.

Bone bonding occurs rapidly with HA particles on the ridge surface, leading to the formation of some bone and dense fibrous connective tissue growing throughout a mound of particles. Bone formation is therefore possible for a few millimeters beyond the normal anatomic contours of bone, utilizing the particles in a "bone-bridging" capacity. This property of the HA material causes bone to grow into defects or onto resorbed areas for augmentation. Otherwise it would not likely occur. HA is characterized as osteoconductive and osteophilic, but not osteogenetic.

Studies have shown that its osteogenetic activity is less than that of hemopoietic marrow.[50] Because of these interesting properties of HA, which seems to encourage dense fibrous-bony growth beyond "normal" bony limits, we can only speculate how much bone height can be obtained by augmentation with HA alone. Patients may easily have 8 to 10 mm of ridge height increase consisting largely of fibrous connective tissue cementing HA particles. However, since many Class IV mandibles are dangerously deficient in height, width, and strength, it seems appropriate to provide a mixture of cancellous bone and marrow with the HA particles. This is particularly true for the "pencil-thin" or *width-deficient* ridge. Stability of a large height increase with HA alone in these patients is questionable, since the ratio of surface area interface to height increase is poor. The same height-deficient but wider mandible would be expected to show satisfactory results with HA alone. Therefore, we are currently recommending HA mixed with bone for Class IV ridge height and *width*-deficient patients who are good candidates for obtaining iliac bone. In these patients it is usually desirable to augment more than 5 to 6 mm. In fact, large augmentations of 10 to 15 mm have been accomplished. Postoperative decrease in ridge height of HA-bone augmentation should be greater than with HA alone, as resorption occurs with the cancellous particles through the first six months.

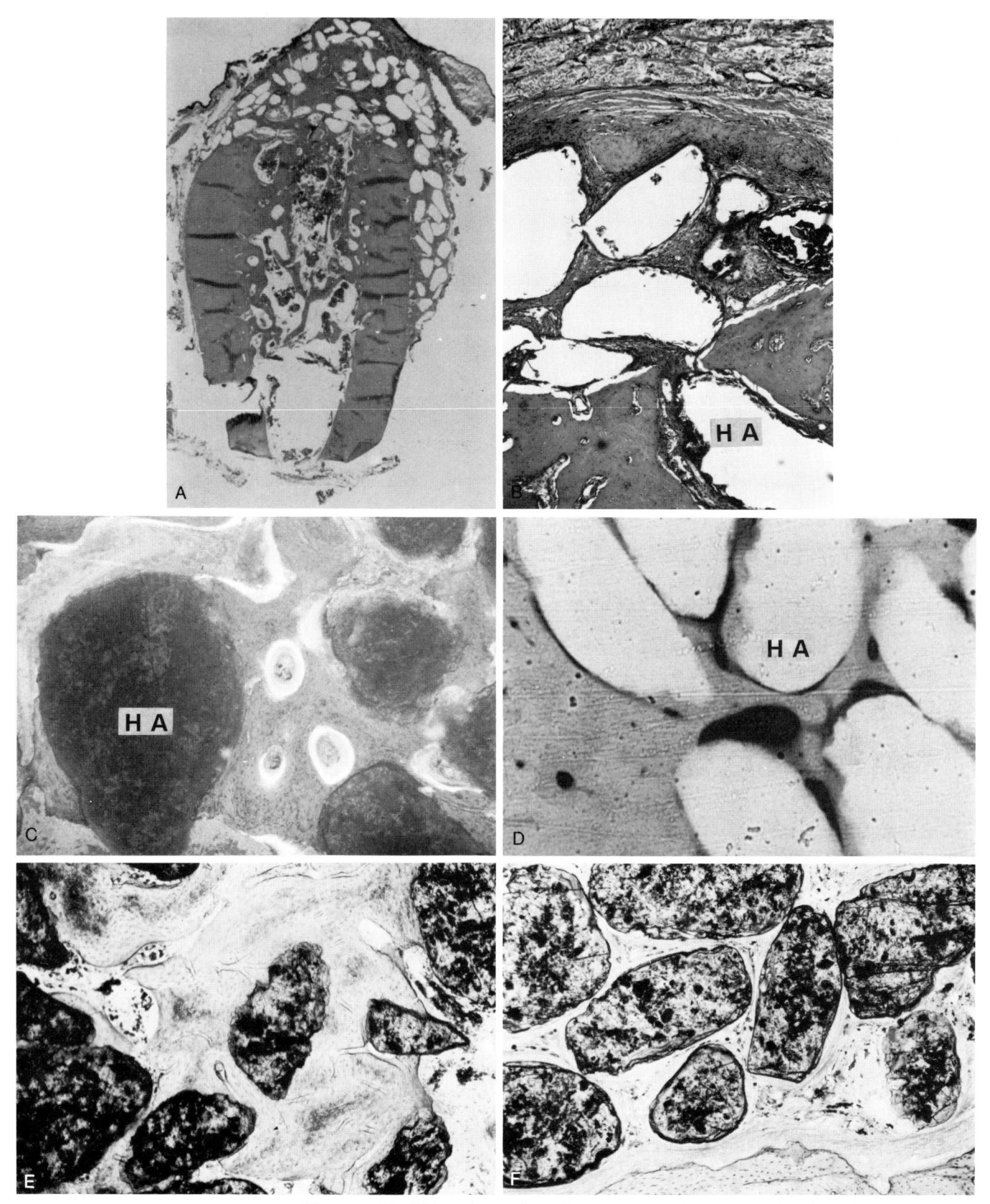

Figure 8–25. HA and cancellous bone augmentation on dog alveolar ridge. *A,* Interparticle bone formation is evident at eight weeks (H & E stain, × 3). *B,* Mature lamellar bone formation is nearly complete from crest to gingival tissue at 16 weeks (H & E, × 40). *C,* Sharp oxytetracycline fluorescence in haversian systems at 16 weeks (ground section, × 40). *D,* Microradiograph of the center of ridge augmentation at 16 weeks (ground section, × 40). *E,* Mature lamellar bone ingrowth in the center of the ridge augmentation at 16 weeks (ground section, × 40). *F,* Augmentation with HA alone on dog alveolar ridge crest. Noninflammatory fibrous tissue interspersed between particles at 16 weeks (ground section, × 40).

Beyond that time ridge height maintenance of both types of patients appears clinically to be very similar.

Preliminary studies by Zide et al. depicting the biomechanical behavior of different ratios of autogenous bone and hydroxylapatite for major continuity defects suggest that ratios of 1:4 to 1:1 (HA to autogenous bone) yield comparable strength with autogenous grafts alone up to six months in dog mandibles.[72] Autogenous bone grafts for cancellous reconstruction of continuity defects are known to undergo significant postoperative resorption. The use of hydroxylapatite in

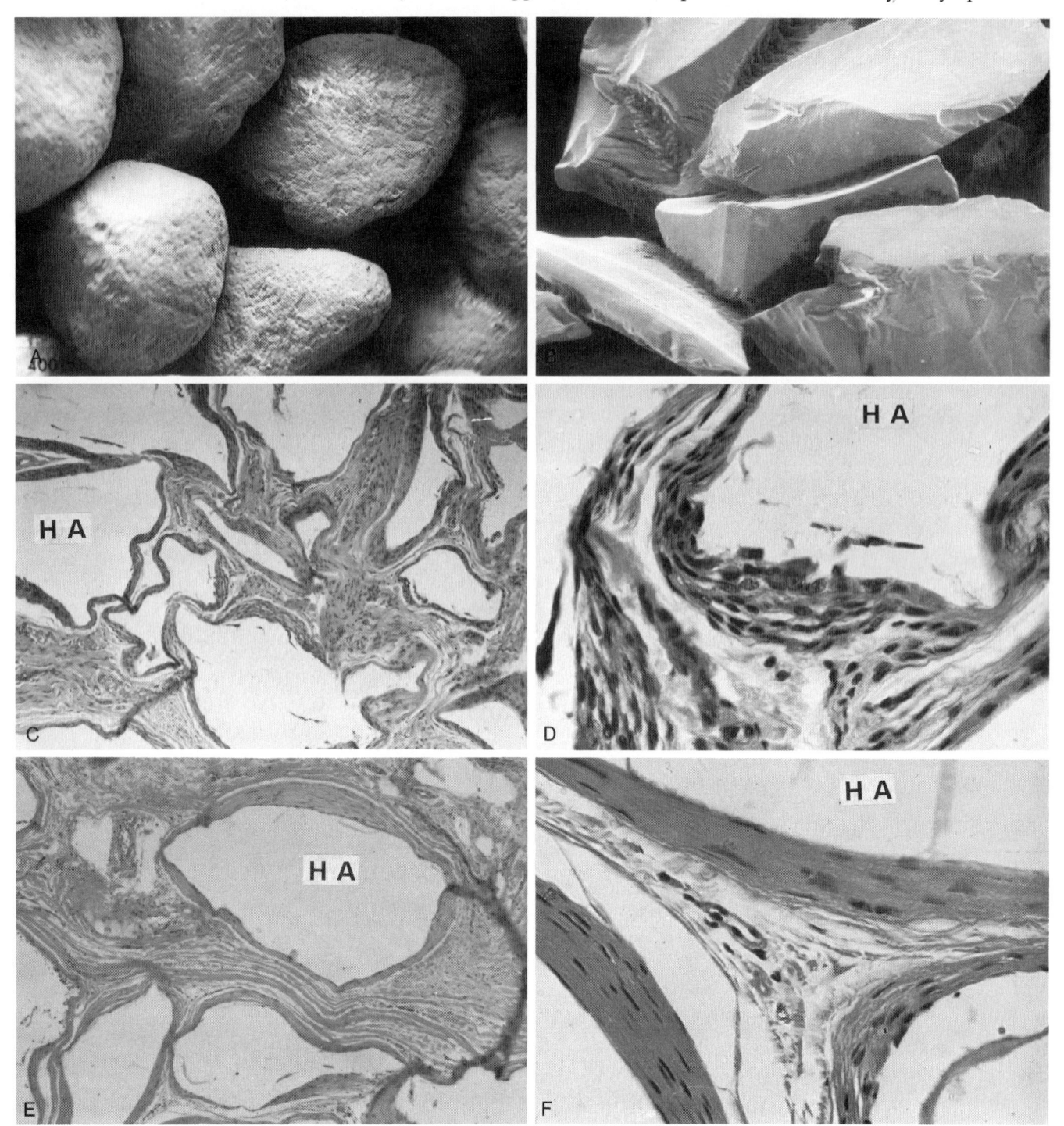

Figure 8–26. Rounded (A), and irregular (B) particles (SEM, × 65). C, Irregular-shaped HA at six months. The connective tissue is moderately vascular and cellular. Histiocytic borders of the particle spaces are likewise cellular (H & E, × 100). D, Higher magnification of interface seen in C (H & E, × 500). E, Rounded HA at six months. Hypocellular noninflammatory fibrous tissue (H & E, × 100). F, Higher magnification of interface seen in E. Fibrous lining membranes have flattened cells (H & E, × 500).

these grafts may limit bone resorption because of the nonresorbability of HA and its biomechanical influence on bone, which may minimize bone resorption as a result of biologic apatite attachment.

Differences in particle shape may affect the inflammatory reaction of the surrounding soft tissue. Matlaga et al.[73] demonstrated that when triangular, pentagonal, and circular rods of various polymeric materials were implanted in rat muscle, the less angular shapes had less inflammation in the surrounding tissue.

The difference in particle shape was confirmed grossly and by scanning electron microscopy, which showed irregular or sharp-edged and rounded or smooth particles (Fig. 8–26A,B). Misiek et al. placed 0.5 cc of both particles randomly in the buccal soft-tissue cheek pouches of 15 beagle dogs.[74] The specimens were removed at intervals of two weeks, six weeks, three months, and six months, viewed for the degree of inflammation present, and then subjectively compared within the same time interval.

Histology revealed no significant difference between the inflammation present in the two- and six-week specimens of both particles. At three months the sharp-edged particle specimens showed more inflammation than the rounded particle specimens, and at six months, the former still had mild to moderate inflammation, while the latter showed little or no inflammation remaining (Fig. 8–26C–F).

These findings suggest that irregular, sharp-edged particles have a tendency to maintain an inflammatory response for a longer time period than smooth, rounded particles implanted under similar circumstances. The continued presence of inflammation may have an adverse effect on stability of HA particles at the soft-tissue interface, particularly under the long-term stress of a dental prosthesis. Thus, the reduced inflammation seen with smooth, rounded particles would indicate superior soft-tissue compatibility. In bone defects, however, differences in particle shape probably have no significance.

The use of HA particles to rebuild a deficient alveolar ridge and placement of mandibular staple bone plates show encouraging results after four years of follow-up.[75] Resorption of the posterior ridge can result in prosthetic overloading of the mandibular staple bone plate. Placement of a nonresorbable material such as HA to level and restore

Figure 8–27. HA-staple combination. *A*, Stabilization pins show correct incision for simultaneous placement of HA and staple bone plate. *B*, Four-year radiograph of simultaneous HA–iliac cancellous bone mixture with staple bone plate.

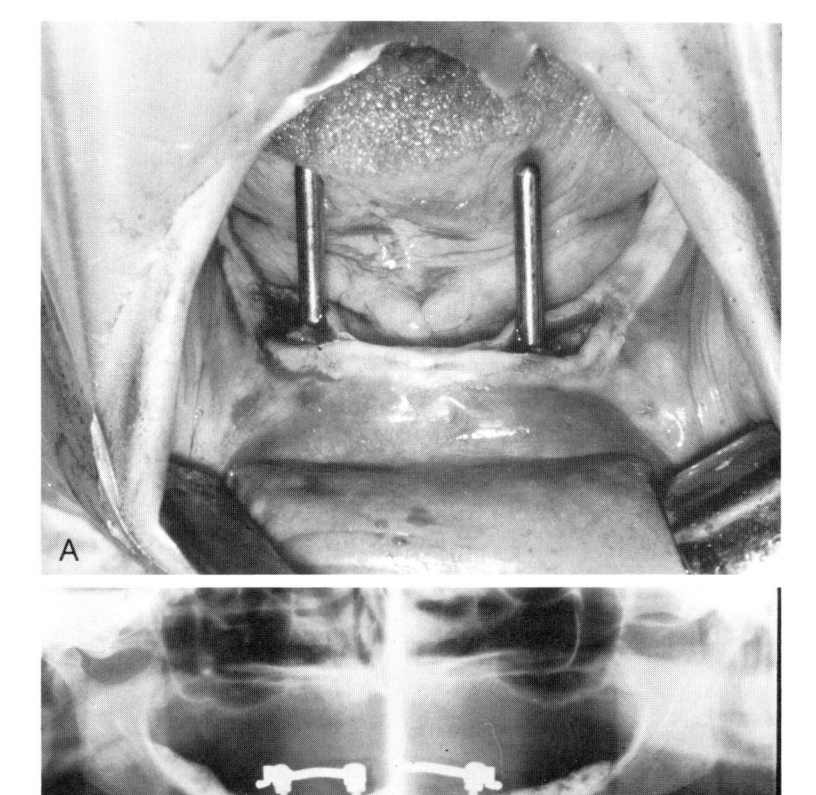

ridge height may also increase posterior ridge stability. Clinical results reported by Kent et al.[62, 75] with simultaneous placement of the staple and HA and by Small[76] with staple placement after HA augmentation are encouraging (Figs. 8–27 to 8–30). The sequence of simultaneous placement is briefly: (1) a ridge crest incision that bisects the attached mucosa from lateral incisor to first molar region, reflection of the mucoperiosteum, and tunneling anteriorly and posteriorly as necessary; (2) placement of the staple using drill guide and jaws or claws clamped directly on the alveolar bone rather than a splint; (3) injection of the HA; (4) placement of a splint secured with the fastener nuts.

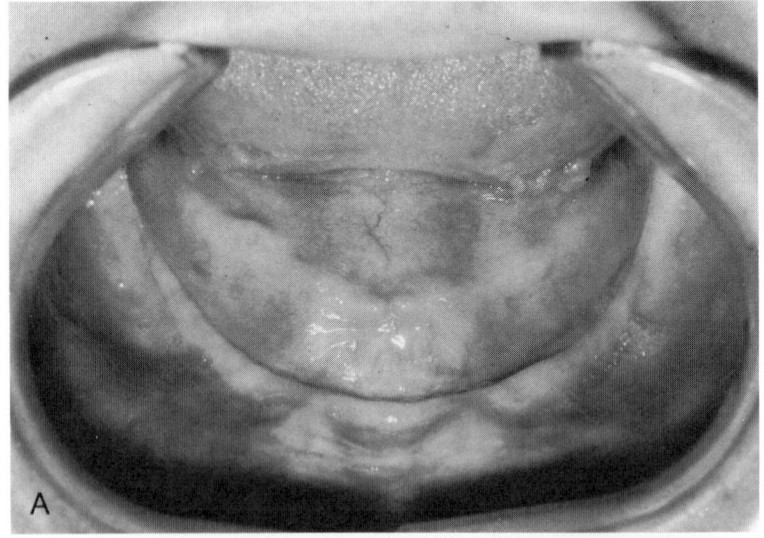

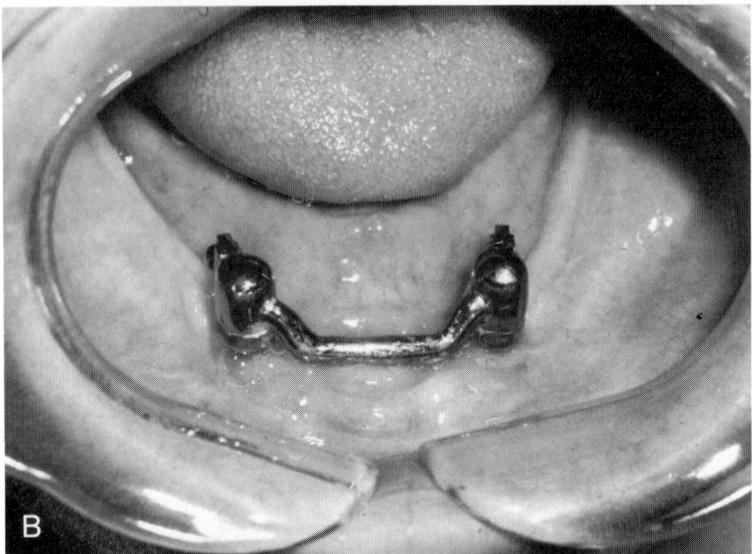

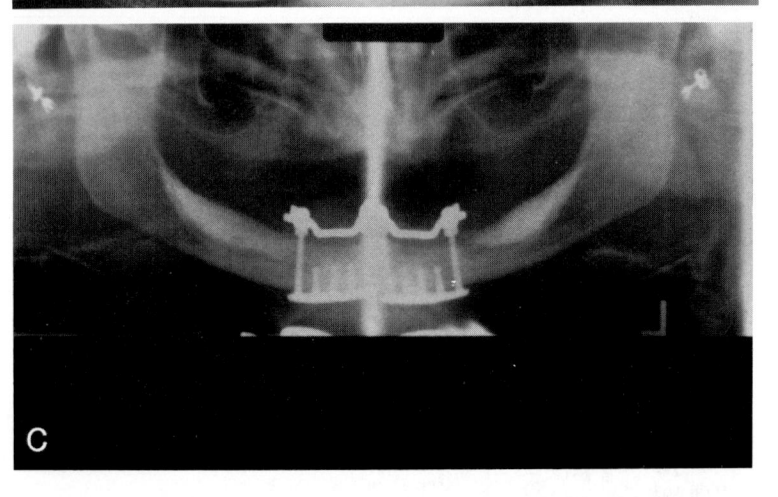

Figure 8–28. Correction of a Class IV ridge deficiency with simultaneous HA-bone and staple bone plate. *A*, Preoperative concave ridge. *B*, 18-month postoperative result shows convex ridge with increased height. *C*, 18-month radiograph.

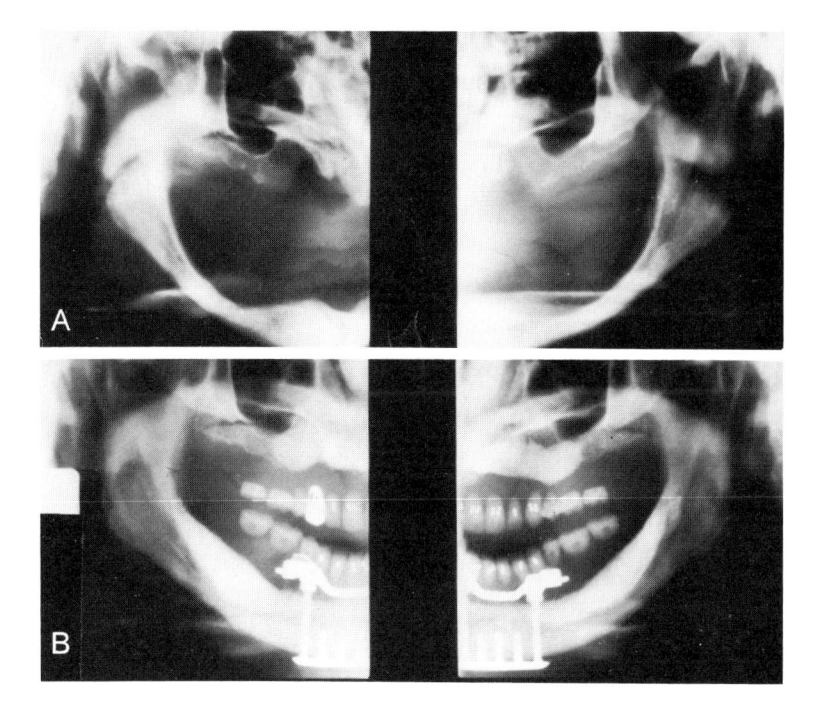

Figure 8–29. A Class IV *wide* mandibular ridge deficiency with severe anterior maxillary resorption in which HA alone was combined with a staple bone plate. *A*, Preoperative radiograph. *B*, Two-year postoperative radiograph.

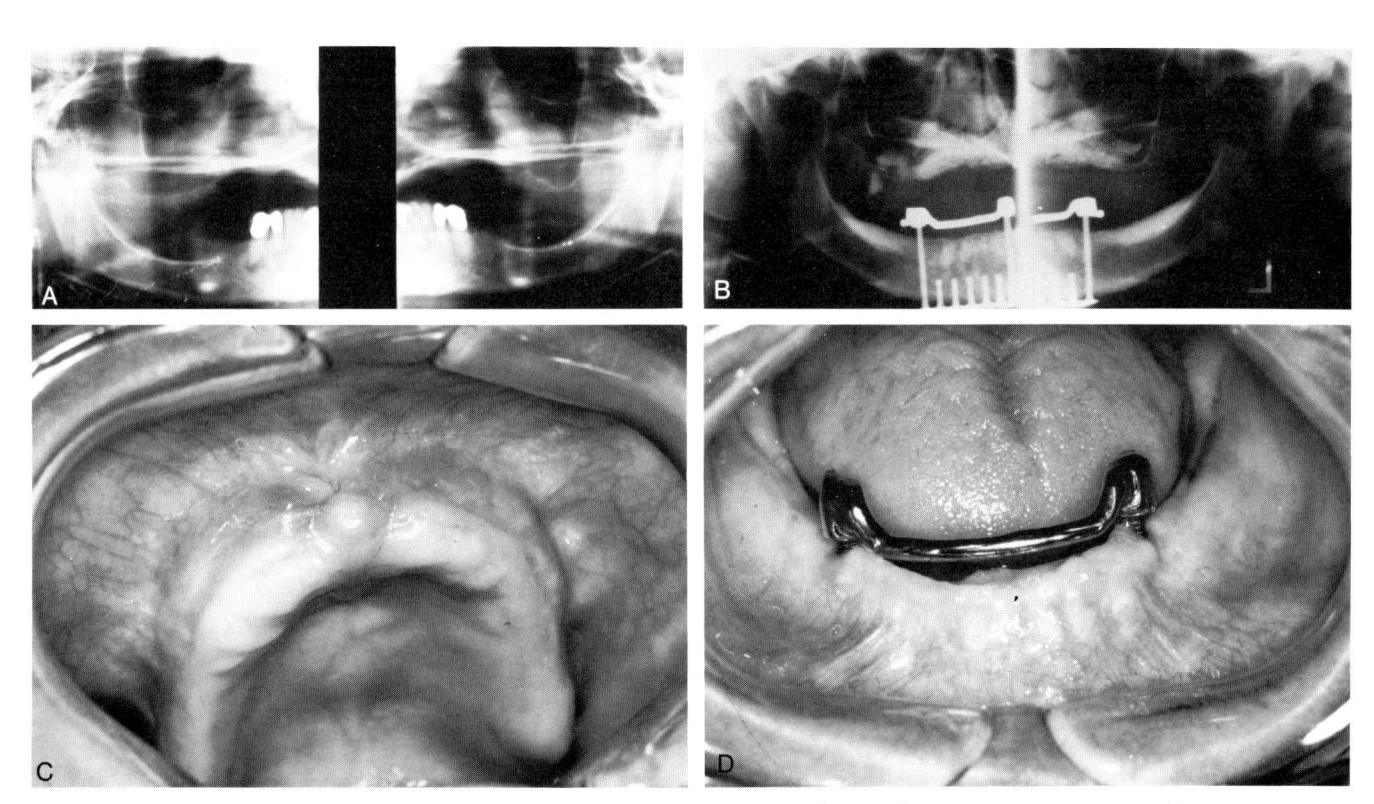

Figure 8–30. Class IV anterior maxillary and Class III posterior mandibular ridge deficiencies with failing anterior teeth. The anterior maxilla was reconstructed with HA and bone. The mandible was reconstructed with HA alone, including tooth sockets, and staple. *A*, Preoperative radiograph. *B*, Postoperative radiograph. *C*, Postoperative maxillary result. *D*, Postoperative mandibular result.

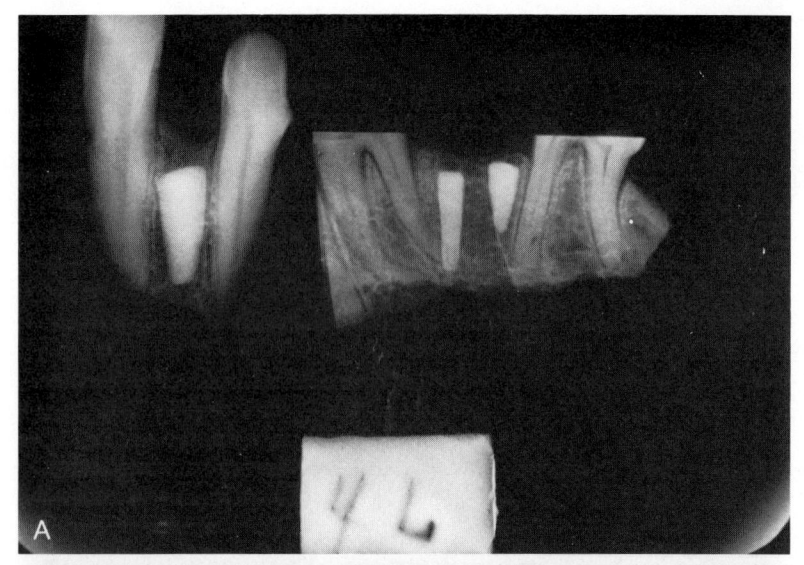

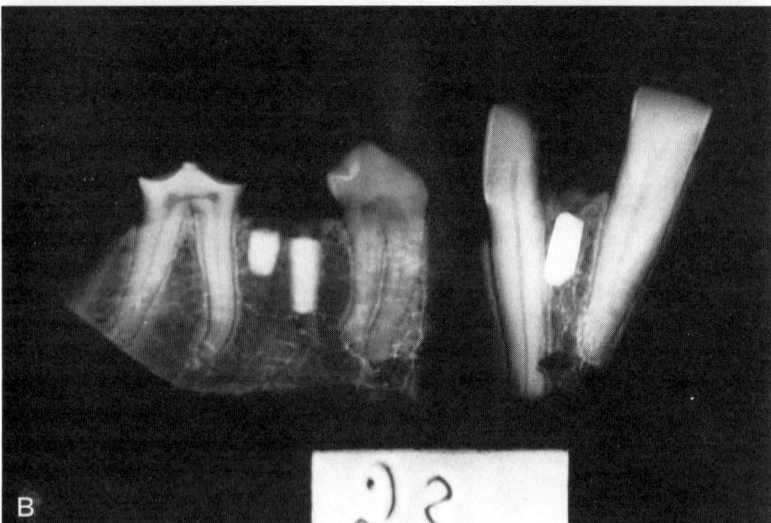

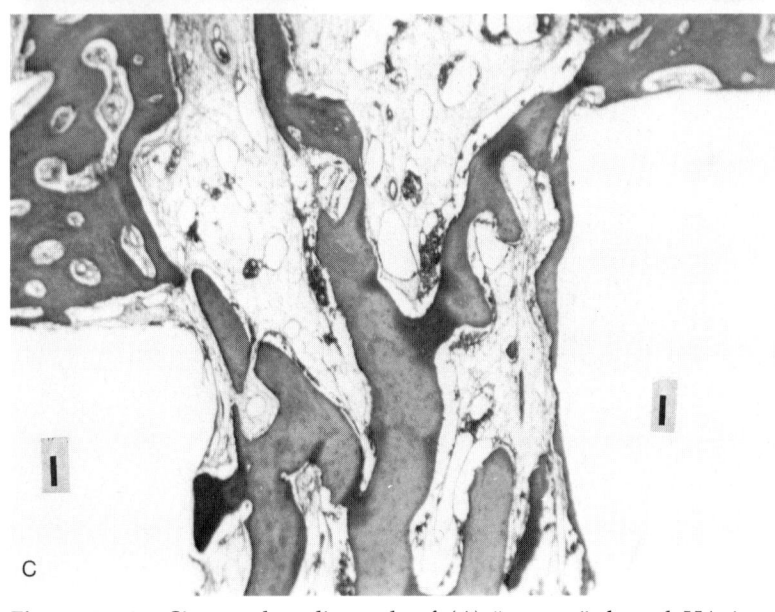

Figure 8–31. Six-month radiograph of (A) "custom"-shaped HA implant and (B) "general"-shaped HA implants. Bone growth over the implant crest and up to the apical base of the general implant is comparable to that with custom implants. C, Crestal interseptal bone surrounding two second premolar implants at six months interfaces with both implant surfaces (I) without intervening soft connective tissue.

ALVEOLAR RIDGE PRESERVATION

Prevention of alveolar bone resorption by a variety of nonresorbable synthetic materials has generated several studies. However, PMMA, vitreous carbon, aluminum oxide, and titanium have resulted in host rejection by fibrous encapsulation.[77] Studies by Boyne and Szutz[78] have suggested that HA root implants are useful in preventing immediate postextraction ridge resorption.

Quinn and Kent compared "general" and "custom"-shaped root implants in baboons.[79] "General" implants were wedged tightly without gingival closure into fresh extraction sockets but extended from 1 to 2 mm below crest level to only half the socket length, while "custom" implants filled the entire sockets.* By one month gingival healing over the implants had occurred. By three months alveolar bone formed over the implant crest, and bone interfaced at the implant apical areas without an intervening fibrous tissue capsule (Fig. 8–31). The importance of implanting HA roots immediately when teeth are extracted was also demonstrated by Quinn and Kent.[79] At seven months in beagle dogs HA roots implanted in fresh extraction sites preserved the alveolus* (Fig. 8–32). The sites were 2 to 3 mm greater in height and width than empty extraction control sites. HA roots implanted in extraction areas three months after tooth removal did not offer alveolar ridge preservation to any greater extent than control sites followed for an additional three months. Maximum preservation of the alveolus with HA implants requires early if not immediate placement when teeth are extracted.

In another study by Block et al., the use of HA particles in fresh extraction sites aided in preservation of ridge size.[80] HA particles and solid HA roots were placed alternating with control sockets. The roots were placed 3 mm beneath the alveolar crest and wedged firmly into position, without gingival coverage. Particles were firmly placed in the sockets and Surgicel was placed subgingivally over the extraction sites to achieve clot-controlled particle position.

At four weeks dense cortical bone was well adapted to the HA-root surface and between particles. Crestal bone growth with normal healthy mucosal coverage occurred in all sockets. Radiographs and clinical examination showed greater height (10 per cent) and alveolar crest width (15 per cent) with the particles than roots from 12 to 16 weeks. At 16 weeks, buccal crestal cortical bone resorbed, leaving an intact mucosa over the roots. Particles appeared to be en-

---

*Durapatite, Sterling Winthrop Lab., Inc., Albany, NY.

cased in bone with less buccal crestal plate resorption. By six months the preservation of width of the alveolar bone in HA root and particle sockets was similar, with no significant differences. From 6 to 12 months, vertical height was 15 per cent greater in particle sockets as compared to roots and controls. At 12 months, control sockets were 30 per cent less in width than the roots or particles. At 18 months ridge form was similarly preserved in both particle and root sockets. The ridge form was maintained by the implant's presence in spite of some crestal and buccal bone resorption.

In a human study by Quinn et al., HA ridge maintainers* were placed in fresh and healed sockets following removal of teeth in both the mandible and maxilla, using contralateral sockets as controls.[81] Implants were selected from metal socket gauges and contoured with diamond cylindrical burs to fit snugly approximately 2 mm below the alveolar bone crest level, since previous animal studies have shown that gingival tissue and ultimately bone cover the implants placed in fresh extraction sockets. The implants were tightly wedged into the sockets using hand pressure (Fig. 8–33).

Dimensional changes in height and width were determined by *triangulation* using India ink tattoo points. The apex of the triangle was placed at the crest of the ridge and the base of the triangle 5 mm below the crest on the facial and lingual sides. Clinical and radiographic examinations were accomplished at three-month intervals.

In 50 patients followed up to 26 months, fresh socket implant sites had twice as much alveolar ridge size preserved as the control sites (Fig. 8–34). These early results suggest that HA root implants placed in *fresh* extraction sockets can maintain alveolar bone height and width while supporting functioning dentures. Although the clinical significance of reporting data through only two years of follow-up may be questioned, it is well-known that a significant amount of resorption occurs within the first six months. Major differences between control sites and previously healed socket implant sites would not be significant, however, for several years.

Recommendations for surgical management of the reconstructive edentulous patient are as follows:

1. Correct minor soft-tissue abnormalities early when ridge height and form are adequate.
2. Perform vestibuloplasties only if alveolar ridge form is satisfactory in height and exhibits a convex contour.

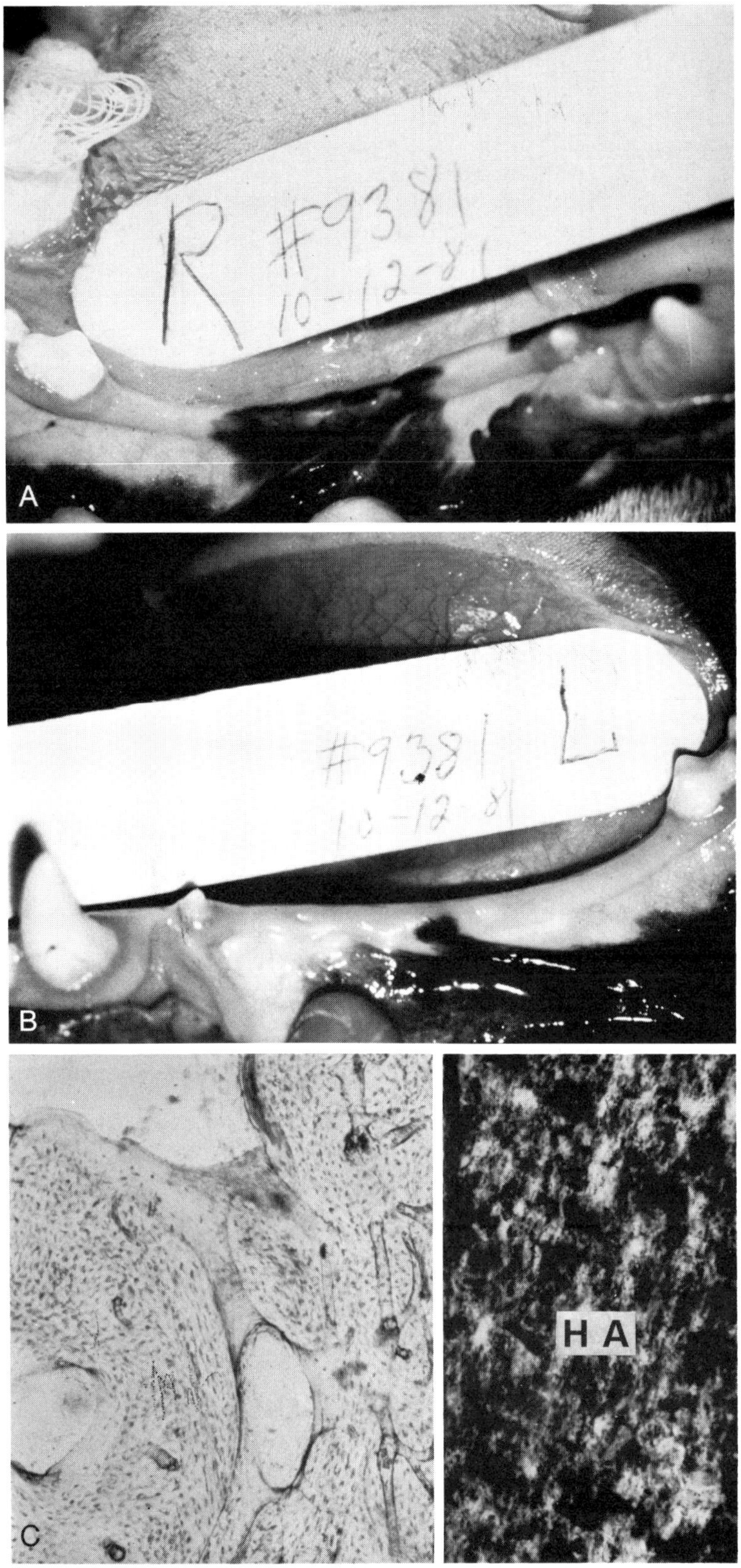

Figure 8–32. Preservation of the dog alveolar ridge with HA ridge maintainers. *A,* Control side at seven months. No implants had been placed when teeth were extracted. *B,* Opposite side at seven months. Implants were placed immediately following extractions. *C,* Undecalcified section of HA-bone interface at seven months.

---

*Calcitite®, RM, Calcitek, Inc., San Diego, CA.

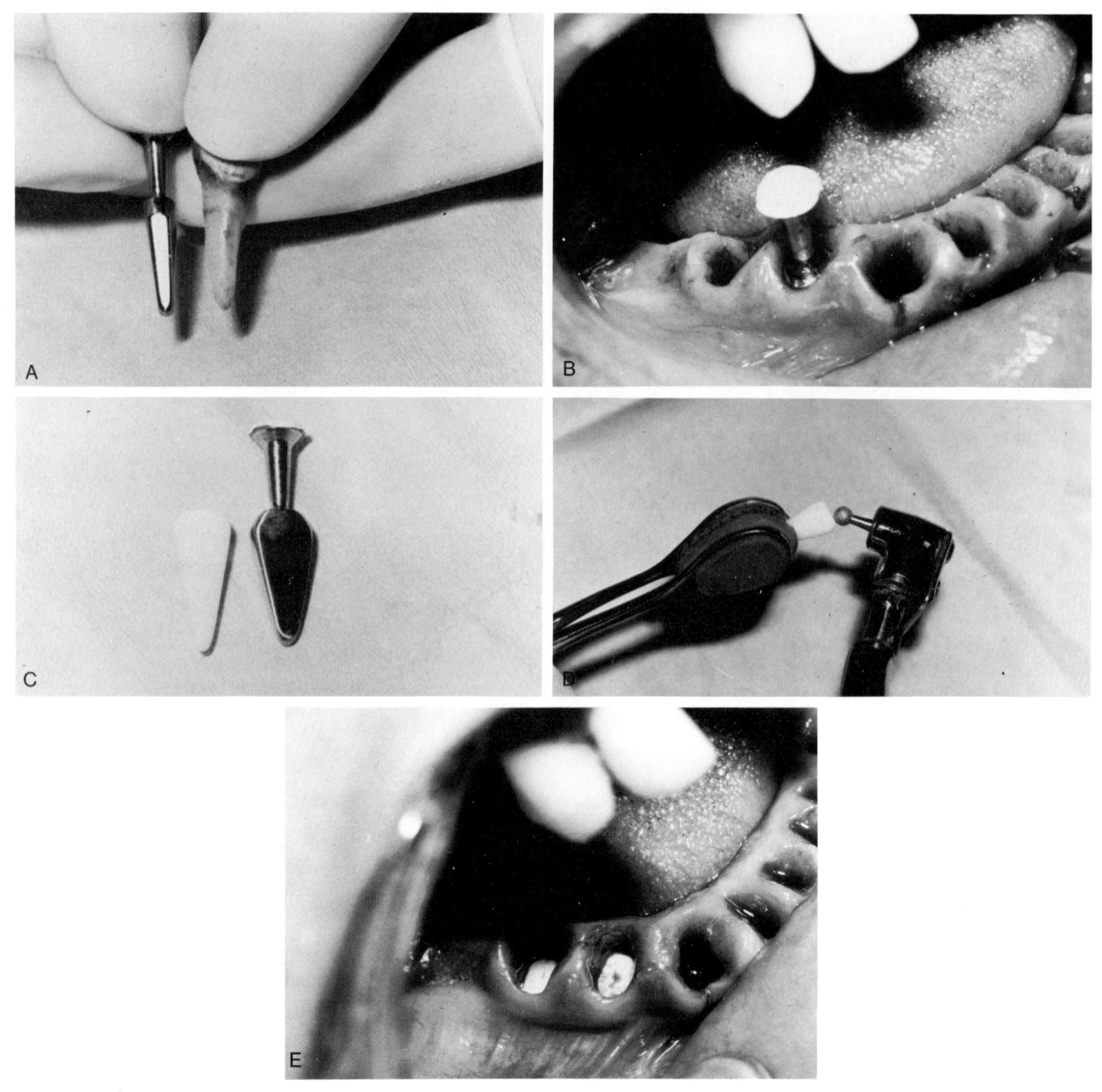

342 / RECONSTRUCTION OF THE ALVEOLAR RIDGE WITH HYDROXYLAPATITE

Figure 8–33. Preservation of alveolar bone, with Calcite HA alveolar ridge maintainers (RM). *A,* The extracted tooth is compared to a metal socket gauge. *B,* The socket gauge is tried into extraction site. *C,* A Calcite RM implant is selected. *D,* The occlusal aspect of implant is contoured with a diamond bur. *E,* Implant placement.

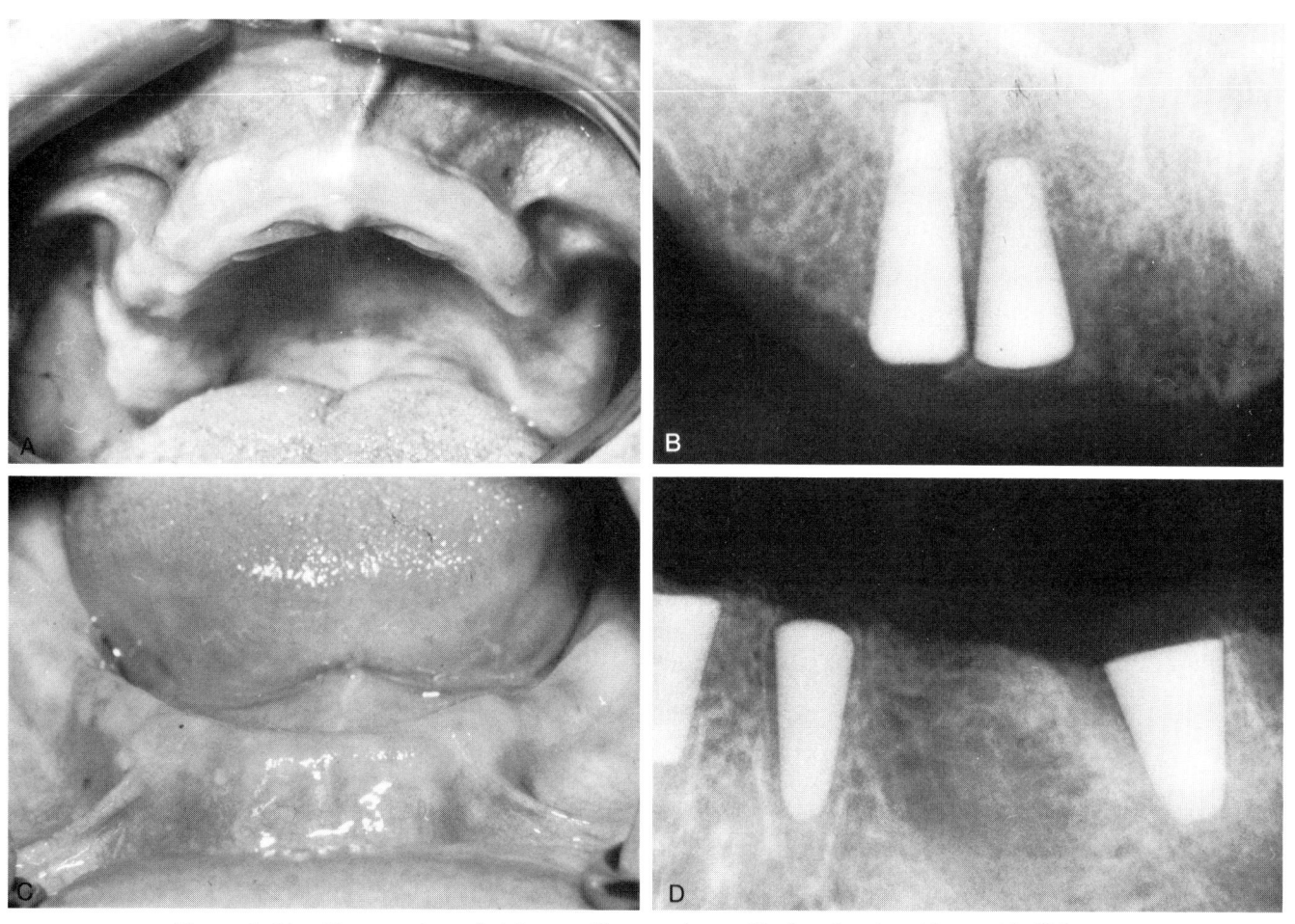

Figure 8–34. Preservation of right maxillary and mandibular alveolar ridges with Calcite RM at 24 months. The left maxillary and mandibular ridges served as controls with no implants.

3. Perform HA augmentation to eliminate undercuts and improve ridge height and contour.

4. Early reports show successful use of HA with mandibular staple, Swiss screws, and subperiosteal implants simultaneously. HA may improve the stability and longevity of the dental implant when used as a filler to restore bone loss around the necks and framework of dental implants (Fig. 8–35). HA has not been used with sufficient experience to recommend placement of blade type or other endosseous dental implants *through* an augmented ridge. The combination of dental implants placed anteriorly and HA placed posteriorly in the mandible seems to be an effective complete restorative measure.

5. HA particles may also be used with rib grafts and horizontal interpositional or visor osteotomy techniques to improve ridge contour, since more permanent increase in ridge width can be obtained.

6. Mucosa, dermis, and skin graft vestibuloplasties or re-epithelialization techniques are possible after two to three months. At this time, a hard, stable HA ridge indicates sufficient fibrovascular tissue bed to receive soft-tissue grafts or allow for re-epithelialization techniques. Most soft-tissue procedures should be delayed until after adequate ridge height and form are obtained, since HA augmentation is more difficult on a previously skin- or mucosa-grafted ridge.

7. Preliminary results with solid HA root implants suggest that preservation of the alveolar ridge is possible while supporting dentures.

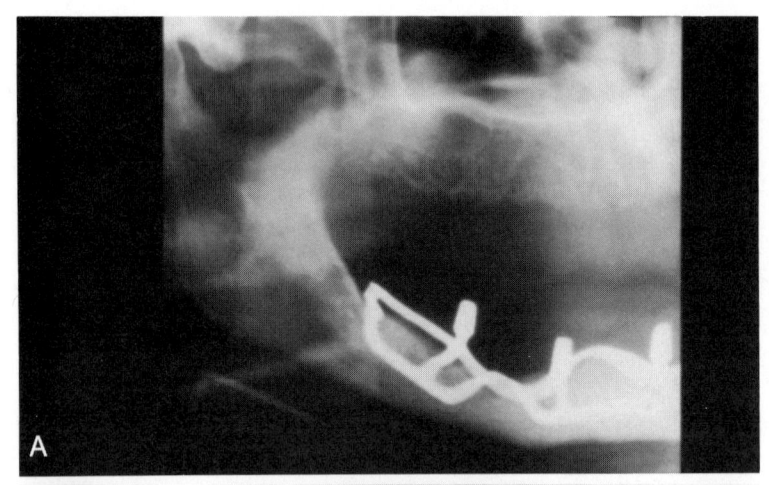

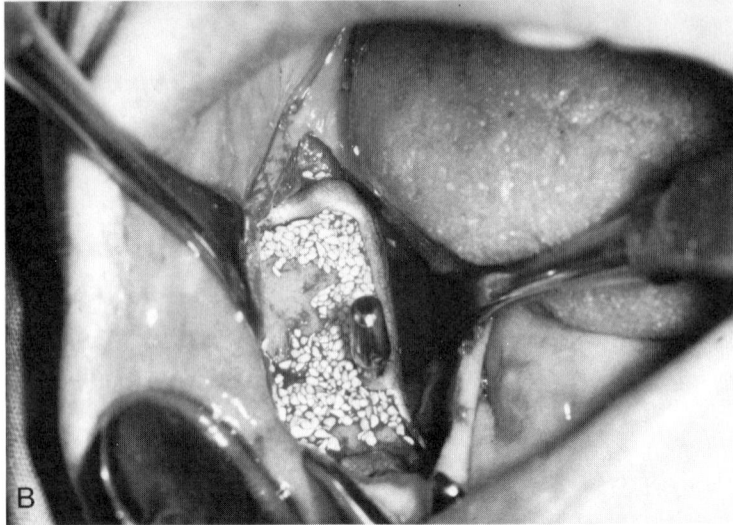

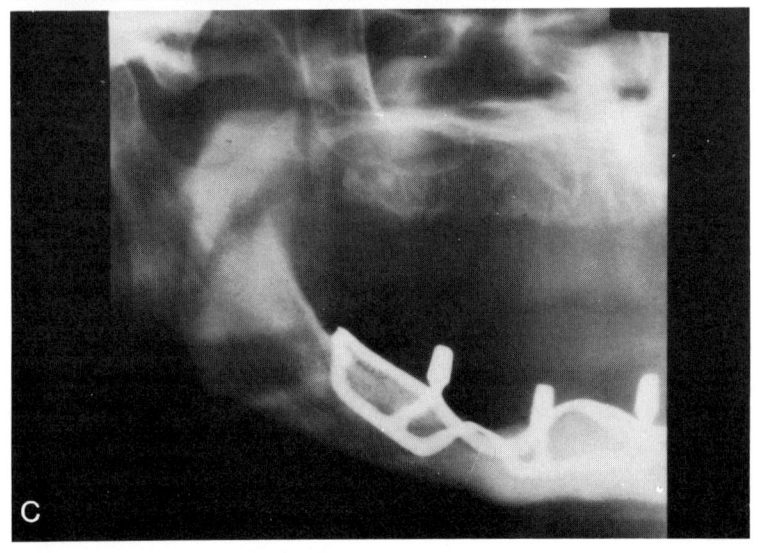

Figure 8–35. *A,* Radiograph of a failing subperiosteal implant with posterior ridge resorption. *B,* Soft connective tissue is removed and HA particles are packed between the implant frame and bone. *C,* Postoperative radiograph.

SUMMARY

The use of particulate, dense, nonresorbable hydroxylapatite for ridge augmentation has demonstrated a significant improvement over other techniques. Denture construction begins as early as four weeks after augmentation. Stability is improved, and relines and remakes are less frequent than in patients who have been augmented with autogenous bone alone. Skin and mucosal graft vestibuloplasties are possible after two months, compared to four to six months after augmentation following autogenous bone grafts alone. In most patients augmentation of alveolar deficient ridges with HA has resulted in a permanently improved ridge height and convex contour. The overlying soft-tissue mucosa is nonmobile, and vestibular depth can be maintained except in severe ridge deficiencies for which postoperative vestibuloplasties are required. HA can be effectively used to gain total reconstruction with staple bone plates.

Animal and clinical studies are in progress to evaluate the use of HA particles and blocks in extraction sockets, clefts, cysts, mandibular continuity defects, interpositional applications in orthognathic surgical procedures, and facial augmentation in which these materials may function alone or combine with autogenous or allogenic bone as a cortical cancellous extender.

BIBLIOGRAPHY

1. Davis WH, et al.: Long term ridge augmentation with rib grafts. J Maxillofac Surg 3:103–106, 1975.
2. Fonseca RJ, et al.: Revascularization and healing of onlay particulate autologous bone grafts in primates. J Oral Surg 38:572, 1980.
3. Baker RD, Terry BC, Davis WH, and Connole PW: Long-term results of alveolar ridge augmentation. J Oral Surg 37:486–489, 1979.
4. Wang JH, Waite DE, and Steinhauser E: Ridge augmentation: An evaluation and follow-up report. J Oral Surg 34:600, 1976.
5. Fazili M, et al.: Follow-up investigation of reconstruction of the alveolar process of the atrophic mandible. Int J Oral Surg 7:400, 1978.
6. Kelley JF, and Friedlander GE: Preprosthetic bone graft augmentation with allogeneic bone: A preliminary report. J Oral Surg 35:268, 1977.
7. Peterson LJ: Augmentation of the mandibular residual ridge by a modified visor osteotomy. J Oral Maxillofac Surg 41:332–338, 1983.
8. Stoelinga PJW, et al.: A reappraisal of the interposed bone graft augmentation of the atrophic mandible. J Maxillofac Surg 11:107–112, 1983.
9. Kent JN, Homsy CA, and Hinds EC: Proplast in dental facial reconstruction. Oral Surg 39:347–359, 1975.
10. McConnel D: Apatite. New York, Springer-Verlag, 1973.
11. Francis MD, and Centner RL: The development of diphosphonates as significant health care products. J Chem Educ 55:760, 1978.
12. Albee FH, and Morrison HF: Studies in bone growth, triple calcium phosphate as a stimulus to osteogenesis. Ann Surg 71:32, 1920.
13. Haldeman KO, and Moore JM: Influence of a local excess of calcium and phosphorous on the healing of fractures. Arch Surg 29:385, 1934.
14. Ray DR, and Ward AA: A preliminary report of studies of basic calcium phosphate in bone replacement. In Surgical Forum. Philadelphia, WB Saunders Co, 1952, p 429.
15. Levitt SR, Crayton PH, Monroe EA, and Condrate RA: Forming method for apatite prosthesis. J Biomed Mater Res 3:683, 1969.
16. Monroe EE, Votava W, Bass DB, and McCullen J: New calcium phosphate ceramic material for bone and tooth implants. J Dent Res 50:860, 1971.
17. Hubbard WG, Hirthe WM, and Mueller KH: Physiological calcium phosphate implants. Proc 26th Ann Conf Eng Med Bio 15:198, 1973.
18. Aoki H, Kato K, Ebihara M, and Inoue M: Studies on the application of apatite to dental materials. J Dent Eng (Japan) 17:200, 1976.
19. Jarcho M, Bolen CH, Thomas MB, Bobick J, Kay JF, and Doremus RH: Hydroxylapatite synthesis and characterization in dense polycrystalline form. J Mater Sci 11:2027, 1976.
20. Rao WR, and Boehm RF: A study of sintered apatites. J Dent Res 53:1351, 1974.
21. Jarcho M, Salsbury RL, Thomas MB, and Doremus RH: Synthesis and fabrication of tricalcium phosphate ceramics for potential prosthetic applications. J Mater Sci 14:142, 1979.
22. Rejda BV, Peelen JGJ, and deGroot K: Tricalcium phosphate as a bone substitute. J Bioeng 1:93, 1977.
23. Roy DM, and Linnehan SK: Hydroxylapatite formed from coral skeletal carbonate by hydrothermal exchange. Nature 247:220, 1974.
24. deGroot K: Bioceramics consisting of calcium phosphate salts. Biomaterials 1:47, 1980.
25. Jarcho M: Calcium phosphate ceramics as hard tissue prosthetics. Clin Orthoped 157:259, 1981.
26. Metsger SD, Driskell TD, and Paulsrud JR: Tricalcium phosphate ceramic, a resorbable bone implant: Review and current status. J Am Dent Assoc 105:1035, 1981.
27. Huffman EO, Cate WE, Deming ME, and Elmore KL: Rates of solution of calcium phosphates in phosphoric acid solutions. Agric Food Chem 5:266, 1957.
28. Mooney RW, and Aia MA: Alkaline earth phosphates. Chem Rev 61:433, 1961.
29. Veldhuis A, Driessen T, Dennissen HW, and deGroot K: A five year evaluation of apatite tooth roots as means to reduce residual ridge resorption. Clin Prevent Dent 6:5–8, 1984.
30. Jarcho M, Kay JF, Gumaer KI, Doremus RH, and Drobeck HP: Tissue, cellular and subcellular events at a bone-ceramic hydroxylapatite interface. J Bioeng 1:79, 1977.
31. Aoki H, Kato J, Ogiso M, and Tabata T: Studies on the application of apatite to dental materials. J Dent Eng (Japan) 18:86, 1977.
32. Sayler K, Holmes R, and Johns D: Replamineform porous hydroxylapatite as bone substitute in craniofacial osseous reconstruction. J Dent Res 56B:173, 1977.
33. Mors WA, and Kaminski EJ: Osteogenesis replacement of tricalcium phosphate ceramic implants in the dog palate. Arch Oral Biol 20:365, 1975.
34. Ferraro JW: Experimental evaluation of ceramic calcium phosphate as a substitute for bone grafts. Plast Reconstr Surg 63:634, 1979.
35. Cameron HU, MacNab I, and Pilliar RM: Evaluation of a biodegradable ceramic. J Biomed Mater Res 11:179, 1977.
36. Shima T, Keller JT, Alvira NM, Mayfield FH, and Dunsker SB: Anterior cervical discectomy and interbody fusion: An experimental study using a synthetic tricalcium phosphate. J Neurosurg 51:533, 1979.
37. Nery EB, and Lynch KL: Preliminary clinical studies of bioceramics in periodontal osseous defects. J Periodontol 49:523, 1978.
38. Nery EB, Lynch KL, Hirthe WM, and Mueller KH: Bioceramic implants in surgically produced infrabony defects. J Periodontol 46:328, 1975.
39. Hassler CR, McCoy LG, and Clarke LC: Studies on the degradability of large tricalcium phosphate segments. Proc 2nd Ann Meet Soc Biomater 1976, p 88.
40. Denissen HW, and deGroot K: Immediate dental root implants from synthetic dense calcium hydroxylapatite. J Prosthet Dent 42:551, 1979.
41. Kato K, Aoki H, Tabata T, and Ogiso M: Biocompatibility of apatite ceramics in mandibles. Biomater Med Dev Art Org 7:291, 1979.
42. Kay JF, Doremus RH, and Jarcho M: Ion micromilling of bone-implant interfaces. Trans 4th Ann Meet Soc Biomater 10th Int Biomater Symp, 1978, p 154.
43. Jasty V, Jarcho M, Gumaer KI, Sauerschell R, and Drobeck HP: Bone tissue response to dense hydroxylapatite disc implants in mongrel dogs: A light and electron microscopic study. Ninth Int Cong Electron Microscopy 2:674, 1978.
44. Jarcho M, Jasty V, Gumaer KI, Kay JF, and Doremus RH: Electron microscopic study of a bone-hydroxylapatite implant interface. Trans

4th Ann Met Soc Biomater 10th Int Biomater Symp, 1978, p 112.
45. Ogiso M, Kaneda H, Arasaki J, Tabata T, and Hidaka T: Epithelial attachment and bone tissue formation on the surface of hydroxylapatite ceramics. First World Biomater Cong (Baden, Austria) 1980, 4.1.5 (abstract).
46. Denissen HW, deGroot K, Kakkes P, van den Hooff A, and Klopper PJ: Animal and human studies of sintered hydroxylapatite as a material for tooth root implants. First World Biomater Cong (Baden, Austria) 1980, 3.8.1 (abstract).
47. Ham AW, and Cormack DH: Histology. 8th ed. Philadelphia, JB Lippincott Co, 1979, p 399.
48. Getter L, Bhaskar SN, Cutright DE, Perez B, Brady JM, Driskell TD, and O'Hara MJ: Three biodegradable calcium phosphate slurry implants in bone. J Oral Surg 30:263, 1972.
49. Grower MF, Horan M, Miller R, and Getter L: Bone inductive potential of biodegradable ceramic in millipore filterchambers. J Dent Res 52:160, 1973.
50. Boyne PJ, Fremming BD, Walsh R, and Jarcho M: Evaluation of a ceramic hydroxylapatite in femoral defects. J Dent Res 57A:108, 1978.
51. McDavid PT, Boone ME, Kafrawy AH, and Mitchell DF: Effect of autogenous marrow and calcitonin on reactions to a ceramic. J Dent Res 58:1478, 1979.
52. Levin MP, Getter L, and Cutright DE: A comparison of iliac marrow and biodegradable ceramic in periodontal defects. J Biomed Mater Res 9:183, 1975.
53. Lemons JE, Ballard JB, Culpepper MI, and Niemann KMW: Porous tricalcium phosphate ceramic for segmental lesions. First World Biomater Cong (Baden, Austria) 1980, 4.10.3 (abstract).
54. Levin MP, Getter L, Adrian J, and Cutright DE: Healing of periodontal defects with ceramic implants. J Clin Periodont 1:197, 1974.
55. Boyne PJ, and Shapton BA: The response of surgical periodontal defects to implantation with a hydroxylapatite ceramic. Trans 4th Ann Meet Soc Biomater 10th Int Biomater Symp, 1978, p 115.
56. Hassler CR, McCoy LG, and Rotaru JH: Long term implants in solid tricalcium phosphate. Proc 27th Ann Conf Eng Med Bio 16:488, 1974.
57. Finn RA, Bell WH, and Brammer JA: Interpositional grafting with autogenous bone and coralline hydroxylapatite. J Maxillofac Surg 8:217, 1980.
58. Piecuch JF, Topazian RG, Skoly S, and Wolfe S: Experimental ridge augmentation with porous hydroxylapatite implants. J Dent Res 62:148, 1983.
59. Niwa S, Sawai K, Takahashi S, Tagai H, Ono M, and Fukuda Y: Experimental studies of the implantation of hydoxylapatite in the medullary canal of rabbits. First World Biomater Cong (Baden, Austria) 1980, 4:10.4 (abstract).
60. Pawluk RJ: Personal communication.
61. Kent JN, Quinn JH, Zide MF, Finger IM, Jarcho M, and Rothstein SS: Correction of alveolar ridge deficiencies with nonresorbable hydroxylapatite. J Am Dent Assoc 105:993–1001, 1982.
62. Kent JN, Quinn JH, Zide MF, Guerra LR, and Boyne P: Alveolar ridge augmentation using nonresorbable hydroxylapatite with or without autogenous cancellous bone. J Oral Maxillofac Surg 41:629–642, 1983.
63. Larson HD, Finger IM, Guerra LR, and Kent JN: Prosthetic management of hydroxylapatite augmented ridges. J Prosthet Dent 49:461–469, 1983.
64. Kent JN: Modifications of HA alveolar ridge reconstruction technique. Unpublished data.
65. Barson RE, and Kent JN: Hydroxylapatite reconstruction of alveolar ridge deficiency with an open technique—a preliminary report. Oral Surg 59:113–119, 1985.
66. Kent JN, Quinn JH, Zide MF, and Jarcho M: Hydroxylapatite augmentation of atrophic alveolar ridge. Biomedical Engineering II—Recent Developments. In Hall CW (ed): Proceedings of the Second Southern Biomedical Engineering Conference. Elmsford, NY, Pergamon Press, pp 77–80.
67. Kent JN, James R, Finger I, Jarcho M, Taggart J, and Cook S: Augmentation of deficient edentulous alveolar ridges with dense polycrystalline hydroxylapatite. First World Biomater Cong (Baden, Austria), April 8–12, 1980.
68. Kent JN, Cook SD, Quinn JH, and Thomas K: Radiographic evaluation of alveolar ridge augmentations with hydroxylapatite. J Dent Res (Abstract 1421). International Association for Dental Research and American Association for Dental Research, New Orleans, Louisiana, March 18–21, 1982.
69. Block MS, and Kent JN: Radiographic evaluation of hydroxylapatite augmentation of deficient mandibular alveolar ridges. J Oral Maxillofac Surg 42:793, 1984.
70. Block MS, and Kent JN: Canine mandibular response to hydroxylapatite combined with bone. J Dent Res (Abstract No. 1388). International Association for Dental Research and American Association for Dental Research, Dallas, Texas, March 15–18, 1984.
71. Chang C, Matukas VJ, and Lemons JE: Histologic study of hydroxylapatite as an implant material for mandibular augmentation. J Oral Maxillofac Surg 41:729–737, 1983.
72. Zide MF, Misiek DJ, Kent JN, and Jarcho M: The evaluation of strength and resorption with different ratios of hydroxylapatite and bone in canine mandibular continuity defects. Unpublished data.
73. Matlaga BF, Yasenchak LP, and Salthouse TN: Tissue response to implanted polymers: The significance of sample shape. J Biomed Mater Res 10:391, 1976.
74. Misiek DJ, Kent JN, and Carr RF: The soft tissue response to different shaped hydroxylapatite particles. J Oral Maxillofac Surg 42:150–160, 1984.
75. Kent JN, Misiek DJ, Silverman H, and Rotskoff K: Mandibular staple bone plate: A multicenter review. Oral Maxillofac Surg 42:421–428, 1984.
76. Small IA: Personal communication.
77. Lavelle C, Wedgwood D, and Riess G: A new implant philosophy. J Prosthet Dent 43:71–77, 1980.
78. Boyne PJ, and Szutz TJ: Fluorescent microscopy of hydroxylapatite implants in alveolar bone maintenance. J Dent Res (abstract 1166). International Association for Dental Research and American Association for Dental Research, Chicago, March, 1981.
79. Quinn JH, and Kent JN: Alveolar ridge maintenance with solid nonporous hydroxylapatite root implants. Oral Surg 58:511–521, 1984.
80. Block MS, Kent JN, and Jarcho M: A comparison of dense, solid hydroxylapatite (HA) roots and particulate HA in dog extraction sites to preserve alveolar bone. J Dent Res (Abstract no. 998). International Association for Dental Research, Las Vegas, March, 1985.
81. Quinn JH, Kent JN, Hunter RG, and Schaffer CM: Preservation of the alveolar ridge with hydroxylapatite tooth root substitutes. J Am Dent Assoc 110:189–193, 1985.

9
RECONSTRUCTION AND REHABILITATION OF CANCER PATIENTS

*Robert E. Marx, D.D.S.,
and Timothy R. Saunders, D.D.S.*

> Repair is not simply the surgeon's ally, it is his life line. Unless the surgeon aids the forces of repair, he will be little more than a surgeon of the last century who has somehow found a modern operating room.
>
> THOMAS K. HUNT
> WALTON VANWINKLE, JR.

Reconstructive surgery to restore functional anatomy in cancer-related defects is challenging. If we strive to rehabilitate cancer victims rather than only replace missing tissue parts, then prosthetic management must follow surgical reconstruction. Bony and soft tissue reconstruction of large, functional defects caused by therapeutic cancer extirpation should be viewed as reconstructive preprosthetic surgery. Other forms of reconstructive preprosthetic surgery encompass augmentation of existing ridges and elimination of mucosal encumbrances, but reconstruction of cancer defects also embraces basic bony continuity, soft-tissue integrity, and facial form. In addition, cancer-related defects are often compounded by radiation damage, surgical scarring, pharyngeal-laryngeal compromise, and tobacco- and/or alcohol-related tissue changes. This group of patients usually has a more comprehensive set of organic and functional obstacles than other groups. The goal of this chapter is to describe the biologic and technical means to gain functional rehabilitation in these patients.

PATIENT ASSESSMENT

SURGICAL CONSIDERATIONS

Anatomy of Cancer Defects

The most common cancer-related defect is seen after hemimandibulectomy and ipsilateral radical neck dissection. Besides the sacrificed bone and lost jaw continuity, the internal jugular vein, sternocleidomastoid muscle, spinal-accessory nerve, and lymphatics within the investing fascia of both the anterior and posterior triangles of the neck are removed. During the extirpative surgery, the cervical branch of the facial nerve, and often the marginal mandibular branch as well, are sacrificed. The results are an atrophied and fibrotic platysma and loss of lower lip control. Such patients characteristically have a concave facial deformity and a thinness of overlying skin (Fig. 9–1). The skin is denervated and adherent to the deep tissues of the neck (digastric muscles, geniohyoid, and even the superior and middle pharyngeal constrictors). This results in im-

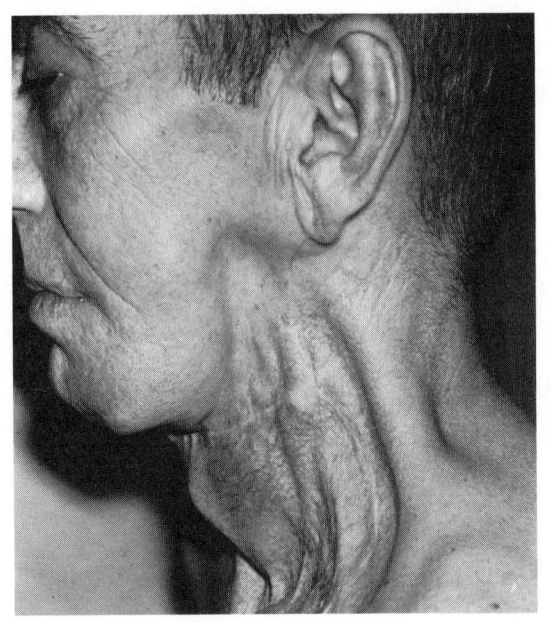

Figure 9–1. Characteristic concave soft- and hard-tissue deformity seen after hemimandibulectomy and radical neck dissection.

mobile skin that is dry and often caked with keratin. The carotid artery is located within scar tissue just below the skin. The ipsilateral shoulder droops owing to paralysis of the denervated trapezius. If radiation has been part of the therapeutic protocol or if the surgical extirpation has scarred the pharyngeal constrictors and stylopharyngeous muscle, dysphagia will result.

In every patient assessment, a list should be made based on anatomic considerations that include (1) structures that are missing, (2) structures that are present but compromised in function or vascularity, and (3) structures that remain with anticipated blood supply and function.

A recent advance in cancer surgery has improved anatomic considerations for reconstruction and rehabilitation. "Functional neck dissection" leaves more structures in the neck with less scarring and disruption of the blood supply (Fig. 9–2). The biologic basis of this new approach is the knowledge that lymphatics do not penetrate the muscle fascia, carotid sheath, or perineurium,[1] therefore allowing incontinuity resection of the fascia and lymphatics of both triangles of the neck pedicled to the carotid sheath.[2] The sternocleidomastoid muscle, spinal-accessory nerve, marginal mandibular nerve, and sometimes the internal jugular vein can be retained. The patient will have less muscular dysfunction, more tissue in the neck, and most importantly greater vascularity. The most important feature of the functional neck dissection is the retention of the sternocleidomastoid muscle. This is retained not because of its functional role of rotating the head to the contralateral side but rather because of its blood supply and perforating vessels to its overlying skin. The functional neck dissection retracts the sternocleidomastoid muscle to slide the resection specimen beneath it and sacrifices its superior thyroid arterial supply and venous drainage. However, it retains dominant occipital vessels and less important vessels from the thyrocervical trunk. This muscle adds bulk and vascularity to the neck and prevents much of the skin atrophy. The difference between patients who have had a full versus functional neck dissection is dramatic (Figs. 9–1 and 9–2).

Knowledge of the extirpative surgery and the ability to assess each patient's anatomy are necessary in order to anticipate the problems in rehabilitation and plan approaches to prevent them.

Hard-Tissue Defects

The most important consideration related to the hard-tissue defect is the status of the remaining condyle and proximal segment. There are three alternative ways of dealing with the ramus and condyle when a tumor exists in the tonsillar and/or retromolar areas.[3] A horizontal ostectomy can be made superior to the lingula, leaving the condyle and coronoid process. Another procedure is the oblique ostectomy, leaving the condyle and condylar neck. The third is a complete disarticulation. None of these approaches is particularly advantageous for reconstruction. Leaving the coronoid process distracts the

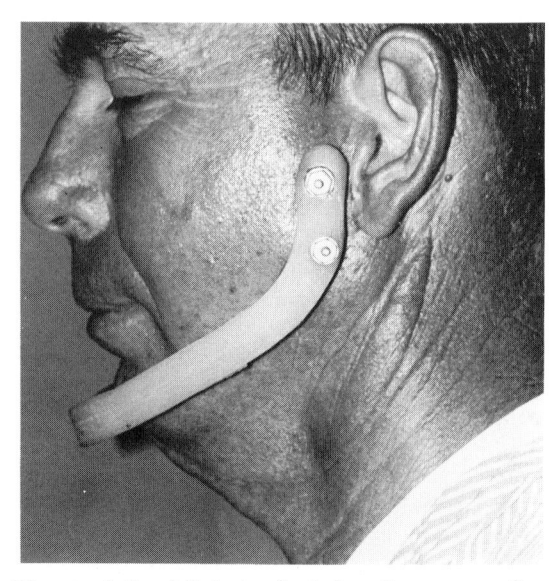

Figure 9–2. Minimized deformity seen after hemimandibulectomy and functional neck dissection.

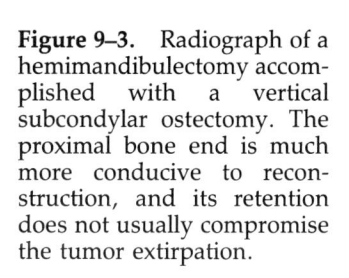

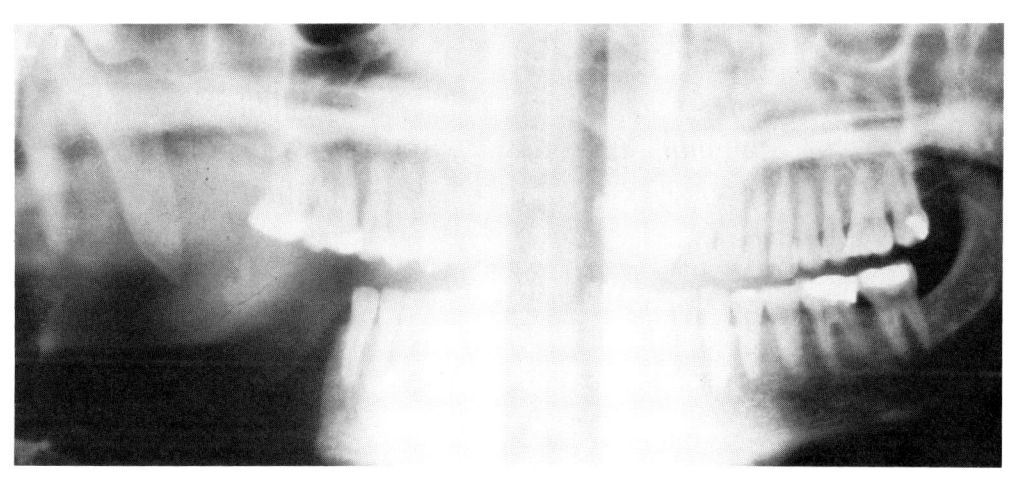

Figure 9–3. Radiograph of a hemimandibulectomy accomplished with a vertical subcondylar ostectomy. The proximal bone end is much more conducive to reconstruction, and its retention does not usually compromise the tumor extirpation.

proximal segment by the pull of the temporalis. The oblique ostectomy eliminates the distraction, but the most fragile and fracture-prone area of the mandible becomes the eventual graft-host interface. This type of extirpative surgery forces the reconstruction to be thin in the area where a bulk of bone is required to resist fracture. Disarticulation sacrifices the actions of the lateral pterygoid muscle. It commits the reconstructed mandible to only rotational movements at a point within or near the temporal fossa.

An ostectomy that best prepares the patient for jaw reconstruction, while still maintaining sound cancer surgery principles, is the vertical subcondylar ostectomy (Fig. 9–3). This ostectomy will retain the condyle in the fossa and maintain the integrity of the lateral pterygoid muscle. It will not become distracted, but will allow for reconstruction of the entire ramus width. This approach has only recently been introduced to cancer surgery, so disarticulations and small proximal segments remain the most widely used. Nevertheless, each type of proximal segmentation can be approached with a different technique to provide a functional and esthetic result. Radiographs that adequately assess the amount and location of the proximal segment are necessary to plan the appropriate surgery. The most difficult cancer-related defect of the mandible to reconstruct is the resected symphysis. Such defects usually present with concomitant soft-tissue retraction and bilaterally displaced proximal segments. These segments are superiorly displaced to a severe degree and medially rotated (Fig. 9–4).

One needs to assess the adequacy of skin and adjacent soft tissues to accommodate a graft in these patients. Careful examination of the mucosa for bone that has eroded through the mucosa from proximal segment distraction is important. In this type of reconstruction, problems include alignment of posterior arches and achievement of a curved arch form across the midline. Fixation devices such as Gunning-type splints cannot be used because they would rest upon the graft itself. Extra-skeletal pin fixation would either require pin placement into the graft or leave the graft without fixation to the proximal segments. Such cases must be planned so that more rigid internal fixation can achieve a curved anterior arch form and chin contour. The surgical incision to expose each ramus should also be planned. A coronoidectomy on each side, plus release of various scars, is necessary to reposition the proximal segments in correct orientation.

Soft-Tissue Defects

The key to successful reconstruction of the jaw rests with the quality and quantity of the

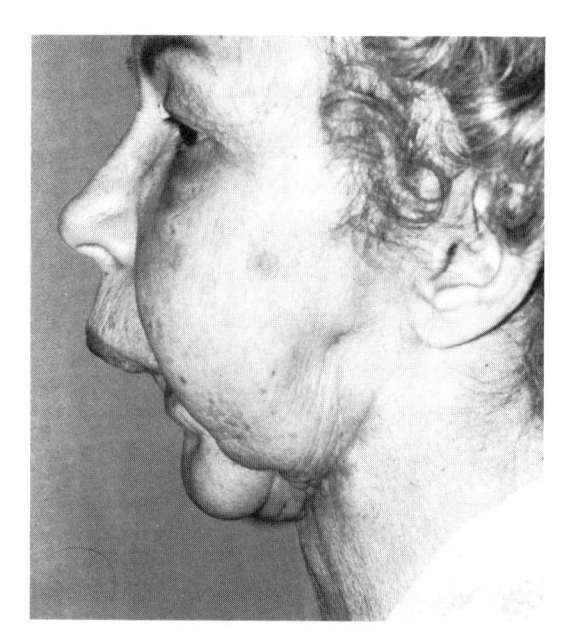

Figure 9–4. Resultant defect after symphysis resection, demonstrating severe chin retraction ("Andy Gump" deformity) and loss of angle form from rotation of proximal segment.

soft-tissue recipient bed. Prior to bony reconstruction, a definitive decision is required as to whether the quality of the tissue needs improvement and whether additional bulk is needed. Since fibroblastic cellularity and vascular density determine the quality of the recipient tissue, surgically scarred and/or irradiated tissue fields are candidates for qualitative improvement. An empirical rule is that only patients who have received more than 5000 rads of irradiation and/or a full radical neck dissection or previous graft attempts are likely to have sufficient tissue scarring to require qualitative improvements.

Patients who require qualitative improvement in the recipient tissue bed should be strongly considered for presurgical hyperbaric oxygen, or any one of several alternative myocutaneous flaps distant from the irradiated field. Each has the ability to improve the vascular and cellular components of the recipient tissue. When qualitative improvement alone is required, hyperbaric oxygen is preferred. It eliminates the morbidity from the donor site and improves all the tissues of the recipient bed. Myocutaneous flaps are vascular flaps with excellent cellularity, but they do not improve the local host tissue *per se*. Placed in heavily scarred or irradiated tissue, they often have difficulty healing to the local tissue because of the vascular compromise within the local tissue. Both methods may need to be employed where qualitative and quantitative improvements are required. Hyperbaric oxygen will not add bulk to the recipient tissue area. For quantitative deficiencies, only myocutaneous flaps are adequate. Other flaps are either insufficiently cellular to provide viable fibroblasts, insufficiently vascular, or insufficiently thick to be useful. The adequacy of the recipient tissue bulk is assessed during the clinical examination. Patients with 1 cm or less of thickness between skin and oral mucosa in the intended graft site should be considered for tissue flaps. This can be estimated with palpation or roughly measured by a needle that is impaled by a rubber stop.

Radiation Effects

Whatever the form of delivery of therapeutic ionizing radiation, the end result is a hypocellular, hypovascular, and measurably hypoxic tissue[4, 5] (Fig. 9–5). Since some form of irradiation is included in most cancer-therapy protocols, this type of compromise within the recipient tissue must be anticipated. Historically, grafts placed into irradiated tissues have had high rates of complications (81 per cent in some reports)[6] and low rates (20 to 60 per cent) of functionally acceptable results.[6, 7] However, in the past few years prereconstruction hyperbaric oxygen has been shown to improve the success rate (90 to 94 per cent) to equal that of grafts placed into nonirradiated tissues.[8] In addition, applications of microvascular surgery have shown initial promise in transplanting vascularized bone and periosteum to jaw defects.[9] Irradiated tissue no longer presents as an insurmountable obstacle to successful reconstruction. Several alternative modalities and techniques are available today that can consistently achieve functionally acceptable results in these patients. Most of these techniques are within the scope of the oral and maxillofacial surgeon.

Timing of Reconstruction

It was once accepted that reconstruction of cancer-related defects should be delayed until a three- to five-year disease-free period passed. The fear was not only that a persistent tumor would once again become clinically evident but that reconstruction would somehow interfere with recognition of such a tumor. This concept is no longer considered valid. With present-day combined surgical, irradiation, and chemotherapeutic approaches, better tumor controls are achieved. In patients who are treated for cure, it is senseless to wait three to five years for a recurrence to develop. Emphasis today is on early reconstruction in cancer patients. The advantage of such early reconstruction is that 60 to 70 per cent of good-candidate

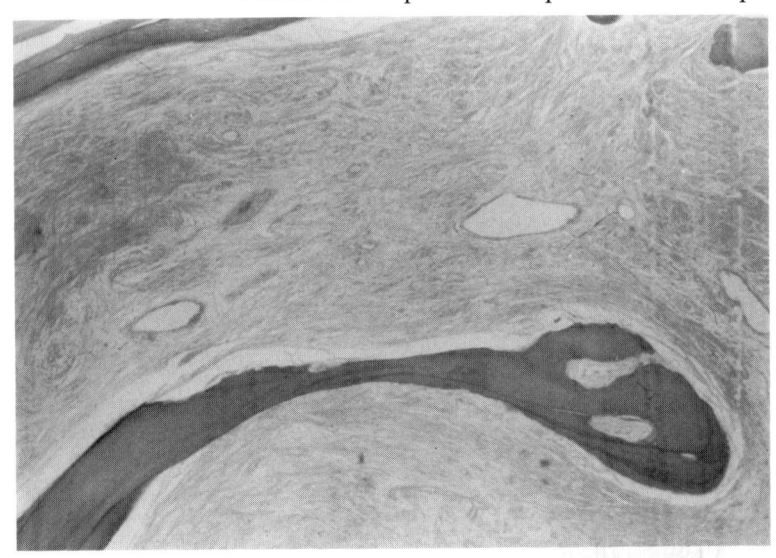

Figure 9–5. Photomicrograph of irradiated recipient tissue and bone. The stroma is one of mummified collagen that is hypocellular and hypovascular. Oxygen tension measurements on this tissue also demonstrate it to be hypoxic (H & E, × 60).

patients remain disease-free for five years or more. Therefore, the impact of facial deformity and masticatory dysfunction on these patients' lifestyles is averted. Our experience has shown that of 94 patients undergoing reconstruction, those who returned to active and productive lifestyles with the fewest difficulties were reconstructed within the first year.

An invalid concept is that early jaw reconstruction obstructs the recognition of persistent tumors or second primaries. It was feared that metallic cribs used in reconstruction would obscure radiographic evidence of tumors invading the mandible. Since most persistent tumors and all second primaries begin as mucosal lesions, radiographic assessment for each is inadequate. Each is best recognized by clinical examination of the mucosa. Because of reconstructive techniques used today that avoid metallic cribs, this concept fails to be creditable. The experience is, in fact, just the reverse. Recurrent disease is more frequently identified and at an earlier time in reconstructed patients. Two teams of surgeons and one or more prosthodontists follow the patient. Each patient receives a more thorough examination on a more frequent basis than do those attending busy cancer clinics, where time may not allow it. Fourteen of our 115 reconstructed patients developed "recurrent tumor"; in 11 of these cases the recurrence was recognized by the reconstructive team. In patients who develop "recurrent tumors" after reconstruction, salvage surgical procedures or salvage irradiation protocols may be used with the same yield as in the nonreconstructed patient. The techniques and principles described in subsequent sections of this chapter show how the grafted bone and soft tissue is reconstructed almost free of foreign bodies. These tissues are then capable of responding to further cancer treatment without increased complications.

Patient selection and assessment are critical to early reconstruction. Cancer surgeons state that 65 per cent of patients who develop clinical evidence of persistent tumor do so in the first year.[10] However, these patients are poor surgical and irradiation cure risks. Most of these patients have T_3 and T_4 lesions with some regional neck metastases on initial presentation. Patients with T_1 and T_2 lesions, or T_3 lesions that are N_0 or N_1 at most, are the best candidates for early reconstruction. If they are in good general health and their cancer therapy has been sufficiently aggressive, then early reconstruction is recommended. The reconstructive team is responsible for making this assessment.

Many patients' views on cancer surgery have changed. Patients now feel that modern medicine has more to offer than masticatory dysfunction and facial deformity. Today's patients are not willing to accept the "you should just be happy to be alive" philosophy that once prevailed.

Reconstruction is best performed within the first year. If accomplished within the first year, the patient's self-image of being a cripple is more thoroughly reversed, and a more complete return to an active lifestyle is observed. Immediate reconstruction is another approach that addresses a patient's unwillingness to accept deformity and dysfunction.[11] Immediate reconstruction best restores form and function but often falls short of the ideal. The main reason is the high incidence of graft infection (20 to 25 per cent), with partial or complete graft loss.[12, 13] Reconstructions that become contaminated with the oral flora and those that have recipient tissues open for longer periods of time are more prone to infection. The added time for reconstruction and blood loss from donor bone harvesting increase the morbidity of the extirpative surgery. Poor experiences reported with immediate jaw reconstructions should make the surgeon cautious about choosing this alternative.[11-13] Immediate reconstruction is indicated when graft contamination can be prevented. Unfortunately, this is rarely possible in cancer surgery.

Prosthodontic Considerations of Mandibular Continuity Defects

Functional Deficit

Defects of the mandible vary greatly in location, size, and extent, and the deficiencies that result also vary. These deficiencies are related to physiologic, cosmetic, and psychological problems. A classification of mandibular defects has been described by Cantor and Curtis.[14] Although this classification system is suggested primarily for edentulous patients, it is also applicable to partially edentulous patients. This system classifies defects based on remaining structures.

Class I mandibular resection defects involve alveolar resection with preservation of mandibular continuity (Fig. 9–6A). Class II resection defects involve loss of mandibular continuity with resection distal to the canine area (Fig. 9–6B). Class III resection defects are associated with a minimum of midline loss of continuity (Fig. 9–6C). Class IV resection defects result from lateral continuity resection where bony augmentation formed pseudoarticulation of bone and soft tissue in

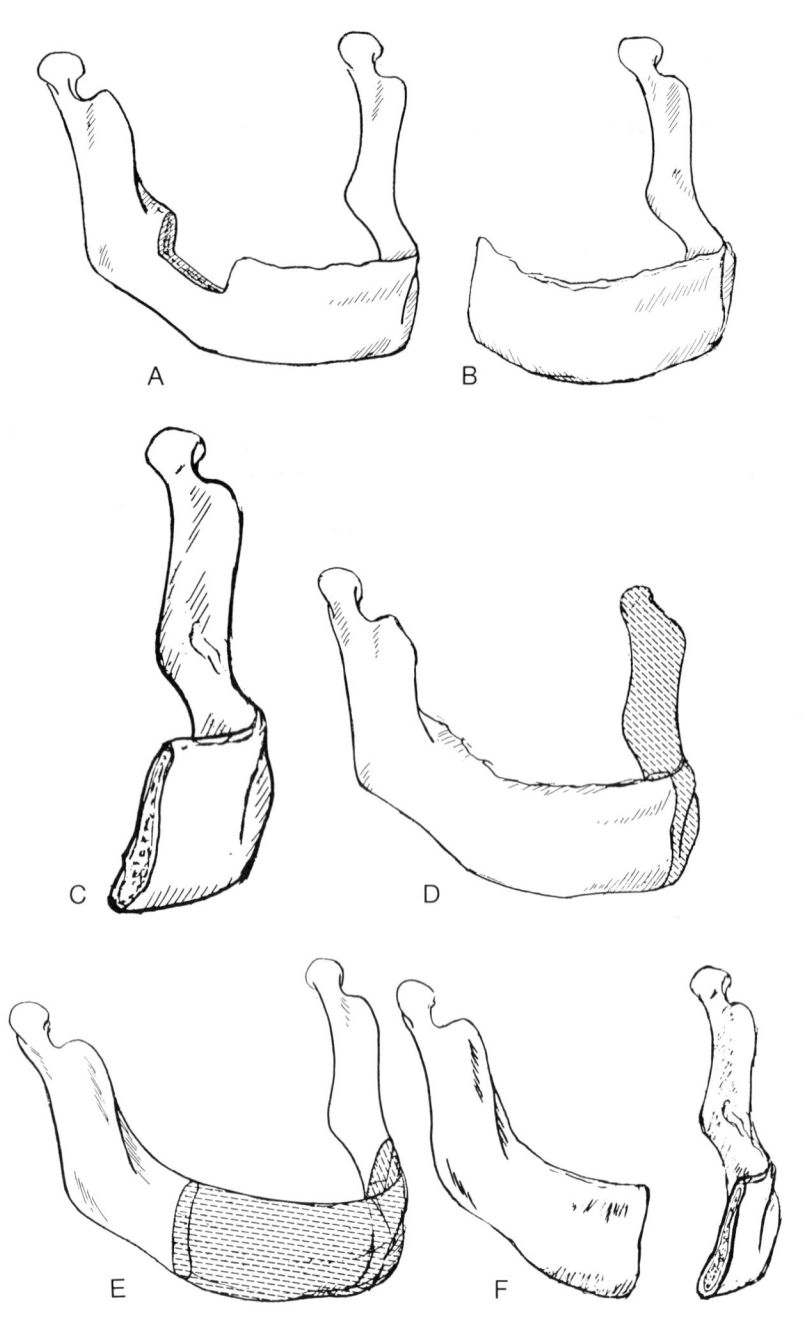

Figure 9-6. *A*, Class I mandibular resection, involving alveolar resection and preservation of mandibular continuity. *B*, Class II mandibular resection, resulting in loss of continuity distal to the canine area. *C*, Class III mandibular resection, involving a minimum of midline loss of continuity. *D*, Class IV resection of lateral portion of mandible with subsequent augmentation to restore form and function. *E*, Class V midline resection with subsequent augmentation similar to Class IV. *F*, Class VI, similar to Class V defect but with no augmentation following resection.

the region of the ascending ramus (Fig. 9-6D). The Class V mandibular continuity resection defect is caused by midline resection with preservation of bilateral temporomandibular articulation. Continuity of these segments was re-established by surgical reconstruction (Fig. 9-6E). Class VI mandibular defects are similar to those of Class V patients; however, mandibular continuity was not restored (Fig. 9-6F).

Patients who require mandibular resection that results in continuity defects are usually more difficult to rehabilitate without bony reconstruction, as viewed by the prosthodontist. As previously stated, this rehabilitation is contingent upon defect location, size, and extent, as well as the presence or absence of teeth and other supporting intraoral structures.

Physiologic concerns are related to mastication, deglutition, phonation, and respiration. Mastication is affected by the loss of mandibular continuity, teeth, bone, and musculature. These defects pose specific problems due to mandibular segment deviation, which is often noted as a medial, inferior, and posterior change in direction. Along with the segment deviation, there is also an alteration in mandibular rotation patterns. Rotation of the mandible, which is usually reproducible in the horizontal axis, often changes to a nonreproducible position following this type of resection[15] (Fig. 9-7).

Deglutition, phonation, and respiration

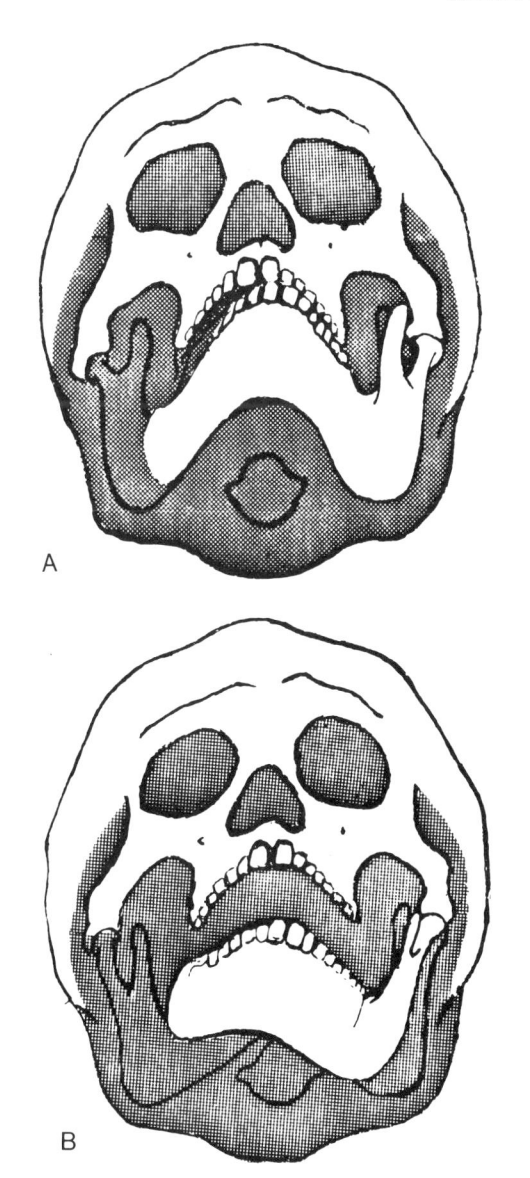

Figure 9–7. *A*, Arch and occlusal relationship relating resected to nonresected mandible to maxilla. *B*, Potential mandibular deviation of the resected arch upon opening movement.

are also affected by mandibular resection. Exact effects depend upon the reaction of hard and soft tissues, the resection of associated neurologic structures, and the undermining of tongue mass to aid in the closure of the surgical defect.

The cosmetic deficiencies associated with mandibular defects are more pronounced than those associated with maxillary defects. The results include cosmetic facial asymmetry, a direct result of mandibular deviation, loss of underlying facial hard and soft tissues, and neurologic weakness or impairment due to surgical resection.

Similarly, the psychological deficiencies associated with mandibular defects are more pronounced than those of maxillary defects. Psychological difficulties result primarily from gross physiologic and cosmetic impairment.

The primary objective of rehabilitation in patients who do not receive bony reconstruction is to retrain muscles controlling mandibular movement whenever possible. The result of this therapy may eliminate the use of a prosthesis to assist in redirecting mandibular movement.

The principles of function of the prosthesis used in patient rehabilitation are specific to the arch to which they are related. These principles are ultimately governed by the remaining maxillary and/or mandibular teeth. If teeth are absent or there are too few for prosthesis support and retention, prosthodontic rehabilitation may be limited or the patient may be rendered untreatable.

Phases of Prosthetic Management

Principles and limitations of prosthodontic treatment will be detailed as they pertain to continuity defects. Also taken into consideration will be the fact that continuity defects often need no complicated prosthodontic support. Generally, three phases of treatment are followed for mandibular continuity defect patients: extirpative surgical, interim, and reconstructive-rehabilitative. Each phase is supported by a specific prosthesis. The extirpative surgical phase utilizes maxillomandibular fixation via tooth-to-tooth, tooth-to-prosthesis, or prosthesis-to-prosthesis fixation; the interim phase utilizes physical therapy exercises and/or the maxillary inclined plane prosthesis; and the reconstructive-rehabilitative phase of treatment uses the mandibular guide flange prosthesis, maxillary occlusal table prosthesis, or no prosthesis support because of specific patient limitations.

Surgical Phase

The treatment of the patient to undergo mandibular extirpative surgery resulting in a continuity defect is initiated presurgically. Maxillomandibular fixation should be considered, using either tooth-to-tooth, tooth-to-prosthesis, or prosthesis-to-prosthesis fixation. The major advantage of fixation is the minimization of mandibular deviation resulting from scar contracture. This minimization of deviation tends to vary, however, from patient to patient depending on the surgical procedures performed and/or the use of radiation therapy.[16, 17] Rigid fixation typically is used for a period of one to two weeks. This is usually followed by elastic fixation for one to two months following surgery.

If the patient can maintain a satisfactory

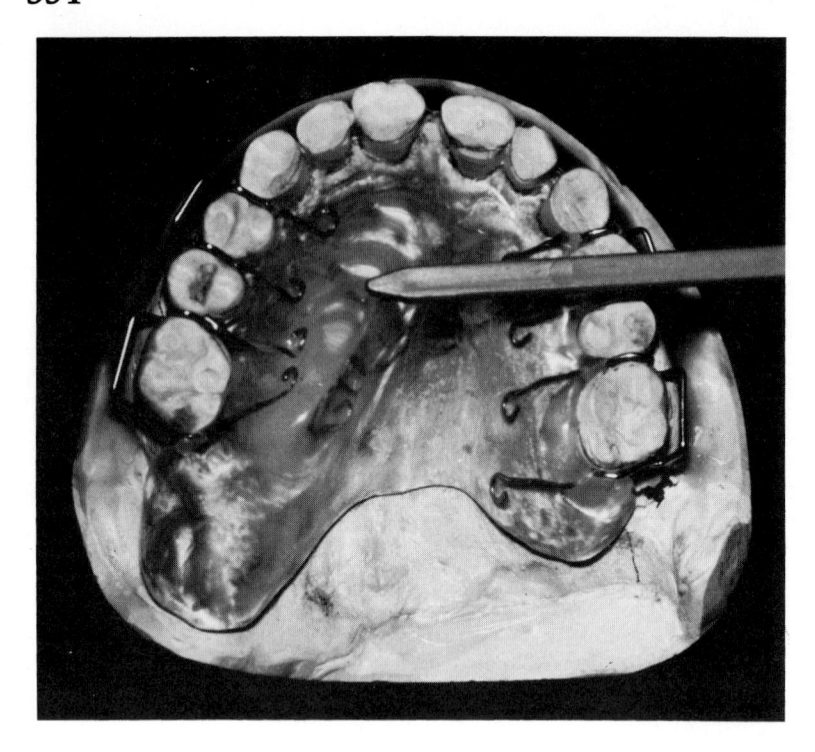

Figure 9–8. Used as a training prosthesis, the maxillary inclined plane helps guide the mandible into a better relationship with the maxilla.

relationship of mandible to maxilla following the removal of fixation, then no additional early rehabilitative prosthodontic support is required. However, if an adequate arch relationship cannot be maintained, additional prosthodontic support is necessary.

Interim Phase

Provided that a sufficient number of teeth remains in both the maxillary and mandibular arches, the maxillary inclined plane prosthesis can be fabricated. This is a training prosthesis designed with a plane inclined from the central palatal area toward the occlusal surfaces of the posterior teeth on the side opposite the mandibular defect (Fig. 9–8). The purpose of this prosthesis is to help guide the deviated mandibular segment into a more satisfactory relationship with the maxilla. The prosthesis is worn for limited periods of time throughout the day; however, it is not worn during meals or while sleeping. If there is no progress in jaw relationship achieved when the prosthesis is removed after two to three months of use, consideration must be given to other treatment alternatives.

Reconstructive-Rehabilitative Phase

The use of the mandibular guide flange prosthesis is considered reconstructive-rehabilitative treatment (Fig. 9–9). However, the use of such a prosthesis is predicated on the presence of maxillary and mandibular teeth. Without maxillary teeth for the mandibular guide flange to oppose, the use of such a prosthesis is not possible. Although the prosthesis may not be worn for extended hours during the day, it is specifically worn

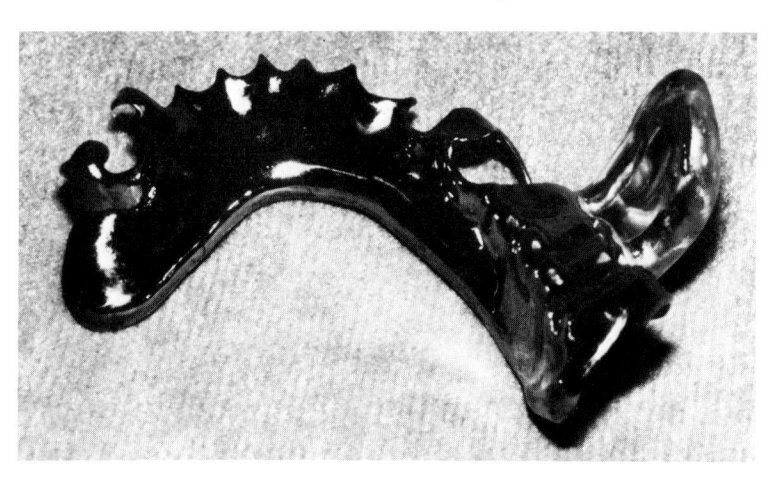

Figure 9–9. The mandibular guide flange is a "holding" prosthesis, helping to maintain maxillary-mandibular alignment.

during meals. Maxillary teeth adjacent to the mandibular flange can be moved as a result of the forces exerted on them. It is therefore necessary to cross-arch stabilize the maxillary teeth to provide adequate support.

Patients who are edentulous or whose remaining teeth may not facilitate the use of the mandibular guide flange prosthesis require additional prosthodontic consideration.

The maxillary occlusal plane or table prosthesis is used for patients who have no remaining maxillary teeth or whose remaining dentition will not support the mandibular guide flange prosthesis. The maxillary occlusal plane prosthesis is an extension of the normal occlusal plane toward the palatal midline (Fig. 9–10). The opposing dentition makes occlusal contact in a midpalatally deviated position. Masticatory function takes place in the same position.

Tongue mass is often reduced by the surgical removal of a tumor, resulting in limitation of function that is evident in the physiologic performance of mastication, deglutition, and phonation. The location and extent of the occlusal plane may aid in improving mastication and phonation by reducing the palatal vault area.

For some patients, a prosthesis cannot be used for rehabilitation purposes. Specific anatomic limitations or a low patient tolerance level does not permit the use of prostheses. In such cases, consideration should be given to the maxillary complete denture prosthesis with palatal vault modification for speech accommodation.

Because there are specific limitations and problems associated with rehabilitation of any intra-oral defect, thought must be given to surgical reconstruction, especially the re-establishment of mandibular continuity. A primary reconstructive goal should be proper alignment of the residual segment or segments with the maxillary arch. Augmentation of the height and width of the segment should also be considered. Reconstruction should allow adequate space for the mandibular and/or maxillary prosthesis and establishment of a more normal mandibular-to-maxillary tooth relationship.

Surgical reconstruction should re-establish adequate labial and lingual vestibular depth and a contour that can properly accommodate a prosthesis. Scar- and tongue-releasing procedures may be required to improve tissue and tongue mobility as well as overall functional capabilities of these patients.

Because each patient presents with individual limitations due to location, size, and extent of defects, the re-establishment of mandibular continuity must strive for ideal surgical reconstruction even though something less than ideal may ultimately result. Once surgical reconstruction has restored integrity to the arch, the patient can be given more conventional prosthodontic treatment (Fig. 9–11). As in the treatment of the maxillary defects, resilient materials* can be employed for mandibular reconstruction.

The process of rehabilitation is time-consuming and often frustrating for both the doctor and the patient. As reviewed, both maxillary and mandibular defect patients must undergo various treatment phases involving the fabrication of different prostheses. The total rehabilitative process may take several months or more to complete. It really never ends, because successful outcome of treatment is seen only when patients are followed on a routine recall basis.

RECONSTRUCTION OF MANDIBULAR CONTINUITY DEFECTS

SURGICAL APPROACH

Biologic Basis of Bony Reconstruction

As compared to other connective tissues, healing of bone and bone grafts is somewhat unique in that healing arises from tissue re-

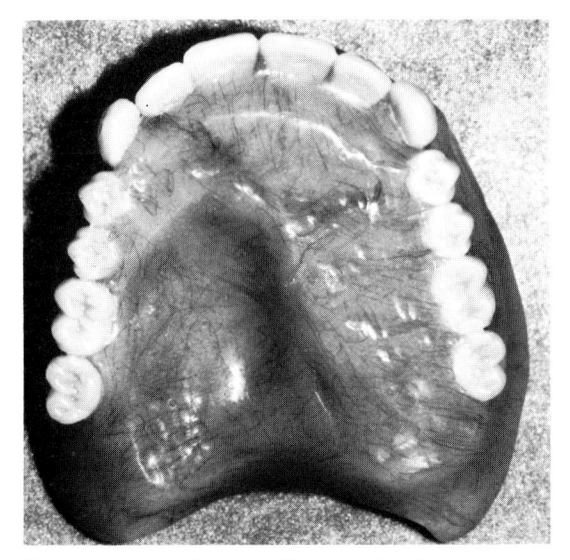

Figure 9–10. The maxillary occlusal table prosthesis allows mastication to occur at a deviated midline position.

---

*Softic 49—Kerr/Sybron Corporation, Romulus, MI.

356 / RECONSTRUCTION AND REHABILITATION OF CANCER PATIENTS

Figure 9–11. Patient augmentation series. *A,* Frontal view of patient following mandibular augmentation, prior to prosthodontic rehabilitation. *B,* Panoramic radiograph of the patient immediately following augmentation and fixation. *C,* Panoramic radiograph of the patient two years following augmentation. *D,* Intraoral view of the patient following augmentation, vestibuloplasty, and skin grafting. *E,* Tissue surface mandibular prosthesis showing definitive resilient liner (Softic 49).

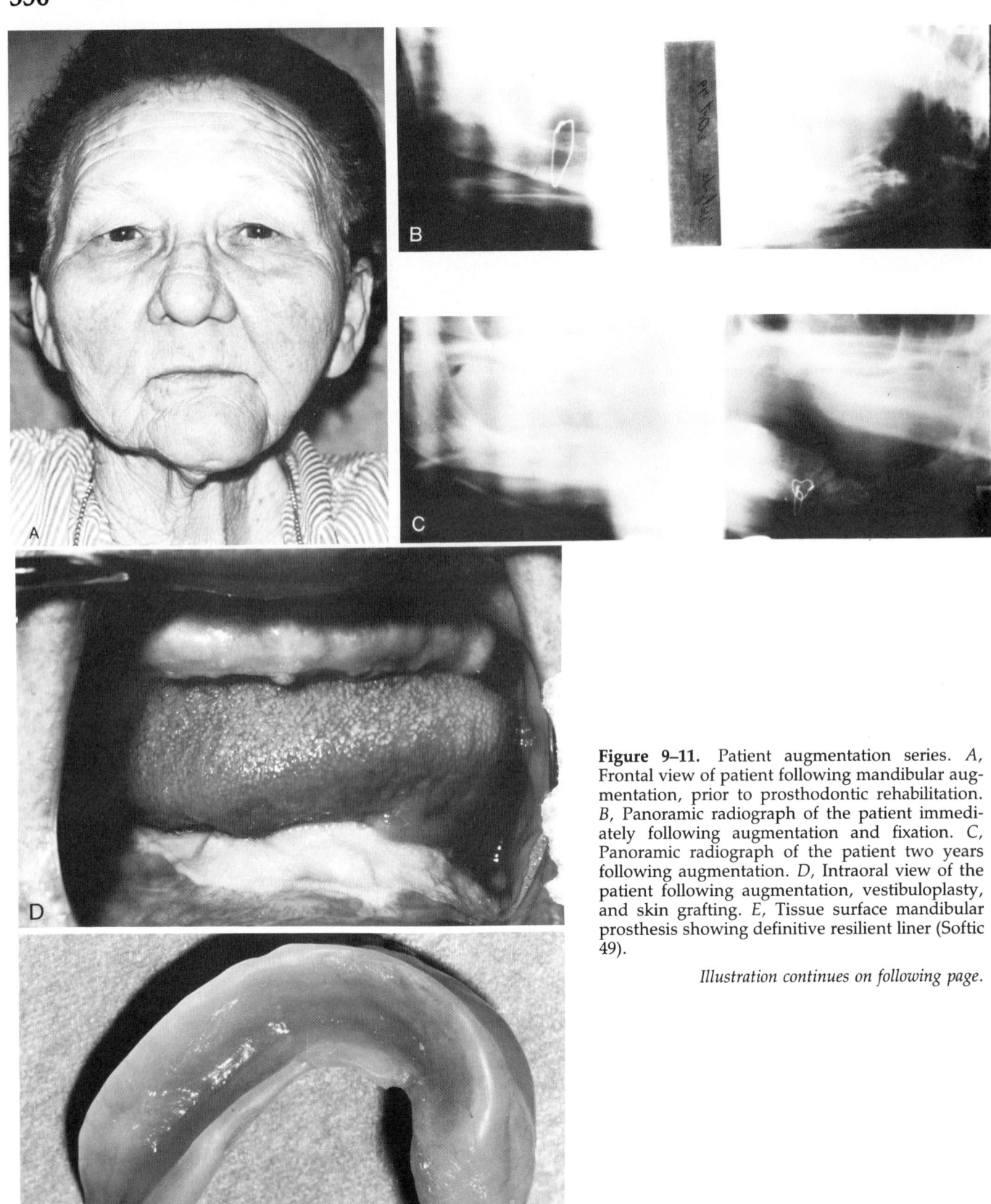

Illustration continues on following page.

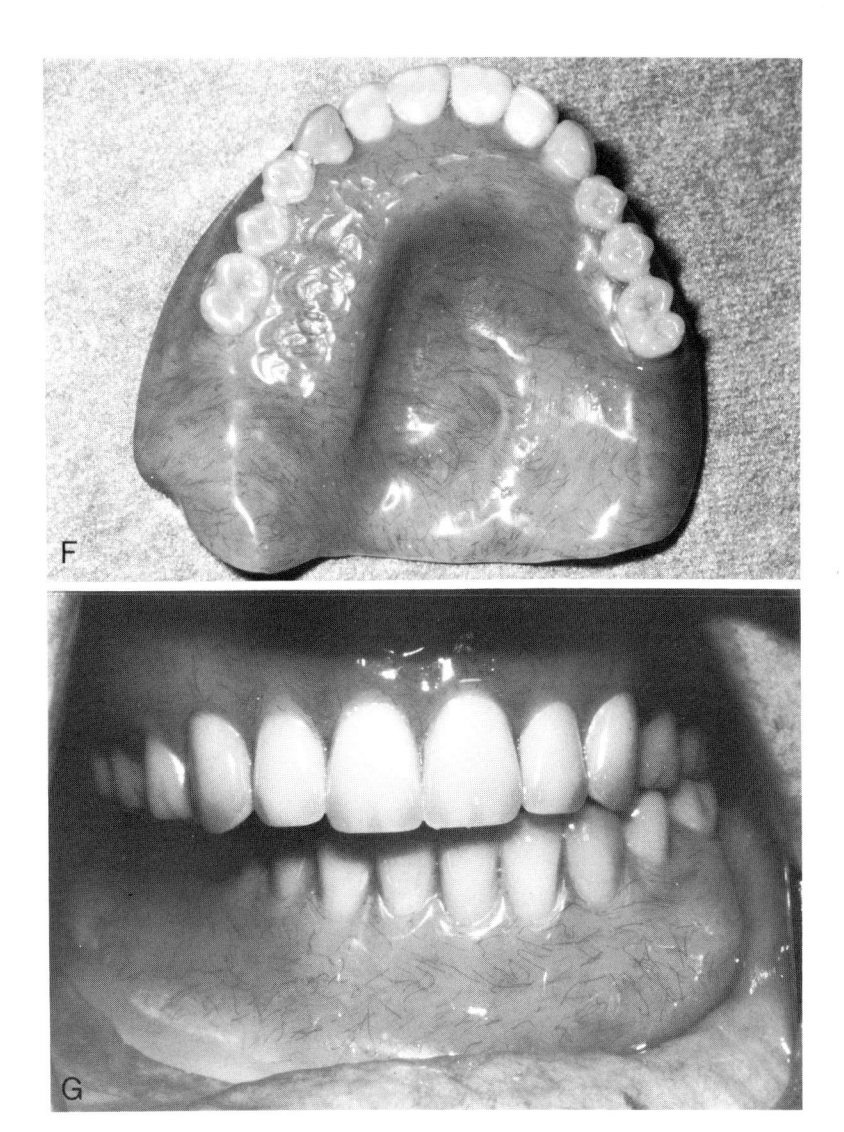

Figure 9–11 *Continued. F,* Occlusal view of maxillary prosthesis showing occlusal table. *G,* Intraoral view of maxillary-mandibular prosthesis. *H,* Frontal view of patient following augmentation and prosthesis placement.

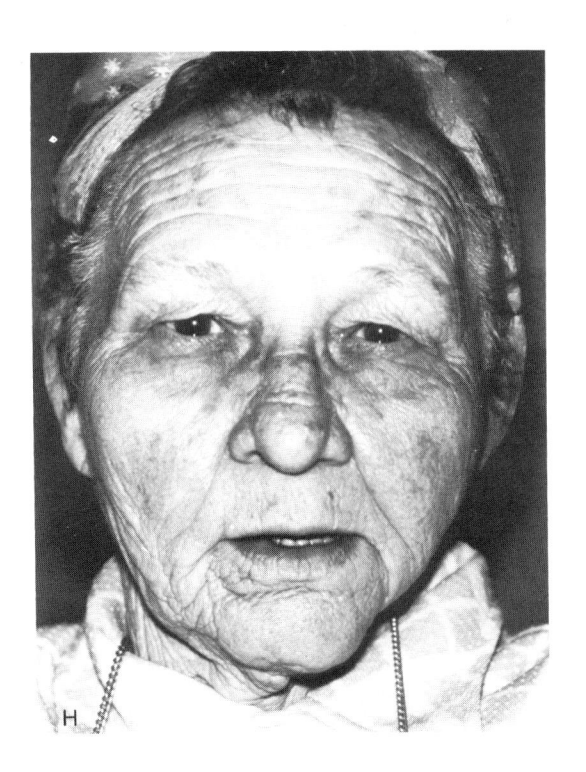

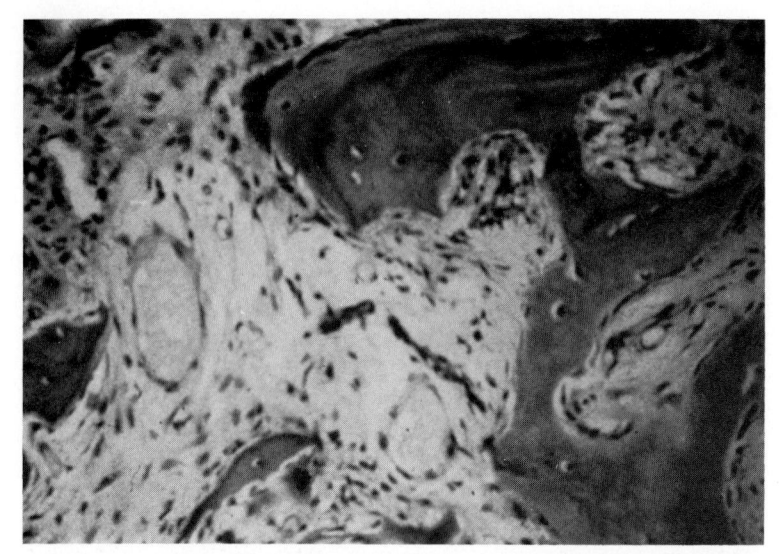

Figure 9–12. Cancellous bone harvested from the ilium. Endosteal osteoblasts and marrow mesenchymal cells are those osteogenic cells rather than osteocytes (H & E, × 60).

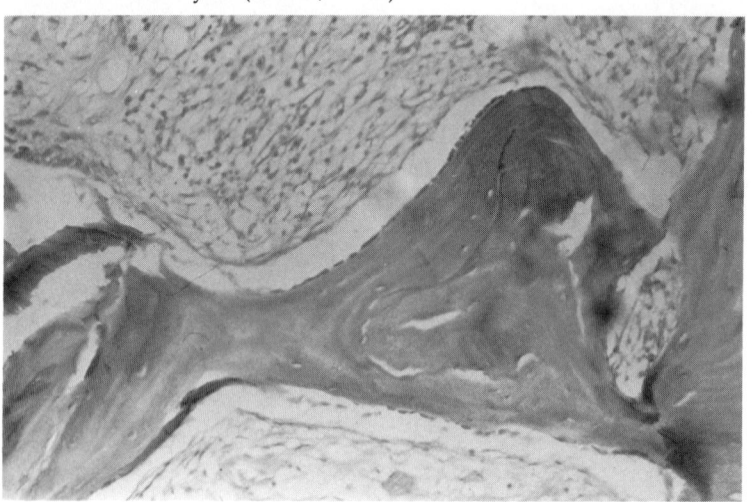

Figure 9–13. Phase-one bone formation around nonviable bone particle from transplanted mineral matrix. Prominent endosteal osteoblast layer seen at periphery of new bone (H & E, × 60).

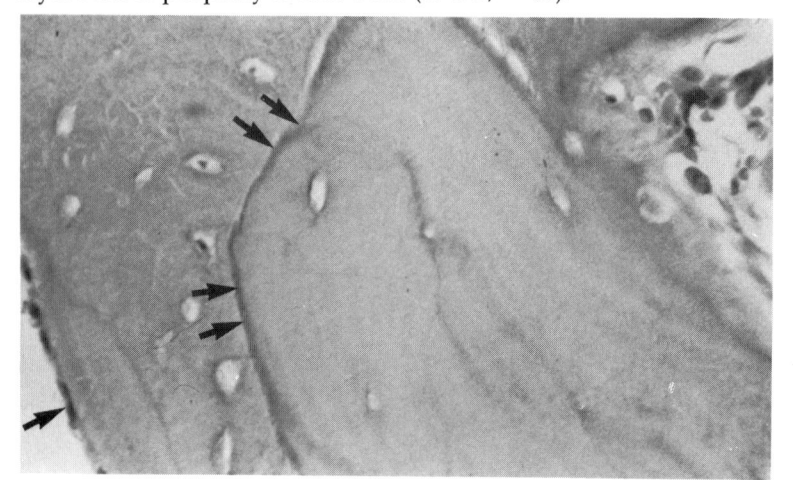

Figure 9–14. Cellular phase-one bone evidenced by nuclei within lacunae produced around nonviable mineral matrix evidenced by empty lacunae. Endosteal osteoblasts (single arrow) began as surface cells of original bone particle transplant (double arrow) (H & E, × 150).

generation rather than from simple tissue repair with scar. It therefore requires both the element of cellular proliferation, as does epithelial healing, and the element of collagen synthesis more common to connective tissue repair.

There is now overwhelming evidence supporting the two-phase theory of osteogenesis[18–20] as originally proposed by Axhausen.[21] This theory states that bone formed in a bone transplant initially arises from transplanted cells that have survived transplantation, have proliferated, and have formed new osteoid (Figs. 9–12 to 9–14). The first phase of bone regeneration forms bone in a random and haphazard fashion dependent on the spatial orientation of the grafted tissue (Fig. 9–14). It also has been shown to be most active within the first four weeks after transplantation and then to wane as the second phase of bone regeneration assumes the dominant role.

This second phase consists of osteogenesis derived from cells of the host connective tissue bed and host bone (Figs. 9–15 and 9–16). The role of the second phase is resorption remodeling, whereby the immature and haphazard bone formed in phase one is replaced by mature osteons with an organized structure (Fig. 9–15). The second phase requires an induction of host fibroblasts, which grow into the grafted tissue. This induction has been shown to be mediated by bone morphogenetic protein (BMP) derived from the mineral matrix of the transplanted bone.[22, 23] Bone morphogenetic protein is an acid-insoluble protein of 23,000 molecular weight that has the ability to affect the genetic machinery of mesenchymal tissues. It directs the differentiation of inducible cells, such as fibroblasts, along osteoblastic lines so that they synthesize type I collagen and form hydroxyapatite salts for bone matrix production (Fig. 9–17). The second phase begins about two weeks after grafting and increases in activity to peak in six weeks to six months. It then slowly decreases but does not cease activity as the graft continues to remodel dynamically.

The first phase of bone regeneration is clinically important because it dictates the quantity of bone that the graft will form. The second phase does not actually produce new bone quantity but rather replaces the bone of phase one. This bone is capable of existing without resorption owing to an organized structure and a functional periosteum (Fig. 9–16). Bone graft techniques need to support both phases of bone regeneration to be successful. Grafts that do not support phase one with transplantation of a sufficient number of viable osteocompetent cells will form

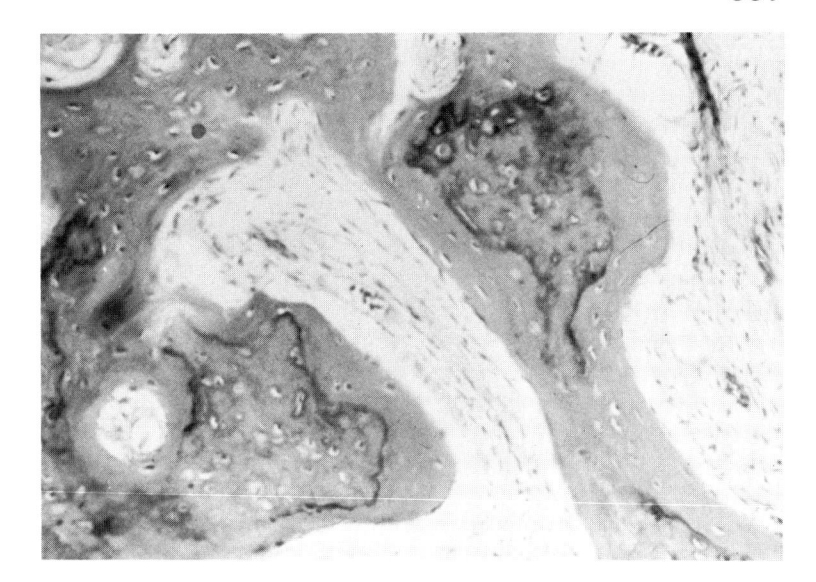

Figure 9–15. Haphazard cellular phase-one bone replaced by phase-two bone derived from mesenchymal elements within the graft (H & E, × 60).

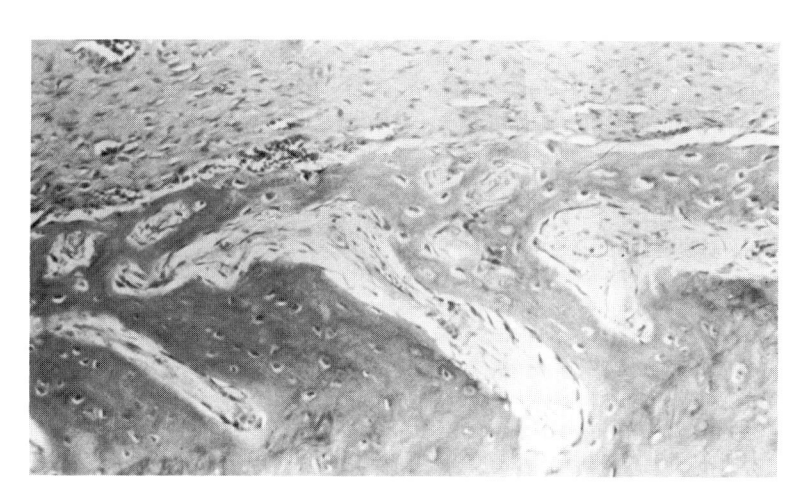

Figure 9–16. Host connective tissue bed acting as a functional periosteum maintaining the osseous content of the graft. (H & E, × 100).

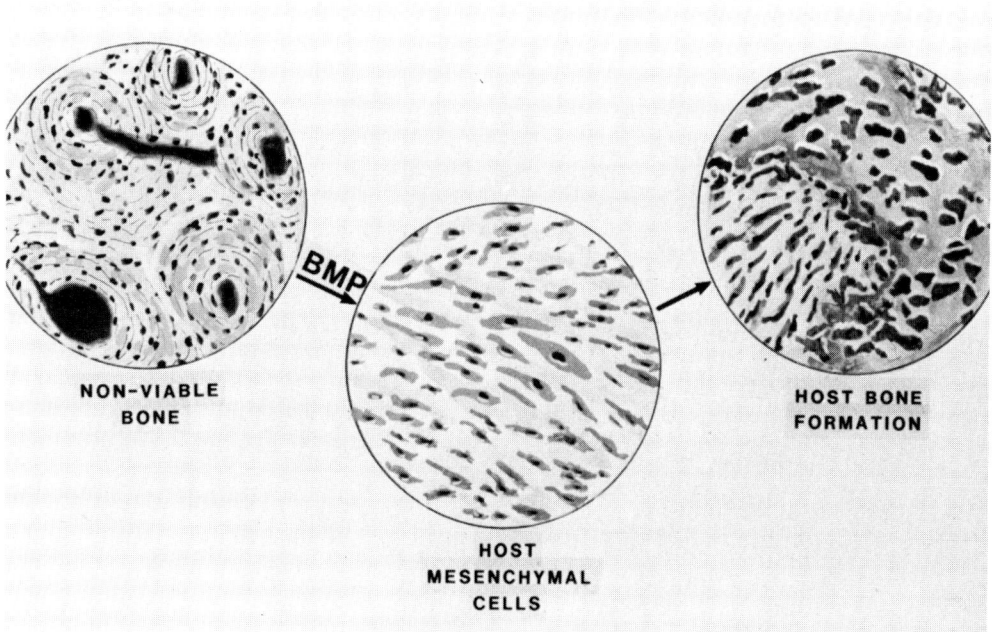

Figure 9–17. Bone induction principle: bone morphogenetic protein–mediated host bone formation from viable or nonviable bone source.

BONE INDUCTION PRINCIPLE

NON-VIABLE BONE → BMP → HOST MESENCHYMAL CELLS → HOST BONE FORMATION

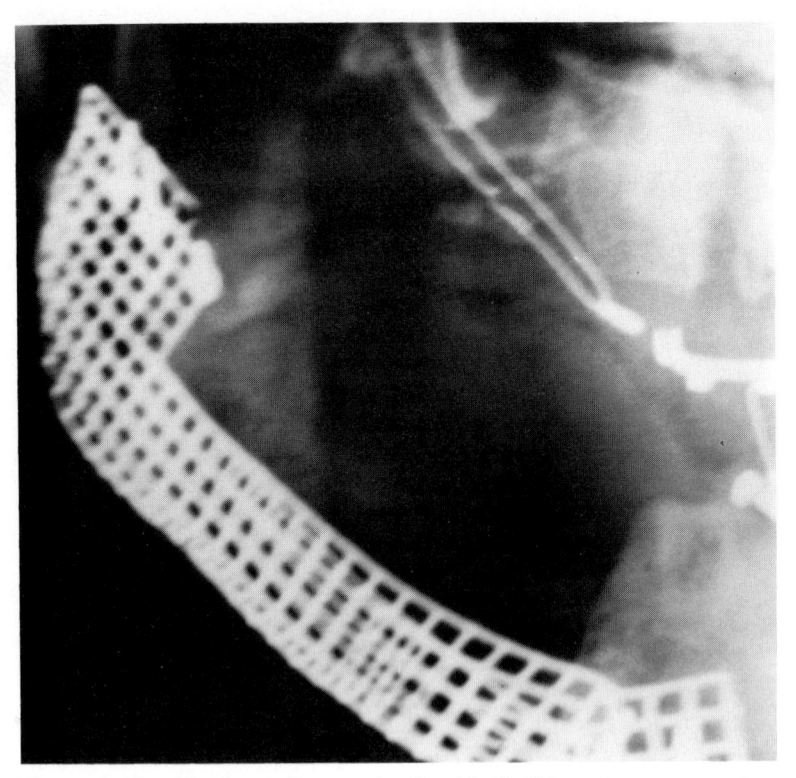

360 / RECONSTRUCTION AND REHABILITATION OF CANCER PATIENTS

Figure 9–18. Rigid stainless steel crib with PBCM graft at two weeks.

a bony ossicle of a reduced size as compared to the original transplanted material.

Friedenstein has shown that the quantity of osteogenesis is directly proportional to the density of cells packed into diffusion chambers.[24] Simmons et al. confirmed this work and identified the osteoprogenitor cells as the endosteal osteoblasts on the bone surfaces of cancellous bone (see Fig. 9–12).[25] The clinician can, therefore, enhance phase-one bone formation by using donor bone with a high cancellous-to-cortical ratio, such as the ilium. Most importantly, he/she can condense the graft material to a high cellular density. Grafts that do not support phase two will evidence resorption of the initial bone ossicle formed in phase one.

The phenomenon of bone graft resorption is familiar to oral and maxillofacial surgeons, especially in reconstructions of cancer-related defects in irradiated patients. This phenomenon was once attributed to the functional matrix theory, which suggested that resorption was induced by metallic cribs that absorbed the functional stresses to the graft. However, this phenomenon was not universally seen in grafts in which metallic cribs were used (Figs. 9–18 and 9–19) but was also seen in many situations in which a crib was not used (Fig. 9–20). This explanation amounted to a misinterpretation of the functional matrix theory as originally proposed by Moss et al.[26, 27] Such bone graft resorption actually occurs because the bone derived from phase one is resorbed without replacement by phase-two bone. This may occur if the recipient tissue bed does not contain a sufficient number of cells capable of induction or if the transplanted bone contains too little BMP to induce host fibroblasts that have grown into the graft. Irradiated tissue is typically hypocellular in inducible fibroblasts (see Fig. 9–5).

Such tissue evidences resorption of bone grafts because there are insufficient numbers of cells to replace phase-one bone and form a periosteum around the graft. The clinician has some control over phase-two bone production. He can derive the maximum contribution from the second phase by ensuring that the recipient bed is as cellular and as vascular as possible. This can be achieved to some degree by limiting the scarring produced by the extirpative surgery. Other techniques include employing a functional neck dissection where possible, transposing uncompromised tissue into the recipient bed with muscle or myocutaneous flaps, or hyperbaric oxygen induction of fibroplasia and angiogenesis prior to reconstruction.

One can also stimulate the second phase by ensuring that sufficient BMP is transplanted within the graft material. How much is sufficient is not exactly known, but Urist has identified the greatest concentration of BMP to be within the mineral cortex of bone.[23] Although we use primarily cancellous bone from the ilium, packed very densely

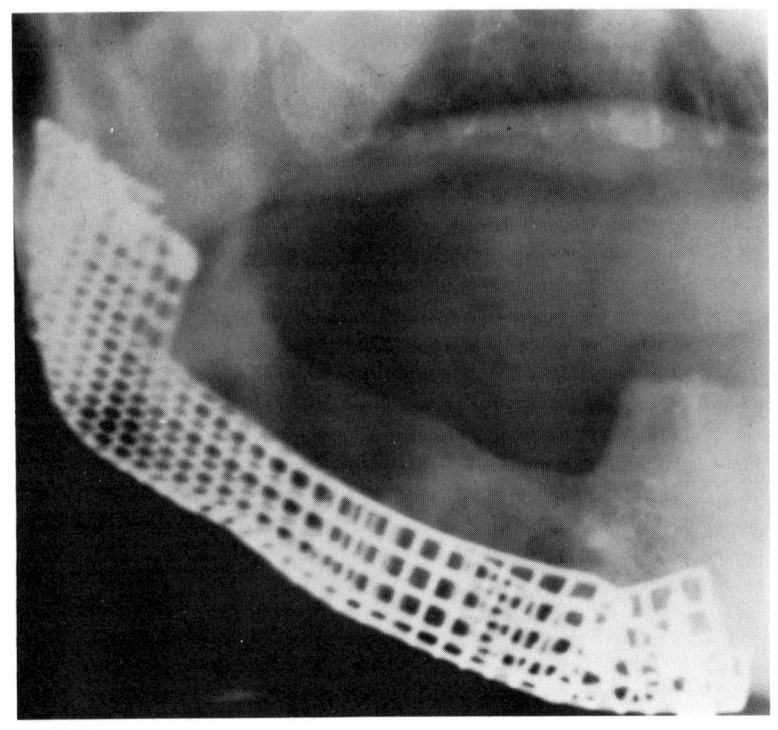

Figure 9–19. Six-year follow-up radiograph of the patient in Figure 9–18, evidencing a well-consolidated graft that has not undergone resorption.

into the recipient bed to support phase one, we also harvest chips of the lateral iliac cortex for a source of BMP within the graft. The addition of cortical chips has not been tested in a controlled fashion, but it does have some theoretical merit and has been associated with excellent clinical results.

The application of the two-phase concept of bone regeneration in facial bone reconstruction is a necessity for consistently successful results. Several steps can be taken to enhance the contributions from each phase. They include preparation of the recipient tissue bed, alteration of the composition of transplanted bone, and alteration of the method of graft placement to improve the quantity of bone produced by the graft as well as the length of time it lasts. In addition, the merits of each clinical bone graft system in use today can be assessed by their ability to take advantage of contributions afforded in each phase of bone regeneration.

Goals of Mandibular Reconstruction

There are currently five basic approaches for reconstructing the resected mandible with autogenous bone grafts: block cortical-cancellous grafts, particulate bone cancellous marrow (PBCM) grafts within alloplastic cribs, PBCM grafts within allogeneic bone cribs, osteomyocutaneous grafts, and microvascular bone periosteal grafts. None is universally successful. Each has some physiologic and technical advantage or disadvantage. The physiologic merits of each system should be assessed in terms of their ability to derive functional bone from both phase-one and phase-two bone regeneration. The technical merits of each system must be evaluated in the context of patient morbidity, simplicity of instrumentation, and feasibility of achieving a high percentage of successful results. In mandibular reconstruction, the following five goals must be worked toward and achieved before the graft can be termed a success.

Restoration of Continuity. The restoration of continuity provides the greatest restoration of function. A continuous mandible restores the mechanical advantage in mastication to nearly normal masticatory efficiency. This can be achieved despite previous extirpation of some muscles of mastication and/or suprahyoid opening muscles. Correction of jaw deviation while restoring continuity will also restore facial symmetry. In addition, reconstruction of a solid continuous mandible without deviation helps alleviate the patient's negative self-image.

Restoration of Alveolar Bone Height. A

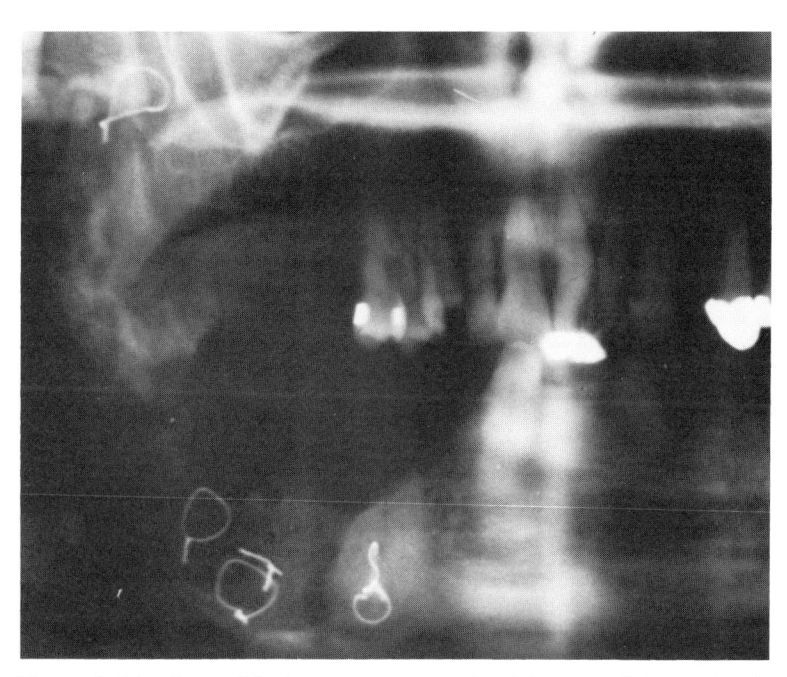

Figure 9–20. Large block autogenous graft without rigid internal crib, evidencing prominent resorption at 18 months particularly noted at graft center.

mandibular reconstruction that fails to restore alveolar bone height is an incomplete success. Complete functional rehabilitation requires a stable denture-bearing surface of adequate alveolar height and width.

Restoration of Osseous Bulk. Too often pencil-thin mandibular grafts are termed "successful" when they are actually incapable of supporting function or a prosthesis. Pathologic fractures are common in these grafts. Restoration of osseous bulk is mandatory if the graft is to accommodate the functional demands placed upon it without resorption or fracture.

Maintenance of Osseous Content (minimum follow-up—18 months). Grafts lacking a phase-two contribution are not dynamic enough to remodel. They may undergo resorption due to function, nonfunction, or poor revascularization and are of little value to the patient. In our experience, bone graft resorption has been unrelated to function, lack of function, or the presence of rigid internal fixation trays or plates. Instead, it has been observed that late resorption is related to a diminished or absent phase-two contribution secondary to a diminished cellularity and/or vascularity of the recipient soft-tissue bed. If resorption occurs unrelated to a procedural complication, such as a wound infection or dehiscence, it occurs within the first 18 months, usually between six months and one year. In our experience, a graft that shows no evidence of resorption by 18 months continues to function without resorption throughout the patient's lifetime.

Restoration of Acceptable Facial Form.
The overall goal in reconstruction of the cancer patient is to enable him or her to return to the mainstream of life. Restoration of function and rehabilitation of the dentition is not always enough because the patient bases much of his self-image on his appearance. Restoration of facial form is necessary if patients are to return to their families and society as participating members.

Basic Surgical Technique

The practical aspects of soft-tissue dissection, prevention of graft infection, handling of the graft, and fixation and immobilization of the graft support the physiologic aspects of bone regeneration. Every effort should be made to place the graft into an infection-free, vascular, recipient tissue rich in inducible fibroblasts.

Several practical considerations appear to be important in the handling of harvested bone grafts. It is advantageous to place the bone into the recipient tissue as soon as possible. The timing of bone harvest and bone placement should be closely coordinated. Once bone has been harvested, it should immediately be placed in a saline solution. At one time, a blood-soaked sponge was thought to be the preferred storage medium; however, work by Marx et al. has shown that saline is the superior storage medium and that products of clotted blood are actually cytotoxic to graft cells.[28] Antibiotic solutions should also be avoided, as they do not protect against wound infection and may also be cytotoxic to graft cells. Studies have shown cancellous marrow cells to be hardy cells capable of 95 per cent survival after four hours storage in saline at operating room temperature.[28]

The practical considerations of the soft tissue dissection should be obvious to all surgeons. The careful handling of soft tissue, the elimination of dead space, and the preservation of vascularity are basic to all surgery. Considerations unique to reconstructing the mandible after cancer surgery include the following:

1. The approach should be strictly transcutaneous. Transoral bone graft placement incorporates the contamination of oral flora, dramatically increasing the potential for infection.

2. The incision should be as low in the neck as possible. This allows for closure without tension after a superior repositioning of the incision line that can occur because the graft adds contour to the tissue. An incision at the level of the superior margin of the larynx is useful (Fig. 9–21). If the upper member of a McFee neck dissection or other horizontal scar is present in the neck, excising the scar is a reasonable approach. The skin incision is made with a scalpel, after which the remainder of the sharp dissection can be done with an electrocautery knife or commercially available "Hot Knives.". We use the standard "Bovie" unit with a tapered tip. Tissue that is held under tension may easily be sectioned with the "Bovie" unit coagulation mode. In this manner we have observed a reduction in blood loss and a more visible surgical field without a significant char effect seen with the cutting mode.

3. Dissect the recipient tissue bed as close to the oral mucosa as possible without perforating into the mouth. Restoring the alveolar bone height and osseous bulk is facilitated in this manner. To achieve this, dissection is carried to the level of the fascia over the digastric muscles and turned superiorly to expose the remaining mandibular segments. Anteriorly, the plane of dissection becomes the fascia overlying the sternohyoid muscle inferiorly and the anterior belly of the digastric superiorly. Dissecting the proximal and distal mandibular segments and reflecting periosteum for a short distance help define the extent of dissection. The soft tissue between the segments is dissected, using each bone end as a rough guide to prevent oral perforation. As the dissection approaches the oral mucosa, one can palpate

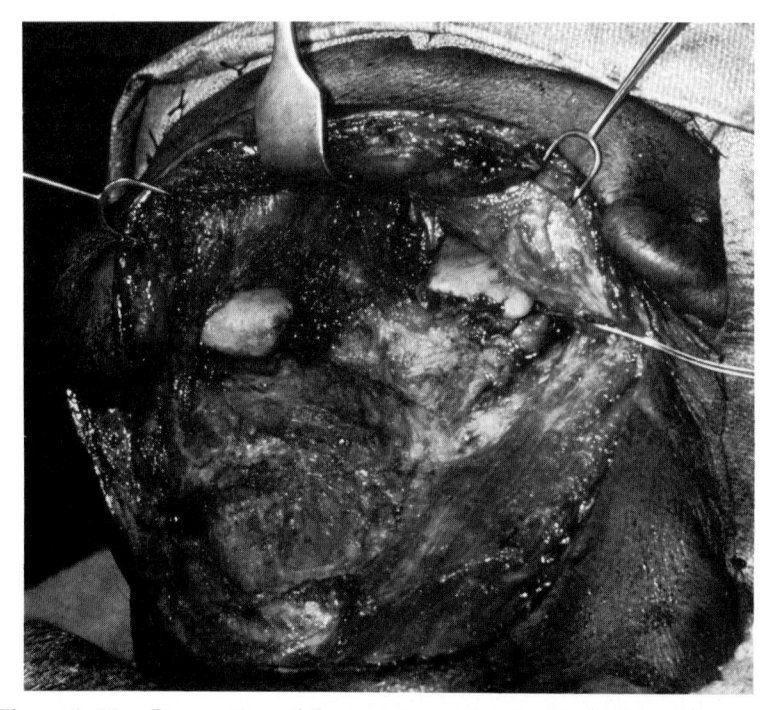

Figure 9–21. Preparation of the recipient tissue bed is facilitated by an incision at the level of the larynx and exposure of the proximal and distal bone segments prior to developing the graft bed between them.

the maxillary teeth or maxillary denture to judge the thickness of remaining mucosa (Fig. 9–21).

4. Remove the coronoid process in every case in which it has not been removed by the extirpative surgery. Removal of the coronoid will eliminate the temporalis pull, which prevents adequate repositioning of the proximal segment. It is advisable to remove the coronoid process rather than to allow it to retract superiorly. If not removed, it will rest in the posterior maxillary vestibule and can interfere with the denture flange. The coronoid can be chipped into small pieces and added to the graft material as a source of BMP.

5. Eliminate dead space by suturing the deep tissue to the graft. Often a subtle dead space medial to the graft can develop a hematoma and infection. To eliminate this medial dead space and to approximate the recipient tissue closely to the graft, one can suture deep tissue to the graft through bur holes placed in the graft or crib.

6. Close without tension in several layers. It is important to eliminate as much of the dead space as one can with the closure. Most studies indicate a higher incidence of wound infection related to dead space by virtue of requiring less of a microflora inoculum to produce a clinical infection.[29] One should begin the closure by closing the deep surface of the cover flap to the deep tissue of the recipient bed at the inferior margin of the graft (Fig. 9–22). This will envelope the graft within connective tissue and should eliminate dead space as well as closely approximate the vascular and cellular elements of the host tissue bed to the graft. The remainder of the cover flap should be closed to the deep tissue of the recipient bed inferior to the graft. Once this is accomplished, there is often a separation of wound edges amounting to several centimeters due to the added contour provided by the graft. One should not attempt to close this by stretching or advancing the superiorly based cover flap. The closure should be accomplished at the expense of the neck tissue inferior to this separation. The superior flap contains much of the vascular pedicle for the graft as well as the facial nerve branches. It should have been dissected close to the oral mucosa; further dissection would risk perforation and resultant contamination. Advancement of the tissue in the neck may be accomplished by undermining inferiorly to the level of the clavicle (Fig. 9–23). One can even continue the undermining dissection, if necessary, past the clavicle onto the anterior chest wall. The dissection should be at a depth that includes the platysma. If the platysma is not recognizable because of denervation atrophy, the plane of undermining should be superficial to the fascia over the strap muscles of the neck. Closure should be accomplished with the head in a relaxed or neutral position. Since much of our dissection for recipient tissue bed preparation is carried out with the head extended, one must remember to change the head position. Most closures can then be accomplished with minimal undermining in the neck.

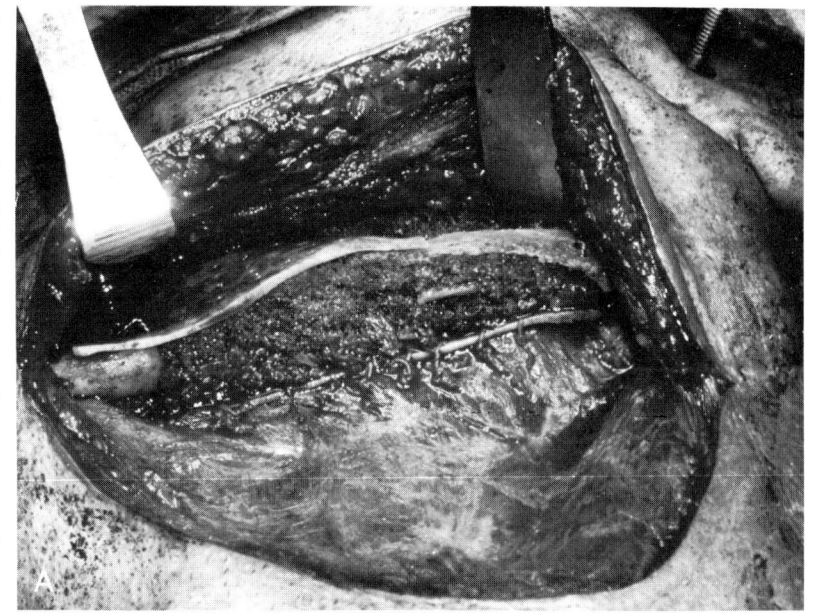

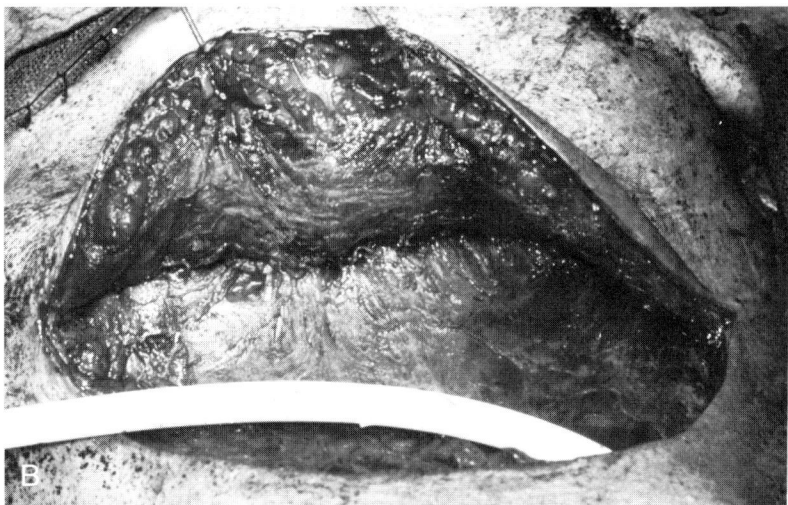

Figure 9–22. *A*, Bone graft in place with retractors reflecting superiorly based cover flap. *B*, Initial level of closure is to envelope the graft by closing the deep surface of the cover flap to the connective tissue at the base of the dissection at the graft's inferior margin.

One can resort to local transposition flaps or a sternocleidomastoid myocutaneous flap for closures in necks that are too scarred to be capable of advancement with undermining alone. The undermined skin can be converted into a rotational transposition flap by extending the incision into the posterior triangle and gradually curving it to extend ver-

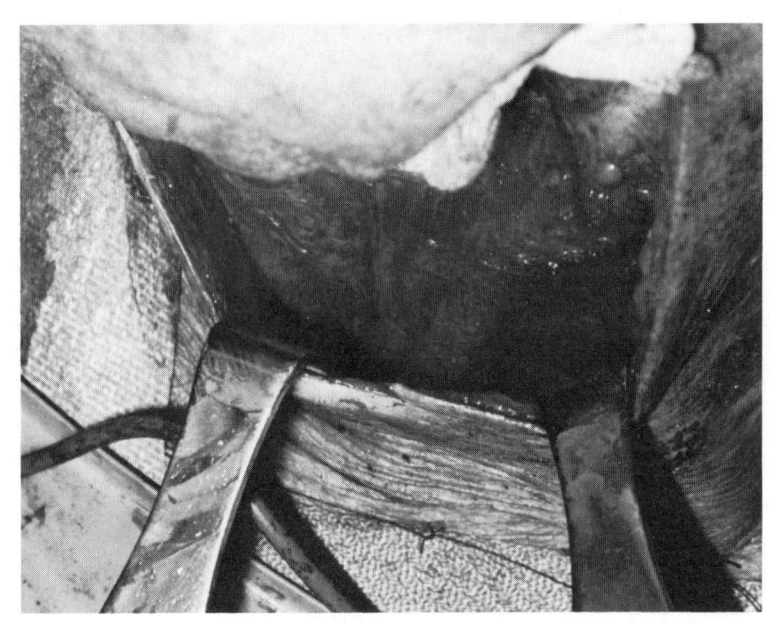

Figure 9–23. Closure often requires undermining tissue in the neck to the level of the clavicle. Advancement of tissue to gain closure should be accomplished at the expense of the inferior neck tissue rather than the superior cover flap.

tically (Fig. 9–24) within the posterior triangle. The flap retains its vascular pedicle and can be advanced along the curvilinear incision to close the superior cover flap. If the sternocleidomastoid is present, it can be used as a mastoid-based myocutaneous flap and can be placed into the wound separation (Fig. 9–25). Details of this flap will be discussed further in this chapter. The decision of whether to employ this flap, however, must be made prior to undermining the skin over the muscle. Such undermining disrupts the perforating vessels from the muscle to the overlying skin and can result in loss of the entire skin paddle.

7. Drain the wound with a continuous-suction drain. Drain it at the most inferior and posterior dependent area of the wound. Because drains serve as a pathway for organisms to enter the wound as well as evacuating drainage, we generally keep the drains in place only until less than 50 ml of drainage is collected over 24 hours. This usually allows us to discontinue the drain between 48 and 72 hours after surgery. A pressure dressing is recommended. It is also advisable to continue the pressure dressing for 24 to 48 hours after the drain is removed, a time when reaccumulation of fluid and blood may occur.

8. Prophylactic systemic antibiotics of the clinician's choice are indicated. We currently use a cephalosporin with high activity against staphyloccocus, but penicillin has also proven to be effective. One should begin the prophylactic coverage with intravenous antibiotics one hour before surgery begins. The intraoperative antibiotic dose should be 3 to 5 million units of penicillin or 3 to 4 grams of cefoxitin or its equivalent. Antibiotics are continued for only three to five days unless a wound complication develops.

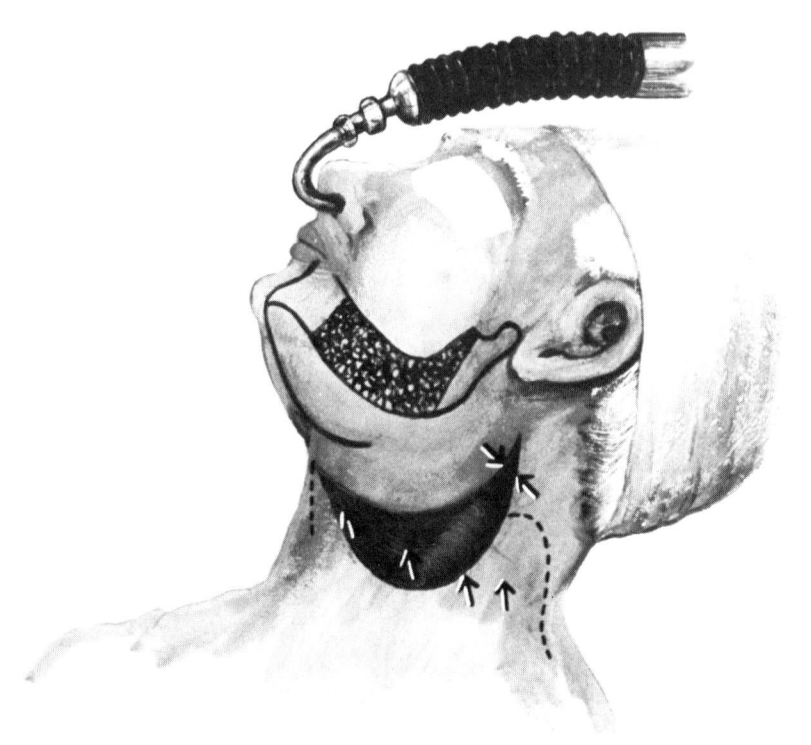

Figure 9–24. Extension of the incision into the posterior triangle in a vertical direction will often allow advancement for closure in difficult cases.

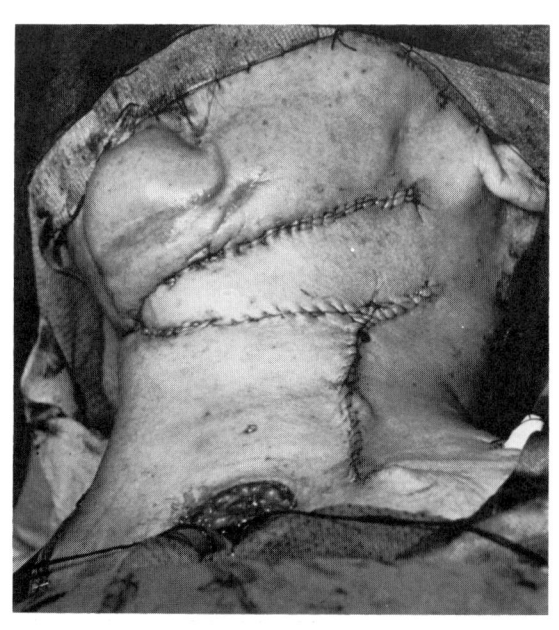

Figure 9–25. Sternocleidomastoid myocutaneous flap can also be placed into a neck wound to gain closure in difficult cases.

9. If oral perforation occurs during the dissection, one should close the opening through the extra-oral wound and irrigate with extensive amounts of saline. An attempt to rotate local tissue into the area of perforation is also of value. We have found muscle transpositions of sternocleidomastoid, digastric, or stylohyoid to be useful. Placement of the bone graft material can then proceed as planned. Closure can be accomplished in the same manner, although a suction drain should not be used. Since no closure is absolutely without seepage, a suction drain will tend to pull saliva and oral organisms into the wound. This situation can best be managed with a Penrose-type drain and pressure dressings. One should also consider extending the antibiotic coverage and using a drug with good activity against anaerobes common to oral flora. It is reasonable to add clindamycin 300 mg q6h if penicillin or one of the cephalosporins is used. If cefoxitin or cefobid is employed, good activity against anaerobes should exist, particularly of the *Bacteroides* genus, which is uncharacteristic of most other cephalosporins. These modifications will not absolutely prevent a graft infection but will somewhat reduce its potential.

Block Autogenous Grafts

Block autogenous grafts are not recommended for reconstruction of cancer-related defects. Although they initially fill the void with mineralized bone and provide a pleasing radiographic picture, their history is associated with nonunions,[30] pathologic fractures,[30, 31] and progressive resorption, particularly noted at the graft center[31] (see Fig. 9–20). Their failure can be seen as an inadequate formation of phase-one bone. The majority of tissue transplanted is mineralized cortical bone. Phase-one bone regeneration is reduced because fewer endosteal osteoblasts are transplanted. The most populous cell transplanted in this graft system is the osteocyte within its lacuna. Osteocytes have been shown to degenerate shortly after transplantation and do not contribute osteogenesis to bone regeneration.[32] In addition, Enneking et al. have shown revascularization of block grafts to be delayed[33] so that the few transplanted osteocompetent cells have a reduced survival potential. Enneking has also described such grafts to develop resorption cavities as revascularization takes place.[34] As each osteon is slowly revascularized, osteoclasts resorb bone.[34, 35] Few graft-derived bone cells (phase one bone) are available to replace this resorbed bone, and induced host fibroblasts are not capable of regenerating new bone as they are of replacing and remodeling existing viable bone (phase two). Since bone resorption precedes any bone apposition, creating large resorption cavities, pathologic fractures can be expected. Their location is predictably in the graft center. Limited bone proliferation from each host bone end creates a relatively weak area in the center.

PBCM Grafts Within Alloplastic Cribs

Particulate bone and cancellous marrow (PBCM) is the most osteogenic graft material a surgeon can employ. An advantage is its ability to transplant sufficient numbers of endosteal osteoblasts, marrow mesenchymal cells capable of induction, and BMP. It therefore derives significant contributions from both phase-one and phase-two bone regeneration. Its particulate form also permits enhanced survival of transplanted cells. This material permits unimpeded diffusion of nutrients prior to vascularization and unimpeded vascular ingrowth. The particulate form does, however, require some type of crib framework.

Several materials have been proposed for containing PBCM grafts. The most popular has been titanium,[36] but many other materials have their advocates: stainless steel,[37] Dacron-polyurethane,[38] and Teflon,[39] among others (see Figs. 9–28 to 9–31). Each manufacturer offers a unique advantage of his crib. Teflon is supposed to be inert and smooth. Dacron-polyurethane is easily contoured and radiolucent so that metal will not interfere with the radiographic assessment of the graft. Stainless steel is "custom made" on small, medium, or large dry specimens and is rigid so that jaw fixation is not required. Titanium is pliable but has enough rigidity to obviate jaw fixation.

However, the most important advantage of each system is that it permits the use of PBCM. Each crib can produce consistently successful results based not on the physical properties of the crib but on the vascularity and cellularity of the host tissue. No one alloplastic crib system has any dramatic advantage over another. The phenomenon of bone resorption within the crib is not related to a crib's depriving the jaw of functional stimulation. The phenomenon is related only to a loss of either phase-one or phase-two bone regeneration (Figs. 9–26 and 9–27). Alloplastic cribs need not be chosen or avoided for this reason. The biggest problem with alloplastic cribs in cancer-related defects is poor tolerance in thin, scarred, and irradi-

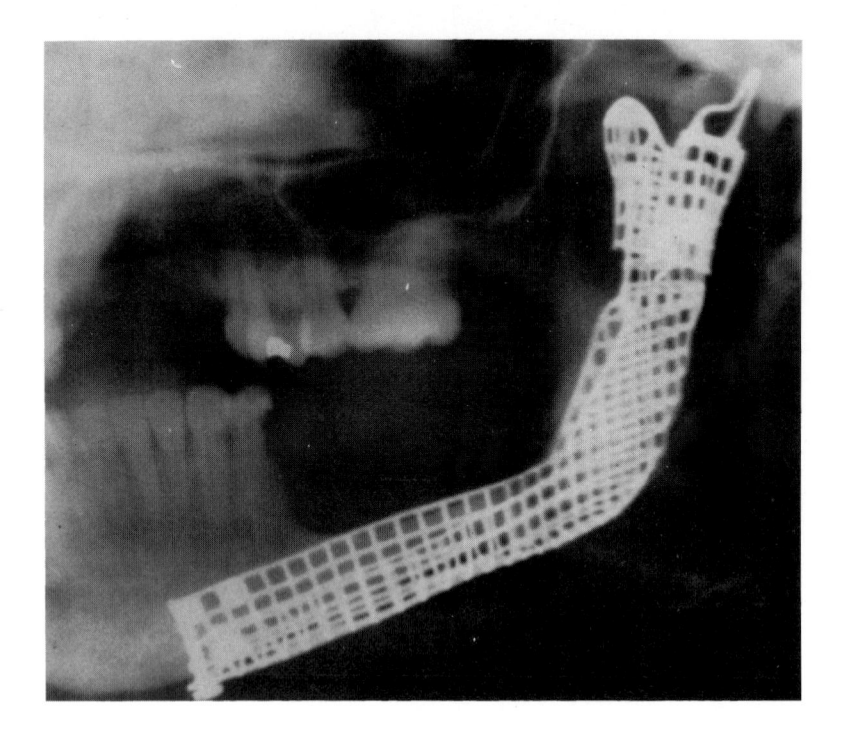

Figure 9–26. Empty crib phenomenon due to lack of phase-one bone formation. In this case osteocompetent cells were rendered nonviable by temporary storage in distilled water.

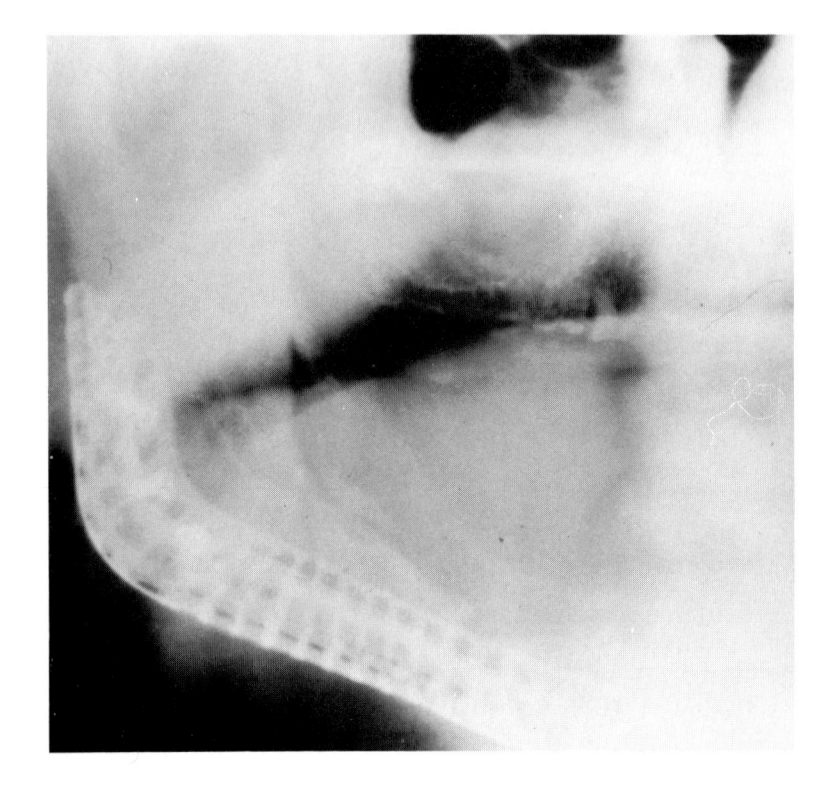

Figure 9–27. Late bone resorption in crib due to lack of phase-two bone replacement of phase-one bone. In this case irradiated tissue bed was deficient in inducible cells to form phase-two bone or a periosteum about the graft.

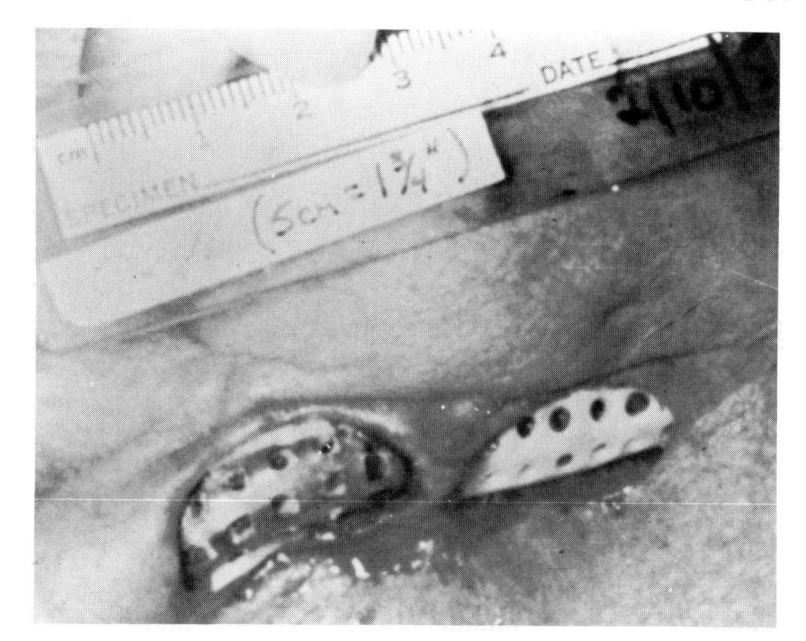

RECONSTRUCTION AND REHABILITATION OF CANCER PATIENTS / **367**

Figure 9–28. Titanium and Teflon crib exposed through cutaneous breakdown of irradiated tissue.

ated tissue. Mucosal or cutaneous breakdown is commonly observed in these patients (Fig. 9–28). When such dehiscence occurs, part or all of the crib must be removed and part or all of the graft may be lost.[40]

The soft-tissue dissection that is required to place alloplastic cribs varies only in the amount of bone exposure required at each remaining bony segment. An added length of bone must be exposed to allow for sufficient overlap and, therefore, stability of the crib. This is important in irradiated patients, in whom most of the blood supply to the residual bone filters through the periosteal pedicle. Fixation to each bony segment requires a minimum of three screws. This will secure the crib without the need for maxillomandibular fixation (see Fig. 9–32). When a proximal segment is missing, cribs will remain stable if five screws are used at the distal segment. In such cases, an acrylic condylar head may be built into the crib framework and will function reasonably well (Figs. 9–31 to 9–34). In defects of the symphysis and body across the midline, alloplas-

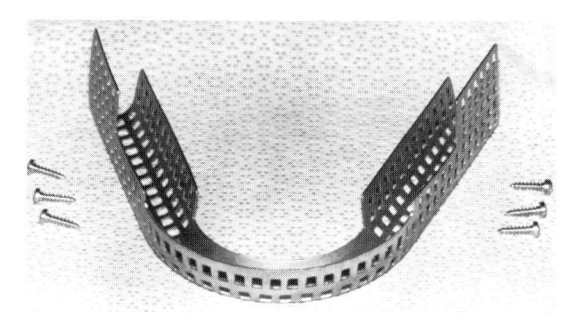

Figure 9–29. Titanium mandibular crib.

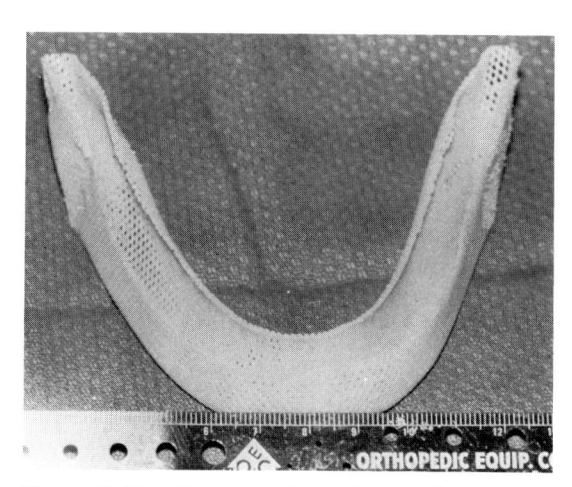

Figure 9–30. Dacron-polyurethane crib.

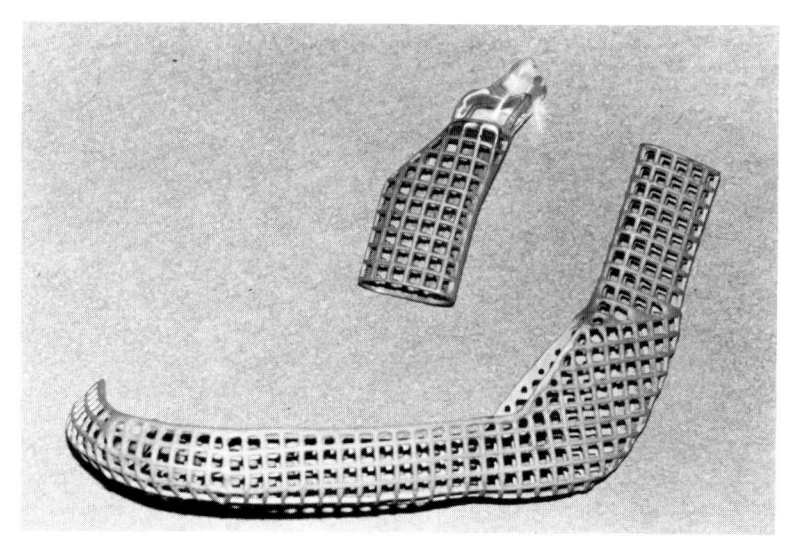

Figure 9–31. Stainless steel hemimandibular crib with acrylic condyle on ramus extension.

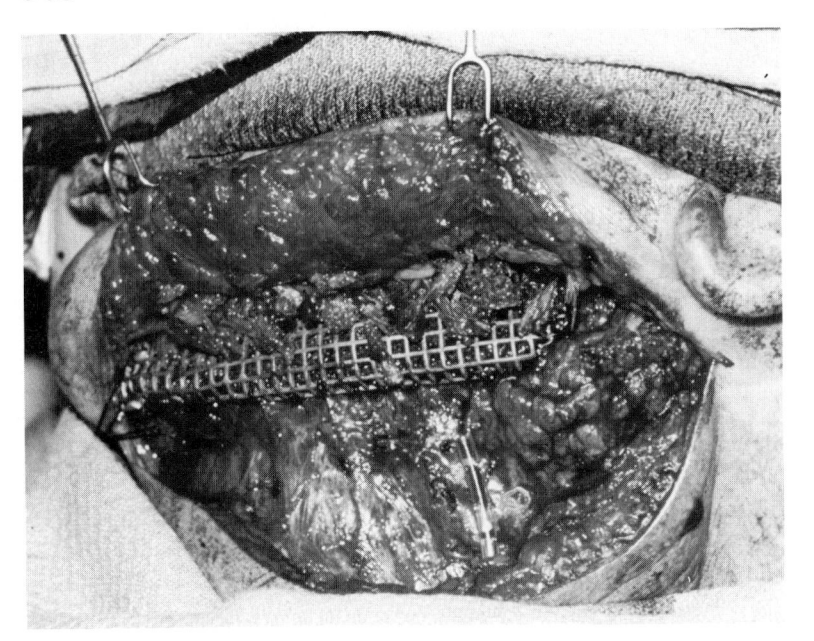

Figure 9–32. Stainless steel hemimandibular crib with PBCM graft in place. Three-screw fixation seen on distal bony segment.

tic cribs can achieve excellent contour and function (Figs. 9–35 to 9–37). In this particular defect, a rigid form with reasonable arch contour is required. Only alloplastic cribs and hollowed-out allogeneic mandibles satisfy this requirement. If sufficient soft tissue is present, an alloplastic crib can serve as well as an allogeneic mandible.

Although metallic and polymer alloplastic cribs suffice in many reconstructions, they do not for the irradiated and scarred tissue common to cancer-related defects. The poor track record of such cribs in these types of defects led us to develop different techniques. We used allogeneic bone as cribs and retained the advantages of PBCM grafts without accepting the disadvantages of nonresorbable foreign bodies.

PBCM Grafts Within Allogeneic Bone Cribs

The ideal crib for reconstruction in cancer-related defects would be one that is both biocompatible and bioresorbable. Allogeneic bone cribs come closest to this ideal. Allogeneic bone processed by the freeze-drying method has low immunogenicity. It is undetectable by current methods of testing clinical immunogenicity (tissue biopsy, regional lymph node biopsy, humoral antibody assessment, and second set grafting) and exhibits superb biocompatibility. This bone is bioresorbable by virtue of its nonviable mineral matrix. Allogeneic bone as well as transplanted cortical and block autogenous bone undergo resorption owing to lack of viable

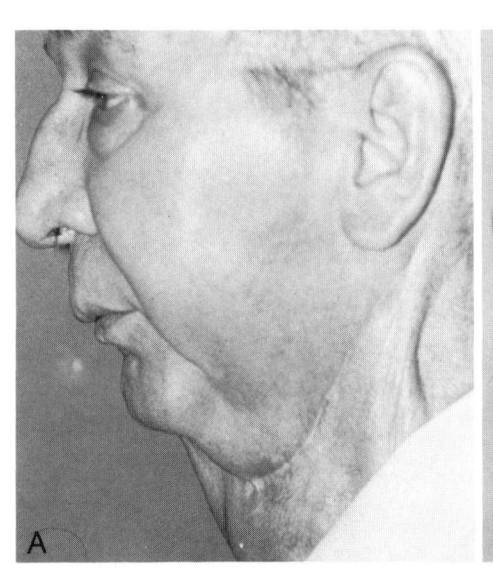

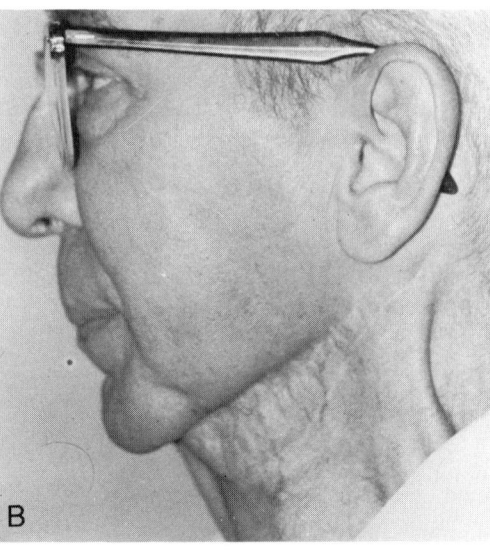

Figure 9–33. *A*, Patient with deformity resulting from hemimandibulectomy, radical neck dissection, and 6400 rads of irradiation. *B*, Patient after reconstruction using stainless steel hemimandibular form. Jaw contour and chin position in normal alignment. Patient also received University of Miami/HBO protocol for reconstruction.

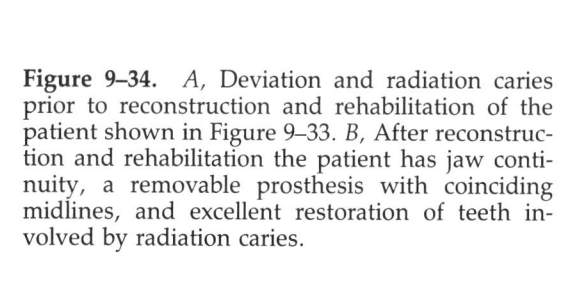

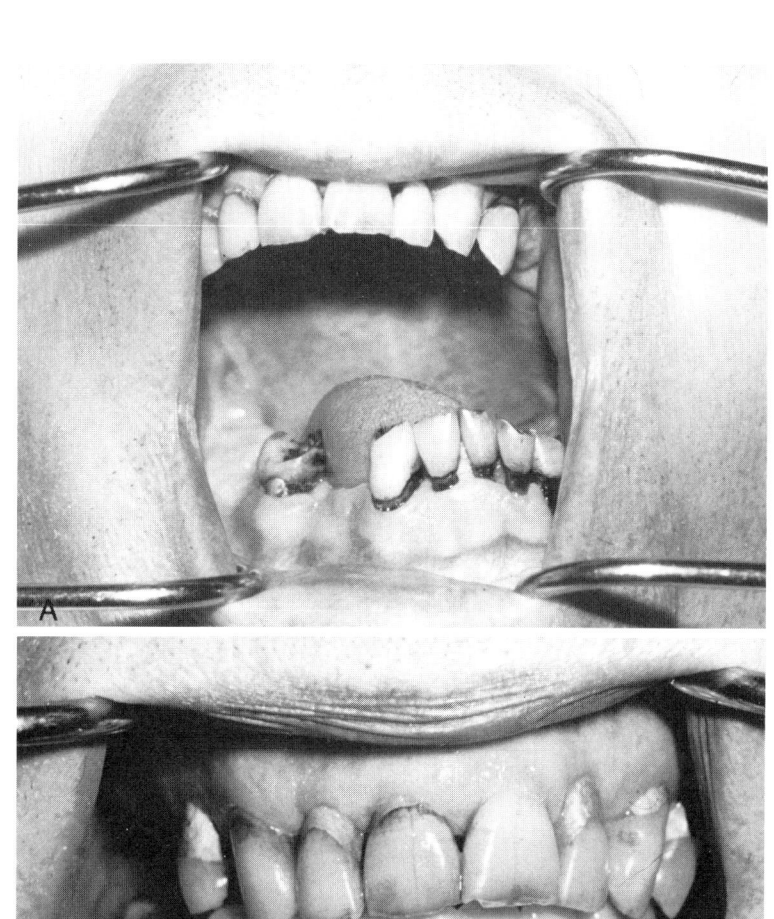

Figure 9–34. *A,* Deviation and radiation caries prior to reconstruction and rehabilitation of the patient shown in Figure 9–33. *B,* After reconstruction and rehabilitation the patient has jaw continuity, a removable prosthesis with coinciding midlines, and excellent restoration of teeth involved by radiation caries.

Technically, allogeneic cribs offer easy contouring at the time of surgery. Each crib may be shaped and manipulated to fit the host bone ends. The cribs provide the desired contours without risking graft devitalization or weakening metal trays. Like alloplastic cribs, they allow a graft of all particulate cancellous bone and marrow and afford a means of condensing the graft material to enhance phase-one bone regenera-

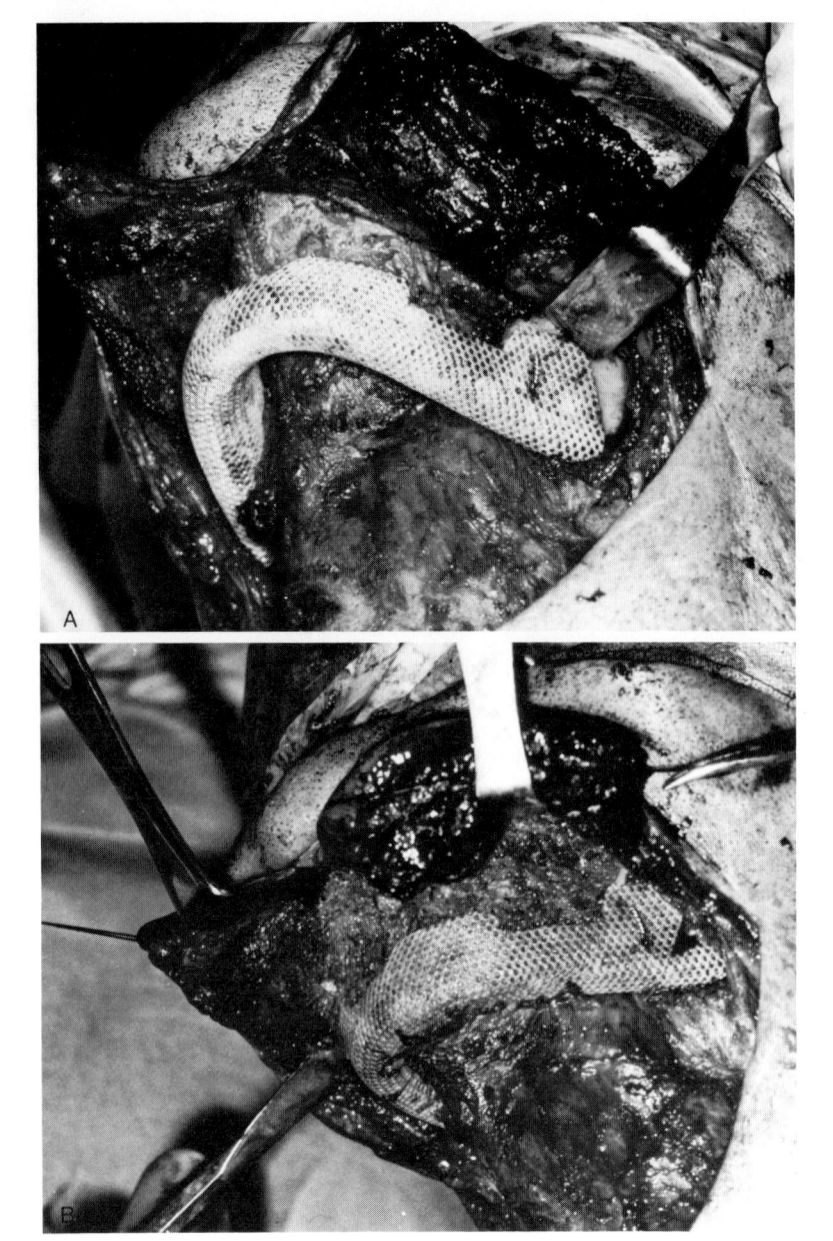

Figure 9–35. *A,* Full mandibular Dacron-polyurethane crib used in large reconstruction of symphysis and mandibular bodies. *B,* Mandibular crib with deep tissue sutured directly to crib in order to eliminate dead space and trough packed with PBCM.

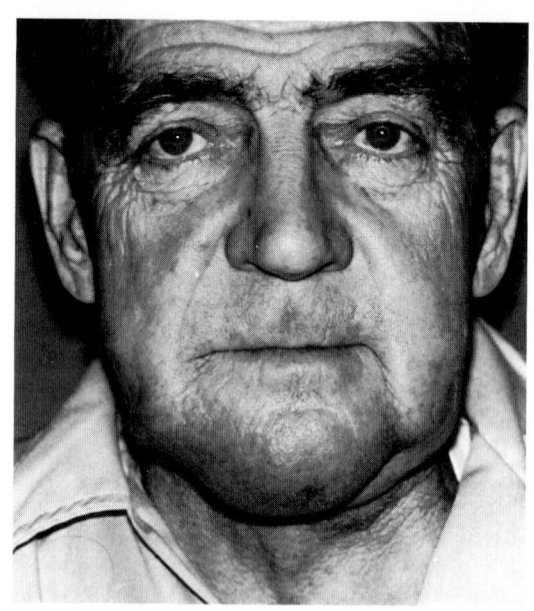

Figure 9–36. Frontal view of the patient in Figure 9–35, demonstrating full mandibular contour and symmetry achieved with this crib-graft system.

osteocytes. Supplanting alloplastic cribs with cribs of allogeneic bone is more than a reduction in foreign-body mass. The biocompatibility of allogeneic bone is an advantage in irradiated tissues because recipient tissue and grafted bone become incorporated rather than remaining inert.[31] Although alloplastic cribs often perforate the skin or mucosa, allogeneic cribs do not. Bioresorbability is another advantage. In 186 cases in which the authors have used allogeneic bone cribs, 144 were in irradiated tissue. All have completed radiographic resorption of the allogeneic crib, and none perforated thin tissue nor required surgical removal.

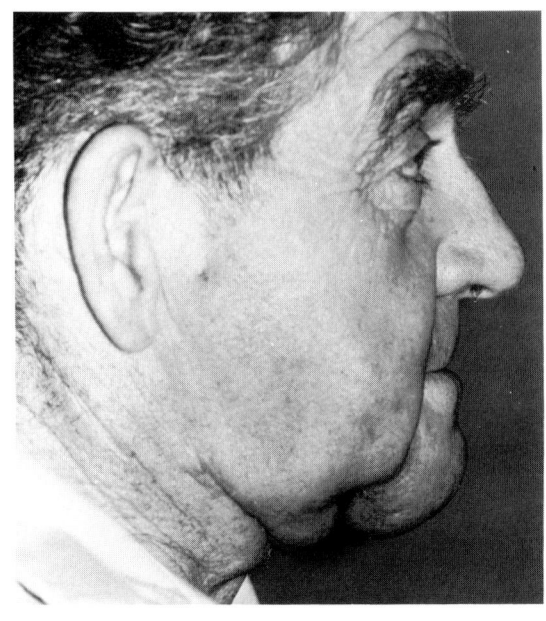

Figure 9–37. Profile view of the patient in Figure 9–35, demonstrating anteroposterior dimension achieved with this crib-graft system.

tion. Using any of the three types of allogeneic bone cribs, one can reconstruct a mandibular continuity defect with a physiologically sound graft supporting both phases of bone regeneration. The three techniques of particulate bone and cancellous marrow grafts within allogeneic cribs are as follows:

Allogeneic Mandibles

An allogeneic mandible is the ideal crib for mandibular reconstruction because of its morphology. It is hollowed out, cut to fit the remaining host bone, and packed densely with autogenous particulate bone and cancellous marrow. We have found it particularly advantageous in reconstructing large mandibular resections that cross the midline.

Allogeneic mandibles are biocompatible and bioresorbable cribs that may take anywhere from six months to two years to completely resorb, depending on the thickness of the cortex. As a rule, all allogeneic bone cribs are thinned down as much as possible. Although allogeneic bone processed by the freeze-dried method retains BMP activity, it is primarily a structural framework for a PBCM graft rather than a source of BMP. In fact, allogeneic mandibles are different from other allogeneic bone specimens; they must be harvested in an unsterile manner. They are subsequently sterilized by irradiation with gamma irradiation, which denatures BMP, or exposed to ethylene oxide, which preserves BMP. Nevertheless, BMP activity from an allogeneic crib source is usually not necessary for phase-two bone regeneration if the autogenous PBCM graft is densely packed with cancellous bone and incorporates some cortical chips. The biggest disadvantage inherent in using allogeneic mandibles is their lack of availability. The current state mortician laws and next-of-kin consents do not frequently allow for cadaver mandible harvest. It is unrealistic to build a reconstructive system on unavailable tissue. Although it provides excellent results, this tissue should be reserved for large defects that cross the midline and particularly in situations in which other allogeneic crib specimens or alloplastic cribs will not suffice.

The technical aspects of recipient tissue preparation are no different when placing an allogeneic mandible crib. The specimen is reconstituted in saline. Reconstitution time recommended by most tissue banks is 12 to 24 hours.[41] However, practicality allows reconstitution to begin the moment one enters the operating room. By the time anesthesia is induced, the sterile field prepared, and the soft-tissue dissection completed, two to four hours of reconstitution time have elapsed. We have used this practical approach and have found adequate rehydration of the specimen and workability of the bone. Although many believe that antibiotic solutions should be added to the reconstitution medium, studies have not shown positive effects from their use and they create the potential for sensitization or hypersensitivity within the recipient.[31]

The mandible graft should be sectioned to fit the host bone proximal segments with overlap for fixation with wires (Figs. 9–38 and 9–39). The graft should be hollowed to an extreme thinness of the buccal cortex, lin-

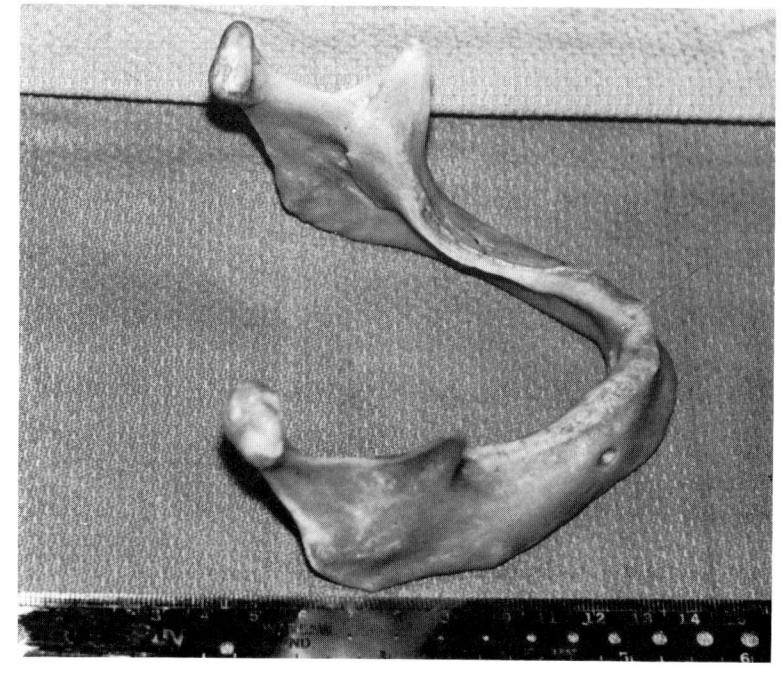

Figure 9–38. Freeze-dried allogeneic mandible from the University of Miami Tissue Bank.

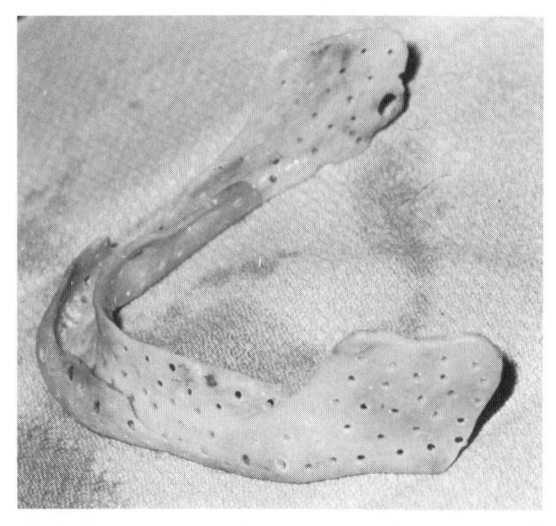

Figure 9–39. Allogeneic mandible perforated and hollowed out into a crib form. Sufficient lateral ramus cortex is preserved to allow overlap for fixation to proximal bone segments.

gual cortex, and inferior border so that the bone becomes translucent (Fig. 9–39). One should have the height of the lingual cortex at the desired vertical height of the graft. The buccal cortex can be reduced in height to allow ease of access for condensing the autogenous PBCM (Fig. 9–39). We also perforate the crib with bur holes to promote vascular ingrowth. We have found that by arranging the bur holes in the same pattern as the five on a die, one can place numerous holes without propagating a fracture line. A row of bur holes is also placed at the inferior border to allow suturing of the deep recipient tissue to the crib. Fixation of the crib to each residual bone segment may be accomplished with a vertical mattress 24-gauge wire (Figs. 9–40 and 9–41) or with screws.

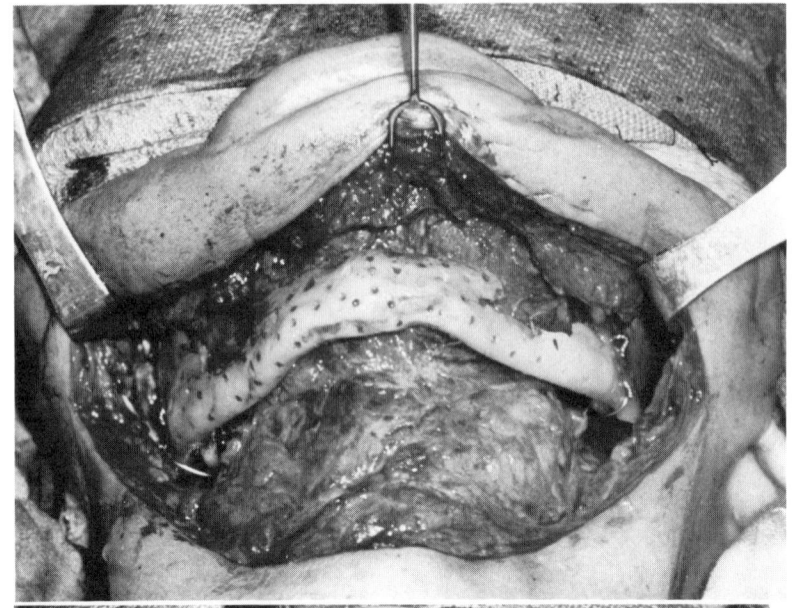

Figure 9–40. Allogeneic mandible crib form fixed in place with vertical mattress wires to host rami.

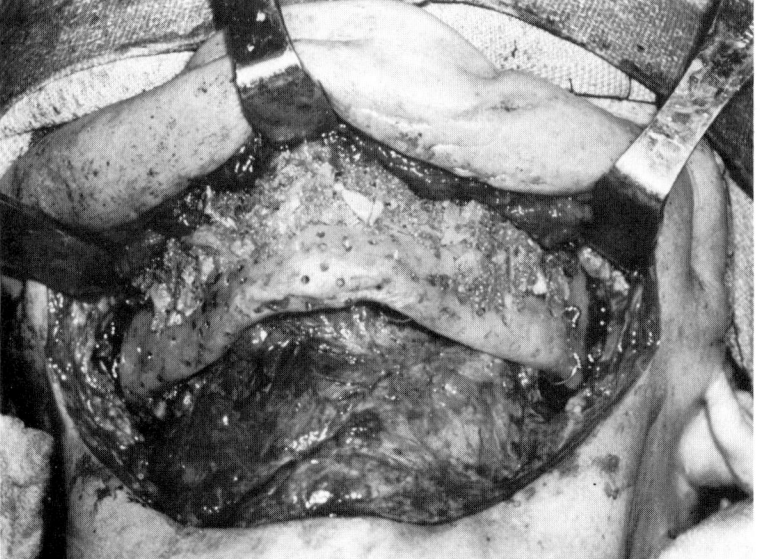

Figure 9–41. Allogeneic mandible crib form with PBCM graft packed within.

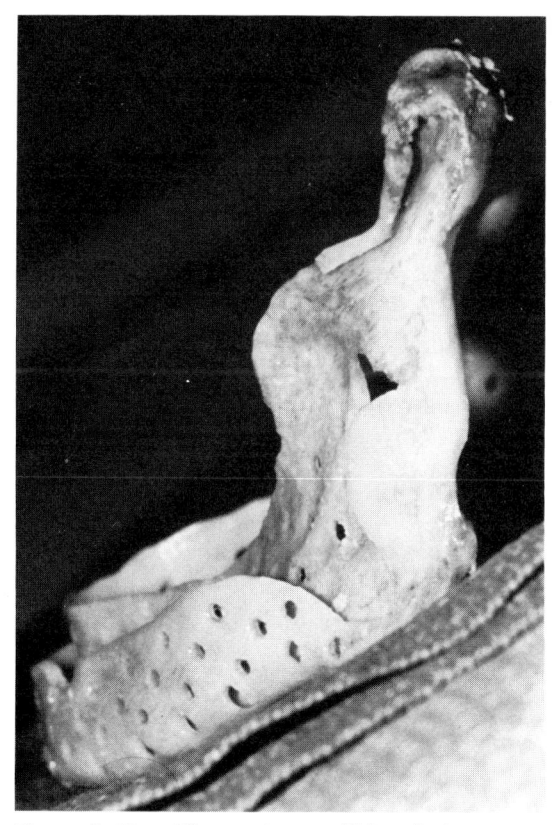

RECONSTRUCTION AND REHABILITATION OF CANCER PATIENTS / **373**

Figure 9–42. Allogeneic mandible crib forms can also make use of the condylar area for required condylar reconstruction.

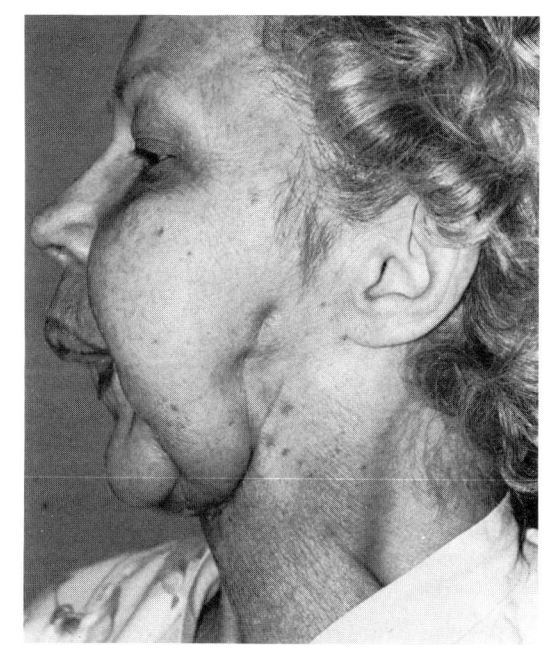

Figure 9–44. Prereconstruction profile view of the patient in Figure 9–43. "Andy Gump"–like deformity created by tissue loss in the neck and chin retraction.

Since indicated defects for allogeneic mandibles are large and include missing bone on each side of the midline, additional fixation is not required. Without suprahyoid function, these patients cannot exert sufficient rotational movement at the graft-host interface to produce a nonunion. Although we have observed suprahyoid and genioglossus muscle reattachments with these grafts, such reattachment occurs after graft consolidation, so that nonunion has not been observed. Where the defect includes one or both condyles, the allogeneic mandible serves as a crib in this area as well (Fig. 9–42). The lateral cortex of the ramus, condylar neck, and pole of the condyle can be removed and hollowed out to accept a PBCM. The graft, when consolidated, should retain a condylar morphology, although it will serve only as a rotational center without translation.

Since allogeneic mandibles are difficult to

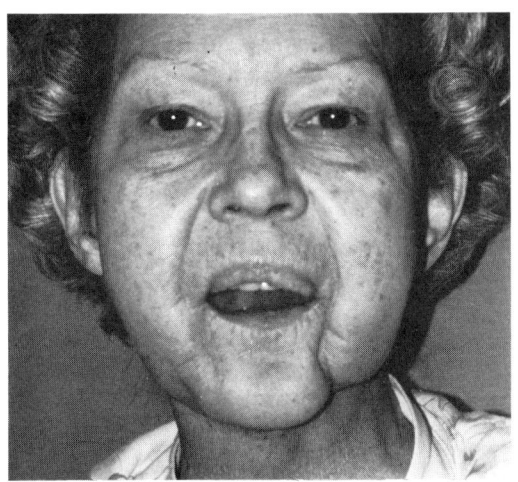

Figure 9–43. Prereconstruction frontal view of patient who has had a mandibular resection from angle to angle and 9200 rads of irradiation.

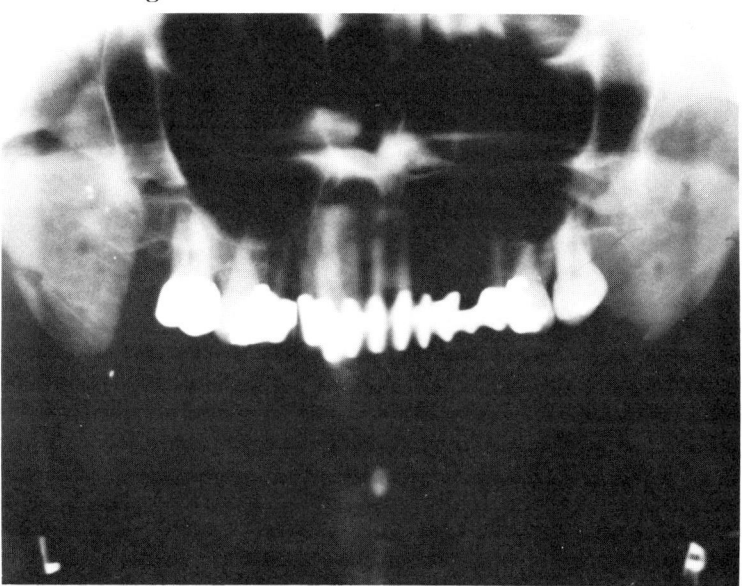

Figure 9–45. Prereconstruction panoramic film of the patient in Figure 9–43, demonstrating continuity defect from angle to angle and anterior-superior rotation of proximal segments.

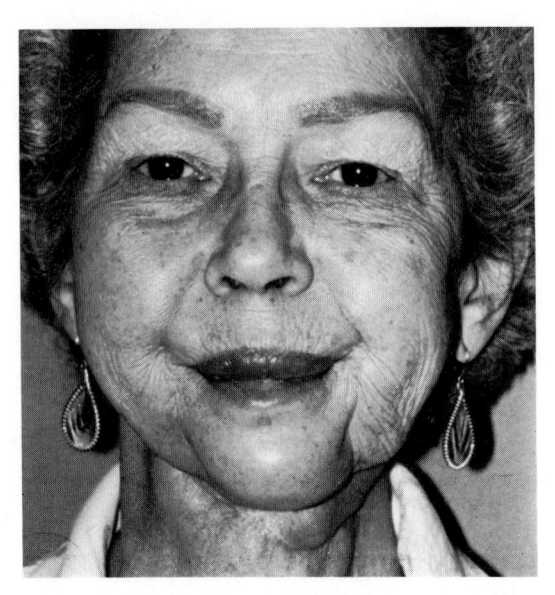

Figure 9–46. Frontal view of the patient in Figure 9–43 after reconstruction using allogeneic mandible crib, PBCM graft, and University of Miami/HBO protocol.

obtain but provide the best morphology for symphysis contour and arch form, their use should be reserved for large defects (Figs. 9–43 to 9–48). We would not recommend their use in hemimandibular reconstruction because other allogeneic bone cribs work well in this situation. One should not attempt to bisect a mandibular specimen into two hemimandibular specimens for use in two different patients. This procedure exposes the specimen to contamination and violates the tissue-banking principle of one specimen for one recipient.

Allogeneic Ilia

In 1965, Manchester published an innovative concept in mandibular reconstruction that may be applied to allogeneic bone cribs.[42] His technique took advantage of the contour similarity between a hemimandible and the ipsilateral iliac crest. He used a sterile pewter template in the shape of a mandible to carve out a large block from the autogenous ilium. The shape, size, and contour were ideal for reconstructing hemimandibulectomy defects. However, the solid block nature of these grafts, with a lack of phase-one bone regeneration, produced functionally inadequate results plagued with resorption. In addition, such large blocks of bone harvested from the iliac crest resulted in increased donor site morbidity, including herniation of abdominal contents through the defect.

The Manchester concept can be applied to an allogeneic bone specimen hollowed out and used as a crib for a PBCM graft. Because it incorporates both phases of bone regeneration and obviates the morbidity of such large block resections of the ilium, this use retains the merits of Manchester's original idea. An ipsilateral allogeneic ilium can be hollowed and fitted to the remaining mandible at the time of graft placement. If one inverts the ilium and views it from the lateral aspect, a hemimandibular form may be easily scribed (Figs. 9–49 and 9–50). We have found it best to design the crib so that the tubercle of the ilium corresponds to the angle of the mandible. The iliac crest contour, from the tubercle posteriorly, will then approximate the contour of the mandible from the angle anteriorly as far as the canine region. A ramus outline and condylar shape may be developed from the ilium below the crest in the area between the tubercle and the anterior margin. The crib is thinned and perforated to enhance revascularization and crib resorption. Its main purpose is to serve as a framework against which an autogenous PBCM graft can be densely packed into a shape that provides the criteria for success discussed earlier: continuity, alveolar height, osseous bulk, and facial form. The advantage of this approach, in addition to its simplicity of technique and its morphologic characteristics, is the availability of the allogeneic bone specimens. Ilia are routinely harvested by tissue banks today. They are harvested in a sterile manner and are com-

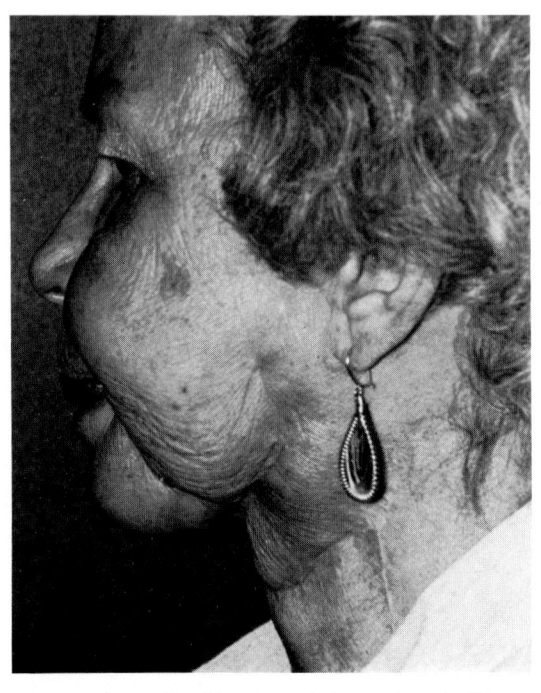

Figure 9–47. Profile view of the patient in Figure 9–43, demonstrating nearly normal chin contour and lip competence.

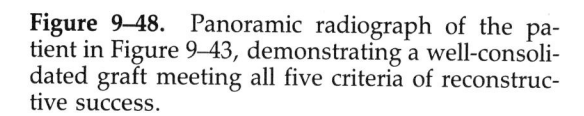

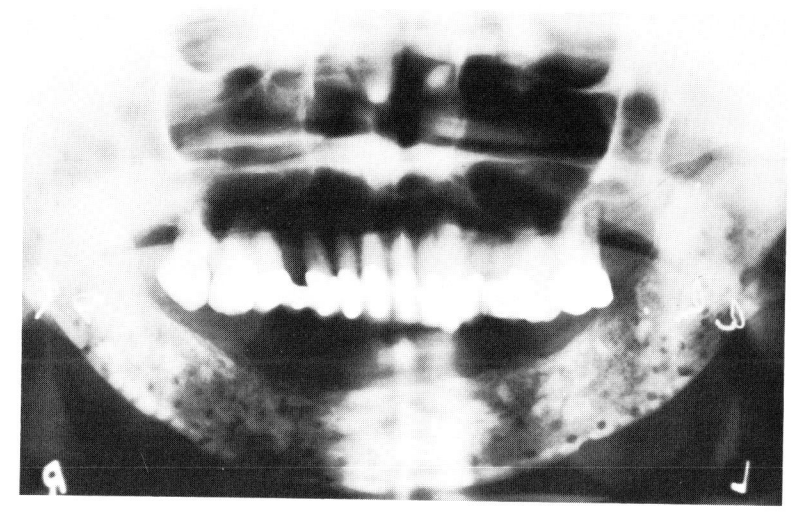

Figure 9–48. Panoramic radiograph of the patient in Figure 9–43, demonstrating a well-consolidated graft meeting all five criteria of reconstructive success.

Figure 9–49. Inverted left ilium with outlined mandibular form for a left hemimandibular crib. Mandibular angle should be scribed on the tubercle of the ilium.

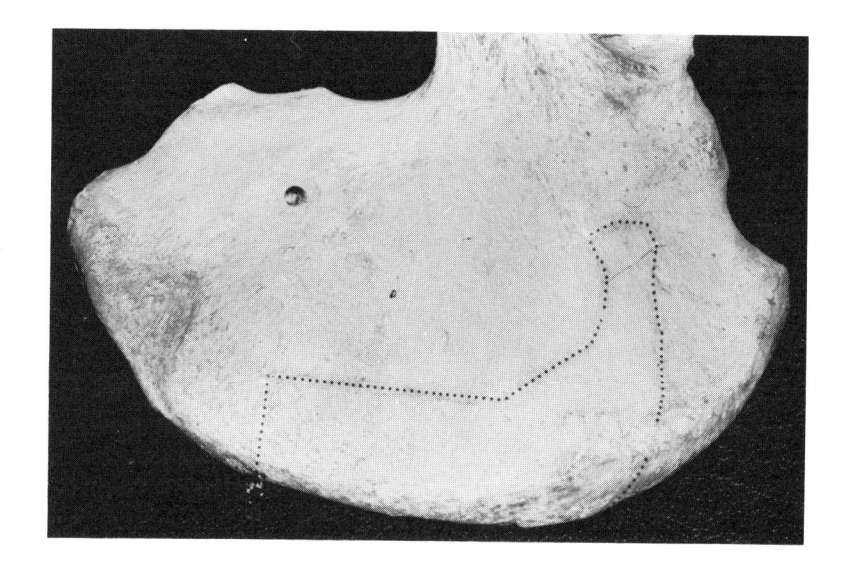

Figure 9–50. Convex curvature of the iliac crest posterior to the tubercle simulates the curvature of the mandible from the angle to the canine region.

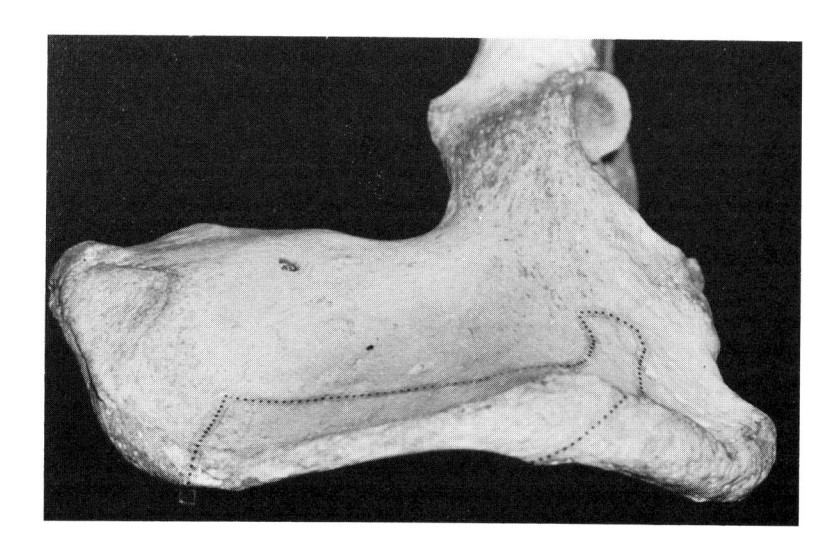

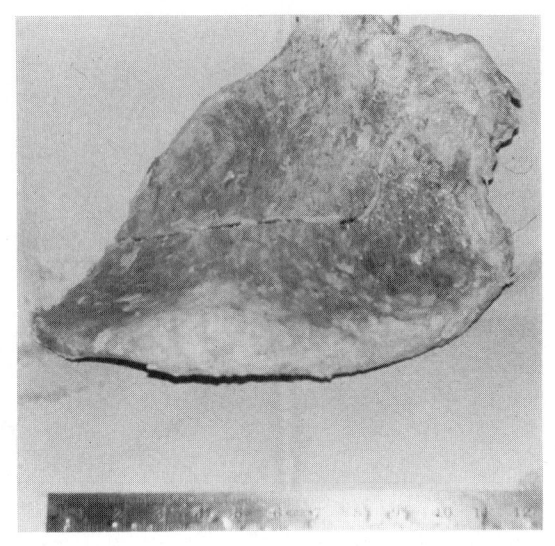

Figure 9–51. Freeze-dried allogeneic ilium specimen from the University of Miami Tissue Bank prior to crib fabrication.

monly available in a freeze-dried form. However, the use of allogeneic ilia in this manner is new to tissue banks. Specimens such as these can easily be obtained but require a special request to the tissue bank.

Once the crib is fashioned, thinned, and perforated, placement into the recipient bed is straightforward (Figs. 9–51 and 9-52). Fixation to each host bone segment may be accomplished with transosseous wires or even screws (Figs. 9–53 and 9–54). Since this specimen is indicated mostly for hemimandibular defects, arch alignment and stability of the distal segment must be ensured during placement. Either maxillomandibular fixation or the reduction rig of the Joe Hall Morris extraskeletal pin fixation device may be used. Since hemimandibular defects retain much of the suprahyoid muscle pull and there is often a sufficient pterygomasseteric sling, sufficient rotational forces can be

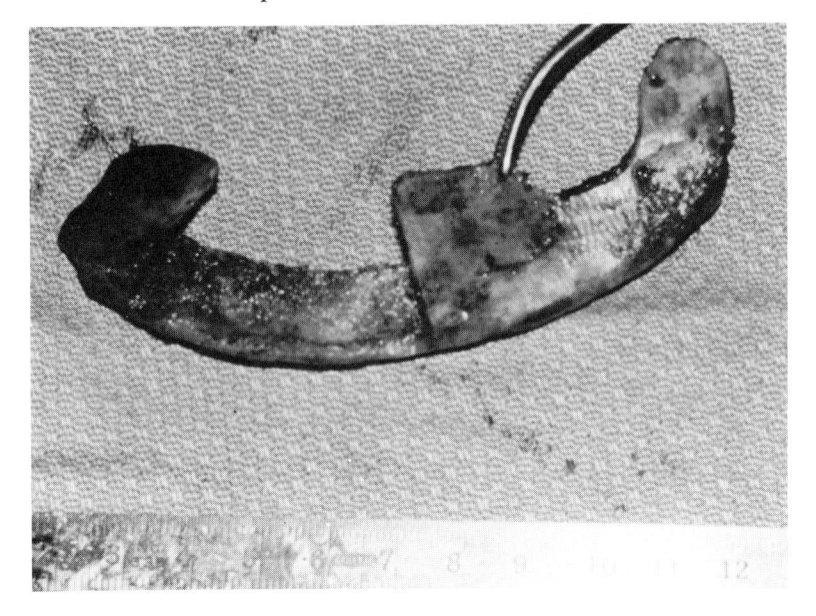

Figure 9–52. Hemimandibular crib developed from the specimen in Figure 9–51.

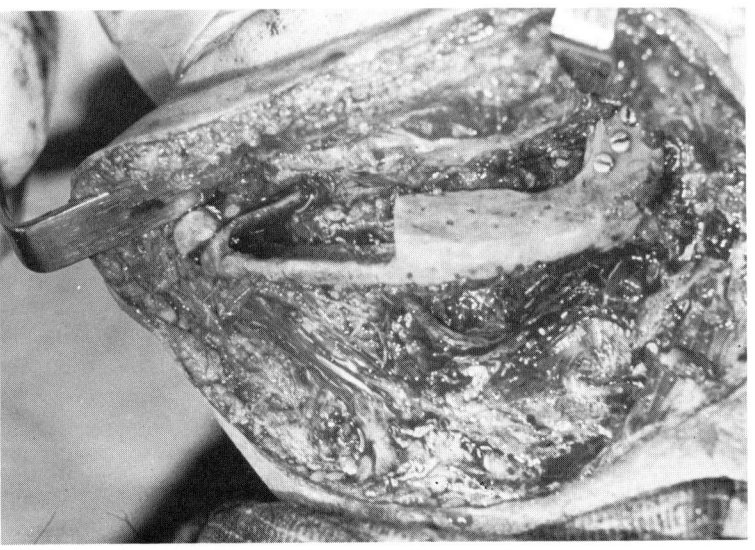

Figure 9–53. Hemimandibular crib fixed to the proximal segment with screws and to the distal segment with wires. Note deep tissues sutured to crib via transosseous bur holes.

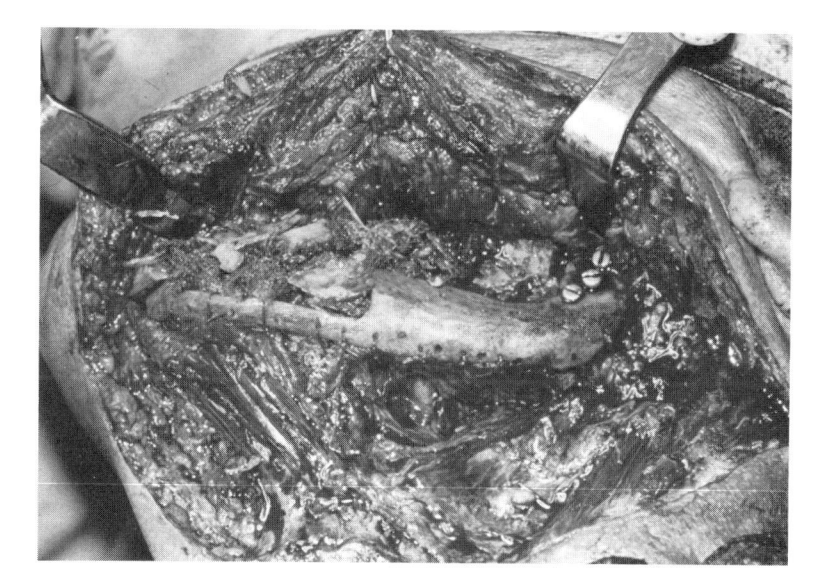

Figure 9–54. PBCM graft material placed into crib through lateral window access.

placed at the graft-host interface. Although ipsilateral allogeneic ilium cribs can be somewhat rigid, it is not recommended that they be used without other fixation.

This technique has been an extremely useful one. It provides a superb facial contour and large volume for a PBCM graft for the most commonly occurring hemimandibular defect (Figs. 9–55 and 9–56). Used in this manner, we have seen long-lasting functional and esthetic results (Figs. 9–57 to 9–60) and have observed resorption of the original allogeneic crib that occurs between 6 and 18 months (Fig. 9–61).

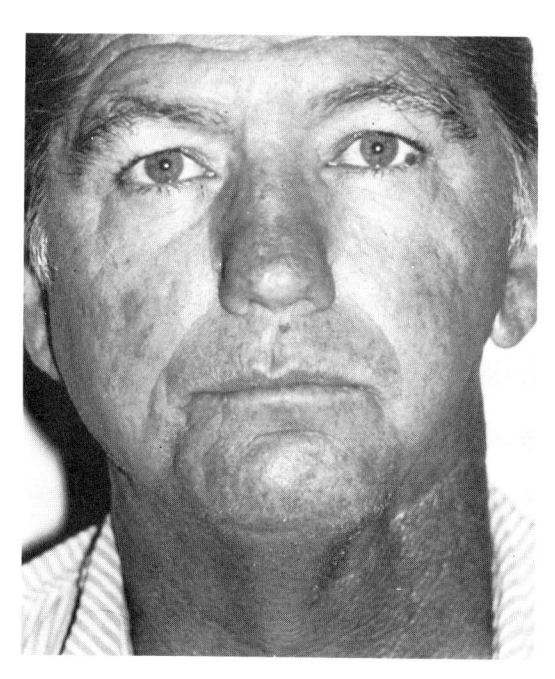

Figure 9–55. Frontal view of hemimandibulectomy patient who also received a functional neck dissection and 5500 rads of irradiation.

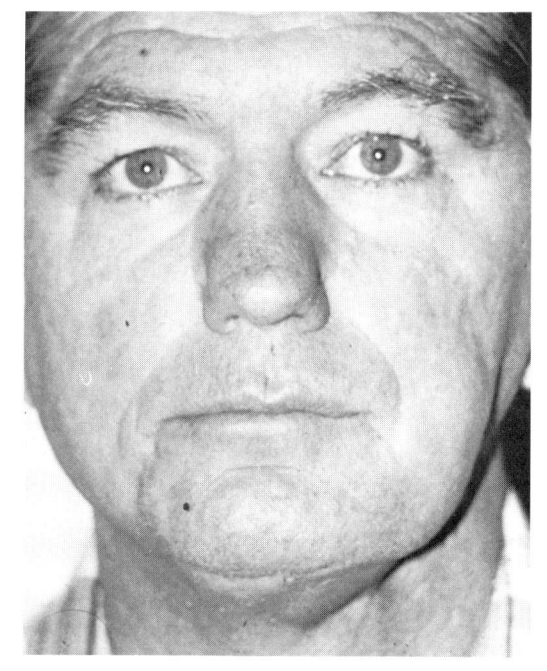

Figure 9–56. Frontal view of the patient in Figure 9–55 after reconstruction using the crib shown in Figure 9–52 and University of Miami/HBO protocol. Full mandibular contour and symmetry are apparent.

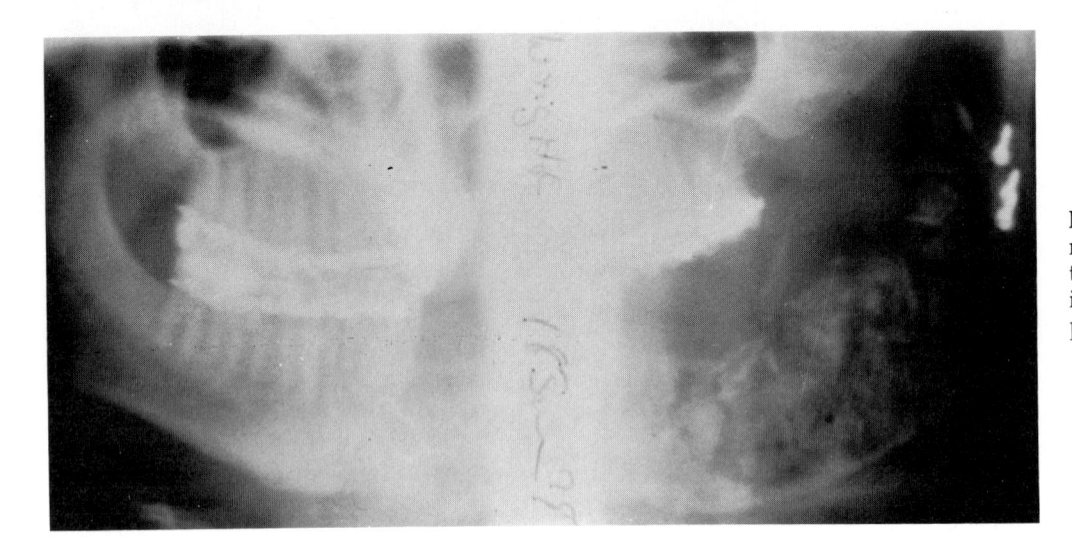

378 / RECONSTRUCTION AND REHABILITATION OF CANCER PATIENTS

Figure 9–57. The particulate nature of a PBCM graft in this allogeneic crib is evident in this two-week postsurgical panoramic radiograph.

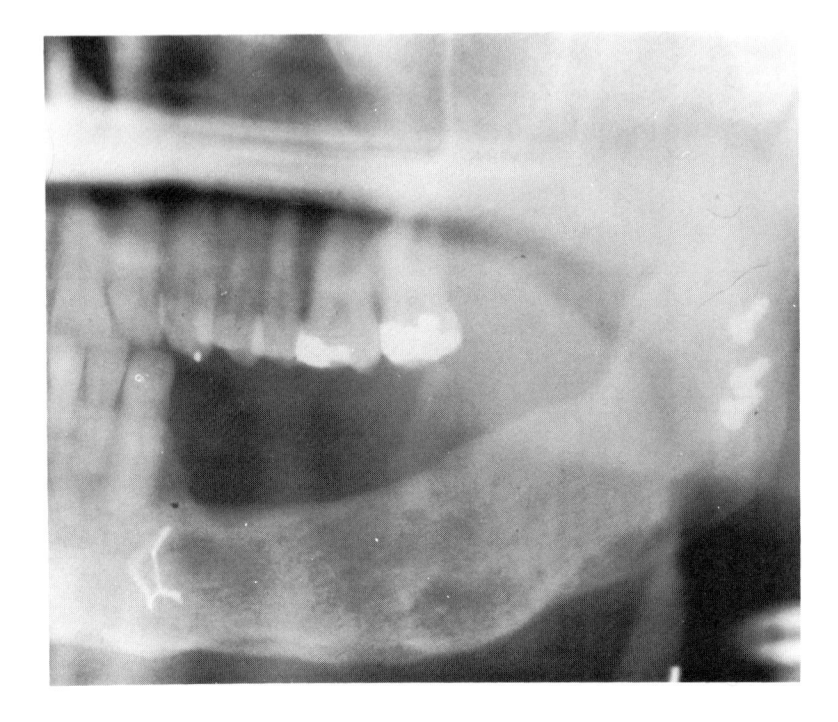

Figure 9–58. Four-year follow-up of this graft indicates a well-consolidated graft without resorption fulfilling all five criteria of success.

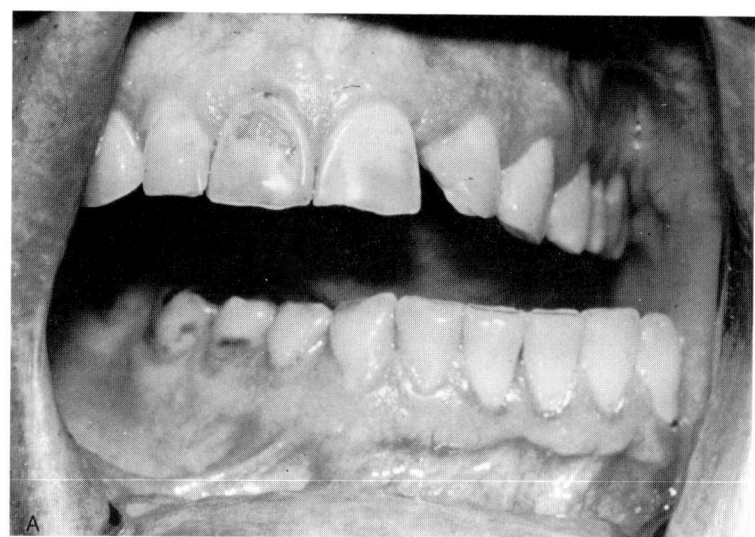

Figure 9–59. *A,* Severe deviation of the mandible toward the resected side prior to reconstruction. *B,* Four-year follow-up with repeatable centric occlusion and centric relation. Midlines coincide.

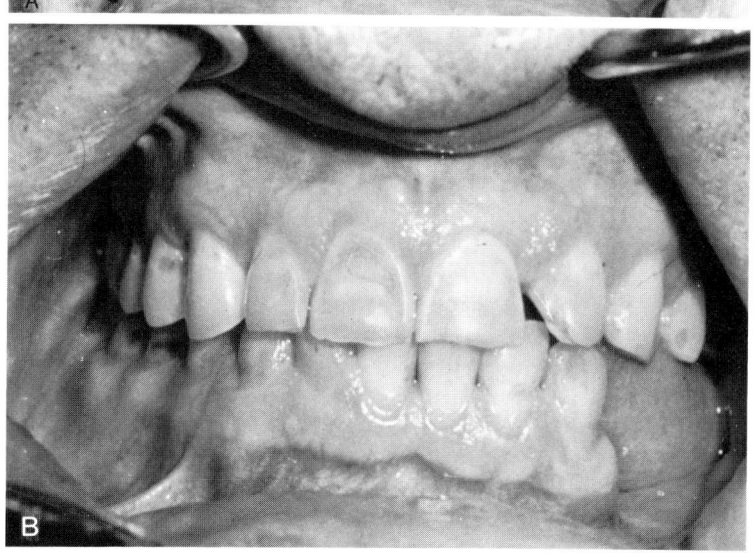

Figure 9–60. Unrestricted opening without deviation.

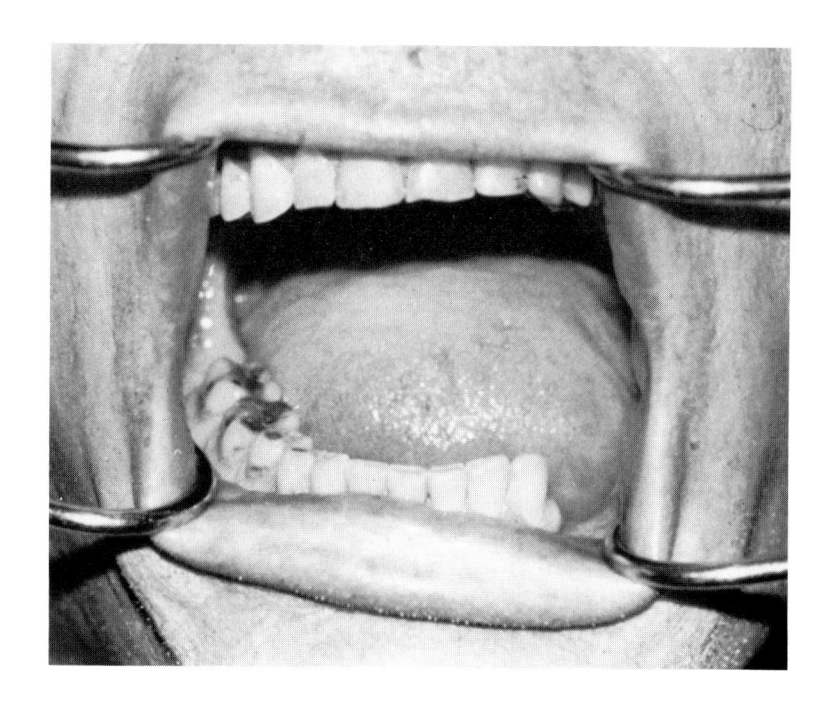

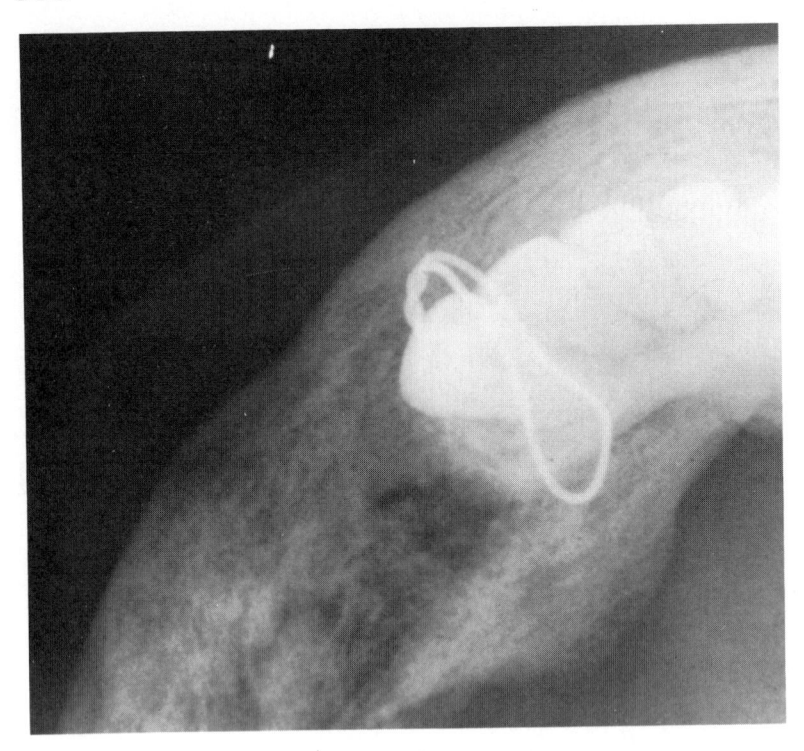

Figure 9–61. One-year follow-up occlusal view demonstrates a well-trabeculated graft without a distinction between graft and host bone. The arch form and buccal-lingual width are excellent. There is no residual allogeneic crib seen at this time.

Allogeneic Split-Rib Segments

A very versatile use of allogeneic bone cribs can be derived by splitting allogeneic ribs longitudinally (Figs. 9–62 and 9–63). After cutting to a proper length and removing the cancellous portion, a thin bendable cortex of bone remains. One can fix half the split rib to form a medial cortex and the other half to form the lateral cortex. Both halves can be fixed to each remaining mandibular segment with a vertical mattress wire. Once the grafts are in position, the contour and shape of the mandible are defined. A PBCM graft may be condensed between the plates of bone, with the allogeneic plates acting as a matrix band (Figs. 9–64 and 9–65).

The height of bone achieved is governed by the superior extent of the soft-tissue dissection. The width of bone is not less than the width of the remaining mandible and usually turns out wider because the allogeneic plates are expanded by the PBCM graft (Figs. 9–66 to 9–70).

Continuity defects, which include a portion of the ramus but have not disarticulated the condyle, require a different orientation of the split-rib segments. In these cases one segment of rib is used to form an inferior border, which is carried to the posterior border of the proximal condylar segment, and the other split-rib segment forms a superior margin from the height of the alveolus to the anterior border of the condylar segment (Figs. 9–70 and 9–71). In traversing the continuity defect, each allogeneic rib segment is

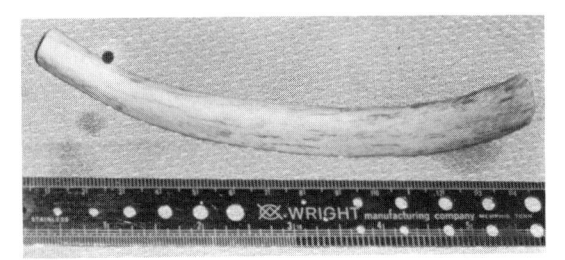

Figure 9–62. Allogeneic rib after reconstitution in sterile saline.

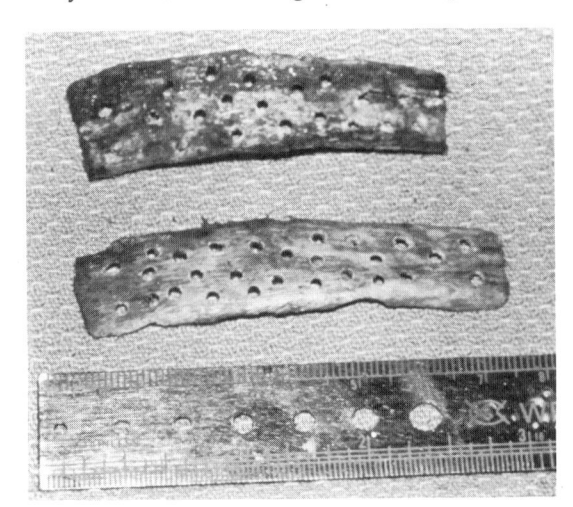

Figure 9–63. Allogeneic rib longitudinally split into two cortices that are thinned and perforated to serve as a crib for a PBCM graft. The longer segment here will serve as the buccal cortex, the shorter segment as the lingual cortex.

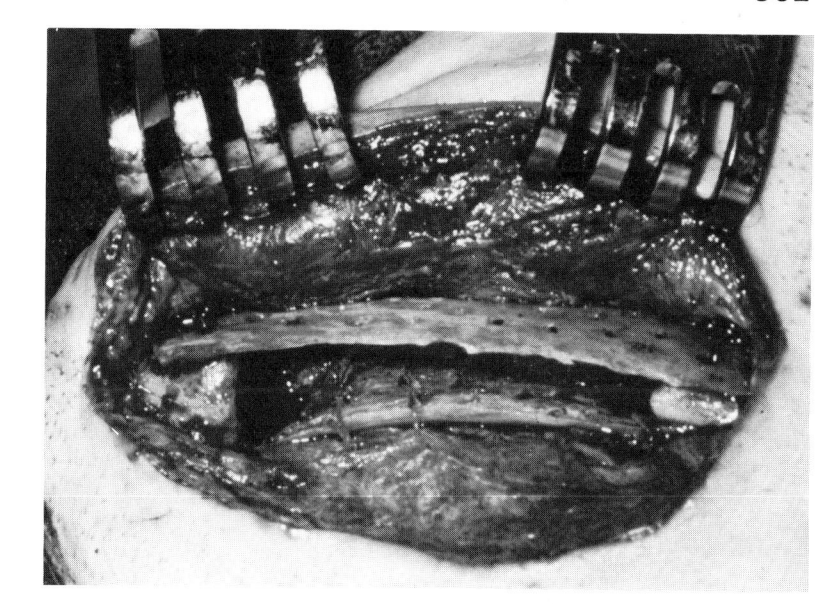

Figure 9–64. The allogeneic split ribs are wired into place with vertical mattress wires. These bone cribs function as a matrix band for the placement of PBCM graft material.

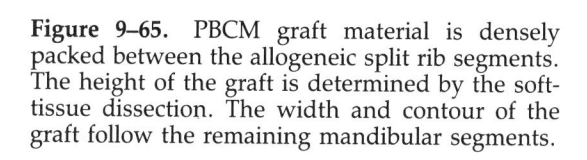

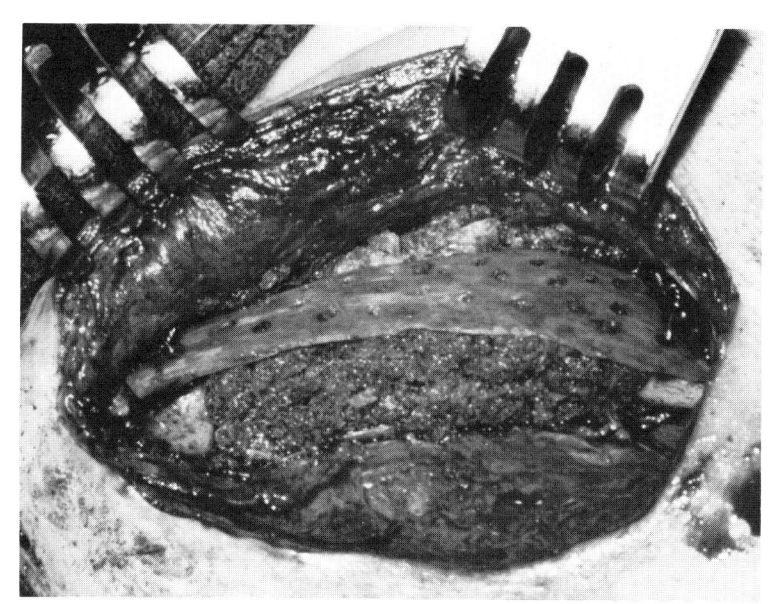

Figure 9–65. PBCM graft material is densely packed between the allogeneic split rib segments. The height of the graft is determined by the soft-tissue dissection. The width and contour of the graft follow the remaining mandibular segments.

Figure 9–66. The particulate nature of a PBCM graft is evident in this early radiograph. The allogeneic split rib cribs placed in a buccal and lingual fashion as in this case are usually not seen on radiographs.

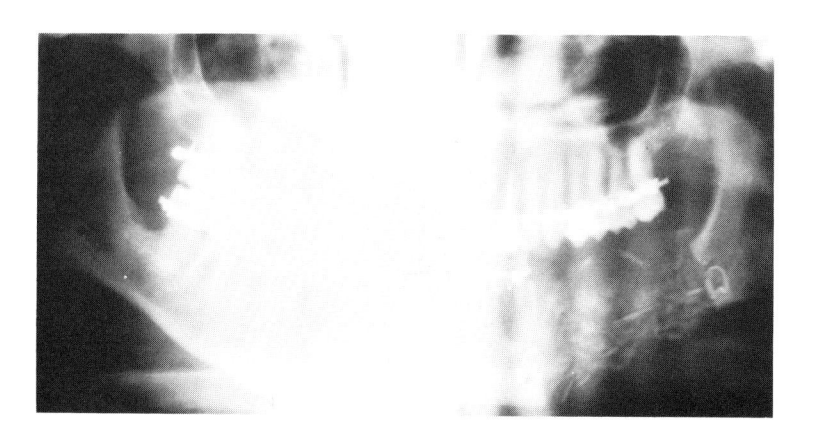

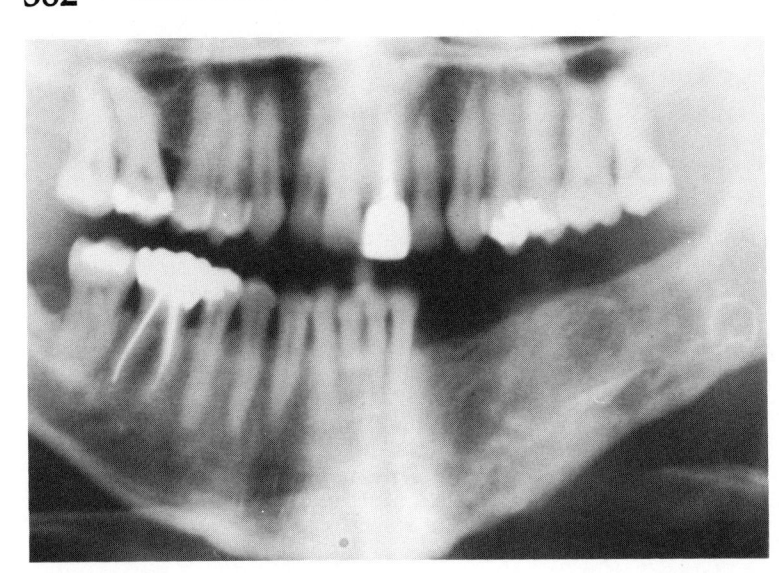

Figure 9–67. A two-year follow-up demonstrates the consolidation of the PBCM graft, as well as an impressive height and contour of bone.

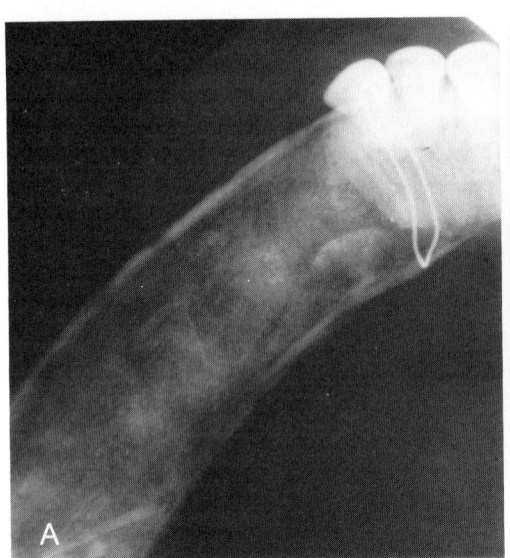

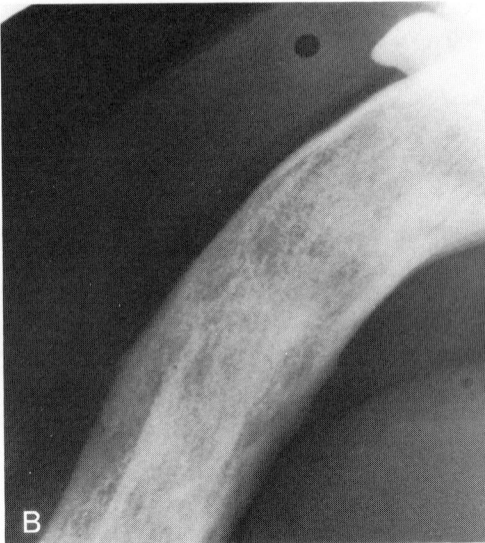

Figure 9–68. *A*, An occlusal view of this graft at two months demonstrates the buccal and lingual allogeneic crib plates and a consolidating PBCM graft between. *B*, An occlusal view at two years shows the allogeneic crib plates to be resorbed and replaced by a much more radiographically dense graft.

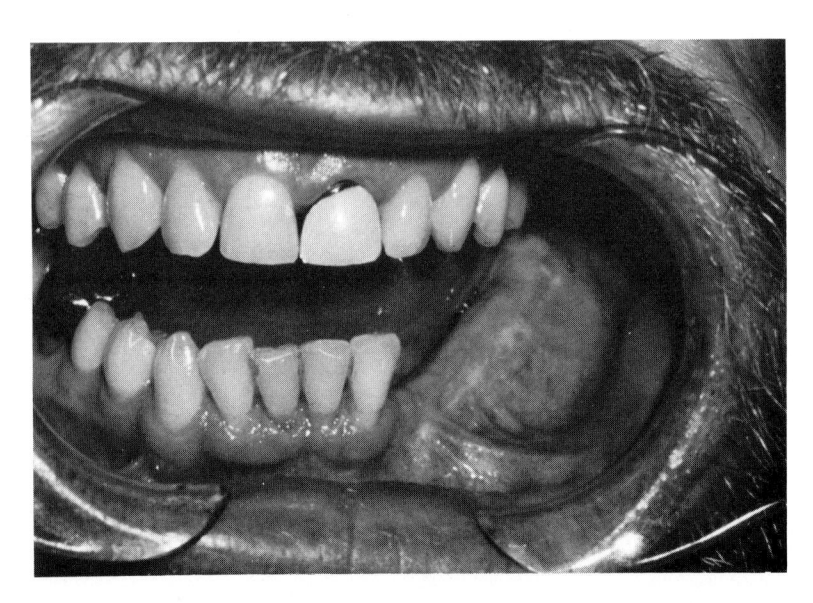

Figure 9–69. Height of the alveolus achieved with this graft system. No vestibuloplasty was required.

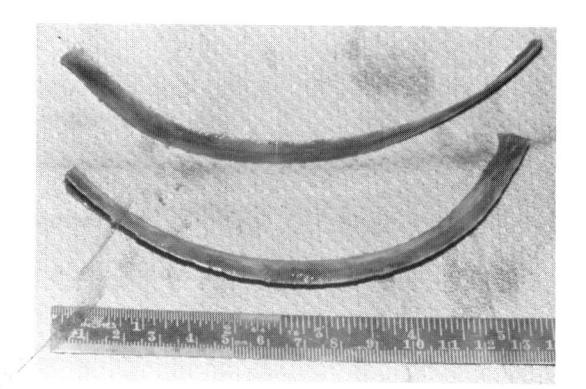

Figure 9–70. Allogeneic split ribs may also be oriented in a superior margin–infer border fashion. The natural curvature of a rib will approximate the angle and ramus contours.

bent to form an angle of the mandible and is sutured to the deep tissues. In this situation the allogeneic bone is fixed to the host mandible by individual transosseous wires. The PBCM graft is placed from the lateral aspect against the medial soft tissue (Fig. 9–72). The contour and height of the graft are defined by the allogeneic rib segments. They, in turn, are defined by the height of the remaining mandible. The advantages of autogenous PBCM grafts and allogeneic bone cribs are realized in these two procedures, as is the straightforward means of achieving an accurate mandibular form. Additionally, allogeneic ribs are the most available and least expensive tissue specimens currently available from tissue banks. Because of the simplicity, versatility, and physiologic advantages of the graft system, it is the preferred approach whenever possible. Allogeneic split-rib segments, oriented to form medial and lateral cortical plates, have particular usefulness in defects of the mandibular body or symphysis. Allogeneic split-rib segments, oriented to form the inferior border and the

Figure 9–71. Allogeneic split ribs oriented to form an angle and ramus by serving as an inferior border and superior margin.

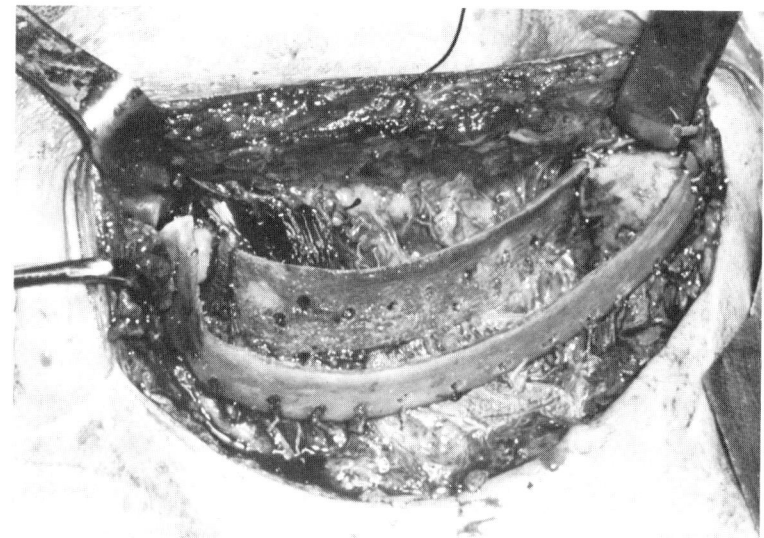

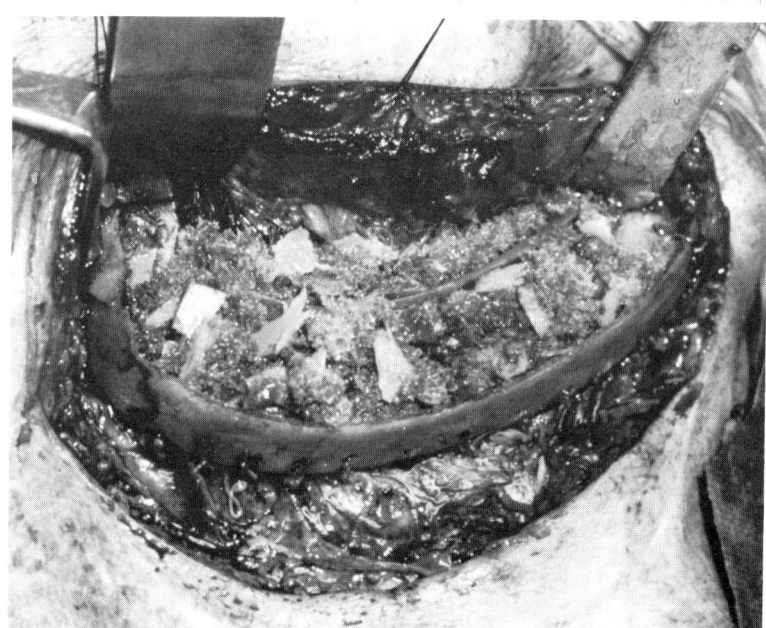

Figure 9–72. PBCM graft material is packed into this crib matrix band from the lateral aspect.

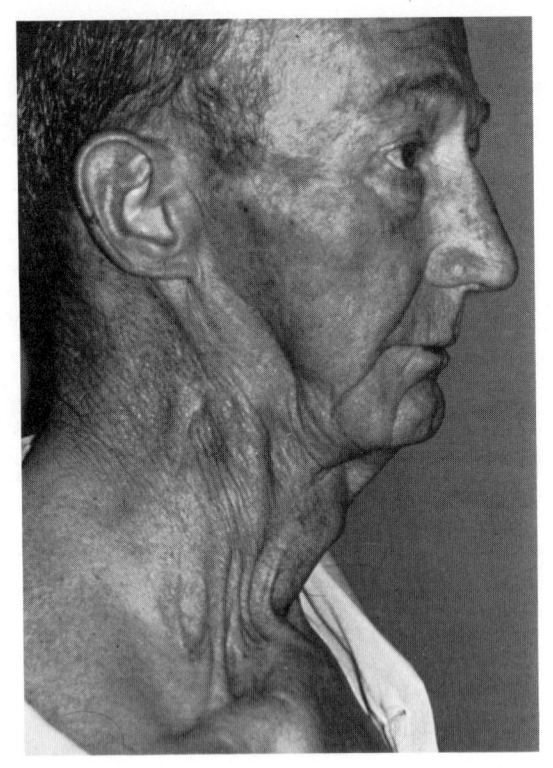

384 / RECONSTRUCTION AND REHABILITATION OF CANCER PATIENTS

Figure 9–73. Patient as seen prior to reconstruction after a hemimandibulectomy, radical neck dissection, and 6600 rads of irradiation.

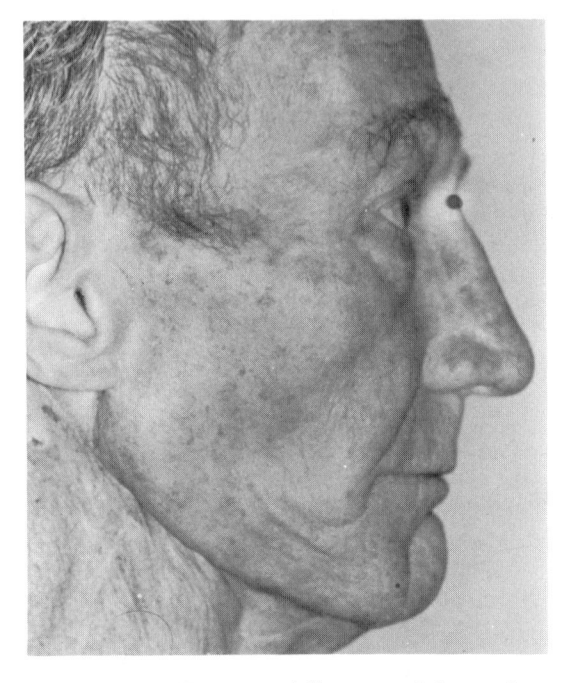

Figure 9–74. Five-year follow-up of the patient in Figure 9–73 indicates an excellent angle form, contour, and chin position achieved with this graft system. Owing to his radiation damage, he also received the University of Miami/HBO protocol.

superior margin of the alveolus, have particular usefulness in restoring the angle and ramus (Figs. 9–73 to 9–75).

When the condyle has been removed during the cancer extirpation, a modified approach can be used for this clinical situation. Any time a condyle is lost, translation of the mandible on that side is also lost. The remaining lateral pterygoid muscle retracts and fibroses. No bone graft or alloplast replacement of the condyle is able to achieve anything more than a pseudarthrosis capable of only rotational movement. Therefore, a goal of condylar replacement is to develop a pseudarthrosis that will exhibit unimpeded rotation and not resorb to change the ramus height or dental occlusion.

A costochondral graft taken from any rib from the fifth through eighth ribs, which is scored and bent to form the inferior border and angle serves this purpose well (Figs. 9–76 and 9–77). Although a solid block graft, it is used in this instance as a crib with a morphologic condylar form. Fixed to the inferior border of the distal segment in this manner, the greatest thickness of the autogenous rib comes to lie in the mediolateral dimension. The costochondral element with a 3-mm cartilage cap can be trimmed to fit into the temporal fossa. An allogeneic split-rib segment is used for the superior margin to complete the matrix band. An autogenous PBCM graft is packed between the two (Figs. 9–78 and 9–79). One must be sure to place part of the PBCM graft material up against the costochondral junction so that sufficient phase-one bone regeneration can take place in that area. In our experience, this technique allows condylar reconstruction without compromising the remainder of the graft (Figs. 9–80 and 9–81).

Both allogeneic and alloplastic cribs allow a high concentration of osteocompetent cells to be condensed into a graft. Allogeneic cribs have an additional advantage of being biocompatible and bioresorbable. Such cribs act as a trough or a matrix band to allow condensation of the PBCM graft material. The work by Friedenstein et al.[24] and Simmons et al.[25] indicates that compressing the PBCM graft material into such cribs enhances the amount of phase-one bone production.

We have found that ideally 8 to 10 cc of PBCM should be compressed into the crib for each centimeter of mandibular length to be reconstructed. Six cc of PBCM per centimeter length is an absolute minimum. Below this level, there is insufficient phase-one bone formation, which can result in cribs that never develop bone ossicles. Bone os-

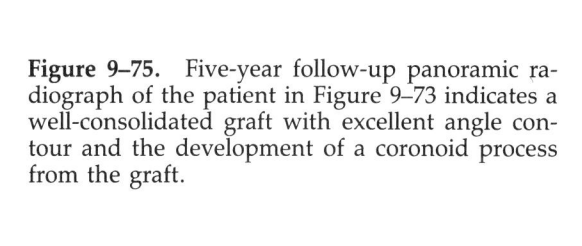

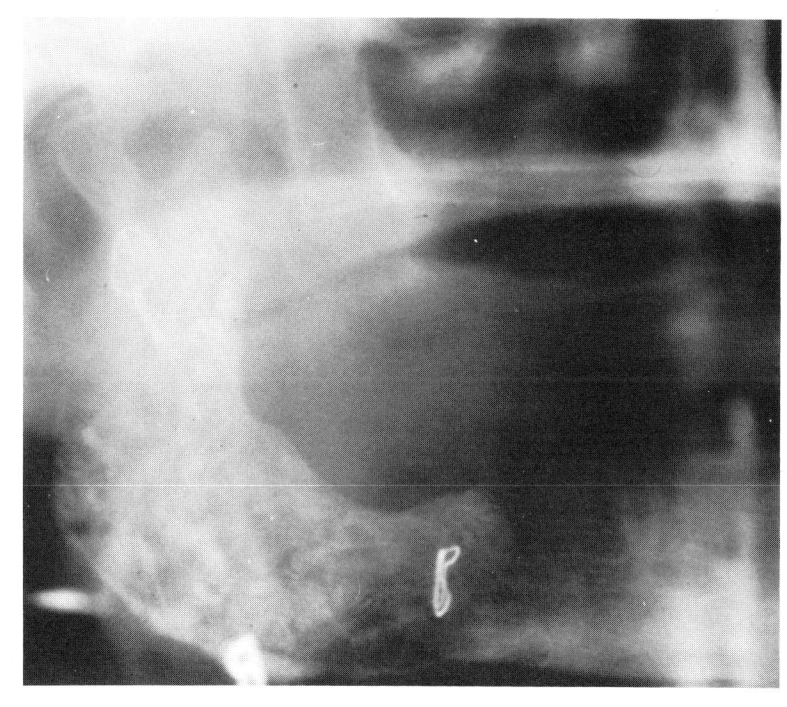

Figure 9–75. Five-year follow-up panoramic radiograph of the patient in Figure 9–73 indicates a well-consolidated graft with excellent angle contour and the development of a coronoid process from the graft.

sicles that quickly resorb have been observed by many.[30, 36, 43] Technically, there are two ways to achieve compression of PBCM into cribs. First, the PBCM is precompressed by placing it into the barrel of a sterile syringe and activating the plunger. Ten cc of bone can be compressed into a volume of 5 cc in this manner. If the barrel is cut open at the base of the needle hub, the apparatus can be used to push the compressed bone into the crib (Figs. 9–82 to 9–84). Once in the crib, an amalgam condenser can further compress the PBCM material (Figs. 9–85 and 9–86). In this way, a sufficient cellular density of viable osteocompetent cells is consistently achieved.

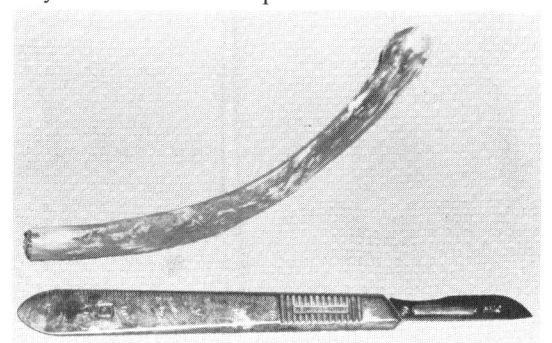

Figure 9–76. An autogenous sixth rib with a 3- to 5-mm cartilage cap can serve as a crib segment, as well as establish an articulation within the temporal fossa.

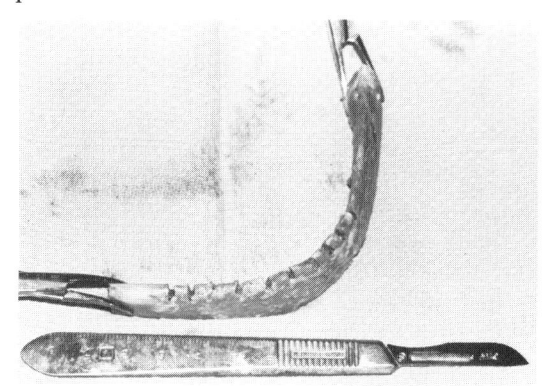

Figure 9–77. The rib can be scored and bent to conform to the contour of the angle and the posterior border of the ramus.

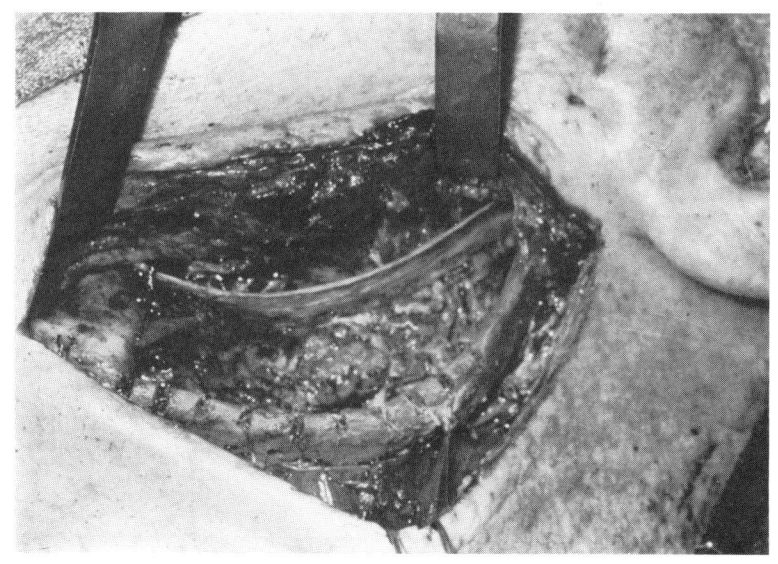

Figure 9–78. Fixed to the inferior border of the distal segment, the rib is bent and sutured to the deep tissues. The cartilagenous cap fits into the temporal fossa.

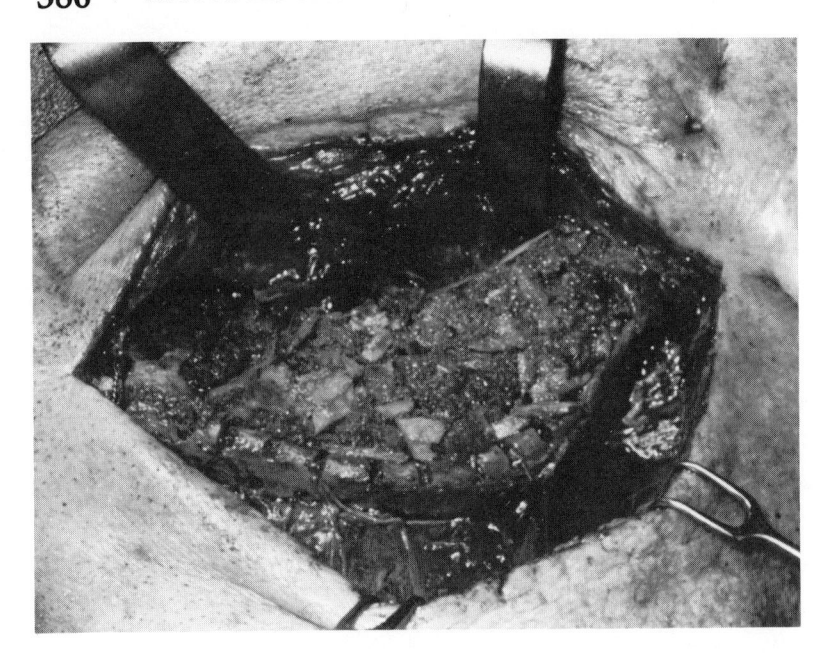

386 / RECONSTRUCTION AND REHABILITATION OF CANCER PATIENTS

Figure 9–79. With a cortical strut of allogeneic or autogenous bone at the superior margin, a PBCM graft is placed into the crib.

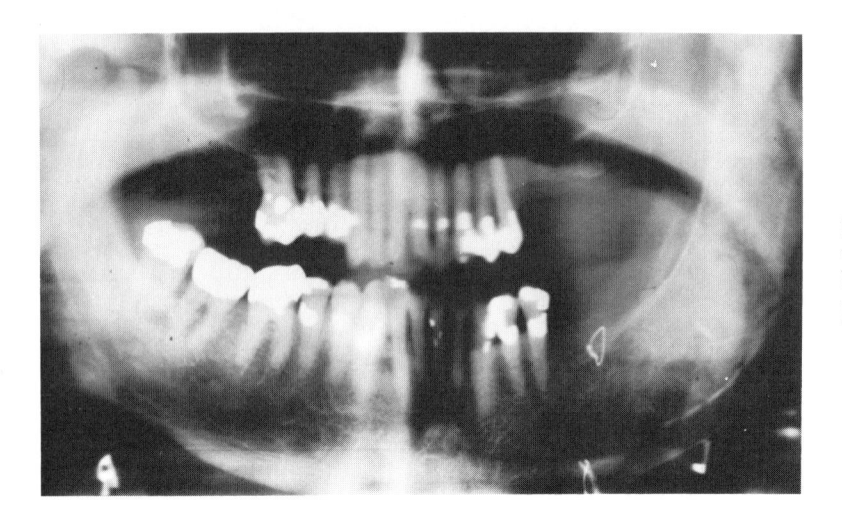

Figure 9–80. Panoramic radiograph evidencing a well-consolidated graft of excellent height and bulk and bone in a condylar form within the temporal fossa.

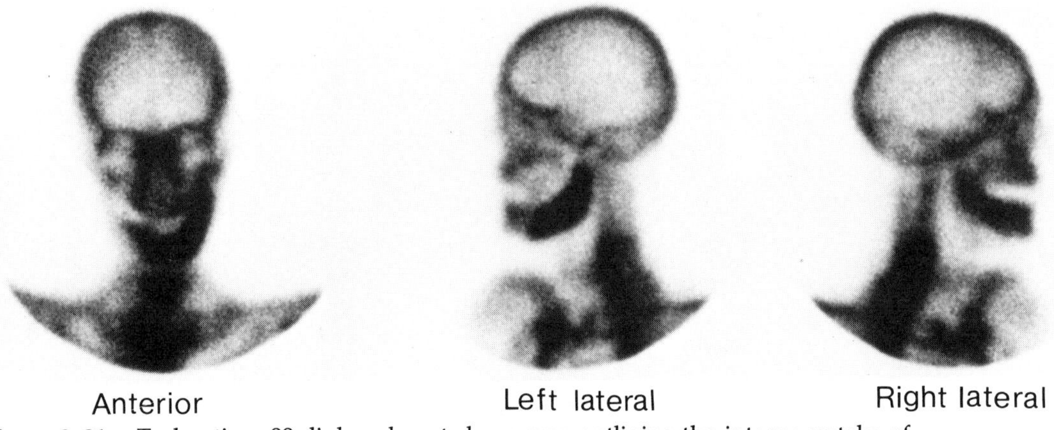

Anterior   Left lateral   Right lateral

Figure 9–81. Technetium-99 diphosphonate bone scan outlining the intense uptake of this graft, suggestive of osteoblastic activity and vascularity.

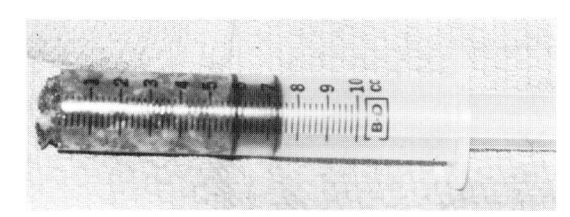

RECONSTRUCTION AND REHABILITATION OF CANCER PATIENTS / **387**

Figure 9–82. Ten cc of PBCM compressed to a volume of 5 cc.

Figure 9–83. Compressed PBCM graft material is placed into the crib by activating the plunger. The bone exits through the cut barrel end where it is further compressed by an amalgam condensor.

Figure 9–84. PBCM graft material is compressed into the crib in a sequential fashion to achieve the maximum cellular density.

Figure 9–85. Sufficient cellular density is achieved when 8 to 10 cc of PBCM graft material is compressed into the crib for each centimeter of length.

Special Considerations in Irradiated Tissues

Irradiated tissues of the head and neck have been shown to be hypovascular, hypocellular, and hypoxic[44-46] (see Fig. 9–5). This "three-H" phenomenon[44,45] defeats both phases of bone regeneration. A hypovascular recipient tissue reduces survival of transplanted osteocompetent cells. Fewer surviv-

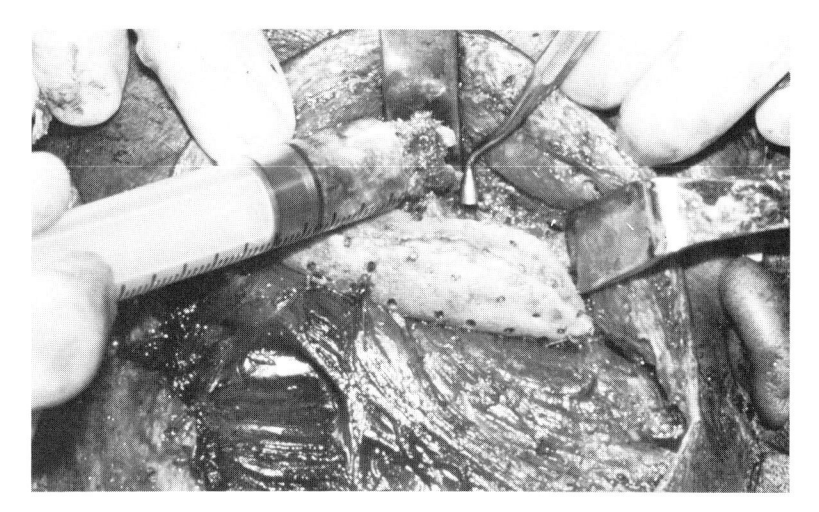

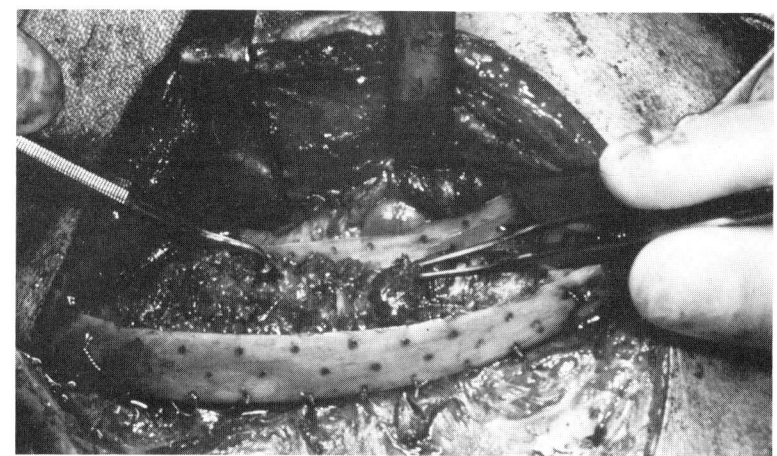

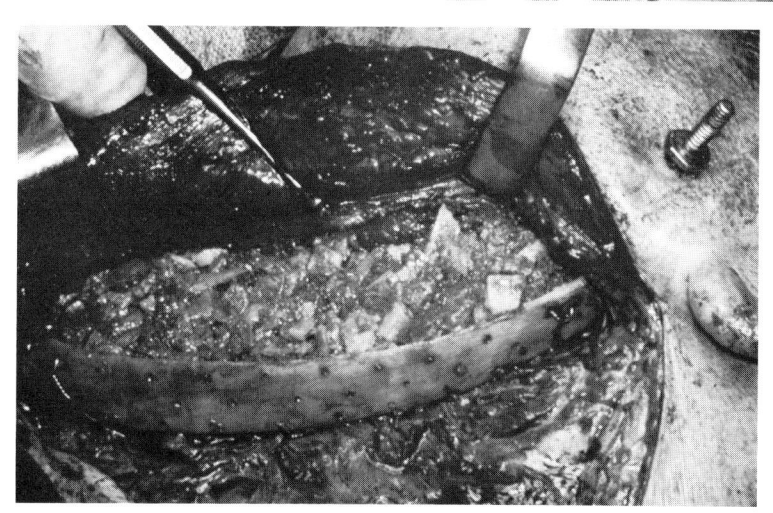

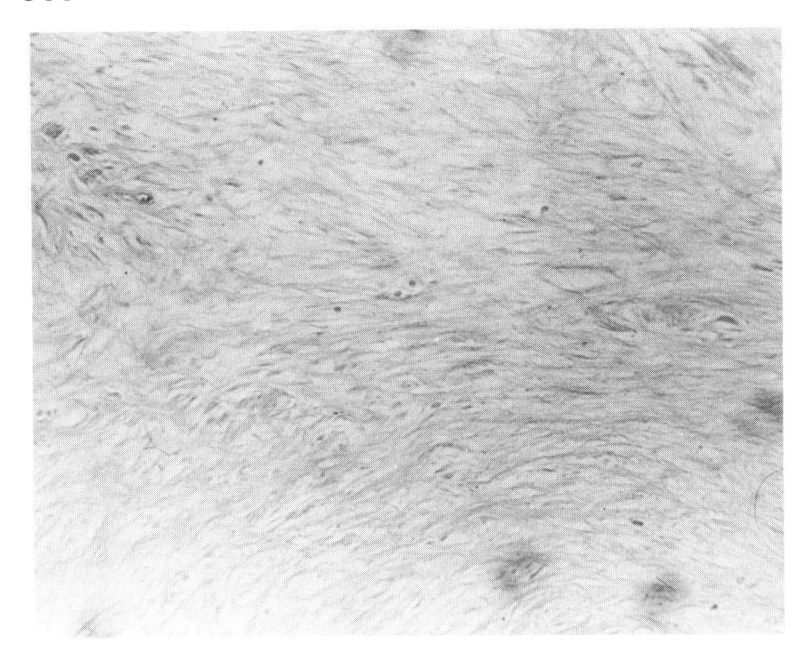

Figure 9–86. Irradiated recipient tissue bed demonstrating a hypocellular, hypovascular stroma. This tissue measured a transcutaneous oxygen reading of only 28 per cent that of nonirradiated tissue.

ing cells reduce the amount of bone formed in phase one. In hypocellular tissues, a reduced number of host fibroblasts are available to grow into grafts and become osteoblasts, and thus replacing phase-one bone with phase-two bone. A reduced number of such cells also reduces the formation of a functioning periosteum around the graft. Hypoxic tissue reflects diminished vascularity, slow cellular turnover, and a diminished capacity to heal after surgery, when metabolic and oxygen demands are markedly increased. Because of these factors, free grafts that depend on transplant cellular survival, proliferation, phase-one bone production, phase-two bone replacement of phase-one bone, and development of a periosteum have a low incidence of success and a high incidence of complications.[6–8, 28]

Recently, three approaches have been suggested to enhance reconstructive success in irradiated patients: osteomyocutaneous grafts, microvascular bone periosteal grafts, and free grafts placed into recipient tissues enhanced by hyperbaric oxygen exposures. The concept in osteomyocutaneous and microvascular bone periosteal grafts is to transplant living osteocytes on a vascular pedicle. By maintaining or anastomosing the nutrient artery and draining veins of the donor bone, osteocytes can maintain their viability. Such grafts would be independent of either phase of bone regeneration and require healing only at each graft-host interface. Exposing the recipient tissue to hyperbaric oxygen prior to bone grafting has been shown to induce an angiogenesis and fibroblastic cellular increase in irradiated tissues[8, 44, 45, 47] (Figs. 9–87 and 9–88). In addition, hyperbaric oxygen–induced increases in baseline tissue oxygen levels of irradiated tissue have been recently documented[47] (Fig. 9–89). Hyperbaric oxygen enhances both phase-one and phase-two bone regeneration in free PBCM grafts.

Osteomyocutaneous Grafts

An osteomyocutaneous graft with potential in mandibular reconstruction consists of

Figure 9–87. The irradiated recipient tissue bed of the patient in Figure 9–86 after 20 hyperbaric oxygen sessions as part of the University of Miami/HBO protocol. The tissue now demonstrates a fibroblastic cellularity, with functional vessels lined by endothelium and containing red blood cells. This tissue measured a transcutaneous oxygen reading of 81 per cent that of nonirradiated tissue.

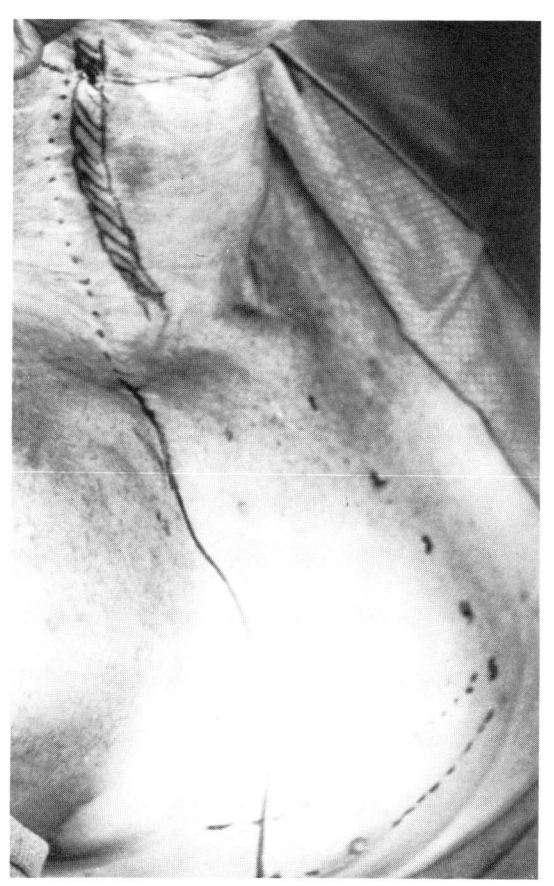

Figure 9-89. Outline of pectoralis major osteomyocutaneous graft harvesting the fourth rib and skin pedicled to the pectoralis major muscle. (Courtesy of Sterling R. Schow, D.M.D., Brooke Army Medical Center, Fort Sam Houston, Texas.)

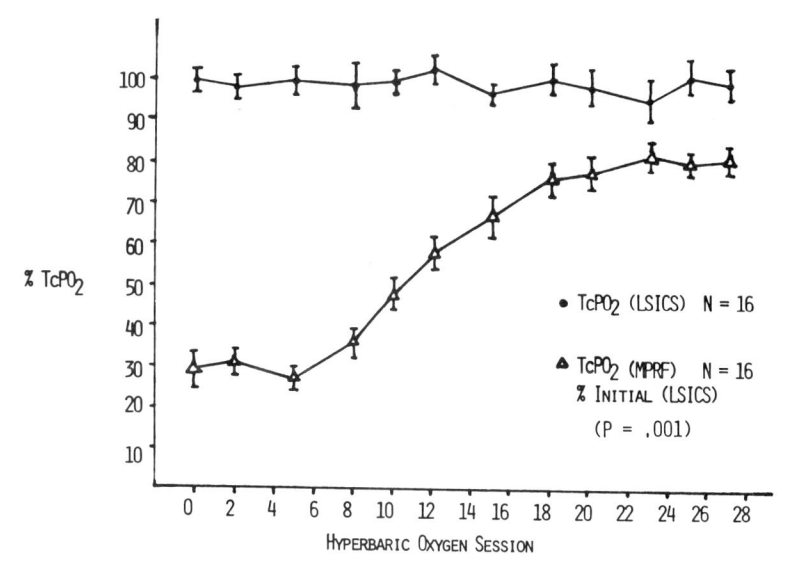

Figure 9-88. Graph of transcutaneous oxygen (TcPO$_2$) measurements normalized to the per cent of the initial reading derived from the left second intercostal space (LCICS) versus the number of hyperbaric oxygen sessions. LCICS is a reference area representing nonirradiated tissue. Its value did not appreciably change over the course of hyperbaric oxygen treatment. The midpart of the radiation field (MPRF) showed three phases: A lag phase of six to eight sessions (phase of collagen synthesis and endothelial cell proliferation), a rapid rise phase (phase of revascularization), and a plateau phase (phase of maximum revascularization and normoxic feedback inhibition of further collagen synthesis and endothelial proliferation).

rib, pectoralis major muscle, and an overlying skin paddle. This flap is based on the tissue overlying the clavicle. The blood supply is derived from the pectoralis supply in the thoracoacromial artery and venous system.[48] The optional skin paddle is taken medial and inferior to the nipple. The rib is usually the fifth, sixth, or seventh. In this graft, the muscle remains attached at the base and is tunneled subcutaneously in the neck. Transosseous wires can then be used to fix the rib to the remaining mandibular segments with an intact vascular pedicle, muscle sheath, and bone periosteal complex. The skin paddle can be used to restore soft-tissue defects or add to the quantity of the recipient bed. The muscle bulk provides soft tissue in the neck to resemble the outlines of a sternocleidomastoid muscle (Figs. 9-90 to 9-92).

Bone, on a vascular pedicle with its own soft tissue, is an attractive concept. In theory, maintaining the blood supply to a segment of bone permits transplanting viable osteocytes and mineral matrix. Such an achievement bypasses the need for either phase-one or phase-two bone regeneration.

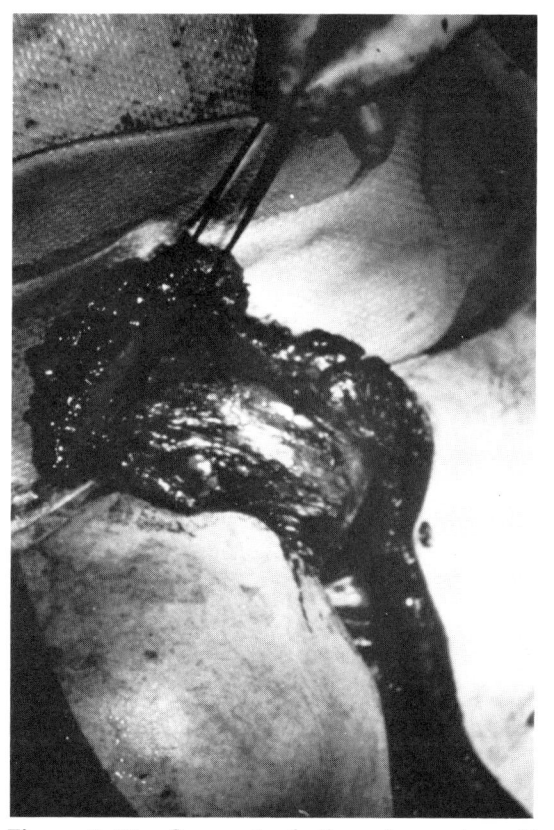

Figure 9-90. Segment of rib and muscle cuff with muscle pedicle. (Courtesy of Sterling R. Schow, D.M.D., Brooke Army Medical Center, Fort Sam Houston, Texas.)

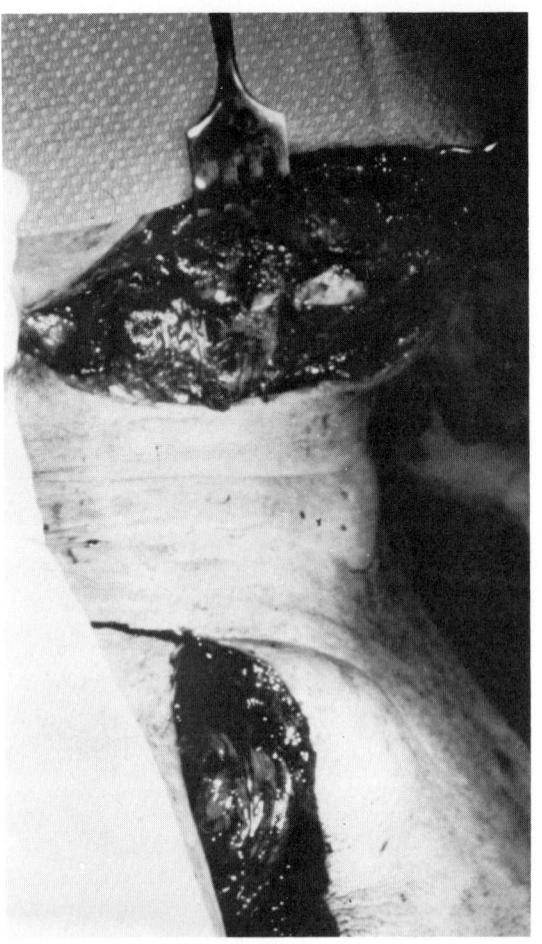

Figure 9–91. Segment of rib and muscle tunneled subcutaneously in the neck and fixed to the recipient bone ends. (Courtesy of Sterling R. Schow, D.M.D., Brooke Army Medical Center, Fort Sam Houston, Texas.)

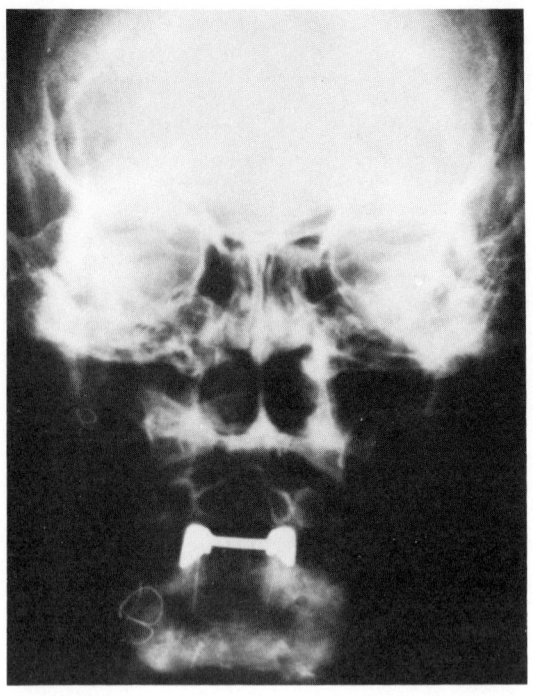

Figure 9–92. Postoperative radiograph of viable rib regaining continuity and facial symmetry. (Courtesy of Sterling R. Schow, D.M.D., Brooke Army Medical Center, Fort Sam Houston, Texas.)

drainage producing congestion, edema, and eventually ischemic necrosis (Figs. 9–93 and 9–94). In irradiated necks, the tunneling procedure often places the flap between the unresilient, irradiated skin and the bony clavi-

The graft should heal by callus formation at each graft-host interface. The longevity of the graft would be assured through the transplantation of viable vascularized periosteum. This would obviate the need for induction of host fibroblasts to assume a periosteum role. Practical experience with this system, however, falls short of the theoretical possibilities. Perforating vessels from the muscle to the periosteum and bone, as well as to the skin paddle, are unpredictable and vary greatly among individuals. Often the bone or skin paddle becomes devitalized. Even when perforating vessels do afford bone viability, often it is not a long enough segment for the common continuity defects of the mandible. Also, the rib cannot be scored or bent to develop a mandibular contour, as devitalization may occur owing to interruption of the periosteal blood supply. The failures associated with these flaps have generally not been due to inadequate arterial supply but rather to inadequate venous

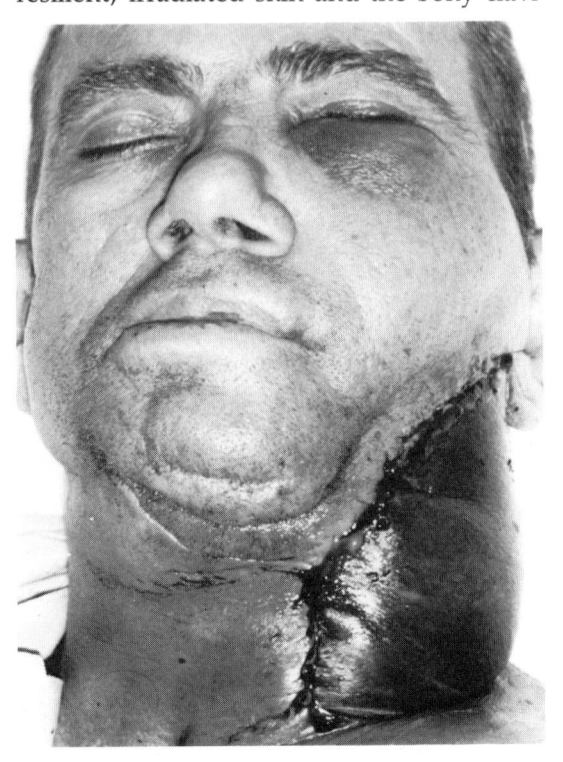

Figure 9–93. Osteomyocutaneous flap undergoing ischemic necrosis 24 hours after placement owing to impeded venous drainage.

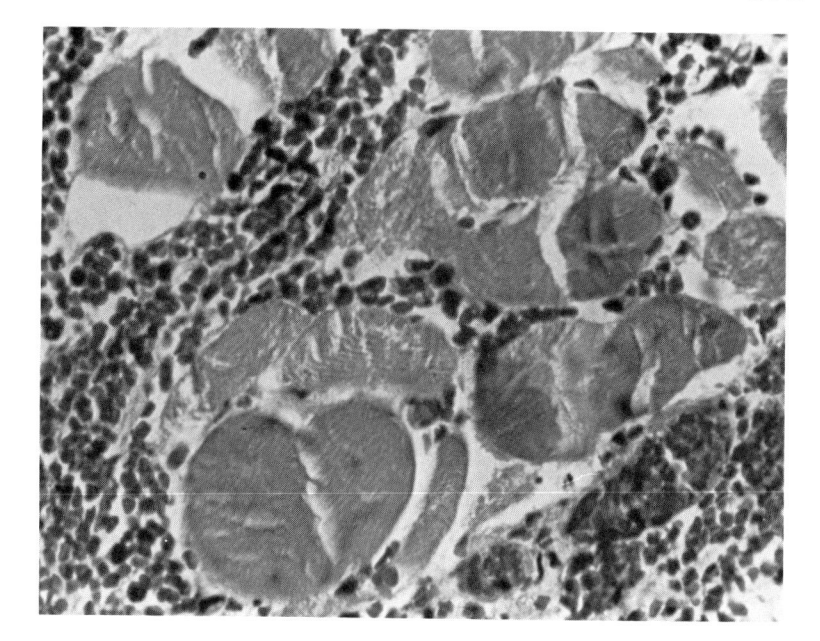

Figure 9–94. Photomicrograph of muscle from the case in Figure 9–93, evidencing muscle degeneration and severe vascular congestion.

cle, obstructing venous drainage (Fig. 9–93). To combat this, some surgeons resect the middle third of the clavicle or fracture it at mid-length. Even a successful graft affords an inadequate bulk of bone to be functionally useful. Such grafts do not meet the five criteria used to determine graft success. The concept, nevertheless, has some merit. Myocutaneous flaps without bone have been shown to be useful for improving quality and quantity of soft-tissue recipient beds. They have also been useful for immediate reconstruction of large soft-tissue defects from extirpative surgery.[49, 50] With bone, their value as a reconstructive system for mandibular defects remains to be demonstrated and their use is currently plagued with unacceptable levels of morbidity.

Microvascular Bone Periosteal Grafts

Microvascular Rib Periosteal Grafts. Since the beginning of microsurgical techniques, transfer of vascularized bone segments for mandibular reconstruction has shown great potential. In dog models and in some early human trials, viability and union of vascularized rib grafts have been reported. Donoff has shown re-establishment of periosteal blood flow in dogs and seems to have achieved the same in humans.[9, 51] The technique requires an intrathoracic harvest of the anterior and middle third of a rib with its nutrient anterior intercostal artery and draining vein. Ariyan and Finseth have shown the blood supply of the anterior third of a rib to be adequate for microvascular free transfers.[52] The harvest of the posterior third of a rib jeopardizes the artery of Adamkiewicz supplying the local segment of spinal cord, thus risking paraplegia. The rib-periosteum composite is transferred to the recipient tissue, where an intact artery and vein have been prepared for anastomosis (Fig. 9–95). Even in irradiated or previously operated necks, useful recipient vessels have not been difficult to locate (Fig. 9–96A). Under the microscope, the anastomosis using 10-0 nylon sutures on a BV750 needle or its equivalent is accomplished (Fig. 9–96B). The graft ends are fitted into place with as much minimal scoring as possible to prevent devitalization. Fixation to the remaining mandibular segments is accomplished with transosseous wires.

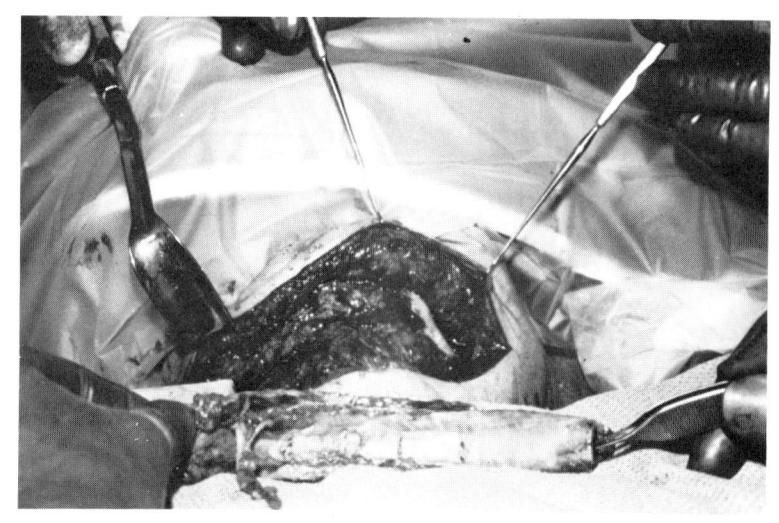

Figure 9–95. Autogenous rib harvested with an intact periosteum, nutrient intercostal artery, and draining vein is transferred to the recipient tissue in the neck. (Courtesy of R. Bruce Donoff, D.M.D., M.D., and Nalton F. Ferraro, D.M.D., M.D., Massachusetts General Hospital, Boston.)

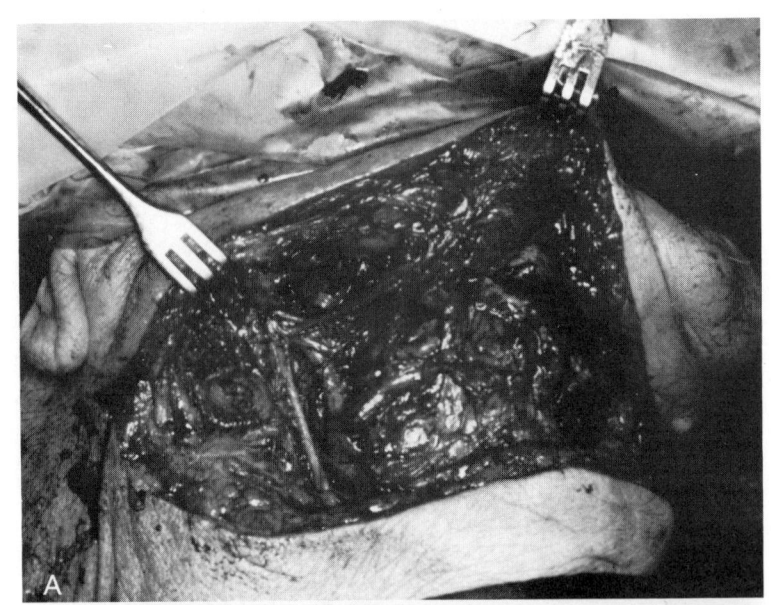

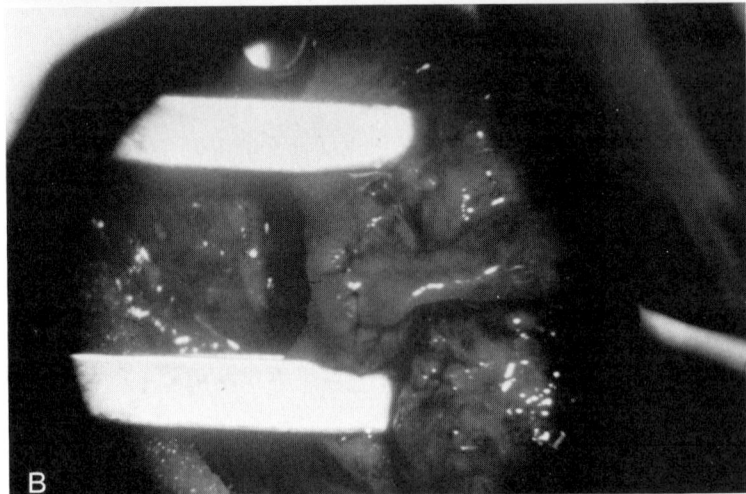

Figure 9–96. *A*, In spite of irradiation, which affects smaller vessels, suitable larger vessels are usually present into which an anastomosis may be accomplished. *B*, An end-to-side microvascular anastomosis is accomplished using 10-0 nylon sutures. (Courtesy of R. Bruce Donoff, D.M.D., M.D., and Nalton F. Ferraro, D.M.D., M.D., Massachusetts General Hospital, Boston.)

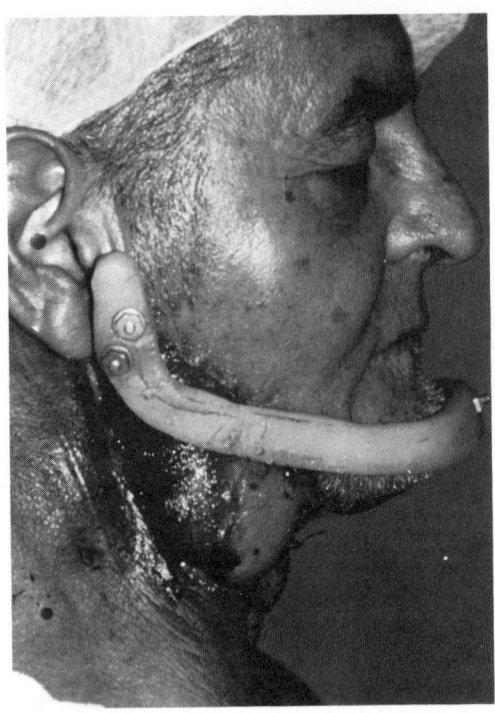

Figure 9–97. Partial or complete necrosis of the flap is possible if the vascular pedicle is disrupted or thromboses.

If successful, such a system offers the possibility of reconstruction without bone regeneration in irradiated and scarred recipient tissue. However, several series have reported some distressing complications.[53, 54] In some cases, the anastomosis fails, leaving a block-type graft within nonviable soft tissue. This usually results in graft loss (Fig. 9–97). The rib harvest requires closed-chest drainage in every case. In 14 cases reported by Serafin et al.,[53] 12 developed pleural effusions and four developed significant pneumonias extending the hospital course. In addition, three developed gastrointestinal bleeds, three developed malunions, two developed orocutaneous fistulae, and two grafts were completely lost. Only one graft of 14 was sufficient to support a prosthesis. Increased blood loss and increased length of both surgery and hospital stays gave Serafin et al. cause to suggest that "significant patient morbidity and pulmonary complications should indicate caution when considering these methods of reconstruction." Nevertheless, microvascular transfer of rib for the resected mandible is an important consideration in compromised recipient tissue. The apparent morbidity must be weighed against the results. The extensive morbidity and marginal results reported by Serafin et al. are being improved and techniques perfected. The future of this graft system depends on the training and expertise of microsurgeons. The inadequacy of a rib, even if the microsurgery is completely successful, is a major problem with this technique (Fig. 9–98).

Microvascular Iliac Crest Grafts. Another microvascular graft under clinical investigation utilizes bone from the ilium with its overlying soft tissue. It is based upon the vascular supply from the deep circumflex iliac artery with its variable concomitant veins (Fig. 9–99). In an effort to improve upon the marginal osseous bulk of a rib, Ryan has investigated this system[55] and found that it demonstrated significant patient morbidity (Figs. 9–100 to 9–102). Morbidity from this

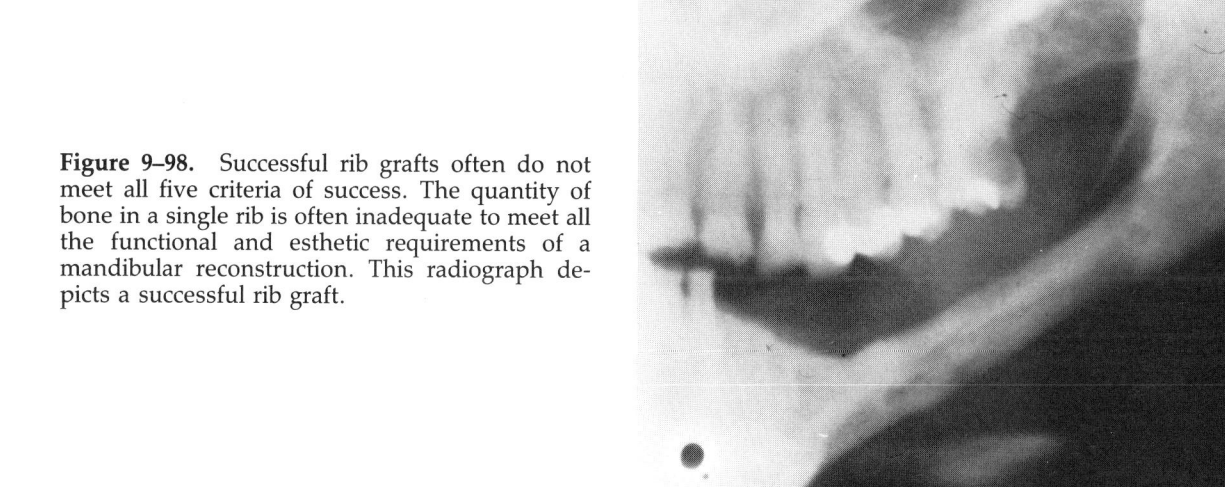

Figure 9-98. Successful rib grafts often do not meet all five criteria of success. The quantity of bone in a single rib is often inadequate to meet all the functional and esthetic requirements of a mandibular reconstruction. This radiograph depicts a successful rib graft.

technique takes the form of delayed ambulation and an extended hospital course. This prolonged recovery is due to the inclusion of portions of the iliacus and gluteus medius muscle cuffs in the donor tissue (Fig. 9-101).

Stone and Franklin have investigated a similar approach for immediate reconstructions in large, hard- and soft-tissue cancer-related defects. Although tissue transplant survival was reported, extensive blood loss and pulmonary emboli occurred.[56] Free transfers of iliac crest are limited in length and ability to be bent into an arch form. Their usefulness is, therefore, limited to hemimandibular defects that do not extend past the canine region. As with microvascular rib-periosteal grafts, technique perfection and further clinical trials are required before this sytem can be used on a wider scale.

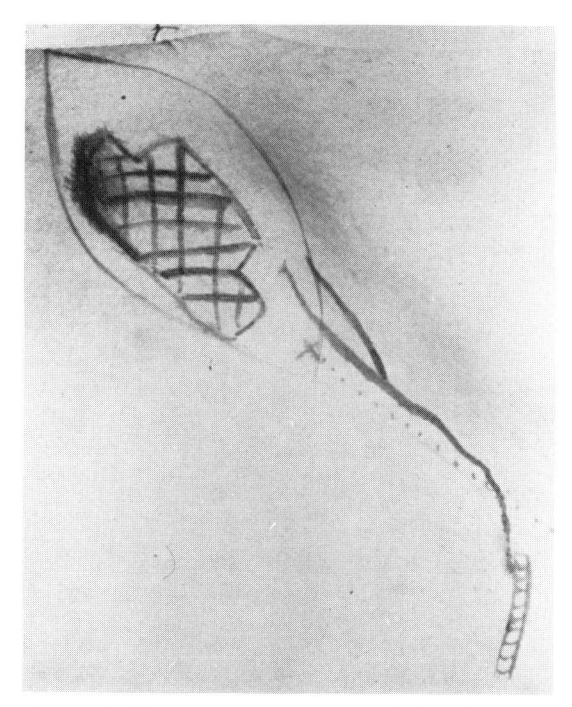

Figure 9-99. Surgical diagram of the deep circumflex iliac arterial course to the medial aspect of the right iliac crest. (Courtesy of Doran E. Ryan, D.D.S., Medical College of Wisconsin, Milwaukee.)

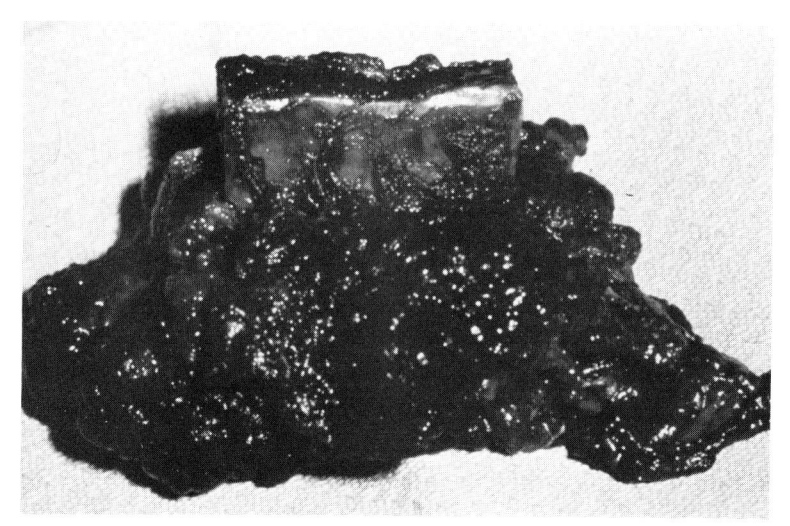

Figure 9-100. Block of right ilium and cuff of gluteus medium muscle harvested for a microvascular free transfer. (Courtesy of Doran E. Ryan, D.D.S., Medical College of Wisconsin, Milwaukee.)

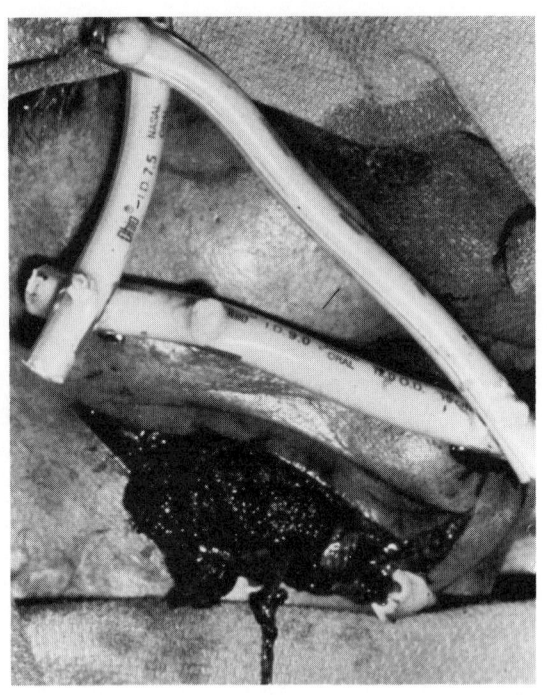

Figure 9–101. Bone block and muscle are transferred to the recipient tissue bed with long vessel length suitable for anastomosis with existing neck vessels. (Courtesy of Doran E. Ryan, D.D.S., Medical College of Wisconsin, Milwaukee.)

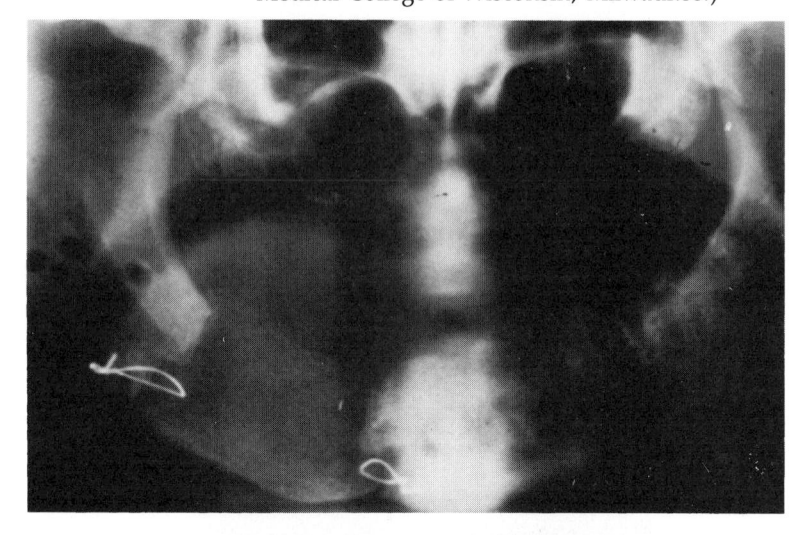

Hyperbaric Oxygen–Enhanced Recipient Tissue

Owing to poor results seen with nonvascularized bone grafts placed into irradiated and scarred tissues[6, 7] and excessive morbidity of microvascular grafts,[53–55] a growing interest in hyperbaric oxygen (HBO) has occurred. Improving compromised recipient tissue so that common and straightforward graft systems may be used with success is an attractive concept.

Early use of hyperbaric oxygen focused on postsurgical application to promote graft survival and enhance osteogenesis.[57, 58] Recently, Marx and Ames have focused the application of HBO on the presurgical phase, indicating that HBO improves the vascularity and cellularity of the recipient tissues.[8] It has been suggested that HBO enhances the contributions from both phases of bone regeneration. Irradiated tissues of the neck demonstrate oxygen tensions between 5 and 15 torr.[47] Nonirradiated tissues demonstrate oxygen tensions between 45 and 55 torr.[47, 49, 50] At depth, HBO improves irradiated tissue oxygen tensions to levels as high as 50 to 150 torr independent of hemoglobin saturation.

Figure 9–102. Panoramic radiograph of successful ilium block microvascular transfer. (Courtesy of Doran E. Ryan, D.D.S., Medical College of Wisconsin, Milwaukee.)

Figure 9–103. Two-week panoramic radiograph of a PBCM graft placed in a patient who had received 7200 rads of irradiation. He was reconstructed using the University of Miami/HBO protocol.

Figure 9–104. A two-year follow-up panoramic film indicates a consolidated graft without resorption, fulfilling all five criteria of a successful reconstruction.

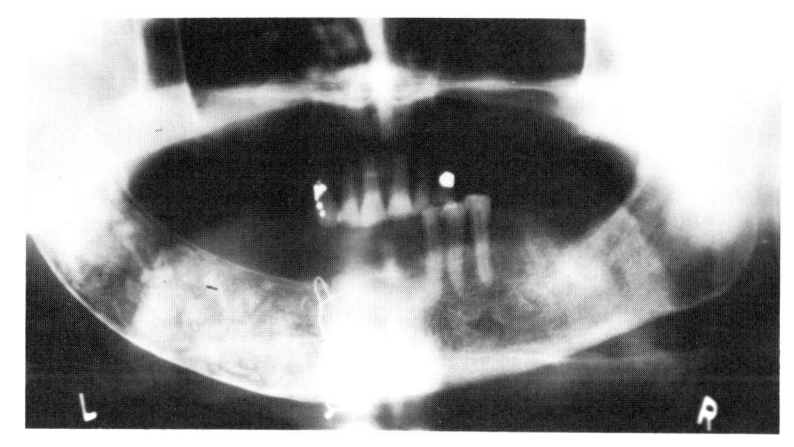

When sea level pressures and room air breathing are restored, oxygen tensions of irradiated tissue fall back to the 5 to 15 torr range. After 8 to 12 sessions of HBO, irradiated tissue oxygen tensions remain above pre-HBO levels after return to sea level pressures. Between the eighth and eighteenth exposures, irradiated tissue oxygen tensions rise to 80 to 85 per cent of those of nonirradiated tissues and seem to plateau at this level (Fig. 9–88), suggesting that the increase in irradiated tissue oxygen tensions is due to HBO-induced angiogenesis. Using a protocol based on these findings, we have accomplished 116 mandibular reconstructions of hemimandibulectomy defects in irradiated patients. One hundred and five have fulfilled the five criteria of success discussed earlier in this chapter, including long-term follow-up without resorption (Figs. 9–103 to 9–111). The University of Miami protocol

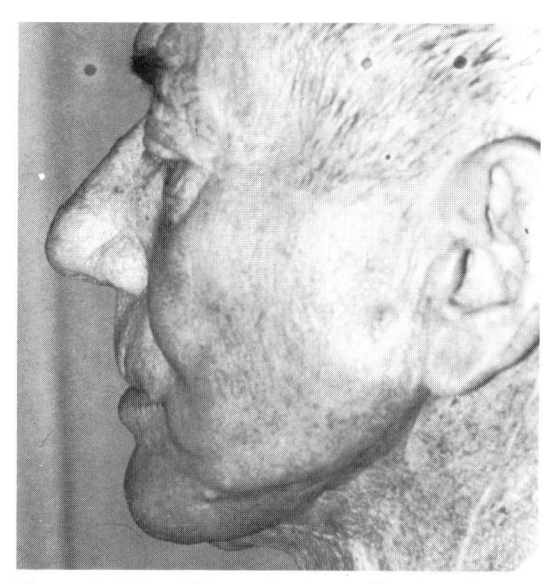

Figure 9–106. This patient's profile view demonstrates excellent contour and chin position.

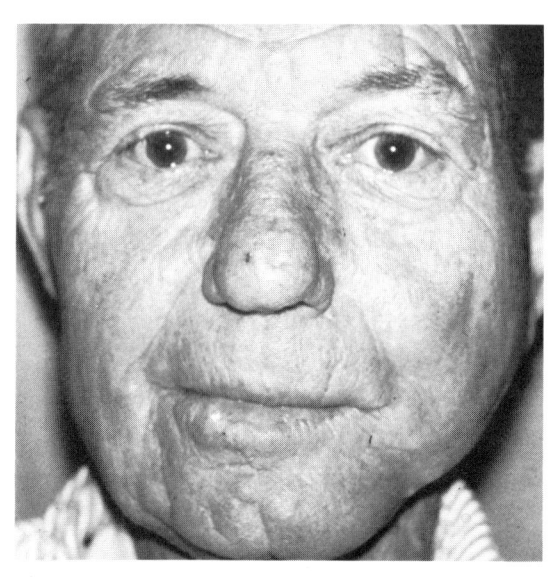

Figure 9–105. This patient's frontal view demonstrates symmetry and cosmetic contour achieved despite tissue deficiency and irradiated tissue.

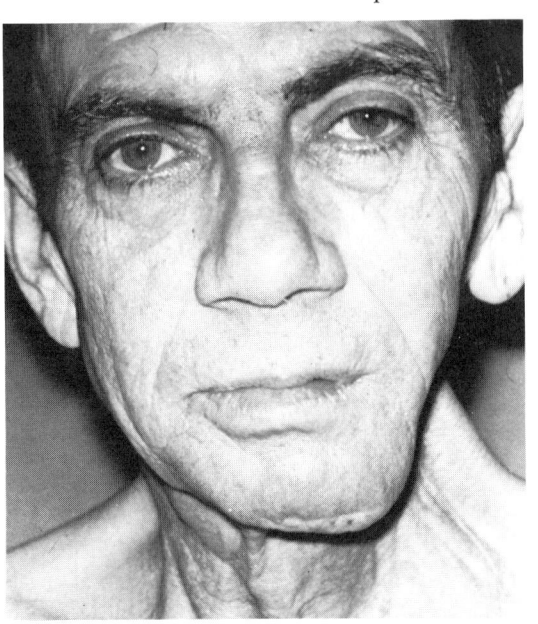

Figure 9–107. Patient seen prior to reconstruction after a hemimandibulectomy, radical neck dissection, and 8000 rads of irradiation.

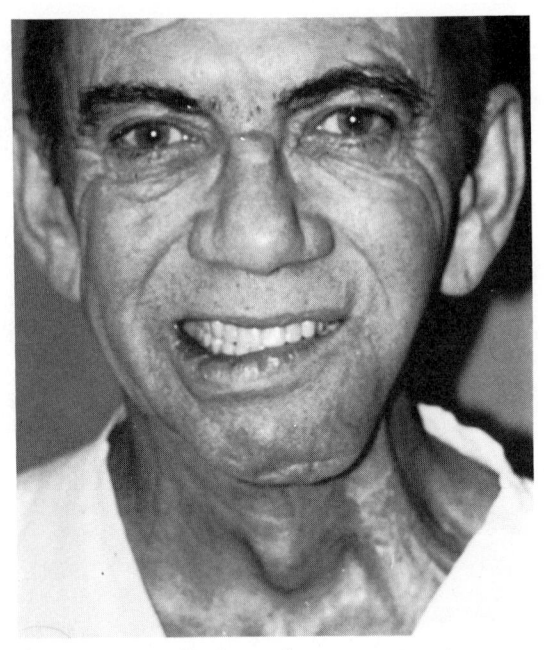

Figure 9–108. Patient after reconstruction supported by the University of Miami/HBO protocol. Despite irradiation, all patients requiring a prosthesis are fitted with one.

consists of (1) 20 presurgical HBO sessions, (2) bone graft reconstruction, (3) 10 postsurgical HBO sessions, (4) necessary ridge extension procedures accomplished 10 weeks after grafting, and (5) functional loading eight weeks after the last surgical procedure. Each HBO session consists of 90 minutes of HBO exposure at 2.4 atmospheres absolute pressure. Sessions may run one per day, five days per week.

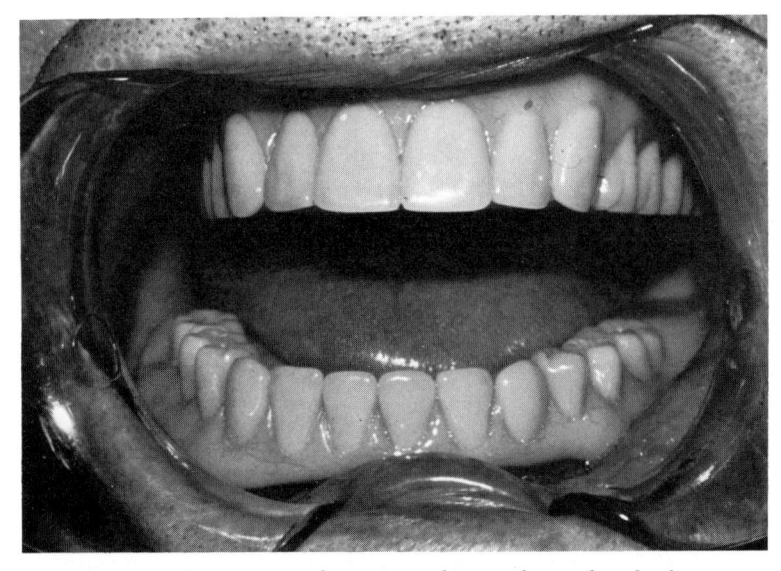

Figure 9–109. Patient's appliances in place with good arch alignment, occlusal relationship, and function without mucosal breakdown.

The actual mechanism by which HBO enhances both phases of bone regeneration goes back to the common pathways of connective tissue repair. The intermittent (once per day) application of HBO allows the fibroblasts within the compromised recipient tissue to produce collagen during HBO exposure. They will still retain the stimulus for collagen synthesis by returning to the hypoxic state after each session. When enough collagen synthesis occurs, endothelial cell proliferation will develop new capillaries so that revascularization of the irradiated tissue can begin. Because it takes several days to synthesize enough collagen to promote angiogenesis, the 6- to 8- session delay before irradiated tissue oxygen tensions rise is an expected observation. Through serial biopsies, Beehner and Marx[47] have shown an HBO-induced fibroblastic neocellularity and neovascularity of irradiated tissues into which bone grafts were placed (Figs. 9–86 to 9–88). The neovascularity promotes enhanced cellular survival of osteoprogenitor cells as well as an early revascularization of the bone graft. Both mechanisms enhance phase-one bone regeneration. The neocellularity increases the population of host cells capable of graft invasion to enhance phase-two remodeling replacement. It also develops a functional periosteum about the graft for long-term stability.

It is clear that HBO has the theoretical mechanisms to support all bone graft systems. Its most advantageous application is to enhance recipient tissues prior to bone grafting. Clinically, HBO has improved reconstruction success rates in irradiated tissues from about 50 per cent to well over 90 per cent.[8, 44, 45] There are many desirable attributes of HBO for the surgeon: HBO does not increase surgical morbidity, HBO does not require special training or instrumentation, and HBO allows the surgeon to use common, straightforward graft systems with success.

The biggest drawback of HBO is that it will not improve the quantity of the soft-tissue recipient bed. If extirpative surgery has left the reconstructive surgeon with a thin tissue space between skin and oral mucosa, a soft-tissue flap for bulk is still required. In addition, HBO chambers are not readily available to all surgeons. However, hyperbaric medicine is an expanding specialty. There are 143 chambers in the United States and over 100 in Western Europe, and additional facilities are under construction.

The contraindications to HBO are few but important. HBO is contraindicated in patients with optic neuritis because of the possibility of exacerbation. It is also contraindicated in active viral or immunosuppressive disorders because of a suspected but unproven immunosuppression by HBO.[59, 60] Patients with active malignancies have in the past been excluded from HBO; it was conjectured that increased oxygen tensions might increase the replication rate of tumors. Recent work strongly suggests this is not true.[61, 62] Harmon and Marx, using a squamous cell carcinoma model, have demonstrated equal tumor growth rates in HBO-exposed and control animals.[62] Patients requiring reconstruction for cancer-related defects have a greater risk of developing second primaries and persistent tumor from the known carcinogens of tobacco, alcohol, and irradiation.[63] These findings indicate that HBO may be used in these patients without adding to their risk.

HBO is a recent advancement in maxillofacial reconstruction. It is growing in popularity because its morbidity is minimal and because application to bone grafting systems does not require special training or instrumentation. It allows surgeons to operate in irradiated and scarred tissue with reduced complications of wound healing. HBO, however, is not a panacea for reconstruction, nor is it so effective that it allows the surgeon to deviate from sound surgical principles and sterile techniques. Our experience with HBO included 14 failures in 154 reconstructions in irradiated tissues. All were related to technical errors that were not preventable or salvageable with HBO.

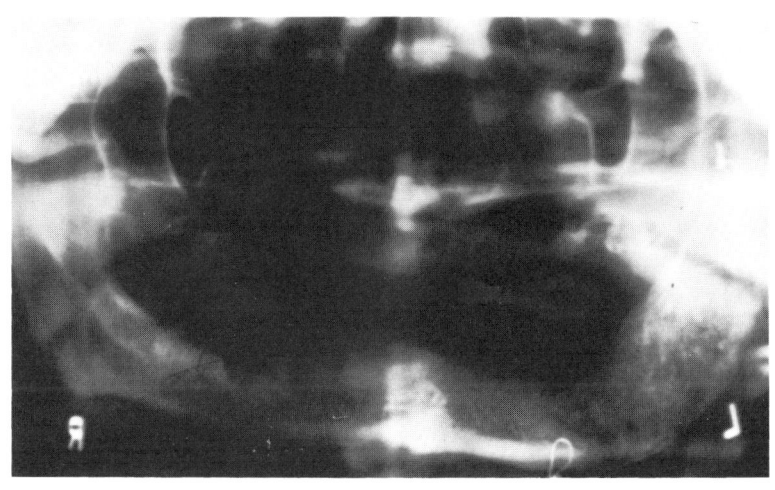

Figure 9–110. Patient's radiograph three years after reconstruction demonstrates a consistent osseous bulk without resorption.

Special Considerations Where Quantitative Soft-Tissue Defects Exist

The vascular and cellular quality of the recipient tissue is important to reconstructive efforts; likewise, the quantitative volume of the recipient tissue is equally important. Not only is it required so that a bone graft can be placed without dehiscence through mucosa or skin, but it also provides facial contour. Although bony reconstruction improves facial contour greatly, it cannot make up for extensive soft-tissue extirpation. As we have stated, local tissue flaps of dermis and skin[64] and deltopectoral flaps are not desirable because their high fat content does not support phase-one or phase-two bone regeneration.[40] Several muscle and myocutaneous flaps have been used to bring vascular and inducible tissue into the intended recipient bed from the irradiated field. The development of these flaps has been a great advantage to the surgeon reconstructing cancer-related defects.

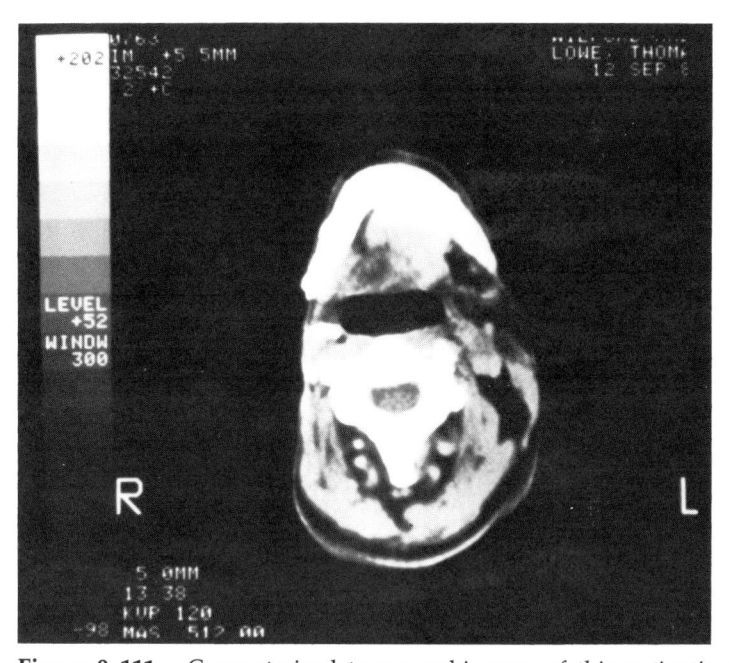

Figure 9–111. Computerized tomographic scan of this patient's graft demonstrates the equal or greater bulk of bone and contour as compared to the unoperated side.

The Sternocleidomastoid Muscular and Myocutaneous Flaps

Many of today's reconstructive indications arise from defects secondary to resections for osteoradionecrosis[44, 45] and from bony defects in which functional neck dissections have preserved the sternocleidomastoid muscle (SCM).[1, 2] This is a convenient local muscle that may be used as a muscular or myocutaneous flap, made possible by a dominant artery arising from the occipital artery in its superior third[49, 50] (Fig. 9–112). The muscle is

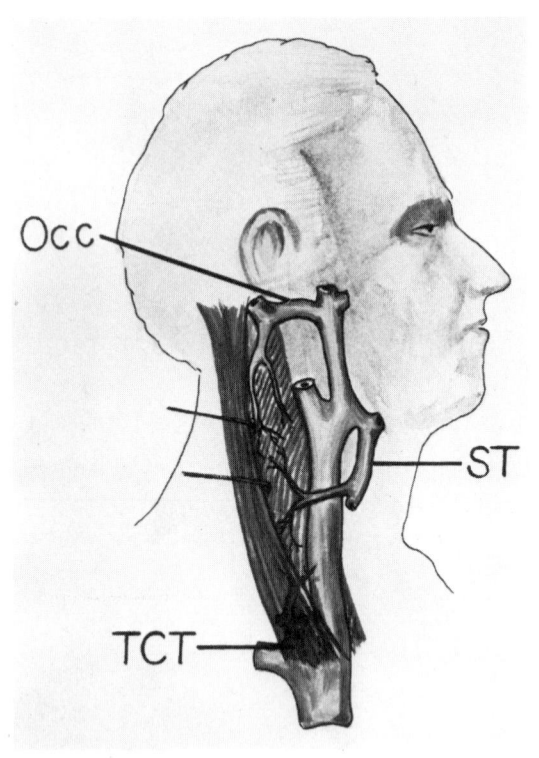

Figure 9–112. Illustration of the vascular anatomy of the sternocleidomastoid muscle. The dominant supply is through the occipital vessels, although the superior thyroid vessels are required to maintain the viability of the inferior 3 to 5 cm. (Occ = Occipital, ST = superior thyroid, TCT = thyrocervical trunk.)

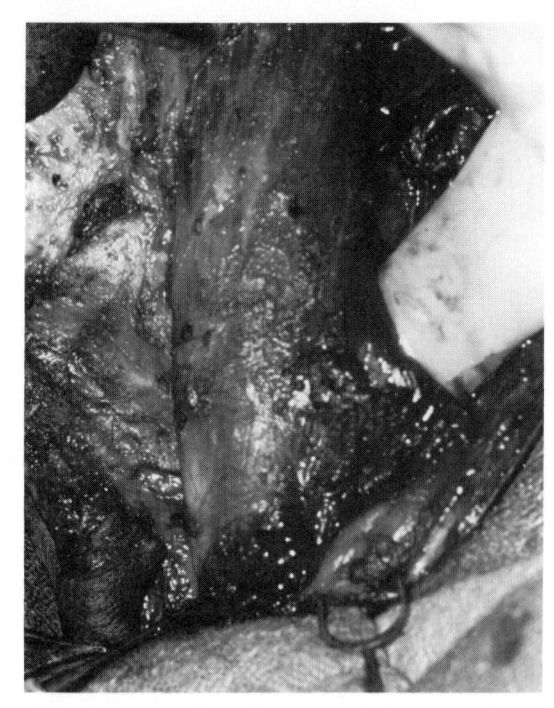

Figure 9–114. Detachment of the sternal and clavicular heads of the sternocleidomastoid muscle is facilitated by an electrocautery knife and the dissection of the muscle free from the carotid sheath.

also supplied by branches off the superior thyroid artery at its middle third, a variable branch from the inferior thyroid, or an unnamed branch off the thyrocervical trunk at its inferior third. Through a rich anastomosis, the dominant occipital branch can maintain the viability of the muscle and overlying skin territory for the entire muscle length except for the inferior 3 to 5 cm (Fig. 9–113). To maintain this lower segment of muscle and overlying skin, preservation of the superior thyroid branches is required.

As a muscular flap, the SCM has been useful in obliterating dead space and providing a vascular tissue in the angle and body regions during bony reconstruction. It also provides a soft-tissue bulk for facial contour around the angle region. During bony recon-

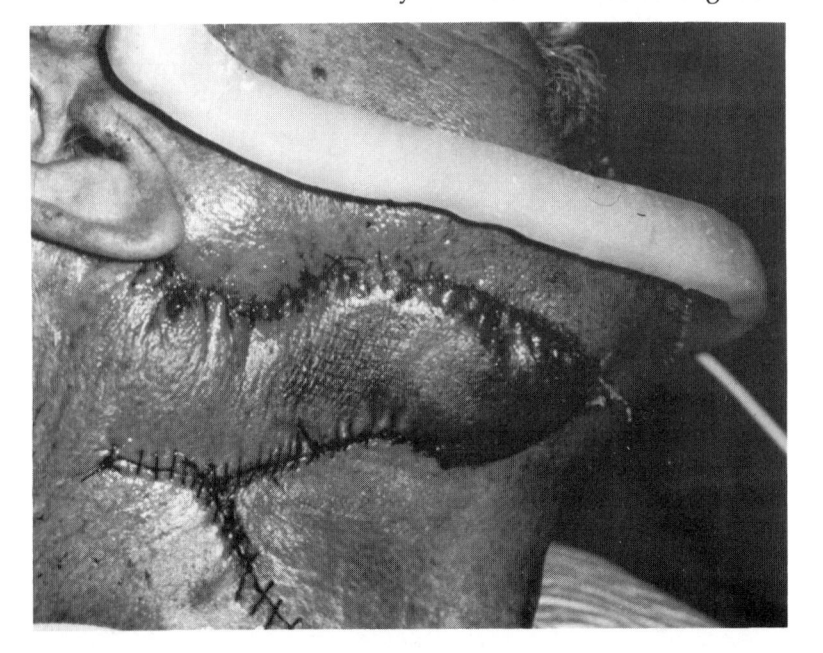

Figure 9–113. Tissue necrosis and vascular congestion evident in a sternocleidomastoid myocutaneous flap in which the superior thyroid vessels were sacrificed.

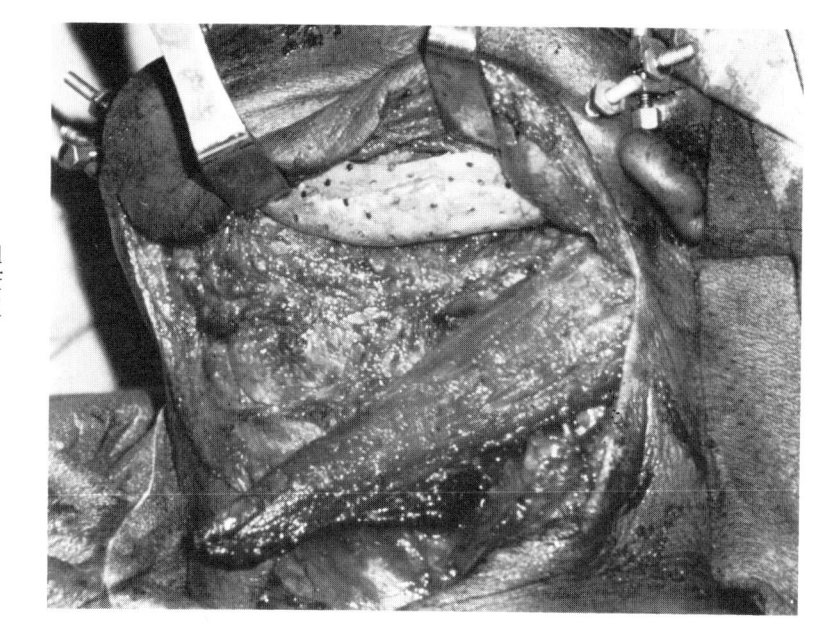

Figure 9–115. Traction suture placed at sternal and clavicular insertions facilitates dissection of muscle from the deep fascia and the carotid sheath.

struction, access to the full length of SCM can be obtained by making an incision over the anterior border from the submandibular incision used to prepare the bone graft bed to the sternoclavicular joint. The skin is separated from the muscle fascia and retracted. Beginning at the anterior border, the muscle is reflected from the deep cervical fascia and carotid sheath by blunt dissection at its inferior third. Placing a gloved finger beneath the muscle in the supraclavicular fossa will allow incision of the muscle from its clavicular and sternal insertions without risking the structures immediately deep to the muscle (Fig. 9–114). With traction sutures placed at the sternal and clavicular heads, the muscle can be separated under direct vision from the carotid sheath and fascia in an avascular plane between these and the deep muscle fascia (Figs. 9–115 and 9–116). Although its inferior vessels require ligation, it is worthwhile to attempt preservation of the superior thyroid vessels for a more assured vascular supply. Based on its mastoid inser-

Figure 9–116. Sternocleidomastoid muscle dissected from the carotid sheath and based on its mastoid origin. A branch of the superior thyroid artery can be seen entering its deep surface at the anterior border.

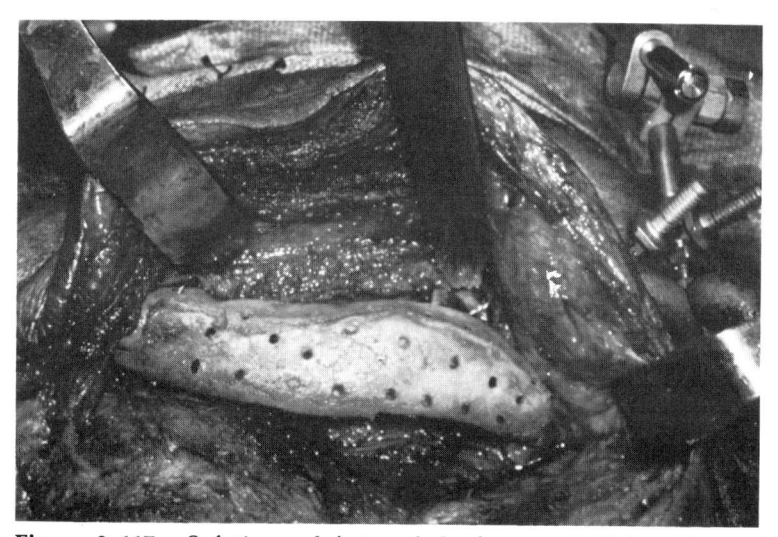

Figure 9–117. Soft-tissue defect and dead space medial to the graft into which the muscle will be transposed.

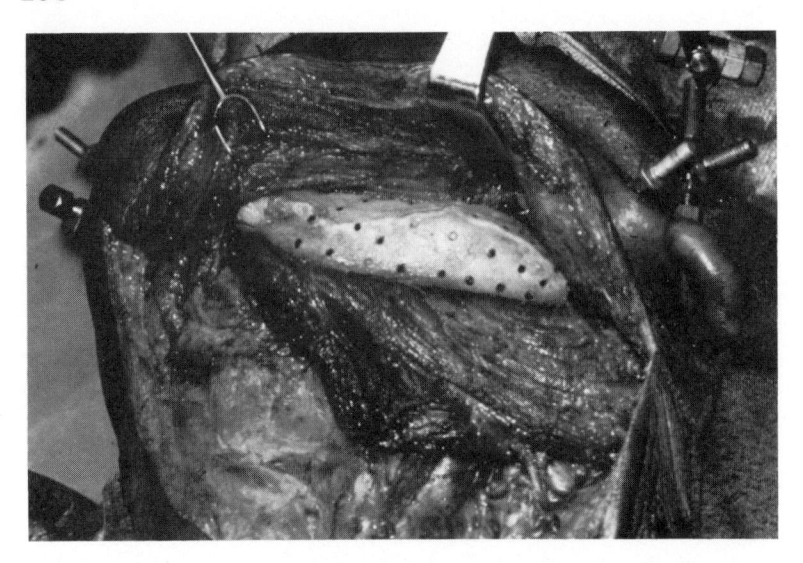

Figure 9–118. Transposed muscle obliterating dead space and providing a vascular tissue bulk in the area. The muscle is sutured to the deep tissue bed and to the allogeneic bone crib.

tion and occipital branches, the SCM can be rotated to obliterate dead space and provide contour from the angle to the canine region (Figs. 9–117 to 9–120). Closure is obtained by reapproximating the overlying skin in a "Y"-shaped closure in the neck.

As a myocutaneous flap, we have found the SCM useful in adding soft-tissue bulk to the angle and body region prior to bony reconstruction. It also provides cover and closure in severely scarred necks at the time of bony reconstruction. A set of perforating vessels from the muscle belly to the overlying skin territory that serves as a myocutaneous flap is an additional anatomic feature of the SCM. Sufficient perforating vessels do exist to transfer a width of skin over the full length of the muscle as wide as the distance from its anterior to its posterior border.[65, 66] The flap is developed by incising the skin in the supraclavicular fossa, over the anterior and posterior borders of the muscle, so that two parallel incisions are formed. Without further retraction or dissection, the skin

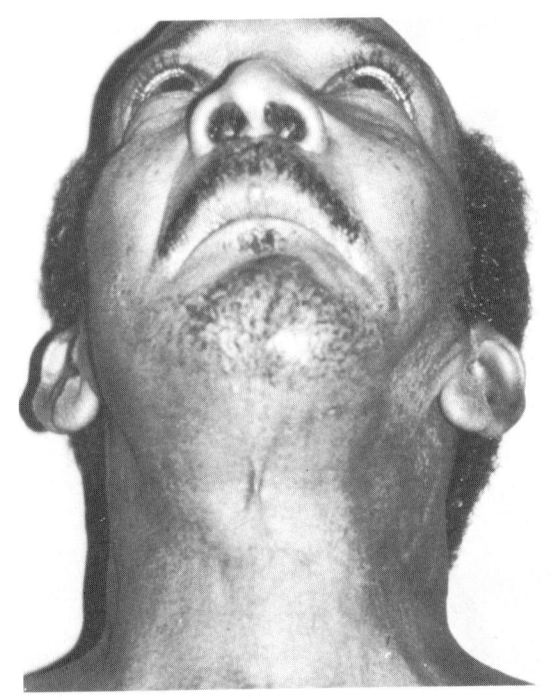

Figure 9–119. Concave facial deformity prior to reconstruction resulting from a hemimandibulectomy, parotidectomy, and functional neck dissection.

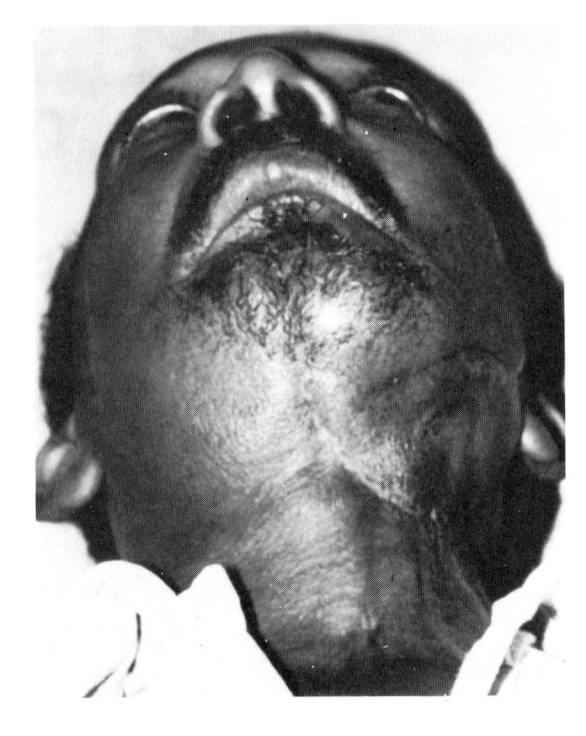

Figure 9–120. After bone graft reconstruction and the sternocleidomastoid muscle transposition, the facial form is greatly improved.

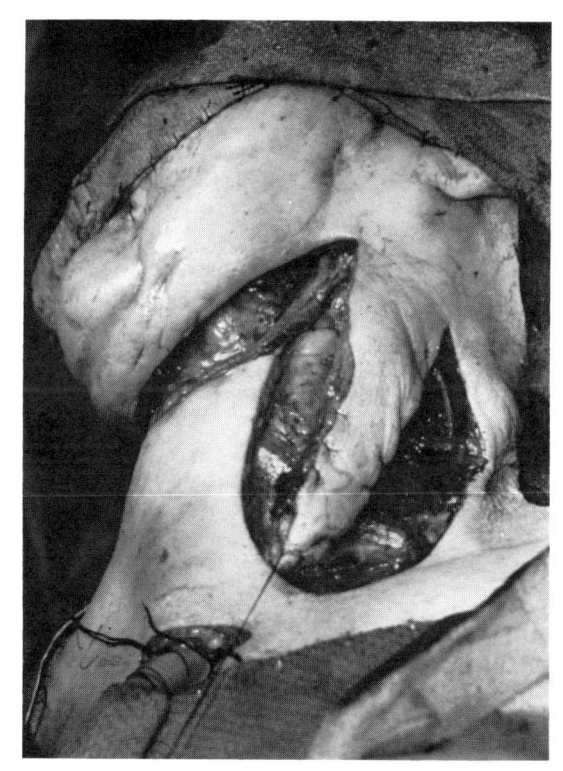

Figure 9–121. The sternocleidomastoid myocutaneous flap requires suturing of the skin edge to each muscle border to prevent shearing of the perforating vessels to the overlying skin by retraction efforts.

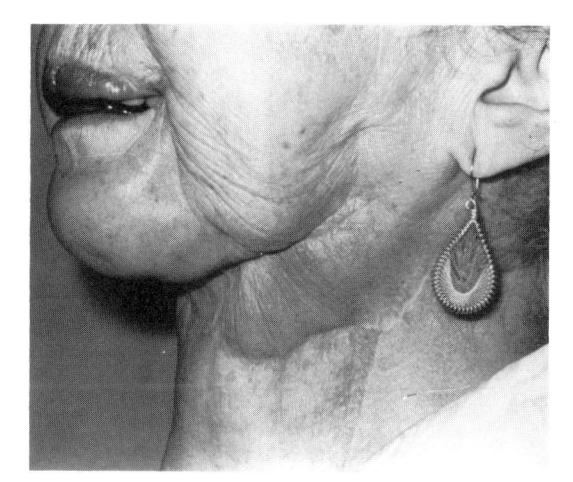

Figure 9–123. Sternocleidomastoid myocutaneous flap after one year with good color match and providing a much greater quantity of epithelialized tissue inferior to the bone graft, preventing scar contracture.

should be sutured to the muscle borders to prevent shearing of the perforating vessels by skin retraction (Fig. 9–121). As the sternal and clavicular insertions are incised and the myocutaneous flap developed in a superior direction, the skin incisions are extended and sutured to their respective muscle borders. In an identical manner to the muscular flap, the SCM myocutaneous flap can be rotated from its mastoid origin and placed into a tissue bed as far anterior as the canine region (Figs. 9–122 to 9–124).

Both flaps have a predictable blood supply and a reliable survival. Each is local tissue with straightforward surgical access and minimal morbidity. Functionally, patients are able to continue rotational, flexion, and extension movements of the head after this surgery.

Figure 9–122. *A*, Sternocleidomastoid myocutaneous flap transposed into neck incision during bony reconstruction in order to close wound. Donor site can be closed primarily by undermining. Spinal accessory nerve seen coursing into posterior triangle of the neck at the base of the donor wound. *B*, Donor site closed in primary fashion.

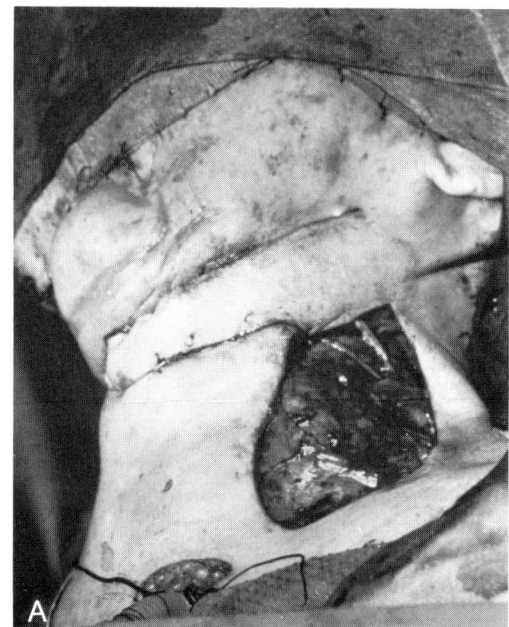

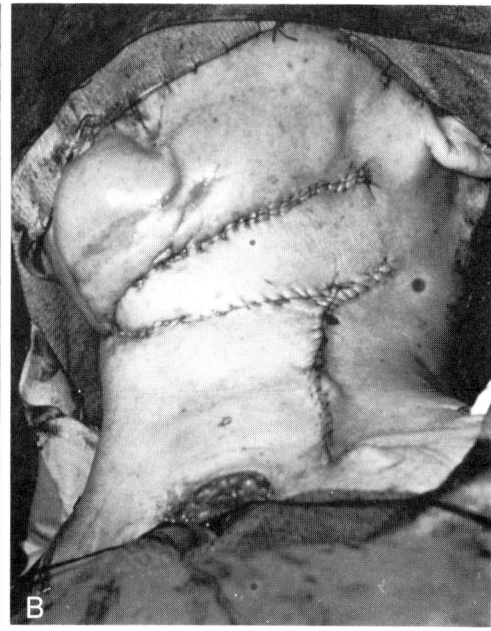

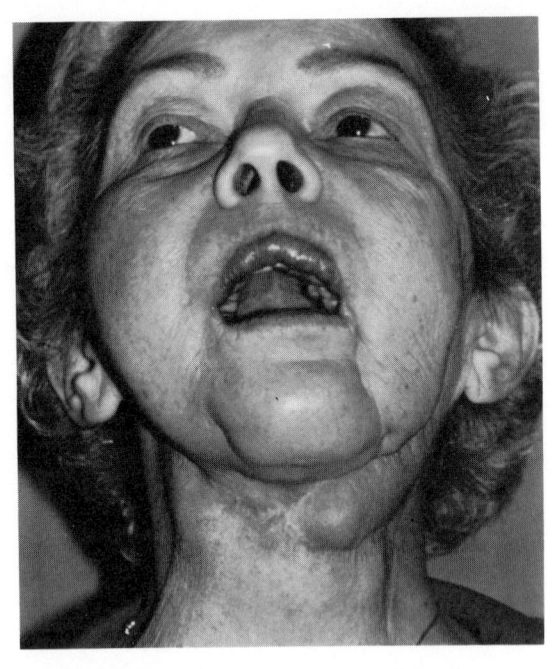

Figure 9–124. The presence of additional tissues in the scarred area immediately inferior to the bone graft allows this patient to fully extend her head.

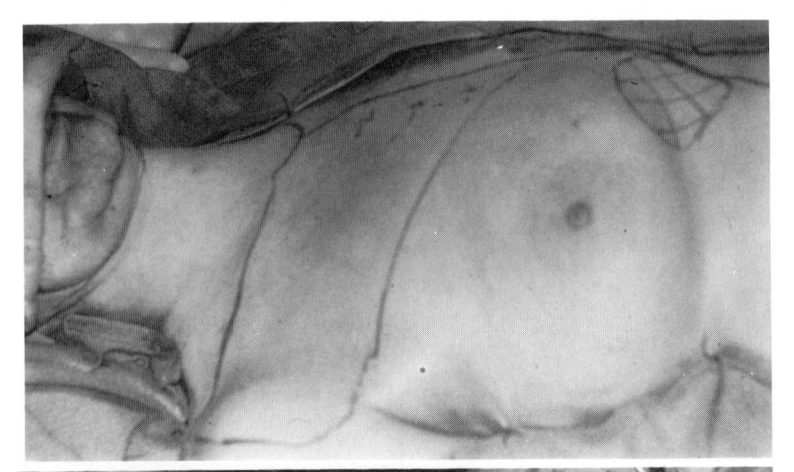

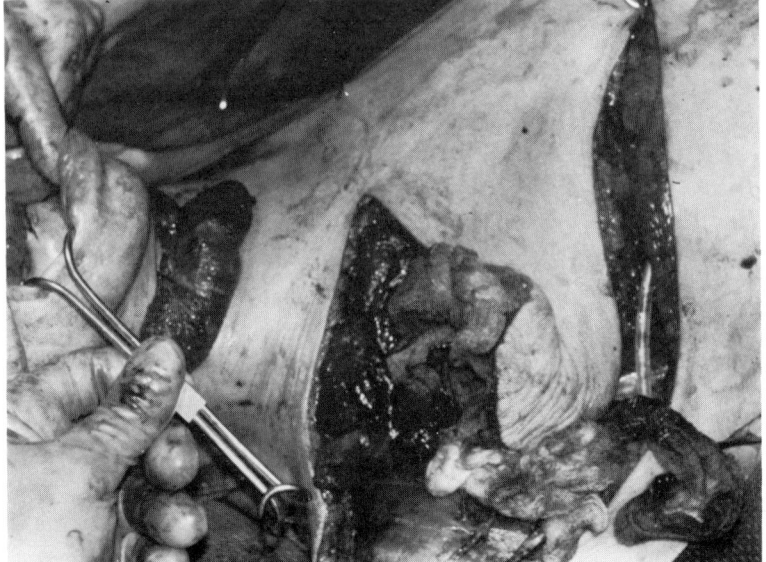

Pectoralis Major Myocutaneous Flaps

A myocutaneous flap from the anterior chest wall is the flap of choice when a vascularized soft-tissue bulk is required in the symphysis area or a larger bulk of tissue is required in the angle region.[67, 68] The pectoralis major (PM) myocutaneous flap is supplied by the pectoral branch of the thoracoacromial artery as it arises from the second division of the axillary artery.[67] Access to the muscle is best achieved by first elevating a standard deltopectoral flap, then continuing the incision medial to the nipple in an inferior direction and scribing a circular skin paddle inferior and medial to the nipple (Figs. 9–125 and 9–126). In this manner, future use of the deltopectoral flap is retained and the entire lengthy incision can be closed in a primary fashion (Fig. 9–127). The flap itself is tunneled in the neck and sutured to the edges of the defect (Fig. 9–128). The skin in this flap must also be sutured to the muscle edges to prevent shearing of the perfor-

Figure 9–125. Outline for a pectoralis major myocutaneous flap approached by development of a deltopectoral skin flap and harvesting a skin paddle inferior and medial to the nipple.

Figure 9–126. The skin paddle pedicled to the pectoralis major muscle has been tunneled through the neck and placed into the floor of the mouth, assisted by a transverse neck incision.

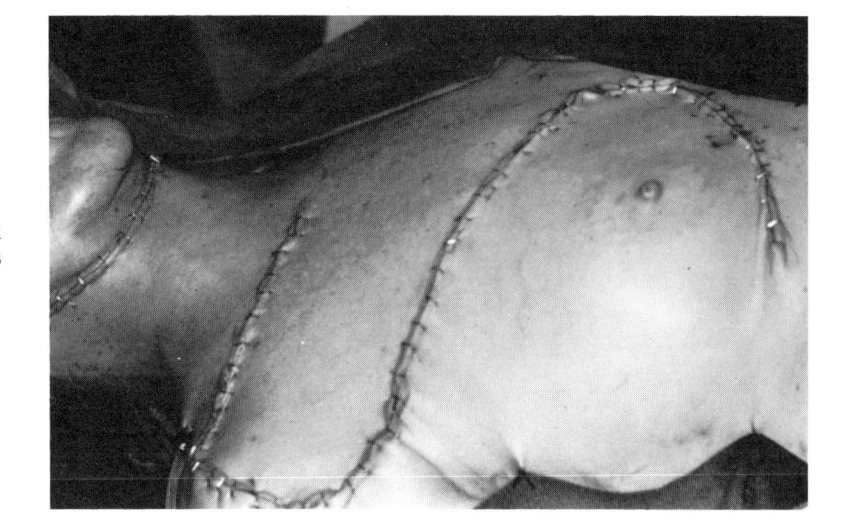

RECONSTRUCTION AND REHABILITATION OF CANCER PATIENTS / **403**

Figure 9–127. The entire defect can be closed primarily. The dentopectoral flap access allows future use of this flap if indicated.

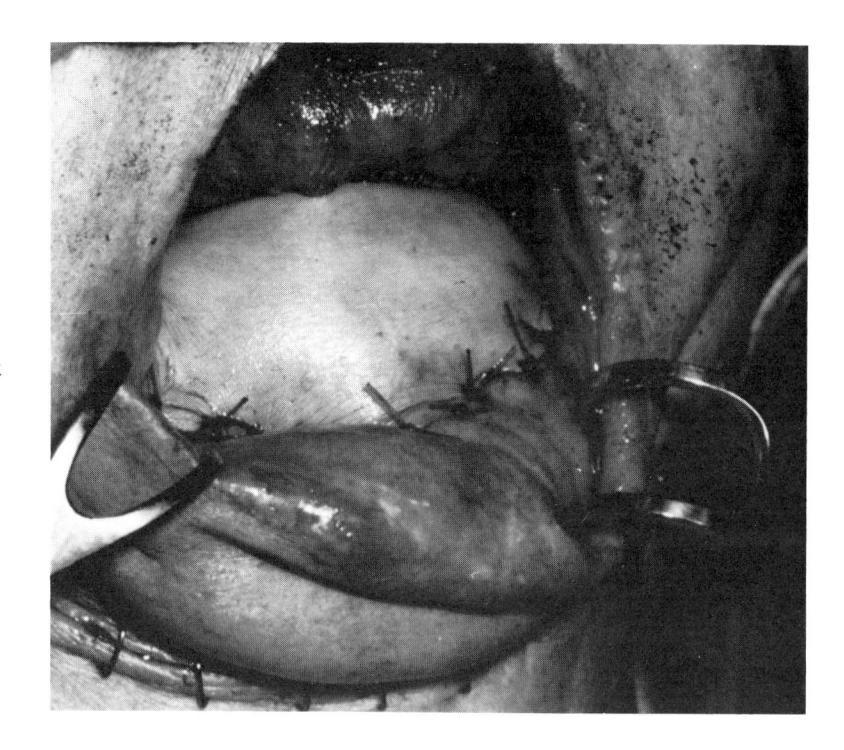

Figure 9–128. Skin paddle and muscle bulk closed into the defect in the floor of the mouth.

ating branches. It is also important to suture the muscle to deep tissue at the recipient site, and the skin paddle to either skin or mucosa. Since this muscle retains much of its innervation, subsequent contraction can separate the muscle from the skin paddle if only a surface closure is achieved. This flap's weakness lies with the potential inadequacy of its venous drainage, as with the osteomyocutaneous flap. Problems have arisen related to venous congestion by a situation analogous to the closed compartment phenomenon. That is, early in the postsurgical course, muscle edema occurs within unresilient irradiated tissues in the neck. This compresses the muscle against the clavicle and results in a loss of some or all of the skin paddle and muscle. When a part of the flap is lost, it is usually the peripheral portion of the skin paddle, creating a dehiscence from the recipient tissue edges and a central island of viable tissue (Fig. 9–129). This flap, however, is more reliable than the osteomyocutaneous flap because the perforating vessels to the overlying skin are more predictable than the perforating vessels to the underlying periosteum and bone. As the flap of choice when an SCM flap will not suffice, it can provide oral lining, skin cover, and/or muscle bulk to the recipient tissue.

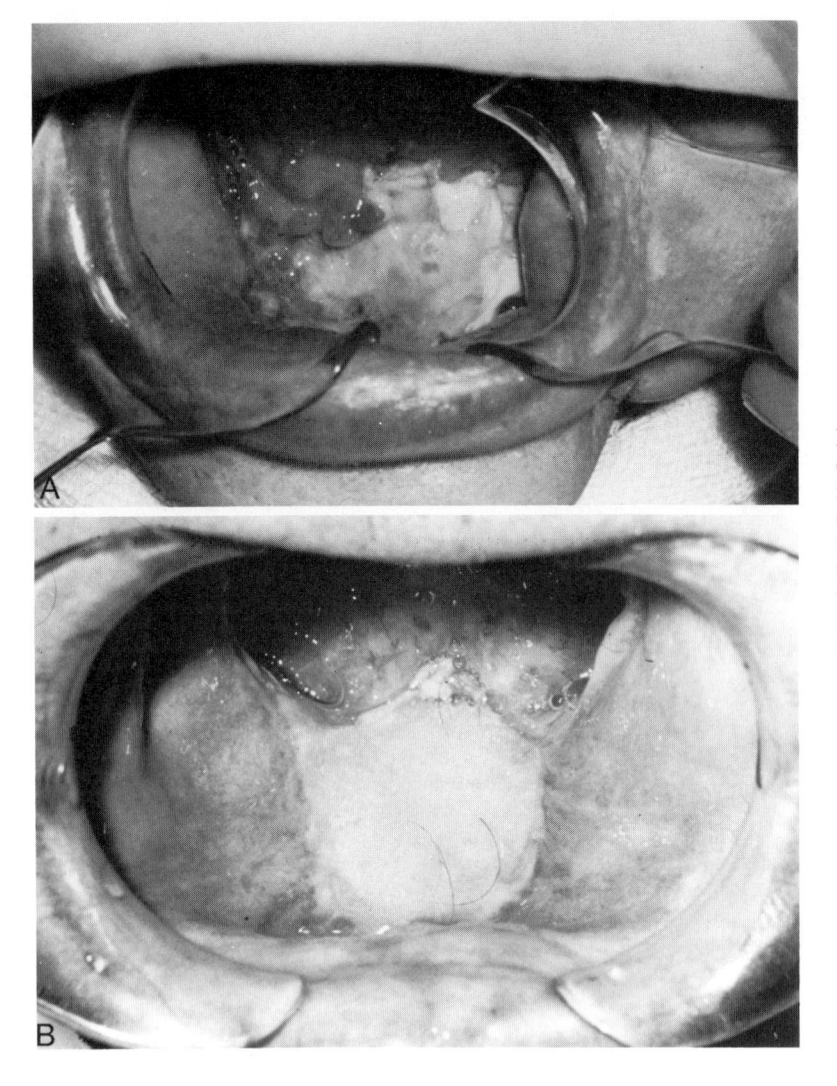

Figure 9–129. *A,* A pectoralis major myocutaneous flap that has undergone ischemic necrosis of its skin paddle. If the muscle remains viable, mucosal epithelium will resurface the area. *B,* A pectoralis major myocutaneous flap that underwent some peripheral skin loss, resulting in a smaller paddle than originally transposed but adequately supplying the needed tissue in the floor of the mouth.

Latissimus Dorsi Myocutaneous Flap

For soft-tissue defects in excess of 10 cm, the latissimus dorsi myocutaneous or microvascular free flap may be the only one with sufficient tissue bulk and area.[68] A skin paddle 12 cm in diameter may be transferred with a broad muscle paddle of nearly limitless size (Fig. 9–130). The blood supply is through the thoracodorsal branch of the subscapular artery as it branches off the third division of the axillary artery. This large muscle and skin paddle may be brought up to the area of the mandible by a

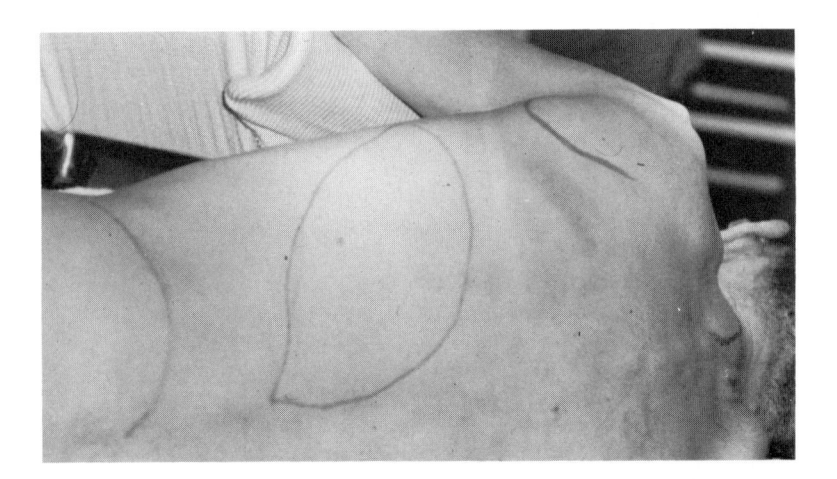

Figure 9–130. Outline of the large skin paddle possible with a transposition of a lattisimus dorsi myocutaneous flap.

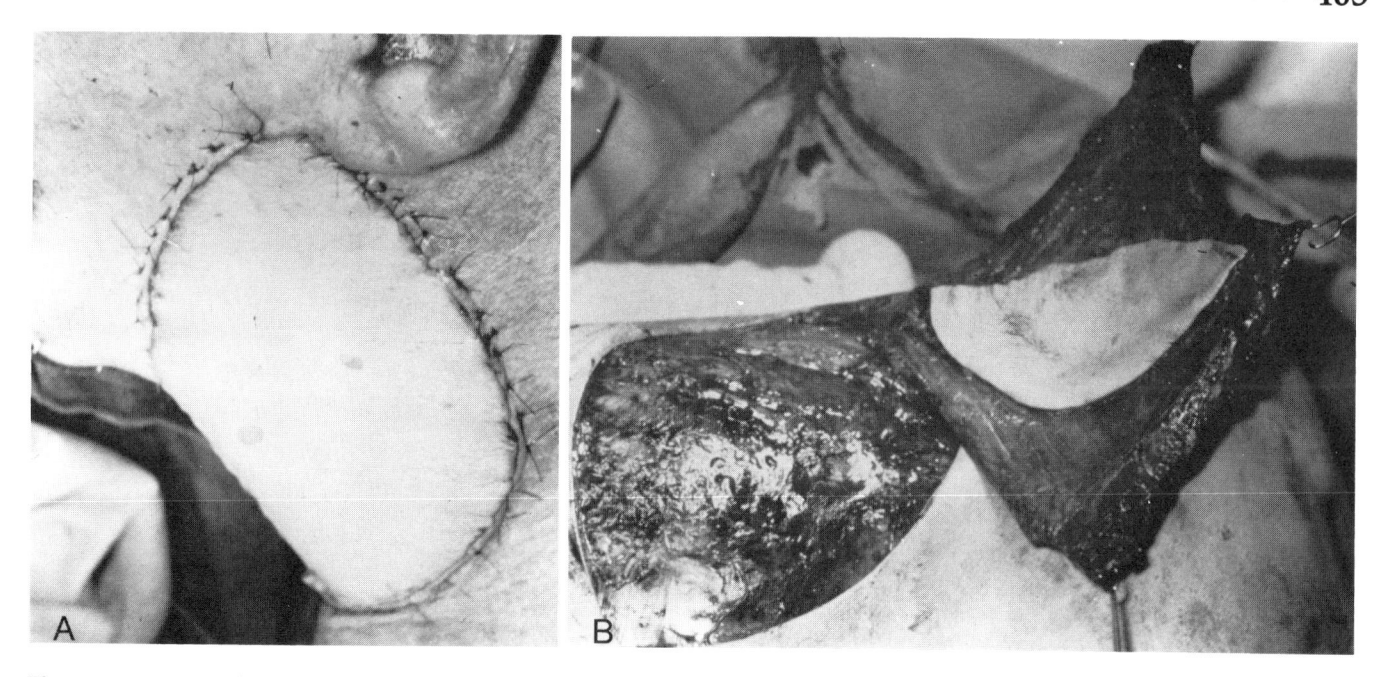

Figure 9–131. *A,* The latissimus dorsi muscle allows transposition of a very large muscle bulk. The muscle is tunneled through the axilla, over the clavicle, and into the facial or neck defect. *B,* This muscle flap is indicated when there are large soft-tissue deficits. Here a 12 × 12 cm skin paddle was used with an 18 × 20 cm muscle segment.

tunnel, through the axilla and over the clavicle (Figs. 9–131 and 9–132), or may be transferred as a free flap with vessel anastomoses. This myocutaneous flap has extensive usage and value in breast reconstruction because of favorable rotation and close approximation. In head and neck defects the results have been more complicated. There have been muscle congestion and venous drainage difficulties caused by inadequate volume in the

Figure 9–132. Loss of the entire skin paddle and one third of the muscle pedicle due to ischemic necrosis from venous congestion.

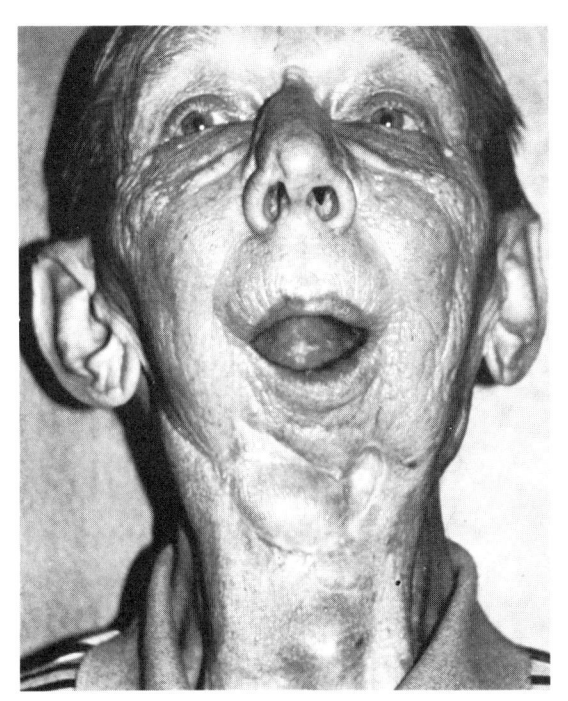

Figure 9–133. Extensive soft-tissue deficit of the skin and anterior neck region proposed for a free microvascular transfer of latissimus dorsi muscle and skin.

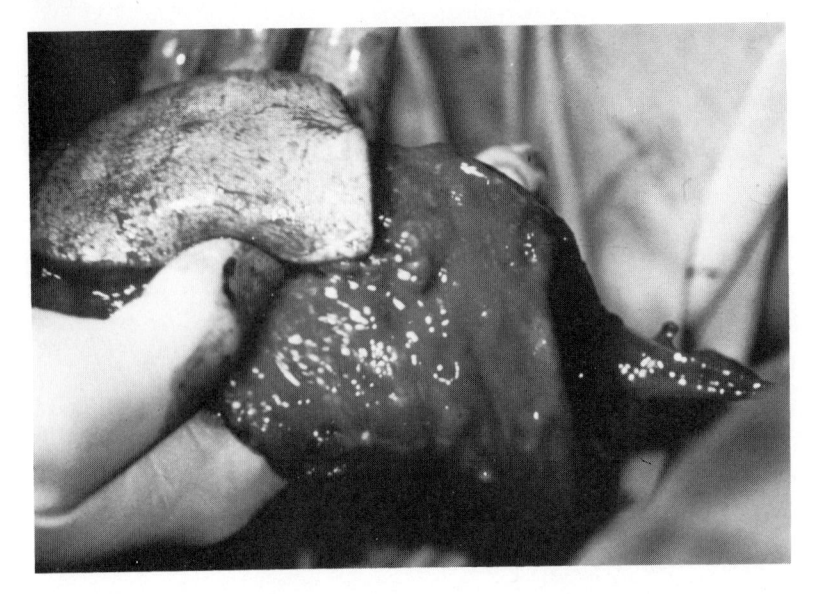

Figure 9–134. Large muscle bulk and skin paddle with isolated thoracodorsal artery and vein.

neck and axillary tunnel. For cancer-related defects of the jaws, this flap is best used as a free microvascular transfer (Fig. 9–133). Because the thoracodorsal artery and vein are large, the prognosis is excellent (Figs. 9–134 and 9–135).

Autogenous Nerve Grafting

The advent of microneural repair has made autogenous nerve grafting a very real consideration in cancer patients. Although it is generally felt that motor nerves can be grafted within a year and sensory nerves grafted at any time after excision,[69] immediate grafting gives the best prognosis for return of function. After several months, it is difficult to find the resected nerve ends. Even if tagged by sutures or wires, they are technically difficult to separate from surrounding scar. Although infection reduces the incidence of success in immediate bone grafts, immediate nerve grafts seem not to be associated with loss due to infection.[70] It has been our practice in selected patients to immediately graft segments of the inferior alveolar nerve and lingual nerve if these were sacrificed during the cancer extirpation.

The sural nerve is the preferred donor nerve for lingual and inferior alveolar nerve grafting because its diameter is the same as or larger than each. Although the greater auricular nerve will suffice, it is smaller in diameter and not thought to encourage full nerve regeneration. The greater auricular

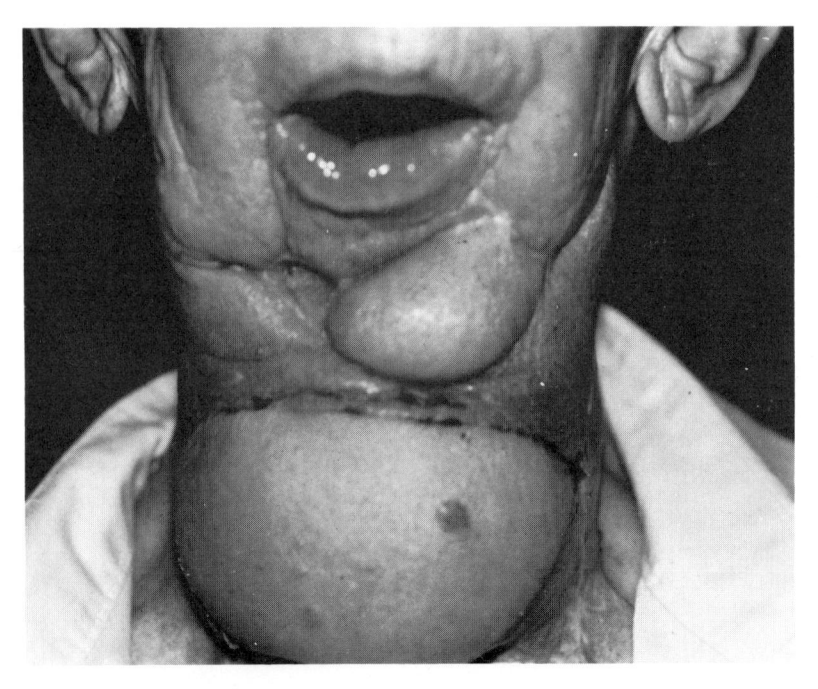

Figure 9–135. Survival of entire muscle and skin in the recipient area, indicating a successful and patent vascular anastomosis.

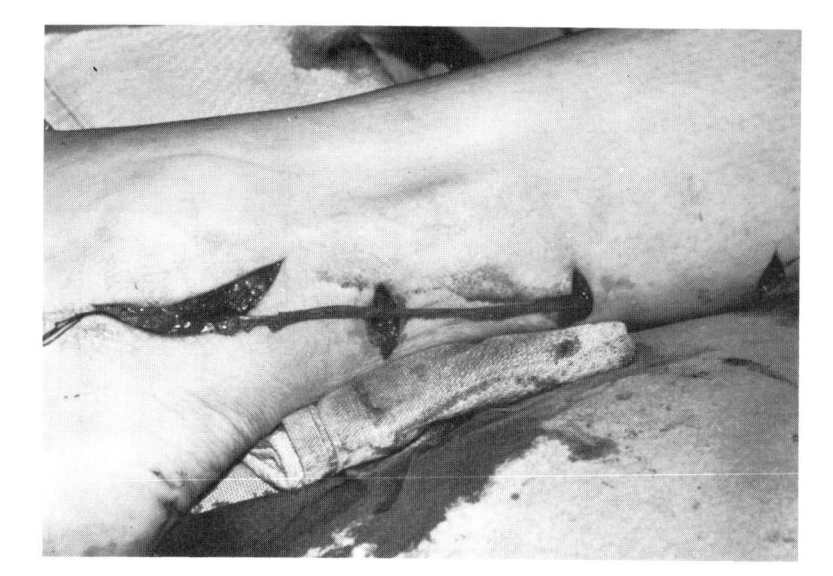

Figure 9–136. Exposure of the sural nerve is made dorsal to the medial malleolus. The nerve is dissected free and harvested through a series of horizontal incisions to the midcalf level.

nerve is an excellent nerve for facial nerve grafting.

The sural nerve becomes superficial midway up the calf as it emerges between the two bellies of the gastrocnemius. Its full length (up to 20 cm) may be harvested from this point to the lateral malleolus. The nerve is harvested using a series of small horizontal incisions along the dorsal aspect of the leg. The nerve is separated from the subcutaneous tissue and pulled through the uppermost incision (Fig. 9–136). The morbidity of this nerve harvest is small, as the sural nerve is solely sensory to the distal third of the leg, lateral aspect of the ankle, and heel. Sacrifice of the sural nerve requires special caution in runners, hikers, and others who walk or run for long distances. The greater auricular nerve is easily found as it becomes superficial to the sternocleidomastoid fascia at the midpoint of the posterior border. The nerve is separated from the subcutaneous tissue and harvested from this point to where it branches over the angle of the mandible (Fig. 9–137).

For lateral margin tumors of the tongue,

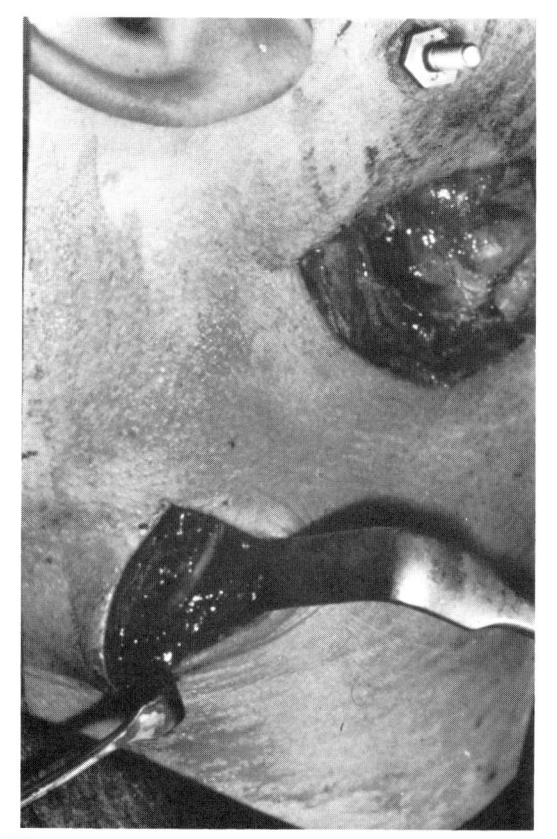

Figure 9–137. Exposure and harvest of the greater auricular nerve are accomplished by an incision over the posterior border of the sternocleidomastoid muscle at its midlength. Eight to nine cm of nerve may be harvested.

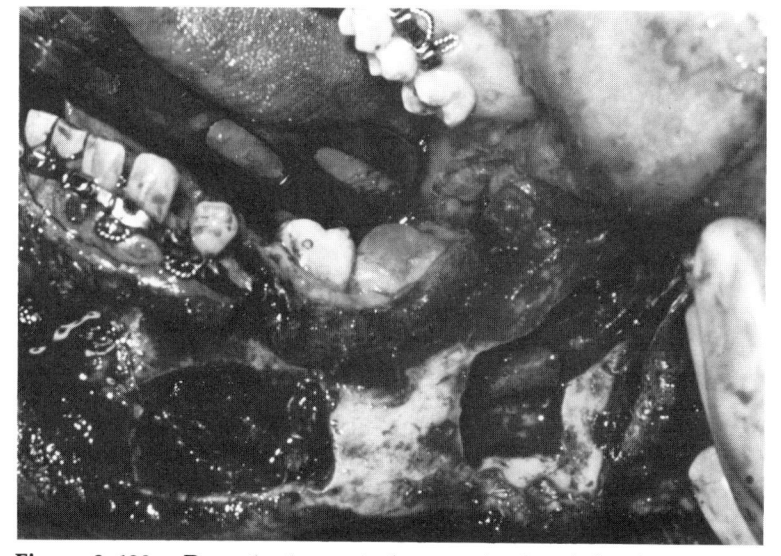

Figure 9–138. Decortication to isolate proximal and distal nerve ends for autogenous nerve graft repair of the inferior alveolar nerve.

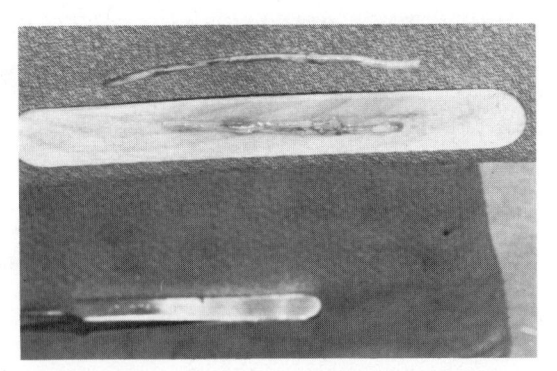

Figure 9–139. Segments of sural nerve for autogenous nerve grafts. The nerve length should be 1.5 times the separation length of the nerve ends.

retromolar trigone, or anterior tonsillar pillar requiring mandibular resection, the inferior alveolar nerve is transected and tagged at the mental foramen just above the lingula. Since these tumors invade the jaws from the lingual, lateral decortication windows proximal and distal to the tumor may be used without disturbing the en bloc principles of cancer resection (Fig. 9–138). The resected nerve ends are tagged as the tumor is resected. The donor nerve harvest should take place simultaneously with the tumor resection. The nerve ends should be prepared for anastomosis so that the nerve graft can be placed as soon as the surgical margins are free of tumor. One should use a length of nerve graft 1.5 times the length of nerve end separation (Fig. 9–139). This can accommodate retraction and ensure an anastomosis free of tension. Since 20 cm or more of sural nerve can be harvested but usually only 8 or 9 cm of usable greater auricular nerve, the sural nerve is preferred (Fig. 9–140).

Anastomosis is accomplished under the microscope to achieve a perineural intrafascicular repair[71] (Figs. 9–140 to 9–142). The nerve grafts are allowed to remain free in the tissue, and the soft tissue can be closed in a routine manner for cancer resection. At times, we have tagged the nerves by suturing a wire just below and parallel to the nerve graft. This helps to more easily identify the nerve at the time of an early bony reconstruction. We have found this to be usually unnecessary, as the nerve will form a sheath of bone about its distal end by osteoconduction of endosteum from the distal bone segment (Fig. 9–143). The inferior alveolar nerve graft comes to lie more medial and superior, putting it in a position that does not risk disturbance by the bony reconstruction. Most bone graft techniques are compatible with this approach to autogenous nerve grafting (Fig. 9–144).

The selection of patients for this consideration is extremely important. The nerve grafting procedure should not compromise the tumor extirpation by violating en bloc resection or compromising tumor-free margins. The procedure needs to be carried out without adding time to surgery. It should not be attempted if the tumor extirpation is expected to be exceedingly long. The indication for nerve grafting is to gain a return of sensation to anatomic structures (lip and tongue) that are most beneficial for the patient. Of the few bone graft patients on whom we have used this approach and whom we have followed for more than a year, sensation has returned to roughly 80 per cent of their unoperated side. They have subjectively welcomed return of sensation and, in general, are better able to control secretions and manage with prosthetic appliances. However, even 80 per cent of full sen-

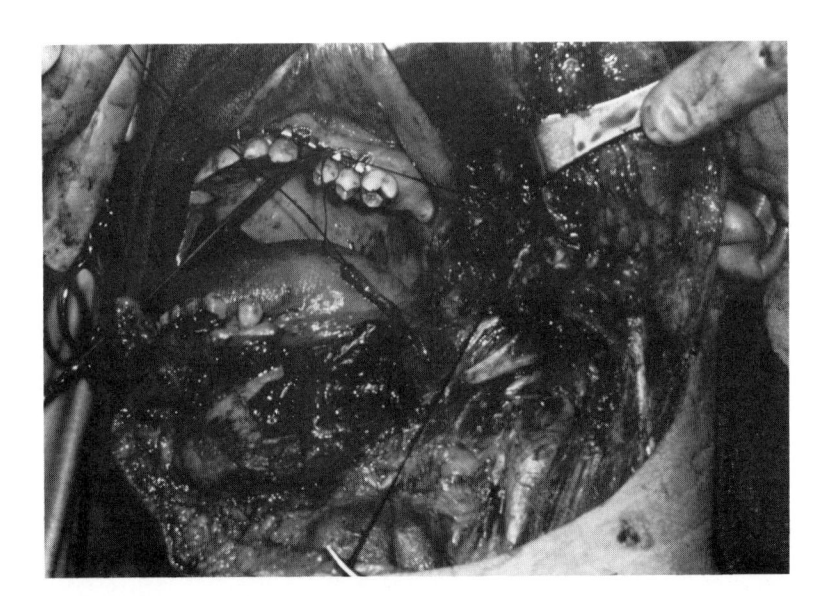

Figure 9–140. After hemimandibulectomy and neck dissection, the proximal and distal nerve stumps of the lingual and inferior alveolar nerve are identified by a suture.

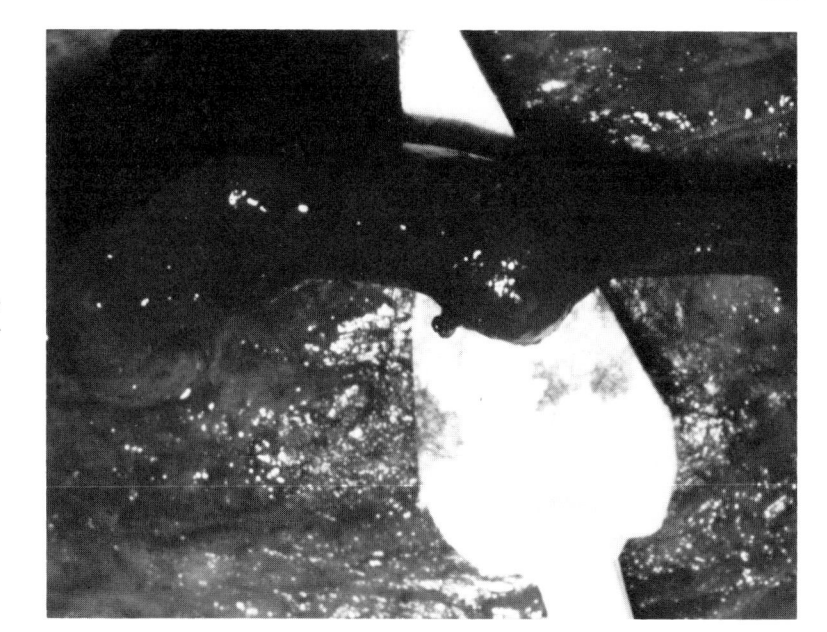

Figure 9–141. The nerve graft–to–host nerve anastomosis is achieved by a perineural intrafascicular repair.

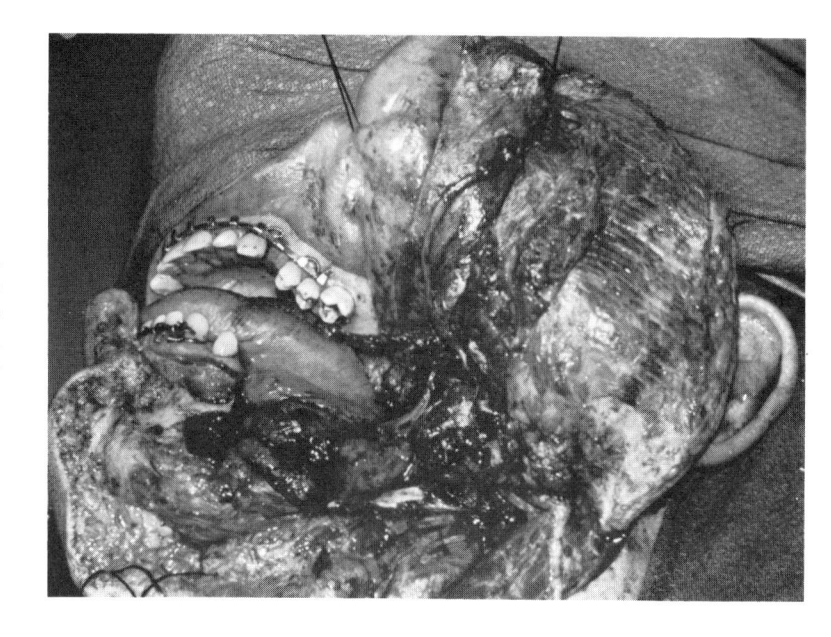

Figure 9–142. Each nerve graft should remain passive within the wound. The nerve grafts here evidence the required length to permit a tension-free closure. A wide-access surgical approach such as this lip-split approach permits unencumbered microscopic surgery.

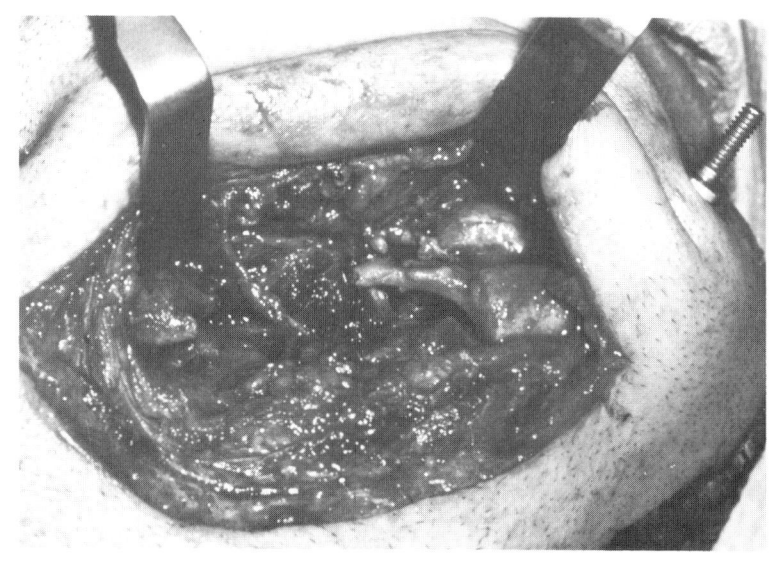

Figure 9–143. Bone formation by osteoconduction along epineural sheath of nerve graft.

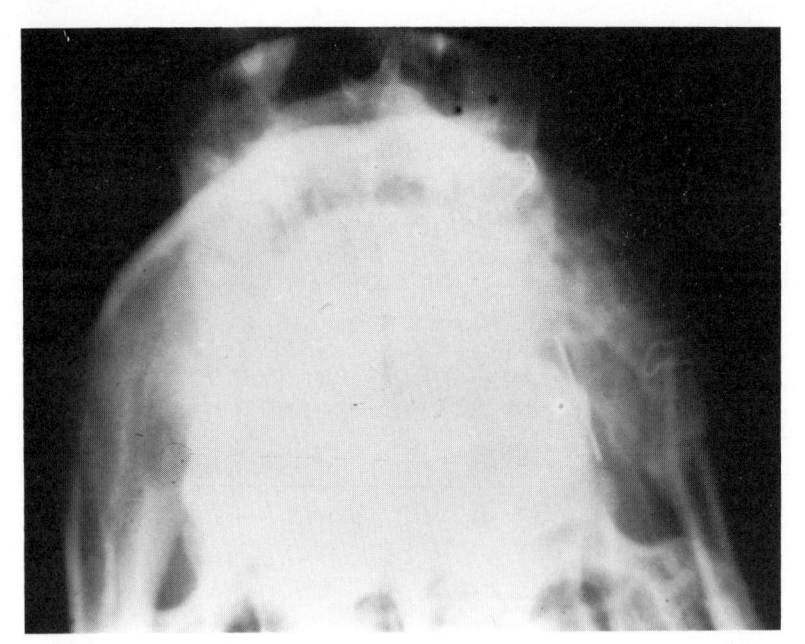

Figure 9–144. Radiograph of bone graft placed three months after autogenous nerve graft. Note the wire which marks the nerve graft as being medial to the bone graft. After one year this patient has had a return of sensation that he describes as 80 per cent that of the unoperated side and exhibits 15 mm two-point discrimination, as compared to 10 mm on the unoperated side.

sation is a paresthesia that some patients find annoying. Further work in this area is required. At the time of this writing, autogenous nerve grafting in cancer-related defects is seen as a promising area to further improve the quality of rehabilitation for patients.

Jaw Fixation Techniques in Reconstruction

Ability to achieve proper fixation in reconstructive surgery is a great advantage in oral and maxillofacial surgery. Grafts that are not adequately immobilized will often separate at the graft-host interface and go on to protrude through mucosa or skin. A fibrous union or a malunion will usually develop. Acceptable fixation may be achieved with any one of three basic approaches: rigid internal fixation, Gunning-type splints, or external skeletal pin fixation. Graft immobilization with any of these three techniques should also achieve arch alignment, vertical dimension, and prevention of distal segment rotation.

Rigid Internal Fixation

This type of fixation is accomplished with metallic cribs of stainless steel and titanium. Allogeneic bone cribs and Dacron-polyurethane cribs are too flexible and thin to be relied upon. Metallic cribs serve well for rigid internal fixation when three screws are placed in each bone segment and sufficient host bone is engaged by crib flanges. Because longevity of the bone ossicle in such cribs is related to the two phases of bone regeneration, rather than to the functional stress absorbed by these cribs, there is no strong indication to remove cribs once they are in place. We routinely leave metallic cribs in original positions and have accomplished vestibuloplasty procedures without exposing the cribs. The advantage of rigid internal fixation is best realized in reconstruction of the symphysis and body regions of the mandible on each side of the midline. The graft immobilization they achieve is absolute, and the patient can function early after surgery. A disadvantage is that they commit the reconstruction to a large foreign-body mass that is often not well-tolerated by thin or irradiated tissue.

Gunning-type Splints

Gunning-type splints may be used by modifying the patient's existing dentures or by processing acrylic bases with an occlusal surface from mounted casts. In either case, a firm male-female interlocking at the occlusal level is required. Holes are placed in the acrylic to fix each to their respective jaw, and an arch bar or individual lug can be embedded into the acrylic for maxillomandibular fixation (Figs. 9–145 and 9–146). The maxillary member should encompass the full arch and be fixed to the maxilla by three skeletal wires. The mandibular member should encompass the remaining alveolar ridge without encroaching on the graft-host margin. We prefer the mandibular member to be at least 2 cm from the bone margin. Two circummandibular wires are sufficient to fix the mandibular member to the mandible.

In the fabrication of Gunning-type splints, the case alignment cannot be done in the laboratory. The ability to reposition a deviated mandible needs to be assessed before splint construction and a check bite obtained in this relationship. Some deviations are heavily scarred and are impossible to reposition into an ideal arch alignment. In these cases, a prereconstruction scar release is required or a less than ideal arch alignment must be accepted.

Gunning-type splints are a superb fixation device and relatively quick and easy to apply. However, they do immobilize the jaws as well as the graft, which provides an airway consideration and impacts on a patient's nutrition. This is a disadvantage in a population of patients whose nutritional intake is better served by unrestricted jaw movement. Such splints may also cause pressure ulcerations on alveolar ridges, es-

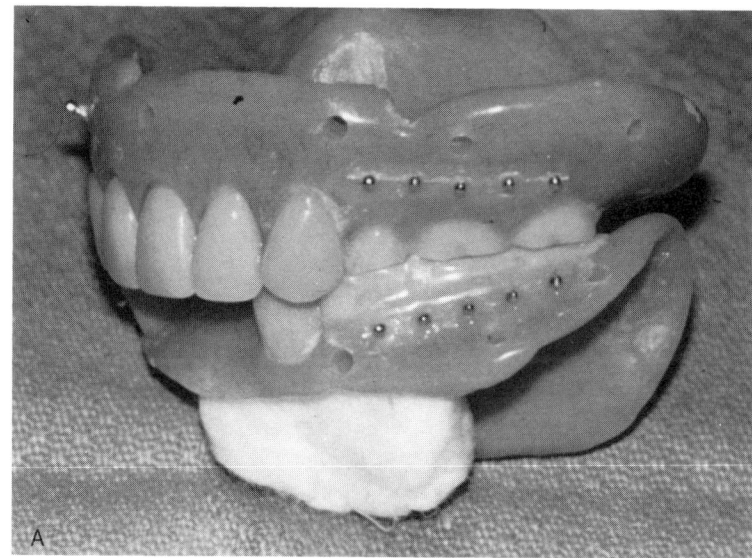

Figure 9–145. *A*, Gunning-type splints made by modifying existing dentures. Maxillo-mandibular fixation is achieved via individual lugs embedded within acrylic. *B*, Gunning-type splints may be fixed to the maxilla via alveolar, piriform rim, zygomatic buttress, or circumzygomatic wires. They are usually fixed to the mandible via circummandibular wires.

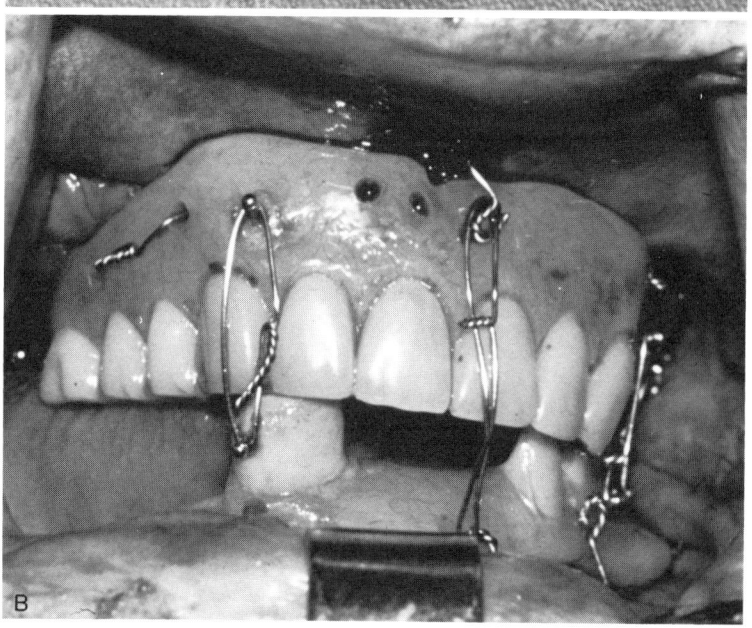

Figure 9–146. Gunning-type splints with embedded arch bars for maxillo-mandibular fixation and midline feeding port.

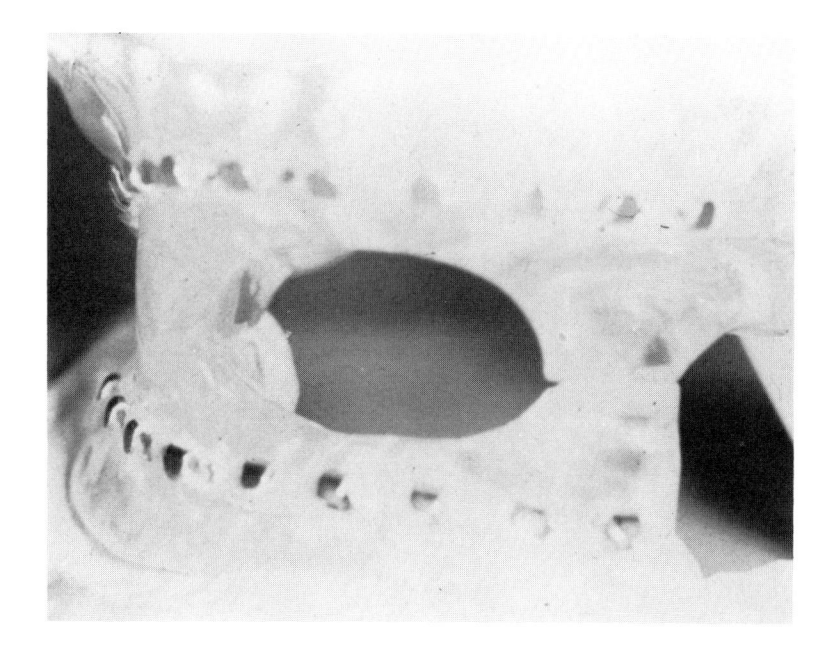

pecially in irradiated mucosa. In addition, these splints do not control the proximal bone segment, but rather rely solely on the graft system used to position and immobilize the proximal segment.

Gunning-type splints are usually used for six to eight weeks. At that time, the maxillomandibular fixation is removed but the splints are left fixed to the arches. If the graft demonstrates good consolidation, and no deviation is seen after one week, the splints are removed completely.

External Skeletal Pin Fixation

External skeletal pin fixation as described by Morris[72] is the most convenient and useful fixation technique for reconstructions in cancer-related defects. One should attempt to place the pins as far from the graft-host interfaces as possible and within tissue that has not been in the field of irradiation. We have not observed complications related to pin placement in irradiated skin or pin-related complications of the bone graft in our experience with this system. The jaws are usually aligned by splints, existing occlusions, or even estimations as the sterile reduction rig is applied. We often place the reduction rig in an inverted position away from the direct operating field (Fig. 9–147). The acrylic phase is applied and the reduction rig removed after all wounds have been closed (Fig. 9–148).

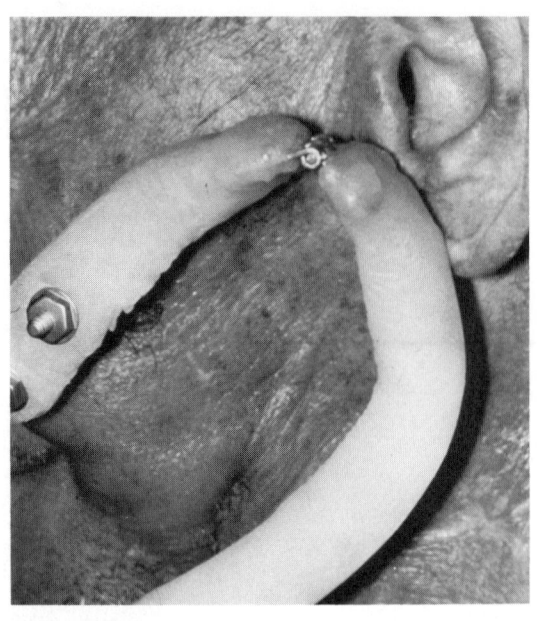

Figure 9–148. Hinge modification of the external skeletal pin fixation acrylic phase. The hinge is embedded in acrylic, connecting zygoma pins to mandibular pins with rotation about the hinge.

We have developed a fixation modification for patients who do not have a remaining proximal segment or have one of insufficient size. It incorporates a simple door hinge placed between an acrylic phase attached to two pins in the zygoma and another acrylic phase attached to mandibular pins (Figs. 9–149 and 9–150). Placement of a ¾ inch by 1 inch brass door hinge, with its center of rotation over the midpoint of the temporal fossa, has provided excellent graft immobilization with rotation at the reconstructed condyle, while still retaining the advantages of the external fixation device.

An advantage of this technique, with or without the hinge modification, is that oral splints and wires become unnecessary. The patient's airway is more secure without maxillomandibular fixation. The patient's nutrition is assisted by nearly normal jaw excursions, and most report a more active lifestyle during their fixation phase. We have used this fixation technique in most reconstructions and have found it adequate without the need for internal fixation or fixation using Gunning-type splints.

RECONSTRUCTION OF THE MAXILLA

SURGICAL APPROACH

Goals of Surgery

The need for bony reconstruction of the maxilla is less than that of the mandible.

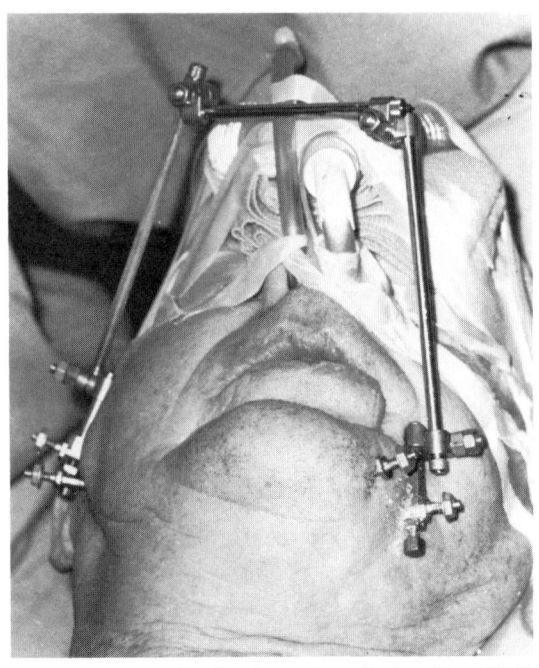

Figure 9–147. Reduction rig of the Joe Hall Morris external skeletal pin fixation device applied in an inverted manner to place it out of the direct surgical field.

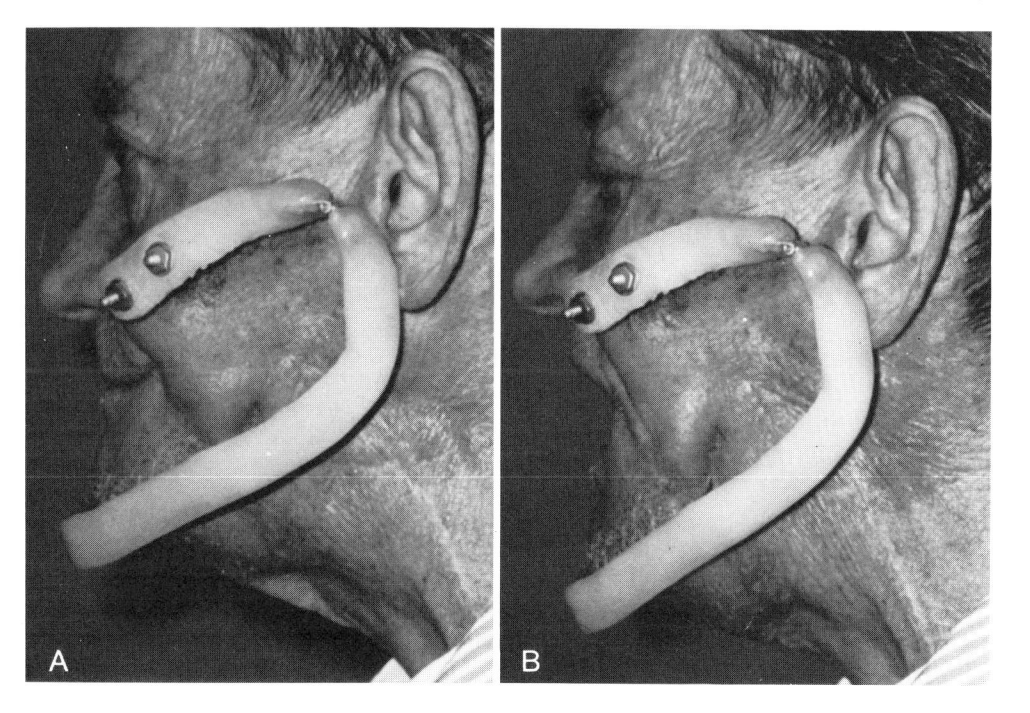

Figure 9–149. *A*, Hinge fixation device with jaw in closed position. *B*, Hinge fixation device allowing unrestricted opening with rotation about the hinge center.

Maxillofacial prostheses, in most instances, have been able to restore acceptable function and facial form to these deformities. Hemimaxillectomy defects that require vomer flaps, palatal flaps, tongue flaps, and other flaps to successfully reconstruct the palate and alveolar ridge can often be better functionally and cosmetically managed by a prosthesis. The investment in multiple tissue flaps and bone grafting to obtain an edentulous ridge is often thought to be too much for too little. However, there are certain instances in which bony reconstruction can add stability to a maxillofacial prosthesis and in which facial form is not obtainable by a prosthesis[73] (Fig. 9–150). These cases usually consist of hemimaxillectomy defects that cause scars and place constraints on the extension of any such prosthesis. Maxillofacial prostheses, in these cases, cannot successfully compete against scar bands in their efforts to provide facial contour. A maxillofacial prosthesis also requires a three-point stability that is often lacking in hemimaxillectomy defects. In function, this instability places torquing forces on the contralateral side. In dentulous cases, these torquing forces on retention clasps contribute to periodontal breakdown and mobility of the teeth. In edentulous cases, unseating of the prosthesis is common and too often accepted as the best that can be accomplished. Therefore, goals in maxillary reconstruction include facial contour enhancement that a prosthesis is unable to achieve. The graft should also strive to create a bony ridge in the buccal mucosa. Although this ridge is too facially located to serve as a functional denture-bearing ridge, it can serve as a lateral buttress to achieve three-point stability for an obturator/prosthesis and a seal.

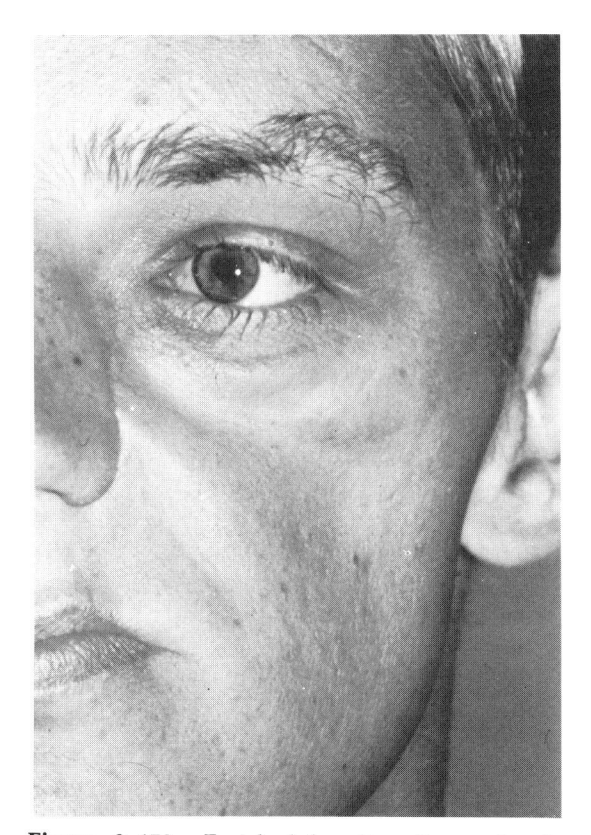

Figure 9–150. Facial deformity after a hemimaxillectomy for a palatal tumor. Restrictive scarring prevented improvement by prosthetic means alone.

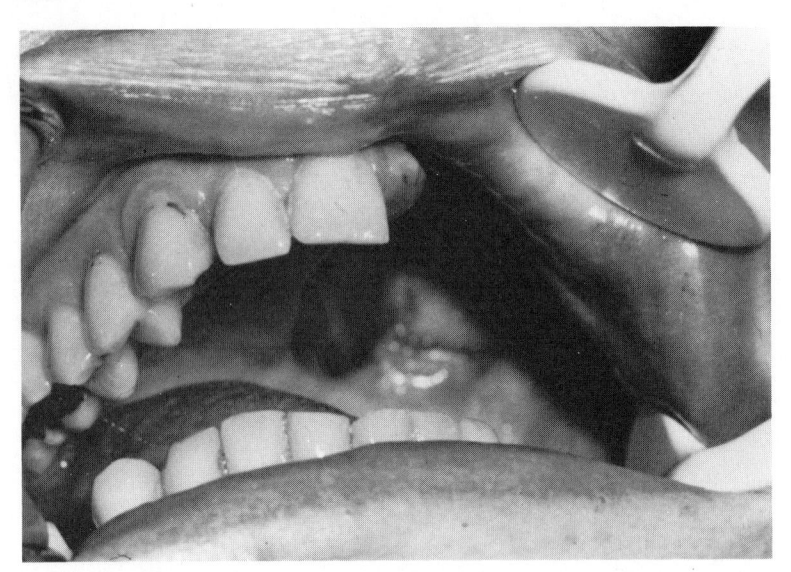

Figure 9–151. Large oral-nasal oral-antral communication resulting from hemimaxillectomy. Difficulty in lip retraction evident here is indicative of the scarring prominent after this surgery.

Soft Tissue Assessment

In the maxilla as in the mandible, the quantity and quality of the recipient bed are the two most critical factors for bony reconstruction. An important assessment is whether or not there is sufficient thickness of facial tissue for a bone graft between the oral mucosa and the facial skin. In hemimaxillectomy surgery, a curtain of buccal mucosa can serve as the deep wall or base of a bone graft. Although scarred, this tissue has sufficient vascularity to support graft survival. Oral-nasal and oral-antral communications should be left open to be obturated by a prosthesis (Fig. 9–151). The facial skin should have enough laxity, or be capable of being advanced to close without tension, over the bone graft. A tense facial skin, over a bone graft that lies between such skin cover and a base of unresilient scarred oral mucosa, will resorb owing to the pressure. Facial contour gained by this graft can then be lost. Deficiencies of facial soft tissue need to be corrected by local flaps before bony reconstruction. The remaining host bone needs to be considered. Most hemimaxillectomy defects leave the body of the zygoma, the infraorbital rim, and the nasal process of the maxilla. This provides a good base on which to fix a bone graft. One can literally "hang" such a graft off the infraorbital rim with medial stabilization at the lateral nasal wall and lateral stabilization at the zygoma. The bone graft comes to lie within a pocket that is developed between the oral mucosa and the overlying skin. The superficial extent, or "build-up," of the bone graft is dictated by the desired facial contour and the limitation of soft tissue. The inferior extent and bulk of bone are dictated by the desired facial contour, limitations of soft tissue, and the requirements of bone that may be used as a point of stabilization for a prosthesis. A post–bone graft vestibuloplasty can create a very acceptable alveolar ridge. The graft is capable of withstanding functional stresses and adding stability to a prosthesis if sufficient graft bulk was achieved.

Technique of Surgery

The best soft-tissue approach we have found is through a modified Weber-Ferguson incision. The lip is left unsplit, with the incision beginning at the superior aspect of the philtrum. The incision is extended around the alar base, superiorly to the lateral nasal crease, and then horizontally at the level of the infraorbital rim or as far laterally as one needs to gain access to the zygoma (Fig. 9–152). The advantage of this approach is to allow wide open access with an assured blood supply through the facial artery and the transverse facial branch off the superficial temporal artery. It also offers the capability of posterior extension and undermining to advance the soft-tissue flap and avoid a closure under tension. The best bone graft material remains the highly osteogenic par-

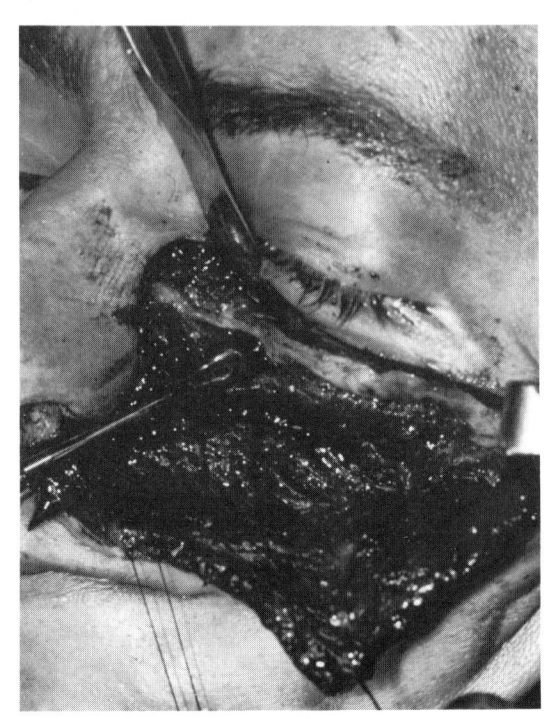

Figure 9–152. Reconstruction of the maxilla is best approached with a Weber-Ferguson–type incision. The graft may be fixed to the zygoma and infraorbital rim.

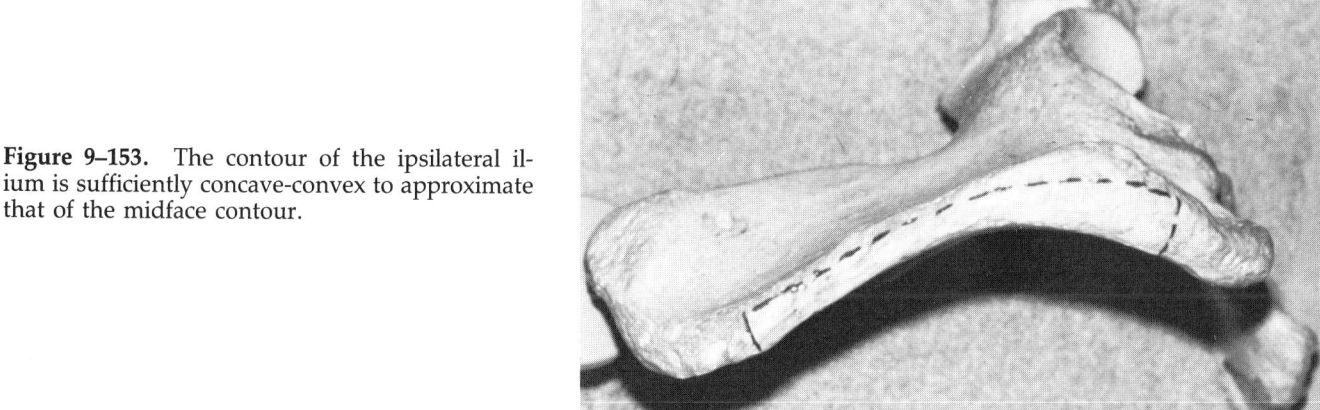

Figure 9–153. The contour of the ipsilateral ilium is sufficiently concave-convex to approximate that of the midface contour.

ticulate bone and cancellous marrow. However, an alloplastic crib becomes unacceptable in such defects, and these grafts will settle in areas of dependence to achieve undesirable results without form. In these cases, we have used either corticocancellous grafts with particulate bone and marrow supplementation, or allogeneic cribs with autogenous particulate bone and cancellous marrow. In corticocancellous grafts, the medial surface of the ipsilateral ilium provides a nearly ideal convex surface approximating the hemifacial convexity (Fig. 9–153). If at least half the rounded portion of the iliac crest is included, it will serve as an excellent form for the supplemental particulate bone and marrow. The graft can then be built out to the desired contour with the particulate bone and cancellous marrow (Fig. 9–154). The rounded trough effect of the iliac crest prevents settling of the graft in dependent areas. In composite grafts, allogeneic ribs may be split longitudinally to span the defect and provide a form for autogenous particulate bone and marrow. It can then be placed between the allogeneic bone and the base of the recipient bed (Fig. 9–155). In either approach, wound closure is achieved by a primary two-layered closure. One must be sure to extend the flap incisions to close the

Figure 9–154. A PBCM graft may be compressed about the ipsilateral ilium crib to achieve a desirable facial contour.

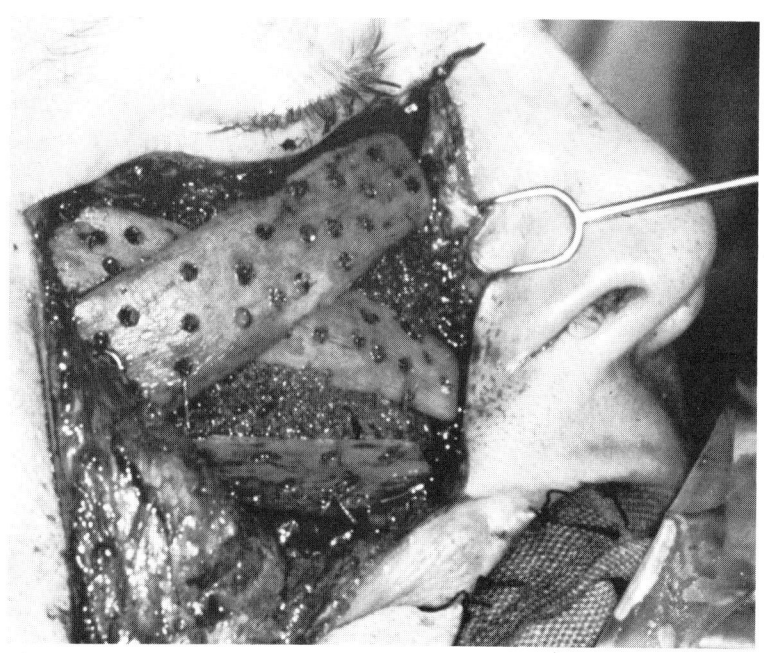

Figure 9–155. Allogeneic split rib segments were used in this reconstruction to support and contain the PBCM graft.

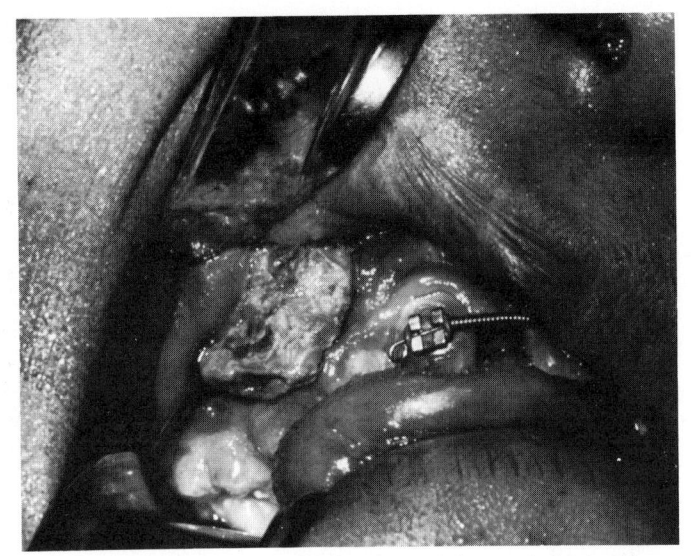

Figure 9–156. Exposed nonviable graft segment due to infection from transoral bone graft placement.

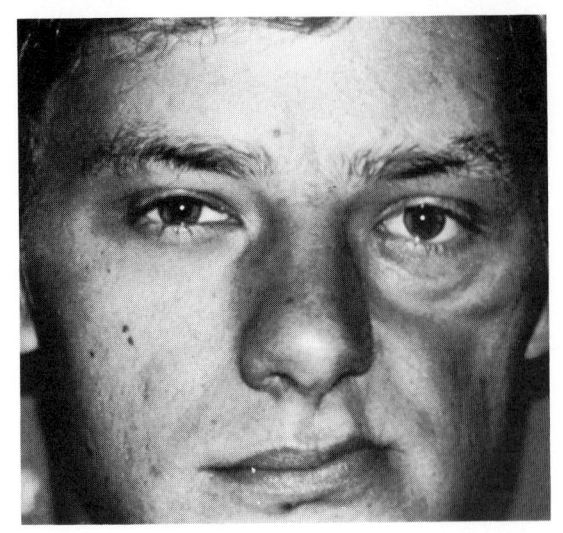

Figure 9–157. Young patient with hemimaxillectomy deformity and prominent retraction of cupid's bow.

greater convexity of facial form without tension. This is best achieved by closing the infraorbital and nasal portions of the modified Weber-Ferguson incision toward the medial canthus of the eye. Such closure usually eliminates dead space so that drains are not required. In individual cases in which dead space exists, small suction drains are recommended for 24 to 48 hours.

In these grafts, one must not attempt transoral bone grafting. Surgical access is limited and so is the ability to build out the graft to a desired or premeasured contour. The closure often ends in the scarred areas of the oral mucosa, leading to dehiscence (Fig. 9–156). These grafts also have a higher incidence of infection due to contamination during placement.

Results of Maxillary Reconstruction

Bone grafts to the maxilla have retained their bony content and support of form and function over the years. Obwegesser has also reported several reconstructions of the hemimaxilla that have retained acceptable facial contour.[83] The concept of progressive resorption of onlay or contour grafts placed into nonfunctional areas such as the maxilla is well-known. The absence of functional stresses was once thought to promote a gradual resorption of such grafts. Grafts that are revascularized early, such as particulate bone and marrow grafts, are thought to resorb more quickly because of their increased cellularity and the fact that osteoclasts arise from the circulation.[35] Grafts that are slow to revascularize, such as cortical, cortico-cancellous, or allogeneic grafts, are thought to remain longer. Onlay grafts to the facial bones, including the mandible, distend their soft-tissue envelope. Although soft tissue has the limited ability to accommodate to an expanded volume, it is by no means 100 per cent expansive. There is always some tissue contraction. The ensuing pressure placed on the underlying bone graft is the more likely cause of the observed resorptions. This would tend to explain the longevity of hemimaxillary reconstructions where an adequate soft-tissue bed exists despite the nonfunctional nature of the graft (Figs. 9–157 to 9–160).

Bony reconstruction of the maxilla where indicated remains a viable approach in the restoration of facial form and potential prosthesis support structure. It is often overlooked in the rehabilitation plans for patients. The results are encouraging for such

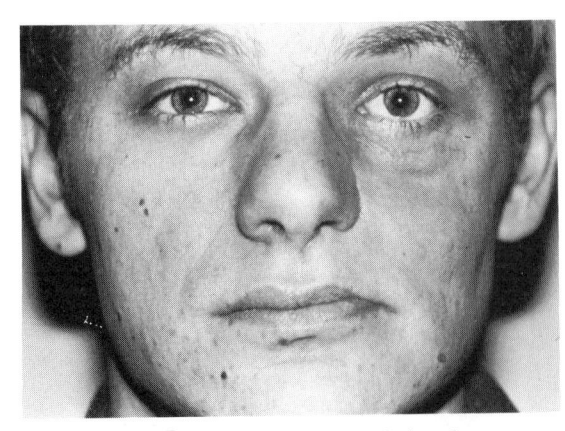

Figure 9–158. Greatly improved facial contour and lip symmetry after bone graft reconstruction of the maxilla.

Figure 9–159. Four-year follow-up of the maxillary graft demonstrates a radiographically well-consolidated graft without resorption and an alveolar ridge contour.

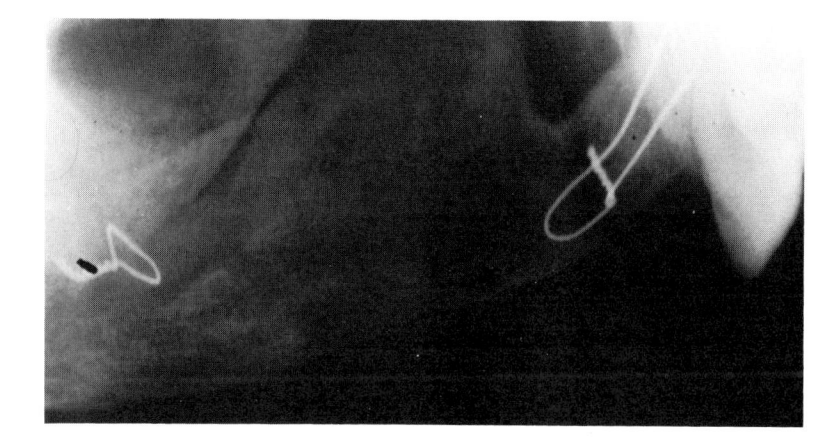

reconstruction in that it can accomplish an improved facial form and functional prosthesis base that will last.

PROSTHETIC MANAGEMENT OF MAXILLARY DEFECTS

Partial or total resection of the maxilla results in various hard- and/or soft-palatal defects. These defects have been classified according to location, size, and extent. Prosthodontic care of patients is for the purpose of prosthesis fabrication as a means of primary defect rehabilitation. Following surgery, the patient frequently encounters specific deficiencies. These deficiencies can be classified into three areas: physiologic, cosmetic, and psychological.

The patient's physiologic deficiencies are related to mastication, deglutition, speech, and respiration. Cosmetic deficiencies are often minor as viewed extraorally and may be noticed only as a result of neurologic and musculature weakness and/or loss of anatomic mass following tumor resection. This may result in some facial weakness and hollowing on the defect side. The patient's psychological deficiency is normally directly related to the physiologic and cosmetic deficiencies encountered. The degree to which this may be a problem has been reviewed by Curtis[73] and Gillis.[74] Their specific findings generally note that the patient's psychological profiles before and after extirpative surgery are similar.

Prosthodontic support and treatment for patients with maxillary defects can also be divided into three phases: extirpative surgical, interim, and reconstructive-rehabilitative. The primary objective of each of these phases of treatment is to obturate the defect. The immediate result is improvement in the physiologic functions of mastication, deglutition, speech, and respiration. In addition, the prosthesis, by virtue of its design, assists in the replacement and support of facial structures and improves some of the patient's cosmetic deficiencies. Psychological support is generally attributed specifically to improvements in physiologic function and amelioration of cosmetic deficiencies.

Extirpative Surgical Phase

The extirpative surgical phase of prosthodontic support is initiated presurgically with specific attention given to the location, size, and extent of the potential defect. After the impressions are made and the casts obtained, the potential defect is outlined in

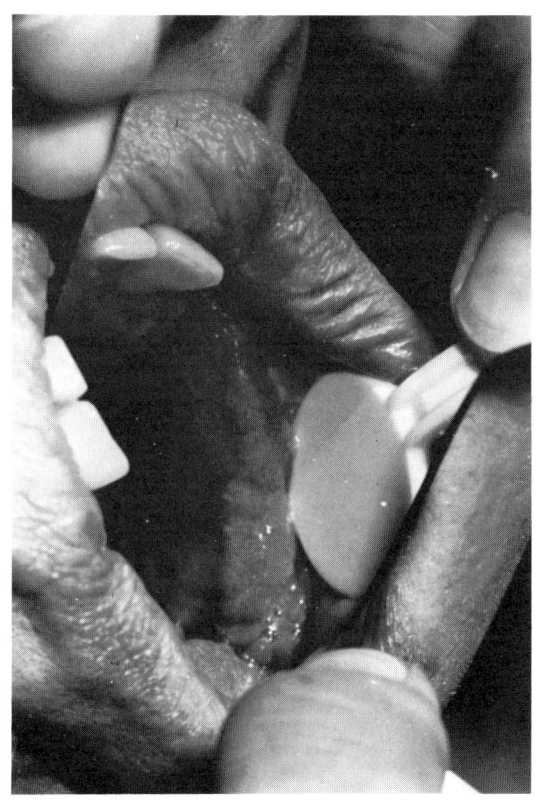

Figure 9–160. Oral view of bone graft after four years.

consultation with the cancer surgeon (Fig. 9–161A). The cast is then modified for surgical obturator fabrication (Fig. 9–161B). The cast base should be extended laterally and posteriorly to accommodate modification for prosthesis fabrication. It is also essential that the cast base be of increased thickness to aid in its modification. These routine procedures are often neglected, causing an increase in laboratory time.

The surgical obturator is normally claspless and is retained by wire ligation. Clasps can be used if desired (Fig. 9–162). If multiple teeth are to remain, it is helpful to have the laboratory block out the master cast at zero degrees, duplicate, wax-up, and process for prosthesis fabrication. Having the surgical obturator processed on such a cast results in ease of insertion at the time of surgery. In most instances, the only modification necessary is the area of resection. It is also advisable to overextend the prosthesis, since it is simpler to reduce the extension than to increase the extension at the time of surgery.

The surgical obturator is usually worn for

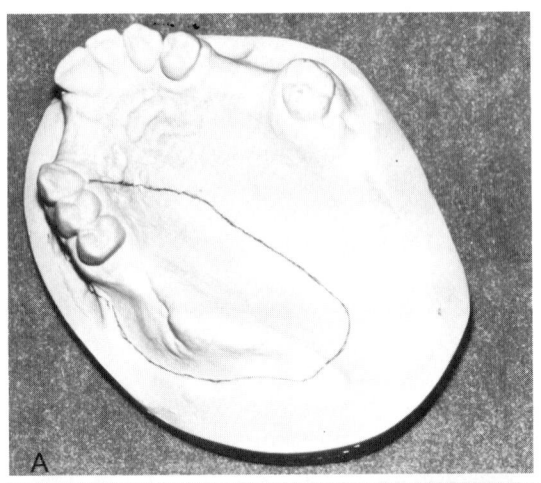

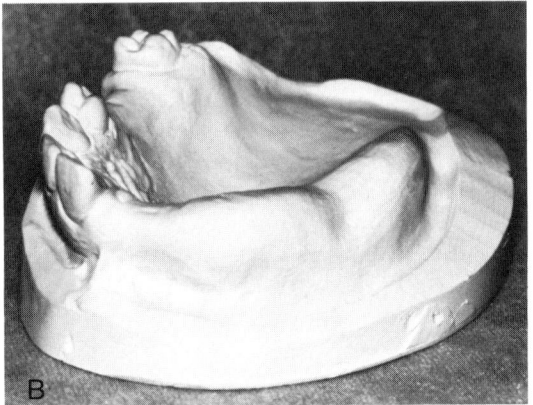

Figure 9–161. *A,* The maxillary cast with outline of proposed surgery resection. *B,* The maxillary cast following modification for prosthesis fabrication.

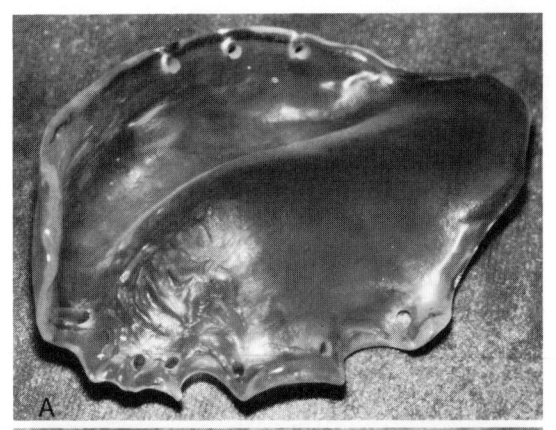

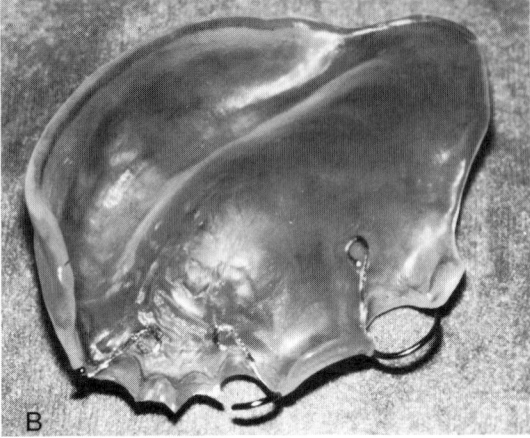

Figure 9–162. *A,* "Claspless" surgical obturator for wire or suture ligation. *B,* "Clasped" surgical obturator secured by remaining natural teeth.

five to seven days. Once removed, it is either modified or replaced by the interim obturator prosthesis. It is advantageous to remove the surgical obturator early in the day. This allows adequate time for fabrication of the interim obturator and insertion of the prosthesis the same day. Gross insertion adjustments, which are normally encountered if no prosthesis is worn for an extended period of time, are thus eliminated.

Interim Phase

The interim obturator prosthesis is generally worn for a period of four to six months while healing occurs. Because this prosthesis is worn during the healing period, stresses transmitted to the supporting tissues, surgerized and nonsurgerized, should be minimized. This can be achieved by several means: prosthesis weight, occlusion, and prosthesis adjustment and modification during the healing phase of treatment.

The weight of the prosthesis can be reduced by processing a hollow-bulb obturator, typically used in patients with large defects. In those instances in which the defect may be less encompassing, the obturator can

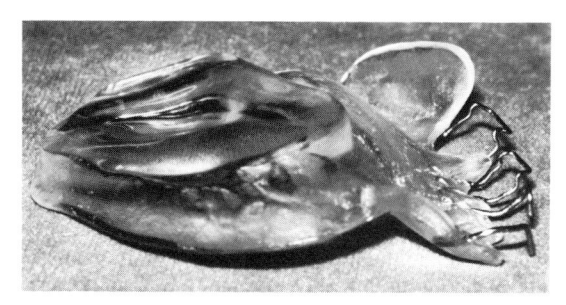

Figure 9–163. Interim solid obturator prosthesis with concave superior surface used to minimize stress by weight reduction.

be processed solidly. It will be reduced concavely on the superior surface, thus reducing obturator mass and weight (Fig. 9–163). Resilient materials may also be considered for use in obturation of the defect (Fig. 9–164).

Because stresses generated during occlusion frequently hinder the healing process, the elimination of teeth on the prosthesis is often advised for the immediate postsurgical period. Teeth can be added for an esthetic, not functional, purpose, with the patient's knowledge.

It is essential to recall the patient during the healing period to provide adjustment or modification of the interim obturator prosthesis. In addition, it is psychologically beneficial for the patient to return periodically during this phase of treatment. Patient problems related to the rehabilitation process can be discussed and supportive care offered.

Reconstructive-Rehabilitative Phase

Once the surgical area has healed and the tissues have adequately stabilized, fabrication of the definitive obturator prosthesis is initiated. This prosthesis obturates the palatal defect and usually replaces the intra-oral anatomic form. If necessary, it is supportive of the facial tissues.

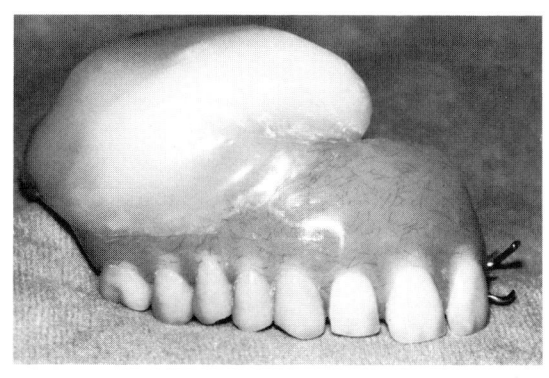

Figure 9–164. "Resilient" (Softic 49) interim obturator prosthesis used to increase potential retention, stability, and comfort for the patient.

Specific considerations given to the definitive obturator should include support, retention, and stability. The materials used for obturator fabrication are either nonresilient (polymethylmethacrylate) or resilient (silicone or plasticized methacrylate) (Fig. 9–165). All resilient materials have been utilized to take advantage of additional areas of retention, increase tissue compatibility, and aid in overall patient comfort.[75–78] Resilient materials are not problem-free but if properly used can be most beneficial.[79] How-

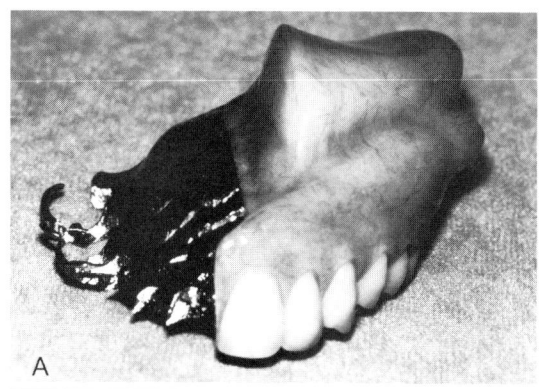

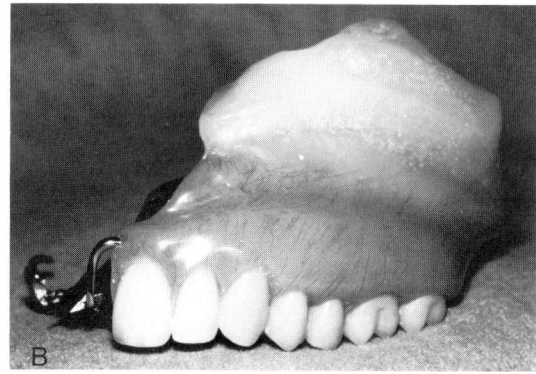

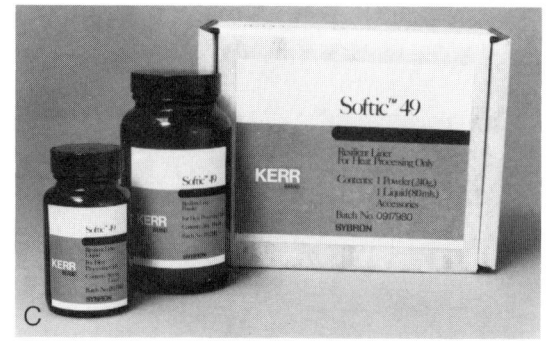

Figure 9–165. *A*, Definitive obturator prosthesis fabricated in hard denture base resin. *B*, Definitive obturator prosthesis fabricated in "resilient" resin (Softic 49). *C*, Softic 49, a definitive resilient lining material, has been the material of choice for our patient population. Softic 49 is the only material that has been well-tolerated by the xerostomic patient; it is nonsupportive of fungal or bacterial growth, tissue-like in its resiliency, superior in bond strength, and requires only routine handling, processing, finishing, and repair procedures.

ever, the success of any treatment is not necessarily due to the material or the treatment methods employed, but rather may be due to the recall and follow-up schedule on which the patient is placed.

Although surgical reconstruction for the rehabilitation of maxillary defects is not often indicated for improvement of physiologic function, it is sometimes indicated for patient cosmesis (Fig. 9–166). It must be emphasized, however, that bone and soft-tissue grafting procedures are specifically for cosmetic improvement of facial symmetry and the support of a prosthesis to rehabilitate the patient's physiologic function. The placement and resulting location of the graft assist the prosthesis by offering some cross-arch stabilization.

Because it is used to support facial tissue symmetry, the bone graft is often located too far laterally to benefit prosthesis support. This does not compromise prosthodontic treatment. The prosthesis approaches the graft site and utilizes the areas as the lateral anatomic limitation for prosthesis extension. If the grafted area is used for positive support for the prosthesis, there will be a dramatic compromise in vestibular contour, prosthesis flange extension, and prosthesis contour.

Extra-Oral Rehabilitation

Extra-oral anatomic areas commonly involved in tumor resection are the auricular, facial, nasal, and orbital. Also involved are those areas that result in communication of extra-oral and intra-oral defects. The resulting postsurgical deficiencies can, like those defects of the maxilla and mandible, be divided into three areas of concern: physiologic, cosmetic, and psychological.

Physiologically, the deficiency is specific to the anatomic structure and/or structures involved in tumor resection and the specific function provided by the resected anatomy.

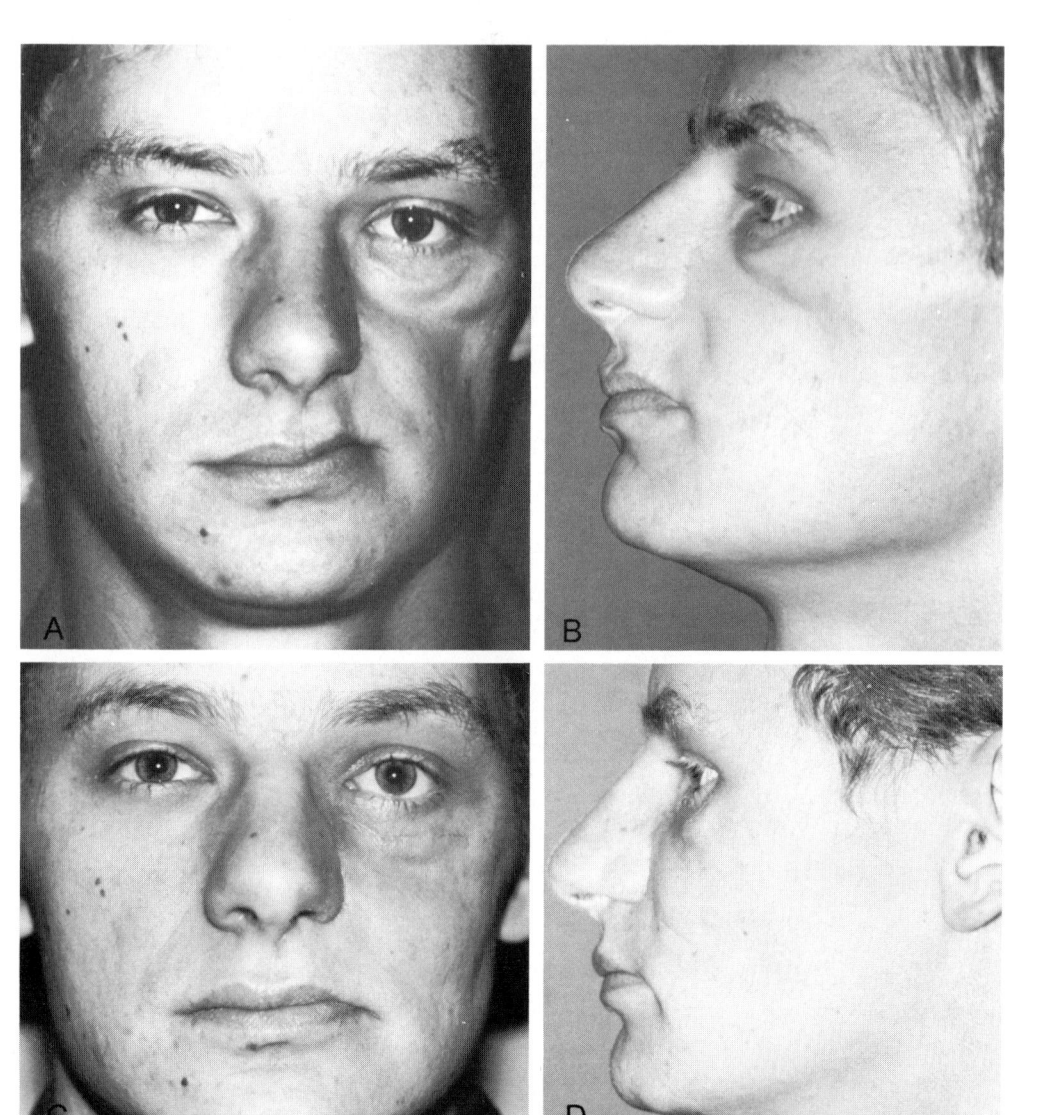

Figure 9–166. Preoperative frontal (*A*) and lateral (*B*) view of patient with facial asymmetry associated with right zygomatic process. Postsurgical frontal (*C*) and lateral (*D*) views of patient with facial asymmetry.

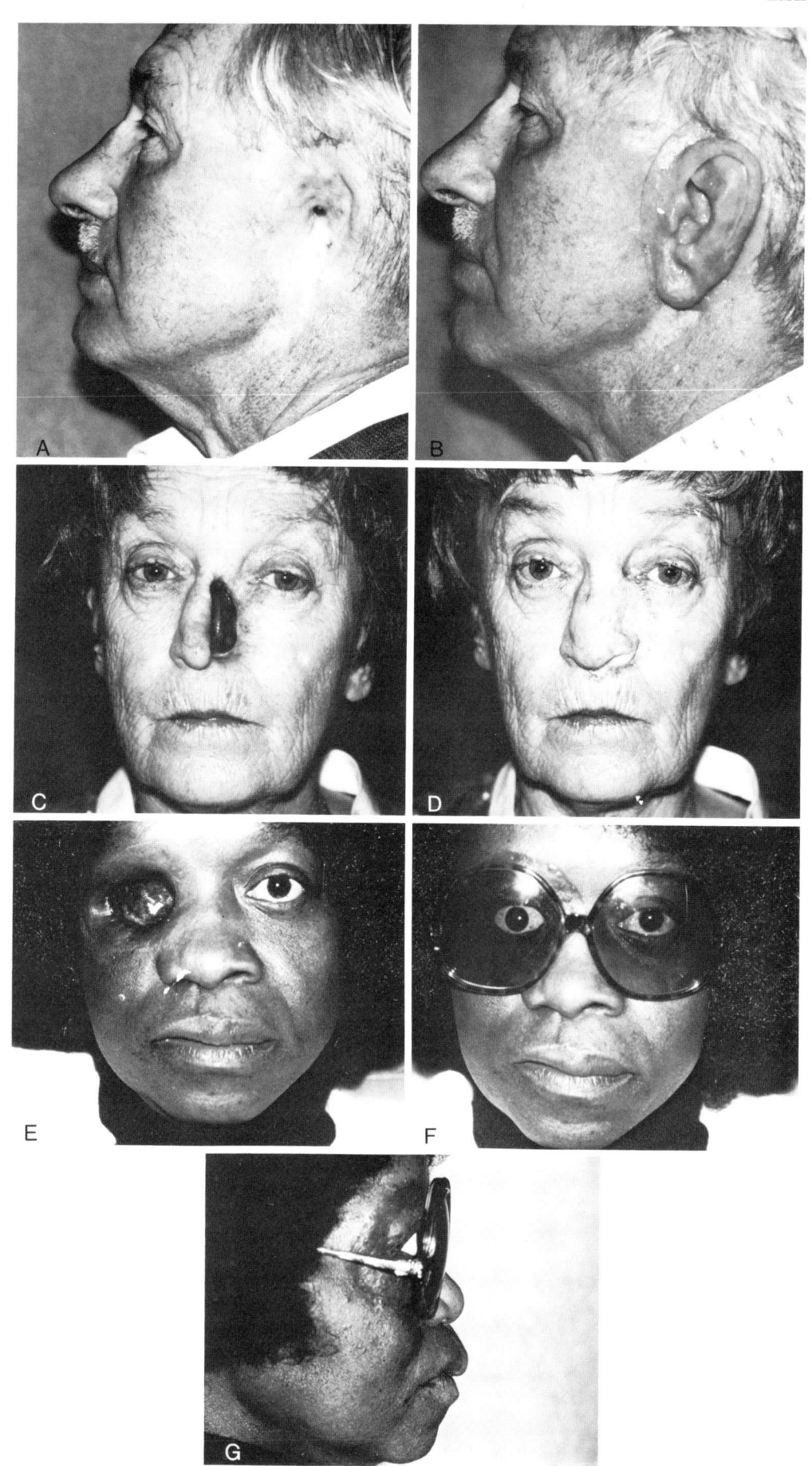

RECONSTRUCTION AND REHABILITATION OF CANCER PATIENTS / **421**

Figure 9–167. *A*, Auricular defect prior to placement of the prosthesis. *B*, Following placement of prosthesis. *C*, Nasal defect prior to placement of the prosthesis. *D*, Following placement of prosthesis. *E*, Orbital defect prior to placement of prosthesis. Frontal view (*F*) and lateral view (*G*) of patient with prosthesis placed.

Cosmetic deficiencies are generally associated with loss of facial integrity and/or facial symmetry. Neuromuscular impairment must also be considered.

Psychological deficiencies are typically related to loss or impairment of normal physiologic function associated with the lost structure(s). The resulting alteration of facial symmetry and neurologic impairment or loss are also potential psychological problems for the patient. The patient's and/or family's expectations of rehabilitation are likewise of primary concern.

The objective of extra-oral rehabilitation is threefold: improvement of physiologic function, when possible, by restoration of the resected structure or structures; cosmetic improvement by restoring or improving extraoral integrity and/or symmetry; and psychological benefit to the patient by hopefully improving the patient's self-image and level of social acceptability (Fig. 9–167).

Associated with any rehabilitative process are certain limitations and problems. The surgical defect itself is often the major limitation. This is specific to the location, size, and extent of the defect. The defect configuration can also pose a problem owing to the varying mass of remaining tissue over which a prosthesis must be constructed (Fig. 9–168).

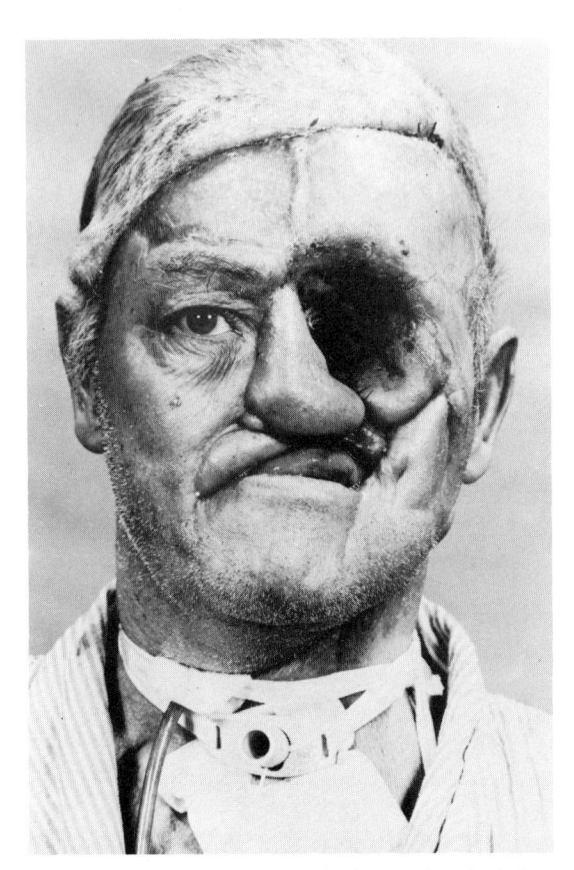

Figure 9–168. Patient with large facial defect with gross tissue irregularities that would cause much difficulty in facial prosthesis fabrication.

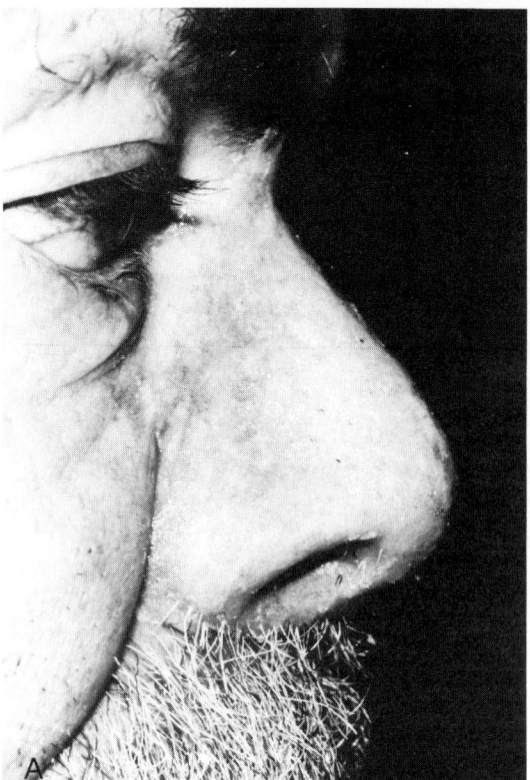

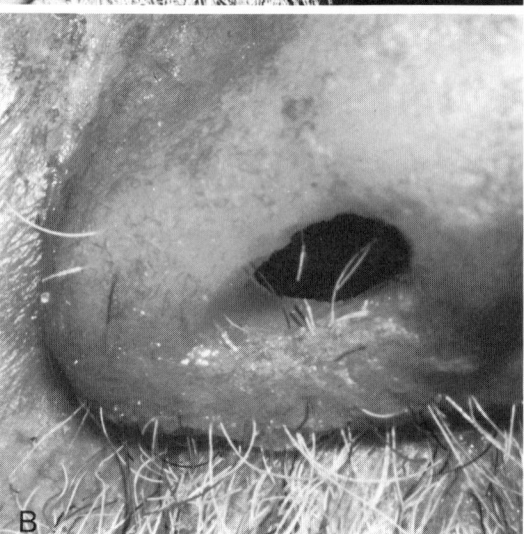

Figure 9–169. *A*, Nasal prosthesis exhibiting marginal separation at the inferior border due to differences in tissue mobility and movement. *B*, Close-up view of same.

In addition, the configuration of the defect governs the manner in which retention of the prosthesis is accomplished.

Marginal adaptation of the prosthesis is limited by the structures to which it must be adapted. These supporting structures can also pose a problem. Because it is necessary to adapt the prosthesis to both movable and nonmovable tissue (Fig. 9–169), marginal leakage may occur as a result of limitations imposed by the adhesives or mechanical mechanism employed for prosthesis securement.

Cosmetic rehabilitation can be limited by the specific material utilized for prosthesis fabrication. No one single material is totally acceptable to date, and silicone is most often considered the material of choice for extra-oral prosthesis fabrication. Various other materials have been used, but all have specific limitations.[17, 79-82] These limitations are associated with material color, texture, form, translucency, ease of manipulation, flexibility, dimensional stability, weight, edge strength, color stability, durability, toxicity, and biocompatibility. Cosmetic limitations also include the inability to restore proper facial symmetry or integrity. Neuromuscular weakness is usually not correctable by prosthesis rehabilitation, and, as previously mentioned, problems are also associated with prosthesis movement.

Extra-oral rehabilitation is not without inherent problems. The success of such treatment may not be specifically associated with prosthesis intervention but is probably more importantly associated with patient support and improvement of self-image.

REHABILITATION PROGRAMS*

Despite the fact that members of the health-care team provide assistance throughout the rehabilitation period, the information they provide the patients is often fragmented, misunderstood, or simply forgotten. Many patients and their families struggle through the long, complex process of rehabilitation without fully understanding what has happened to them, what is going to happen to them, or the reasons why certain phenomena occur. Feeling confused, abandoned, and frightened, they desperately seek information. For these reasons, two patient rehabilitation programs were developed to provide the patients and their families with the necessary follow-up information.

The two slide-tape programs are entitled "Your Obturator Prosthesis" and "Your Mandibular Prosthesis." The opening statement of each 15-minute presentation discusses the surgery performed for the removal of a tumor that resulted in a surgical defect (Fig. 9–170). Various postoperative problems associated with surgery are discussed in detail. These include *physiologic problems* (mastication, deglutition, phonation, and respiration), *cosmetic problems* (facial asymmetry, neuromuscular impairment, and loss of tooth/teeth support and function), and *psychological problems* (specifically resulting from physiologic and cosmetic deficiencies).

The various prostheses used to rehabilitate these patients are accurately described, emphasizing their assets as well as their limitations (Fig. 9–171). Stress to supporting tissue, mastication, speech quality, leakage, and cosmetics are discussed. Patients are informed of the average treatment time associated with their respective rehabilitative process.

A major thrust of both programs is to educate patients in the care of the oral cavity and the maintenance of the prosthesis. Instructions are given regarding inserting, wearing, and removing the prosthesis. Oral and prosthetic hygiene and dietary suggestions are presented. Emphasis is placed on

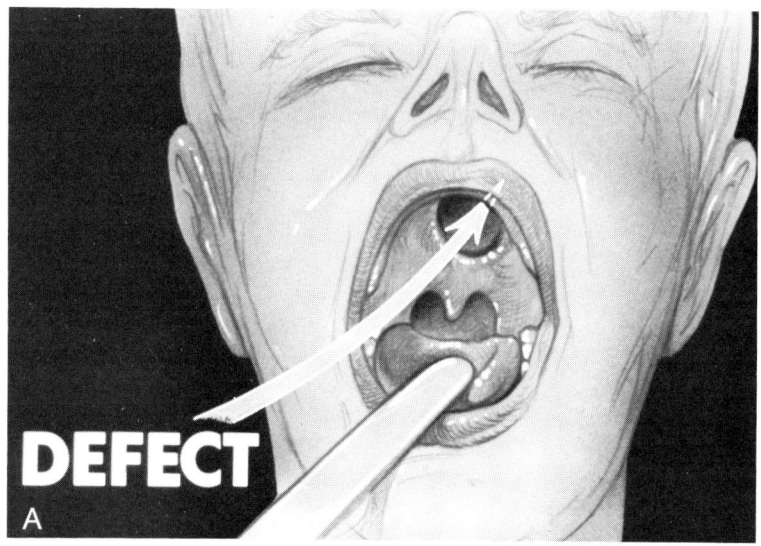

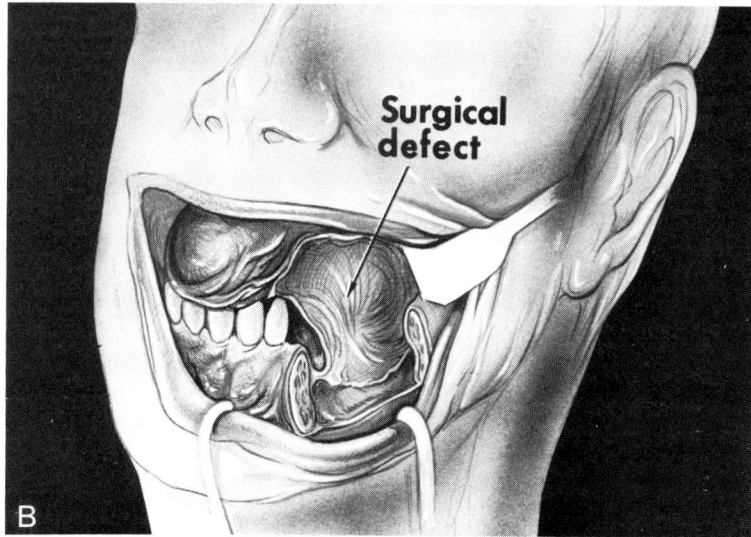

Figure 9–170. *A*, Graphic representation of the surgical deficiency resulting from partial maxillectomy. *B*, Graphic representation of the surgical deficiency resulting from partial mandibulectomy.

---

*Supported by National Cancer Institute Contract CN 45120 C. Programs obtained by contacting Mr. Reginold Yule, Audiovisual Center, Mayo Clinic, 200 First St. S.W., Rochester, Minnesota 55901; tel. 507-282-2511, ext. 2328.

424 / RECONSTRUCTION AND REHABILITATION OF CANCER PATIENTS

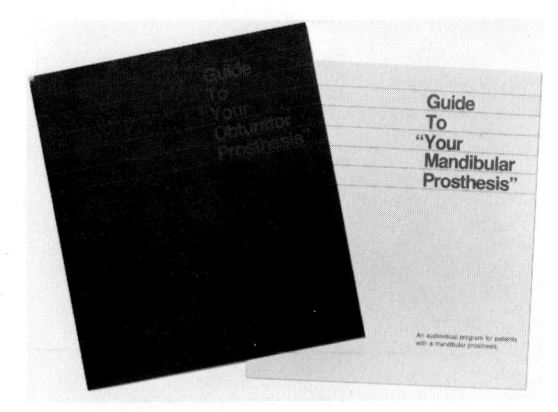

Figure 9–172. Patient education "guide" booklets for maxillary and mandibular defect patients.

ined. It is the patient's relentless dedication to each of these items that determines the success of prosthodontic rehabilitation and the resumption of a normal life.

Booklets that reiterate all the information presented in the slide-tape series are a part of each program (Fig. 9–172).

REHABILITATION (VERSUS) RECONSTRUCTION

When patients and their families successfully pass through the stages of cancer surgery, surgical reconstruction, and prosthetic rehabilitation, each member of the health care team feels a sense of accomplishment and success. It would be naive to think that this population of patients has no further need for health care support beyond routine follow-up. Most of these patients bring us a comprehensive set of problems that were once secondary to their cancer-related deformity but are now of primary concern. Two of the foremost problems are continued alcohol intake to the point of alcoholism and continued tobacco use. Others include xerostomia, dietary inadequacies, caries, and job placement.

ALCOHOLISM

In our experience the positive outlook after rehabilitation of a cancer-related deformity has made a difference in the success of alcohol rehabilitation programs. Of 44 patients who underwent alcohol rehabilitation programs after surgical prosthetic rehabilitation, 27 have successfully completed the program and remained in control for more than 18 months. Twenty-one of these 44 patients had previously failed alcohol rehabilitation courses one or more times. This represents an improvement in the overall yield for

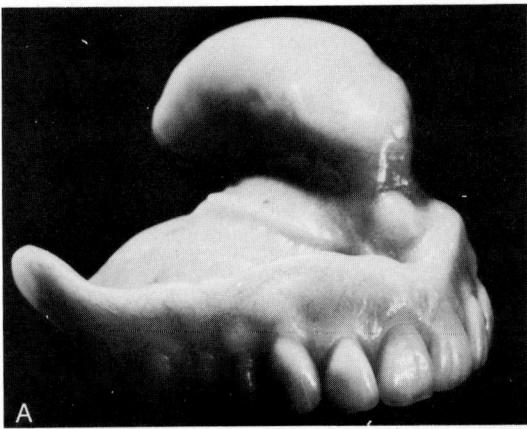

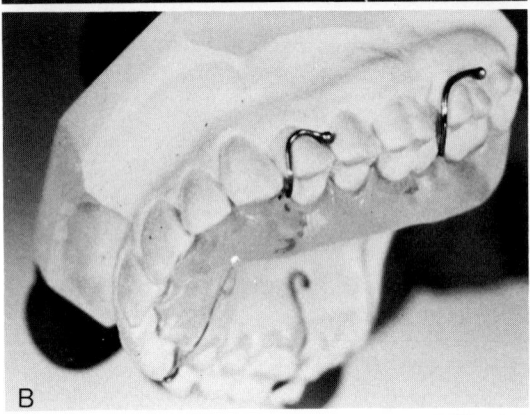

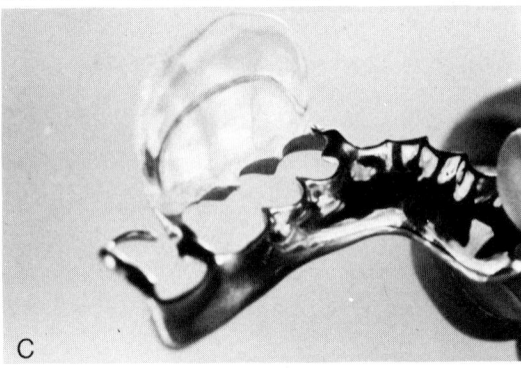

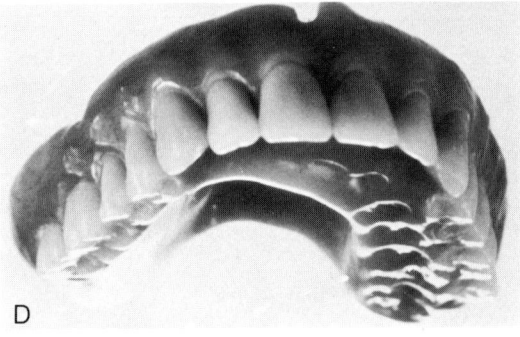

Figure 9–171. *A,* Definitive obturator prosthesis for the edentulous patient. *B,* Maxillary inclined plane used as a patient training aid. *C,* Mandibular guide flange prosthesis. *D,* Maxillary occlusal plane prosthesis.

the patient's long-term observation, necessitating periodic recall appointments when both the tissue and the prosthesis are exam-

this alcohol rehabilitation program of 25 to 35 per cent. It is reasonable to counsel patients at this time to seriously change destructive lifestyle habits and offer referrals to specific programs.

Continued Tobacco Use

It is unrealistic to expect this patient population to be able to completely abstain from tobacco use. We have attempted psychological and psychiatric counseling, as well as hypnosis programs, with disappointing results. In 92 consecutive patients whom we have reconstructed, 80 (87 per cent) continued to smoke to some degree. Twenty-nine of these patients claimed to have completely quit, but 23 of these were observed smoking at some time in their follow-up. This is indicative of the tremendous dependency this habit can create.

In a practical sense, it is reasonable to compromise with these patients and provide them with more attainable goals. We impress upon them the need to quit in an absolute manner and our support in any structured program designed to achieve this. However, we offer them a reduction to 10 cigarettes or less per day as the maximum harmful dose and a sufficient dose for them to prevent withdrawal symptoms. In our experience they seem to be able to live within this framework without gradually lapsing into greater consumption of cigarettes. On each follow-up visit, the potential of second primaries and persistent disease is discussed, along with the risks of heart disease and other illnesses. We now will often give them a reprint of the article by Silverman et al.[10] regarding tobacco usage and the development of second primaries. This contrasts the 25 to 30 per cent incidence of second primaries within five years in those who continue to smoke to the 4 to 6 per cent incidence in those who have quit. It also suggests a reduced incidence in those who reduce their exposure. We sometimes show photographs of patients who have developed second primaries or discuss patients that the individual knew during his reconstructive course who have developed second primaries in a "scared straight" approach. Beyond this informed patient approach, the individual must make the decision and commitment on his or her own.

Xerostomia

Xerostomia remains a persistent problem that neither reconstruction nor hyperbaric oxygen can improve. In fact, with reconstruction and a functional denture prosthesis, the demand for salivary lubrication is increased as patients graduate to more solid diets. Patients often find it reassuring and convenient to carry a cup or a thermos of water. During meals they must accept the need to increase their fluid intake. Many patients prefer saliva substitutes that lubricate the mucous membranes for hours, thus freeing them from the need to carry a water source. The wetting properties of several saliva substitutes also allow patients to tolerate a prosthesis better. Several formulas available today[83] afford patients improved swallowing and additional comfort. In addition, the development of resilient denture base materials by Saunders[84] has made conventional prostheses more functional and comfortable in irradiated patients with xerostomia.

Dietary Inadequacies

Diet is too often an overlooked portion of a patient's follow-up care. Habit patterns established prior to reconstruction and reinforced by alcohol dependence often lead to an imbalanced nutritional intake. Dietary supplements and vitamins alone will not suffice. It is recommended that the patient be seen by a dietician and the surgeon-prosthodontist. It is important that they work with each other to arrive at a balanced intake that is palatable to the patient and realistically achievable within the limits of his/her residual compromise in function.

Dental Maintenance

Those patients with remaining teeth require on-going maintenance care and prophylaxis. Although dental health should be made optimum prior to reconstructive efforts, continued radiation caries and periodontal disease are all too common. Fluoride carriers and instructions in the use of home fluoride applications have proven to be somewhat effective in reducing radiation caries in compliant patients.[85] Plaque control instructions and periodontal care should also be part of the follow-up management. The best surgical reconstructions and prosthetic rehabilitations are a gross compromise of normal function. The additional loss of teeth or any tissue adds further to this compromise of function. Ongoing dental maintenance will often prevent a functionally satisfying result from becoming a useless prosthesis and/or bone graft.

Social Job Placement

Since our goal is to return patients to the mainstream of life after the devastation of major extirpative surgery, assistance in job placement, volunteer work, or intrafamily activities is often required. To help our patients overcome one of the final obstacles to a complete rehabilitation, one should not hesitate to support their applications for work and activities with volunteer organizations, and/or encourage their families to involve them more deeply in their activities.

PERSPECTIVE

Patient rehabilitation made possible by surgical reconstruction is a continuum of progress. Just as the days prior to sterile technique and antibiotics seem barbaric to us today, so will these so-called advanced techniques seem barbaric to our professional successors in the future. If there is any lasting advancement in reconstruction identified in the preceding pages, it is the deeper understanding we have for the biologic processes of tissue healing, which essentially do not change. Relevant to this are the words that follow the quotation at the beginning of this chapter:

"The knowledge to use, foster, and perhaps even control, many of the forces of repair is now within the grasp of every surgeon; it is his to use, if he is willing."

Thomas K. Hunt
Walton VanWinkle, Jr.

BIBLIOGRAPHY

1. Calearo CV, and Teatini G: Functional neck dissection, anatomical grounds, surgical technique, clinical observations. Ann Otol Rhinol Laryngol 92:215–222, 1983.
2. Lingeman RE, Helmus C, Stephens R, and Ulm J: Neck dissection: Radical or conservative. Ann Otol Rhinol Laryngol 86:737–744, 1977.
3. Spiesal B, and Tschopp HM: Surgery of the jaws. In Naumann HH (ed): Head and Neck Surgery. Philadelphia, WB Saunders Co, 1980, pp 133–159.
4. Silver IA: The measurement of oxygen tension in healing tissue. In Herzog H (ed): Progress in Respiratory Research. Basel, S Karger, 1969, p 124.
5. Stevens MR, and Marx RE: Complete resolution of osteoradionecrosis with a new protocol combining hyperbaric oxygen and resection. Proceedings of the 63rd Meeting of the American Association of Oral and Maxillofacial Surgeons, 1981.
6. Adamo AR, and Szal RL: Timing, results and complications of mandibular reconstructive surgery: Report of 32 cases. J Oral Surg 37:755–759, 1979.
7. Obwegesser HB, and Sailer HF: Experience with intra-oral resection and immediate reconstruction in cases of radio-osteomyelitis of the mandible. J Maxillofac Surg 6:257–261, 1978.
8. Marx RE, and Ames JR: The use of hyperbaric oxygen therapy in bony reconstruction of the irradiated and tissue-deficient patient. J Oral Surg 40:412–420, 1982.
9. Donoff RB, and May JW: Microvascular mandibular reconstruction. J Oral Maxillofac Surg 40:122–126, 1982.
10. Silverman S, Greenspan D, and Gorsky M: Tobacco usage in patients with head and neck carcinomas: A follow-up on habit changes and second primary oral/oropharyngeal cancers. J Am Dent Assoc 106:33–35, 1983.
11. Bear SE, Green RK, and Wentz WW: Stainless steel wire mesh—an aid in difficult oral surgery problems. J Oral Surg 29:27–31, 1971.
12. Adekeye EO: Ameloblastomas of the jaws: A survey of 109 Nigerian patients. J Oral Surg 38:36–41, 1980.
13. Obwegesser HL: Simultaneous resection and reconstruction of parts of the mandible via the intraoral route in patients with and without gross infection. Oral Surg 21:693–705, 1966.
14. Cantor R, and Curtis TA: Prosthetic management of edentulous mandibulectomy patients. Part I: Anatomic, physiologic, and psychologic considerations. Prosthet Dent 25:446, 1971.
15. Curtis TA, Taylor RC, and Rositano SA: Physical problems in obtaining records of the maxillofacial patient. Prosthet Dent 34:539, 1975.
16. Aramany M, and Myers E: Dental occlusion and arch relationship in segmented resection of the mandible. In Sisson GA, and Tardy ME (eds): Plastic and Reconstructive Surgery of the Face and Neck. Proceedings of the Second International Symposium. New York, Grune & Stratton, Inc, 1977.
17. Beumer J III, Curtis TA, and Firtell DA: Maxillofacial Rehabilitation: Prosthodontic and Surgical Consideration. St Louis, The CV Mosby Co, 1979.
18. Burwell RG: Studies in the transplantation of bone. The fresh composite hemograft-autograft of cancellous bone. J Bone Joint Surg 46B:110–154, 1964.
19. Gray JC, and Elves MW: Early osteogenesis in compact bone isografts: A quantitative study of contributions of the different graft cells. Calcif Tissue Int 29:225–237, 1979.
20. Elves MW: Newer knowledge of immunology of bone and cartilage. Clin Orthop 120:232–236, 1976.
21. Axhausen W: The osteogenetic phases of regeneration of bone, a historical and experimental study. J Bone Joint Surg 38A:593–601, 1956.
22. Urist MR: The substratum for bone morphogenesis. Develop Biol (Suppl) 4:125–129, 1970.
23. Urist MR: Osteoinduction in undemineralized bone implants modified by chemical inhibitors of endogenous matrix enzymes. Clin Orthop 87:132–138, 1972.
24. Friedenstein AJ, Piatetzky-Shapiro II, and Petrakova KV: Osteogenesis in transplants of bone marrow cells. J Embryol Exp Morphol 16:381–386, 1966.
25. Simmons DJ, Lester PA, and Ellsasser JC: Survival of osteocompetent marrow cells in vitro and the effect of PHA-stimulation on osteoinduction in composite bone grafts. Proc Soc Exp Biol Med 148:986–1003, 1975.
26. Moss ML, and Salentigin L: The capsular matrix. Am J Orthod 565:474–490, 1969.
27. Moss ML, and Ranow RM: The role of the func-

28. Marx RE, Snyder RM, and Kline SN: Cellular survival of human marrow during placement of marrow cancellous bone grafts. J Oral Surg 37:712–718, 1979.
29. Cruz NI, Cestero HJ, and Cora ML: Management of contaminated bone grafts. Plast Reconstr Surg 68:411–414, 1981.
30. Boyne PJ: Restoration of osseous defects in maxillofacial casualties. J Am Dent Assoc 78:767–770, 1969.
31. Marx RE, Kline SN, Johnson RP, Malinin TI, Matthews JG, and Gambill V: The use of freeze-dried allogeneic bone in oral and maxillofacial surgery. J Oral Surg 39:264–274, 1981.
32. Gray JC, and Elves MW: Donor cells' contribution to osteogenesis in experimental cancellous bone grafts. Clin Orthop 163:261–271, 1982.
33. Enneking WF, Burchardt H, Puhl J, and Prostrowski G: Physical and biologic aspects of repair in dog cortical bone transplants. J Bone Joint Surg 57A:237–246, 1975.
34. Enneking WF, and Morris JL: Human autologous cortical bone transplants. Clin Orthop 87:28–39, 1972.
35. Bonucci E: New knowledge on the origin, function and fate of osteoclasts. Clin Orthop 158:252–261, 1981.
36. Boyne PJ, and Zarem H: Osseous reconstruction of the resected mandible. Am J Surg 132:49–53, 1976.
37. Salyer KE, Newsom HT, Holmes R, and Hahn G: Mandibular reconstruction. Am J Surg 134:461–464, 1977.
38. Leake DL, and Habol MB: Osteoneogenesis: A new method for facial reconstruction. J Surg Res 18:331–336, 1975.
39. Small I, Brown S, and Kobernick S: Teflon and Silastic for mandibular replacement; experimental studies and reports of cases. J Oral Surg 22:377–381, 1964.
40. Marx RE, and Kline SN: Principles and methods of osseous reconstruction. Int Adv Surg Oncol 6L:167–228, 1983.
41. Malinin TI: University of Miami Tissue Bank: Collection of postmortem tissues for clinical use and laboratory investigation. Transplant Proc 8(Suppl 1):53–58, 1976.
42. Manchester WM: Immediate reconstruction of the mandible and temporomandibular joint. Br J Plast Surg 18:291–300, 1977.
43. Kelly JF: Maxillofacial missile wounds: Evaluation of long-term results of rehabilitation and reconstruction. J Oral Surg 31:438–447, 1973.
44. Marx RE: Osteoradionecrosis: A new concept of its pathophysiology. J Oral Maxillofac Surg 41: 283–288, 1983.
45. Marx RE: A new concept in the treatment of osteoradionecrosis. J Oral Maxillofac Surg 41: 351–357, 1983.
46. Sheffield PJ, and Workman WT: Continuous tissue oxygen monitoring of hyperbaric oxygen therapy patients by the transcutaneous method. Sixth Annual Conference on Clinical Application of Hyperbaric Oxygen. Long Beach, CA, June 10–12, 1981.
47. Beehner MR, and Marx RE: Hyperbaric oxygen–induced angiogenesis and fibroplasia in human irradiated tissues. Proceedings of the 65th Meeting of the American Association of Oral and Maxillofacial Surgeons, Las Vegas, 1983.
48. Ariyan S: Further experiences with the pectoralis major myocutaneous flap for the immediate repair of defects from excision of head and neck cancers. Plast Reconstr Surg 64:605–612, 1979.
49. Ariyan S: One-stage reconstruction for defects of the mouth using a sternomastoid myocutaneous flap. Plast Reconst Surgery 63:618–625, 1979.
50. Ariyan S: The pectoralis major myocutaneous flap. A versatile flap for reconstruction in the head and neck. Plast Reconstr Surg 63:73–79, 1979.
51. Donoff RB, and May JW: Microvascular transfer of rib. J Dent Res 59(Special Issue A):459, 1980.
52. Ariyan S, and Finseth FJ: The anterior chest approach for obtaining free osteocutaneous rib grafts. Plast Reconstr Surg 62:676–681, 1978.
53. Serafin D, Riefkohl R, Thomas I, and Georgiade NG: Vascularized rib periosteal and osteocutaneous reconstruction of the maxilla and mandible: An assessment. Plast Reconstr Surg 66(5): 718–727, 1980.
54. Daniel RK: Commentary on reconstruction of mandibular defects with revascularized free rib grafts by T Harashima, H Nakajima, and T Imai (the voice of polite dissent). Plast Reconstr Surg 62:775, 1978.
55. Ryan DE: Microvascular free transfers of ilium for mandibular reconstruction. Proceedings of the Society of Air Force Clinical Surgeons Meeting, San Antonio, TX, May, 1983.
56. Stone JD, and Franklin JD: Immediate mandibular reconstruction using free osseous myocutaneous groin flaps. Proceedings of the 62nd Annual Meeting of the American Association of Oral and Maxillofacial Surgeons, 1980.
57. Wilcox JW, and Kolodny SC: Acceleration of healing maxillary and mandibular osteotomies by use of hyperbaric oxygen. Oral Surg 41:423–426, 1976.
58. Mainous EG, Boyne PJ, Hart GB, and Terry BC: Restoration of resected mandible by grafting with combination of mandible homograft and autogenous iliac marrow, and postoperative treatment with hyperbaric oxygenation. Oral Surg 35:13–16, 1973.
59. Hansbrough JF, Pracentine JG, and Eiseman B: Immunosuppression by hyperbaric oxygen. Surgery 87:662–668, 1980.
60. Ayers LN, Tierney DF, and Imagawa D: Shortened survival of mice with influenza when given oxygen at one atmosphere. Am Rev Respir Dis 107:955–961, 1973.
61. McCredie JA, Inch WR, Kruuv J, and Watson TA: Effects of hyperbaric oxygen on growth and metastasis of the C3HBA tumor in the mouse. Cancer 19:1537–1542, 1966.
62. Harmon FW, and Marx RE: The effect of hyperbaric oxygen on carcinogenesis and tumor growth rate. Proceedings of the 65th Annual Meeting of the American Association of Oral and Maxillofacial Surgeons, 1983.
63. Mashberg A, Garfinkel L, and Harris S: Alcohol as a primary risk factor in oral squamous carcinoma. CA 31:146–155, 1981.
64. Rush BF, Swaminathan AP, and Jefferis KR: The use of cervical flaps from irradiated necks in immediate reconstruction. Am J Surg 134:465–468, 1977.
65. Sasaki CT: The sternocleidomastoid myocutaneous flap. Arch Otolaryngol 106:74–76, 1980.
66. Jabaley ME, Heckley FR, Wallace WH, and Knott LW: Sternocleidomastoid regional flaps: A new look at an old concept. Br J Plast Surg 32: 106–113, 1979.
67. McCraw JB, Dibbel DG, and Carraway JH: Clinical definition of independent myocutaneous vascular territories. Plast Reconstr Surg 60:341–349, 1977.
68. Bartlett SP, May JW, and Yaremchik MJ: The lattisimus dorsi muscle: A fresh cadaver study of the primary neurovascular pedicle. Plast Reconstr Surg 67:631–636, 1981.
69. Woodburne RT: Essentials of Human Anatomy.

3rd ed. New York, Oxford University Press, 1965, pp 163, 189–190.
70. Grabb WC: Median and ulnar nerve suture: An experimental study comparing primary and secondary repair in monkey. J Bone Joint Surg 50A:964–969, 1968.
71. Donoff RB: The applications of microsurgery in oral and maxillofacial surgery. In Irby WB, and Shelton DW (eds): Current Advances in Oral and Maxillofacial Surgery. Vol IV. St. Louis, The CV Mosby Co, 1983, pp 156–183.
72. Morris JH: Biphase connector, external skeletal splint for reduction and fixation of mandibular fractures. Oral Surg 2:1382–1398, 1949.
73. Curtis TA: Treatment planning for intraoral maxillofacial prosthetics for cancer patients. Prosthet Dent 18:70, 1967.
74. Gillis RE Jr: An Investigation of the Psychological Factors Involved in Maxillofacial Surgery and Prosthetic Rehabilitation. Thesis, Mayo Graduate School of Medicine (University of Minnesota), Rochester, Minnesota, 1977.
75. Zarb GA: The maxillary resection and its prosthetic replacement. J Prosthet Dent 18:268, 1967.
76. Hahn GW: A comfortable silicone bulb obturator with or without dentures. J Prosthet Dent 28:313, 1972.
77. Ohyama T, Gold HO, and Pruzansky S: Maxillary obturator with silicone-lined hollow extension. J Prosthet Dent 34:336, 1975.
78. Parr GR: A combination obturator. J Prosthet Dent 41:329, 1979.
79. Bauer RW, Cheng A, Saunders TR, and Pierson WP: American Dental Association: Council on Dental Materials, Instruments, and Devices. Acceptance Program for Resilient Definitive Denture Liners, August, 1983.
80. Rahn AO, and Boucher LJ: Maxillofacial Prosthetics: Principles and Concepts. Philadelphia, WB Saunders Co, 1970.
81. Chalian VA, Drane JB, and Standish SM: Maxillofacial Prosthetics: Multidisciplinary Practice. Baltimore, The Williams & Wilkins Co, 1971.
82. Laney WR: Maxillofacial Prosthetics: Postgraduate Dental Handbook Series. Vol. 4. Littleton, MA, PSG Publishing Company, Inc, 1979.
83. Obwegesser HL: Late reconstruction of large maxillary defects after tumor resection. J Maxillofac Surg 1:19–29, 1973.
84. Saunders TR: Development, utilization, and evaluation of educational programs for patients with maxillary and mandibular defects. J Prosthet Dent 42:665, 1979.
85. Stamps JT, Williams EO, and Saunders TR: A review of the irradiated patient: Dental treatment considerations. Milit Med 147:224–228, 1982.

10
RECONSTRUCTIVE SURGERY FOR MAXILLOFACIAL INJURIES

Donald Osbon, D.D.S.

Injuries of the maxillofacial region vary in severity from minor, superficial injuries to more complex types with avulsion of portions of both soft tissue and underlying osseous structures. Patients with these injuries are apprehensive and exhibit concern over wounds involving the facial region. An increasing number of complex and complicated trauma patterns occur from injuries sustained in high-speed land and air transportation and as a result of missile wounds. Treatment of these facial injuries should be directed toward minimizing loss of function and preventing facial disfigurement. Avulsion injuries of the maxilla and mandible often result in a continuity defect with subsequent loss of masticatory function (Fig. 10–1). Many maxillary injuries can be restored successfully by prosthetic means, but continuity defects of the mandible require extensive bone and soft tissue reconstruction. The objectives of that reconstruction are to re-establish general continuity with sufficient bone to support a prosthesis and to correct alveolar and vestibular deficiencies for prosthetic reconstruction. Every effort should be made to restore the normal function of the jaws with satisfactory occlusion of the teeth, utilizing the remaining dentition or providing a functional prosthesis.

Although immediate definitive treatment of maxillofacial wounds reduces the mutilating effect, a significant number of patients will require prolonged and extensive reconstructive procedures. In a survey of 9,439 patients with maxillofacial injuries in the Vietnam conflict, 9.4 per cent exhibited avulsion of a significant portion of the mandible, and long-term reconstructive therapy was required to effect optimum results.[1] Treatment must be predicated on thorough examination and evaluation and must be organized to prevent duplication of effort and repetition of operative procedures. Reconstruction actually starts with the initial treat-

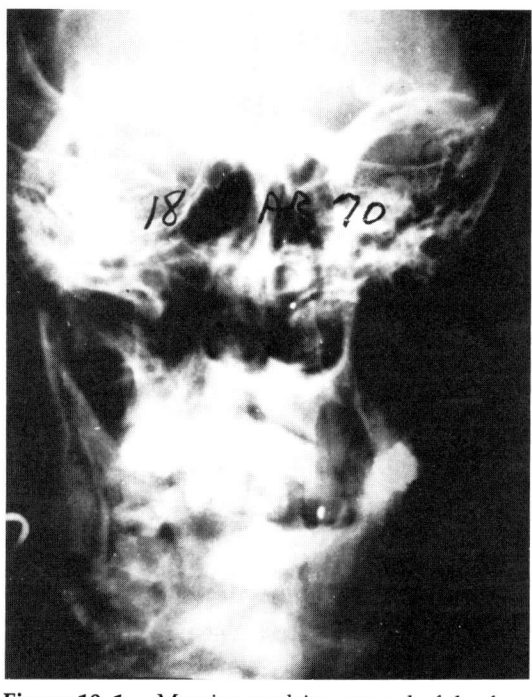

Figure 10–1. Massive avulsive wound of the face with loss of continuity of the mandible.

429

ment which, if carefully performed, will prevent unnecessary scarring and reduce the need for major reconstruction. In those patients with more destructive wounds requiring multiple procedures, subsequent treatment should be organized into intermediate and reconstructive phases.

EARLY CARE

Patients with maxillofacial injuries may also have multiple body injuries consisting of wounds of the head, chest, abdomen, and extremities. The first priority must always be given to life-saving procedures such as the establishment and maintenance of a patent airway, arrest of hemorrhage, recognition and treatment of shock, recognition and treatment of associated head injuries, and treatment of severe trauma to the extremities, thorax, and abdomen. Thorough triage with a complete physical examination should establish the priority of treatment. Since maxillofacial injuries are generally not life-endangering, they will usually have a low treatment priority.

MANAGEMENT OF WOUNDS

Wound Preparation

The majority of maxillofacial wounds are contaminated and require cleaning and preparation using vigorous irrigation (Fig. 10–2). Irrigation should be accomplished using several liters of isotonic saline or sterile water in conjunction with surgical soap solution applied with a brush or sponge. The use of the water jet lavage is extremely helpful in the debridement of wounds containing particles of foreign matter that may be overlooked on visual inspection of the wound. If debris is permitted to remain in the tissues, a permanent tattoo will result. This is difficult to eradicate at a later procedure and may complicate reconstruction. A minimum of 15 to 30 minutes should be devoted to wound preparation.

Soft Tissue

Timing is extremely important in management of soft tissue wounds of the face. Primary closure of these wounds is best accomplished within the first 24 hours following injury for optimum results with minimal scar formation. The facial area has a remarkably good blood supply that allows for primary closure of these wounds. Thorough but conservative debridement, hemostasis, careful tissue handling, and meticulous closure of tissues in layers to as normal a position as possible will afford the best results. Most wounds contain some devitalized tissue. Conservative wound margin trimming, in conjunction with undermining and plastic modification of laceration lines, will usually permit primary closure.

Violation of oral and mucous membrane must be corrected by suturing techniques that permit primary closure of the oral mucosa and by providing a water-tight seal to the oral cavity. A monofilament suture material that prevents submucosal penetration of the contaminated oral fluids should be used.

Avulsive wounds in the perioral region with tissue deficiencies should be managed by suturing the mucous membrane to the skin in preparation for later reconstruction. This permits primary healing and prevents the development of excessive scarring. Areas of avulsed cutaneous tissues should be covered by a medicated, moist dressing in preparation for future coverage by graft or flap.

Bone

Conservative management of fragments of bone is extremely important in comminuted and avulsed injuries. Soft tissue attachment to bony fragments must not be stripped away in an attempt to accomplish fixation by internal wiring or plating. Often these fragments can be molded into position and maintained by a proper soft tissue closure

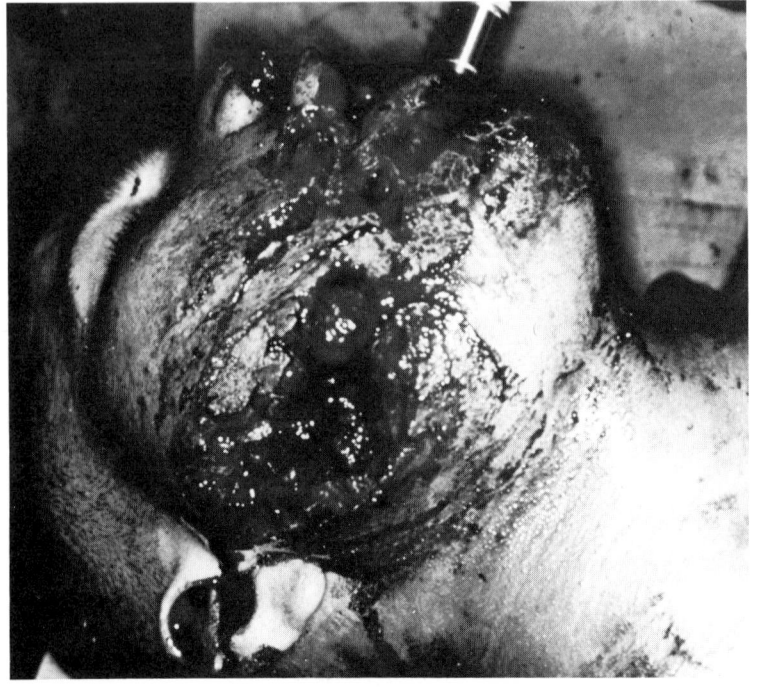

Figure 10–2. Massive through-and-through missile wound with gross contamination.

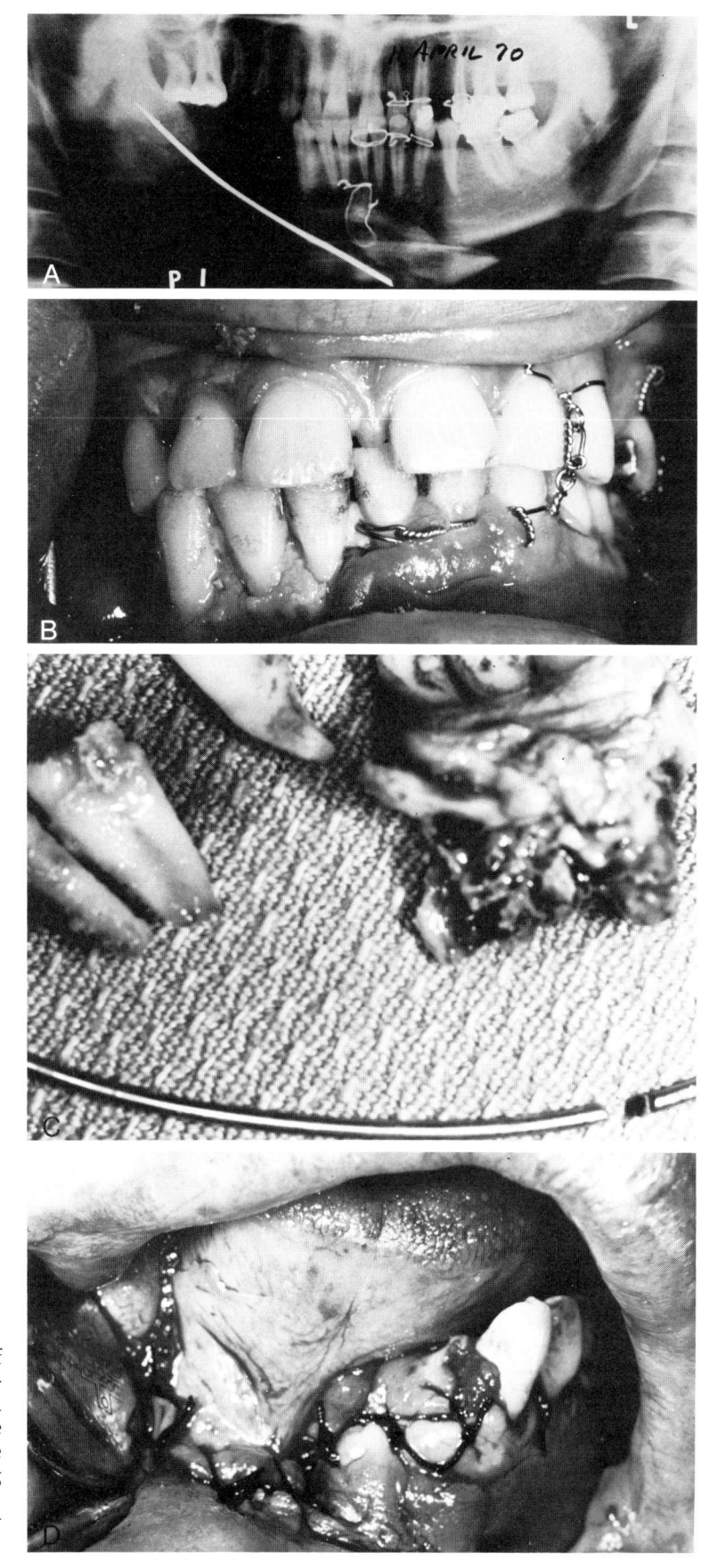

Figure 10–3. *A,* Continuity wound of the mandible with Steinmann pin distracting fragments. *B,* Retained teeth and necrotic bone resulting from inadequate debridement. *C,* Teeth, necrotic bone fragments, and Steinmann pin following sequestrectomy three weeks after injury. *D,* Primary closure following secondary debridement.

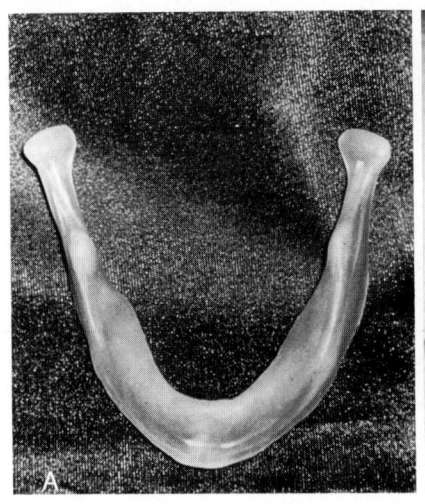

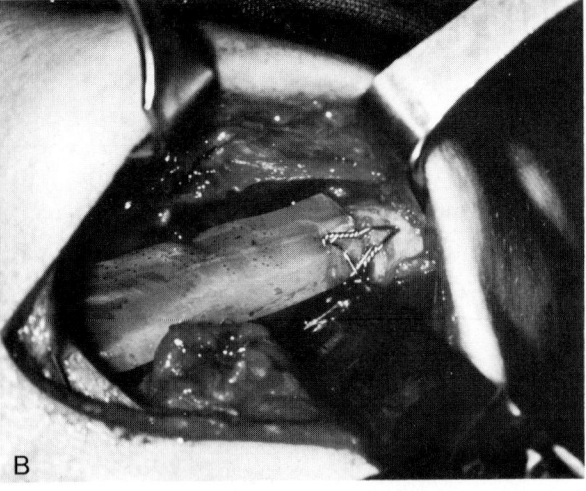

Figure 10–4. *A,* Prefabricated Silastic mandible. *B,* A segment of Silastic mandible used to preserve the soft tissue bed and prevent collapse of mandibular fragments.

and major fragment stabilization. Bone fragments can be stabilized in most cases with the use of maxillomandibular fixation.

Overzealous use of embedded metallic and acrylic devices for transosseous fixation or maintenance of intrabony space will cause wound breakdown, infection, and osseous sequestration (Fig. 10–3). If internal fixation is used, it should be simple and small and not compromise the blood supply to the fragments.[2] Prefabricated Silastic mandibles adapted to fit the osseous defect have been used successfully to maintain space and facial contour in selected cases. They are well-tolerated, preserve a well-formed recipient soft tissue bed, and prevent collapse and distortion of surrounding structures[3] (Fig. 10–4).

Biphasic extraskeletal pin fixation can be used to stabilize unsupported fragments of bone and provides proper alignment of the fragments in avulsive injuries. This appliance is applicable in a variety of locations and situations. It furnishes long-term stability and restores functional and cosmetic anatomy.

Intra-oral

Injuries of the oral structures may vary in severity from lacerations of the oral mucosa and lips to avulsive wounds of the palate, alveolar process, and floor of the mouth. In extensive injuries involving oral cutaneous cummunication, a water-tight mucosal closure is imperative (Fig. 10–5). Prior to soft tissue closure, all fractured teeth that cannot be salvaged or used for immobilization should be removed to reduce the incidence of infection and wound breakdown with fracture nonunion. Teeth should not be removed if it means sacrificing large segments of alveolar bone. Wounds in the floor of the mouth often involve fractures of the mandible with exposed bone and lacerations of the floor of the mouth and tongue. Hemorrhage, edema, and potential airway obstruction are significant problems in these cases. Patients may require a tracheostomy to ensure a patent airway. Lacerations of the tongue should be closed in layers, making every effort to identify and remove fragments of teeth or bone that may be lodged in the tongue.

In avulsive injuries of the palate, an effort should be made to mobilize the remaining palatal mucosa and suture it to the buccal or alveolar mucosa. If there is insufficient tissue for coverage of a palatal defect, an acrylic splint should be fabricated to cover the defect and permit as much granulation of mucosa as possible. Definitive repair should be planned at a later date and may consist of multiple procedures.

Figure 10–5. Primary debridement and water-tight repair of oral mucosa.

Importance of proper early intra-oral care cannot be overemphasized. Breakdown of the oral mucosa in oral cutaneous wounds will almost surely result in an oral cutaneous fistula. Success is dependent on the correct placement of the proper suture material. Gut suture material should be avoided because it does not remain securely tied for a sufficient time.

Drains

Many injuries about the face will require drainage of remaining dead spaces to minimize hematoma formation. Wounds involving only the cheeks, lips, or upper face should be closed in a manner that eliminates all dead spaces. In such cases, drains are not required; however, wounds involving the floor of the mouth, base of the tongue, retromandibular area, infratemporal fossa, and neck will universally have some dead spaces involved and require drainage. Proper placement of a drain is most important with wounds involving the mandible and loss of osseous structure and involvement of the oral cavity. After closure of the oral mucosa, the periosteum should be closed into and over the space occupied by the mandible. A Penrose drain should be placed superficial to the periosteal repair. There is a tendency for breakdown of the tissues with formation of an oral cutaneous fistula if the drain is placed to bone.

INTERMEDIATE CARE

Intermediate care encompasses a variable time span, and the status of the patient relative to future treatment needs is of utmost importance during this phase. Treatment accomplished in the early phase should be reviewed and evaluated and major modifications instituted only if initial efforts are obviously unsuccessful. Additional diagnostic and planning procedures may be necessary at this time, including impressions of the dental arches.

Airway adequacy should be assessed and a decision made concerning the retention of a tracheostomy tube. This is dependent on the future surgical needs of the patient and his ability to handle secretions and diet with the jaws in fixation.

If immobilization of facial fractures was not performed during the early phase, it should be accomplished at this time. If fractures are not immobilized as early as possible, movement of fragments interrupts soft tissue healing, prevents closure of the mouth, and leads to dehydration of the oral tissues. Intra-oral splints may also be used in the definitive reduction and fixation of fracture segments. In edentulous patients, or those with badly comminuted fractures, consideration should be given to the application of biphasic external pin fixation if it was not accomplished in the early treatment phase.

Proper wound care during the intermediate phase is extremely important but is often overlooked. Examples are suture and drain removal, dressing change, irrigations, oral hygiene, and professional observation of the wound status.

Review of the antibiotic program is a necessity. Resistant organisms can develop at this stage and establish chronic soft and hard tissue infections that are extremely difficult to eradicate. When there is drainage, therapy should be reviewed and revised on the basis of culture and sensitivity testing. In addition, it may be necessary to remove fractured or infected teeth, debride necrotic bone or soft tissue, or perform incision and drainage with irrigation of deep necrotic wounds. Antibiotic therapy cannot be effective to alter the course of infection in the absence of correct local wound care.

The general supportive care of the patient during this phase is of the utmost importance. A well-balanced, high-calorie liquid diet with adequate intake should be taken as soon as possible. Oral hygiene care must be emphasized to both the patient and the nursing personnel. The goal of treatment activities during the intermediate phase should be one of coordination as opposed to definitive treatment.

RECONSTRUCTIVE CARE

The late or reconstructive stage of treatment will involve those patients who have a residual defect or have developed some complication in treatment. Both hard and soft tissue management must be included in reconstructive planning. If a continuity defect of bone exists, preparation should be made for bone grafting at the earliest practical time. Sufficient soft tissue is necessary to provide coverage of deficient areas, provide adequate soft tissue for reception of osseous grafts, and restore continuity of the oral structures. The remaining dentition requires optimal maintenance. It will be used to provide an additional source of stabilization during reconstruction and to support the final prosthesis.

Bone Grafting

Functions of a Bone Graft

Restoration of a traumatically avulsed mandible has been a major clinical concern for surgeons for many years. The mandible is the most difficult of the facial bones to reconstruct surgically. A successful bone graft to the mandible should serve the following functions:

Restore Normal Continuity and Function. The restoration of continuity of the mandible provides the patient with the functions of eating, swallowing, and improved speech. The patient can then be restored to nearly normal masticatory function utilizing the remaining dentition or an indicated prosthesis.

Restore an Overall Satisfactory Appearance to the Face. A continuity defect of the mandible results in jaw deviation with considerable facial asymmetry. Restoration of that continuity also restores the patient's self-image and allows him to become a functioning member of society again.

Form Allostructural Framework for Immobilization and Weld Donor Tissue to the Host Bed. The graft or its support system should provide sufficient immobilization for successful regeneration. Movement at the host-graft interface may occur owing to lack of adequate fixation and immobilization; the result will be nonunion.

Furnish a Source of Viable Osteogenic Cells. This is necessary to provide and maintain sufficient osseous content and bulk to the restoration. Contributions of both phases of bone regeneration are necessary to ensure adequate bulk and height of the mandible and alveolar ridge. Minimal resorption should take place to maintain adequate alveolar height and width for prosthetic rehabilitation.

Act as a Precursor for the Bone Induction Principle. The bone graft must provide a sufficient cellular matrix to induce the second phase of bone regeneration, thereby inducing bone production and maturation and remodeling of the graft.

Principles of Bone Grafting

Regardless of the type of bone graft system or the procedure selected, certain basic principles are applicable to all cases.[4]

State of Health and Nutrition. The patient's state of health should be optimized by attention to nutritional and systemic conditions before surgery. Improved healing and fewer postsurgical complications are benefits of adequate nutrition during the preoperative and postoperative periods. Dietary treatment is complicated in bone graft cases that require long periods of maxillomandibular fixation, thus compromising ingestion and mastication. It has been reported that approximately 150 gm of protein plus 3000 nonprotein calories should be provided daily during convalescence from surgery.[5] Therefore, it is extremely important that the patient be well-prepared prior to surgery.

Aseptic Technique. Every effort must be made to provide strict asepsis during grafting of a continuity defect of the mandible. The surgical approach should be extraoral to prevent contamination by the oral flora, which markedly increases the incidence of infection. Special attention should be given to the draping of the patient to further reduce the possibility of contamination from the oral cavity.

Graft Bed. The recipient tissue bed must consist of healthy tissue that is free of infection and scar tissue that has a good blood supply. Scar tissue from previous wounds should be excised whenever possible to ensure that the quality and quantity of the recipient tissue are adequate. The submandibular incision should be placed as low as possible in the neck. It will move superiorly owing to the increased contour of the face as a result of the graft. The incision should be undermined on the surface of the platysma muscle and the dissection carried out to the level of the fascia over the digastric muscles. The dissection should then proceed to expose the ends of the proximal and distal mandibular segments. The tissue between the segments is then dissected carefully to prevent oral perforation. Scar tissue due to previous trauma may make this difficult. It may be helpful to have an assistant reach under the drape and into the mouth to place a finger in the edentulous area. Every effort should be made to dissect the tissue as close to the oral mucosa as possible to allow for restoration of the alveolar bone height.

Handling of the Graft. The graft must be handled carefully to prevent contamination and mechanical injury. Every effort should be made to place the graft into the recipient tissue as soon as possible after harvest. After the bone has been harvested, it should immediately be placed in saline solution[6] (see Fig. 10–7). Although antibiotic solutions are indicated with allogeneic bone, they should not be used for autogenous bone, since they may be cytotoxic to graft cells. If a corticocancellous graft is used, it should be decorticated and placed in apposition to well-vascularized cancellous host bone.

Fixation and Immobilization of the Graft. One of the major reasons for graft failure is improper fixation and immobilization. The graft is secured with transosseous wires placed in a mattress or figure-of-eight configuration (Fig. 10–6D and F). Maxillomandibular fixation should be utilized if the patient has remaining teeth. If there are no teeth proximal to the canine area on the side of the defect, a lingual splint should be fabricated with an extension arm engaging the maxillary teeth above the defect. This prevents torquing of the mandible with increased tension at the graft-host interfaces. Additional tension can be relieved by removing the coronoid process. This will also eliminate the temporalis influence on the proximal fragment. In edentulous patients, Gunning type splints should be utilized. Extraskeletal pin fixation may be used to supplement the immobilization and in rare cases may provide the only immobilization.

Wound Closure. The wound should be closed carefully in layers without tension (Fig. 10–6F). Special effort should be made to eliminate any dead space to prevent hematoma formation around the graft. If the deep tissues are inadequate to cover the graft, they should be sutured to the graft or to a crib supporting the graft. The layers of tissue that were established during the initial dissection should be carefully reapproximated. If necessary, additional undermining is done to eliminate all tension. The wound should be drained through a dependent stab incision (Fig. 10–6G). A drain should be placed superficial to the soft tissue over the graft but not in direct contact with the graft.

Antibiotics. Systemic antibiotics are utilized for all bone grafts. Penicillin is the first choice, although the cephalosporins have also proven to be effective. Intravenous antibiotics are started the morning of surgery with 4 million units of penicillin every four hours and continued for seven days unless an infection develops.

Restoration of Function. The ultimate objective of bone grafting continuity defects of the mandible is the restoration of function. Every effort must be made to provide an environment that will restore the normal functions of mastication, speaking, and swallowing with the natural dentition or a satisfactory prosthesis.

Methods of Mandibular Reconstruction

Autogenous bone has been used extensively for years in the restoration of continuity defects, bone cavities, contour defects, and disarticulation defects of the mandible. It has the advantage of being readily obtainable from a number of sources in the body. The iliac crest is an excellent source of autogenous bone, and various shapes of corticocancellous grafts can be obtained in solid or particulate form. Autogenous hematopoietic marrow and autogenous cancellous bone containing marrow appear to be the only types of bone graft material that are capable of actively inducing osteogenesis. Boyne[7–9] was instrumental in developing a technique using autogenous particulate cancellous bone and marrow. A large portion of the graft remains viable and stimulates osteogenesis. It also leads to bony proliferation and rapid union. The graft material is supported by a metallic crib that provides form and structural support for the graft and stability to the mandibular fragments. The metallic crib may be precast or formed at surgery from commercially available panels. However, the metal framework can be difficult to fabricate and adjust during surgery and may have to be removed after the graft is healed.

Resected ribs are another source of bone, although there is less hematopoietic marrow in rib bone than in the iliac crest. Ribs usually regenerate within approximately six months and may be useful in augmentation cases of the alveolar ridge and temporomandibular joint, in arthroplasties, and in young children.

In recent years, researchers have attempted to provide an allogeneic bone implant that is equal to or possibly even superior to fresh autogenous bone for use in the repair of large defects. Urist and associates[10–12] reported that a specially prepared decalcified or surface decalcified allogeneic bone or dentin would induce differentiation of mesenchymal cells into osteoblasts followed by the stimulation of the cells to form new bone. Surface decalcified allogeneic bone was used by others[3, 4, 13–15] in combination with particulate autogenous cancellous bone and marrow for successful restoration of continuity defects of the mandible. Originally the lyophilized allogeneic bone was exposed to small doses of Co-60 gamma radiation and surface decalcification to reduce antigenicity and facilitate storage for an extended period of time. It has since been shown that surface decalcification is unnecessary.

Current Graft Systems

At the present time there are three graft systems indicated for reconstruction of the

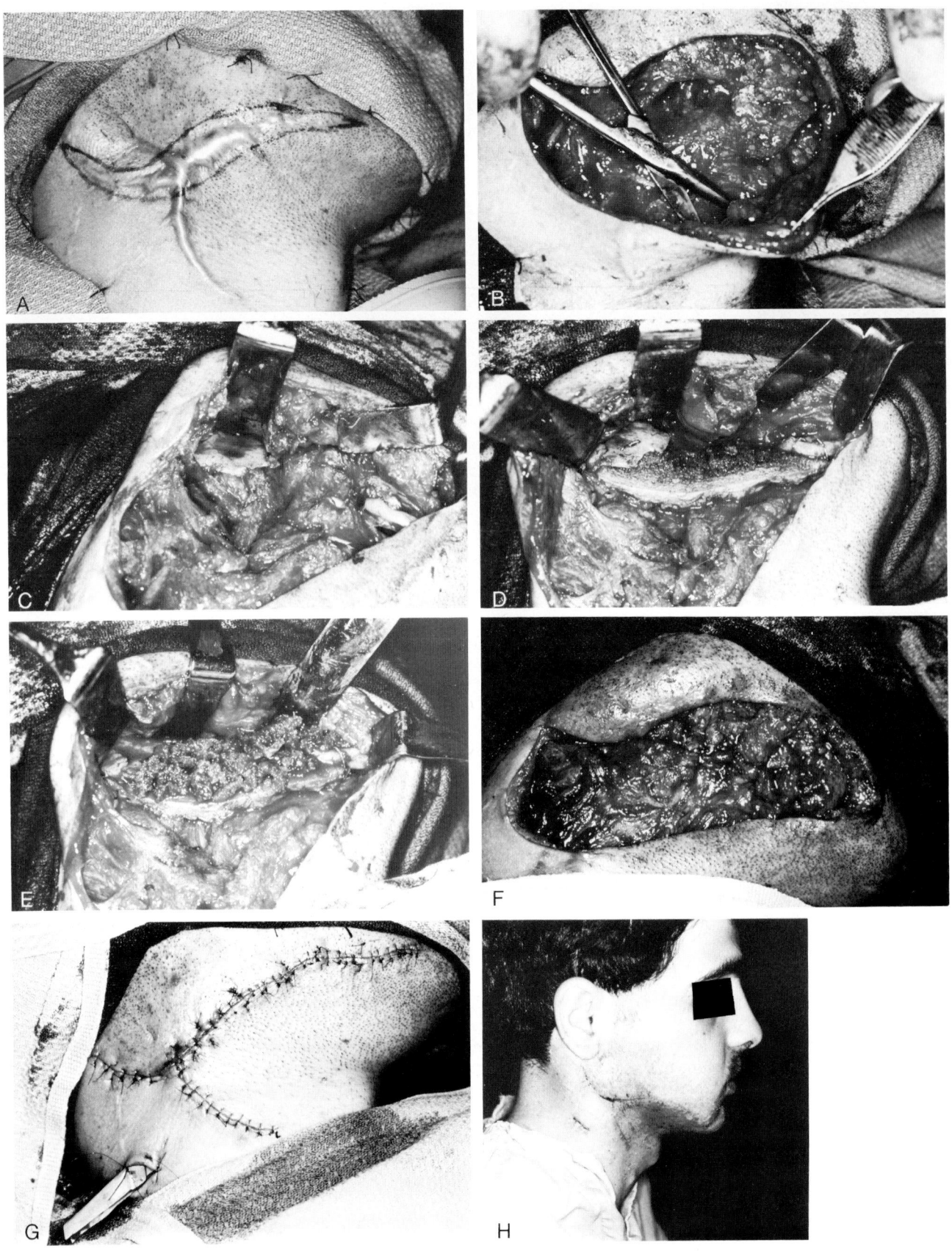

Figure 10–6. *A*, Scar tissue from previous wound outlined for excision. *B*, Generous undermining and establishment of soft tissue planes. *C*, Development of the soft tissue bed with exposure of proximal and distal bone. *D*, Corticocancellous solid graft secured on lingual aspect. *E*, Additional particulate cancellous bone and marrow packed in the defect. *F*, Layer closure eliminating dead space. *G*, Final closure with drain placed in dependent area. *H*, Improved facial contour one week after surgery.

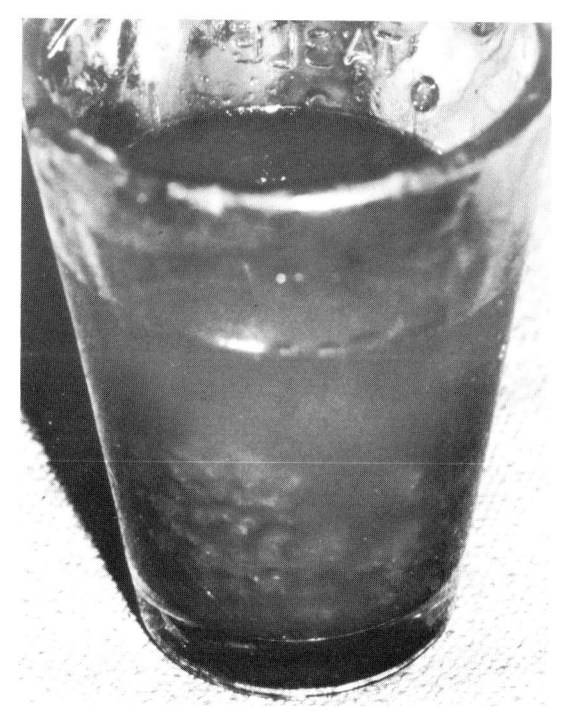

RECONSTRUCTIVE SURGERY FOR MAXILLOFACIAL INJURIES / 437

Figure 10–7. Autogenous particulate cancellous bone and marrow from iliac crest in saline solution.

trauma-induced continuity defect of the mandible. These include solid corticocancellous grafts using iliac crest or rib, particulate cancellous bone and marrow within alloplastic cribs, particulate cancellous bone, and marrow grafts within allogeneic bone cribs. In addition, two other systems should be mentioned, although indications for their use in the traumatized patient are limited; these are the osteomyocutaneous grafts and microvascular bone periosteal grafts.

All of the graft systems have advantages and disadvantages, both physiologically and technically. Each patient should be evaluated to ensure utilization of the system that will offer the best chance of success.

Solid Autogenous Corticocancellous Graft

The success of any graft system depends on careful planning followed by meticulous attention to detail during the surgical procedure. This is particularly true of the solid corticocancellous graft. If managed properly, this graft system is extremely dependable and will satisfy all of the principles outlined previously. The anterior portion of the iliac crest provides the best source for the solid graft, and its use is usually limited to defects of 6 cm or less.

The graft should be taken from either the lateral or medial aspect of the ilium, avoiding a through-and-through defect. Generally, use of the lateral aspect is less traumatic to the patient and reduces the postoperative morbidity (Fig. 10–8). The graft should be placed on the medial aspect of the mandible with approximately 1.5- to 2-cm overlap to allow for morticing of the graft to the proximal and distal segments (Fig. 10–9). The medial surfaces of the host segments should be contoured to permit close apposition at the interface and provide a bleeding surface. Immobilization by fixation of the graft to the segments is critical. This should be accomplished with through-and-through mattress wires or figure-of-eight wires to provide complete immobilization. Once the graft is secured, additional particulate cancellous bone and marrow should be packed over the lateral aspect of the graft, particularly at the interface areas. This step is critical to the success of the solid graft. If additional particulate bone is not provided, there will be few endosteal osteoblasts and marrow mesenchymal cells; therefore, phase one regeneration is almost absent. Wound closure is completed as previously described.

The autogenous rib graft is another form of solid graft that may be used in certain cases requiring a particular shape or additional length of the graft. Indications for the use of a solid rib graft are very limited because the graft resorbs rapidly with very little satisfactory bone replacement. If ribs are used, consideration should be given to splitting and combining them with other sections of rib or particulate cancellous bone and marrow from the ilium.

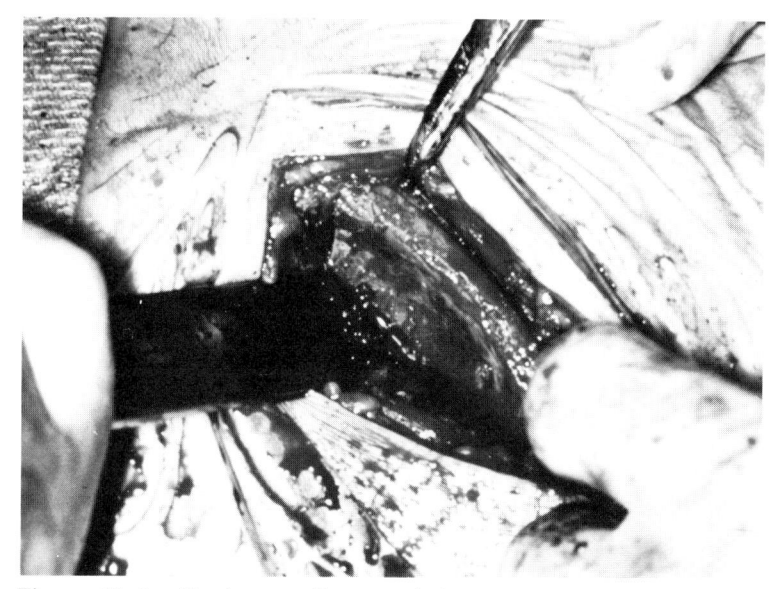

Figure 10–8. Corticocancellous graft harvested from lateral aspect of ilium.

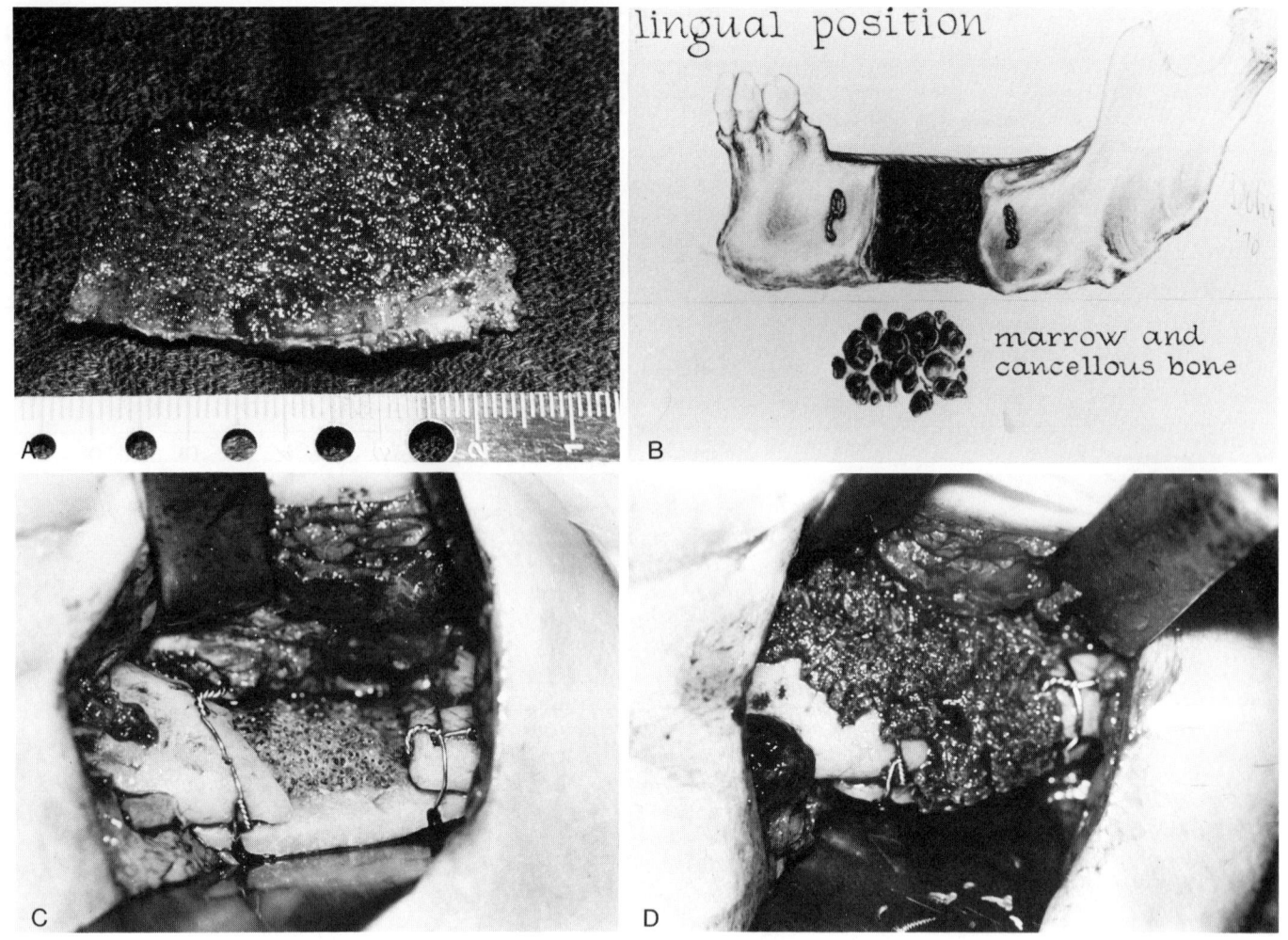

Figure 10–9. *A,* Corticocancellous solid iliac crest graft prior to contouring. *B* to *D,* Placement of the graft on the lingual aspect of the mandible, secured with direct wires, then packed with additional particulate cancellous bone and marrow.

Particulate Cancellous Bone and Marrow Grafts Within Alloplastic Cribs

This graft system is extremely adaptable and provides an excellent method for reconstruction of traumatic defects of the mandible. Since the graft consists of only particulate bone and cancellous marrow, there are many osteoblasts and mesenchymal cells that survive transplantation. Revascularization takes place rapidly without the interference of large cortical areas that must be resorbed.

The primary disadvantage of this system is the lack of allostructural support within the graft. Therefore, some type of alloplastic crib is necessary to hold and support the particulate cancellous bone and marrow. Various types of chrome cobalt alloy cribs have been advocated, including a cast Vitallium mesh crib with adaptable wrought segments at each end for attachment to the host fragments (Fig. 10–10). Boyne later advocated the use of preformed titanium trays.[9] The cribs provide support for the bone and final form and shape of the graft. The cribs adapt well to the various contours of the mandible and can be fabricated to any length. Except in rare instances, they should not provide the sole method of immobilization of the graft and should be used in conjunction with maxillomandibular fixation or extraskeletal fixation.

A major disadvantage of the metallic crib is that it is often necessary to remove the crib prior to prosthetic rehabilitation of the patient. It is seldom possible to reconstruct the soft tissues of the oral cavity with the crib in place. In some instances, areas deficient in bone were noted when the crib was removed and some surgeons have reported total loss of bone in certain areas of the crib.

In recent years a Dacron/urethane tray has been developed.[16] These are semirigid, lightweight, porous, and radiolucent and can be shaped with scissors at the time of surgery. The trays are biocompatible and can be autoclaved for sterilization; however, they still may interfere with the placement of a prosthesis and require removal at a later date.[17]

Particulate Cancellous Bone and Marrow in Allogeneic Cribs

Cribs of allogeneic bone offer many advantages over the alloplastic cribs. Allogeneic bone is completely biocompatible and is well-incorporated into the surrounding tissue. Since cells of lyophilized bone do not survive, the function of the allogeneic bone in the osteogenic process is purely passive. No active osteogenic stimulation occurs, but new bone from the host grows over the absorbable surfaces of the graft. The active portion of the process, or phase one of regeneration, is stimulated by the particulate cancellous bone and marrow contained in the allogeneic crib. Allogeneic bone is also biodegradable, and the cribs will undergo complete resorption and replacement over an extended period of time.

The allogeneic bone crib has the added advantage of being easily manipulated and contoured. The allogeneic bone acts only as a crib and can be thinned and shaped to permit insertion of additional particulate cancellous bone and marrow. The allogeneic bone is adaptable and can be used in a number of different forms.

Allogeneic Mandibles. The ideal crib for mandibular reconstruction is the allogeneic mandible.[3] This is particularly true in cases

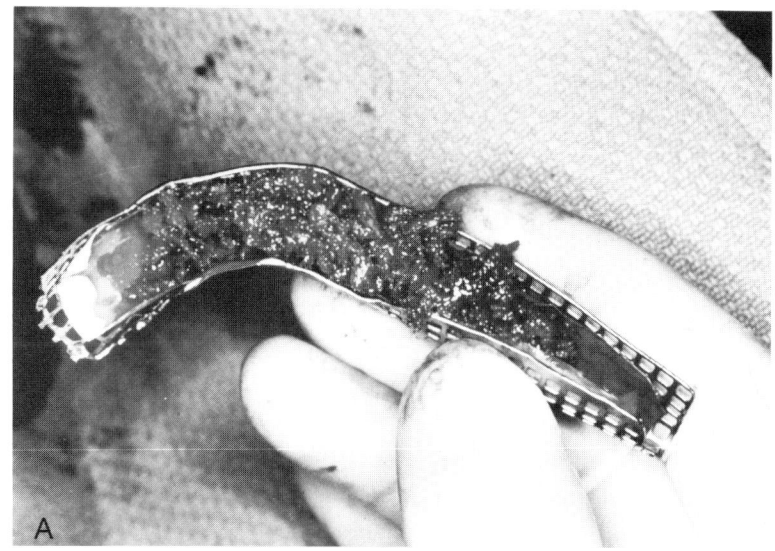

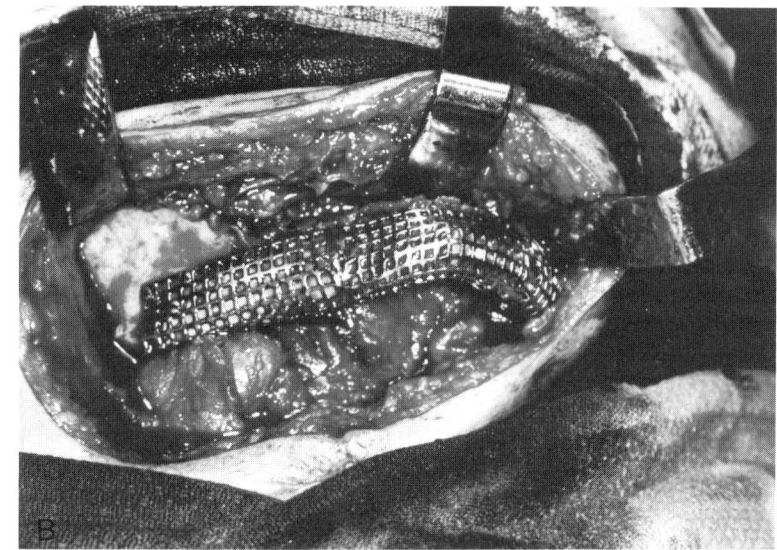

Figure 10–10. *A,* Cast Vitallium crib with adaptable wrought segments at each end contoured to replace the symphysis. *B,* Crib secured to bone segments and packed with particulate cancellous bone and marrow. *C* and *D,* Restoration of the normal contour of the mandible with the crib.

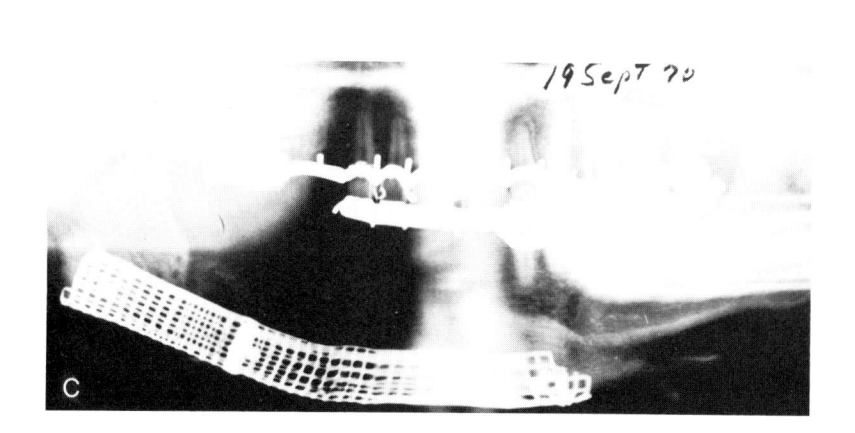

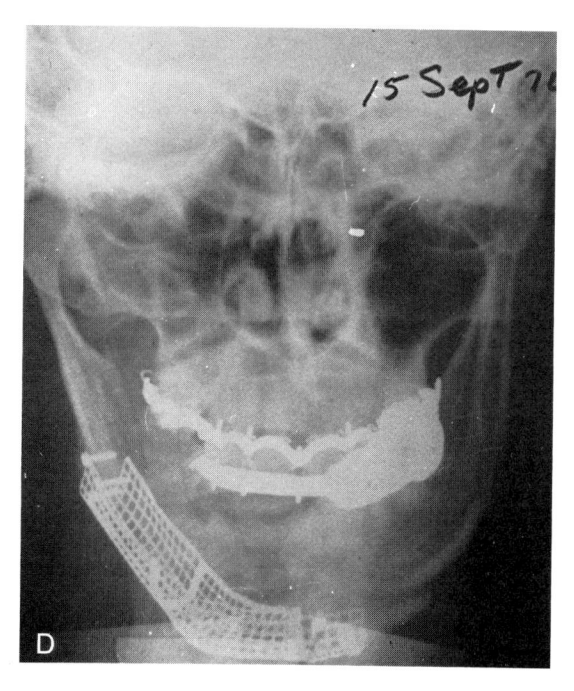

involving restoration of the angle or symphysis, or both. When replacing a condyle, the allogeneic condyle should be reduced in size and covered with an alloplastic material. An alternative is the insertion of an alloplastic fossa implant to ensure free movement of the condyle after the period of fixation. The coronoid process should be removed from the graft and the alveolar height reduced to eliminate excessive tension of the oral mucosa over the graft. The mandible is hollowed out and packed tightly with autogenous particulate cancellous bone and marrow. It should be adapted to the host segment or segments overlapping on the lingual side, if possible. The graft should then be securely wired to the end of the segment to complete the immobilization (Fig. 10–11).

The biggest disadvantage of using allogeneic mandibles as cribs is the difficulty in obtaining them. Although all allogeneic bone is somewhat difficult to obtain, this is particularly true of mandibles, and an alternative choice must therefore be available.

Allogeneic Split Rib Segments. At the present time, allogeneic ribs are the least expensive tissue specimens and the most readily available from tissue banks. Many ribs are thin and friable and not very flexible. If they are split, however, they can be contoured to restore the normal curvature of the mandible. The split halves are measured to allow for overlap at the host segments and secured with wire to the medial and lateral aspects of the segments, forming two sides of a box. Particulate cancellous bone and marrow are then packed between the split halves of allogeneic rib against the soft tissue recipient bed in the superior and inferior aspects. A variation of this technique is made possible by rotating the split ribs 90 degrees to form the inferior and superior surfaces. This modification is particularly useful in the restoration of the angle of the mandible. Both techniques allow for extensive packing of the particulate cancellous bone and marrow.

Costochondral Rib Grafts. In those situations in which it is necessary to replace the condyle, the technique is modified to include the use of an autogenous costochondral rib graft.[18] The cartilage is trimmed to fit the condylar fossa, leaving a 3- to 5-mm cap of cartilage to prevent bony union and form a pseudarthrosis. The solid rib is rotated, with the flat surface forming the angle and lower border of the mandible. In this position, the greatest width of the autogenous rib lies in a mediolateral position. The bulk of the graft can then be made up by using a split allogeneic rib for the superior margin, with autogenous particulate cancellous bone and marrow packed between the two. An alternative to this utilizes a second autogenous rib. It is decorticated and segmented and secured to the costochondral graft to add bulk and viable cells. This has the advantage of avoiding a third operative site at the iliac crest; however, there is increased resorption of the graft with this variation (Fig. 10–12).

Allogeneic Ilia. The crest of the ilium has been used for many years for mandibular reconstruction. There is a striking contour sim-

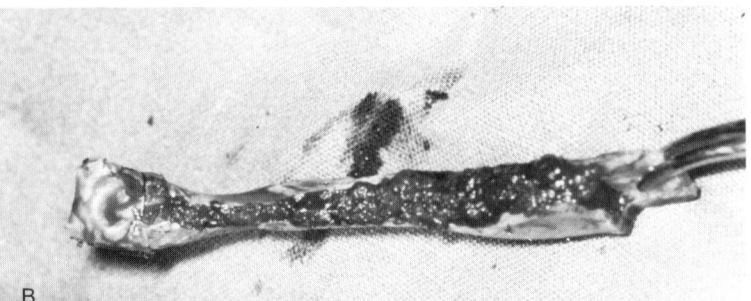

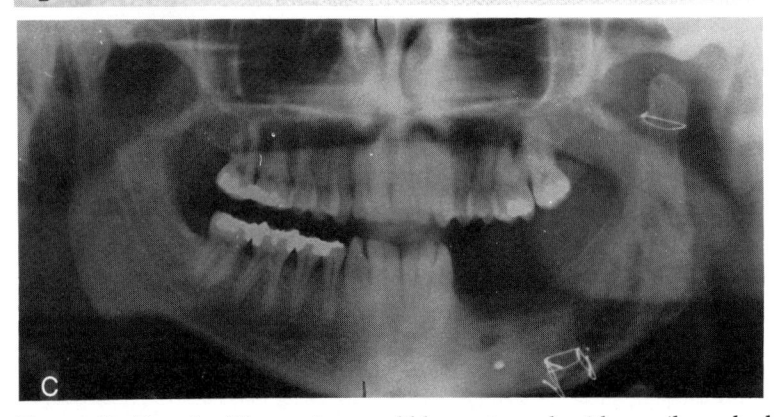

Figure 10–11. *A*, Allogeneic mandible contoured with a crib packed with particulate cancellous bone and marrow. *B*, Occlusal view of composite graft packed with particulate cancellous bone and marrow contoured for immobilization on the lingual aspect of the hooded fragment. The condyle is covered with thin Silastic. *C*, Composite graft in place one year after insertion; minimal resorption is evident.

ilarity between a hemimandible and the ipsilateral iliac crest. A solid graft has been used for reconstruction of the hemimandible. Many of these grafts exhibited extensive resorption, and the donor site morbidity was unacceptable. This same concept can be applied, however, using allogeneic bone iliac crest that can be contoured to form a crib. The crib can then be thinned, shaped, and secured to the segments of the mandible and packed with particulate cancellous bone and marrow. Since ilia are available in most tissue banks, this tissue appears to be a practical alternate to the allogeneic mandible.

Osteomyocutaneous Grafts

The other techniques that have been advocated for mandibular reconstruction are primarily indicated for patients who have had radiation therapy. Osteomyocutaneous grafts consist of bone on a vascular pedicle with its own soft tissue.[19-22] With this concept, viable osteocytes are transplanted, and the blood supply is maintained to the segment of bone. Grafts that have been advocated include one consisting of a segment of rib, pectoralis major muscle, and overlying skin.[23, 24] The rib is usually the sixth or seventh. Another type of osteomyocutaneous graft utilizes the medial third of the clavicle with the sternocleidomastoid muscle attachment pedicled off the origin of the muscle at the mastoid process.[25] Theoretically, the graft should heal as a fracture, although in both cases the bone may be inadequate in both length and bulk. The morbidity of both procedures is considerable and, at this time, there is very limited practical application for the restoration of mandibular defects secondary to trauma with osteomyocutaneous grafts.

Microvascular Anastomosis Grafts.

Another bone grafting method that has shown definite potential is the transfer of vascularized bone segments.[26-28] This technique would be useful in those patients with a poor blood supply to a heavily scarred tissue bed or in irradiated patients. Donoff and May[29] reported success in re-establishing periosteal blood flow in dogs, and in some humans, using vascularized rib grafts. The technique requires an intrathoracic harvest of the anterior and middle third of a rib with the anterior intercostal artery and draining vein. Recipient vessels are located in the neck, and the anastomosis is completed under the microscope between those and the vessels accompanying the rib graft. The bone graft is then positioned and immobi-

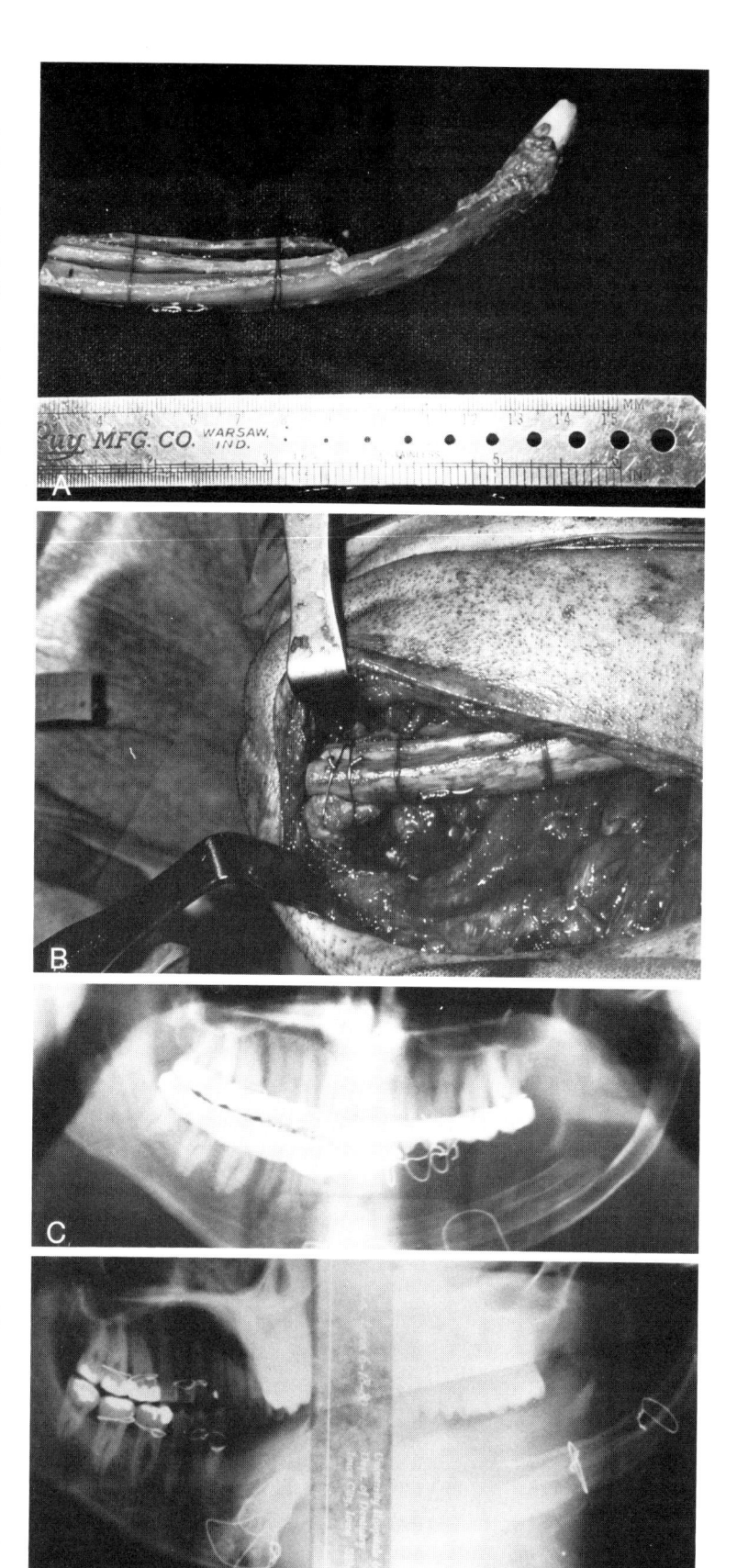

Figure 10–12. *A*, Autogenous ribs contoured to fit the mandible and restore the condyle with costochondral graft. *B*, Graft secured to remaining segment of mandible with direct wires. *C*, Graft in place restoring normal contour of mandible. *D*, Graft after five years with allogeneic bone augmentation to provide additional bulk and strength.

lized with transosseous wires. The blood supply appears to be adequate in most cases for the microvascular free transfer.

However, this grafting method is not without complications. Careful consideration should be given to its application. There have been cases reported of failure of the anastomosis resulting in loss of the graft. Since the rib harvest requires closed chest drainage, pleural effusions and pneumonias are a definite possibility. Other sources of free flaps containing bone have been reported but with varied success.[19] Even though free flaps survive completely, many cases have developed wound dehiscence, fistulization, or abscess formation several weeks to several months following repair.[30] The degree of morbidity and the marginal results reported fail to justify the use of this method in reconstruction of the traumatized patient.[16]

Reconstruction of the Maxilla

Reconstruction of the maxilla following traumatic injuries is far less common than that of the mandible. Most defects in the maxilla are restored successfully with a maxillofacial prosthesis. Avulsive wounds, such as those caused by missiles, may produce extensive scars or oral-nasal, and/or oral-antral communications. Each case must be evaluated individually to determine the best way to restore acceptable function and facial form to these deformities. In some cases, bone grafting is indicated and may involve restoration of the alveolar ridge or a portion of the maxilla.

Soft tissue repair, particularly of the intraoral areas, is extremely important. Whenever an oral-nasal or oral-antral fistula can be repaired to eliminate the need for an obturator, it should be accomplished (Fig. 10–13). However, the soft tissue loss should be evaluated carefully and if the communications are large, the patient may be better off with a well-designed obturator appliance. Soft tissue modifications in the form of vestibuloplasties may improve the extent and quality of the bony supporting denture base. In those patients who are edentulous with inadequate support and retention for an obturator, consideration should be given to utilizing the osseointegration system.[31, 32] This provides strategically located metal implants that can provide stability and retention to the prosthesis.

Complications of Bone Graft Reconstruction

When undertaking major reconstruction procedures of the maxillofacial area, it is important to appreciate the potential complications at the donor and recipient sites.[1, 17] Some complications are predictable and unavoidable, whereas others can be eliminated with careful planning and attention to detail. The reconstructive surgeon must realize the potential for their development and institute measures to avoid them.

Donor Site

Iliac Crest. The most common complication following harvest of a graft from the iliac crest is pain, particularly on ambulation. The degree of discomfort is directly associated with the trauma of the surgery and the amount of soft tissue reflection. A traumatic reflection of a bony flap, with periosteum and musculature attached, permits removal of particulate cancellous bone and marrow with a minimum of postoperative discomfort. A postoperative hematoma may develop, but in most cases it can be prevented by controlling bleeding with bone wax and drainage of the wound postoperatively. Infection occurs rarely and should be managed with antibiotic therapy, drainage, and frequent irrigations. A postoperative paralytic ileus may rarely occur secondary to a retroperitoneal hematoma. A temporary ileus may occur as a normal postoperative sequela.

Rib Resection. There is considerable postoperative morbidity with the harvesting of a rib graft. The patient routinely experiences pain, particularly with deep breathing, and there is a tendency toward restriction of lung expansion. The most common complication of rib resection is pneumothorax. If it occurs, it is treated with a chest tube and careful postoperative management.

Recipient Site

Infection in the recipient site is a major concern in the reconstruction of the traumatized patient. This is particularly true in considering the reconstruction of war wounds. When wound infection develops in the graft site of continuity defect cases, a large percentage result in failure of the graft.[6] Every effort must be made to eliminate those factors that contribute to developing infections. Adequate debridement of the bone segments or the recipient soft tissue bed should be accomplished before attempting a graft. A minimum of three months should have

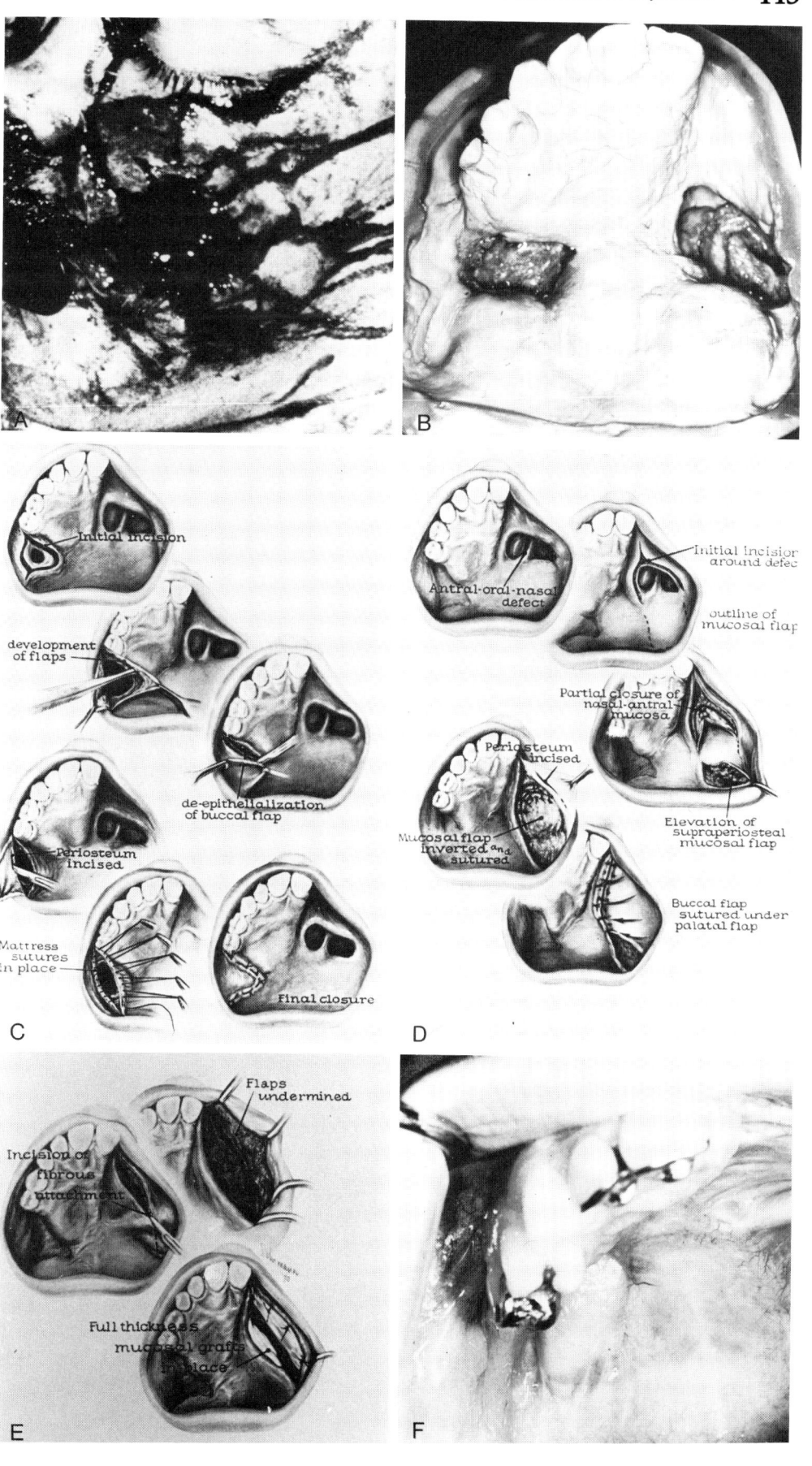

Figure 10–13. *A*, Through-and-through missile wound of the face with partial avulsion of the palate. *B*, Bilateral oral-nasal-antral communications of the palate requiring repair in stages. *C*, Stage 1 repair of the defect of the right palate using an envelope buccal flap. *D*, Stage 2 repair of defect of the left palate using double flaps to provide an epithelial surface for the nasal floor. *E*, Stage 3 sulcus extension with mucosal grafts to eliminate scar contracture prior to construction of a prosthesis. *F*, Completed restoration of the palate ready for insertion of the prosthesis. (From Laskin DM: Oral and Maxillofacial Surgery. Vol 3. St. Louis, CV Mosby Co, in press).

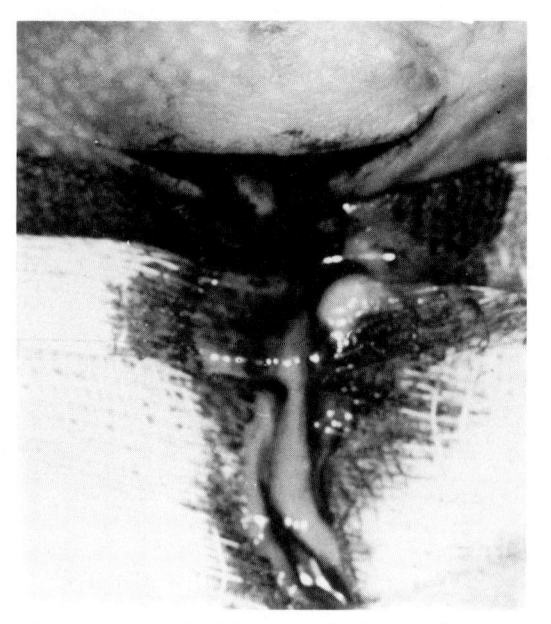

Figure 10–14. Incision and drainage of infection following graft to mandible.

elapsed after injury or after resolution of a postoperative infection. Nonvital teeth and foreign bodies should be removed from close proximity to the graft site.

As discussed previously, every effort should be made to prevent hematoma formation in and around the graft. The hematoma becomes a potential culture medium for bacteria, and its presence interferes with the early nutrition of the graft. The best method of prevention is the careful closure of the wound with the elimination of any dead space. If infection occurs then early aggressive management is necessary.

Perforation of the oral mucosa creates a significant complication. The wound is contaminated, markedly increasing the possibility of infection. Intra-oral perforation that is not recognized at the time of surgery or dehiscence that occurs later also creates postoperative problems. A perforation occurring at the time of surgery should be repaired carefully with a water-tight closure. If the perforation occurs in a particulate cancellous bone and marrow graft with a metallic crib, prognosis for retention of the crib is poor. In those cases in which adequate soft tissue flaps are not established and the tissues are under tension in the closure over the crib, dehiscence may occur. Treatment should consist of daily irrigations, with no attempt to close the soft tissues. Another disturbing complication is that of aseptic necrosis, which occurs without clinical signs of infection and may be associated with instability of the graft-host interface.

Soft Tissue Reconstruction

Reconstruction of soft tissue injury begins with initial management at the time of injury. Primary repair of soft tissue injuries is indicated in the early treatment phase whenever possible.[33] Wounds respond best when treated within a few hours of injury. Primary closure should be accomplished within the first 24 hours, although it may be longer, depending on the amount of contamination and the extent of the wound. Successful repair is the result of meticulous attention to detail utilizing a systemic treatment plan. Minimal careful treatment should be performed and anatomic relations restored to as normal a position as possible. In some cases, secondary repair and scar revision may be necessary during the intermediate and late treatment phases.

Extensive soft tissue injuries of the face with underlying osseous injury should not be repaired until reduction and fixation of the underlying facial fractures are accomplished. In compound fractures, treatment should be accomplished from the inside out and from the bottom up. Oral soft tissue wounds should be repaired prior to the application of maxillomandibular fixation or insertion of splints. The repositioning of bone fragments may be performed through the external wound, thereby anatomically forming a foundation for assembling the soft tissues. If definitive reduction of fractures cannot be accomplished early, temporary suturing of the principal parts should be accomplished. Definitive repair of soft tissue can then be completed after final reduction of the fractures.

Water-tight closure of the oral mucosa is a primary consideration during the initial treatment. This may result in considerable distortion of the oral structures, preventing normal function and interfering with the construction and wearing of a prosthesis. This principle should not be compromised, since there are several procedures to correct the deformity after successful restoration of the osseous defect.

Ridge Extension Procedures

Loss of soft tissue or scarring in the floor of the mouth may result in obliteration or distortion of the alveolar ridge. Augmentation of the ridge area will often be needed. Additionally, a variety of procedures have been described to provide ridge extension by lowering the floor of the mouth and by vestibuloplasty in either the maxilla or the mandi-

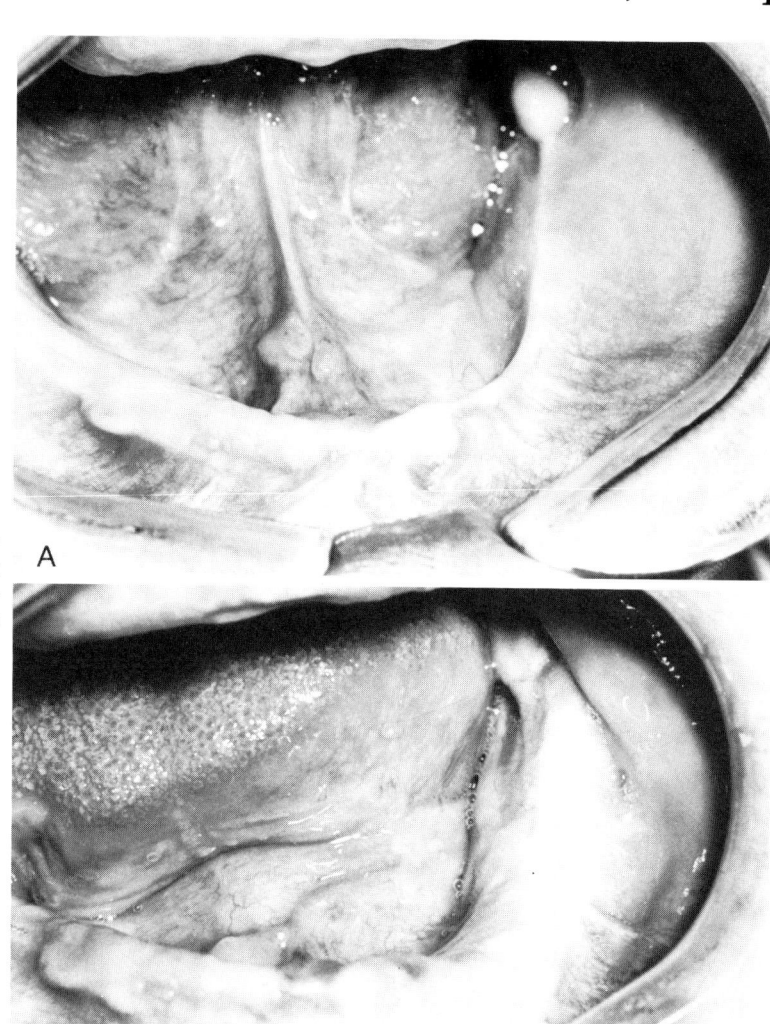

Figure 10–15. *A,* Unfavorable position of soft tissues in relation to grafted mandibular alveolar ridge. *B,* Mandibular ridge following vestibuloplasty with lowering of the floor of the mouth and mucosal grafting.

ble, utilizing skin or free mucosal grafts. Although these procedures were developed to aid the prosthodontist in incidences of advanced atrophy of the maxilla or mandible, they can be readily applied to treatment of avulsion wounds. A detailed discussion and description of these procedures are found elsewhere in this text.

SUMMARY

The majority of patients' maxillofacial injuries can be treated successfully with early definitive care; however, those patients with avulsive wounds of the soft tissue or bone may require long-term reconstructive surgery. The treatment must be predicated on thorough examination, organized planning, and continuing evaluation of the patient's status through the various stages of treatment. Certain factors stand out as significant influences in the success or failure of bone graft reconstruction.

Timing is important to reconstruction of an avulsed wound. The soft tissue and vascular damage present in injuries often extends far beyond the avulsive defect itself, and the wounds are usually contaminated. This results in prolonged healing and considerable scarring; therefore, it is essential to allow time for recovery of vascularity, ensure asepsis, and develop suppleness of the tissues prior to grafting.

It must be emphasized that attention to detail in the overall management of these patients must not be compromised. The basic principles of bone grafting outlined early in the chapter must be adhered to for consistently satisfactory results. Although we can look forward to the continued development of new materials and techniques in the future, increased success will continue to depend on the surgeon's adherence to these recognized principles.

BIBLIOGRAPHY

1. Adamo AK, and Szal RL: Timing, results and complications of mandibular reconstructive surgery: Report of 32 cases. J Oral Surg 37:755–763 1979.
2. Osbon DB: Facial trauma. In Irby WB (ed): Current Advances in Oral Surgery. St. Louis, CV Mosby Co, 1974, pp 214–241.
3. Osbon DB, Lilly GE, Thompson CW, and Jost T: Bone grafts with surface decalcified allogeneic and particulate autologous bone: Report of cases. J Oral Surg 35:276–284, 1977.
4. Osbon DB: Intermediate and reconstructive care of maxillofacial missile wounds. J Oral Surg 31:429–437, 1973.
5. Randall HT: Surgical nutrition: Parenteral and oral. In Kinney JM, Egdahl RH, and Zuidema GD (eds): Manual of Preoperative and Postoperative Care. Philadelphia, WB Saunders Co, 1971, pp 75–108.
6. Marx RE, Snyder RM, and Kline SN: Cellular survival of human marrow during placement of marrow-cancellous bone grafts. J Oral Surg 37:712–717, 1979.
7. Boyne PJ: Restoration of osseous defects in maxillofacial casualties. J Am Dent Assoc 78:767, 1969.
8. Boyne PJ: Autogenous cancellous bone and marrow transplants. Clin Orthop 73:199, 1970.
9. Boyne PJ: Tissue transplantations. In Kruger GO (ed): Textbook of Oral Surgery. 5th ed. St. Louis, CV Mosby Co, 1979, pp 286–309.
10. Urist MR: Bone formation by autoinduction. Science 150:893, 1965.
11. Urist MR, Silverman BF, Büring K, et al.: The bone induction principle. Clin Orthop 53:243, 1967.
12. Dubic FL, and Urist MR: Accessibility of the bone induction principle in surface decalcified bone implants. Clin Orthop 55:225, 1967.
13. Jones JC, Lilly GE, Hackett PB, and Osbon DB: Mandibular bone grafts with surface decalcified bone. J Oral Surg 30:269, 1972.
14. Pike RL, and Boyne PJ: Composite autogenous marrow and surface decalcified implants in mandibular defects. J Oral Surg 31:905, 1973.
15. Pike RL, and Boyne PJ: Use of surface-decalcified allogeneic bone and autogenous marrow in extensive mandibular defects. J Oral Surg 32:177, 1974.
16. Leake D, and Habal MB: Mandibular reconstruction and craniofacial fairing. Br J Oral Surg 16:198–206, 1979.
17. Kelly JF: Management of war injuries to the jaws and related structures. Washington DC, US Government Printing Office, 1977, pp 140–144.
18. MacIntosh RB, and Henny FA: A spectrum of application of autogenous costochondral grafts. J Maxillofac Surg 5:257–267, 1977.
19. Baker SR: Reconstruction of mandibular defects with the revascularized free tensor fascia lata osteomyocutaneous flap. Arch Otolaryngol 107:414–418, 1981.
20. Cuono CB, and Ariyan S: Immediate reconstruction of a composite mandibular defect with a regional osteomusculocutaneous flap. Plast Reconstr Surg 65:477–484, 1980.
21. Panje W, and Cutting C: Trapezius osteomyocutaneous island flap for reconstruction of the anterior floor of the mouth and the mandible. Head Neck Surg 3:66–71, 1980.
22. Green MF, Gibson JR, Bryson JR, and Thomson E: A one-stage correction of mandibular defects using a split sternum pectoralis major osteomusculocutaneous transfer. Br J Plast Surg 34:11–16, 1981.
23. Ariyan S: The viability of rib grafts transplanted with the periosteal blood supply. Plast Reconstr Surg 65:40–51, 1980.
24. Bell MS, and Barron PT: The rib-pectoralis major osteomyocutaneous flap. Ann Plast Surg 6:347–353, 1981.
25. Barnes DR, Ossoff RH, Pecaro B, and Sisson GA: Immediate reconstruction of mandibular defects with a composite sternocleidomastoid musculoclavicular graft. Arch Otolaryngol 107:711–714, 1981.
26. McKee DM: Microvascular bone transplantation. Clin Plast Surg 5:283–292, 1978.
27. Salibian AH, Rappaport I, Furnas DW, and Achauer BM: Microvascular reconstruction of the mandible. Am J Surg 140:499–502, 1980.
28. Panje WR: Free compound groin flap reconstruction of anterior mandibular defect. Arch Otolaryngol 107:17–22, 1981.
29. Donoff RB, and May JW: Microvascular mandibular reconstruction. J Oral Maxillofac Surg 40:122–126, 1982.
30. Serafin D, Riefkohl R, Thomas I, and Georgiade NG: Vascularized rib-periosteal and osteocutaneous reconstruction of the maxilla and mandible: An assessment. Plast Reconstr Surg 66:718–727, 1980.
31. Branemark PI, Hansson BO, Adell R, Breine U, Lindstrom J, Hallen O, and Ohman A: Osseointegrated implants in the treatment of the edentulous jaw. Experience from a 10-year period. Scand J Plast Reconstr Surg 16:1–132, 1977.
32. Breine U, and Branemark PI: Reconstruction of alveolar jaw bone. An experimental and clinical study of immediate and preformed autologous bone grafts in combination with osseointegrated implants. Scand J Plast Reconstr Surg 14:23–48, 1980.
33. Marx RE, Kline SN, Johnson RP, Malinin TI, Mathews JG, and Gambill V: The use of freeze-dried allogeneic bone in oral and maxillofacial surgery. J Oral Surg 39:264–274, 1981.

11

RECONSTRUCTIVE SURGERY FOR THE PATIENT WITH FACIAL CLEFTS

*Deborah Zeitler, D.D.S., M.S.,
Raymond J. Fonseca, D.M.D.,
James B. Troxell, D.D.S., M.S.,
and William LaVelle, D.D.S., M.S.*

The patient with facial clefting presents many surgical and prosthodontic challenges. Treatment of these patients requires coordinated long-term efforts among many health professionals. The goal of the surgical and prosthodontic treatment of patients with clefts is to provide for normal function and esthetic appearance. The treatment may involve fixed or removable prosthodontics, vestibuloplasty, alveolar cleft grafting, or orthognathic surgery. It is important to consider the proper sequencing of therapy in order to achieve the optimum result.

LITERATURE REVIEW

INCIDENCE OF CLEFT LIP AND PALATE

Clefts of the orofacial structures are among the most common of all congenital malformations, occurring in approximately one of 800 births. There have been many epidemiologic studies analyzing the incidence of cleft lip and/or cleft palate in many countries of the world.[1] Since isolated cleft palate is an epidemiologically and embryologically distinct entity from cleft lip, with or without cleft palate, the incidences must be analyzed separately (Table 11–1). Of all clefts, cleft lip, with or without cleft palate, accounts for 60 to 75 per cent, whereas isolated cleft palate accounts for 25 to 40 per cent. The incidence of both categories of clefts is increasing over time.[1,2]

The incidence of cleft lip, with or without cleft palate, is approximately one case per 1,000 births in the United States. This rate of occurrence is much lower in the American black population and much higher in Orientals and certain American Indian groups. In certain Scandinavian studies, the incidence

TABLE 11–1. INCIDENCE OF CLEFT LIP, CLEFT LIP AND PALATE, AND ISOLATED CLEFT PALATE

	RATE PER 1000	MALE TO FEMALE RATIO	SUBCATEGORIES	PER CENT
Cleft palate only	0.5	1:2	Soft palate only Hard and soft palate	25 75
Cleft lip, cleft palate, or both	1.0	2:1	Unilateral lip only Bilateral lip only Unilateral lip and palate Bilateral lip and palate	26 4 49 21

From Fonseca RJ, and Zeitler DL: Management of Dentofacial Deformities in the Cleft Patient. In Bell WH: Surgical Correction of Dentofacial Deformities: New Concepts. Philadelphia, WB Saunders Co, 1985, p 526.

is closer to two cases per 1,000 births.[1] Cleft lip, with or without cleft palate, is twice as common in males as in females. Twenty-six per cent of cases in this category have a unilateral cleft lip only, whereas 4 per cent have bilateral cleft lip only. Forty-nine per cent of cases have unilateral cleft lip and palate, and 21 per cent have bilateral cleft lip and palate.[1]

Isolated cleft palate occurs at a rate of 0.5 cases per 1,000 births, irrespective of race. It is twice as common in females as in males. The genetic heterogeneity appears to be considerably greater for isolated cleft palate than for cleft lip, with or without cleft palate.[1]

Genetic and environmental factors have been implicated, and clefting is apparent by the third month of intrauterine development.

Maxillofacial Growth in Children with Clefts

Many studies have been reported concerning maxillofacial growth in children with cleft lip and/or palate. Patients who have not had surgical repair of their clefts show a variety of relationships, depending on the type of clefts. Cephalometric comparisons of patients with unrepaired clefts of the palate show that they have maxillae and mandibles that are in a more posterior position and a steeper mandibular plane than those of normal subjects. However, the unoperated cleft palate patients tended to have a normal relationship between the mandible and maxilla.[3] Patients who have had no surgical repair of their unilateral cleft lip and palate show a similar tendency for maxillary and mandibular retrusion and a steep mandibular plane. Unoperated bilateral cleft lip and palate patients, however, show maxillary protrusion due to the anterior position of the premaxilla. Both of these groups exhibit a tendency toward anterior collapse of the maxilla on the cleft side, normal to excessive posterior maxillary width, and a superior rolling of the alveolus adjacent to the cleft.[4, 5]

Many longitudinal studies have followed the maxillofacial growth of children with clefts after their primary repair. The early, soft tissue profile of children with unilateral cleft lip and palate is convex, but this convexity decreases with growth and results in a straighter profile than in the noncleft population. The soft tissue lip is long and the nose less prominent but longer than normal.[6]

Growth in width of the maxilla is markedly decreased after palatal surgery. This results in an increased incidence of posterior crossbite in patients with repaired clefts compared with patients with unrepaired clefts and with normal subjects. Total maxillary arch length may be fairly normal, with a tissue deficiency in the anterior alveolus on the cleft side.[6]

Growth of the cleft maxilla appears to slow immediately after primary repair surgery and then to accelerate.[6] This results in maxillary growth similar to that in patients who have had no primary repair. Most studies indicate that patients with repaired lips and/or palates show decreased vertical and horizontal growth of the maxilla, rotation of the palatal plane in a clockwise direction, decreased vertical growth of the ramus steep mandibular plane, and a tendency toward mandibular retrusion.[7–11]

Maxillofacial growth rates in cleft patients do not differ significantly from normal.[12] Facial proportions, however, do differ significantly from normal. In addition to patients who conform to the average findings discussed above, there are many patients with clefts who develop significant skeletal malrelationships with anterior open bite, Class III malocclusions, and posterior crossbite.

DIAGNOSIS AND TREATMENT PLANNING

Special Problems of the Cleft Patient

There are several conditions common to patients with cleft lip and palate that require special surgical and prosthodontic management. A very important problem, unique to cleft patients, is the presence of an alveolar cleft. This anomaly, when left unrepaired, contributes to many problems. An oro-nasal fistula may be present, which could cause hypernasal speech and allow the passage of fluids from the mouth into the nose. Teeth will erupt into malposed positions in the region of the cleft and may erupt out of bony support. The cleft divides the maxilla into separate segments that are individually mobile. This may prevent stabilization of fixed long-term transpalatal retention. (Fig. 11–1).

Teeth in the region of the cleft may be congenitally missing or malformed; supernumerary teeth are also common. These conditions may require full-coverage fixed or removable prosthetic replacement.

Children with clefts often wear removable palatal appliances for many years before reaching an age at which fixed bridges may be inserted. This makes papillary hyperpla-

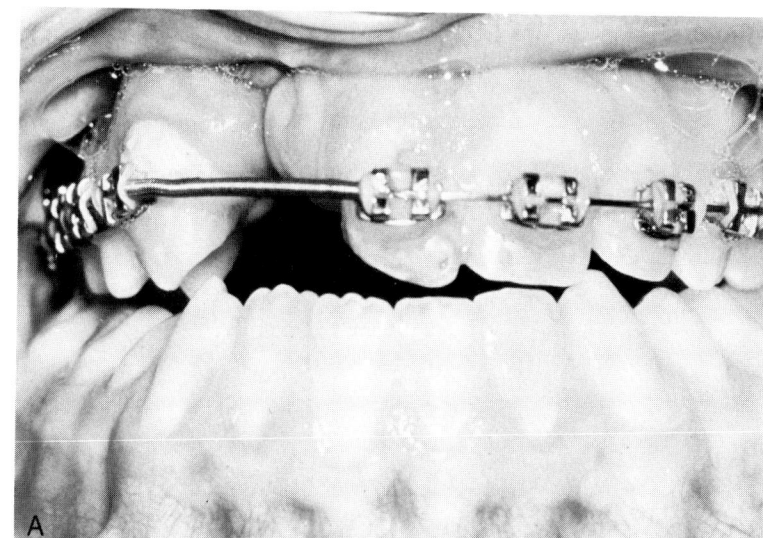

Figure 11–1. *A*, Patient with unilateral alveolar cleft undergoing orthodontic treatment prior to grafting. *B*, Palatal view showing oro-nasal fistula.

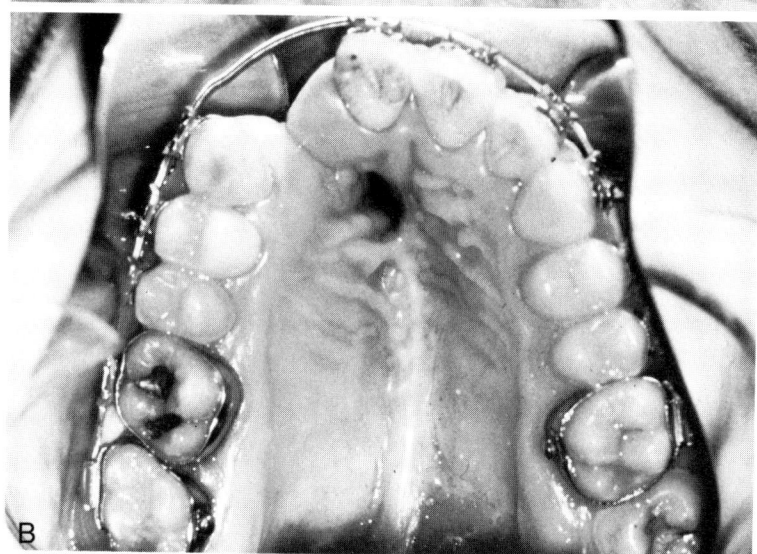

sia of the palatal soft tissues a common malady that must be recognized and treated prior to the insertion of final fixed or removable prostheses (Fig. 11–2). It is important to treat papillary hyperplasia prior to any surgery that involves suturing of palatal mucosal flaps. The palatal tissue on the maxillary incisors may require gingivectomy for oral hygiene considerations as well as for preparation for fixed prostheses (Fig. 11–3).

Owing to primary lip closure, as well as secondary procedures, scarring of the maxillary lateral vestibule often occurs and may be severe (Fig. 11–4). This may require corrective procedures to deepen the vestibule prior to construction of a prosthesis. This is especially true in patients with bilateral clefts.

Because of the altered anatomic structures secondary to the cleft deformities, preoperative, intraoperative, and postoperative adjustments should be evaluated. A close cooperative effort among surgeons, speech pathologists, anesthesiologists, orthodontists, psychologists, and various dental specialists is required to coordinate and optimize the surgical result. Special considerations in diagnosis and treatment planning should be observed, including associated congenital anomalies, alteration or compromise in circulation to the anticipated surgical site, changes in the velopharyngeal mechanism, preoperative and postoperative orthodontic therapy, alterations in nasolabial esthetics and function, and additional surgical fixation for immobilization.

Associated Congenital Anomalies

Patients with cleft lip and/or palate have an increased incidence of associated malformations, some of which may have an influence on the eventual treatment of the pa-

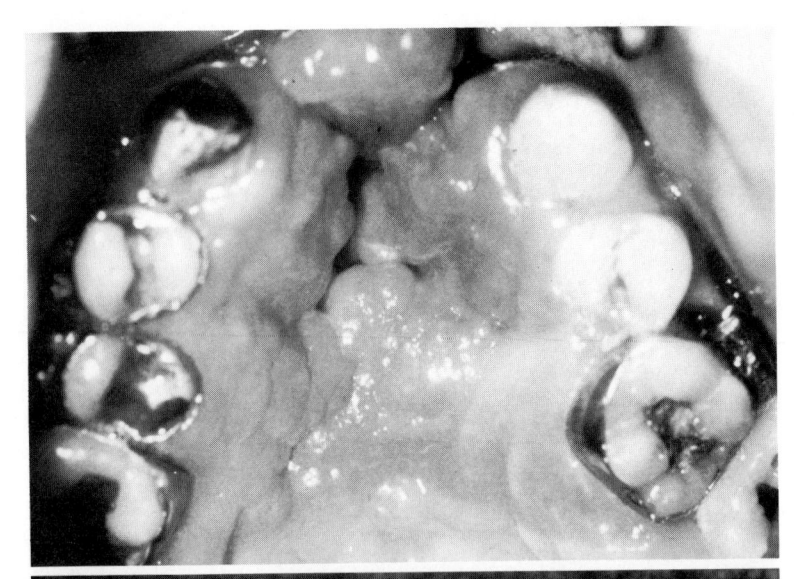

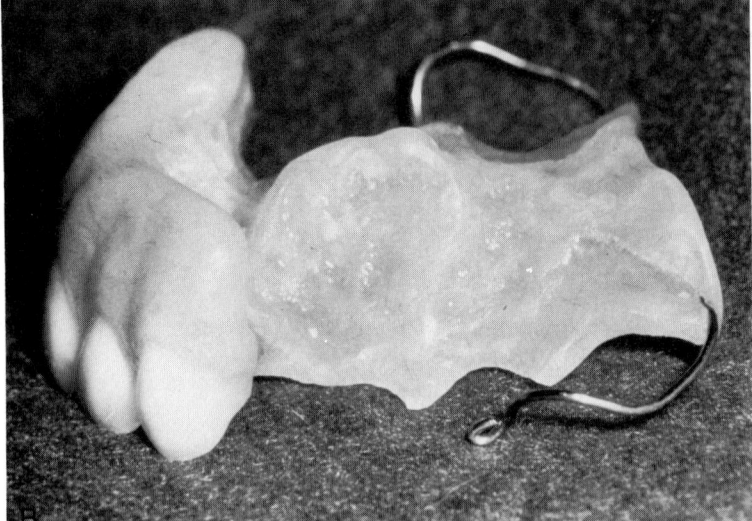

Figure 11–2. *A*, Inflammatory papillary hyperplasia related to long-term use of temporary partial denture. *B*, Temporary partial denture.

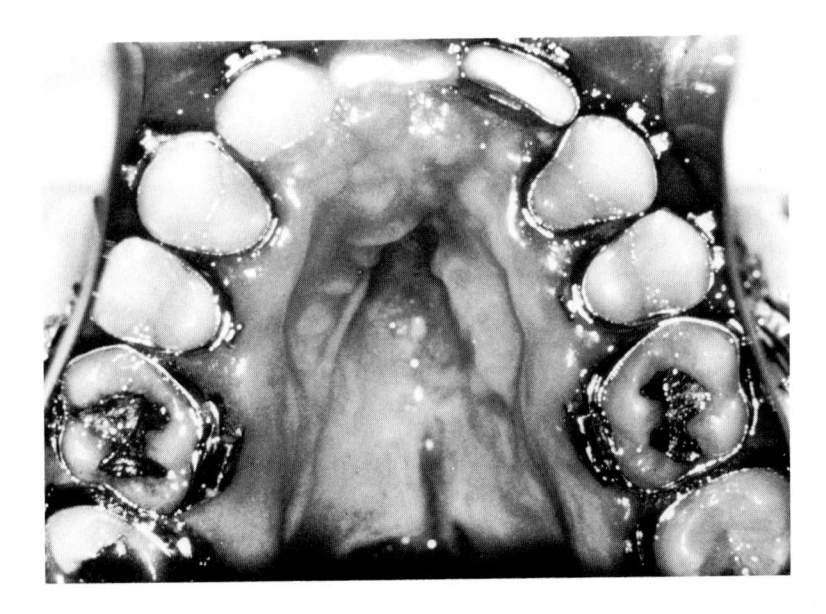

Figure 11–3. Hyperplasia of gingiva on palatal aspect of incisors.

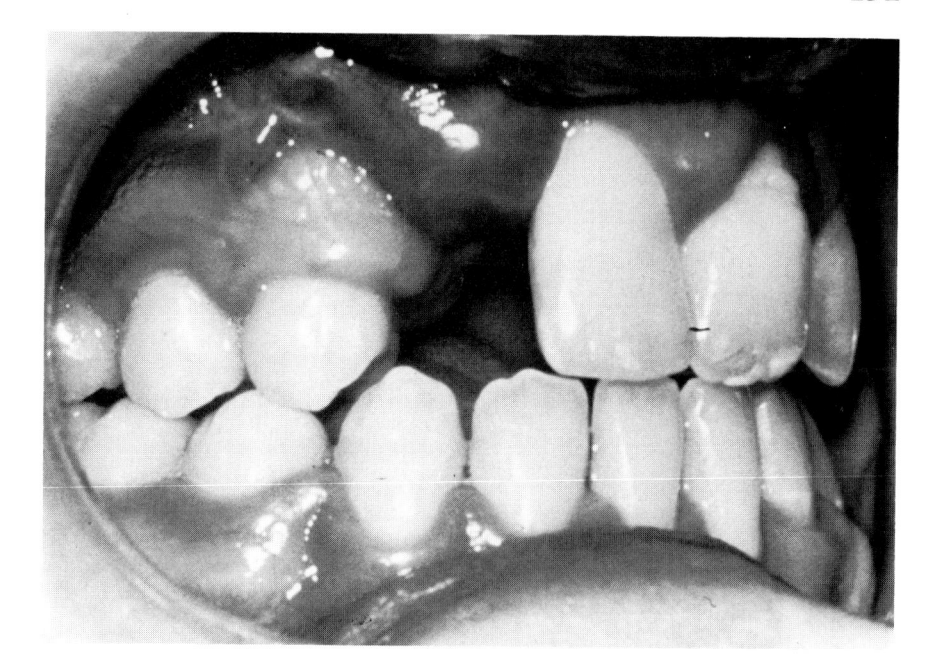

Figure 11–4. Nonkeratinized, mobile tissue in the region of a cleft following pedicle flap closure of the cleft.

tient. Multiple anomalies frequently occur in aborted fetuses with cleft lip and palate. A significant loss of these individuals with multiple malformations occurs during the prenatal and perinatal periods.[2]

In a recent study of 110 cleft patients in a clinic population, 49 had associated anomalies. The relative incidence of associated anomalies was higher for the black patients than for the white patients. The concomitant malformations found in this group included congenital heart disease, limb and skeletal anomalies, and genital abnormalities.[13] Another study of patients in a metropolitan cleft lip and palate clinic found a 6.7 per cent prevalence of congenital heart disease. This represents a ten-fold increase over the prevalence in the general population.[14]

Most cleft patients referred for orthognathic surgery probably have had multiple surgical procedures previously, and associated malformations would have been diagnosed. However, the frequent occurrence of associated anomalies, particularly congenital heart disease, highlights the need for a careful history and physical examination to identify any major malformations that would complicate the patient's perioperative course.

ANATOMIC CONSIDERATIONS

The blood supply to the maxilla has been examined in near-term fetuses with normal and cleft palates. In two studies, Maher[15, 16] has found that the posterior, superior alveolar artery courses to the midline, helping to supply the premaxilla as well as the posterior maxilla. The greater palatine artery, in its course anteriorly, anastomoses with the lateral nasal septal artery, the superior alveolar artery, the labial branches of the facial artery, and the contralateral greater palatine artery. These anastomoses occur in both cleft and noncleft samples, although variability in both groups exists.

Significant buccal and/or palatal scarring (Fig. 11–5) frequently occurs in the patients who have had multiple procedures for repair of their clefts.[17] In addition to the implications for vascular supply, this scarring may

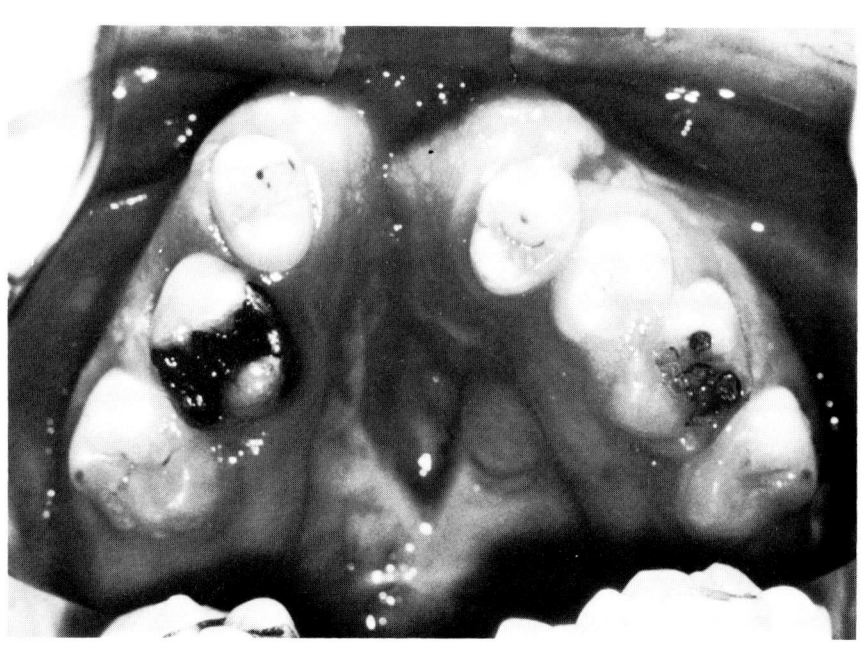

Figure 11–5. Severe scarring, as seen in this palate, may limit movement of maxillary segments during orthognathic surgery.

cause difficulties in achieving mobility of the maxillary segments during maxillary osteotomies.[18]

Prosthodontic Timing

It is not unusual for patients with a cleft of the alveolus to have missing teeth. There may be premature loss of one or several anterior maxillary teeth. Definitive prosthetic rehabilitation of the dental arch should be performed after surgical-orthodontic correction is complete but should occur prior to the final soft tissue labial and/or nasal surgery. Once a surgical-orthodontic procedure is complete and intermaxillary fixation is released, a transpalatal arch retainer with acrylic teeth can be used to help maintain the surgical result and to contribute to the facial esthetics. Six months after surgery, a fixed prosthetic appliance can be inserted if desired.

PRESURGICAL WORK-UP

The evaluation of the cleft patient being considered for reconstructive surgery should begin the same way as with other patients. First, the patient's chief complaint, expectations, and dental history should be obtained, with special attention to the patient's previous surgeries and anesthetic complications or problems. A head and neck examination will help to identify problems that may require special management preoperatively, intraoperatively, or postoperatively. A brief assessment of velopharyngeal competence by the surgeon should be followed by a thorough assessment by a speech pathologist in order to document the preoperative condition. All patients with pharyngeal flaps should be evaluated for the size of the lateral ports (Fig. 11–6). If general anesthesia will be required, an anesthesia consultation is important to assure that a nasoendotracheal tube of appropriate size will pass beside the pharyngeal flap if nasal intubation is necessary. If there is doubt, a tube may be passed through the nasopharynx under local anesthesia in the clinic. If the ports of the pharyngeal flap are too small to allow for passage of an endotracheal tube, they can be increased in size using laser surgery prior to the definitive cleft repair.

The soft tissue in the oral cavity should be evaluated for the degree of labial and palatal scarring, labial or palatal fistulas, and health of the tissue in the region of the alveolar cleft and hard palate. Measurements of lip length, incisor display, overjet, overbite, and midline deviations should be recorded and Angle class of occlusion, crossbite, and other dental conditions should be noted. Along with the clinical examination, impressions of the arches, photographs of the face and teeth, and a radiographic examination are necessary. In addition to a lateral cephalogram and panoramic radiograph for all patients, periapical radiographs should be made of the alveolar cleft region. The radiographs should be evaluated for missing and supernumerary teeth, impacted teeth, and bone height on teeth adjacent to the cleft.

When indicated, the cephalometric evaluation of the patient with a cleft does not differ from that of a noncleft patient. Routine measurements and observations of the patient in adjusted natural position should be made to compare the maxillary and mandibular positions to the cranial base and to each other. It also helps to identify the tooth positions in relationship to the bone structures and to each other, and to do a soft tissue profile evaluation. Natural horizontal and vertical reference lines are utilized to facilitate the cephalometric examination.

SURGICAL CONSIDERATIONS

Historical Perspectives

Alveolar Cleft Grafting

The first attempts at grafting bone to alveolar clefts were made in 1908 and 1914, but

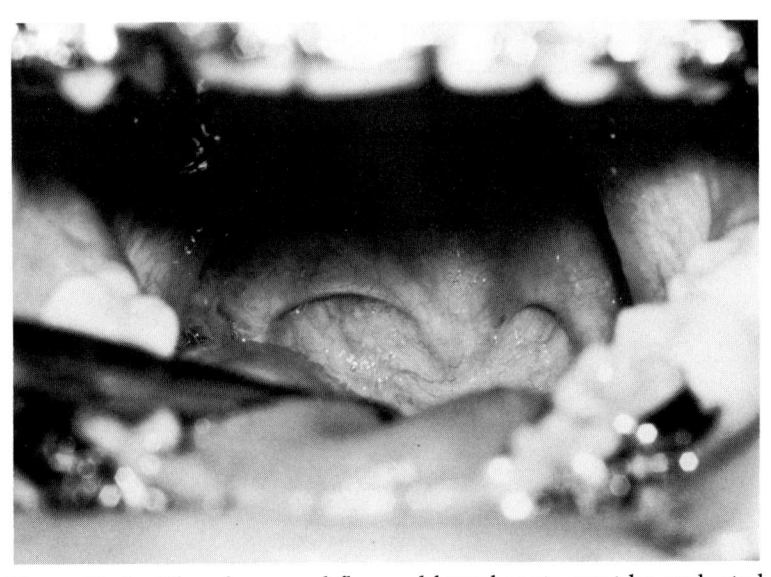

Figure 11–6. The pharyngeal flap and lateral ports must be evaluated if a nasoendotracheal tube will be used.

the modern era of alveolar cleft grafting began in the 1950's.[19-21] Follow-up studies of bone grafting in infancy have shown that maxillary growth is inhibited by this early intervention. However, if bone grafting of the alveolar cleft is delayed until most of maxillary growth is complete, many advantages may be realized.

Studies appeared in the 1970's that suggested if bone graft repair of alveolar clefts was delayed until the age of the mixed dentition (about 8 to 14 years), good function would result and there would be much less effect on growth and development. Boyne and Sands[22] reported the results of alveolar cleft grafting on 10 patients. Their recommended operation time was between ages nine and eleven, before the canine teeth had fully erupted. The procedure involved grafting autologous cancellous bone and marrow to clefts in patients not requiring orthognathic surgery. The oro-nasal soft tissue communication was closed during the procedure. Canine teeth erupted into the grafted areas in eight patients.

Grafting between the ages of 7 and 12 years will establish a solid alveolus for stabilization of the maxillary segments. The oronasal fistula will be closed. The bone in the cleft area will allow for the normal eruption of teeth (in particular, the maxillary canine) into an area of excellent periodontal support. Teeth may be moved orthodontically into or through the grafted bone. A normal appearance to the alveolus will result and allow for the insertion of a fixed prosthesis, if necessary. A high percentage of successful results may be expected.

Total Maxillary Osteotomies with Simultaneous Alveolar Cleft Grafts

In 1927, Wassmund[23] performed the circular detachment of the maxilla at the LeFort I level. Axhausen[24] was the first to advance the maxilla at the LeFort I in 1934. In 1942 Schuchardt[25] used weights to advance the maxilla but stated that this procedure could not be used for patients with clefts.

In 1969 Obwegeser[26] described the use of the LeFort I osteotomy at a relatively high level for advancements of up to 20 mm. This technique was shown for a patient with a cleft of the lip and palate. Obwegeser cautioned that such movements may significantly impair blood flow through the greater palatine arteries.

There have been recent articles describing the techniques of osteotomy with bone grafting[18] and osteotomy with lip revision.[27]

The concept of combining alveolar cleft grafting with osteotomy provides closure of the oro-nasal defect, stabilization of the arch, and correction of the dentofacial deformity in one surgical procedure. By combining lip revision with maxillary advancement, maximal esthetic improvement and the best muscle balance may be achieved.

TIMING OF SURGERY

Development of the dentition in patients with cleft lip and/or palate is delayed when compared with normal subjects. This delay is evident in both arches but is more pronounced in the cleft segment. This phenomenon may be due to nutrition, surgery, and/or genetics.[28] Although the dentition is delayed in development, the growth rate of the maxilla and mandible in cleft patients is not significantly different from that of normal patients.[12]

When a graft to an alveolar cleft is indicated, the timing of the surgery is important. The graft should be delayed until the majority of midfacial growth is complete. On the other hand, it is important to perform the procedure before the eruption of the maxillary canine. This will allow the canine to erupt into a solid alveolus rather than into the cleft without bony support (Fig. 11-7). This means that the timing of the alveolar cleft graft should be individualized and should occur sometime between the ages of 7 and 12. Expansion of the maxilla should be performed prior to bone grafting of the alveolus, since it is more easily achieved and the resultant wider cleft allows for greater access during surgery.

The timing of orthognathic surgery for the cleft patient is similar to the timing for the patient without a cleft. Mandibular sagittal excesses should be operated upon after cessation of growth, whereas maxillary and mandibular sagittal deficiency can be corrected earlier. Operations in the maxillary arch require careful observation of the location of unerupted teeth, since the horizontal osteotomy is in the vicinity of these teeth.

IMMOBILIZATION

Immobilization is required following maxillary and/or mandibular orthognathic surgical procedures on a cleft patient. Unlike the patient without a cleft deformity (in whom immobilization may not be indicated following maxillary advancement), the scarring of the soft tissue in the surgical area of the pa-

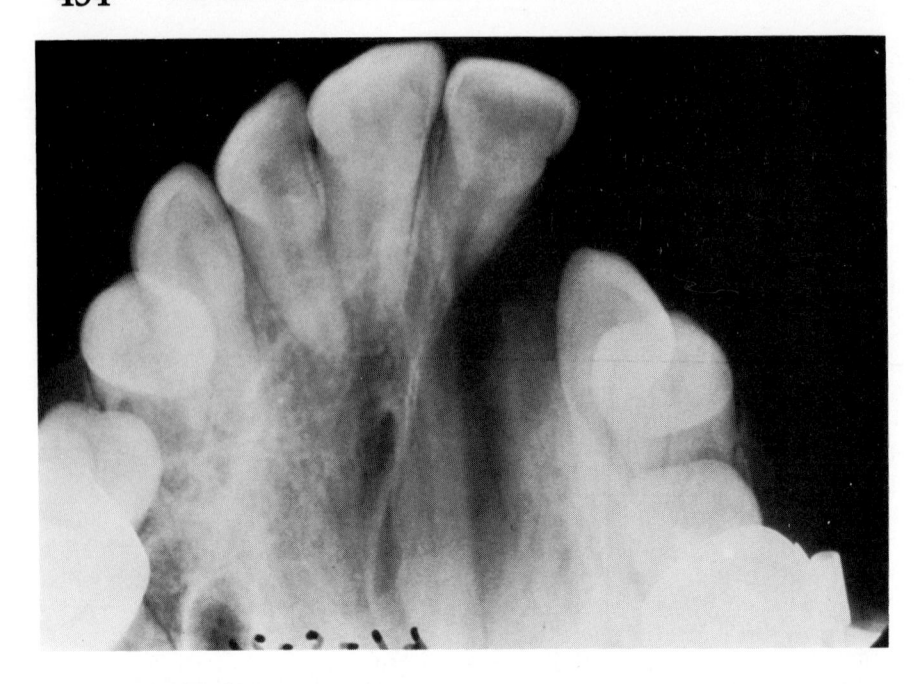

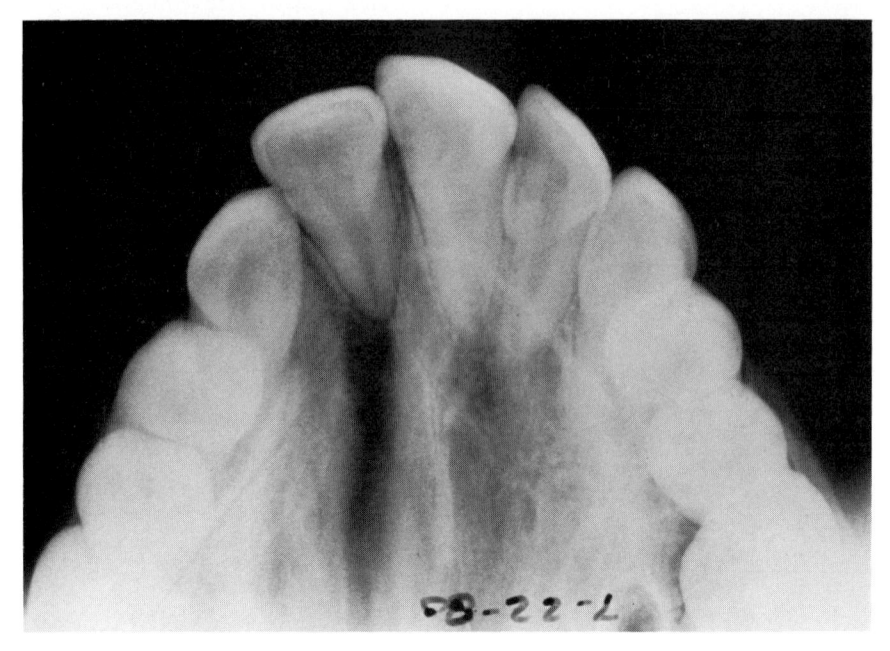

Figure 11–7. *Top*, Canine in region of cleft prior to graft. *Bottom*, Canine erupting into healed bone graft.

tient tends to make relapse a distinct possibility. Usually in these patients, there are multiple maxillary segments because of residual alveolar and palatal clefts. The use of autologous and/or allogeneic bone grafts in these cleft areas is recommended to help achieve intra-arch stability while also establishing continuity with the clefted alveolar ridge. The length of maxillomandibular fixation in the cleft patient should be between six and eight weeks, with skeletal fixation utilized for those patients with extreme movements or movements that were difficult to achieve at the time of surgery.

Surgical Techniques

Technique for Repairing Unilateral Clefts

After general anesthesia is given in the operating room, the patient is prepared and draped for simultaneous procurement of the iliac crest graft and the alveolar cleft procedure. Either an oral or a nasal endotracheal tube may be used. An oral anode tube is used most frequently because it allows complete access to the maxilla, nasal floor, and upper lip and will not kink when head positions are changed. Also, an oral tube will not disturb a pharyngeal flap.

The iliac crest procedure is performed as described in the literature.[29, 30] No cortical bone is taken; the graft consists of cancellous bone and marrow. Approximately 20 cc should be obtained, the amount varying with the cleft size. The graft is kept in normal saline, as recommended by Marx.[31]

After placement of a throat pack, the unilateral cleft is examined. Then, epinephrine solution is infiltrated along the cleft for hemostasis and ease in dissection. A 25-gauge needle is used to probe the bony margins of the cleft both palatally and labially. After the width of the bony defect has been determined, a pericoronal incision is made in the sulcus from either the first or the second molar to the corresponding tooth on the opposite side of the arch (Fig. 11–8). An incision is then made along the palatal aspect of the cleft through mucosa to bone (Fig. 11–9). The incision is beveled to preserve palatal mucosa and to avoid the need for inversion of a large amount of tissue into the floor of the nose. The interdental papillae of the teeth adjacent to the cleft are reflected to improve visualization. An incision over the crest of the ridge is made anterior and posterior to the cleft (Fig. 11–10). Careful reflection and handling of this tissue are important because it will be used in the four-cornered closure. Often, the anterior extent

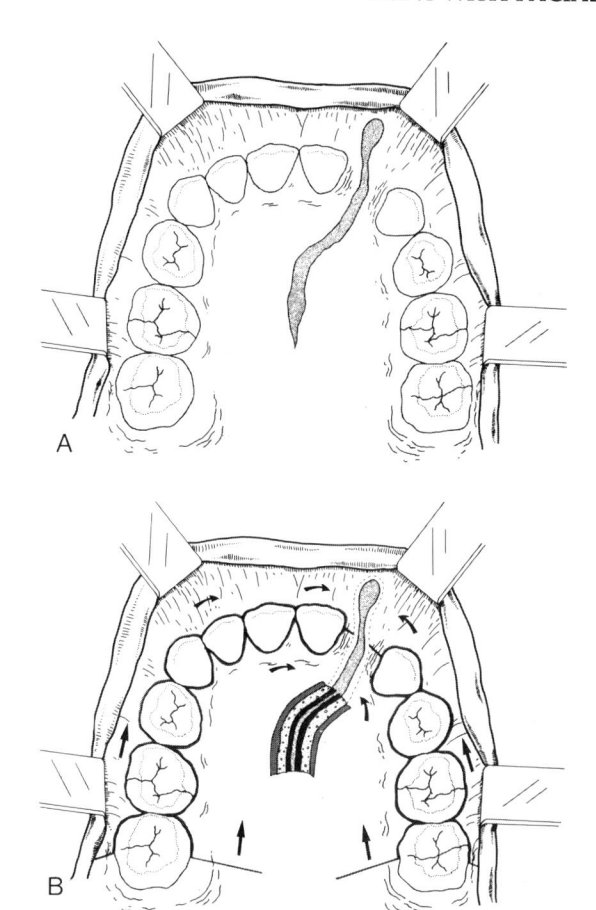

Figure 11–9. Palatal incision for unilateral cleft.

of the bony cleft is not clearly demarcated, and the superior extent of the incision is tapered into the submucosal tissue. After adequate reflection of soft tissue, the margins of the nasal mucosa are approximated with

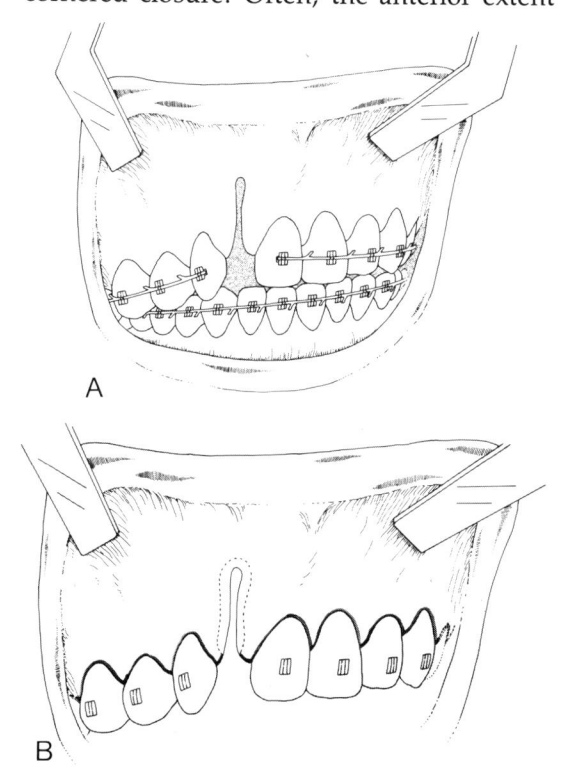

Figure 11–8. Buccal incision for unilateral cleft.

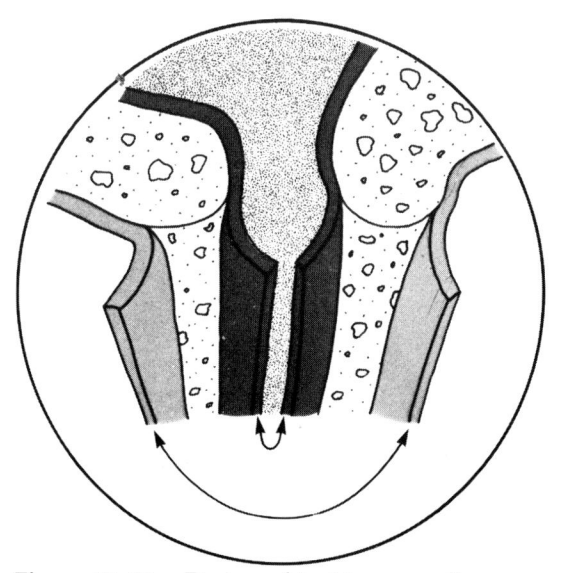

Figure 11–10. Design of incision over the crest of the alveolar ridge.

456 / RECONSTRUCTIVE SURGERY FOR THE PATIENT WITH FACIAL CLEFTS

4-0 Vicryl* suture material on a P-2 cutting needle (Fig. 11–11). A careful check of the closure in the region of the oronasal fistula must be done because an epithelium-lined tract may jeopardize the closure. The nasal soft tissues are repositioned superiorly to form the floor of the nose.

Vertical releasing incisions are made on the palatal and labial aspects in the molar regions. Full mucoperiosteal flaps are then reflected on the palatal and labial aspects of the alveolus, and relaxation of the labial flaps is gained by periosteum-releasing incisions. Generally, a tension-free closure can

---
*Polyglactin 910 synthetic absorbable suture made by Ehicon, Inc.

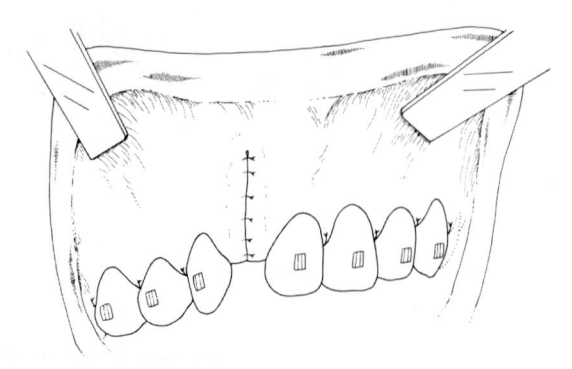

Figure 11–12. Closure of labial tissues by advancement of flaps.

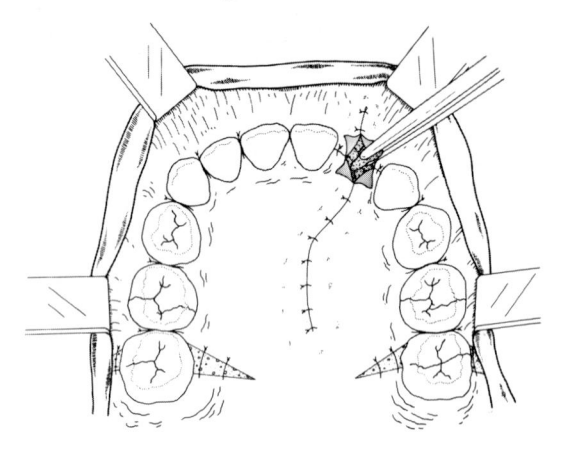

Figure 11–13. Palatal closure.

be obtained by advancement of the papillae one tooth toward the midline. The palatal closure is begun with 4-0 Supramid* suture material (Figs. 11–12 and 11–13). The bone graft is packed into the prepared site. Closure is completed with a four-corner suture over the graft site and multiple simple interrupted sutures to approximate the remainder of the incision (Fig. 11–14). Alternatively,

---
*Polyamide synthetic nonabsorbable suture made by S. Jackson, Inc.

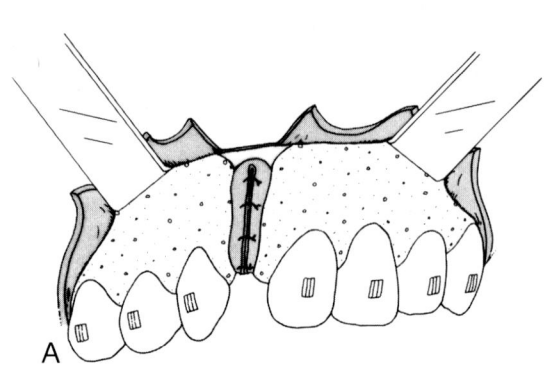

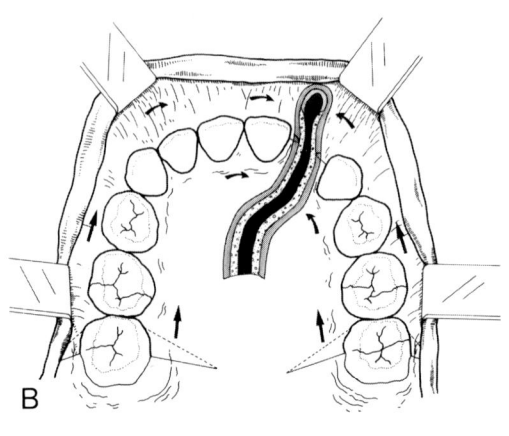

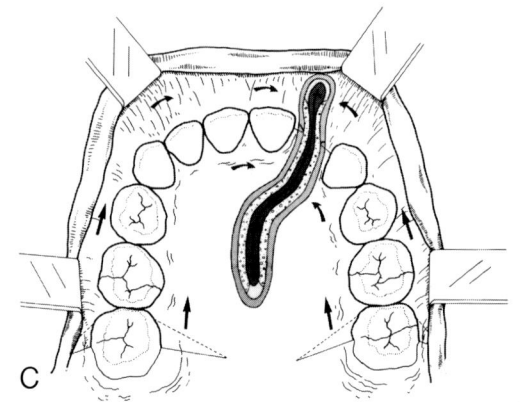

Figure 11–11. Method of suturing nasal mucosa.

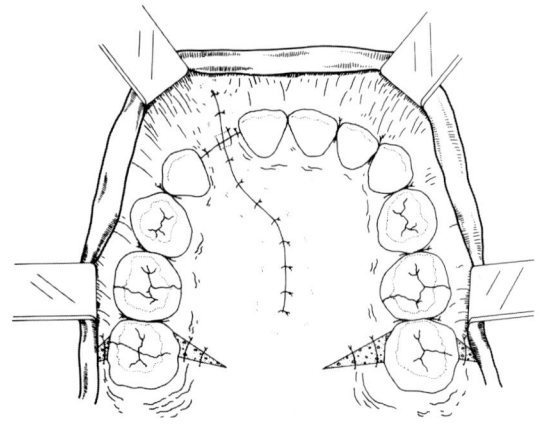

Figure 11–14. Four-corner suture.

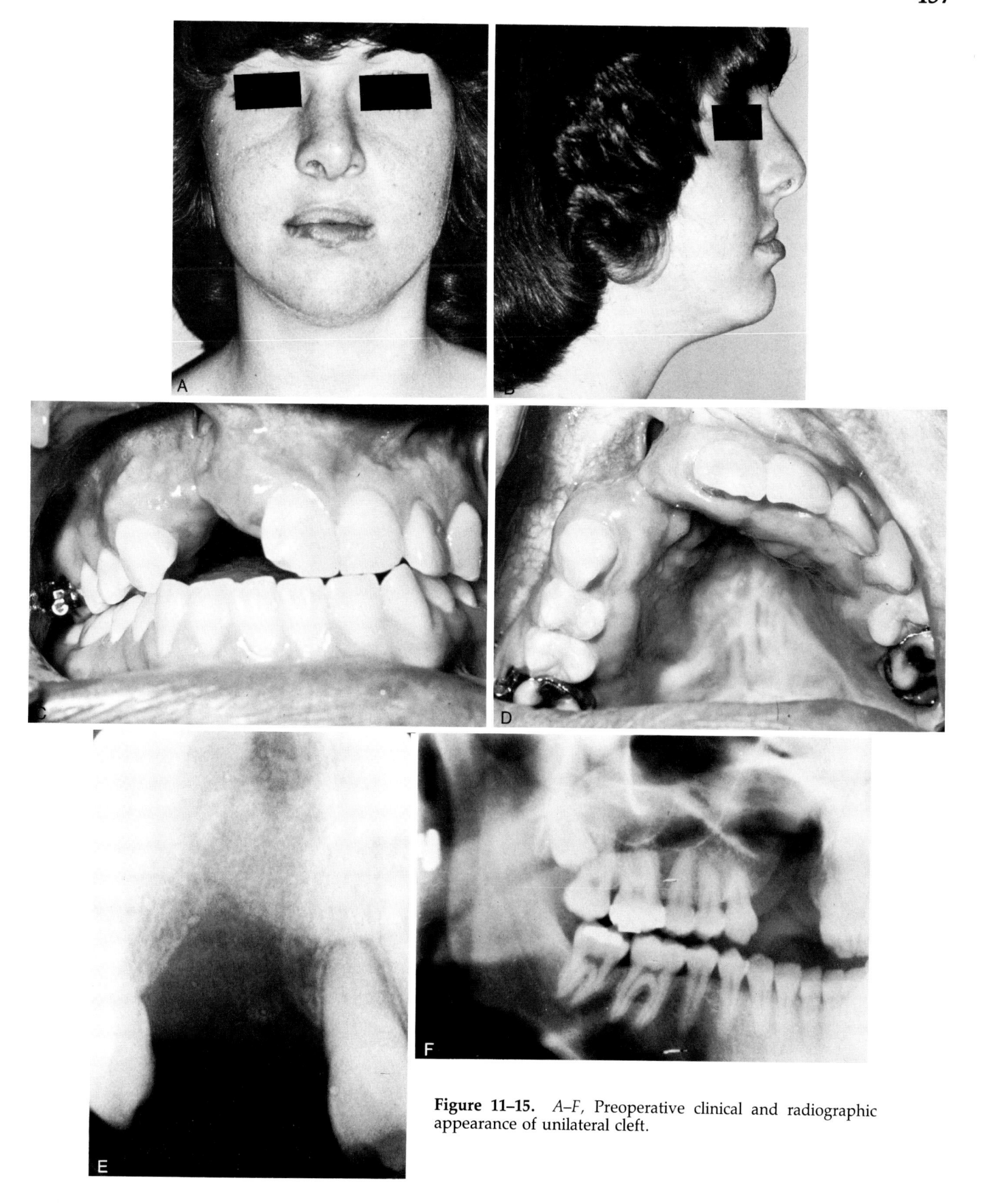

Figure 11–15. *A–F,* Preoperative clinical and radiographic appearance of unilateral cleft.

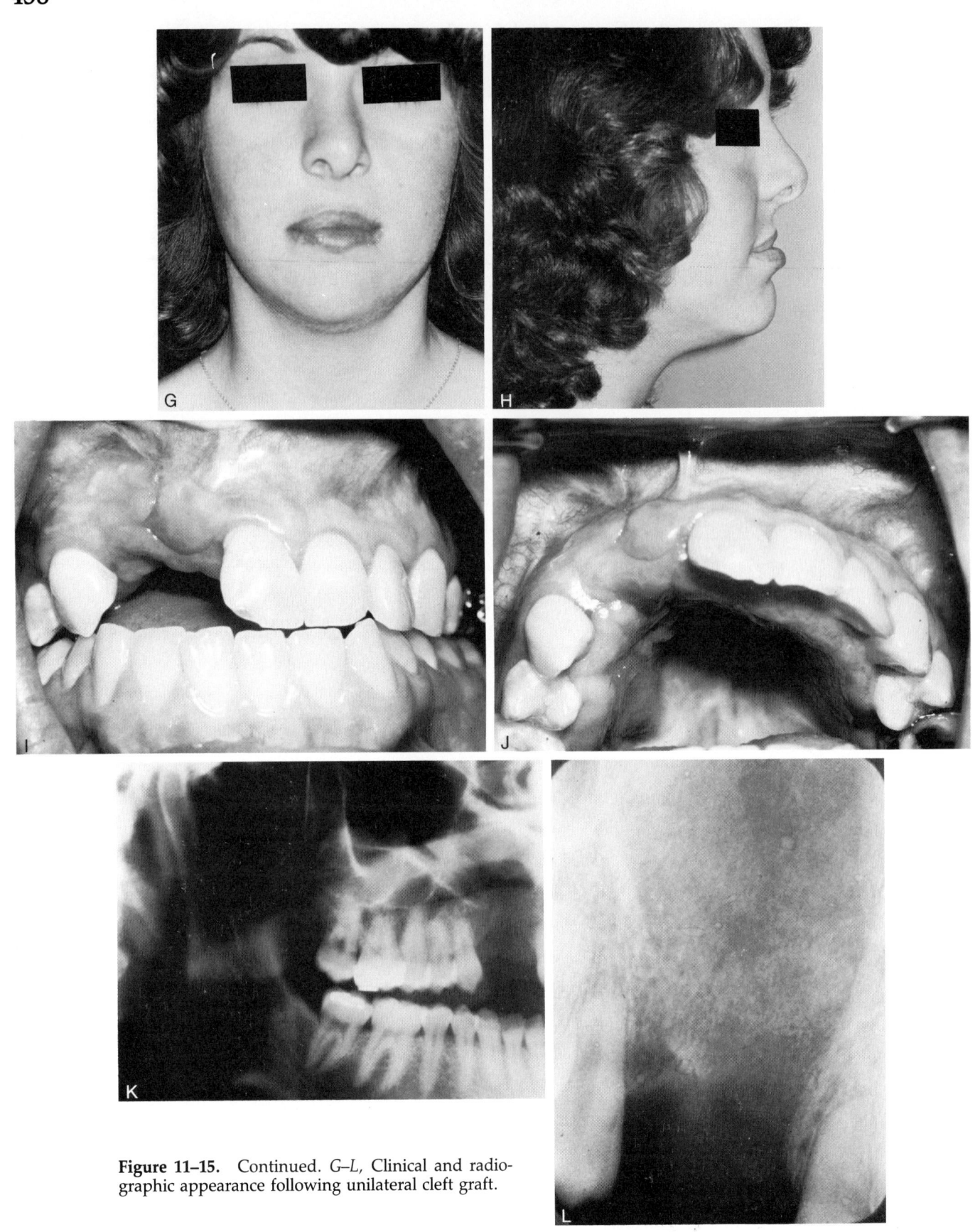

458 / RECONSTRUCTIVE SURGERY FOR THE PATIENT WITH FACIAL CLEFTS

Figure 11–15. Continued. *G–L,* Clinical and radiographic appearance following unilateral cleft graft.

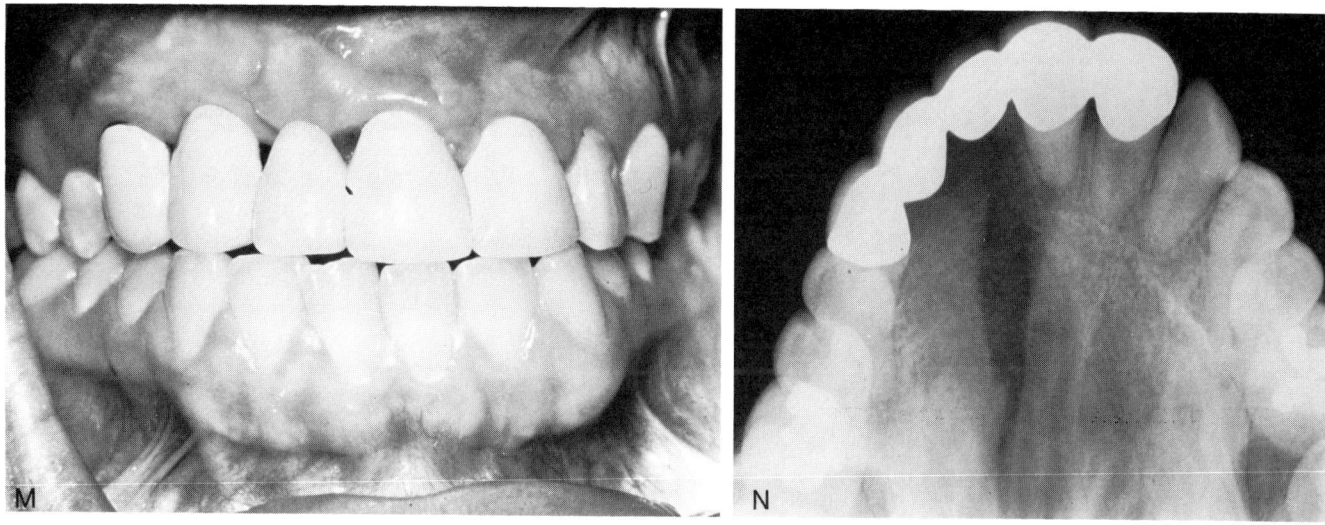

Figure 11–15. Continued. M–N, Appearance following reconstruction with a fixed prosthesis.

a pedicle flap from the lip may be rotated over the areas of the cleft alveolus to aid in closure. A prefabricated acrylic splint may be ligated to a tooth on each side of the arch with 0.018-inch wire. Patients are routinely given preoperative and postoperative antibiotics and steroids. Decongestants are given postoperatively as needed. A humidifier at the bedside helps keep the patient's nasal mucosa moist. The splint and sutures may be removed after 14 days (Fig. 11–15).

Technique for Repairing Bilateral Clefts

The bilateral alveolar cleft graft procedure is similar to the unilateral repair. Both clefts are grafted in one stage. The incisions and flaps are developed in the same fashion except in the premaxillary region, where only a mucoperiosteal tissue cuff sufficient for closure is reflected from the posterior aspect of the premaxilla (Fig. 11–16). The "nasal floor" tissue is reflected and closed bilaterally (Fig. 11–17). Periosteal and vertical releasing incisions are important in the bilateral procedures because the premaxillary tissue cuff does not advance easily (Fig. 11–18). After the graft is placed, the oral closure is begun. Two four-corner sutures are tied, and the remainder of the wound is closed with simple interrupted sutures (Fig. 11–19). Two pedicle flaps may be used for closure if necessary. The blood supply to the premaxilla must be protected by minimal soft tissue reflection from this segment. The position of the premaxilla may be altered during this procedure, if desired (Fig. 11–20).

Orthognathic Surgery

Since patients with cleft lip and/or palate present with a variety of dentofacial deformities, total arch procedures involving either the mandible or maxilla, or both, are often indicated. The presence of either a unilateral or a bilateral alveolar cleft will modify the surgical approach to the maxilla.

Isolated mandibular surgery performed in the cleft patient does not require special consideration. The only modification made by the authors is to utilize only the sagittal split osteotomy for all mandibular advancements and retrusions in cleft patients. This decision is based on the premise that the operation affords increased stability with positive and direct fixation of the osteotomized segments because maxillomandibular fixation is often difficult to achieve owing to an incomplete maxillary dentition in the cleft patient. Other mandibular procedures such as the transoral vertical ramus osteotomy can be successfully utilized for cleft patients with the above deformities. Maxillary surgical procedures for advancement with or without superior or inferior repositioning of the maxilla require special consideration. These procedures are usually concomitant with alveolar cleft bone grafting in which autologous iliac cancellous bone is utilized. The presence of a unilateral or bilateral cleft will alter the surgical design.

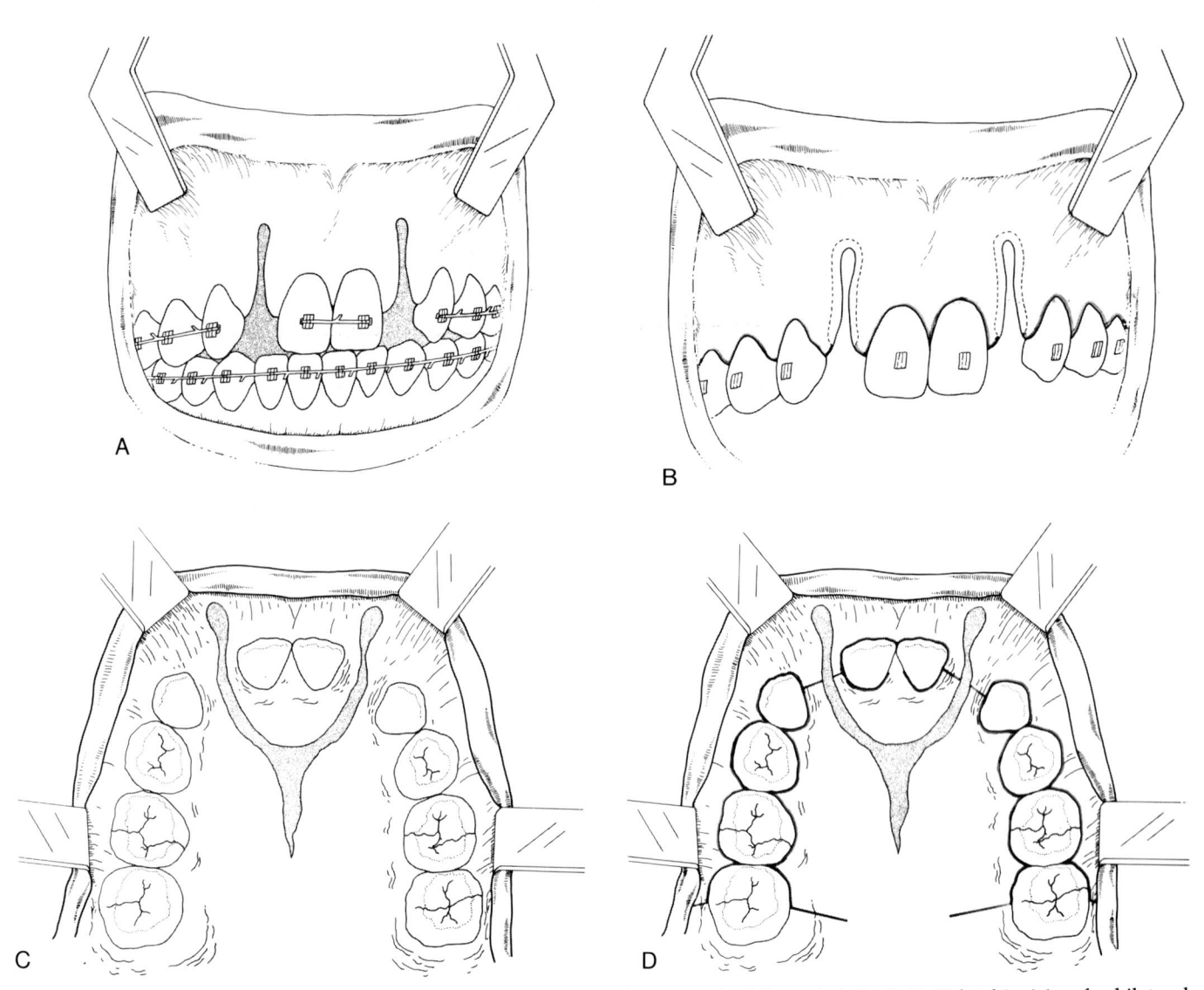

460 / RECONSTRUCTIVE SURGERY FOR THE PATIENT WITH FACIAL CLEFTS

Figure 11–16. *A–B*, Buccal incision for bilateral cleft. *C–D*, Palatal incision for bilateral cleft.

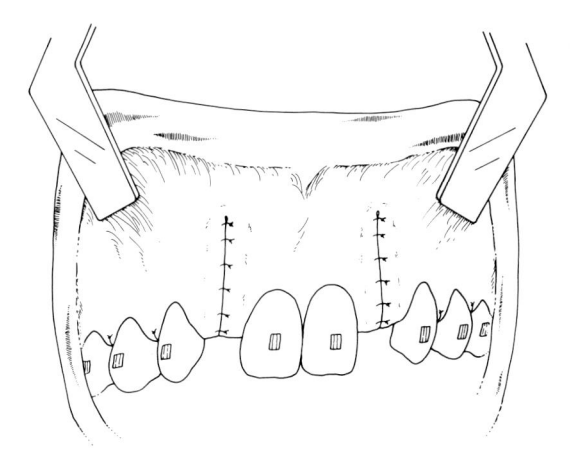

Figure 11–18. Labial closure after graft placement.

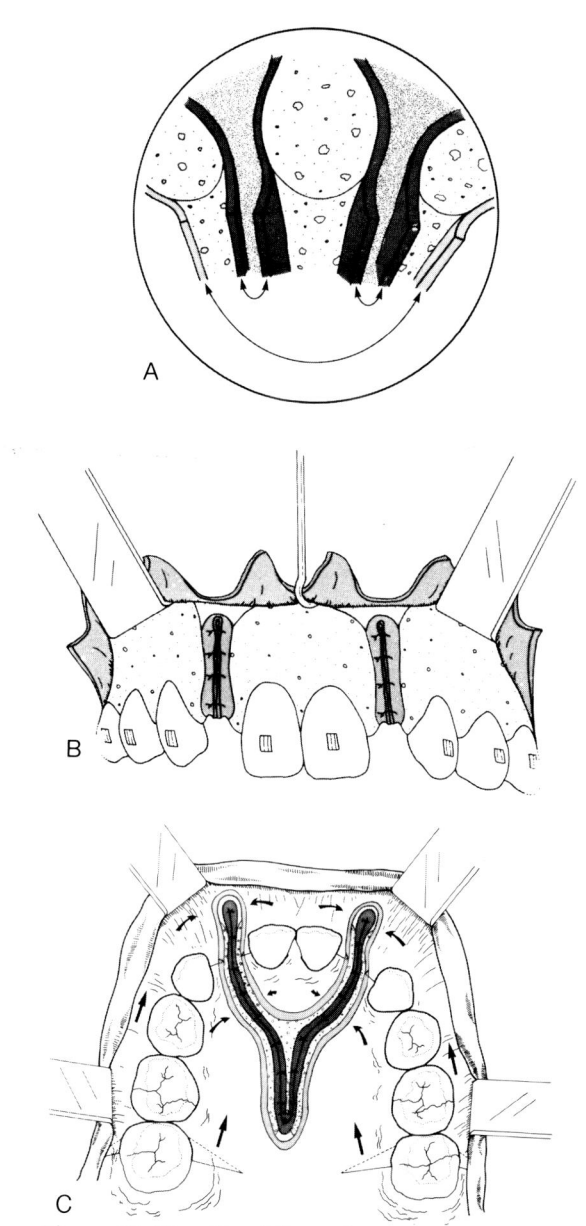

Figure 11–17. Nasal floor closure.

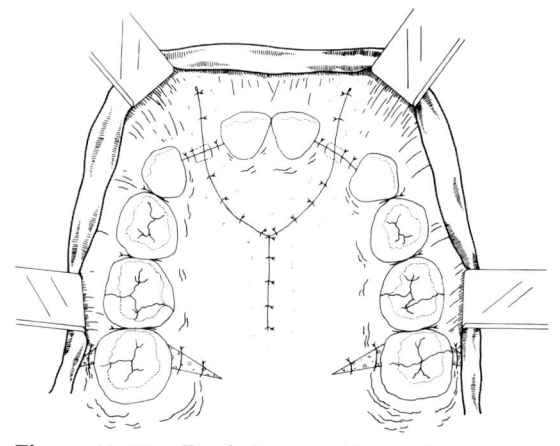

Figure 11–19. Final closure with two four-corner sutures.

tion of the tuberosity of the maxilla and pterygoid plates (Fig. 11–22). If a superior movement of the maxilla is planned, then a predicted amount of bone is removed from the lateral and buccal maxillary wall.

The mucoperiosteum is dissected from the nasal septum on the side of the cleft and is elevated from the opposite nasal floor. Then the nasal septum is osteotomized from the maxilla with a vomer chisel. The lateral wall of the nose is then osteotomized to the junction of the palatine bone. The maxillary tuberosities are separated from the pterygoid plates with a curved pterygoid osteotome, ensuring inferior placement of the osteotome at the fissure to avoid transection of the maxillary artery.

A horizontal incision is made just below the level of the nasal floor in the cleft area. This is done to free the lateral nasal mucoperiosteum and nasal septal mucoperios-

Maxillary Advancement with a Unilateral Alveolar Cleft

In the presence of a unilateral cleft, a circumvestibular incision can be used (Fig. 11–21). This incision should extend through the oro-nasal fistula at its midportion. The lateral walls of the maxilla are exposed bilaterally, and the mucoperiosteum is elevated along the lateral wall of the nose. A periosteal elevator is used to protect the nasal mucosa. The labial and buccal bone along the lateral wall of the nose and maxillary sinus is then osteotomized posteriorly to the junc-

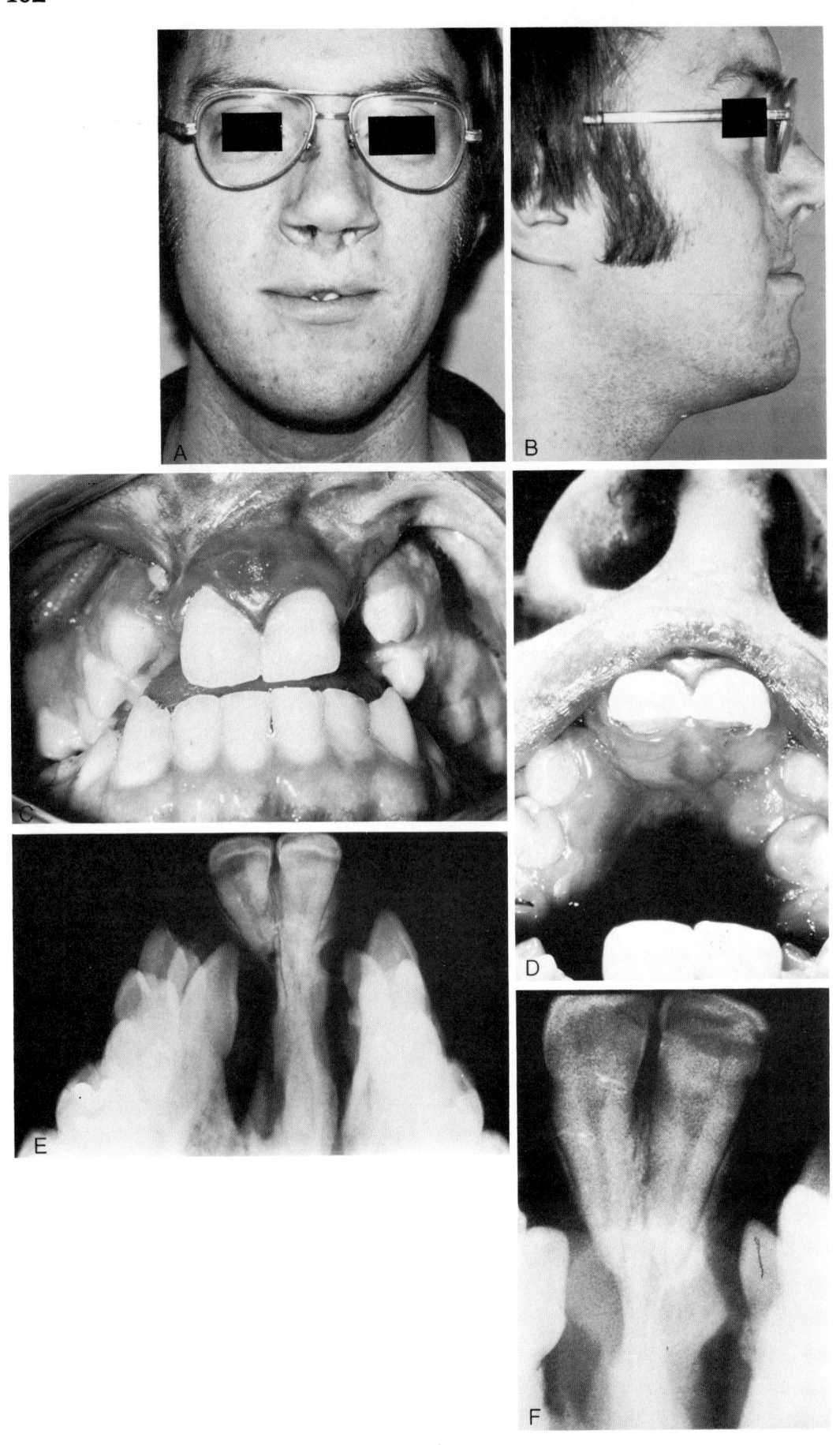

462 / RECONSTRUCTIVE SURGERY FOR THE PATIENT WITH FACIAL CLEFTS

Figure 11–20. *A–F,* Preoperative clinical and radiographic appearance of bilateral cleft.

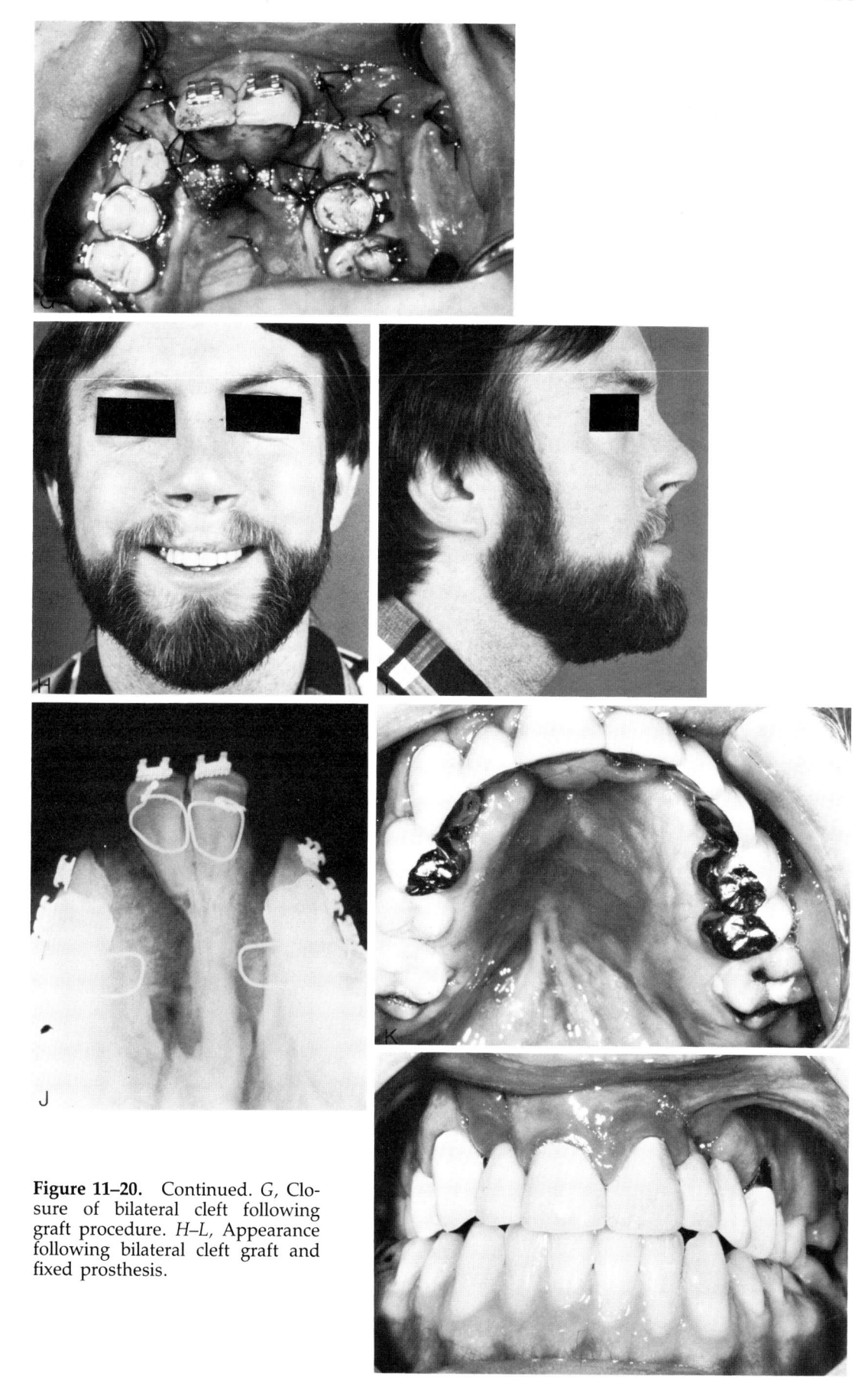

Figure 11–20. Continued. *G*, Closure of bilateral cleft following graft procedure. *H–L*, Appearance following bilateral cleft graft and fixed prosthesis.

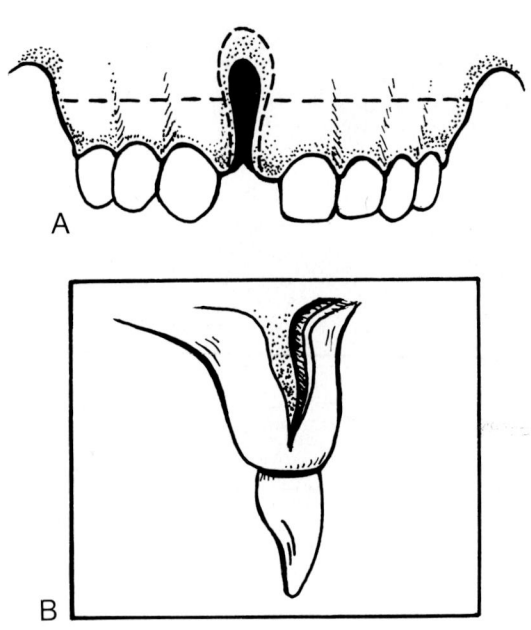

Figure 11–21. *A*, Design of incision for maxillary advancement with unilateral cleft graft. *B*, Incision carried over alveolus.

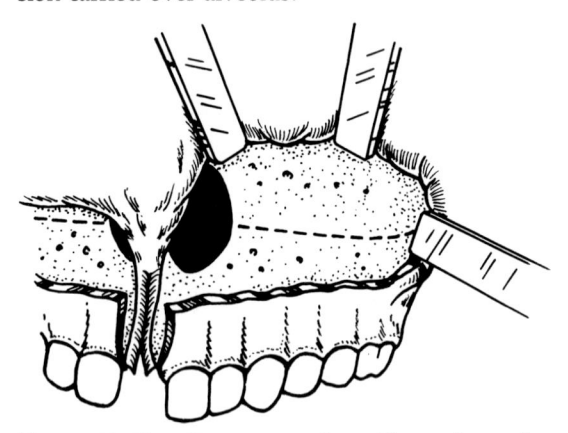

Figure 11–22. Osteotomy of maxilla performed.

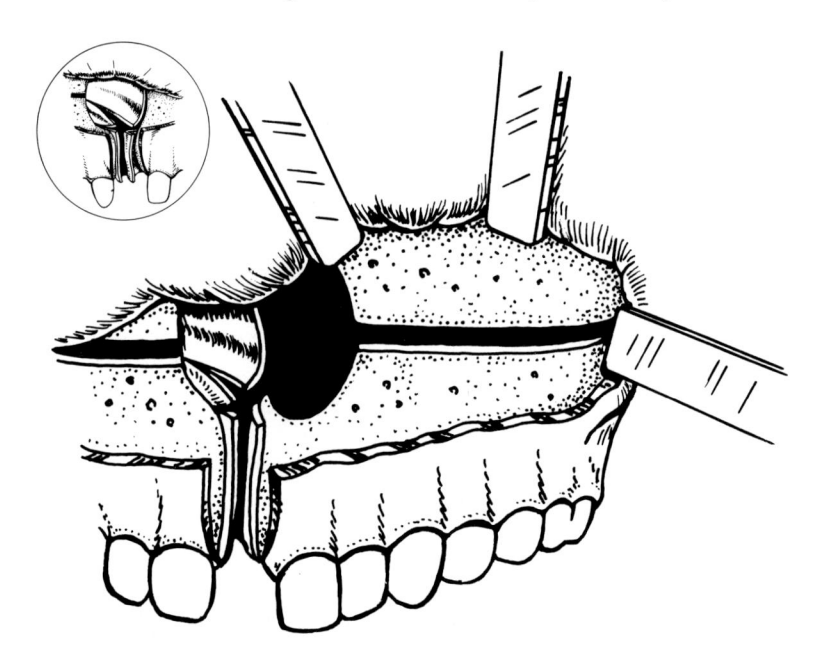

Figure 11–23. Incision to separate nasal from palatal mucosa.

teum from their continuation into the cleft area. These flaps will later become the soft tissue lining of the nasal floor. These incisions should be made prior to downfracturing to avoid tearing the mucoperiosteum (Fig. 11–23).

The maxilla is then downfractured and the segments are mobilized and placed into the surgical splint. The nasal floor is closed by suturing the mucoperiosteal flaps from the lateral nasal wall and nasal septum (Fig. 11–24). To facilitate suturing of the palatal mucosa, the splint is removed.

The splint is inserted and maxillomandibular fixation is applied. Direct osseous wires are tightened bilaterally at the maxillary buttress and piriform rim areas. An additional wire is placed in the superior hole at the piriform rim and suspended to the maxillary archwire. Autologous cancellous bone from the iliac crest is placed along the osteotomy site and in the alveolar cleft area (Fig. 11–25). Blocks of corticocancellous bone may be placed between the maxillary tuberosities and pterygoid plates or in a step created anterior to the buttress to hold the maxilla in the advanced position. The soft tissues over the alveolar cleft can be closed by direct approximation of the residual soft tissues adjacent to the cleft or by rotation of a labial finger flap into the soft tissue defect if the amount of tissue is inadequate (Figs. 11–26 to 11–28). If eruption of a tooth is expected in the area of the finger flap and attached gingiva is not present, then a free gingival graft should be performed prior to the eruption of the tooth (Fig. 11–28).

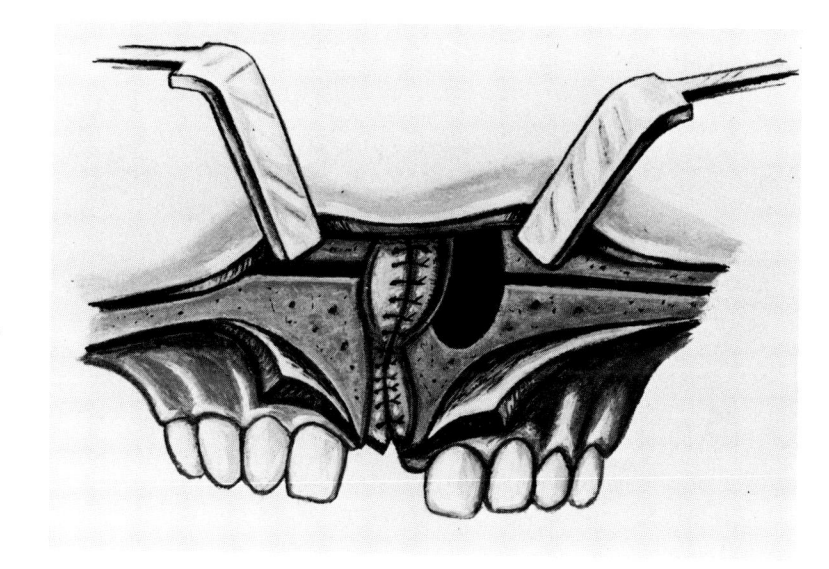

Figure 11-24. Closure of nasal floor.

Maxillary Advancement with Bilateral Alveolar Clefts

The maxilla usually cannot be approached with predictable success utilizing the downfracture technique with a horizontal vestibular incision with bilateral clefts. The blood supply to the premaxillary segment is predominantly derived from the labial soft tissues. Hence, interruption of this blood supply might severely compromise the vitality of this segment.

Utilizing horizontal incisions, extending from the posterior margin of the cleft area to the maxillary buttress, the lateral wall of the maxilla is identified (Fig. 11-29). The nasal mucoperiosteum is then elevated from the lateral nasal wall. An osteotomy is extended from the piriform rim to the maxillopterygoid junction. A small guarded osteotome is then used to osteotomize the lateral nasal wall posteriorly to the palatine bone. A

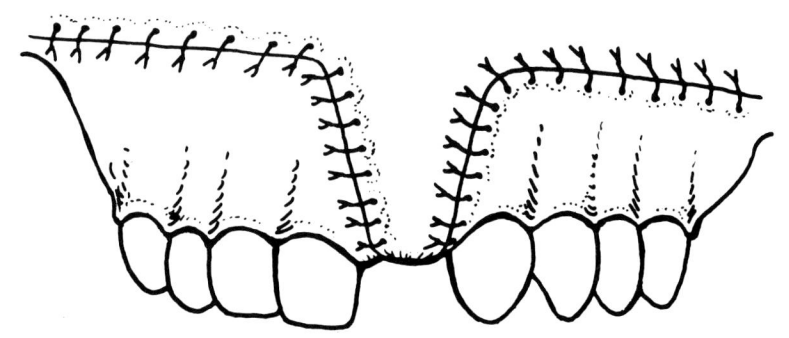

Figure 11-26. Labial closure.

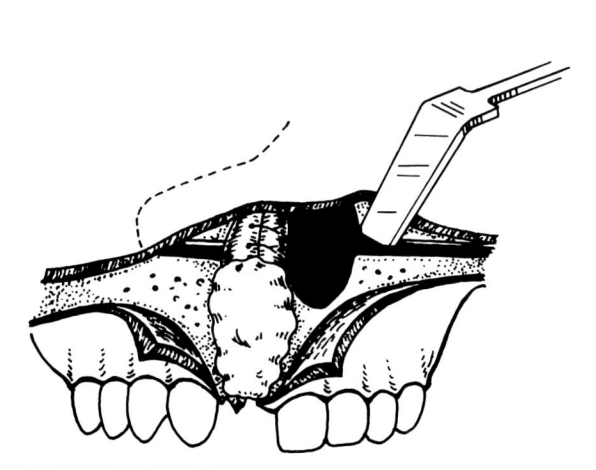

Figure 11-25. Placement of cancellous bone in cleft with outline of closure using pedicle flap.

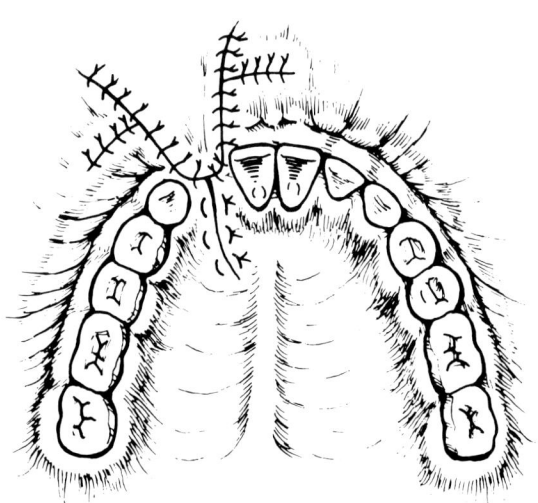

Figure 11-27. Palatal closure.

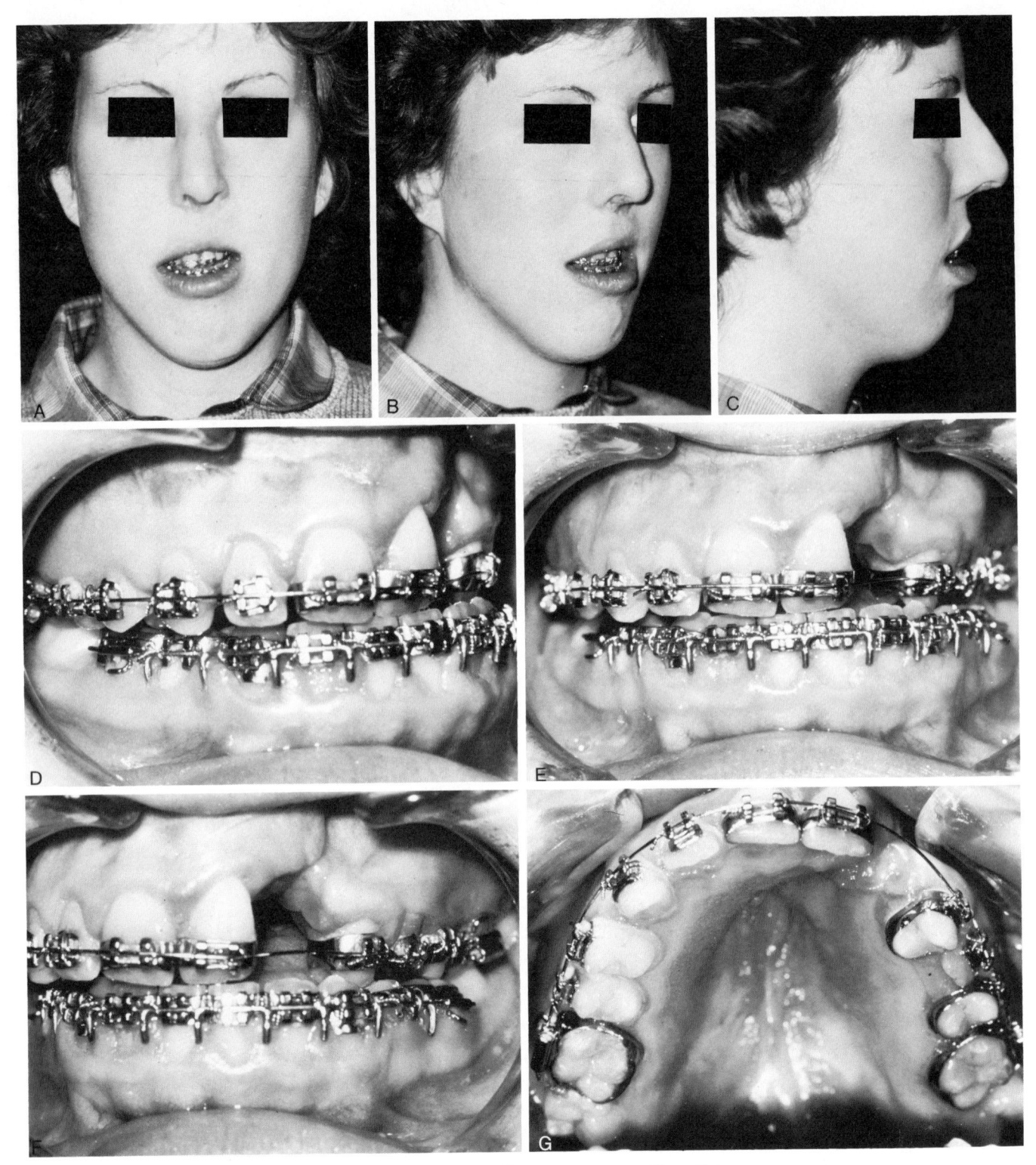

466 / RECONSTRUCTIVE SURGERY FOR THE PATIENT WITH FACIAL CLEFTS

Figure 11–28. *A–G,* Preoperative appearance prior to maxillary osteotomy with unilateral cleft graft.

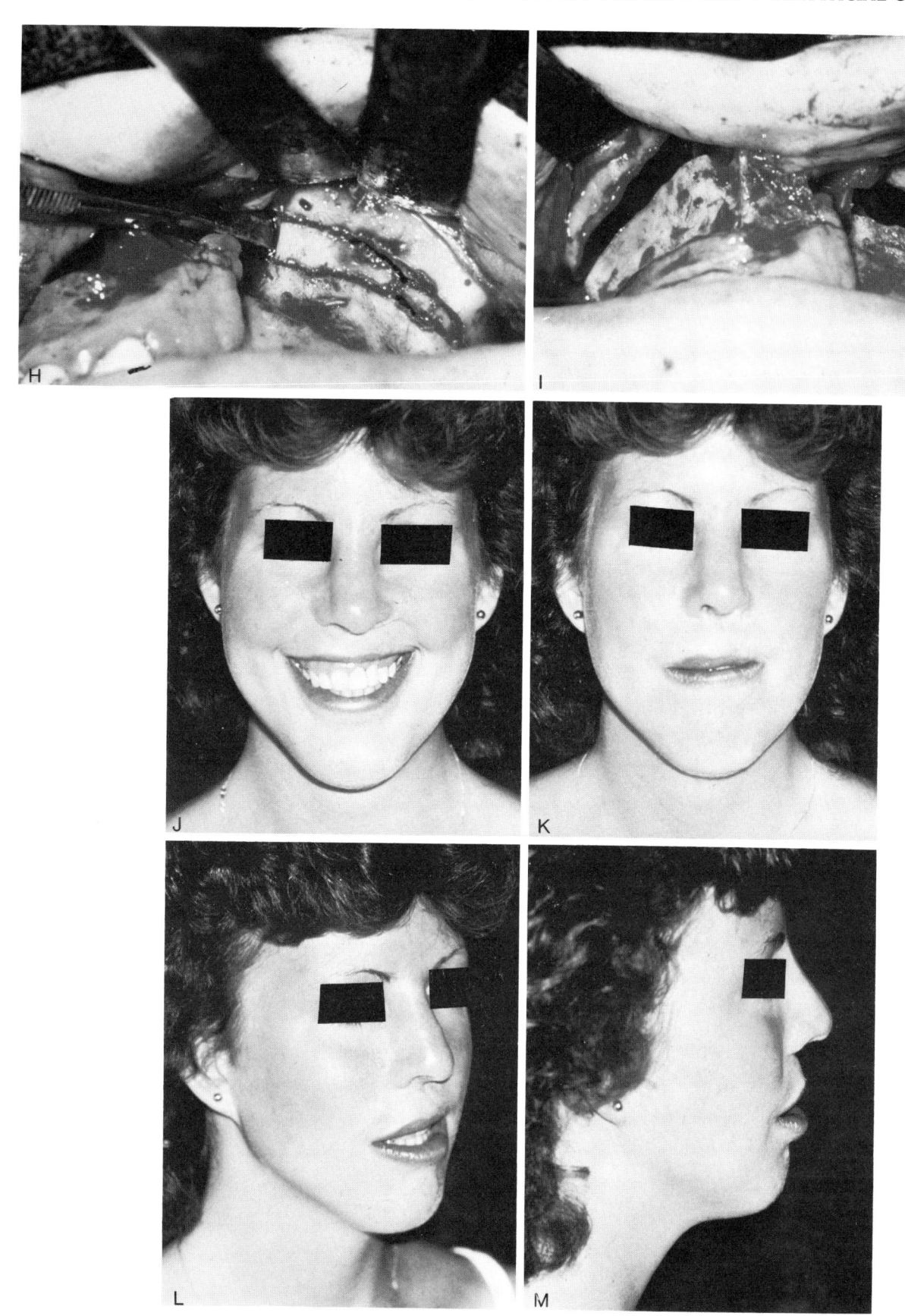

RECONSTRUCTIVE SURGERY FOR THE PATIENT WITH FACIAL CLEFTS / 467

Figure 11–28. *Continued. H,* Osteotomy performed. *I,* Ostectomy performed. *J–Q,* Appearance following maxillary osteotomy, unilateral cleft graft, and restoration with a fixed prosthesis.

Illustration continued on following page.

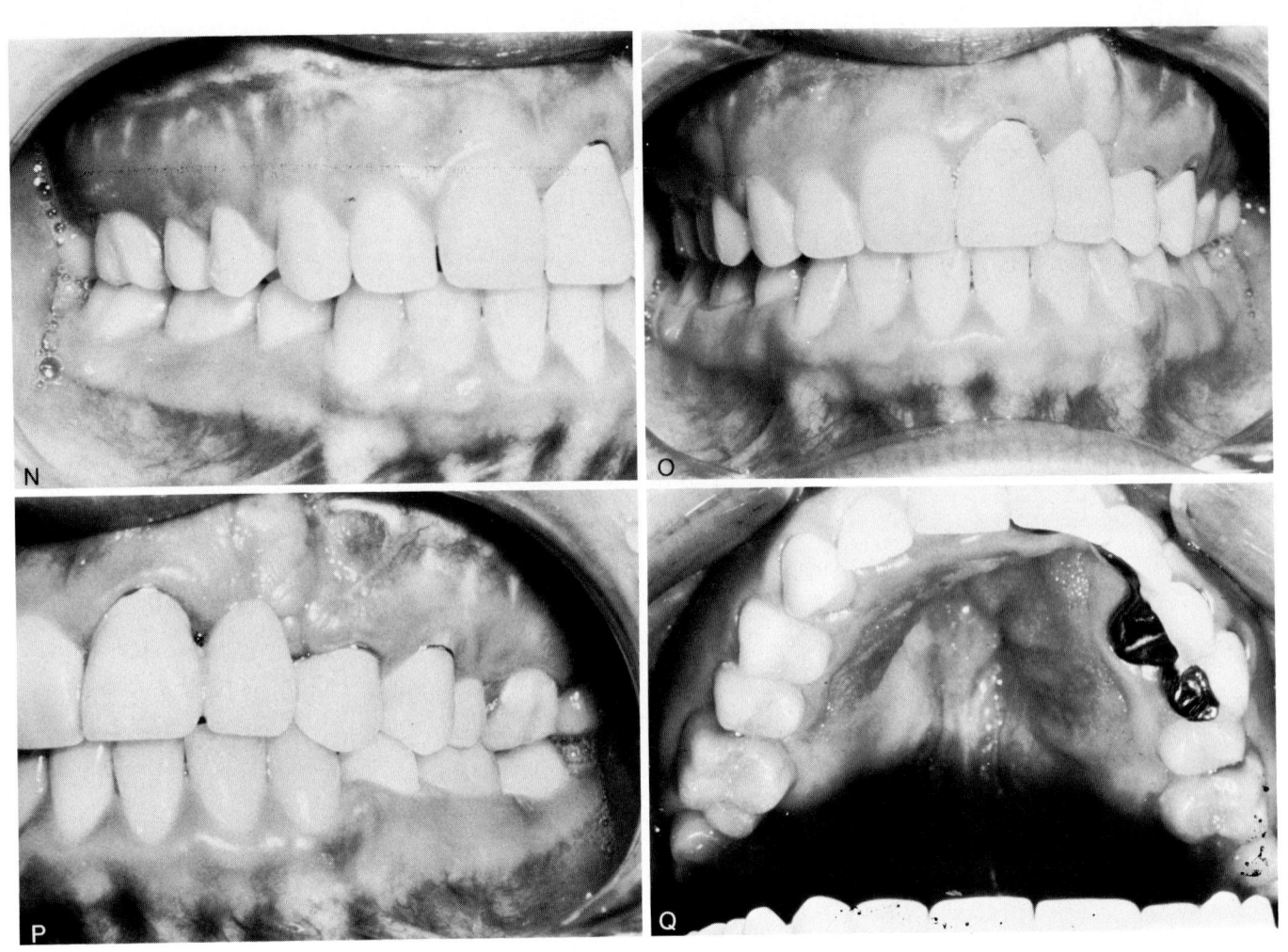

Figure 11–28. *Continued.*

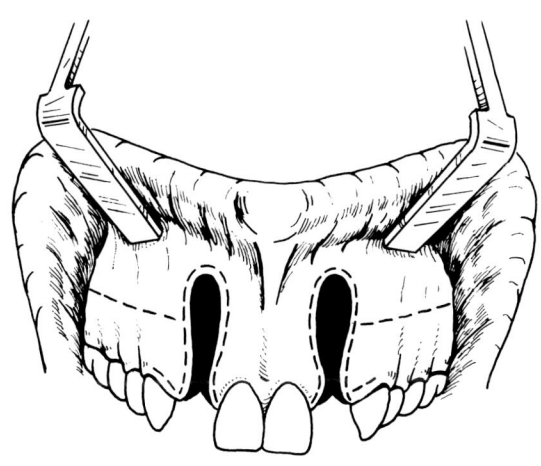

RECONSTRUCTIVE SURGERY FOR THE PATIENT WITH FACIAL CLEFTS / **469**

Figure 11–29. Outline of incision for maxillary advancement with bilateral cleft graft.

curved pterygoid osteotome is placed at the junction of the maxillary tuberosity and pterygoid plate and malleted until a separation is achieved. These procedures are then repeated on the contralateral side. The two posterior segments are then downfractured in an inferior and medial direction. If any osteotomy is necessary, it is accomplished from this downfractured position.

The mucoperiosteum is reflected from the lateral nasal walls and the nasal septum through the cleft area. This allows adequate mobilization of the maxillary segments for advancement. The vomer can be sectioned from this approach as well.

The palatal soft tissue is developed and sutured at this time (Fig. 11–30). The occlusal splint is then positioned, and maxillomandibular fixation is applied. Direct intraosseous wires are placed bilaterally in the buttress and piriform rim areas. Piriform rim suspension wires are also used as previously described.

Bone grafts (autologous cancellous iliac crest grafts taken simultaneously by a second operating team) are inserted in the cleft areas. These grafts are used to augment the osteotomy sites and to provide osseous continuity over the clefted area (Fig. 11–31). Corticocancellous blocks of bone are used to position the maxilla anteriorly by placing them between the maxillary tuberosities and

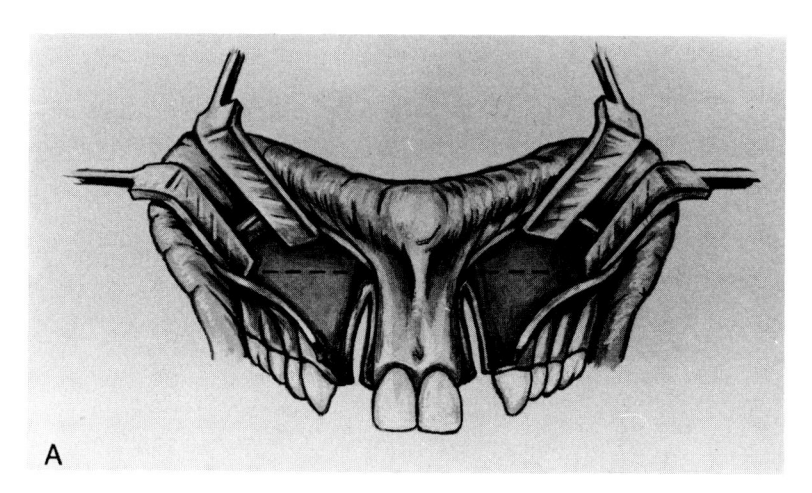

Figure 11–30. Osteotomy performed and palatal mucosa sutured.

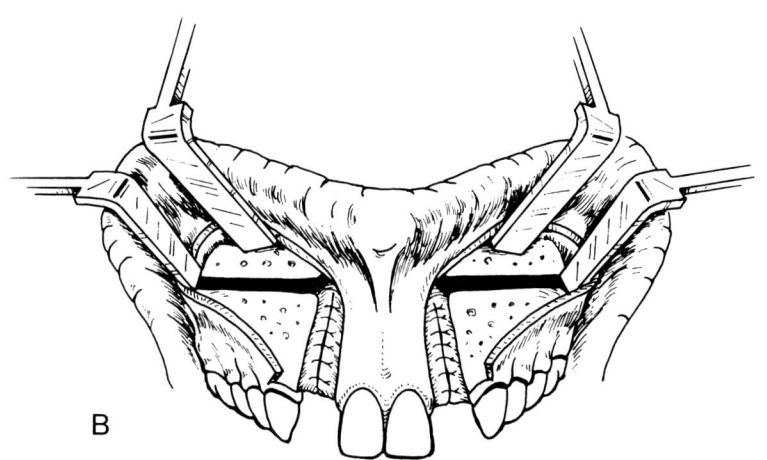

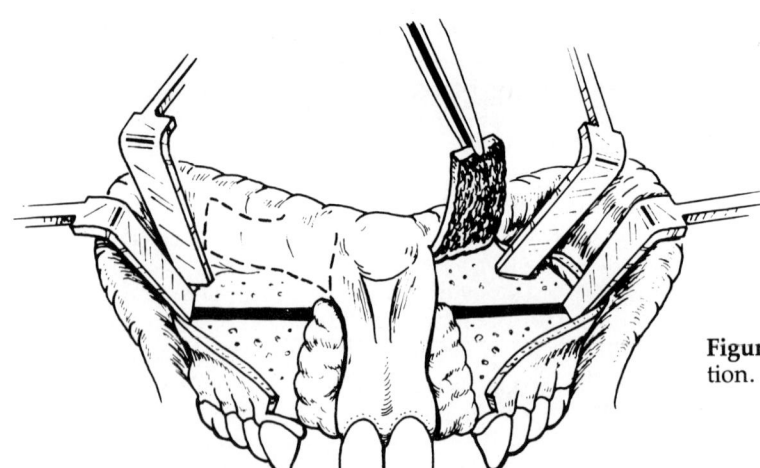

Figure 11–31. Graft of cancellous bone in position.

pterygoid plates. Labial flaps are then elevated utilizing either direct approximation of adjacent soft tissue or rotation of a labial finger flap (Figs. 11–32 to 11–34).

Simultaneous Maxillomandibular Surgery

Severe dentofacial deformities in cleft patients often require combined maxillary and mandibular osteotomies. With the improvements in hypotensive anesthetic and surgical techniques, both arches can be approached simultaneously with predictable success. The maxillary surgical techniques of simultaneous maxillary advancement with either a unilateral or bilateral cleft have been discussed in this chapter.

The sequencing of the osteotomies intraoperatively is worthy of note. If the ilium is to be used for a source of autologous bone, then two surgical teams should start the procedure simultaneously. The cancellous bone will then be available for grafting at approximately the same time it is required at the oral recipient site. The mandible should be approached first. The osteotomies, but not the split of the mandible, should be performed bilaterally. After this is complete, the maxilla is osteotomized, mobilized, and segmented. An interim splint with intermaxillary fixation is then utilized to position the maxilla in its predicted location. Intraosseous wires are then tightened, and the interim splint is removed. The sagittal split of the mandible is completed, and the final splint is inserted. Intermaxillary fixation is then applied and the proximal segments of the mandible are wired into place. Finally, all soft tissue incisions are sutured.

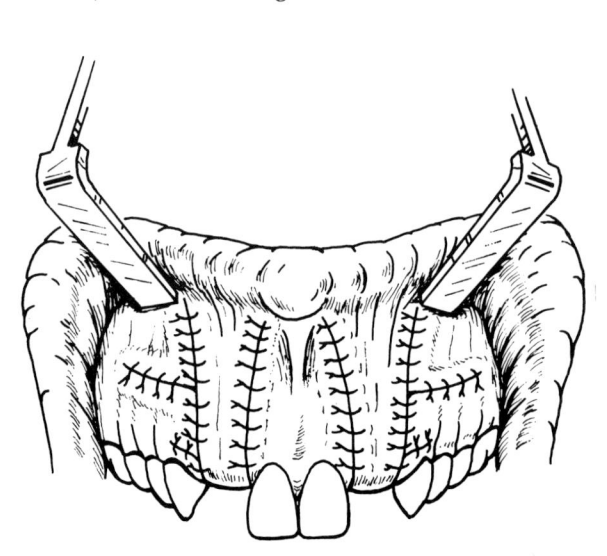

Figure 11–32. Closure with pedicle flaps.

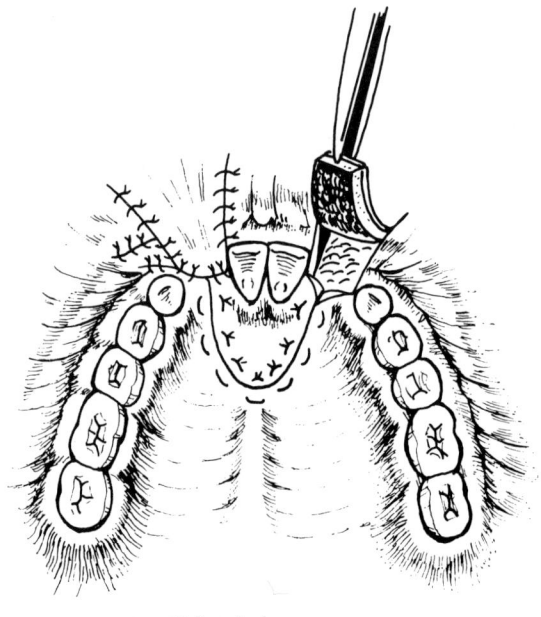

Figure 11–33. Palatal closure.

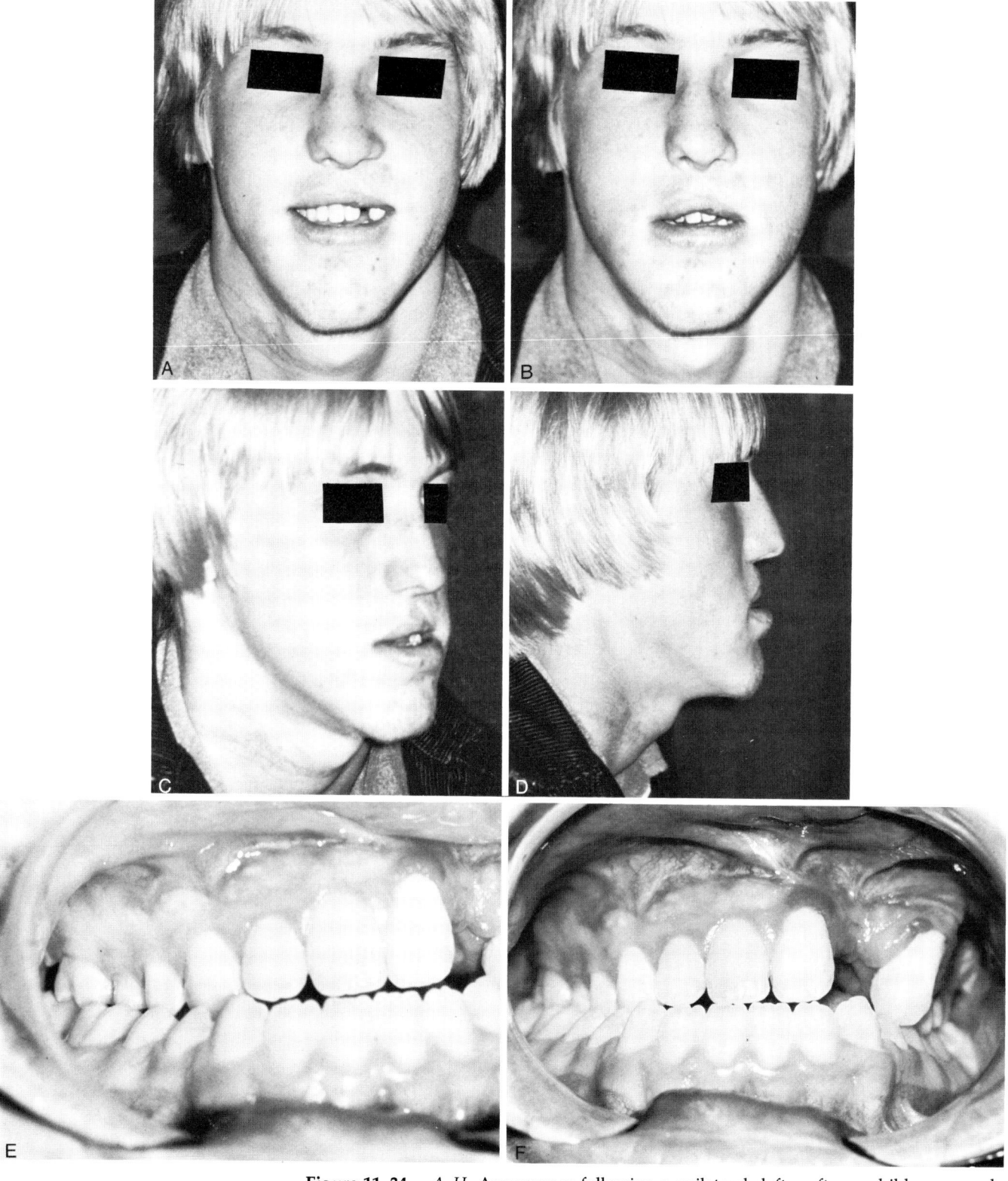

RECONSTRUCTIVE SURGERY FOR THE PATIENT WITH FACIAL CLEFTS / **471**

Figure 11–34. *A–H,* Appearance following a unilateral cleft graft as a child, now ready for maxillary and mandibular osteotomies.

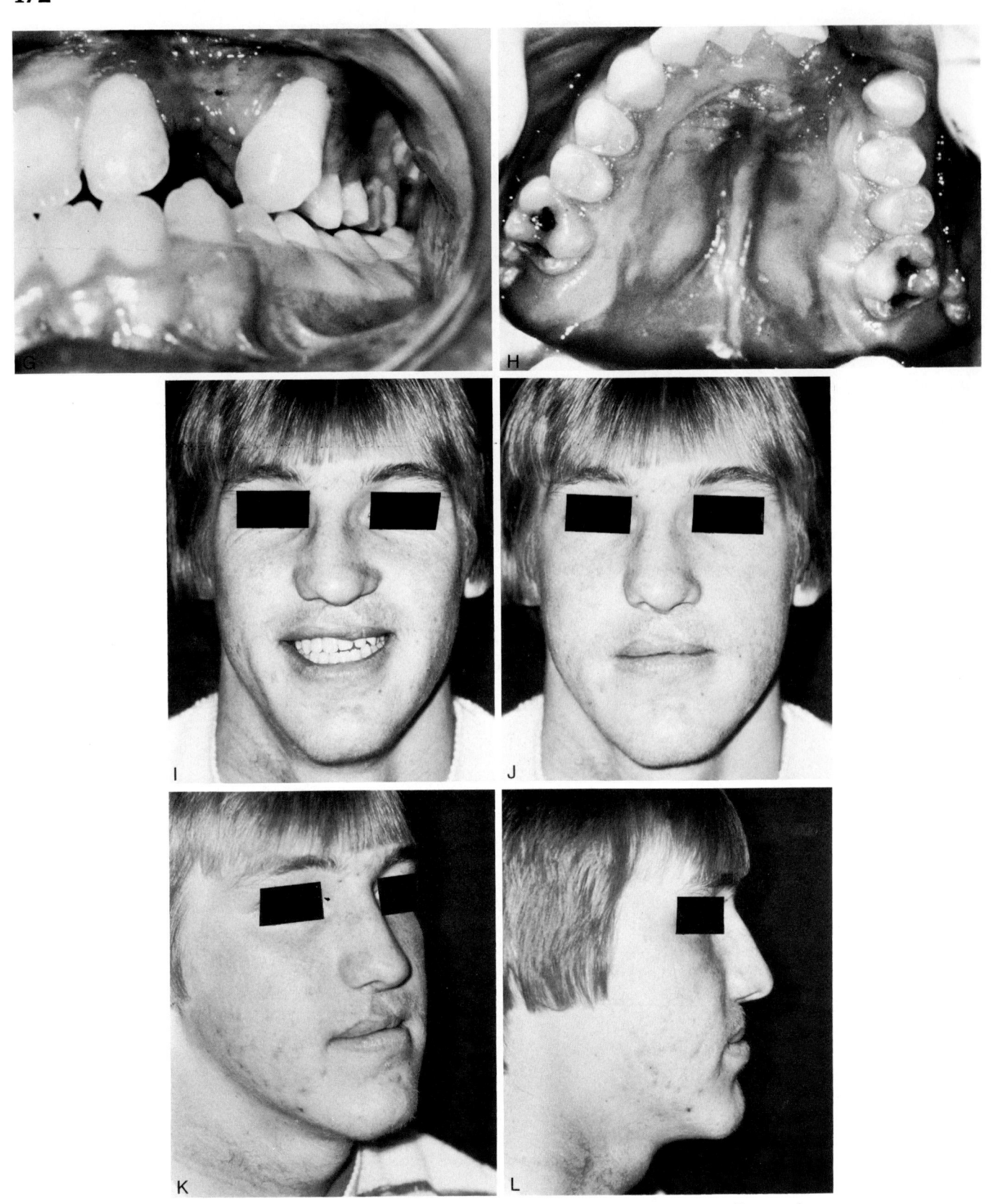

472 / RECONSTRUCTIVE SURGERY FOR THE PATIENT WITH FACIAL CLEFTS

Figure 11–34. Continued. *I–P,* Appearance following simultaneous maxillary and mandibular osteotomies.

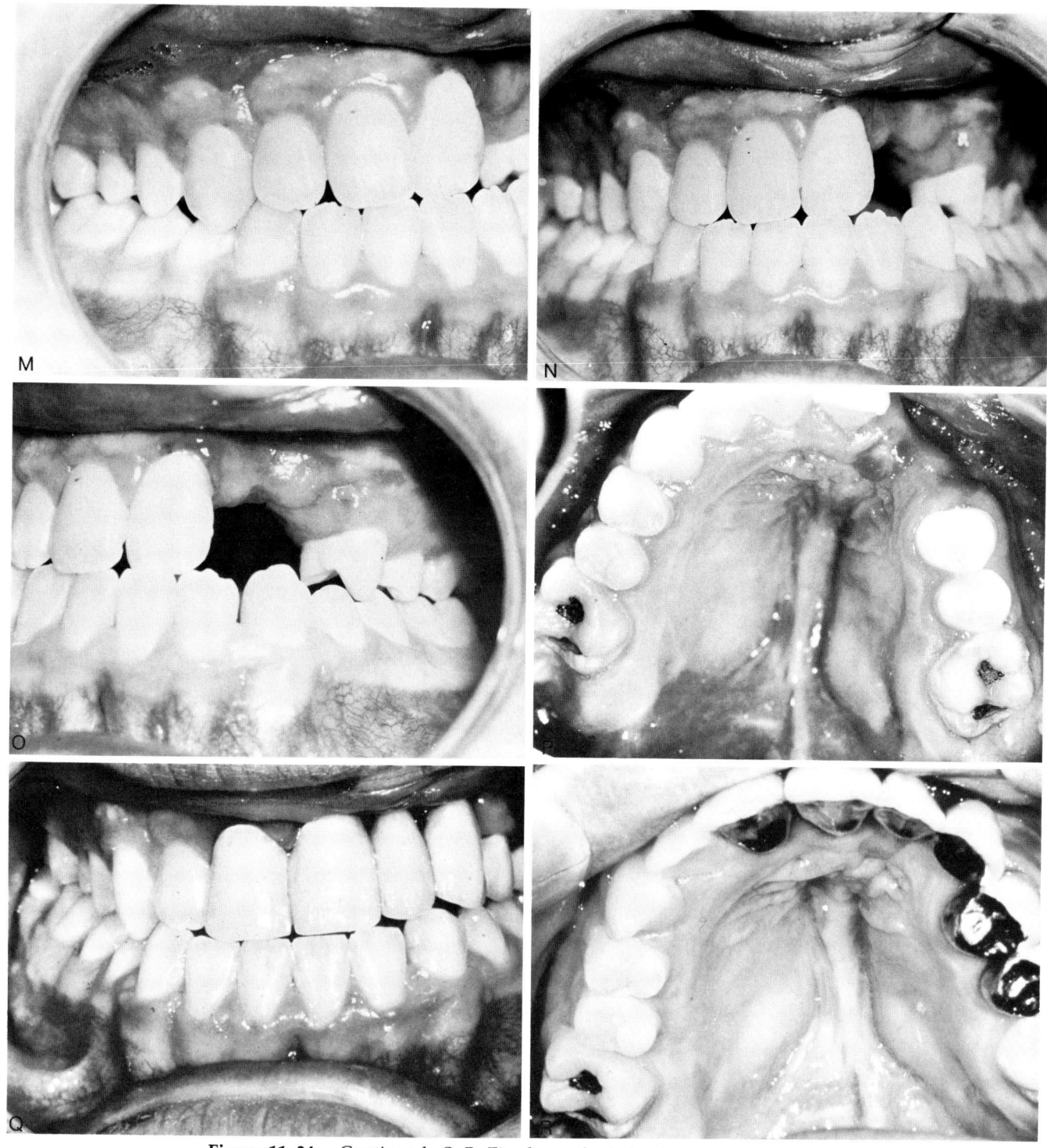

Figure 11–34. Continued. *Q–R*, Fixed prosthesis in place.

BIBLIOGRAPHY

1. Edwards M, and Watson ACH (eds): Advancements in the Management of Cleft Palate. Edinburgh, Churchill Livingstone, 1980.
2. Ross RB, and Johnston MC: Cleft Lip and Palate. Baltimore, Williams and Wilkins, 1972.
3. Bishara SE: Cephalometric evaluation of facial growth in operated and non-operated individuals with isolated clefts of the palate. Cleft Palate J 10:239, 1973.
4. Bishara SE, Krause CJ, Olin WH, Weston D, Van Ness J, and Felling C: Facial and dental relationships of individuals with unoperated clefts of the lip and/or palate. Cleft Palate J 13:238, 1976.
5. Bishara SE, Olin WH, and Krause CJ: Cephalometric findings in two cases with unrepaired bilateral cleft lip and palate. Cleft Palate J 15:233, 1978.
6. Mapes AH, Mazaheri M, Harding RL, Meier JA, and Canter HE: A longitudinal analysis of the maxillary growth increments of cleft lip and palate patients (CLP). Cleft Palate J 11:450, 1974.
7. Horowitz SL, Graf B, Bettex M, Vinkka H, and Gerstman LJ: Factor analysis of craniofacial morphology in complete bilateral cleft lip and palate. Cleft Palate J 17:234, 1980.
8. Johnson GP: Craniofacial analysis of patients with complete clefts of the lip and palate. Cleft Palate J 17:17, 1980.
9. Maue-Dickson W: The craniofacial complex in cleft lip/palate: An updated review of anatomy and function. Cleft Palate J 16:291, 1979.
10. Shibasaki Y, and Ross RB: Facial growth in children with isolated cleft palate. Cleft Palate J 6:290, 1969.
11. Vora JM, and Joshi MR: Mandibular growth in surgically repaired cleft lip and cleft palate individuals. Angle Orthod 47:304, 1977.
12. Nakamura S, Savara BS, and Thomas DR: Facial growth of children with cleft lip and/or palate. Cleft Palate J 9:119, 1972.
13. Siegel B: A racial comparison of cleft patients in a clinic population: Associated anomalies and recurrence rates. Cleft Palate J 16:193, 1979.
14. Geis N, Seto B, Bartoshesky L, Lewis MB, and Pashayan HM: The prevalence of congenital heart disease among the population of a metropolitan cleft lip and palate clinic. Cleft Palate J 18:19, 1981.
15. Maher WP: Distribution of palatal and other arteries in cleft and non-cleft human palates. Cleft Palate J 14:1, 1977.
16. Maher WP: Artery distribution in the prenatal human maxilla. Cleft Palate J 18:51, 1981.
17. Drommer R: Selective angiographic studies prior to LeFort I osteotomy in patients with cleft lip and palate. J Maxillofac Surg 7:264, 1979.
18. Tideman H, Stoelinga P, and Gallia L: LeFort I advancement with segmental palatal osteotomies in patients with cleft palates. J Oral Surg 38:196, 1980.
19. Brauer RO, and Cronin TD: Maxillary orthopedics and anterior palate repair with bone grafting. Cleft Palate J 1:31, 1964.
20. Georgiade NC, Pickrell KL, and Quinn GW: Varying concepts in bone grafting of alveolar palatal defects. Cleft Palate J 1:43, 1964.
21. Horton CE, Crawford HH, Adamson JE, Buxton S, Cooper R, and Kanter J: The prevention of maxillary collapse in congenital lip and palate cases. Cleft Palate J 1:25, 1964.
22. Boyne PJ, and Sands NR: Secondary bone grafting of residual alveolar and palatal clefts. J Oral Surg 30:87, 1972.
23. Wassmund M: Lehrbuch der praktischen Chirurgie des Mundes und der Kiefer. Bd 1. Leipzig, 1935.
24. Axhausen G: Zur Behandlung Veralteter Disloziert Geheilter Oberkieferbruche. Dtsch Zahn-Mund-Kieferhk 1:334, 1934.
25. Schuchardt K: Ein Beitrag zur chirurgischen Kieferorthopadie unter Berucksichtigung ihrer Bedeutung fur die Behandlung angeborener und erworbener Kieferdeformitaten bei Soldaten. Dtsch Zahn-Mund-Kieferhk 9:73, 1942.
26. Obwegeser HL: Surgical correction of small or retrodisplaced maxillae. The "dish-face" deformity. Plast Reconstr Surg 43:351, 1969.
27. Schendel SA, and Delaire J: Functional musculoskeletal correction of secondary unilateral cleft lip deformities: Combined lip-nose correction and LeFort I osteotomy. J Maxillofac Surg 9:108, 1981.
28. Fletcher SG, Berkowitz S, Bradley DP, Burdi AR, Koch L, and Maue-Dickson W: Cleft lip and palate research: An updated state of the art. Cleft Palate J 14:261, 1977.
29. Farhood VW, Ryan DE, and Johnson RP: A modified approach to the ilium to obtain graft material. J Oral Surg 36:784, 1978.
30. Mrazik J, Amato C, Leban S, and Mashberg A: The ilium as a source of autogeneous bone for grafting: Clinical considerations. J Oral Surg 38:29, 1980.
31. Marx RE, Snyder RM, and Kline SN: Cellular survival of human marrow during placement of marrow-cancellous bone grafts. J Oral Surg 37:712, 1979.

# 12

RECONSTRUCTIVE ORAL AND MAXILLOFACIAL SURGERY FOR THE TOTALLY AND PARTIALLY EDENTULOUS PATIENT WITH DENTOFACIAL AND DENTOALVEOLAR DEFORMITIES

David E. Frost, D.D.S., M.S.,*
Raymond J. Foneseca, D.M.D.,
and Timothy A. Turvey, D.D.S.

The advances of restorative and preventive dentistry over the past 30 years have greatly increased the life expectancy of the dentition, although there are an estimated 25 to 30 million edentulous adults in the United States. Estimates suggest that 5 per cent of the American population are severely handicapped with dentofacial deformities, indicating that a large group of patients must exist with developmental malrelationships of the jaws that are not correctable by conventional prosthetic management. This large group of patients, excluded from the atrophic group (see Chapter 6 for their treatment), could greatly benefit from reconstructive oral and maxillofacial procedures.

Rehabilitation of these patients has been relegated to compromised prosthetic care for many years by the limitations of the prosthesis itself. Frequently the rehabilitation is limited because of unrecognized, undiagnosed, or untreated dentofacial and dentoalveolar deformities. The prosthetic esthetic result will be improved, the management of the edentulous state made easier, and the overall prosthetic function improved if the proper jaw relations are established through surgical positioning of the underlying bony base.

Functional and esthetic rehabilitation of the edentulous patient with a dentofacial deformity has some differences from the management of a patient with teeth having a similar deformity. Volumes of literature exist which discuss diagnosis, treatment planning, and surgical approaches to these patients.[1, 2] There are subtle differences in surgical techniques which will be discussed with each procedure. The major problem in treatment of these patients arises in the diagnosis and treatment planning for the total correction. Unlike the dentate patient, soft tissue position, jaw position, lip-tooth relations, and cephalometric norms are of little

---

*Dr. David E. Frost's contribution to this chapter, including illustrations, has been published with the permission of the United States Air Force.

475

value, or are misleading, in the edentulous patient, unless proper jaw position and vertical relations are established. The conventional data base established in orthognathic surgical management of the dentofacial deformity is of little overall value for the edentulous patient.

TOTALLY EDENTULOUS PATIENT

Diagnosis and Treatment Planning

A determination of the patient's desires and expectations from treatment is critical for planning treatment, and this should be done at the initial visit. It is imperative that the surgical team member as well as the prosthetic member be involved in the initial evaluation and in each step of the treatment plan. As has been seen recently in dentofacial and craniofacial deformity corrections, team communication and understanding of the limitations of each specialty are the largest areas of treatment breakdown.

Treatment plans require consideration of alveolar atrophy and prosthetic management (see Chapters 3 and 6) as well as jaw malrelations. Intregrated management with a prosthodontist or restorative dentist is necessary to evaluate and plan sequentially for all ramifications of the deformity. Not infrequently a diagnostic mounting will be necessary to fully evaluate the skeletal malrelationships in three dimensions. This is best accomplished by the prosthodontist. While fabrication of occlusal rims, face-bow transfer records, and centric relation mountings for the edentulous patient is not technically difficult, experience in these procedures is a definite aid. The prosthodontist is the best suited member of the health care team for this task. The mounted casts can be evaluated much like a mounted set of dentate models. The complete evaluation will be discussed further in this chapter.

Radiographic analysis should consist of a lateral cephalogram, made with a maxillary occlusal rim in place, and a panoramic radiograph. Other specialized radiographs may be required for specific indications in selected individuals (i.e., posteroanterior cephalogram in asymmetry cases). The use of properly fabricated occlusal rims will give proper support to the lips with the jaws in their pretreatment position as well as eliminate some of the pseudoskeletal malrelationships that may develop secondary to overclosure of the mandible.

Evaluation of the skeletal relationships from the radiographs will be somewhat more difficult than in the usual orthognathic case. However, the overlying soft tissue evaluation will be nearer to the patient's normal with teeth if the occlusal rims are in place and the radiographs are made with the proper vertical relationships. Although no extensive tables of cephalometric norms exist for edentulous patients, they would be of less overall value than the norms for dentate patients.[3-5] The continued dynamic state of resorption that exists in these patients would make the values vary appreciably. However, the soft tissue profile and basic bony landmarks give ideas as to the type of deformity that exists apart from the resorption and atrophy.

Facial evaluation of the patient should be conducted with the jaw held in the proper vertical position. In general, patients should be evaluated from the full face and profile positions. Proportions of the facial thirds, balance of facial thirds and asymmetry should be noted. The prosthodontist will be able to aid in determination of lip support expected by a prosthesis, the amount of vertical change possible with a prosthesis, and acceptability of minor jaw malpositions. It should be remembered with the totally edentulous patient that a degree of freedom exists that is not normally present in the dentate patient. Therefore a slight malrelationship, usually secondary to resorption, may be acceptable prosthetically. This final determination, as well as final positioning of the jaws, rests with the well-informed restorative dentist or prosthodontist.

Determination of the anteroposterior position of the prosthetic teeth will aid in determining anteroposterior position of the maxilla and mandible. Mavroskoufis and Ritchie[6] have postulated that this position is 10.2 mm anterior to the middle of the incisive papilla. There is disagreement as to this figure, however; Morrow et al.[7] find this distance to vary from 5 to 7 mm, depending upon tooth form. For treatment planning and prediction tracing purposes, 8 mm has been found to be a workable distance.

Surgical Procedures

Maxillary Deficiency—Vertical

This problem and its treatment are discussed in Chapter 6.

Maxillary Deficiency—Anteroposterior

Masking prosthetic procedures, such as addition to the maxillary anterior denture flange, have a definite limit to their usefulness. This procedure can be used to correct the minimally deficient maxilla or the maxilla that is posteriorly positioned minimally and secondary to atrophy. The true skeletal hypoplasia should be approached at the appropriate level with an osteotomy of the type used for dentate patients with similar dentofacial deformities.[1]

Specific refinements of the LeFort I total maxillary osteotomy are appropriate for the totally edentulous patient. These would include incision position, grafting for stabilization, splint fabrication, and others.

The surgical incision can be placed somewhat lower to avoid a scar at the depth of the vestibule which may interfere with adequate prosthetic rehabilitation. It is important to remember when placing the incision that if a splint is necessary to stabilize the jaws, as in a two-jaw procedure, the flange of the splint may interfere with suturing if the incision is too low. While fabricating the splint, it is advisable to keep the flange as short as possible while still maintaining stability.

Stabilization of the anteriorly placed maxilla is made easier and more stable with bone grafts to the pterygoid fissure or with a modification of the LeFort I osteotomy at the buttress region[8] (Fig. 12–1). The modification allows for a change in the bone cut to allow for grafting in a more anterior and readily examinable position. Grafting can successfully stabilize the maxilla. Currently allogeneic bone is readily available, is biologically acceptable, and is stable without requiring a second operative site.[9, 10] However, autologous bone is equally acceptable and could make consolidation more rapid. Future material, such as block hydroxyapatite, is a possible alternative as well.

The usual technique of transosseous wiring at the buttress and pyriform region will generally suffice to stabilize an edentulous maxilla. Frequently the bone is so thin in the atrophic patient that a horizontal mattress wire of double light gauge wire may decrease the chance of pulling through the bone. Minibone plates adequately stabilize the dentate maxilla, but their usefulness in the edentulous patient is decreased owing to the possible interference with the flange of the final prosthesis.

If a stent is utilized to position the maxilla, it can also be used to place the patient into maxillomandibular fixation. While this is not usually necessary in a single jaw operation to the maxilla, it may be necessary in a combined jaw case. If so, stabilization of the stent can be accomplished with either a midpalatal screw, circumzygomatic wires to

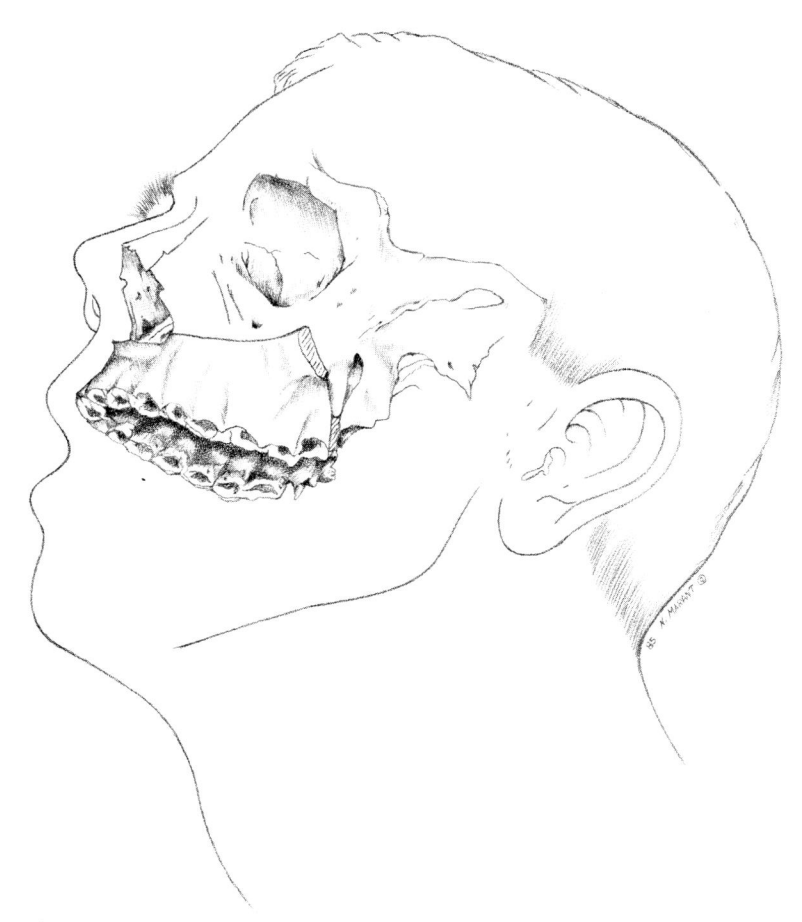

Figure 12–1. Modification of the LeFort I osteotomy cuts to allow for block graft at the buttress area.

the stent, infraorbital wires to the stent, peralveolar wires or pins, or transnasal wires. All techniques have been used successfully.

Maxillary Excess—Anteroposterior

Esthetics and function are best served by bony removal or repositioning to eliminate the oversupported, protruding upper lip associated with maxillary excess. The simplified approach to remove the anterior facial flange of the prosthesis does little to decrease the lip prominence and may make denture stability and retention unacceptable.

Anterior alveoloplasty is used to reduce mild maxillary excess. Collapsing the facial cortical plate after removal of intraseptal bone or more radical alveoloplasties have been suggested, but the increased rate of resorption associated with these techniques makes their advisability questionable.

Biologically sound techniques, such as segmental maxillary osteotomies, have been used for decades to treat dentate patients.[1] They were advocated as an approach to maxillary sagittal excess by West and Burk.[11] This technique does not sacrifice the anterior alveolar bone or invade the cortical plate, which might speed the resorptive process. An acceptable esthetic and functional result can be predictably achieved. The surgical approach is similar to that in dentate patients. Rarely would a fixation appliance be necessary. A surgical stent will aid in securing the proper position of the alveolus, much as an interocclusal splint would help key the position of a dentate segmental osteotomy. Placement of incisions that might interfere with prosthetic care should be considered, and efforts to avoid a vestibular incision should be made.

Mandibular Excess—Anteroposterior

The procedure of choice for the totally edentulous patient with mandibular sagittal excess is the transoral vertical ramus osteotomy. The intra-oral sagittal split osteotomy, although very useful in dentate patients, has the drawback of the placement of the anterior lateral DalPont osteotomy. Frequently, the mandible in the edentulous patient is very thin in this area and the amount of bony interface after the osteotomy is unsatisfactory. This is especially so if there has been a degree of proximal segment rotation. Also, as the mandible is positioned posteriorly, the anterior superior aspect of the DalPont modification should be trimmed so that there is no interference with the denture flange postoperatively. A short DalPont extension is recommended if the sagittal split osteotomy is to be used to correct this deformity in the edentulous atrophic mandible.

Advantages of the transoral vertical ramus osteotomy are relative ease, less potential danger to the inferior alveolar neurovascular bundle, and a more favorable position of the proximal segment for prosthetic follow-up or care. The disadvantages include the potential for condylar sag and clockwise rotation of the mandibular distal segment. These problems are admittedly minimal in the dentate patient and become less so in the edentulous patient.

The surgical procedure consists of a soft tissue incision over the external oblique ridge from midway on the anterior border of the ascending ramus to the region where the mandibular second molar was previously located. A subperiosteal reflection of the lateral and posterior border of the mandible is accomplished. A J-periosteal elevator is introduced on the lateral aspect of the mandible to strip the attachment of the medial pterygoid. The sigmoid notch is identified and appropriate retractors are placed. Then, with the use of an oscillating saw, a vertical osteotomy is performed from the depth of the sigmoid notch to the angle of the mandible (Fig. 12–2). If preferred, an inverted L-osteotomy may be used (Fig. 12–3). Either technique will allow for the sliding of the distal segment within the proximal segments, shortening the functional length of the mandible in the sagittal plane by the desired amount. Before stabilizing the segments, the proximal segment is distracted and the medial pterygoid is stripped completely from this and the distal segment.

The desired intermaxillary fixation is applied and then the proximal segment is positioned in the fossa passively. A wire is passed so that it will passively position the condyle in the fossa while maintaining the proximal segment adapted to the mandibular ramus (Fig. 12–4).

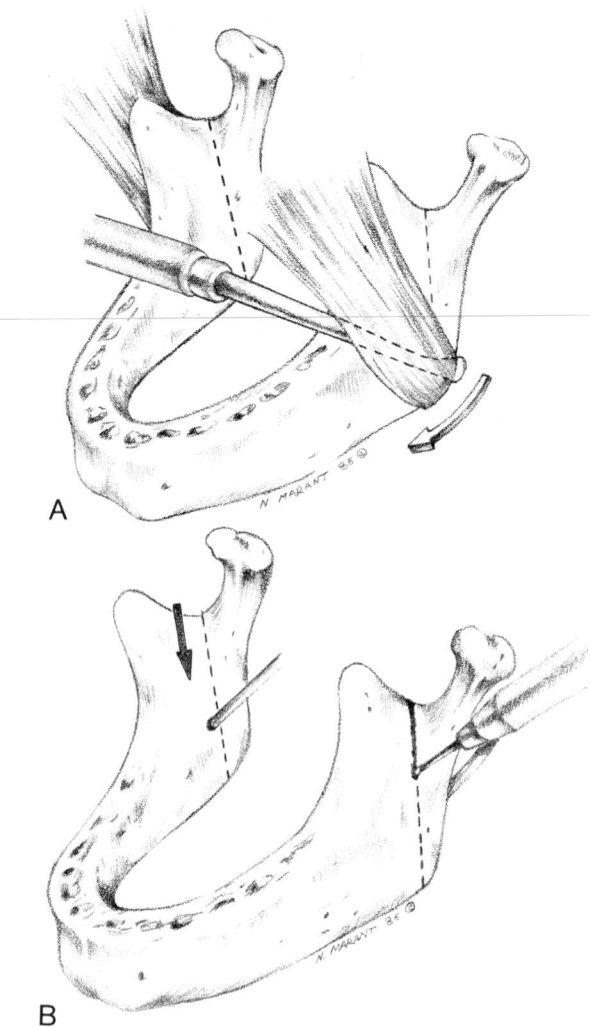

Figure 12–2. *A*, J-periosteal elevator to release muscle attachment. *B*, Transoral vertical ramus osteotomy for mandibular posterior repositioning.

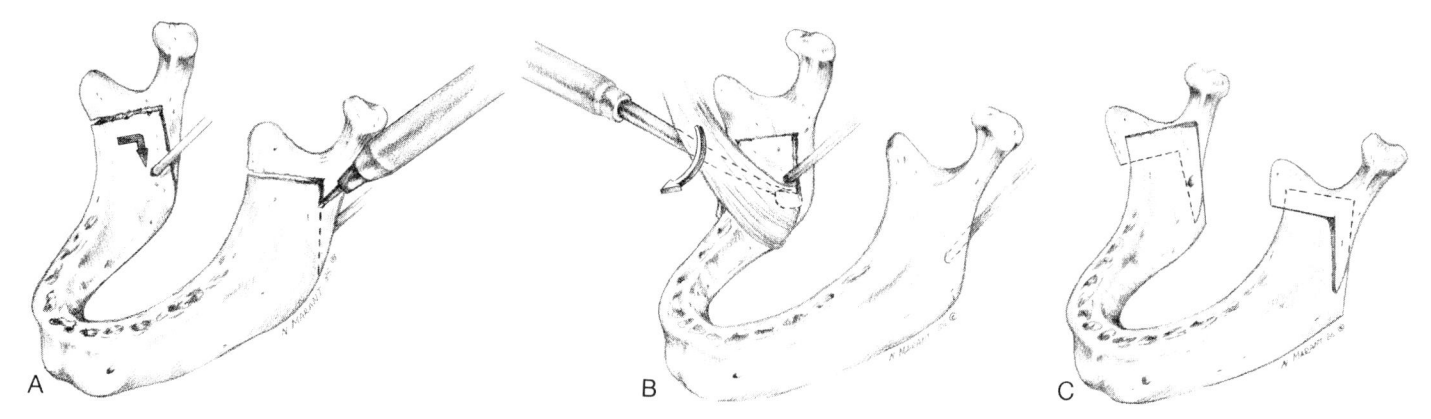

Figure 12–3. *A*, Inverted L-osteotomy. *B*, J-periosteal elevator to release sling for posterior repositioning. *C*, Overlap of inverted L-osteostomy.

An alternative technique of stabilization would be to use a lag screw system. This system requires decortication of the medial aspect of the proximal segment, allowing this segment to rest passively against the ramus without undue torque on the condyle. Then using standard techniques for placement of lag screws, the proximal segment can be screwed to the distal segment, eliminating the need for maxillomandibular fixation (Fig. 12–5).

Closure in standard fashion is performed and prosthetic care can be accomplished approximately four to six weeks later. If Gunning type splints are required, maxillomandibular fixation should be maintained for at least six weeks and followed by a period of muscular rehabilitation prior to definitive prosthetic care.

Mandibular Deficiency—Anteroposterior

The standard of care for treatment of patients with the dentofacial deformity of mandibular sagittal deficiency has become the intra-oral sagittal split ramus osteotomy with one of its many modifications.

The procedure remains essentially the same for the totally edentulous patient and is described in a number of publications.[12-17] To accommodate prosthetic care, the incision is made more lateral than usual, decreasing the chance of a scar band under the prosthesis. This mucoperiosteal incision is made halfway up the ascending ramus along the external oblique ridge to the level of the first or second molar. The lateral dissection is

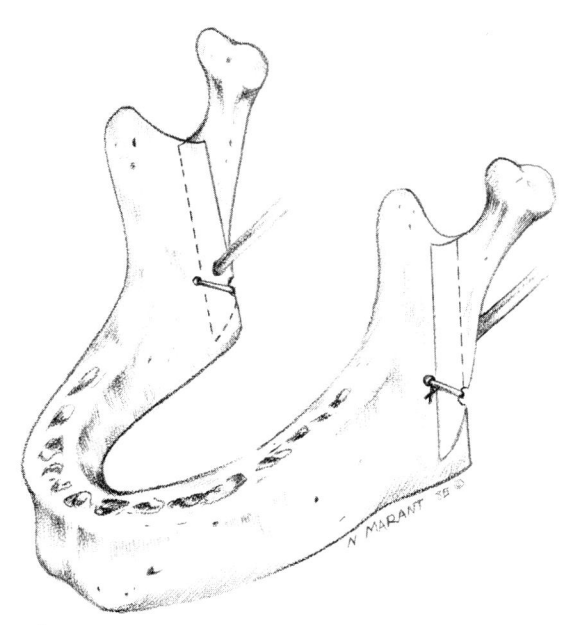

Figure 12–4. Wire placement to aid in securing the proximal segment of the transoral vertical ramus osteotomy.

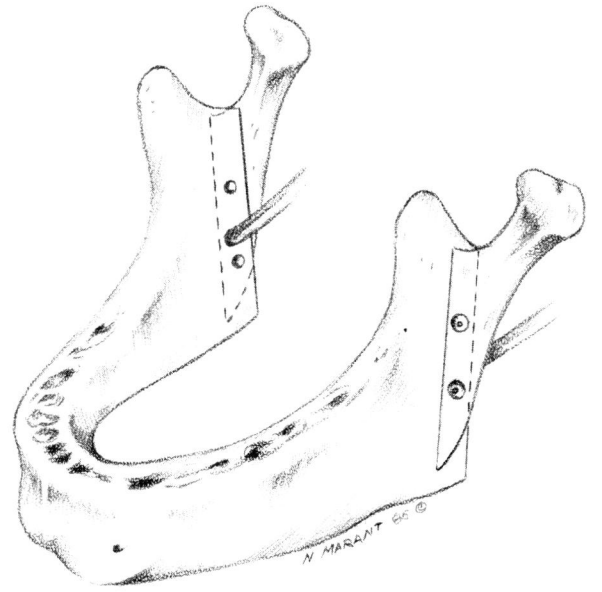

Figure 12–5. Lag screws for stabilization of the proximal segment in transoral vertical ramus osteotomy.

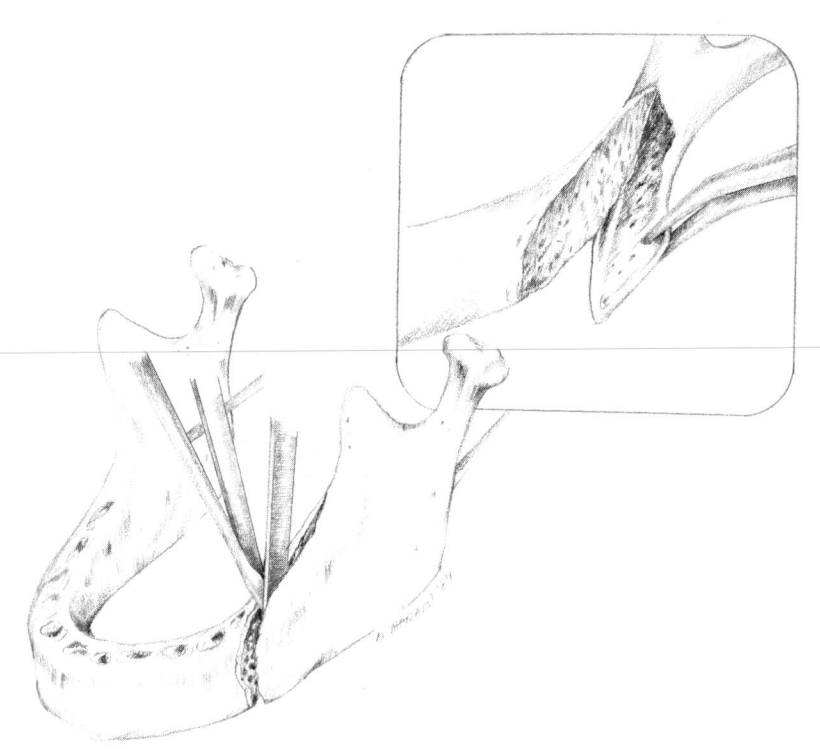

Figure 12–6. Sagittal split osteotomy, with split being completed with multiple spatula osteotomes.

done subperiosteally to the antigonial notch, and the mucoperiosteum is reflected superiorly until the coronoid process and the sigmoid notch are identified and exposed. The sigmoid notch is exposed medially. A retractor is placed above the lingula and subperiosteally so as to protect the neurovascular bundle.

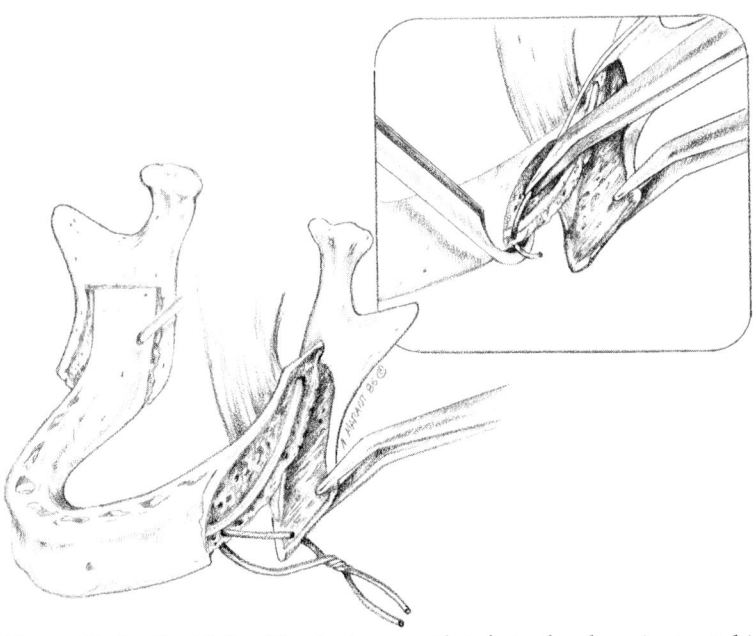

Figure 12–7. Sagittal split osteotomy with inferior border wire to stabilize and secure the proximal segment.

The bone cuts begin with a horizontal osteotomy of the medial aspect of the mandible approximately halfway between the lingula and the sigmoid notch. The bone cut is carried only through the medial cortical plate. No attempt is made to carry this cut to the posterior border of the mandible. Next the bone cut is carried down to the lateral aspect of the mandible where it is changed to a vertical osteotomy and is extended to the inferior border. These cuts are also carried only through the cortex; however, at the inferior border it should be carried completely through the inferior cortex.

The split is started by gradually splitting the lateral cortex from the medial cortex and cancellous portion of the mandible, using small cutting osteotomes. The osteotomes can be used to gradually torque the segments open, sequentially increasing in size (Fig. 12–6). Care is taken to identify the neurovascular bundle (NVB) within the split at this time. Once the NVB has been identified, the larger osteotome can be inserted below the NVB and greater torque applied to complete the sagittal split. The J-periosteal elevator is then introduced between the bone segments, and the medial pterygoid muscle fibers are completely stripped off the distal segment of the mandible.

Stabilization of the segments can be achieved in any one of many ways. A set of previously prepared Gunning splints that are indexed to the desired new position of the mandible can be placed and temporary intermaxillary fixation is placed. A channel retractor (Fig. 12–7) is then introduced between the segments and hooked under the inferior border of the distal segment. A bur hole is placed below the NVB and into the channel retractor. Then a 25-gauge stainless steel wire is passed into the hole and into the retractor's curve. This will cause the wire to curve facially and then be retrieved. Another hole is placed low in the proximal segment and anterior to the distal segment wire. This will allow for a distal vector of force on the condylar segment, assuring that it is seated in the fossa as well as preventing any "kick-up" of the proximal segment. An added advantage of this inferior border wire is that it will not interfere with prosthetic rehabilitation. The wires are then tightened together, cut short, and twisted to bone.[12]

The incision is closed in a single layer and routine postoperative care is completed. Closure with an over-and-over suture will not cause as much wound edge eversion, is easier than the often recommended horizontal mattress, and will leave less scar band in the area of the prosthesis periphery. If this technique is utilized, the Gunning splints with intermaxillary fixation must be maintained for a minimum of eight weeks. The prosthetic Gunning splints should be made with the lateral border short so that they will not interfere with suturing of the incision. After the eight weeks of intermaxillary fixation, muscle rehabilitation is done for approximately four weeks and then prosthetic care may begin.[18]

An alternative exists to intermaxillary fixation. This consists of stabilization of the mandible with lag screws. Advantages of this technique are rapid mobilization, which, in the older patient, might be of advantage in muscle rehabilitation, more rapid prosthetic rehabilitation, and direct positive stabilization. Finally, the fixation screws are away from the stress-bearing area, as would be an inferior border wire.

Disadvantages include the need for a small skin incision and the slightly increased danger to the facial nerve, possible compression of the inferior alveolar nerve, and positive placement of the condyle in the final position. This latter drawback allows for no "settling" of the condyle. This is a potential problem in the dentate patient. In the totally edentulous, no such critical "settling" occurs. The compression to the inferior alveolar nerve has not been seen to be a problem, and the scar and danger to the facial nerve are minimal.

Surgical placement of the lag screws begins after the sagittal split is completed (Fig. 12-8). The NVB is completely freed if visible, and all bone spicules are removed from the inner aspects of both segments. This is necessary to prevent any possible damage due to the positive seating effect the lag screws will have. The mandible is then advanced to the predetermined position utilizing the Gunning splints. The proximal segments are positively pushed up and back into the fossa and a large bone clamp is placed along the anterior ascending ramus, over both the medial and lateral segments.

A stab incision is made over the lateral aspect of the mandible. The dissection is carried through the facial tissues in a blunt fashion, and a bur guide is introduced. Using a Smedburg drill, the first hole is drilled, placing it above the NVB and through both cortical plates. The hole is drilled again with the next larger bur but this time only through the lateral cortex. This is followed by a hand tap to prepare the hole for the screw. The tap is sized for the medial (smaller) hole and the screw length is determined and introduced through the skin. It is tightened completely. Two other screws are introduced in a similar fashion, with care being taken to avoid the NVB. Closure of the oral and skin wound is completed in the usual fashion, the stents are removed, and the patient is allowed to function. Prosthetic fabrication can begin at approximately six weeks after removal of intermaxillary fixation.

Although there are other procedures that may be applied to the surgical correction of dentofacial deformities in the edentulous patient, the LeFort I, transoral vertical ramus, and intra-oral sagittal split osteotomies are usually the ideal procedures for these patients. The interested surgeon who finds an unusual problem should refer to one of the numerous standard orthognathic surgery textbooks for the variations and alternatives to treatment.[1,2]

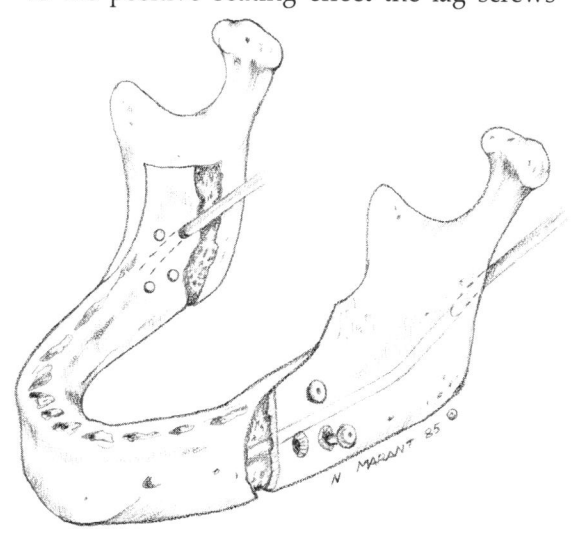

Figure 12-8. Sagittal split osteotomy stabilized with lag screws. Biocortical screws can be used as well.

Combined Jaw Surgery

Patients with deformities involving both arches frequently require simultaneous maxillary and mandibular surgery. The surgical techniques required to obtain a correction of these deformities have been previously described.

The preoperative evaluation should include an assessment of the patient in all three planes of space; sagittal, transverse, and vertical. As previously mentioned, centric relation mountings with occlusal rims and a proper vertical dimension are necessary to determine the amount and direction of movement anticipated prior to surgery.

Intraoperatively, the sequencing of the various procedures should be identical to that for a dentate patient requiring combined arch surgery, making sure not to lose a frame of reference. Stabilization of the patient requires skeletal fixation (circummandibular pyriform aperture and buttress wires are usually adequate).

PARTIALLY DENTATE PATIENTS

Diagnosis and Treatment Planning

The partially dentate patient presents many interesting problems for the reconstructive surgeon. As has been discussed in the previous section, a cooperative team approach is in order when dealing with these patients. However, in these cases the team expands from the restorative specialist and surgeon to include orthodontist, periodontist, and endodontist, if needed. These patients require multifaceted surgical procedures to totally rehabilitate them. They need good treatment plans with rational and objective approaches to the areas of rehabilitation. Therefore, the restorative dentist/prosthodontist should have primary management of the patient and should be closely involved in the surgical and orthodontic planning.

A conservative approach to maxillofacial surgery with an aggressive approach to selective tooth removal is desirable in these patients. Periodontal evaluation and therapy are first performed along with extraction of hopeless teeth. Maintenance dentistry follows, and a final prosthodontic treatment plan should be developed during this period.

The time involved in this phase enables the team to further evaluate patient motivation. Because of proven dental neglect by the majority of these patients, this is a necessary procedure. It would be a disservice to the patient to enter into a lengthy, costly, and elaborate treatment plan that is doomed to failure because of poor hygiene and patient motivation.

Orthodontic care to align teeth and preparation for segmental surgery are then performed. Continued periodontal evaluation is carried out, and a final decision about each tooth is made.

Facial esthetics and cephalometric evaluation are performed as usual for any patient with a dentofacial deformity. Routine dentofacial deformities are handled as appropriate for their deformity and as described in a number of other texts.[1] This generally includes anteroposterior, vertical, and transverse disharmonies of the total jaws. Localized segmental problems will be discussed below.

A final prosthetic surgical treatment plan is developed. This will include decisions about vertical supereruption of posterior teeth, anterior maxillary vertical excess, excessively tipped segments of the maxilla or mandible, as well as individual tooth positions that may be more effectively handled surgically than orthodontically.

In general, it is advisable not to attempt surgical procedures for problems that would normally be corrected orthodontically. In particular this would include closure of diastemas, rotational procedures, and uprighting of individual teeth. Conventional orthodontics can easily manage the majority of these procedures without requiring surgery or endangering an already compromised dentition.

The wide variations in individual treatment possibilities make total discussion of all possible segmental surgical procedures impossible. Therefore, the interested clinician with an unusual problem is referred to the standard orthognathic surgical texts for ideas. It is important to realize that within the broad confines of good surgical techniques, many possible solutions exist for the patient with dentofacial and dentoalveolar deformities requiring surgical preparation prior to prosthetic care.

Surgical Considerations

When planning surgery for the partially edentulous patient, general principles of orthognathic reconstruction should be applied for good results. Flap design should permit maximum blood perfusion through the segments. Segments should be moved within biologic reason and without significant torquing. Attention to soft tissue flaps during surgery is critical, and all means should be taken to assure that flaps are not strangulated by the movement of the segments. In general, segments should be stabilized with wires and splints. Intermaxillary fixation may also be necessary for immobilization, depending on the type of movement that has occurred.

Splint design is another critical factor. We prefer an occlusal index that is thin and away from the gingival tissues. This allows for accurate repositioning of segments at surgery, stabilization of segments postsurgically, and maintenance of good hygiene while the splint is worn. It does not require the strength or rigidity of a partial denture and should be designed accordingly. Tissue-bearing splints should be avoided except in posterior edentulous areas that have opposing teeth. In these situations, it is best to have the splint in contact with the opposing ridge tissue to maintain the inter-ridge height. Lingual or palatal flanges should not be used because they may potentially interfere with blood perfusion through dento-osseous segments. They should also be kept away from the incisions.

After the segmental surgery is completed and adequate healing time has elapsed, the final extractions, necessary tooth preparation, and fixed partial and removable partial or overlay prosthetic replacement can be completed. Where possible, all but hopeless teeth are left until this stage. This enables the surgeon to utilize these teeth for stabilization and immobilization.

POSTSURGICAL MANAGEMENT

Patients are given intravenous antibiotics and steroids at the time of surgery and are maintained on them until discontinuance of the I.V. Oral antibiotics are usually continued for 7 to 10 days. Topical and systemic decongestants are frequently used postsurgically, especially when maxillary osteotomies have been performed. These drugs reduce secretions and help maintain the patency of the airway.

Diet becomes a critical factor for many of these patients. If intermaxillary fixation is applied, high-protein liquids must be consumed. Otherwise, soft mechanical diets may be ingested. Eighteen hundred calories daily is the minimal goal for each patient, and their weight is monitored closely. In general, a minimal weight loss is tolerated well by most patients, but it is important to encourage maintenance of normal weight during the immediate postsurgical phase.

The even distribution of occlusal forces is the key to successful postsurgical management of patients with mutilated dentitions. Carefully constructed, well-balanced splints are generally worn until complete consolidation of segments has occurred. These splints are usually ligated to the arch that has been segmented at the time of surgery. If both arches are segmented, the splint is placed on the one with the most segments.

The judicious use of elastic force should be employed to assist in rehabilitation of jaw movements postsurgically. Additionally, elastics may be utilized to effect movement of segments during the postoperative phase. Elastic therapy may also perpetuate the movement of segments during the postoperative period and should be monitored carefully. If elastic force is employed to assist in rehabilitating jaw movement, it is best to employ its use from skeletal wires rather than teeth. If it is used to move segments, it should be discontinued once the movement is accomplished.

When segments are consolidated, a temporary prosthesis should be placed which will evenly distribute occlusal forces. Under no circumstances should a splint be removed without a temporary prosthesis being inserted immediately. Without proper retention or even distribution of occlusal forces, segments that were moved at surgery may change position quickly. Additionally, segments that have been consolidated postsurgically may loosen if traumatized by uneven occlusal forces.

SUMMARY

Dentofacial and dentoalveolar deformities are frequently compounded in their treatment when a patient is partially or totally edentulous. Successful management of these patients requires meticulous treatment planning and attention to detail in the surgical as well as the adjunctive phases of their treatment. The restorative general dentist or prosthodontist should head the team that is required to effectively coordinate their treatment. The oral and maxillofacial surgeon should enter into many facets of treatment of these patients. The surgical procedures discussed in this chapter are in no way complete; however, they have been shown to be biologically sound and clinically well accepted over many years of use. The advanced prosthetic and rehabilitation team will be able to extrapolate and develop rational approaches to the many varied problems their patients present.

CASE PRESENTATIONS

CASE I

This 43-year-old man desired rehabilitation of his multiple missing teeth and was referred by his orthodontist for evaluation. The patient had been referred to the orthodontist by his general practitioner who was reluctant to institute prosthetic treatment in view of the patient's malocclusion and ridge relationships. Limited time and resources contributed to the premature loss of his original teeth. The patient expressed a preference for permanent bridges rather than removable prostheses, which he had worn for 15 years. Additionally, he indicated that he was now in a position that would permit time and financial resources for a complex treatment plan.

The patient was aware that his mandible was prominent and that he was in anterior crossbite. He also understood the difficulty that these situations presented for prosthetic rehabilitation. On several occasions he had attempted to have other prostheses fabricated but was told that his skeletal and dentoalveolar structures precluded satisfactory construction without surgery.

Facial examination and cephalometric and study model analysis indicated three-dimensional maxillary deficiency. His facial vertical dimension was short with teeth in occlusion, and his occlusal freeway space was estimated at 7 mm. Paranasal deficiency was noted as well as mandibular pseudoprognathism when the patient was in occlusion. At resting jaw position, none of the maxillary central incisors was visible, and at full smile only half of the crowns were exposed (Fig. 12–9).

Occlusal examination and study model examination revealed a Class III relationship with complete crossbite. The patient had worn maxillary and mandibular removable prostheses for 15 years, constructed to facilitate his crossbite.

Oral hygiene was excellent and mild periodontal disease was present. Fixed gingival tissues were noted to present in adequate quantities around all remaining teeth (Fig. 12–10).

Feasibility model surgery conducted on a semiadjustable articulator from a face bow transfer indicated that a two-piece maxillary osteotomy with an interdental cut between the maxillary incisors would permit the maxilla to be displaced forward and to be widened 9 mm. In addition to being advanced, the maxilla was also downgrafted to improve the tooth relationship with the lip and to achieve improved skeletal balance with the mandible, nasal bones, and frontal bone.

The surgery was performed, and autogenous bone harvested from the ilium was grafted into the surgical defects. Additional bone was onlayed to the maxilla to improve midfacial esthetics. A conventional LeFort I downfracture procedure was utilized with two para midline osteotomies for widening. An occlusal acrylic wafer with bilateral posterior mandibular tissue-bearing flanges was placed at surgery and left the entire eight weeks of intermaxillary fixation. Additionally, an 0.036-inch auxiliary wire was used at surgery to stabilize the expanded maxilla. This was effective in the dentulous areas of the maxilla only. All of the segments were also wired directly to the intact bone above the osteotomy cut.

When the intermaxillary fixation was released, the occlusal wafer remained wired to the maxillary teeth. Light skeletal elastics were worn to guide mandibular movements. After two weeks of function, the maxilla was stable and the patient was returned to the orthodontist for detailing of his occlusion. A maxillary and mandibular temporary removable splint was constructed which evenly distributed occlusal forces and permitted orthodontic movement to continue. These were inserted as soon as the occlusal splint was removed. Six

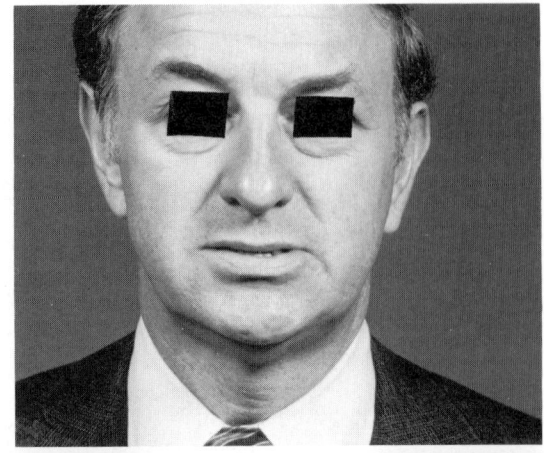

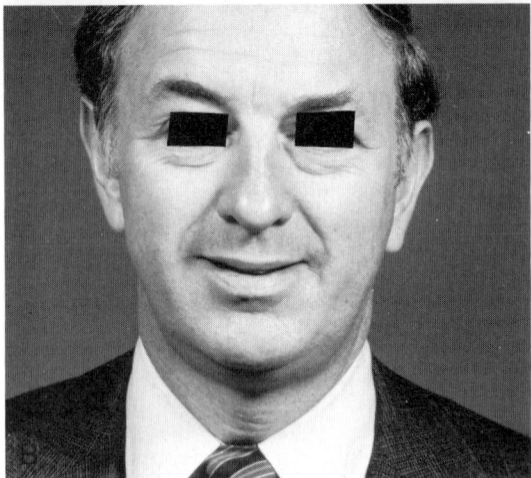

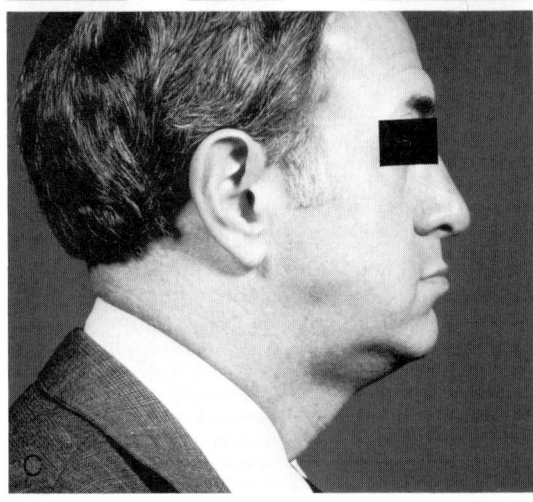

Figure 12–9. Preoperative clinical photographs of Case I. *A* shows overclosure with patient biting into occlusion. *B*, Rest position in proper vertical dimension. *C*, Profile view overclosed into occlusion.

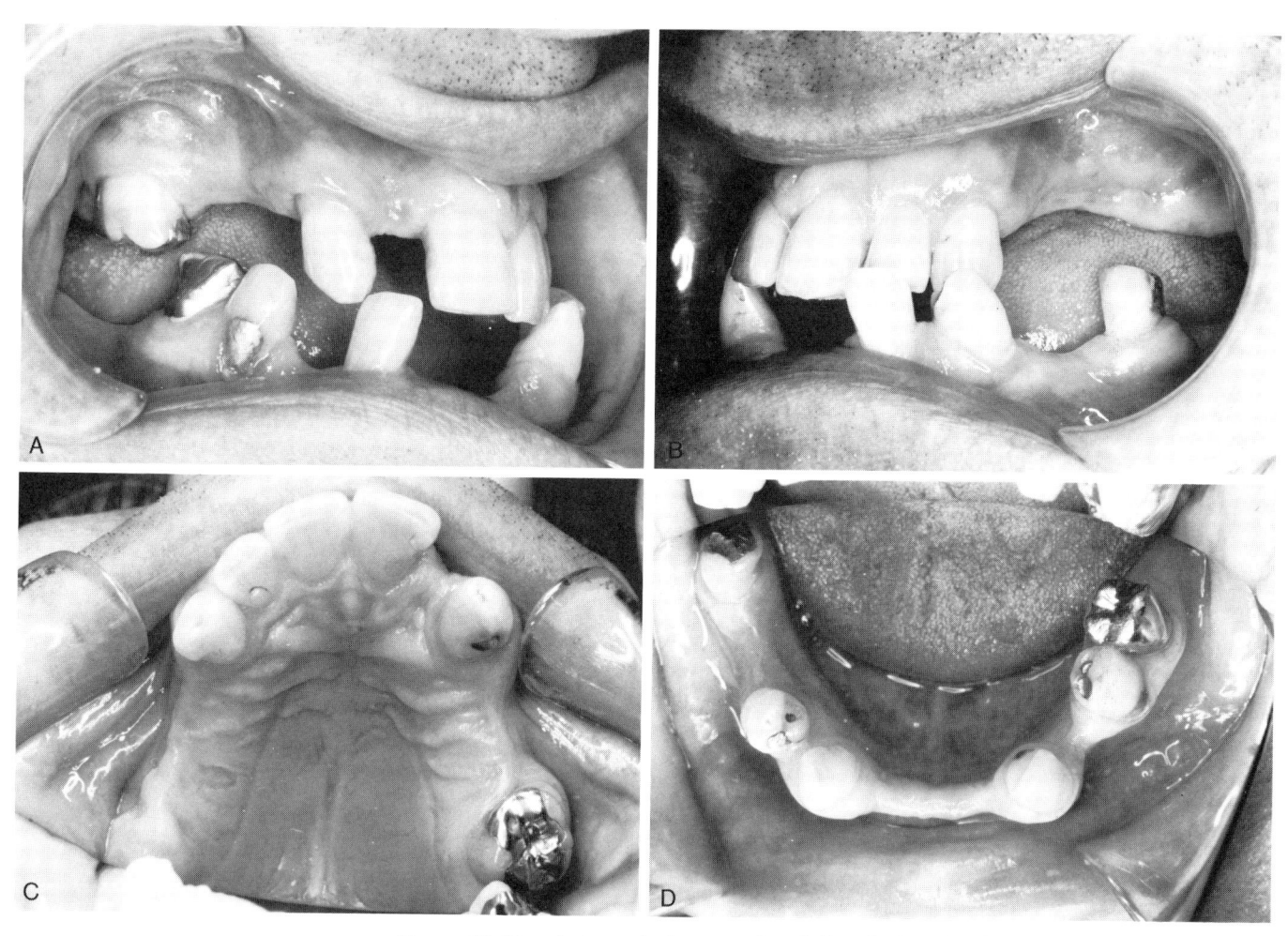

RECONSTRUCTIVE SURGERY FOR THE EDENTULOUS PATIENT / **485**

Figure 12–10. Intra-oral photographs of Case I. *A* and *B* demonstrate multiple missing teeth and overclosure. *C* and *D* are occlusal views of maxillary and mandibular arches.

486 / RECONSTRUCTIVE SURGERY FOR THE EDENTULOUS PATIENT

months following surgery, the patient's maxilla remained completely stable and he was debanded and placed in retainers. Another temporary prosthesis was constructed and the patient wore this for four additional months. This was done to assure dental stability prior to fabrication of the permanent prosthesis.

Two years following surgery the patient continues to do well. His improved facial and occlusal balance remains stable (Fig. 12–11). Permanent prostheses were placed in all quadrants except the left posterior maxilla. A removable partial denture with precision attachments was used because of the lack of posterior abutments in this quadrant. Impeccable attention to balanced occlusal forces postsurgically contributed to the rapid consolidation of the patient's maxilla and the overall stability of the result.

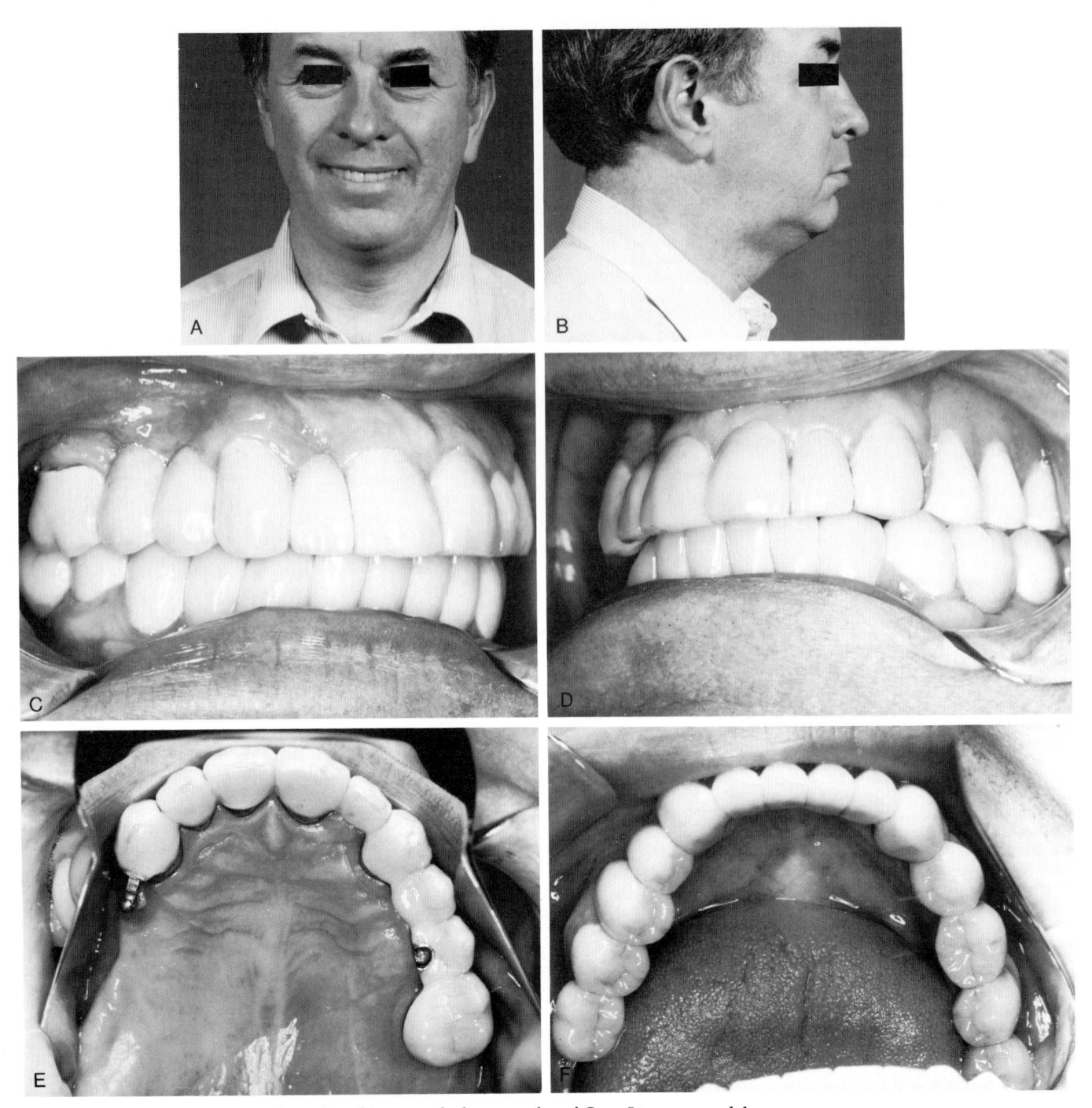

Figure 12–11. Postoperative clinical and intra-oral photographs of Case I two years following surgery.

CASE II

A 34-year-old professional man desired prosthetic reconstruction of his mutilated dentition. The patient indicated that the only dental treatment available to him previously was extractions and this was the reason for his condition. The patient had no facial esthetic concerns but was concerned about his occlusion and dental esthetics.

Facial examination revealed normal features consistent with his physical stature. Intra-orally, he was missing posterior mandibular teeth bilaterally and his maxillary posterior teeth had overerupted and moved buccally, almost occluding with the mandibular ridges. Anterior crossbite was also present, and the mandibular right lateral incisor had been impacted and was removed. The maxillary left central incisor was missing and he had a three-unit bridge in place. The patient's oral hygiene was excellent and there was minimal evidence of periodontal disease. When first seen, orthodontic appliances were on his mandibular teeth.

Because of the ridge malrelationships and anterior crossbite, the prosthodontist was limited in his approach to reconstruction. Orthodontic treatment was also limited because of the absence of posterior mandibular anchorage and the bilateral overeruption of the posterior maxilla.

Radiographs revealed good periodontal support of his remaining teeth. The cephalometric radiograph confirmed that the anterior crossbite resulted from the position of his dentoalveolus and was not due to mandibular prognathism (Fig. 12–12).

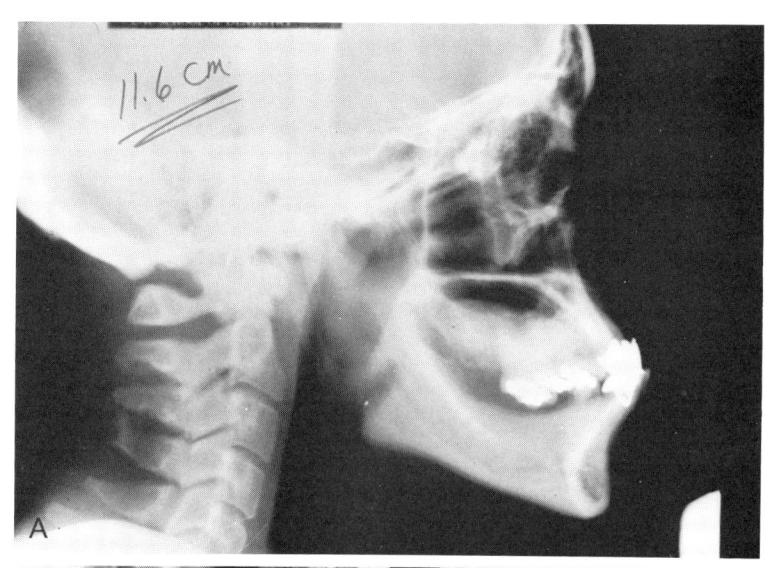

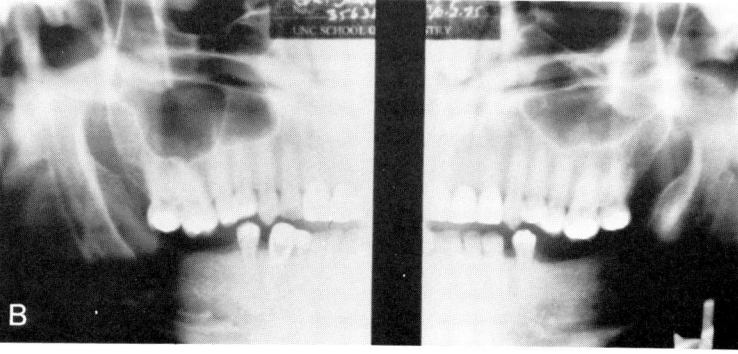

Study models were mounted on an articulator in centric relation. Feasibility model surgery indicated that the posterior maxilla could be raised bilaterally and moved medially to achieve better ridge relationships. The anterior crossbite could be corrected with a four-tooth mandibular subapical osteotomy (Figs. 12–13 and 12–14). Periapical radiographs indicated that interdental osteotomies could be safely performed between the maxillary premolars bilaterally, through the missing mandibular lateral incisor space and the left mandibular cuspid-premolar site. Both the prosthodontist and the orthodontist agreed that the position of the segments following the mock surgery would facilitate prosthetic rehabilitation.

An occlusal splint was fabricated to facilitate repositioning and stabilizing of the segments. Free-end saddle extensions of the splint contacted the mandibular edentulous ridges and supported the repositioned posterior maxillary segments bilaterally.

The surgery was performed and the occlusal splint was stabilized to the mandible with two circummandibular wires. All dentoalveolar segments were wired directly, and intermaxillary fixation was applied for six weeks. This was accomplished by placing a continuous maxillary arch bar on the maxilla and utilizing orthodontic appliances on the

Figure 12–12. Case II. Radiographs revealed good periodontal support of his remaining teeth. Cephalometric radiograph confirmed that the anterior crossbite resulted from the position of his dentoalveolus and was not due to mandibular prognathism.

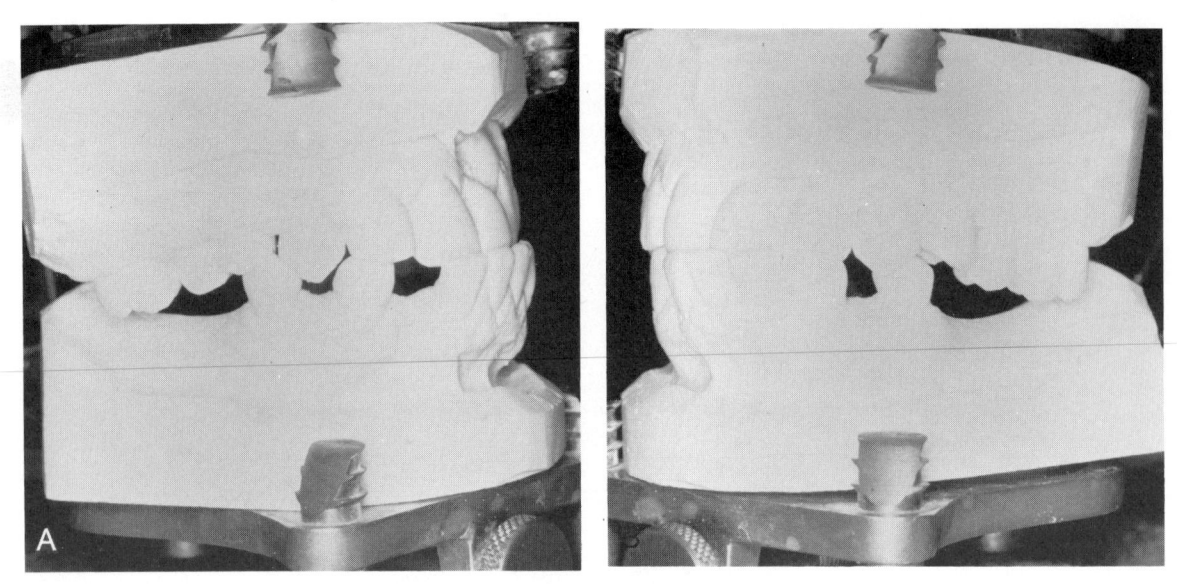

488 / RECONSTRUCTIVE SURGERY FOR THE EDENTULOUS PATIENT

Figure 12–13. Case II. Study models mounted on an articulator in centric relation.

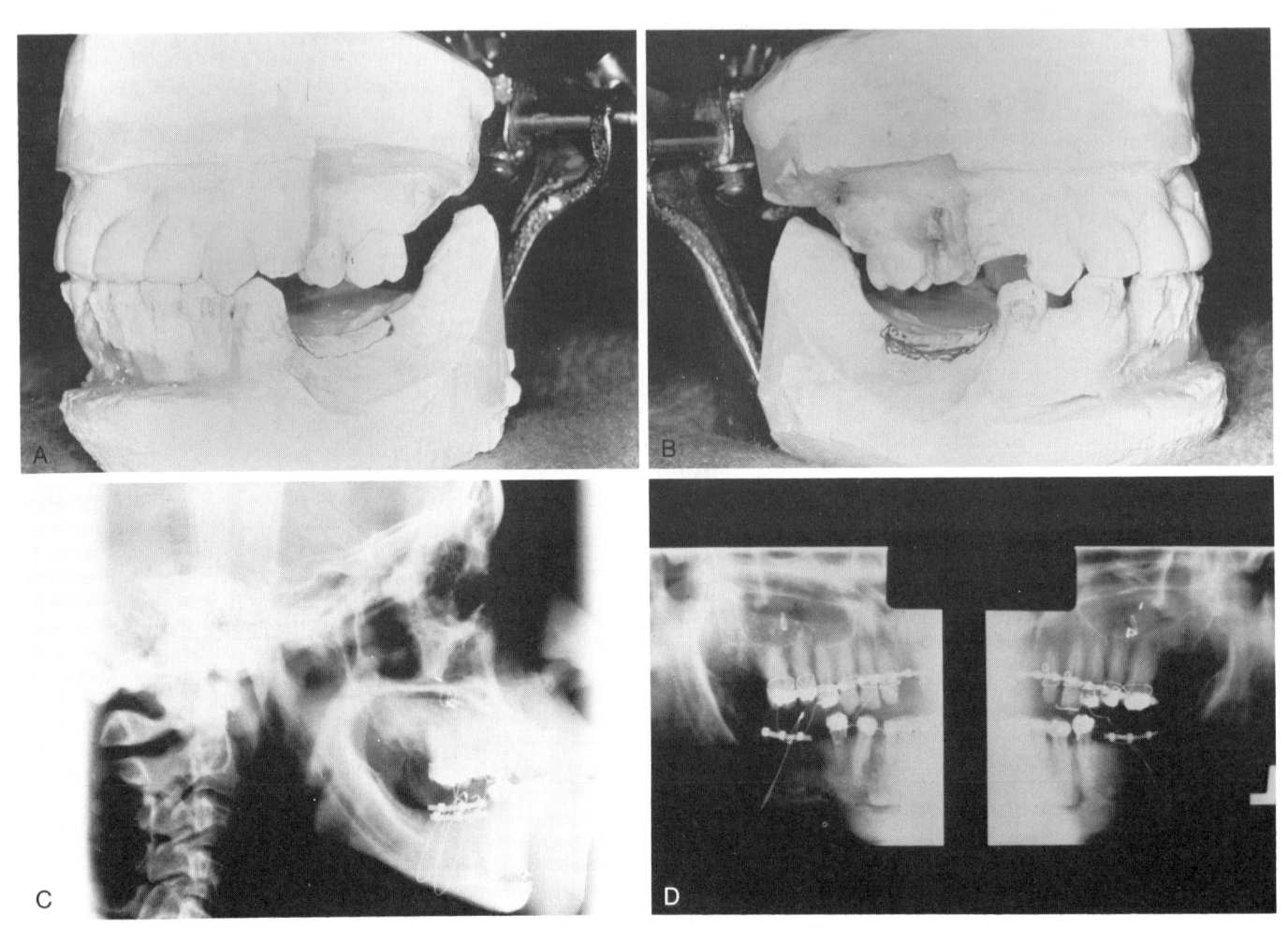

Figure 12–14. *A* and *B*, Model surgery consisting of bilateral posterior maxillary osteotomies and anterior mandibular subapical osteotomy. *C* and *D*, Radiographs revealing osteotomy sites.

mandibular teeth. Additionally, arch bars were placed on the splint in the edentulous posterior mandibular areas. When intermaxillary fixation was released, a temporary mandibular partial denture was inserted immediately to maintain the position of the posterior maxilla until complete consolidation of the segments occurred. Prosthetic rehabilitation was delayed six months until complete consolidation occurred and final orthodontic movement was completed. A three-unit anterior maxillary bridge was then constructed. A precision attachment mandibular partial denture and a

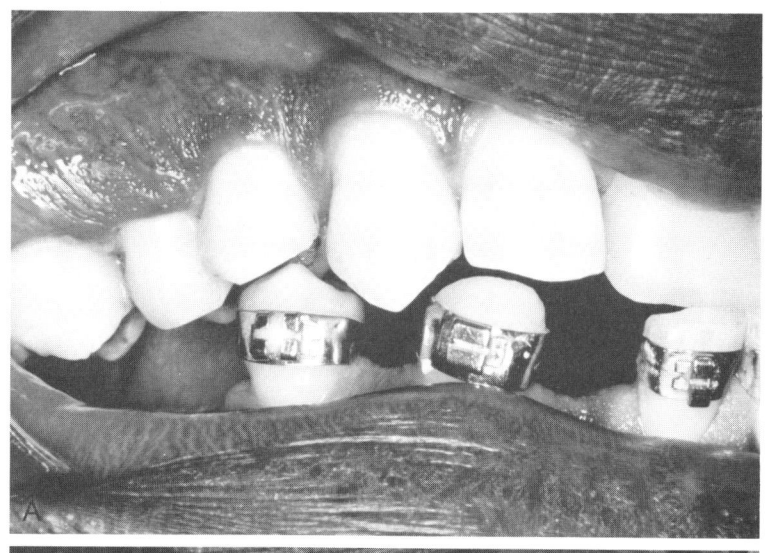

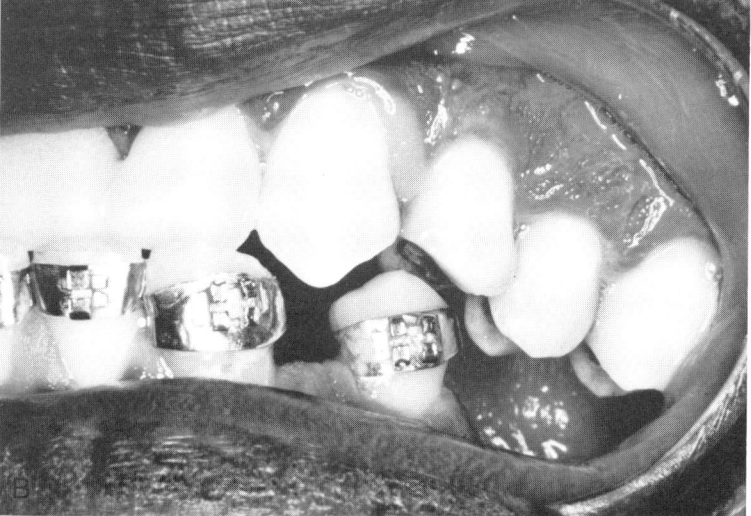

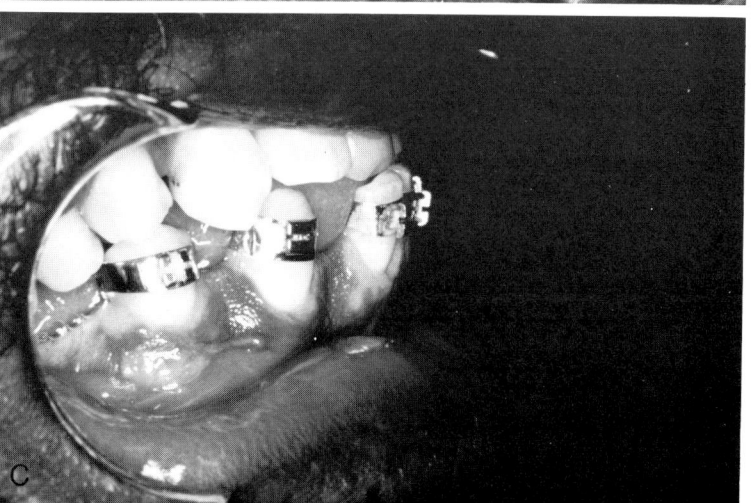

Figure 12–15. Preoperative intra-oral photographs showing hypereruption of posterior maxillary teeth and anterior crossbite.

490 / RECONSTRUCTIVE SURGERY FOR THE EDENTULOUS PATIENT

three-unit bridge were then meticulously constructed to replace the missing mandibular teeth. Five years after surgery, the patient continues to be seen for regular maintenance check-ups. He has been pleased with the appearance and function of his prosthesis (Fig. 12–15 preoperative, Fig. 12–16 postoperative).

The maintenance of the position of the posterior maxillary segments postsurgically with a temporary partial denture was critical to the success of this case. Repositioned posterior maxillary segments may move quickly if left unsupported. They must be retained until the permanent prosthesis is placed.

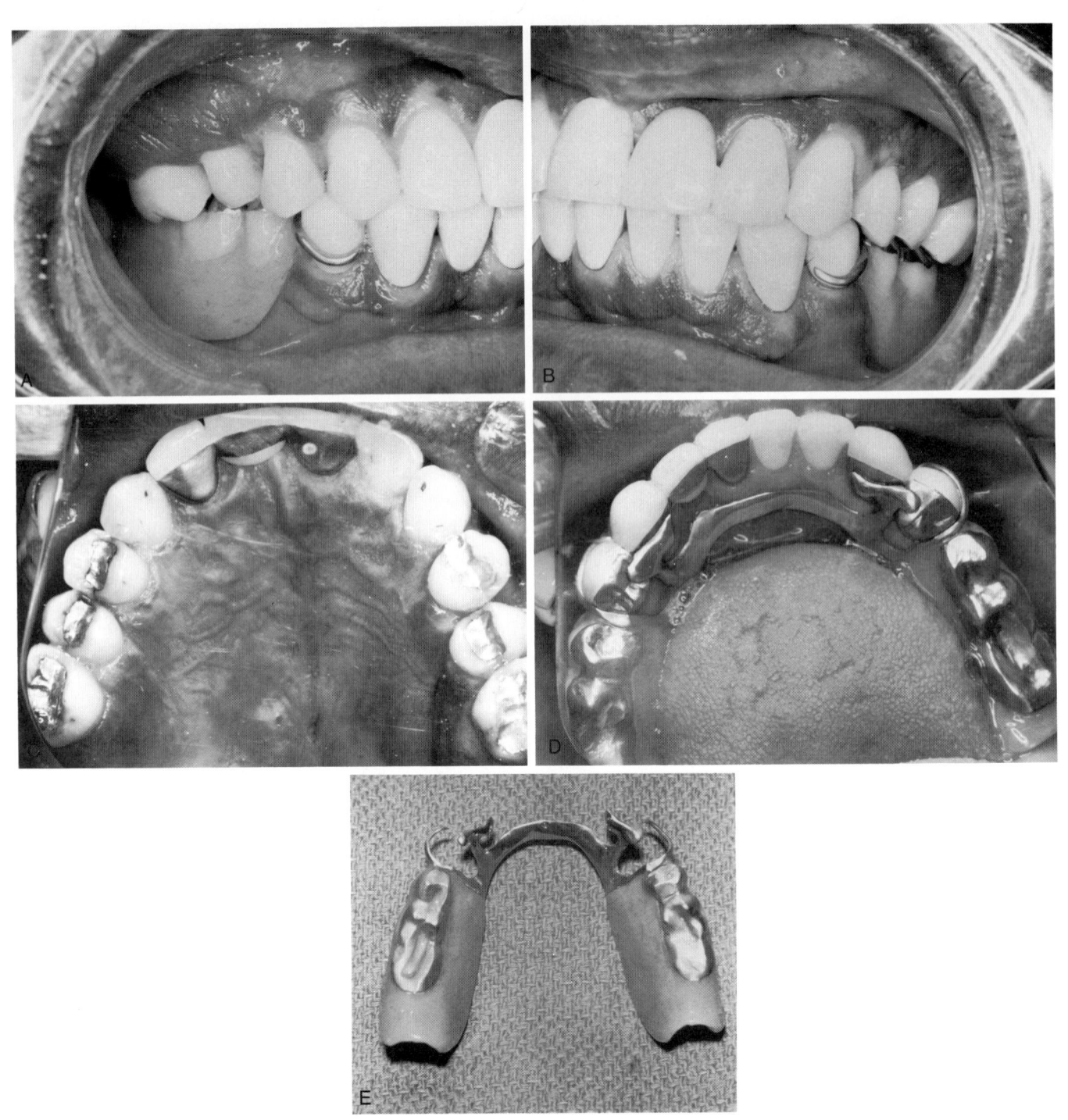

Figure 12–16. Postoperative result of Case II, showing good occlusion and prosthetic rehabilitation.

CASE III

This 34-year-old woman was originally seen by a prosthodontist who referred her because of the anticipated difficulty in fitting a prosthesis. She was concerned about her appearance and the condition of her dentition. Of specific concern was the protrusive relationship of her lips and the amount of gingiva she exposed at repose and during animation. She related that she never cared for the appearance of her teeth and therefore neglected them.

Facial examination revealed vertical maxillary excess and severe bimaxillary protrusion. All of her maxillary incisors and a portion of gingiva were exposed at resting lip posture. At full smile, gross exposure of gingiva was evident. Her profile exam indicated everted upper and lower lips consistent with bimaxillary protrusion. Her anterior facial height was also excessive (Fig. 12–17).

Oral examination revealed a mutilated dentition and evidence of advanced periodontal disease. Maxillary excess and mandibular dentoalveolar excess were present. The posterior edentulous maxillary and mandibular ridges were contacting when the patient occluded, and mandibular lingual tori were also present. Her skeletal and alveolar ridge relationships were not compatible with denture fabrication. Periodontal evaluation indicated that none of her remaining teeth were salvagable (Fig. 12–18).

The treatment plan called for removal of the remaining teeth and eventual construction of complete dentures. A decision on the management of her ridge relationships to facilitate denture construction was reduced to two choices. A radical alveolectomy was a possibility; this would require removal of most of her maxillary, and a portion of her mandibular, alveolar bone. This choice would leave skeletal bone only to support her denture and would ignore her lower face esthetics. Feasibility model surgery done on study casts indicated that excellent ridge relationships could be achieved by performing a three-piece maxillary osteotomy, leveling the segments by moving them up and back, and a mandibular subapical osteotomy with retropositioning. Since the latter approach would maintain most of the alveolus and would reposition the skeleton into a more favorable functional and esthetic relationship, we considered it the preferred choice.

Rather than removing her teeth prior to or at the time of surgery, it was elected to maintain them for the surgical procedure. This permitted more accurate repositioning of her segments, since an occlusal index could be used, and it also provided a more predictable means of fixation. The surgery was performed under general anesthesia and the technical aspects of surgery were conducted uneventfully. A single occlusal acrylic index was used to position the segments in the desired relationship, and intermaxillary fixation was placed for four weeks. The splints were stabilized with pyriform and circummandibular wires. The edentulous posterior maxillary segments were stabilized with direct fixation and were supported with ridge extensions from the occlusal splint. These extensions covered the ridge only and did not impinge on palatal or buccal tissues. The mandibular subapical segment was stabilized with two Kirschner wires (Fig. 12–19). At the end of four weeks, the intermaxillary fixation was removed and her segments were slightly mobile. Four weeks following the release of intermaxillary fixation, the segments tightened. At this time the teeth were extracted and the mandibular tori were removed. The tori were not removed during her initial surgery to minimize tissue dissection and thus maintain blood perfusion into the anterior mandibular dentoalveolus. By the ninth postoperative week, no movement of the segments could be appreciated.

It is of interest to note that several maxillary anterior teeth discolored postsurgically but never developed other symptoms of pulpal pathology. The osteotomies were conducted, as usual, away from the apices of the teeth. Probably the discoloration occurred because of the altered hemodynamics associated with advanced periodontal disease and inflammation. When her teeth were removed, an immediate temporary denture was placed. She functioned with this for five months and then final dentures were constructed.

Eighteen months after surgery the patient's ridge relationships remain stable, and she functions well with her prosthesis. The patient is delighted with her facial change and the result of her dentures (Fig. 12–20).

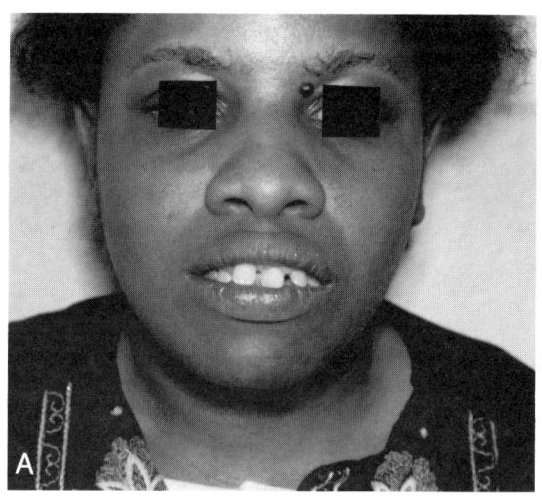

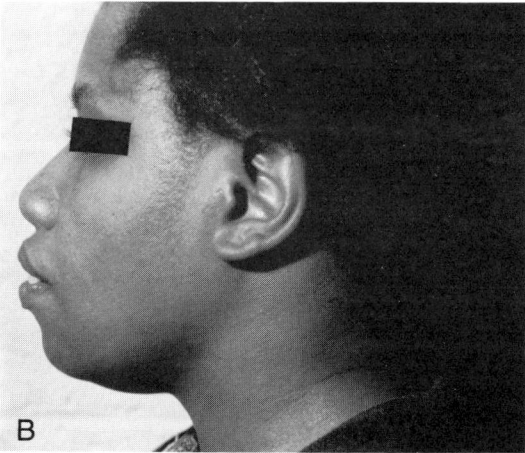

Figure 12–17. Case III. Clinical photographs demonstrating bimaxillary protrusion and excessive lower anterior facial height.

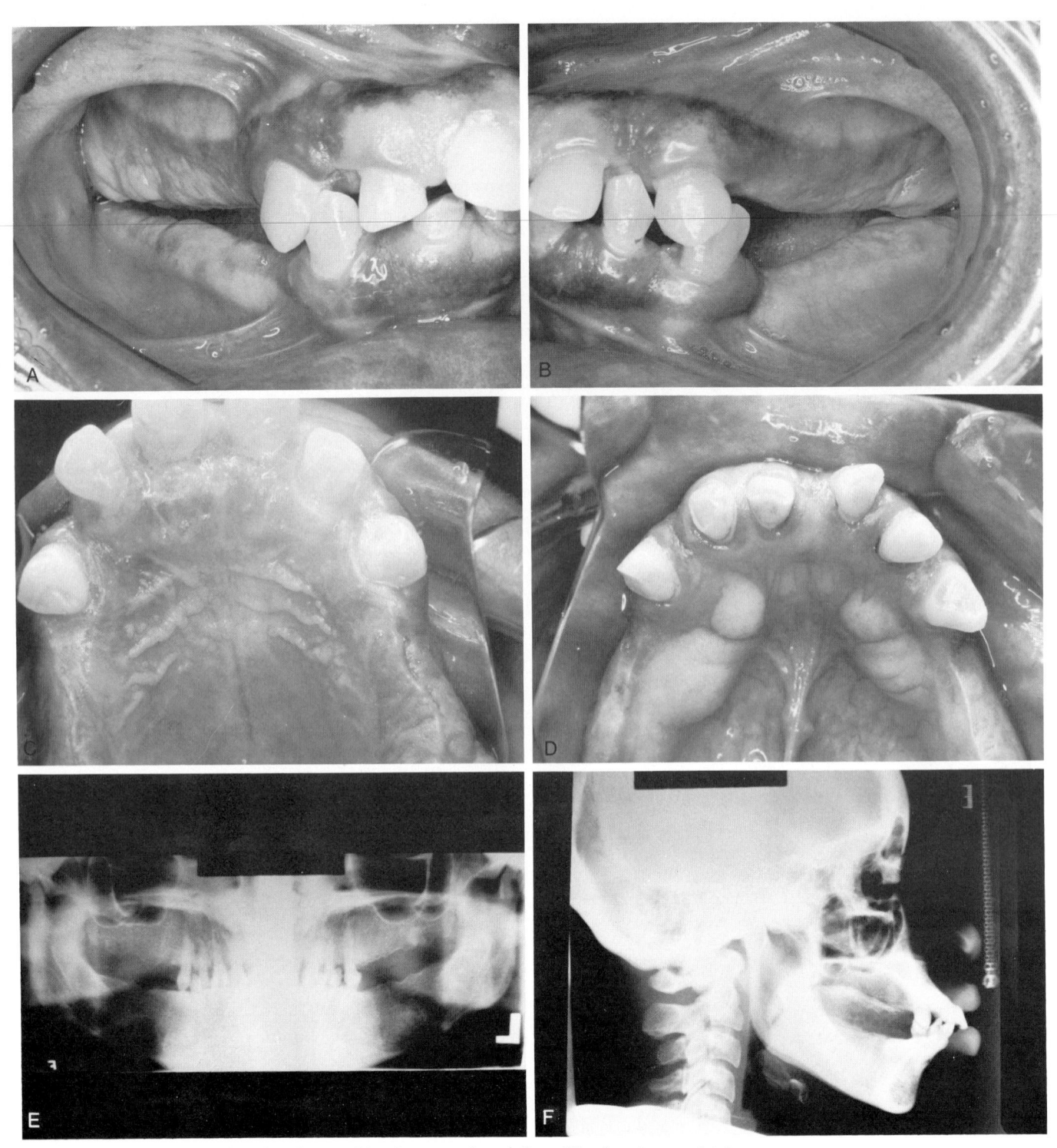

492 / RECONSTRUCTIVE SURGERY FOR THE EDENTULOUS PATIENT

Figure 12–18. Intra-oral and radiographic photographs of Case III, showing multiple missing teeth and bimaxillary protrusion.

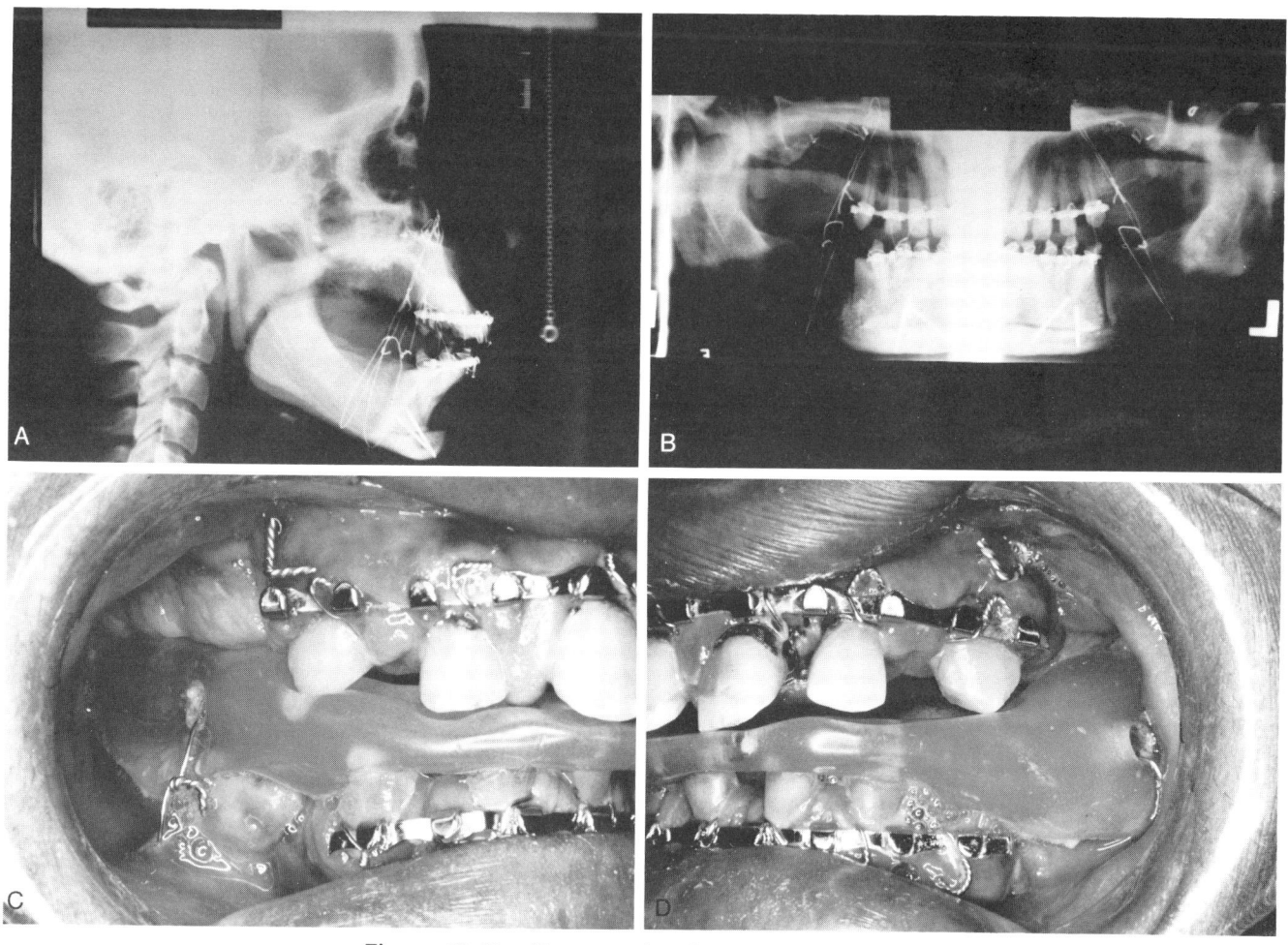

Figure 12–19. Postoperative fixation utilizing skeletal suspension wires, Kirschner wires, and intermaxillary fixation.

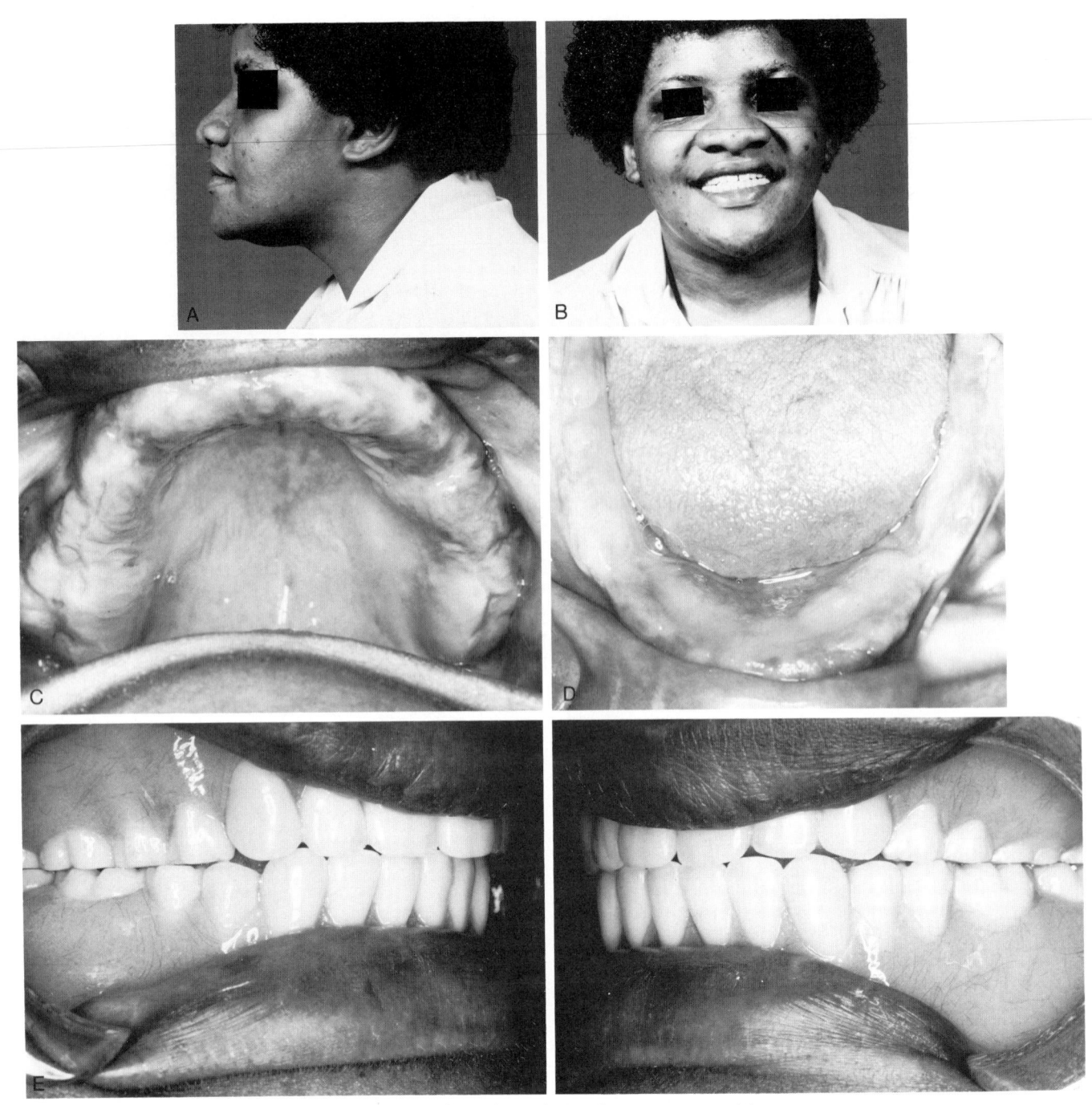

494 / RECONSTRUCTIVE SURGERY FOR THE EDENTULOUS PATIENT

Figure 12–20. Eighteen months after surgery, the ridge relationships remain stable, and she functions well with a prosthesis.

CASE IV

This 35-year-old woman presented for removal of her remaining teeth and construction of complete dentures. She expressed disinterest in salvaging any teeth and indicated that she had undergone extensive orthodontic and periodontal therapy in the past. She said that over the previous five years she lost complete interest in her teeth and now she just wanted them removed.

Facial examination revealed mandibular deficiency, both sagittally and vertically. She had a deep labiomental fold and her maxillary anterior teeth were protrusive (Fig. 12–21). Her oral hygiene was deplorable; she had heavy deposits of plaque and calculus throughout her entire dentition. Her gingival tissues were inflamed and had receded around all of her teeth. Class III mobility was detectable in all four quadrants and she claimed that she wouldn't brush any more because of pain. A Class II malocclusion was present with 12 mm of overjet. The six mandibular anterior teeth had orthodontic appliances in place and these teeth contacted her palatal tissues when she occluded (Fig. 12–22).

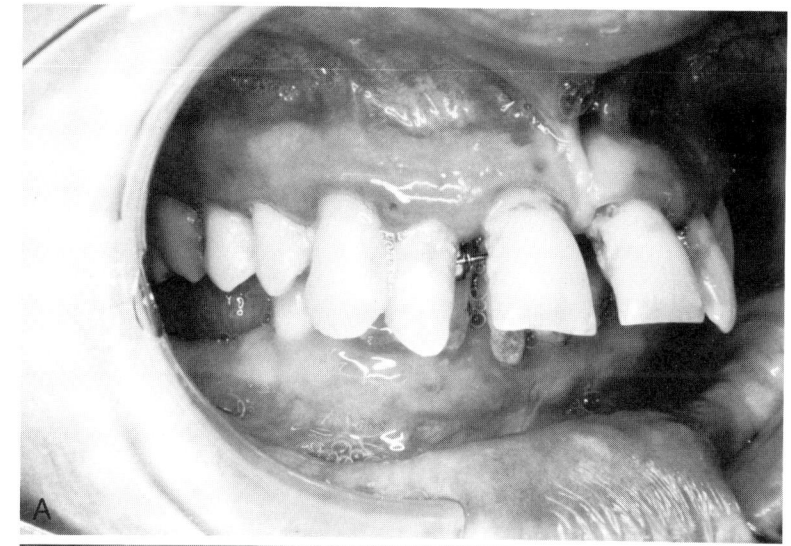

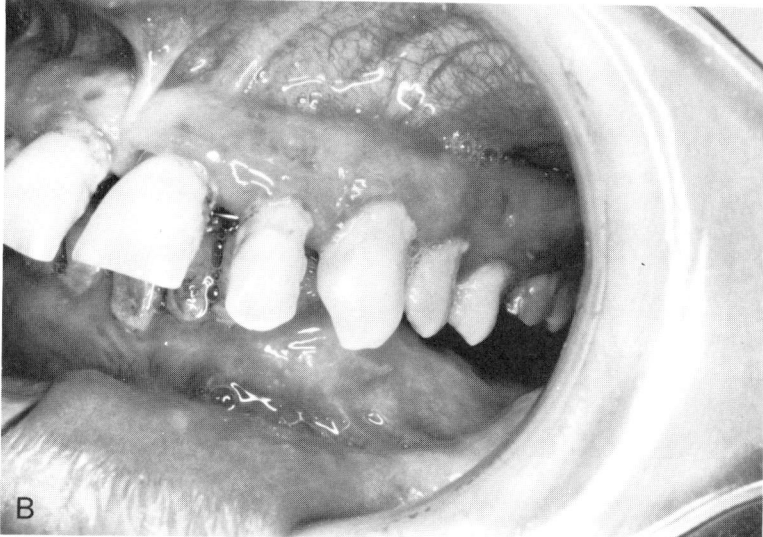

Figure 12–22. The six mandibular anterior teeth had orthodontic appliances in place, and these contacted her palatal tissues when she occluded.

Radiographs indicated severe bone loss around all teeth. Her cephalometric tracing confirmed mandibular deficiency and a short lower facial third. Her skeletal condition and ridge relationships would make prosthetic construction difficult (Fig. 12–23).

Contact was made with the patient's former orthodontist, who supplied records from eight years previously. At that time he and a periodontist were attempting to improve the patient's cooperation and motivation. According to his records, the patient discontinued therapy and never returned for debanding.

Prosthodontic consultation agreed that full-mouth extraction was indicated and that construction of complete dentures would be limited by the mandibular deficiency and collapsed vertical dimension. Improved ridge relationships would facilitate denture construction and function.

Because the patient had several areas of acute infection, it was decided to perform a partial odon-

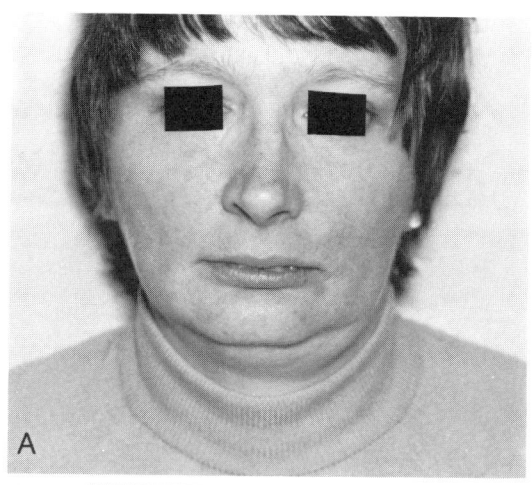

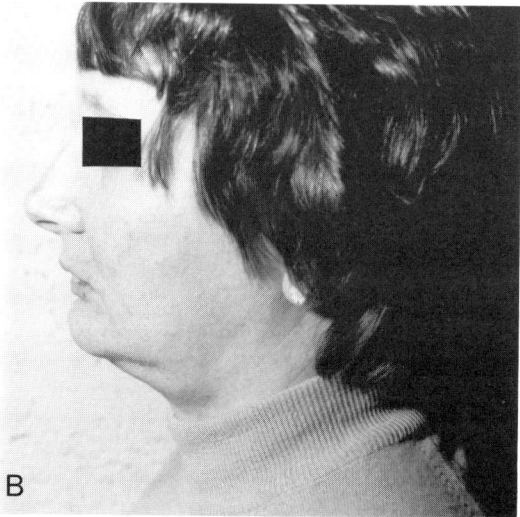

Figure 12–21. Case IV. Facial examination revealed mandibular deficiency, both sagittally and vertically.

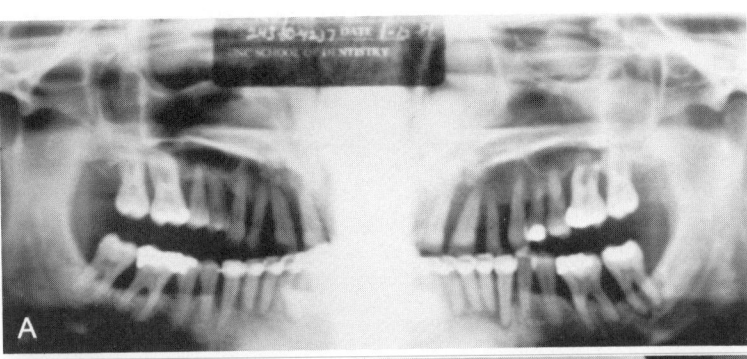

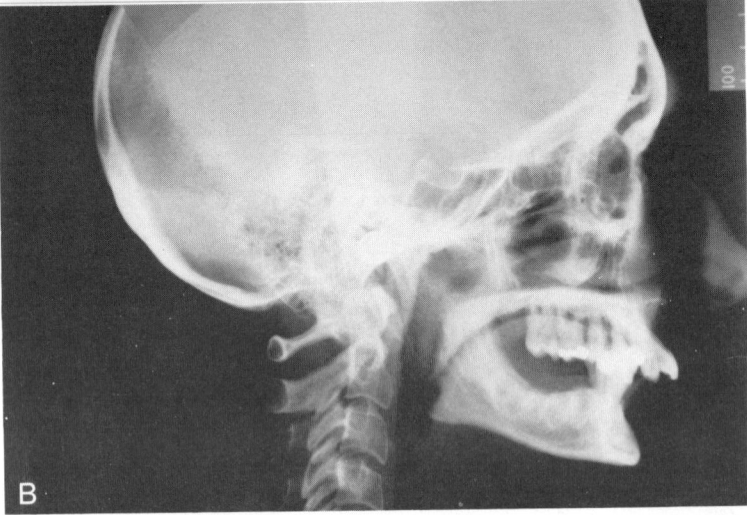

496 / RECONSTRUCTIVE SURGERY FOR THE EDENTULOUS PATIENT

Figure 12–23. Radiographs indicated severe bone loss around her teeth. Her cephalometric tracing confirmed mandibular deficiency and a short lower facial third.

tectomy to relieve her pain. The intention was to leave some teeth in each quadrant to help position and stabilize her mandible when the mandibular advancement was performed. Closer examination revealed rampant periodontal abscesses requiring removal of all teeth except the cuspids in each quadrant and two terminal molars in the right maxilla. This was performed and the mandibular advancement was delayed four weeks to allow the extraction areas to heal.

Mock surgery performed on the study casts and cephalometric tracings indicated that mandibular

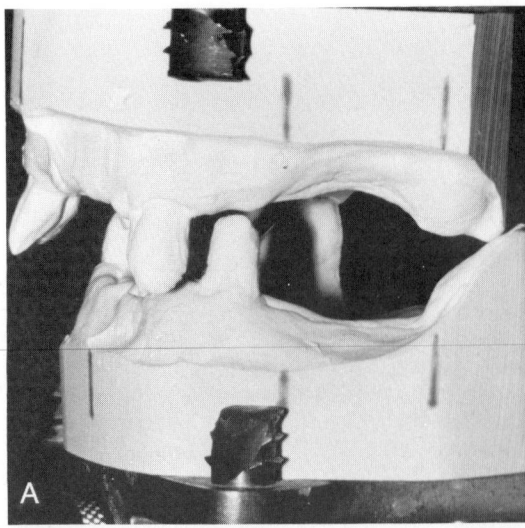

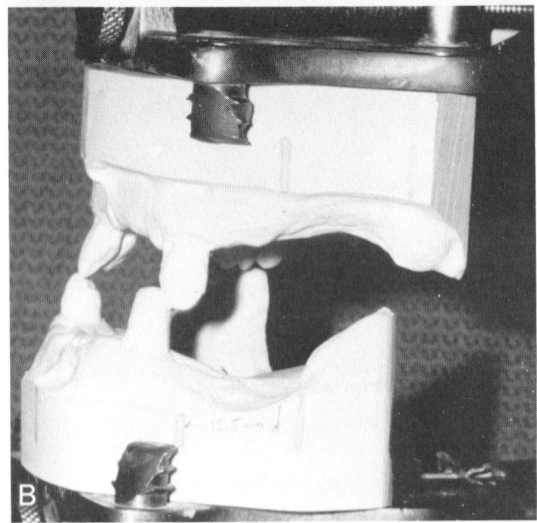

Figure 12–24. Mock model surgery indicated that a mandibular advancement of 15 mm with a clockwise rotation would result in a good ridge relationship.

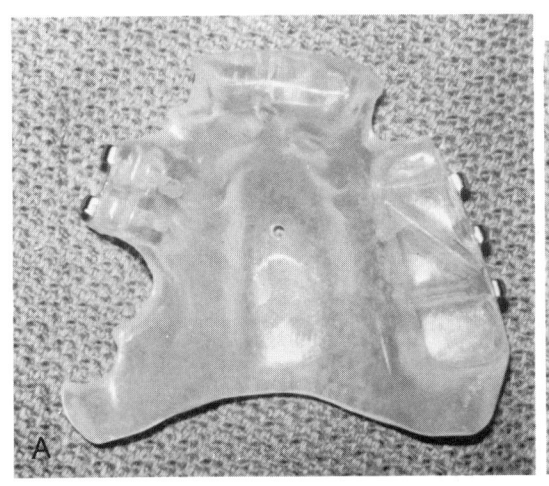

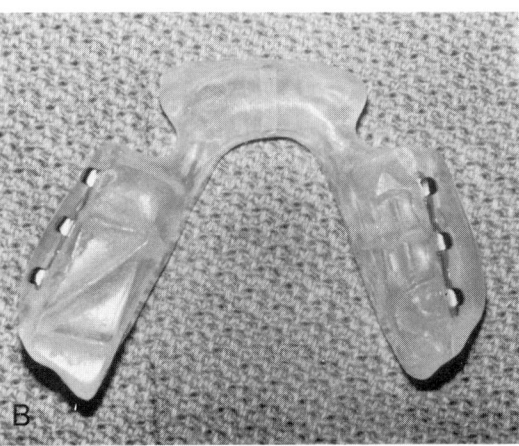

Figure 12–25. Maxillary and mandibular splints were fabricated to key at the correct mandibular position.

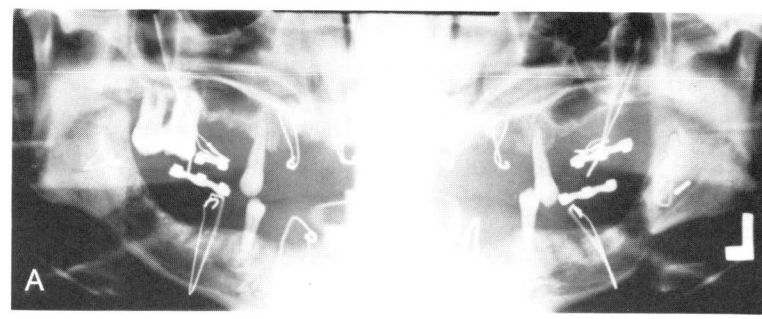

RECONSTRUCTIVE SURGERY FOR THE EDENTULOUS PATIENT / **497**

Figure 12–26. Skeletal fixation was the primary source of stabilization.

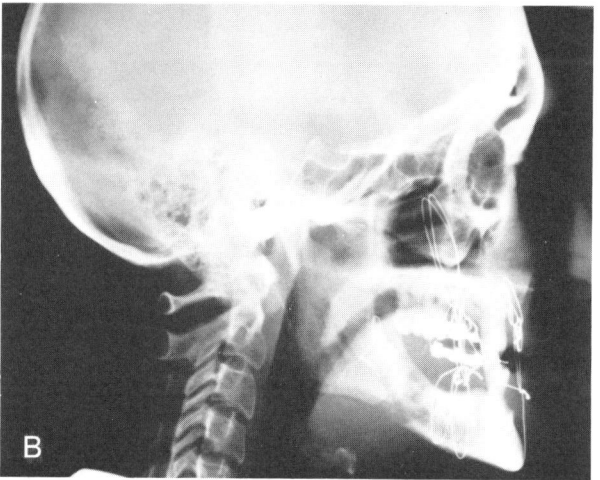

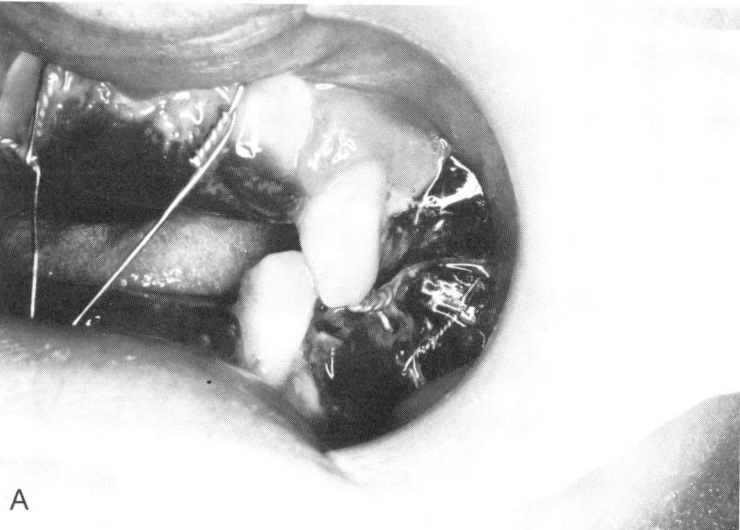

Figure 12–27. When the fixation was released, the splints were left in place and the patient functioned with elastics from her skeletal wires for another four weeks.

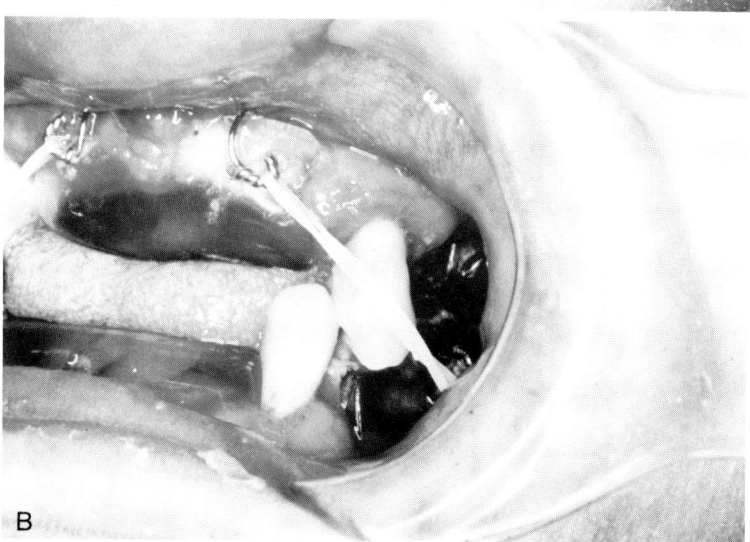

advancement of 15 mm with clockwise rotation to elongate the lower facial third would result in good ridge relationships and facial esthetics (Fig. 12–24). In order to position and stabilize the mandible, maxillary and mandibular splints were fabricated to key at the correct mandibular position. The keyed areas of the splints were the cusp tips of the cuspid and the occlusal surfaces of the splints (Fig. 12–25).

The surgery was performed with a sagittal osteotomy of the mandibular ramus bilaterally. Intermaxillary fixation was applied with arch bars that were placed on the splint. The mandibular splint was secured with three circummandibular wires and the maxillary splint with two circumzygomatic wires and two pyriform wires. Skeletal fixation was the primary source of stabilization (Fig. 12–26).

Intermaxillary fixation was maintained for eight weeks and additionally, the patient wore a cervical collar to help maintain the position of her mandible. When the fixation was released, the splints were left in place and the patient functioned with elastics from her skeletal wires for another four weeks (Fig. 12–27). During this time, the patient's splints continued to occlude properly. There was minimal skeletal movement that did not interfere with the ridge relationships obtained at surgery.

Once the surgical splints were removed, dentures were constructed with locking posterior bite rims and anterior teeth only. These were worn for several months to maintain good mandibular function and position. Final denture construction was delayed six months to assure consolidation of the mandible.

Currently the patient has functioned well with complete dentures for two years. She is pleased with her appearance and her ability to master denture wearing (Fig. 12–28). According to the prosthodontists, denture construction was facilitated by the reconstructed ridge relationships. Mandibular advancement is prone to relapse, especially when the dentition is not reliable for stabilization. Maintenance of the mandibular position in this case was facilitated by skeletal fixation. Preservation of some teeth and construction of keyed splints were also important adjunctive measures utilized.

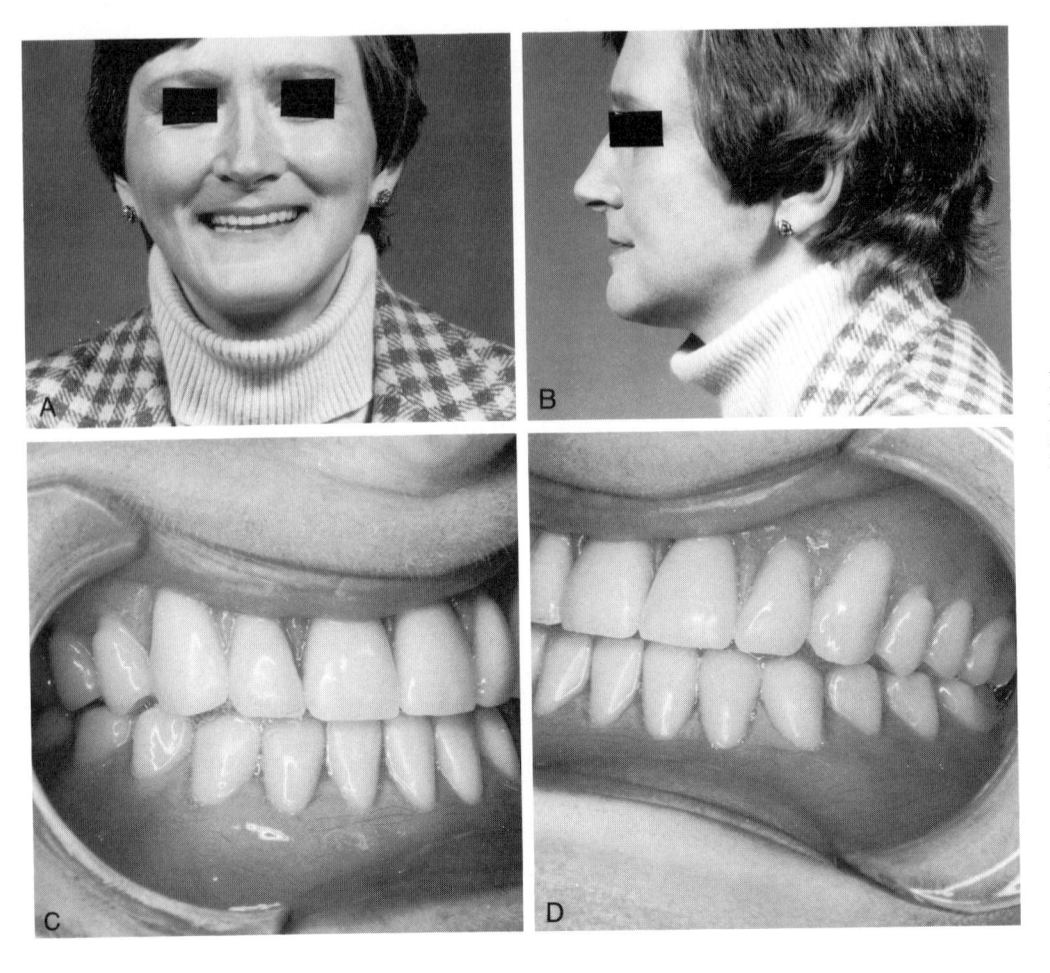

Figure 12–28. Patient two years after surgery, with good esthetic and functional results.

RECONSTRUCTIVE SURGERY FOR THE EDENTULOUS PATIENT / **499**

CASE V

This 56-year-old white male presented to the Veterans Administration Hospital in Iowa City, Iowa, in 1981 with a chief complaint of inability to wear his upper and lower dentures. Clinical examination revealed maxillary and mandibular arches that had adequate amounts of bony and soft tissue available for denture construction (Figs. 12–29 and 12–30). Radiographic analysis of the patient, including a lateral cephalometric analysis, revealed mandibular prognathism with significant anteroposterior discrepancy of the maxillary and mandibular ridges (Fig. 12–31). Treatment was planned for a sagittal split setback of the mandible of 9 mm. The amount of movement to be performed in this case was determined by an articulated study model analysis with occlusal rims fabricated to establish an ideal vertical dimension. Once the ideal anteroposterior relationship was established, Gunning splints were fabricated (Fig. 12–32).

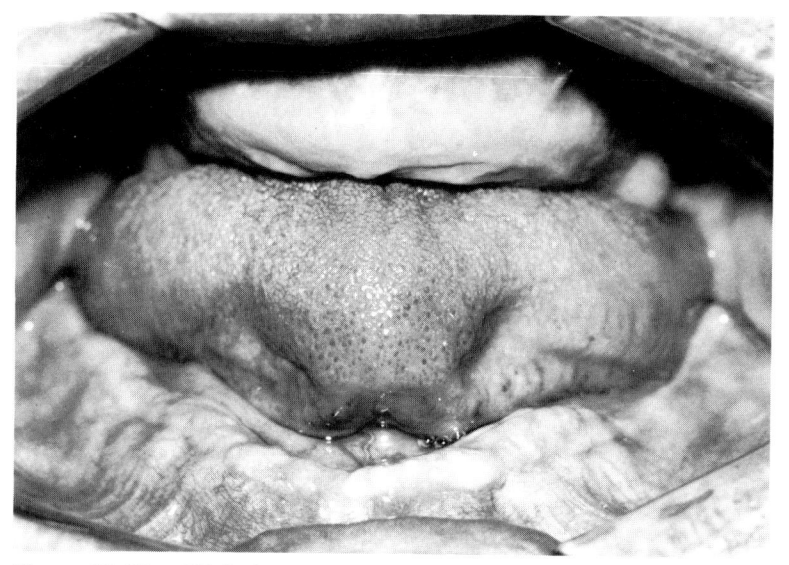

Figure 12–30. Clinical examination revealed maxillary and mandibular arches that had adequate amounts of bony and soft tissue.

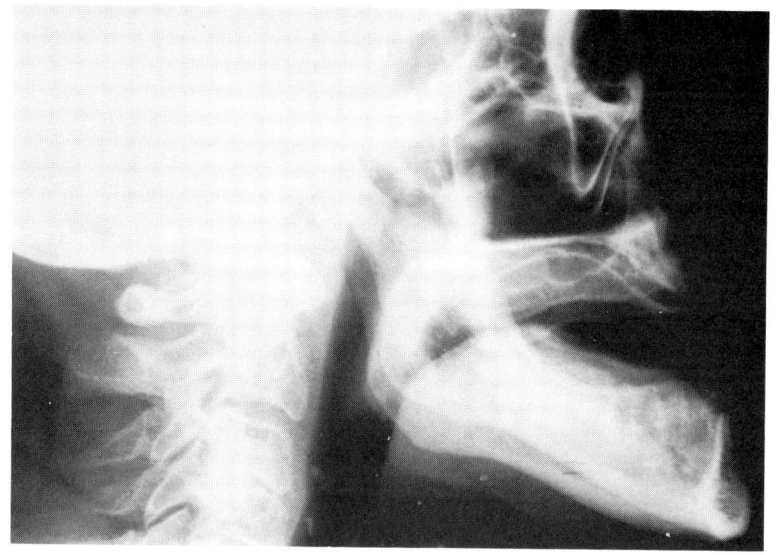

Figure 12–31. Lateral cephalometric analysis revealed mandibular prognathism.

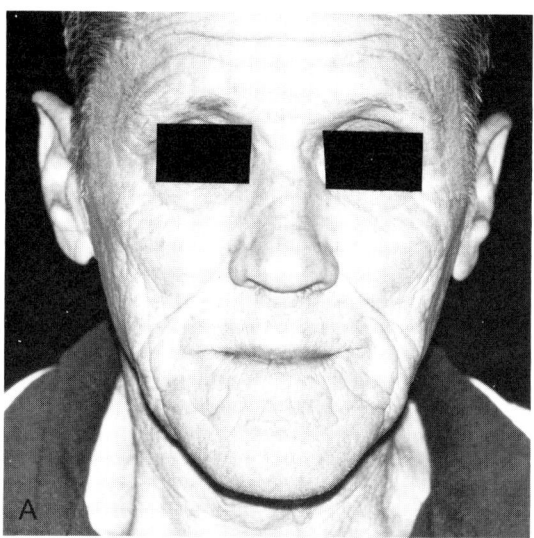

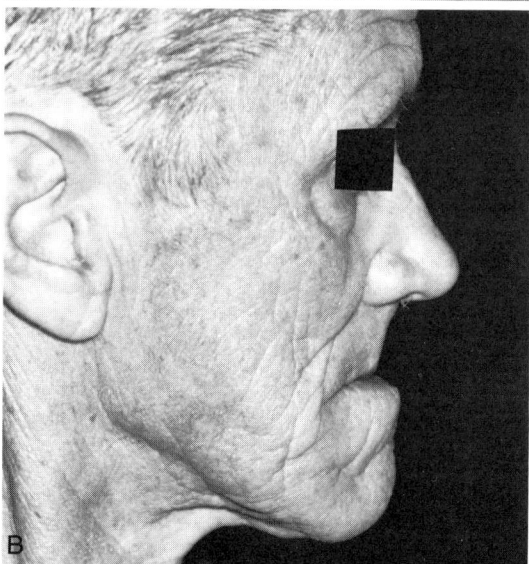

Figure 12–29. Case V. Clinical presentation prior to surgery.

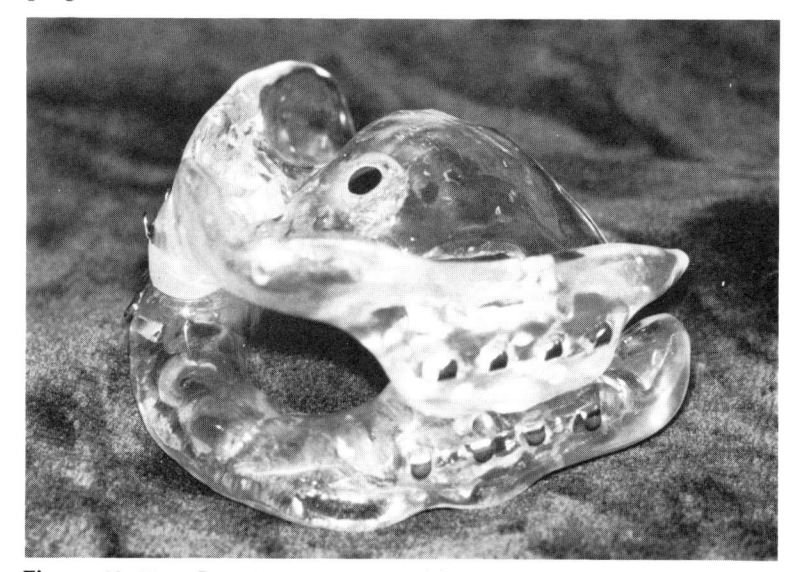

Figure 12–32. Gunning splints fabricated to establish an optimal anteroposterior relationship.

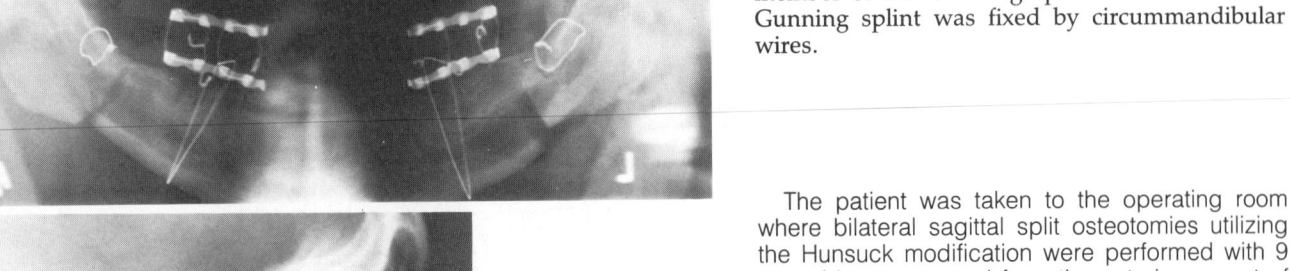

500 / RECONSTRUCTIVE SURGERY FOR THE EDENTULOUS PATIENT

Figure 12–33. Orthopedic 5/8-inch threaded screws were used for stabilization of the upper member of the Gunning splint. The mandibular Gunning splint was fixed by circummandibular wires.

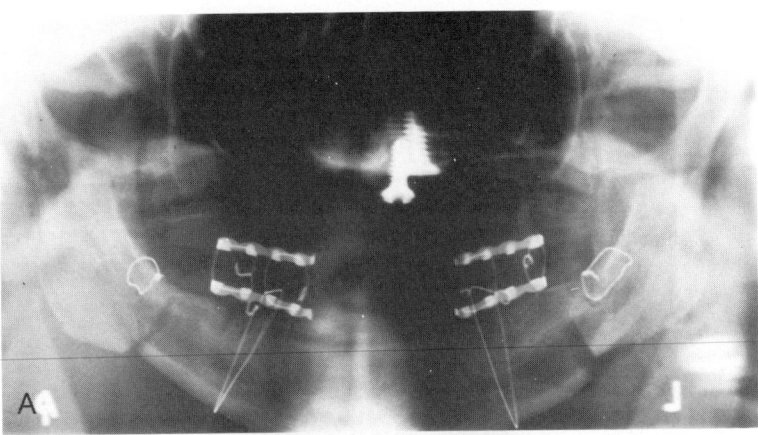

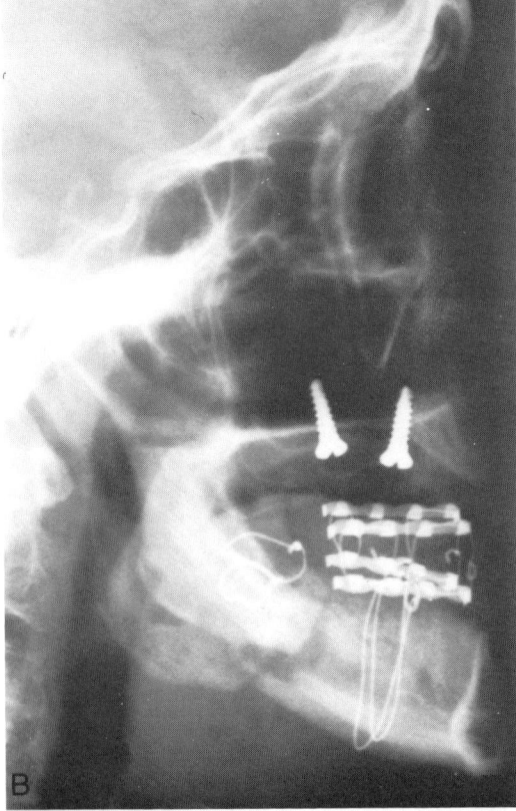

The patient was taken to the operating room where bilateral sagittal split osteotomies utilizing the Hunsuck modification were performed with 9 mm of bone removed from the anterior aspect of the proximal segment. The upper member of the Gunning splint was fixed to the maxilla with two palatal screws in the midportion of the palate, one being placed at the anterior aspect of the junction of the alveolar and palatal shelves and one more posteriorly in the midpalatal region. Orthopedic 5/8-inch threaded screws were used for stabilization. The lower member of the Gunning splint was fixed to the mandible utilizing circummandibular wires in the midbody area of the mandible (Fig. 12–33). The maxillary and mandibular Gunning splints were then fixed to each other with 25-gauge stainless steel wires that were looped around arch bars that had been embedded into the Gunning splints with acrylic. A superior border wire was placed on both proximal segments to maintain good approximation of the proximal segments to the distal segments and to allow for good condylar positioning of the segments (Fig. 12-34). The postoperative course was uneventful. He was discharged from the hospital on the third postoperative day and seen routinely at weekly intervals, and the Gunning splints were removed eight weeks postoperatively. Good occlusal and facial proportions were achieved (Figs. 12–35 and 12–36). He subsequently had maxillary and mandibular dentures fabricated in a Class I ridge relationship with a good vertical dimension (Fig. 12–37).

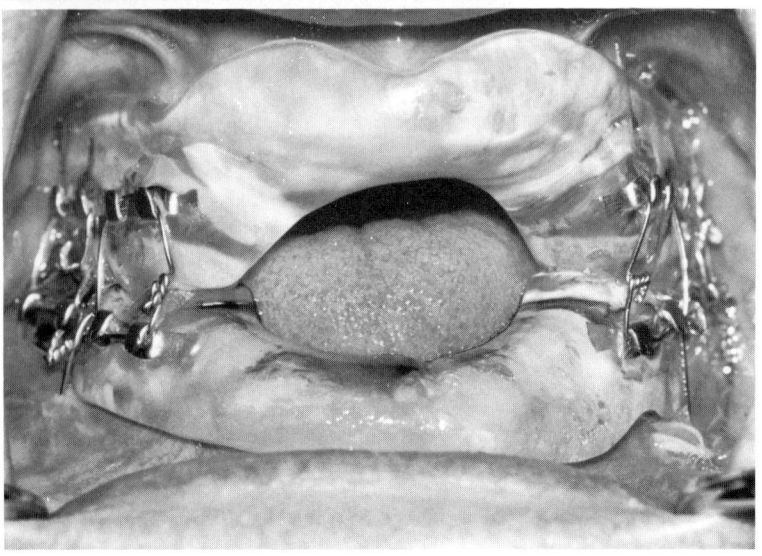

Figure 12–34. Intermaxillary fixation was established using 25-gauge stainless steel wire loops.

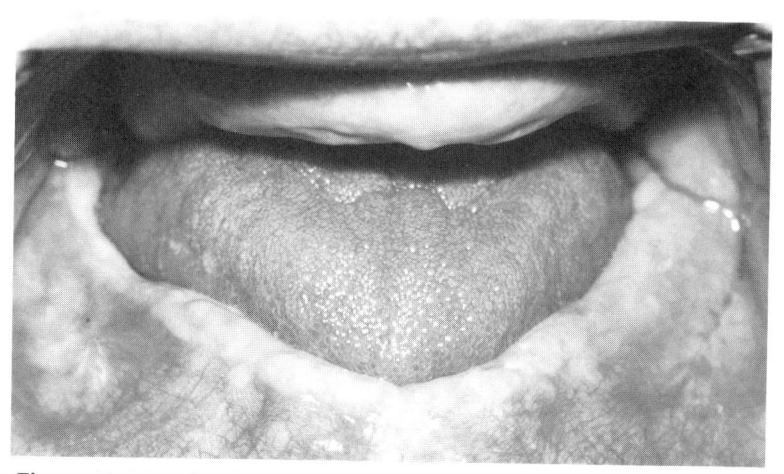

RECONSTRUCTIVE SURGERY FOR THE EDENTULOUS PATIENT / **501**

Figure 12–36. Good occlusal proportions were achieved.

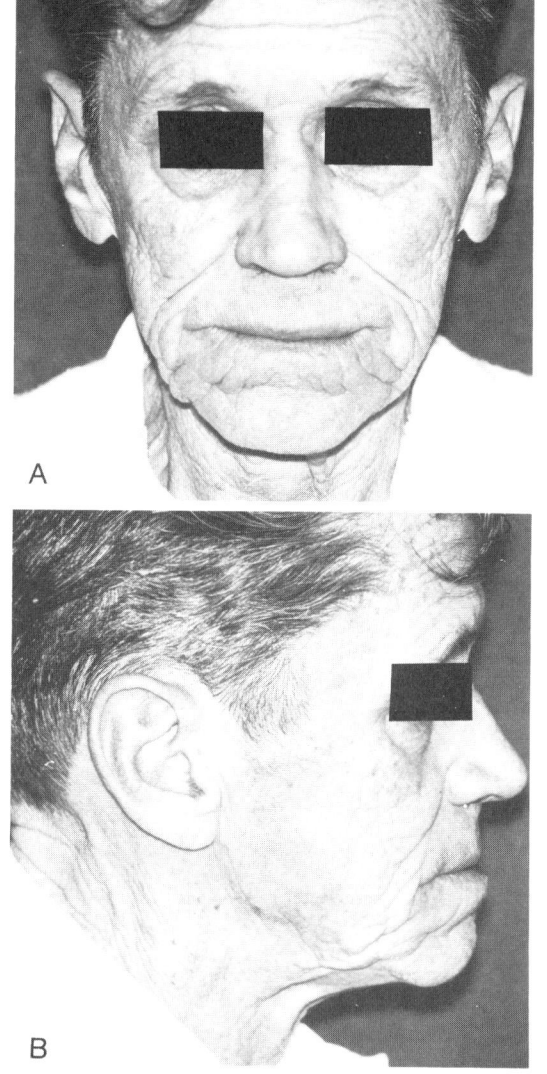

Figure 12–35. Three-year postoperative follow-up revealed a stable satisfactory facial relationship.

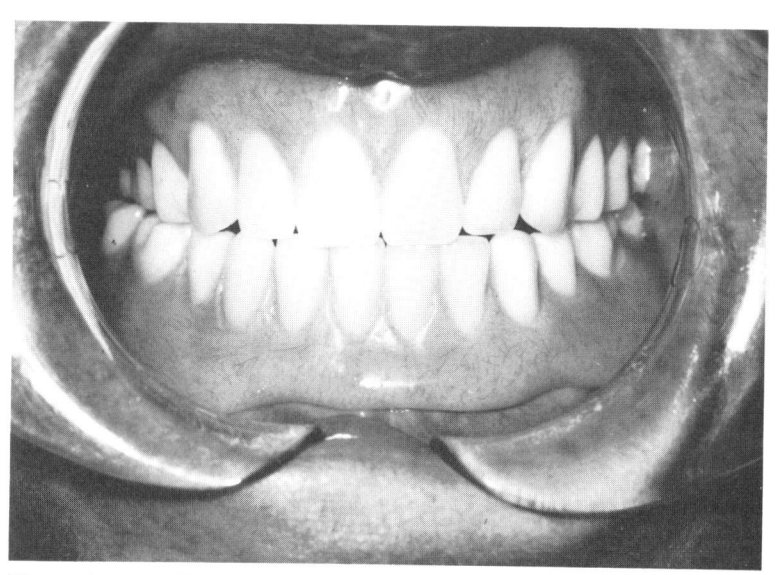

Figure 12–37. Dentures were fabricated in a Class I ridge relationship with a good vertical dimension.

502 / RECONSTRUCTIVE SURGERY FOR THE EDENTULOUS PATIENT

CASE VI

This 47-year-old white female presented to The University of North Carolina oral surgery clinic in January of 1977 with a chief complaint of disliking the protrusive appearance of her upper anterior teeth. Clinical examination revealed a healthy woman who had a rather protrusive appearance of the upper lip with acute nasolabial angle. Intra-oral examination revealed approximately 50 per cent overbite with an 8-mm overjet. The patient was missing multiple maxillary and mandibular teeth (Figs. 12–38 and 12–39). Cephalometric analysis correlated with our clinical impression that maxillary dental alveolar protrusion was the main contributing factor to her skeletal and dental alveolar problem. It was decided that an anterior maxillary osteotomy would be performed, moving the maxilla up 4 mm and back 8 mm to achieve an ideal overjet-overbite relationship.

The patient was hospitalized for an anterior maxillary osteotomy, which was performed under general anesthesia in the operating room. The mobilized anterior maxilla was approached by three vertical incisions in the labial vestibule and a midline palatal incision. Once the maxilla was mobilized, it was moved in the posterior superior direction and fixed to the remaining molar teeth with an occlusal and palatal coverage splint. There was no intermaxillary fixation used at the time. The patient had excellent postoperative healing with an ideal overjet-overbite relationship. The nasolabial angle was satisfactory postoperatively and she had partial dentures fabricated in her new relationship (Figs. 12–40 and 12–41).

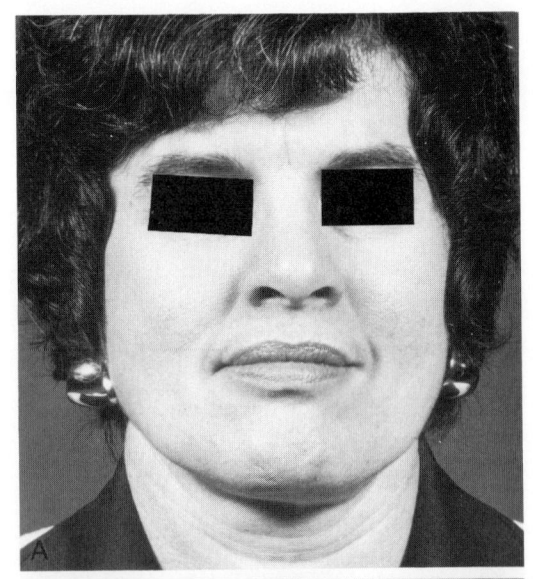

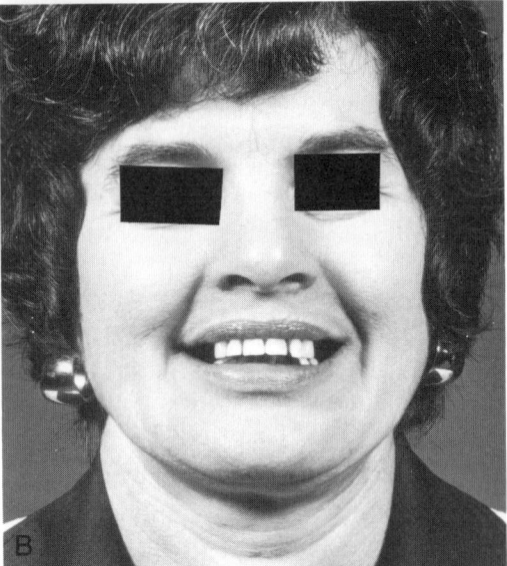

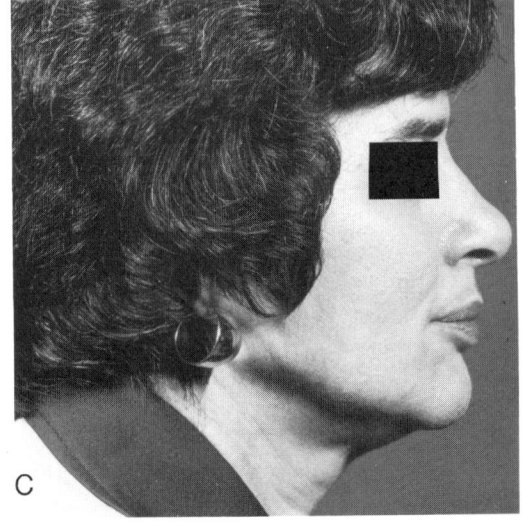

Figure 12–38. Case VI. Clinical appearance revealed a rather protrusive upper lip and acute nasolabial angle.

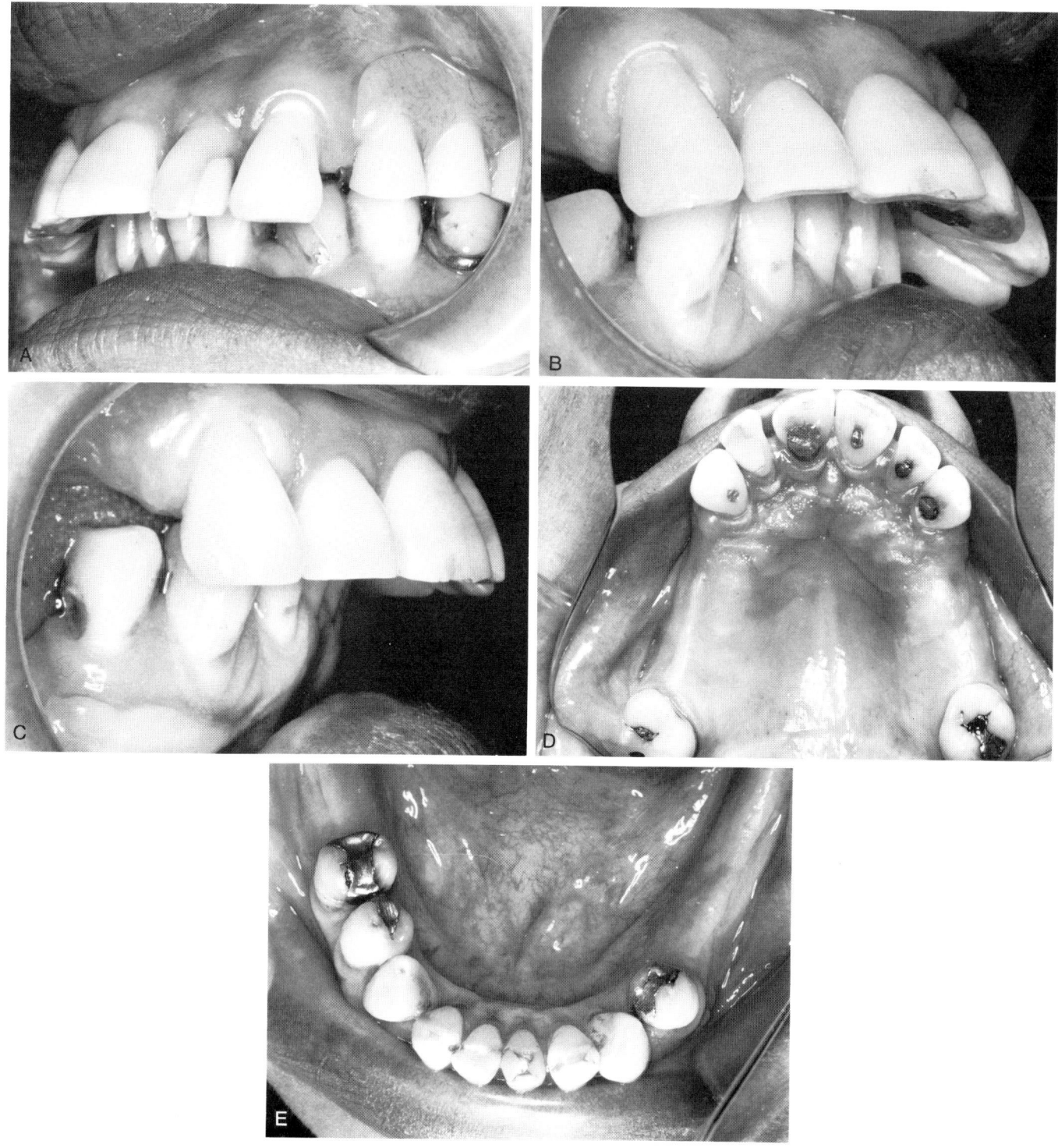

RECONSTRUCTIVE SURGERY FOR THE EDENTULOUS PATIENT / 503

Figure 12–39. The patient had multiple missing teeth and protrusive anterior maxillary teeth.

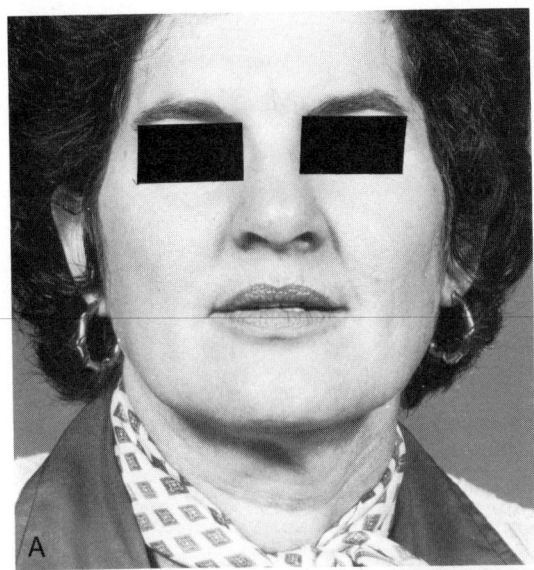

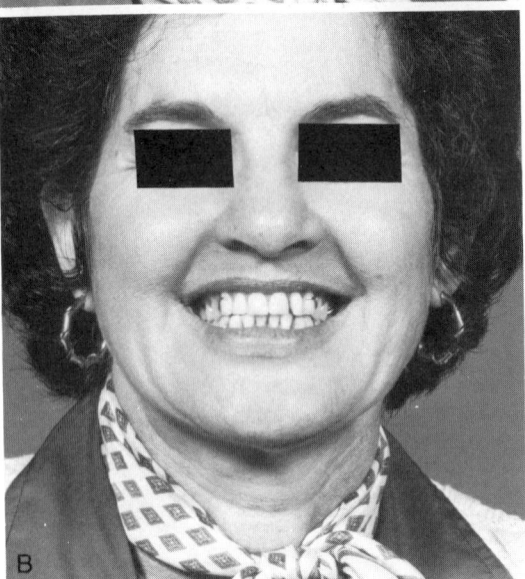

504 / RECONSTRUCTIVE SURGERY FOR THE EDENTULOUS PATIENT

Figure 12–40. Postoperatively she had good facial balance.

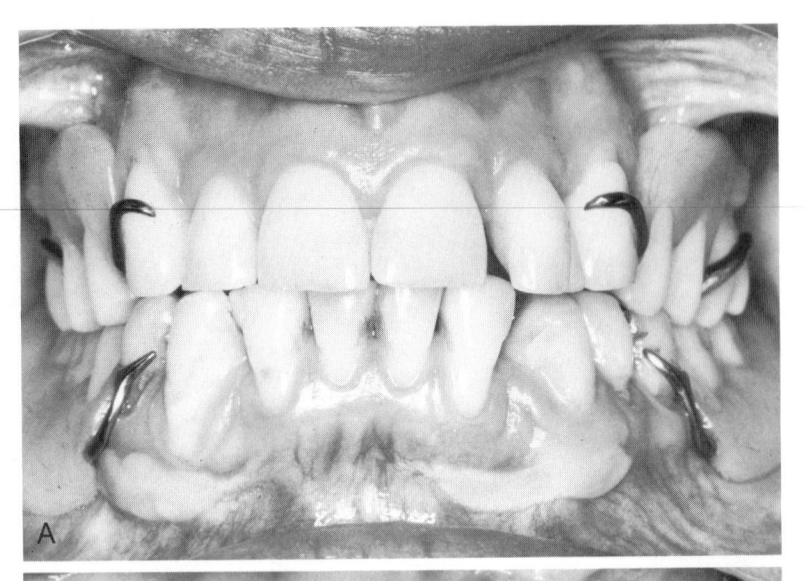

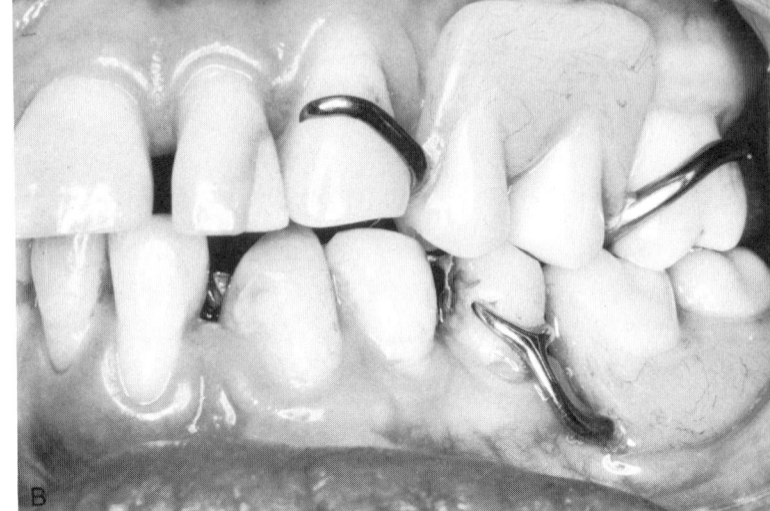

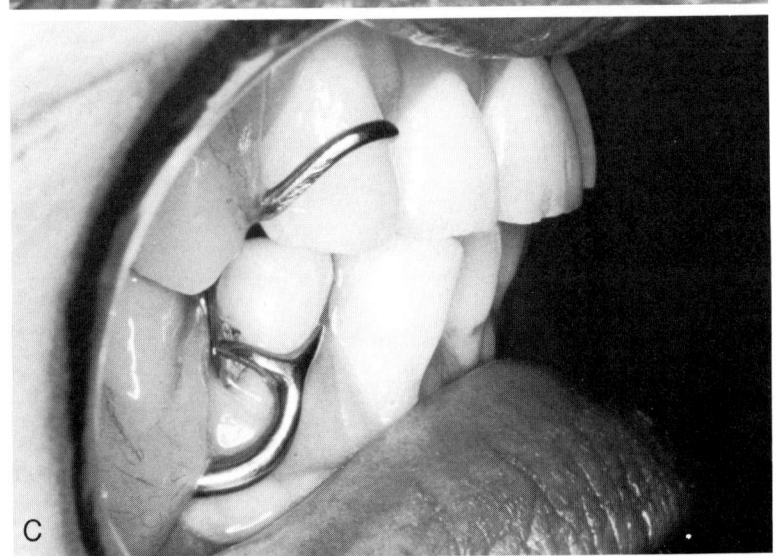

Figure 12–41. The nasolabial angle was satisfactory postoperatively, and she had partial dentures fabricated in her new relationship.

CASE VII

This 57-year-old white female presented to the oral surgery clinic at The University of North Carolina in April, 1979. Her chief complaint was an overly prominent chin and a sunken appearance of her perioral area (Figs. 12–42 and 12–43). Clinical and cephalometric examinations revealed a prognathic mandible, which we felt could be satisfactorily treated with bilateral intra-oral vertical ramus osteotomies and a setback of the mandible of approximately 11 mm.

The patient was hospitalized for her surgery and was taken to the operating room where under general anesthesia bilateral intra-oral vertical ramus osteotomies were performed. The patient was placed in intermaxillary fixation with Gunning splints. The proximal segments were not wired into place. The patient was discharged from the hospital on the second postoperative day, and subsequent postoperative visits revealed uneventful healing. She was released from intermaxillary fixation on the eighth postoperative week with good mandibular range of motion. Subsequent prosthetic follow-up included maxillary and mandibular dentures with good facial and occlusal results (Figs. 12–44 and 12–45).

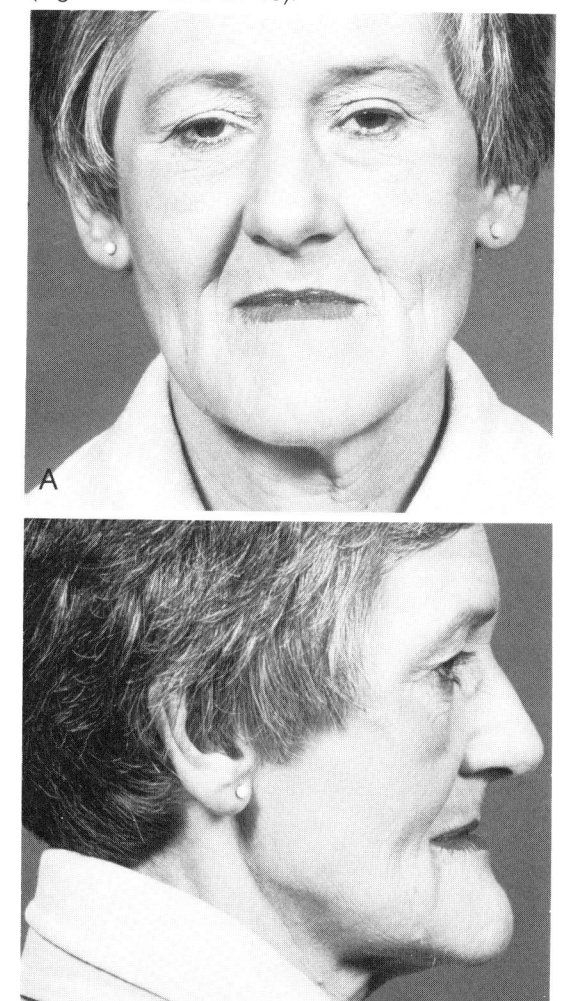

Figure 12–42. Case VII. The patient presented with sunken midfacial area with a concave profile and prominent chin.

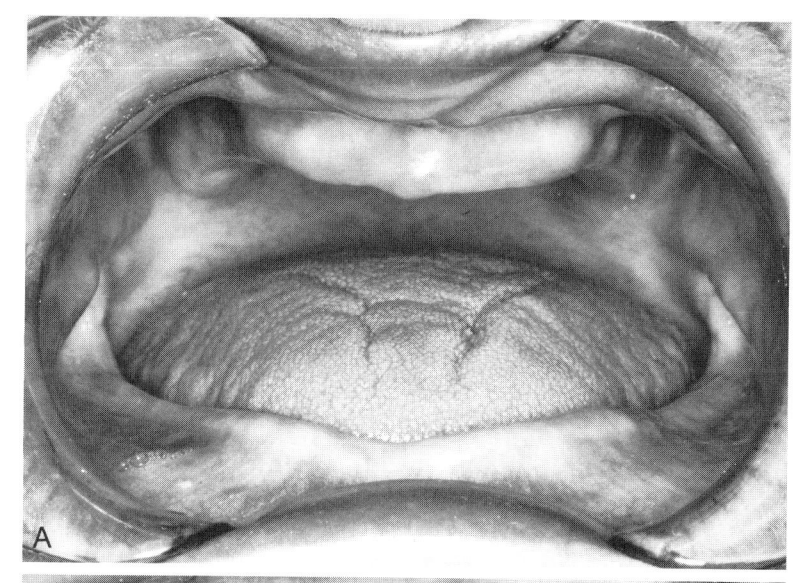

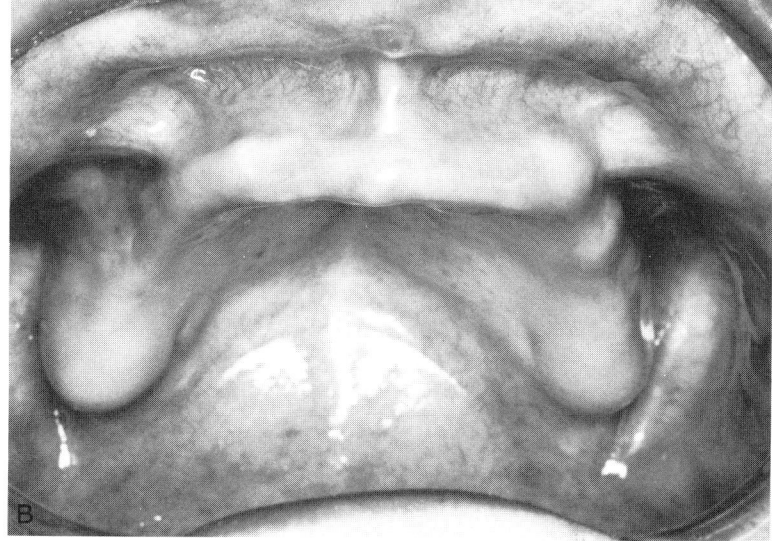

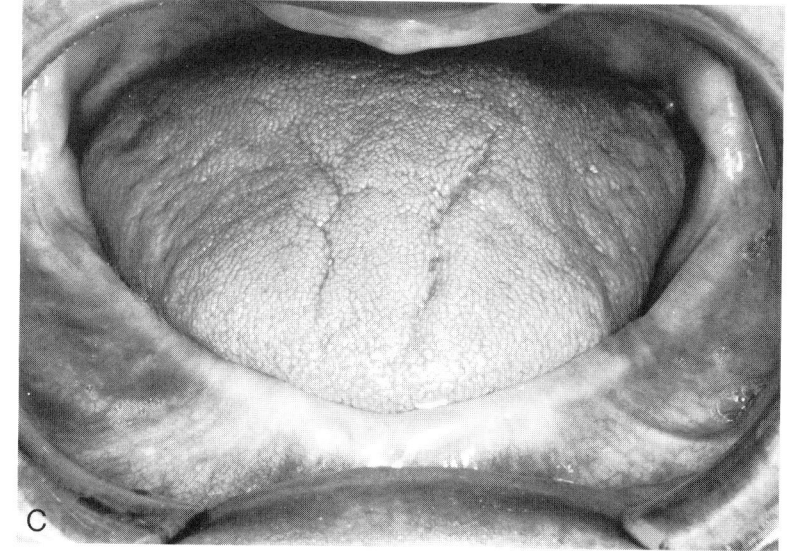

Figure 12–43. Interarch relationship revealed a Class III ridge relationship.

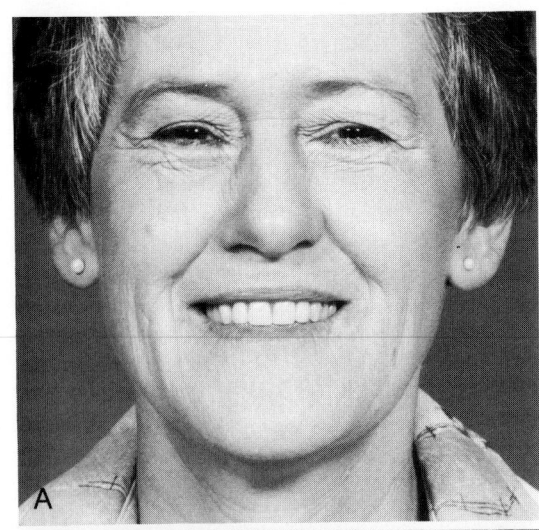

506 / RECONSTRUCTIVE SURGERY FOR THE EDENTULOUS PATIENT

Figure 12–44. Clinical photographs two years postoperatively show good facial balance.

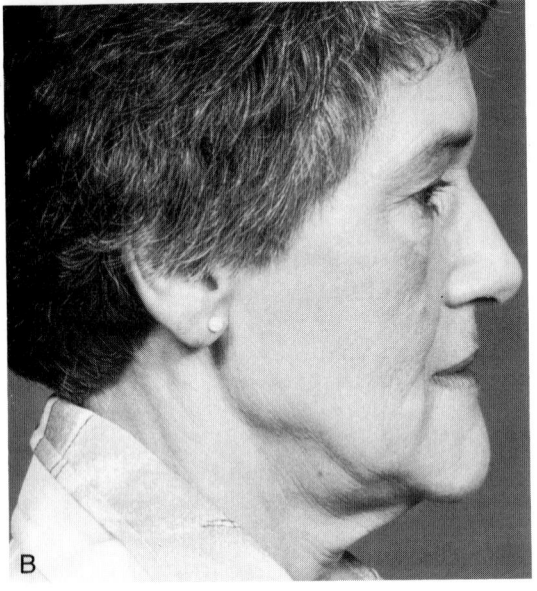

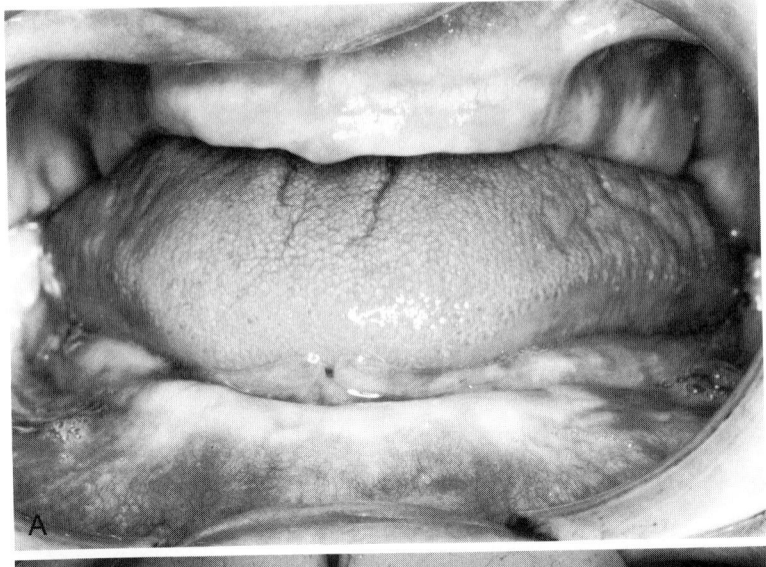

Figure 12–45. Good prosthetic rehabilitation and ridge relationship.

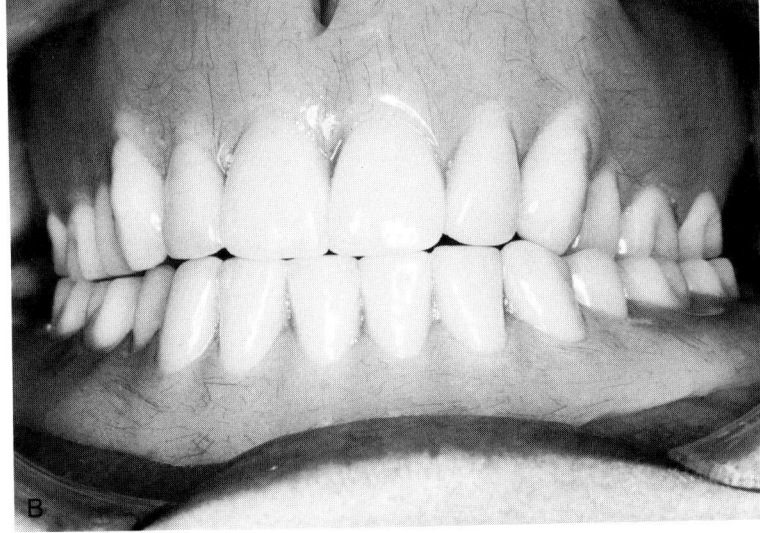

BIBLIOGRAPHY

1. Bell WH, Proffit WR, and White RJ: Surgical Correction of Dentofacial Deformities. Vols I and II. Philadelphia, WB Saunders Co, 1980.
2. Epker BN, and Wolford LM: Dentofacial Deformities—Surgical-Orthodontic Correction. St. Louis, CV Mosby Co, 1980.
3. Atwood DA: Cephalometric study of the clinical rest position of the mandible: Variability in the rate of bone loss. J Prosthet Dent 7:544, 1957.
4. Atwood DA: Reduction of residual ridges: A major oral disease entity. J Prosthet Dent 26:226, 1971.
5. Atwood DA, and Coy WA: Clinical, cephalometric, and densitometric study of reduction of residual ridges. J Prosthet Dent 26:280, 1971.
6. Mavroskoufis F, and Ritchie GM: Nasal width and incisive papilla as guides for the selection and arrangement of maxillary anterior teeth. J Prosthet Dent 45:592, 1981.
7. Morrow RM, Rudd KD, and Eissmann HF: Dental Laboratory Procedures—Complete Dentures. St. Louis, CV Mosby Co, 1980.
8. Araujo A, Schendel SA, Wolford LM, and Epker BN: Total maxillary advancement with and without bone grafting. J Oral Surg 36:849–858, 1978.
9. Frost DE, Fonseca RJ, and Burkes EJ: Healing of interpositional allogeneic lyophilized bone grafts following total maxillary osteotomy. J Oral Maxillofac Surg 40:776–786, 1982.
10. Stroud SW, Fonseca RJ, Sanders GW, and Burkes EJ: Healing of interpositional autologous bone grafts following total maxillary osteotomy. J Oral Surg 38:878–885, 1980.
11. West RA, and Burk JL: Maxillary osteotomies for preprosthetic surgery. J Oral Surg 32:13, 1974.
12. Booth DF: Control of the proximal segment by lower border wiring in the sagittal split osteotomy. J Maxillofac Surg 9:126–128, 1981.
13. DalPont G: Retromolar osteotomy for correction of prognathism. J Oral Surg 19:42, 1961.
14. Epker BN: Modifications in the sagittal osteotomy of the mandible. J Oral Surg 35:157, 1977.
15. Hunsuck EE: Modified intraoral sagittal splitting technic for correction of mandibular prognathism. J Oral Surg 26:250, 1968.
16. Obwegeser H: In Starshak TJ, and Sanders B: Preprosthetic Oral and Maxillofacial Surgery. St. Louis, CV Mosby Co, 1980.
17. Trauner R, and Obwegeser H: Surgical correction of mandibular prognathism and retrognathia with consideration of genioplasty. 1. Surgical procedures to correct mandibular prognathism and reshaping of the chin. Oral Surg 10:677, 1957.
18. Bell WH, Gonyea W, Finn RA, Storum KA, Johnston C, and Throckmorton GS: Muscular rehabilitation after orthognathic surgery. Oral Surg 56:229–235, 1983.

INDEX

NOTE: Page numbers in *italics* indicate figures; "t" following page number indicates "table."

AAA (Autolyzed antigen-extracted allogeneic) bone, 30
Abutment neck, on subperiosteal implant framework, definition of, 271
Abutment operation, for Branemark implants, 218
Acid-base problems, as contraindication for transmucosal implants, 55
Acrylic splint, as template in mandibular staple bone plate implant, 180, *180*, 181
  use in staple bone plate procedure, 182, 184
Acrylic tray construction, for stent method in vestibuloplasty with skin graft, 73, *73*
Activation, in remodeling, 2, *2*
  rate of, alterations in, 3, *3–4*
Acute rejection, of graft, definition of, 23
Alcoholism, cancer patients with, rehabilitation of, 424–425
Alkaline phosphatase activity, in edentulous bone loss, 15
Allergy, to implant component, 55
Allogeneic bone, autolyzed antigen-extracted (AAA), definition of, 30
  for reconstructive cribs, 368, 370
  lyophilized, as substitute for autogenous bone transplant, 30
Allogeneic ilia, 374–379. See also *Ilia, allogeneic.*
Allogeneic mandible, 371–374. See also *Mandible, allogeneic.*
Allografts. See also *Bone allografts.*
  definition of, 20
  first- and second-set immune reactions to, 27
  freeze-dried, 30
  frozen, 30
  immunogenicity of, 25–26
    humoral component of, 26–27
  primary, stages of rejection in, *24*
  rejection, clinical diagnosis of, 24
  secondary, stages of rejection in, *24*

Alloplastic cribs, 365, 367–368, *366–368*, *370*. See also *Cribs, alloplastic.*
Alloplastic materials, in fresh extraction sockets, 61
Alpha alumina oxide, 296. See also *Sapphire, single crystal.*
Aluminum oxide, host rejection of, as implant material, 340
Alveolar clefts, grafts to, 453
  problems from, 448
Alveolar nerve, inferior, immediate grafting for, 406
  position of graft of, 408
  potential for damage to, with visor osteotomy, 146
  transected and tagged during tumor removal, 408
Alveolar neurovascular bundle, decompression of, in modified visor osteotomy, 147, *148*
Alveolar ridge
  and removable prosthesis, 43
  atrophy of, 3
  augmentation of, after injury, 444–445, *445*
  correcting localized contour defects in, 56
  deficiency classification and treatment of, 312t
  disuse atrophy of, 8–9
  edentulous, 305
    natural history of, 48–49
  height restoration of, as goal of mandibular reconstruction, 361
  loss of, on mandible, 142
  management of, history of, 305–307
  net gain to contour of, following graft, particle size and, 32
  placement of holes for staple bone plate in relation to, 181
  preservation of, 340–344. See also *Resorption.*
    and hydroxylapatite maintainer as fresh socket implant, 341, *342*, *343*

Alveolar ridge (*Continued*)
  preservation of, during recontouring, 62
    with hydroxylapatite particles vs solid hydroxylapatite roots, 340–341
  pseudoaugmentation of, with palatal vault osteotomy, 128
  reconstruction procedures, *306*
  recontouring of, for TPS Screw Implant, *238*, 240
  secondary, 62
  resorption of, and Branemark implants success rate, 221
  sensitivity of, to systemic disorders, 4
  stability of, and hydroxylapatite augmentation, 337–338
Alveolar ridge reconstruction
  for Class III deficiency, results of, *327*
  for Class IV deficiency, hydroxylapatite-bone mixture recommendations for, 334
    results of, *328*, *330*
  procedures for, *306*
  radiographic studies of, 332
  surgical technique for major deficiencies, 315, *317*, 318, *319–324*, 322, 324–325
  surgical technique for minor deficiencies, 314–315, *316*
  with hydroxylapatite, 305–346
    LSU studies of, *327*, *328*, *330–331*, *332*
    complications found in, 329, 332t
    summaries of, 331t
    summary of, 344–345
Alveolectomy technique, and edentulous bone loss, 8
Alveoloplasties, and denture fit, 152
  anterior, to reduce mild maxillary excess, 477
  with tooth removal, 61–62
Amalgam condenser, to compress PBCM material, 385
American Society of Anesthesiologists, classes of patient evaluation by, 49, 50t

509

Anastomosis, development between bed and skin graft, effect of, 34
  of microvascular grafts, for mandibular reconstruction after injury, 441–442
  of nerve graft, 408, 409
Anatomic factors, and patient's reaction to dentures, 42–46
Andy Gump deformity, 349, 373
Anemias, as contraindication for transmucosal implants, 55
Anesthesia
  for direct bone impression phase of subperiosteal implant, 272
  for mandibular anterior vestibuloplasty with free mucosal graft, 93, 94
  for onlay bone grafting procedure, 119
  for titanium plasma spray implant, 237
  local, for crestally pedicled mucosal graft, 91
  planning for, in cleft patients, 452
Anesthesiologist, and vestibuloplasty with skin graft and LFM, 74
Ankyloglossia, correction of, 66
Anosmia, iodophor solution and, 182
Anteroposterior (A-P) arch discrepancies, correction of, with rib graft, 122
Antibiotic solution, allogeneic mandible crib reconstituted in, 371
  and bone graft storage, 362
  bone grafts reconstituted with, 153
Antibiotics
  after alveolar ridge reconstruction, 313, 325
  after bone graft for maxillofacial injury reconstruction, 435
  after crestally pedicled mucosal graft, 92
  after mandibular prosthetic reconstruction, 152–153
  after mandibular reconstruction, 364
  after mandibular staple bone plate implant, 186
  after maxillary prosthetic reconstruction, 136
  after surgical deformity correction in partially edentulous patients, 483
  after vestibuloplasty with skin graft, 86
    problems with prophylactic use of, 51–52
  prophylactic use of, as contraindication for transmucosal implants, 53
  review of, for maxillofacial intermediate care, 433
  use after accidental oral perforation in mandibular reconstruction, 365
Antibodies, circulating cytotoxic, testing for, in transplant recipient, 23
  production of, pattern altered by bone marrow removal, 26
  response of, to single bone allograft, in mice, 27
Anticoagulant therapy, chronic dicoumarol, as contraindication of transmucosal implants, 54–55
  as relative contraindication for soft tissue procedures, 52
Antigens, transplantation, 20
  definition of, 19
  detection of, in bone cells, 26
  source of, in grafts, 24
Antihistamines, after maxillary prosthetic reconstruction, 136
Antilymphocyte serum (ALS), immunosuppression of bone graft recipient with, 29
Antrum, implant proximity to, 173

Apatite, biologic, in bone-hydroxylapatite implant band, 310
Arch discrepancies, anteroposterior (A-P), correction of, with rib graft, 122
Ascites, and edentulous bone loss, 14
Aseptic technique, for bone grafts, 434
Atrophic ridges, osseous reconstruction of, 117–165. See also *Mandible, atrophic; Maxilla, atrophic.*
Atrophy, definition of, 1
Auricular defect, prosthesis placement for, 421
Auricular nerve, greater, as donor nerve for grafting, 406
  harvesting, 407, 407
  vs sural nerve, for graft, 408
Autogenous corticocancellous grafts, for mandibular reconstruction after injury, 437, 437, 438
Autogenous nerve grafting, 406–410
Autografts, bone. See *Bone grafts.*
  definition of, 20
  stages of rejection in, 24
Autolyzed antigen-extracted allogeneic (AAA) bone, definition of, 30
Autopolymerizing methyl methacrylate, 112

BMP. See *Bone morphogenetic protein.*
Band keratopathy, and edentulous bone loss, 14
Bayonet handpiece, position of, for use in ramus frame implantation, 284
Bioceram Zestplant, 296–297, 297, 298
Biocompatibility, of implant materials, definition of, 200
Biologic apatite, in bone-hydroxylapatite implant band, 310
Biphasic extraskeletal pin fixation, to stabilize bone fragments, 432, 433
Bite registration trays, preparation of, 274
Blade implants, success of, 168
Blade-vent implants, endosteal, 174, 178, 245–254
  armamentarium for, 247–248
  bony preparation for, 250
  contouring, to fit arch, 248
  contraindications for, 245
  design of, 246, 246–247
  determining size and shape of, 248
  effect of failure of, 254
  immediate postinsertion radiograph of, 252, 253
  indications for, 246
  mobility of, eliminating, 250
  proper seating of, 251, 251, 252
  survival rate of, 254
  technique for, 248–252, 249–253, 254
  temporization of, 252
Bleeding
  and methods of stent fixation, 103
  as airway hazard, 103
  from lingual area, effect of, 82
  from mylohyoid muscle, 97
  pattern of, at skin graft donor site, 33
Block bone autografts, for mandibular reconstruction, problems with, 361, 365
Blocking, in bone transplant, 26
Blood, preventing accumulation of, under skin graft, 89, 90
Blood count, for patient with edentulous bone loss, 14

Blood supply, mandibular effect of edentulous bone loss on, 11
  poor, to palatal bone, as hazard of palatal vault osteotomy, 128
Blood vessels, inosculation of, following skin grafts, 34
Body proportions, for patient with edentulous bone loss, 13
Bonding, bone-implant, implant material used and, 199
  of calcium-phosphate implants, 309–310, 310
Bone
  bare, decortication of, and skin graft success, 35
  cancellous, from ilium, 358
  denuded, skin graft process on, 78
  exposed on lingual of mandible, during vestibuloplasty with skin graft, 87
  formation of, estimating rate of, 15
  frozen, use of thawed, in graft, 27
  healing of, 355, 358
  immunobiology of, 25–31
  internal fixation of, after maxillofacial injury, 432
  management of, in maxillofacial injury, 430, 431, 432
  necrosis of, temperature for occurrence of, 214
  egeneration of. See *Osteogenesis.*
  removal of, for Hollow-Basket implants, 255
  resorption of. See *Resorption.*
  single crystal sapphires as stimulators of, 297
  tumors of, as contraindication for transmucosal implants, 55
  turnover of, in skeletal envelopes, normal progress of, 2
    rate of, determination of, 6, 6
  vitality of, and mechanical stimulation, 311
Bone allografts
  advantages of, for mandible reconstruction, 143
  characteristics of, 32
  chip size of, and alveolar ridge contour net gain, 32
  disadvantages of, 32
  exposition of, 153
  fetal, with bone paste, 29
  for maxillofacial injury reconstruction, 435
  healing of, immunosuppression to improve, 29
  histocompatibility antigens in, 27
  immune response to, effect on healing, 28–29
    histopathology of, 28
  in cleft areas for intra-arch stability, 454
  in place of autogenous bone, 25–26
  in utero studies of, 29
  interpositional, in anterior maxillary osteotomy, 136
    meshed palatal mucosal grafts over, 152
    overlaying with autologous cancellous bone, 126
  modified osteotomies with, infection following, 153
  on edentulous ridge, 31
  onlay, vs onlay bone autografts, on atrophic maxilla, 119
  preferred for anterior osteotomy, with posterior onlay graft, 151

Bone allografts (*Continued*)
  rejection of, 28
    cell-bound, 27
  secondary osteogenic phase in, 28
  treatment of, to destroy antigenicity, 30
  types of, 29–30
Bone augmentation, and timing of skin graft, 57
  and tongue position, 45
  as surgical option to improve denture function, 47
Bone autografts
  advantages for mandible reconstruction, 143
  block, for mandibular reconstruction, problems with, *361*, 365
  cancellous, history of, vs calcium phosphate implants, 311
  for mandibular reconstruction after injury, 435
  for total onlay graft for mandible reconstruction, 144
  in cleft areas for intra-arch stability, 454
  interpositional, in anterior maxillary osteotomy, 136
  on edentulous ridge, 31
  onlay, vs onlay bone allografts, on atrophic maxilla, 119
  patient's cost of acquiring, 25
  types of, for resected mandible reconstruction, 361
Bone biopsy, in examination for edentulous bone loss, 15
Bone blocks, autogenous, for mandibular reconstruction, problems with, *361*, 365
  corticocancellous, in osteotomy site, 151
  insertion between maxilla and pterygoid plates, in total maxillary osteotomy, 124, *126*
Bone bonding, with hydroxylapatite particles, 334
Bone chips. See also *Particulate bone and cancellous marrow grafts.*
  autologous, size of, and alveolar ridge contour net gain, 32
  cortical, as source of bone morphogenetic protein, 361
  packing in onlay bone grafting, 122, *122*
  packing of, on rib graft and mandible, 144, *144–145*
  storage of, 121
Bone density, decreased, drugs associated with, 7t
  measurement of, 14–15
  of white women, 1
Bone disease, systemic
  active, serum phosphate levels in, 15
  and edentulous bone loss, 4
  common types of, 4t
  evaluation for, 12t
  serum calcium levels in, 15
  treatment of, 15–16
Bone grafts, 25–33. See also *Bone allografts; Rib grafts.*
  and two-phase theory of osteogenesis, 358, 360
  availability of material for, 25
  avoiding stress on, from chewing, 136
  choices of, for mandible reconstruction, 143
  complications of, 442, 444
  donor site surgery, 162–164
  donor site variables in, 32

Bone grafts (*Continued*)
  exposure of, and use of allogeneic bone, 153
    treatment of, 153
  fixation and immobilization of, 435, *436*
  for maxillary defects, and prosthodontic treatment, 420
  for maxillofacial injury reconstruction, 434–444
  functions of, 434
  handling of, 434
  healing and revascularization of, 31–33
  incorporation of, into host skeleton, 28
  interposed augmentation of, on atrophic mandible, 145–147
    techniques for, 146
  interpositional, for correction of maxillary atrophy, 123
  in anterior maxillary osteotomy, 136, *136*
    placement of, 124, *126*
    total maxillary osteotomy with, 122–126, 123t
    vs onlay, 33
  lymph node activity following, 27
  marrow-depleted, 26
  maxillofacial, minimizing contamination in, 33
  nerve grafts and, 408
  on vascular pedicle with soft tissue, 389, *389–390*
  onlay, case study of, 156, *156, 157*
    drawbacks of, 305–306
    for maxillary reconstruction, 118t, 118–122
    indications for, 119
    resorption of, 416
    surgical procedures for, 119–122
  posterior, anterior osteotomy with, 150–152
  total, for mandibular reconstruction, 143–145, *144–145*
  pretreatment of, to reduce immunogenicity of, 29
  principles of, 434–435
  prior to implant use, 213
  recipient site variables in, 32–33
  reconstitution of, with antibiotic solution, 153
  resorption of, 361
  storage of, 362
  timing of harvest and placement of, 362
  to alveolar clefts, child's age and, 453
  history of, 452–453
  transoral, problems with, for maxillary reconstruction, 416, *416*
  wound closure after, 435
Bone growth chamber, *214*
Bone implant materials, mechanical properties of, 308t
Bone implants, definition of, 30
  deproteinized, as substitute for autogenous bone graft, 30
Bone impressions, direct, 271–276
  inspection of, 275, *275*
  obtaining, for subperiosteal implant, 274–275
Bone induction principle, 359
Bone loss, edentulous, 1–17. See also *Edentulous bone loss.*
Bone marrow. See *Marrow.*
Bone mill, *326*
Bone morphogenetic protein (BMP)
  and resorption, 360
  coronoid as source of, 363

Bone morphogenetic protein (BMP) (*Continued*)
  in allogeneic mandible cribs, 371
  in osteogenesis, 358
  maintained in AAA bone, 30
  within mineral cortex of bone, 360–361
Bone paste, for intrauterine repair of human skeletal anomalies, 29
Bone-implant bonding, implant material used and, 199
  of calcium phosphate implants, 309–310, *310*
Bone-implant interface, 197
  connective tissue at, problems from, 202
  hydroxylapatite implant and, *310*
  polycarbonate plug for analysis of, *209*
  surface ratio improved with plasma spray, 255
Bony matrix, immunogenicity of, 26
Boplant, definition of, 30
Bossing, and edentulous bone loss, 14
Bovine bone, as alternative to autogenous bone, 30
Brachycephalic face, and edentulous bone loss, 7–8, *8*, 14
Branemark implants, 199, 211–224, *224*. See also *Osseointegrated implant system.*
  abutment operation for, 218
  clinical studies of, control of patients in, 220
    overview of, 219–220
    patient selection for, 220
    summary of, 220
    conclusion for, 223–224
  experimental analysis of, 211–216
    summary of, 216
  factors contributing to success rate of, 168
  failure indications for, 221–222
  fractures of, 221–222
  general aspects of, 222–223
  handling of, 217
  healing-in of, 218
  indications and contraindications for, 220
  insertion of, *217*, 217–218
  instruments for installation of, *218*
  methodologic aspects of, 216–219
    summary of, 220
  physical characteristics of, *216*, 216–217
  prosthetic treatment for, 218–219, *219*
  removal of, 223
  results of treatment with, 220–222
    psychiatric comments on, 222
  sinus penetrating, success rate of, 221
Bridging phenomenon, in skin grafts, definition of, 33
Bruxism, and edentulous bone loss, 9
  and trauma to implant, 55
Buccal frenum correction, 65–66
Buccal inlay vestibuloplasties, maxillary, 114
Buccal mucosa, as support for maxillary bone graft, 414
Buccolabial dissection, in vestibuloplasty with skin graft, 77–79, *78*
Bur holds, and total maxillary osteotomy, 124
Buttons, for suture ends in mouth floor lowering, 90, *90*

Calcification, and calcium phosphate implants, 308, *309*
Calcitonin, coating of, on TCP [(Ca$_3$(PO$_4$)$_2$] implants, and implant success, 311

Calcitonin (*Continued*)
 serum levels of, in edentulous bone loss, 15
Calcium, low intake of, and alveolar bone loss, 7
 serum levels of, in edentulous bone loss, 15
 urinary levels, in edentulous bone loss, 15
Calcium ions, from implants, studies of, 308–309
Calcium phosphate biomaterials. See also *Hydroxylapatite*.
 biologic profile of, 308–312
 characteristics of ideal, 312
 dense ceramic of, scanning electronmicrograph of, *307*
 dense vs porous, 312
 history of, 306–307
 mechanical properties of, 307–308, 308t
 porous bioresorbable, for hard-tissue prosthetics, 308
 preparation and properties of, 307–308
Calcium phosphate implants
 bonding to bone, 309–310, *310*
 factors affecting success of, 310
 healing rates of, 311
 osteogenicity of, 310–311
 porous, problems with, 311, *311*
 vascular system within, 311
 vs cancellous bone autografts, 311
Cancellous bone
 autologous, overlaying interpositional bone allografts with, 126
 from ilium, *358*
 in bilateral cleft graft, *470*
 packing of, on rib graft and mandible, *144*, 144–145
Cancellous bone grafts
 appropriate uses of, 32
 iliac crest as source of, 162
 procedure for obtaining, from iliac crest, 162
 vs cortical, host response to, 32
Cancellous marrow cells, survival rate after harvest, 362
Cancellous-to-cortical ratio, high, for phase-one osteogenesis enhancement, 360
Cancer
 anatomy of defect after surgery for, 347–348
 early reconstruction after treatment for, choosing candidates for, 351
 hard-tissue defects from, 348–349
 immediate reconstruction after treatment for, problems with, 351
 problems compounding defects from, 347
 radiation treatment of, effects from, 350, *350*
 soft-tissue defects from, 349–350
 surgical reconstruction after treatment for, goals of, 355
 timing of reconstruction after treatment for, 350–351
Cancer patients
 extra-oral rehabilitation for, 420–423, *421*
  limitations and problems of, 422, *422*
  objective of, *421*, 422
 irradiated, osteomyocutaneous grafts for, 388–391, *389*, *390*. See also *Irradiated tissue*.
 reconstruction and rehabilitation of, 347–428

Cancer patients (*Continued*)
 rehabilitation programs for, 423–424
 rehabilitation vs reconstruction of, 424–426
Capillaries, in split-thickness skin graft, 34
Cardiovascular examination, for patient with edentulous bone loss, 14
Casts, diagnostic evaluation of mounted, for edentulous patients with deformities, 476
Catgut suture material, 82
 and suture abscess, 87
Ceka attachment, for denture to mandibular staple bone plate, 187
Cement line, definition of, 2
Cephalosporin, prophylactic treatment with, after mandibular reconstruction, 364
Ceramics, biocompatibility of, as implant material, 200
 pore size of, and bony ingrowth, 200
 strength of, as implant material, 200
Channel burs, proper use of, in blade-vent implants, 247, 248–249, *249*
Cheilosis, and edentulous bone loss, 14
Chest radiograph, for patient with edentulous bone loss, 14
Children, with clefts, maxillofacial growth in, 448
Chin, sensory disturbances in, following modified visor osteotomy, 149
Chin droop, and buccolabial dissection, *78*, *79*
 avoiding, following vestibuloplasty with skin graft, 87
 vestibuloplasties and, 92, *93*
Chloride, in oral cavity, 199
Chromosomes, coding of, for production of cell surface antigens, 21
Chronic rejection, of graft, definition of, 23–24
Chvostek sign, positive, and edentulous bone loss, 14
Circulating cytotoxic antibodies, testing for, in transplant recipients, 23
Circumalveolar fixation, stent outline for, *100*
Circummandibular ligatures, 84, *85*
 and stent removal, 86
 in placing and securing stent, 85
Circumnasal floor method, for stent fixation, 101, *101*, 102, 103
Circumpalatal fixation, stent outline for, *100*
Cleft lip, incidence of, 447t, 447–448
Cleft palate, incidence of, 447t, 447–448
Cleft patients, special problems of, 448–449, 449–451
Clefts, facial, 447–474
 anatomic considerations in treatment of, 451, 451–452
 bilateral, surgical technique for repairing, 459, 460–463
 bilateral alveolar, maxillary advancement with, 465, 469–470, 469–473
 congenital anomalies associated with, 449, 451
 diagnosis and treatment planning for, 448–452
 literature review for, 447–448
 maxillofacial growth in children with, 448
 presurgical work-up for, 452
 surgical considerations for, 452–473
 unilateral, surgical technique for repairing, 454–456, 455–459, 459

Cleft (*Continued*)
 facial, unilateral alveolar, maxillary advancement with, 461, *464–468*
Clenching, and edentulous bone loss, 9
Clindamycin, use after accidental oral perforation in mandibular reconstruction, 365
Closure. See also *Sutures*.
 for bilateral cleft repair, *461*
 for bone graft for maxillofacial injury reconstruction, 435
 for intra-oral sagittal split ramus osteotomy, 480
 for mandibular reconstruction after cancer surgery, 363, *363*, *364*
 for maxillary advancement with bilateral cleft graft, *470*
 for maxillary advancement with unilateral cleft graft, 4656
 for maxillary reconstruction, 415–416
 for transmandibular implant, 206, *207*
 water-tight, of oral mucosa, 444
Collagen, production of, by fibroblasts during hyperbaric oxygen exposure, 396
Coloration, of skin grafts, 36
Composite grafts, for maxillary reconstruction, allogeneic ribs for, 415, *415*
Condenser, amalgam, to compress PBCM material, 385
Condyle, goal of replacement, in cancer patient, 384
 reconstruction of, allogeneic mandible cribs for, 373, *373*
Congenital anomalies, associated with facial clefts, 449, 451
Congenital heart disease, occurrence of, in cleft patients, 451
Connective tissue, interface of, between implant and bone, 197
Connector bar superstructure, immediate placement of, after TPS implantation, 234
Connectors, on subperiosteal implant framework, definition of, 271
Contamination, metallic, avoidance of, for Branemark implants, 217
Contour grafts, in maxilla, resorption of, 416
Contraction, in oral tissue transplantation, 35–36
Core-Vent Attachment (C-VA), 227–228, *228*
Core-Vent Implant System, *224*, 224–231
 cementing process for, *230*
 diagnosis and treatment plan, 224
 modification of, *225*
 physical description of, 225–226
 restoration phase of, 226–231
 splinting of, with Titanium Screw Inserts, 230
 summary of, 231
 surgical phase of, 224–226
 verification of osseointegration of, 226
Coronoid process, removal of, in mandibular reconstruction after cancer surgery, 363
 to relieve tension, 435
Cortical bone grafts, vs cancellous, host response to, 32
Cortical chips, as source of bone morphogenetic protein, 361
Corticocancellous bone grafts, iliac crest as source of, 162
 for maxillary reconstruction, ipsilateral ilium for, 415

INDEX / 513

Corticocancellous bone grafts (*Continued*)
  procedure for obtaining, from iliac crest, 162
Corticosteroid use, as relative contraindication for soft tissue procedures, 51
  continuous, as absolute contraindication for transmucosal implants, 53
  for swelling, 87
Cosmetic implants, definition of, 199
Costochondral graft, split-rib for, 384, *385*, *386*
Creatinine, urinary levels of, in edentulous bone loss, 15
Creeping substitution (osteoconduction), definition of, 25
  occurrence of, in graft healing, 31–32
Crestal bone, preservation of, in tooth extraction, 61
  reduction of, in secondary alveolar recontouring, 62
Crestal tissue, removal in vestibuloplasty with skin graft, 81–82
  removal of redundant, 62
Cribs
  allogeneic bone, advantage of, in irradiated tissue, 370
    characteristics of ideal, 368
    compression of PBCM graft material in, 384–385, *387*
    contouring of, 370
    particulate bone and cancellous marrow grafts with, 368–397
  allogeneic ilia, resorption of, 377, *380*
  allogeneic mandible, fixation of, *372*, 372–373
    for condylar reconstruction, 373, *373*
    resorption of, 371
  allogeneic split-rib segments for, 380–385, *380*, *381*
    fixation of, in cancer patient, *381*, 383
  alloplastic,
    fixation of, 367, *368*
    materials for, 365, *367*
    particulate bone and cancellous marrow grafts with, 365, *366–368*, *367–368*, 370
    for injury repair, 438, *439*
    problem with, 365, *367*, *367*
    removal of, 438
    soft-tissue dissection for placement of, 367
    unaccptable for maxillary reconstruction, 415
    unsuited for patients with irradiated or scarred tissue, 368
  metallic, and resorption, *360*, 360, *361*
    for bone graft support, 435
    for rigid internal fixation, 410
    removal of, no indication for, 410
Crossbite, in case presentation, 484, 487
Cross-cut fissure bur, measuring, *284*
Cryosurgery, and epulis fissuratum removal, 66
C-VA (Core-Vent Attachment), 227–228, *228*
Cytotoxic antibodies, circulating, testing for, in transplant recipient, 23

Dacron/urethane tray, 438–439
Dalbo attachment, for denture to mandibular staple bone plate, 186
Dead space
  after maxillofacial injury, drains for, 433
  elimination of
    after maxillary reconstruction, 416

Dead space (*Continued*)
  elimination of, during bone graft closure, 435
    during mandibular reconstruction, 363
    to prevent hematoma, 444
    with deep tissue sutures, in cancer patient reconstruction, 370
    with sternocleidomastoid muscle flap, 399, 400, *400*
Decongestants, after maxillary prosthetic reconstruction, 136
Definitive obturator prosthesis, 419, *419*
  materials for, 419–420
Dental implants. See *Implants*.
Dentistry, goal of, 117
Dentition. See *Teeth*.
Dentoalveolar and dentofacial deformities, edentulous patients with, reconstruction of, 475–507
Denture patients, initial interview for, 42, *42*, *43*
Dentures
  adjustments to, after mandibular staple bone plate insertion, 186
  after secondary epithelialization procedure, 106, 107
  and edentulous bone loss, 9
  and hamular notch, 64
  completion of, after TPS Screw implantation, 243, *244*, 245
  constant use of, after buccal inlay vestibuloplasty, 114
  construction of
    after alveolar ridge reconstruction, 313
    after buccal inlay vestibuloplasty, 113
    after hydroxylapatite augmentation, 325, 329
    after mandibular anterior vestibuloplasty, 97
    after submucous vestibuloplasty, 106
    after transmandibular implant, 208–209
    after vestibuloplasty with skin graft, 86, 90
  conventional, factors determining success of, 41–46
  fit of, and need for alveoloplasty, 152
  function and dense hydroxylapatite implants, 308
  inadequate space for, treatment of, 46
  long-term use of, effect of, 44
  mandibular, improved retention of, with skin-lined pockets, 108
    stability of, and vestibule depth in mylohyoid origin area, 97, *97*
  unstable, surgical solution for, 48
  modification of, to make Gunning-type splints, *411*
  patient's attitude toward, 41
  postponement of wearing, and resorption after visor osteotomy, 149
  removal of, prior to alveolar ridge reconstruction, 312–313
  stable seating area for, as objective of VSG, 70, *70*
  submucosal fibrosis secondary to irritation from, removal of, 66
  surgery to improve structure for. See *Reconstructive surgery, preprosthetic*.
  surgical alteration of soft tissue for, 69
  with ramus frame implant, temporization of, 286–287
Depomethylprednisolone, after mandibular prosthetic reconstruction, 152–153

Deproteinized bone implants, as substitute for autogenous bone graft, 30
Depth gauge, 235–236, *235*, 240
Dermatome, description of use of, 74–75, *75*
Dexamethasone, prior to ramus frame implantation, 282
Dexon, for sutures, 82
  and suture abscess, 87
Diabetes mellitus, and oral fungal infections, 44
  as contraindication for transmucosal implants, 53
  and recipient beds for skin grafts, 34
Diamond excision, for frena removal, 65, *65*
Dichloromethylene diphosphonate, resorption inhibited by, 43
Diet
  after Branemark implants insertion, 218
  after maxillary prosthetic reconstruction, 136
  after subperiosteal implant, 278
  after surgical deformity correction in partially edentulous patients, 483
  and alveolar bone loss, 7
  and recovery from bone graft surgery, 434
  inadequacies in, in cancer patient rehabilitation, 425
Disarticulation, complete, for cancer treatment in tonsillar or retromolar areas, 348, 349
Displacement forces, mechanical resistance to, as objective of VSG, 70
Dividers, stainless steel, 293
Dogs, study of fibula allograft in, 28
Dolder bar, 243, *243*, *244*
  position of, for transmandibular implant, 206, *208*
  to splint TPS Screw implant, 237
Dolichocephalic face, and edentulous bone loss, 7–8, *8*
Donor site
  complications in, following graft harvest, 442
  for palatal mucosal graft, 107–108, *107*, *108*
  surgery at, for bone grafts, 162–164
  surgical technique in vestibuloplasty with skin graft, 74–75
  variables of, in bone grafting, 32
Drains
  after accidental oral perforation in mandibular reconstruction, 365
  after bone graft for maxillofacial injury reconstruction, 435, *436*
  after mandibular reconstruction, 364
  after maxillary reconstruction, 416
  for maxillofacial injury, 433
  at iliac crest donor site after surgery, 162
  following rib harvest for microvascular rib periosteal grafts, 392
Draping patient, for vestibuloplasty with skin graft, 77
Drill guide, 203, *203*
  use for transmandibular implant, 205–206, *205*, *206*
Drill machine. See also *Twist drill*.
  technique of using gradually larger, for implant insertion, *217*
  use to minimize temperature increase during implant insertion, 214
Dysphagia, from cancer therapy, 348

Edema, in mouth floor, and bleeding, 97
  steroids for prevention of, after mandibular prosthetic reconstruction, 153
Edentulous bone loss (EBL), 1–17
  anatomic considerations in, 9–11
  and need for patient history, 49
  and soft tissue alterations, 48–49
  and soft tissue chin support loss, 93, *93*
  anterior maxillary, vestibuloplasty combined with osteotomy to correct, 133, *134*
  evaluation of patients with, 11–16, 12t
  factors influencing, 3–9
    generalized, 4–7
    local, 7–9
  impact on mandible and maxilla, *10*
  in white women, 1
  physiology of, 1–3
  severe anterior, *119*
Edentulous patients
  surgery on, history of, 47
  with dentofacial and dentoalveolar deformities, 475–507
    case presentations of, 483–506
    diagnosis and treatment planning for, 476
    summary of, 483
  with mandible continuity defect, prosthesis for, 355
Edentulous ridge
  evaluating reconstruction for, 413
  gingival scar on crest of, 36
  histologic response to bone graft, 31
  vascular response to bone graft, 31
Education, of cancer patients, 423–424
  of patient prior to implant, 181
Elastic therapy, after surgical deformity correction in partially edentulous patients, 483
Elasticity, of implant materials, 201–202
Elderly patients, and recipient beds for skin grafts, 34
Eloxal cassette, autoclavable, 233
Endocrine system, disorders of, and edentulous bone loss, 6–7
  as contraindication for transmucosal implants, 55
  in patient evaluation for edentulous bone loss, 12–13
Endosteal blade-vent implants, *174*, *178*, *245–254*. See also Blade-vent implants, endosteal.
Endosteal Hollow-Basket Implant System, *174*, *178*, *254*, 254–269. See also Hollow-Basket Implant System.
Endosteal dental implants. See also Branemark implants; Core-Vent Implant System; Titanium Plasma Spray (TPS) Implant System.
  early problems with, 254
  relation to inferior alveolar canal, 173
Endosteum, bone remodeling in, 2
Enhancement, in bone transplant, definition of, 26
Epinephrine solution, for hemostasis in buccolabial dissection, 77
  in unilateral cleft repair, 455
  use prior to lingual dissection, 79
Epithelialization procedures, contraindications for, 50–52, 51t
  secondary, for maxilla reconstruction, 58, *106*, 106–107
Epulis fissuratum, management prior to vestibuloplasty with skin graft, 72

Epulis fissuratum (*Continued*)
  maxillary secondary epithelialization for, 106
  removal of, 66, *107*
Equilibration, importance of, to success of ramus frame, 282
  occlusal, and ramus frame implant success, 287
Esthetics, and prognathism treatment, 46
Exophthalmos, and edentulous bone loss, 14
External skeletal pin fixation, for cancer patient reconstruction, 412, *412*, *413*
Extirpative surgical phase, of prosthodontic treatment for maxillary defects, 417–418
Extra-oral osseointegrated implants, 223
Extra-oral rehabilitation for cancer patients, 420–423, *421*

Face
  atypical pain in, as contraindication for transmucosal implants, 55
  evaluation of, for edentulous patients with dentofacial and dentoalveolar deformities, 476
  morphology of, and edentulous bone loss, 7–8, *8*
  restoration of form of, as goal in reconstruction of cancer patient, 362
Facial clefts, reconstruction of, 447–474. See also *Clefts, facial*.
Facial pouch, split-thickness skin-lined, and buccal inlay success, 109–110
Fat, as undesirable bed for skin graft, 33
  separating genioglossi and geniohyoids, *81*
FDBA (Freeze-dried bone allografts), 30
Fenestrations, in implants, 255, *255*
Fetal allogeneic bone transplantation, with bone paste, 29
Finger dissection, for lingual dissection, 80, *81*
First-set rejection, of graft, definition of, 23
Fistula, oral cutaneous, drain placement to bone and, 433
  oral-nasal, and torus removal, 67
  closure of, in unilateral cleft repair, 456
  in cleft patients, 448, *449*
Fixation, problems with devices for, in resected symphysis reconstruction, 349
  rigid internal, in cancer patient reconstruction, 410
  skeletal, to maintain mandibular position, in case presentation, *497*, 498
  transpalatal, stent for, 103
Fluoride, in human plaque, 201
  in oral cavity, 199
  to reduce radiation caries, 425
Formation, in remodeling, 2, *2*
Fractures, facial, immobilization of, 433
  soft tissue repair after, 444
  in buccal and lingual cortices, waiting period following, and implants, 251
Free grafting, and tongue position, 45
  as surgical option to improve denture function, 46
  mucosal, 92–97
  oral mucosa, advantages of, 36
Freeze-dried bone allografts, 30

Frena, abnormal lingual, removal techniques for, 65–66
Frozen allografts, 30
Functional implants, fully, definition of, 199
Functional neck dissection, vs radical neck dissection, 348, *348*

Gastrointestinal system, diseases of, as contraindication for transmucosal implants, 55
  in patient evaluation for edentulous bone loss, 13, 14
Gauze dressings, on skin graft donor site, 76
Genial tubercles, management prior to vestibuloplasty with skin graft, 72
Genioglossus muscles, accidental detachment during VSG, 87
  and geniohyoids, identifying separation of, 80–81, *81*
  need for vestibular depth in area of, 87
  sectioning of, and swallowing difficulties, 81
Geniohyoid muscles, and genioglossi, identifying separation of, 80–81, *81*
Gingiva, and atrophic maxillary ridge, 119
  hyperplasia of, *450*
  on alveolar ridge, following extraction, 44
Gingivitis, problems with, after Branemark implants, 222
Glossitis, and edentulous bone loss, 14
Glycoproteins, antigens as, 20
  graft success related to, 19
Gold, as implant material, research on, 212
Gold-platinum alloy, as implant material, 201, *202*
  components of, 202
  mechanical values of, 203
Graft expander, 108, *108*
Grafted skin, characteristics of, 35–36
Grafting systems, desired characteristics of, 31
Grafts. See also *Bone grafts; Skin grafts*.
  donor-recipient matching for, 22–23
  free, and tongue position, 45
    as surgical option to improve denture function, 46
  oral mucosal, advantages of, 36
  healing processes of, 31
  host sensitization and effector response to, 23
  immobilization of, goals of, 410
  labiobuccal, 91
  osteomyocutaneous, for irradiated cancer patients, 388–391, *389*, *390*
    for mandibular reconstruction after injury, 441
  rejection of, diagnosis and prevention of, 24
    factors affecting recipient, 24
    immunobiology of, 23–24
  success of, and three-H phenomenon in irradiated tissue, 387–397, *388*
  to irradiated tissue, 350
  total onlay, for mandible reconstruction, 143–145, *144–145*
  transplantation of, biological aspects of, 19–39
  types of, 20, *20*

INDEX / 515

Granulation tissue
　after hydroxylapatite augmentation of alveolar ridge, 329
　after stent removal, 86
　buccolabial, development of, after vestibuloplasty with skin graft, 90
　from denture movement, 107
　long-standing, as undesirable bed for skin graft, 34
　support for growth of, and skin graft success, 33
Gunning splints
　for bone graft fixation after maxillofacial injury, 435
　for immobilizing jaw, 410, *411*, 412
　　disadvantages of, 410, 412
　for stabilization after osteotomy, 480, 481
　in case presentation, *499*, 500, *500*

HA, 305–346. See also *Hydroxylapatite*.
H-2 antigens, in mice, 20
Hair, growth of, on split-thickness skin grafts, 33
　in skin graft, following vestibuloplasty with skin graft, 87
　lack of facial and/or body, and edentulous bone loss, 13–14
Hair follicles, and skin grafts, 36
Hamular notch deepening, closure following, 64–65
　procedure for, 64–65, *65*
　success of, 58
Hard palate, freeing of, 129, *131*
Hard tissue augmentation procedures, contraindications for, 52–53, 53t
Haversian system, bone remodeling in, 2
Heat chamber, for study of bone necrosis, 214, *215*
Hematologic disorders, as relative contraindication for soft tissue procedures, 52
Hematoma, efforts to prevent, near graft, 444
　separating skin graft from bed, 34, *35*
Hemimandibulectomy, anatomical results of, 347–348, *348*
　for palatal tumor, facial deformity after, *413*
　patient with deformity from, following reconstruction, *368*, *369*, 377–380
Hemophilia, as contraindication for transmucosal implants, 53
Hemostasis, lidocaine and epinephrine solution for, in onlay bone grafting, 121
Hepatomegaly, and edentulous bone loss, 14
Heterogeneic individuals, definition of, 19
Heterografts, as substitutes for bone autografts, 30–31
　definition of, 20
Hexachlorophene, donor site preparation with, 74
　for surgical preparation of mouth before staple implant, 182
Histocompatibility antigens, 20
　detection of, in bone cells, 26
　source of, in grafts, 24
Histocompatibility (HLA) complex, major, 20–22
　functions of regions of, *22*
　in man vs mouse, 21, *21*

Histology, and calcium phosphate implants, 308, *309*
HLA phenotypes, relationship of, with human diseases, 22
HLA-D locus compatibility, evaluation to match living related donors, 23
HLA-D region, in MHC, genetics of immune response controlled by, 21
Hollow-Basket Implant System, *174*, *178*, *254*, 254–269
　bone removal reduction in, 255
　indications as to bone quantities, 256
　occlusal views of, *256*
　safety margin for, from vital structures, 255
　summary for, 269
　type "C," *256*, 256–258, *257*, 260
　type "E," *258*, 258–259
　　insertion of, *259*, 260
　type "F," 266–269, *267*–*269*
　　loading of, 268
　　site preparation for, 267, *267*–268, *268*
　　site selection for, 267
　type "H," 259–262, *260*–*263*
　　final seating of, 262
　　site preparation for, 260, 261, *261*
　　use and instruction for, 259
　type "K," 262–265, *264*–*266*
　　seating of, 265, *265*
　　site preparation for, 262–264, *264*
　　stability of, 267
　　sutures for, 265
　vs solid body implants, 256
Homografts. See also *Allografts*.
　definition of, 20
Horizontal ostectomy, for cancer treatment in tonsillar or retromolar areas, 348
Host tissue. See *Recipient tissue bed*.
Human diseases, relationship of HLA phenotypes with, 22
Human leukocyte antigens (HLA), 20
Human plaque, fluoride in, 201
Humoral immune system, human A and B loci antigens recognized by, 21
Hydrocolloid, irreversible, duplication of surgical stent with, 111, *112*
Hydrocortisone cream, postoperative use of, in vestibuloplasty with skin graft, 86
Hydroxylapatite ($Ca_{10}(PO_4)_6(OH)_2$), 307
　alveolar ridge reconstruction with, 305–346
　and Stage III mandible, 57
　augmentation with, and mobile mass removal, 329
　　of mandible, 47
　　recommendations for, 344
　　results of, *324*
　　secondary epithelialization over, 107
　biocompatibility of, 200
　ceramic forms of, 307
　dense form vs porous ceramics, bioresorption of, 307
　elasticity modulus of, 202
　fine powders of, 307
　in fresh extraction sockets, 61
　potential of, for reducing resorption, 56
　properties of, 334
　to restore Stage IV mandible, 57
Hydroxylapatite-autogenous bone mixture, vs hydroxylapatite only augmentation, 324–325, *326*
Hydroxylapatite implants, stability of, and fibrous tissue growth, 200
　interface with bone, *310*

Hydroxylapatite only augmentation, studies of placement, 334
　vs hydroxylapatite with bone augmentation, and resorption, 332
Hydroxylapatite particles, in anterior osteotomy with posterior onlay graft, 151
　confinement of, 314, *315*
　displacement of, 329, *333*
　migration of, modified mucosal dissection to reduce, 318, *319*–*321*
　shape of, and soft tissue inflammation, *336*, *337*
Hydroxylapatite ridge maintainers, as fresh socket implants, 341, *342*, *343*
Hydroxylapatite root implants, general vs custom-shaped, 340, *340*
　ratios for, and resorption, 336–337
Hydroxyproline, urinary levels of, in edentulous bone loss, 15
Hyperacute (secondary) rejection, of graft, definition of, 23
Hyperbaric oxygen therapy. See also *University of Miami/HBO protocol*.
　advantages of and drawback to, 396
　contraindications to, 396–397
　exposure of irradiated recipient tissue to, *388*, *388*, *389*
　to improve recipient tissue bed, 350
　for irradiated cancer patients, 32, 394–397, *394*–*397*
　transcutaneous oxygen measurements vs number of sessions, graph of, *389*
Hyperkeratosis, formation by skin, 70, *71*
Hyperparathyroidism, serum calcium and serum phosphate levels in, 15
Hyperplasia, potential for, around staple bone plate, 181, 186
Hyperreflexia, and edentulous bone loss, 14
Hypersensitivity, to implant component, as contraindication for transmucosal implants, 55
Hypertrophic scarring, prevention of, 91
Hypocellular recipient tissue, and graft success potential, 387–388
Hypoparathyroidism, serum calcium levels in, 15
Hyporeflexia, and edentulous bone loss, 14
Hypovascular recipient tissue, and graft success potential, 387–388
Hypoxic recipient tissue, and graft success potential, 387–388

Ia antigens, 21
Ilia, allogeneic
　advantages of, for cribs, 374
　crib from, resorption of, 377, *380*
　for PBCM grafts with allogeneic cribs, 374–379
　　results of, 377, *377*–*380*
　freeze-dried, *376*
　hemimandibular crib from, *376*
　placement and fixation of, *376*, 376–377, *377*
　shaping of, 374, *375*
　cancellous bone from, *358*
　ipsilateral, for corticocancellous grafts for maxillary reconstruction, 415
　medial approach to, for bone graft, 162, *163*
Iliac crest
　allogeneic, as crib for mandibular reconstruction after injury, 440–441

Iliac crest (Continued)
  and bone graft donor site surgery, 162
    complications in, 442
  augmentation method with, problems
    with, 47
  harvesting grafts from, 437, 437, 438
Iliac crest grafts
  for unilateral cleft patient, 455
  in case presentation, 484
  mandible reconstruction with, prior to
    placement of staple bone plate, 187,
    187–189, 189, 191
  microvascular, for irradiated cancer patients, 392–393, 393, 394
Immobilization, following orthognathic
  surgery on cleft patient, 453–454
Immune response, gene product antigen,
  recognition by, 21
  to bone allografts, effect on healing,
    28–29
  histopathology of, 28
Immunity, transfer of, through plasma
  serum, lymph or spleen cells, 27
Immunogenicity
  and thawing of frozen bone, 27
  cell-mediated component of, 27–31
  definition of, 25
  efforts to decrease, in oral transplant
    surgery, 25
  of bony matrix, 26
  reduction of, through pretreatment of
    bone graft, 29
  retained in frozen bone allograft, 30
Immunosuppression, and skin grafts, 24
  drugs used in, 24
  to improve healing of allogeneic bone,
    29
Implant-bone interface. See *Bone-implant interface.*
Implant(s)
  and age of patient, 49
  as surgical option to improve denture
    function, 47
  bearing capacity of, definition of, 202
  blade-vent, 174, 178, 245–254. See also
    Blade-vent implants, endosteal.
  Branemark, 199, 211–224, 224. See also
    Branemark implants.
  candidate selection for, 169–175
  categories of, 199
  complications associated with, 168
  definition of, 25, 30
  density analysis from radiographs of
    bone tissue around, 216, 216
  determining size of, 173–174
  history of, 167
  history of research on, 211
  importance of bed for, research on,
    213–214
  in preprosthetic reconstructive surgery,
    167–304
  insertion of, surgical trauma at, research on, 214–215
  loading of, research on, 215–216
  macro- and microstructure of, research
    on, 212–213
  mandibular staple bone plate, 175,
    179–197, 199. See also *Mandibular staple bone plate implants.*
  manufacture and handling of, 213
  materials for, 199–202
    biocompatibility of, 200–201
    elasticity of, 201–202
    strength of, 199–200
  medical-legal considerations of, 50

Implants (Continued)
  objective criteria for success of, 223
  osseointegrated. See *Osseointegrated implant system.*
  pathologic abnormality correction prior
    to, 174, 176
  preoperative study of, with casts, 175
  radiographs as aid in planning for, 171,
    171–175, 173–175
  ramus frame, 281–296. See also *Ramus frame implants.*
  shearing strength of adjacent bone to,
    202
  stresses on, 212
  subperiosteal, 269–281, 270. See also
    Subperiosteal mandibular implants.
  success of, definition of, 167–168
  surface of, microroughness of, 212, 213
    for bonding, 234
  transmucosal, contraindications for,
    53–55, 54t
  vitreous carbon, 168
Impression caps, in TPS Screw Implant
  system, 236
Impression trays, laboratory fabrication
  of, 278, 279
  preparation of, 274
Impressions, following TPS Screw implantation, 241, 242
  following vestibuloplasty with skin
    graft, 71
  for acrylic tray construction, 73
Incision(s)
  crestal, in buccolabial dissection, 77, 77
  for alveolar ridge reconstruction for minor deficiencies, 314–315, 316
  for cleft repair
    bilateral, 460
      with maxillary advancement, 469
    unilateral, 455, 455
      with maxillary advancement, 461,
        464
  for direct bone impression phase of
    subperiosteal implant, 272, 273
  for graft procedures
    anterior osteotomy with posterior onlay, 150, 151
    for bone in maxillofacial injury reconstruction, 434
    maxillary osteotomy with interpositional, 124, 124
    onlay bone, 120, 121
    total onlay mandibular, 143–144, 144
  for implant procedures
    blade-vent, 248, 249
    Hollow-Basket "H," 260
    mandibular staple bone plate, 182,
      182, 183
    midcrestal mucoperiosteal, for Hollow-Basket "E," 258
    RA-2 ramus frame, 292–293
    ramus frame, 282, 283
    TPS screw, 237, 238, 239
    transmandibular, 204, 205
  for intra-oral sagittal split ramus osteotomy, for edentulous patients, 479–480
  for maxillary ridge augmentation with
    hydroxylapatite, 315, 317
  for secondary epithelialization procedure, 106, 107
  for vestibuloplasties
    buccal inlay, 111, 111
    maxillary, 100, 101
    mylohyoid area, 97, 97
    submucous, 105

Incision(s) (Continued)
  horizontal ridge crest, for open technique hydroxylapatite mandibular
    augmentation, 318, 322
  in lingual dissection, 79–80, 80
  in modified visor osteotomy, 147
  modified Weber-Ferguson, for maxillary
    reconstruction, 414, 414
  placement of, in mandibular reconstruction after cancer surgery, 362, 362
  to correct anteroposterior deficiency of
    maxilla, 477
Infection
  after mandibular prosthetic reconstruction, 153
  as disadvantage in subperiosteal implant, 47
  control of, near staple bone plate supported by natural dentition, 192
  dead space during mandibular reconstruction and, 363
  in recipient tissue bed, after maxillofacial injury reconstruction, 442
Inferior alveolar nerve, immediate grafting
  for, 406
  position of graft for, 408
Injuries, intra-oral, early care of, 432–433
  maxillofacial. See also *Maxillofacial injuries.*
  reconstructive surgery for, 429–446
Instruments, for endosteal blade-vent implants, 247, 247–248
  for ramus frame implants, 283
  for transmandibular implants, 203
Interim phase, of treatment for mandibular defects in cancer patients, 354
  of treatment for maxillary defects,
    418–419
Interpositional bone grafts, 122–126. See
  also *Bone grafts, interpositional.*
Interpositional osteotomies, disadvantages
  of, 306
Iodophor, contraindication in skin grafts,
  74
  for surgical preparation of mouth before
    staple implant, 182
Ipsilateral radical neck dissection,
  347–348, 348
Irradiated tissue, 387–397, 388. See also
  Radiation treatment.
  advantage of allogeneic bone cribs in,
    370
  as bed for implant, 33, 214
  cribs unsuited for, 368
  hyperbaric oxygen to enhance, 32,
    394–397, 394–397
  oxygen tensions of, vs nonirradiated
    tissue, 394
  revascularization of, after hyperbaric
    oxygen sessions, 396
Irrigation, of maxillofacial injury, 430
Isogeneic individuals, definition of, 19
Isografts, definition of, 20
ITI Endosteal Hollow-Basket Implant Systems, 254, 254–269. See also *Hollow-Basket Implant System.*

Jaw fixation techniques, in cancer patient
  reconstruction, 410–412
Jaw surgery, combined. See also *Maxillomandibular surgery, simultaneous.*
  for deformity correction in edentulous
    patients, 481–482

INDEX / 517

Job placement, in rehabilitation of cancer patients, 426
Joe Hall Morris external skeletal pin fixation device, 412

Keratinization, of mucosa, 44
Kiel bone, definition of, 30

Labial closure, in maxillary advancement with unilateral cleft graft, 465
Labial frenum correction, 65–66
Labiobuccal grafts, 91
Laboratory, instructions for, concerning subperiosteal implant, 278
  materials needed by, to construct subperiosteal implant framework, 279
Laboratory examinations, for patient with edentulous bone loss, 14–15
Lag screws, for stabilization of mandible, 481
Lamellar bone, activation on surface of, 2
Lamina dura, loss of, in systemic disorders, 4
Lateral femoral cutaneous nerve, avoiding, during iliac crest donor site surgery, 162
Latissimus dorsi myocutaneous flap, to correct soft tissue defects, 404–406, 404–406
  problems with, 405, 405–406
LeFort I osteotomy
  for totally edentulous patient, 477
  in case presentation, 484
  interpositional graft to site of, biologic acceptance of, 123
  modified, for maxilla reconstruction, 58
Leukocyte migration test, to study immune response to allografted bone, 26
Lew Lock pin, 288, 290
Lew Passive Attachments, holes for, 228
LFM. See *Mouth floor, lowering of.*
Life expectancy, role in treatment planning for reconstructive preprosthetic surgery, 49–50
Ligatures, circummandibular, 84, 85
  and stent removal, 86
  in placing and securing stent, 85
Lingual area, dissection of, in vestibuloplasty with skin graft, 79–81
  incision for, 79–80, 80
  effect of bleeding from, 82
Lingual nerve, avoiding during lingual dissection, 80
  immediate grafting for, 406
  paresthesia of, 87
Lingual sulcus, postoperative condition of, 99
Lingual swelling, minimizing, and hemostasis, 87
Lip, cleft. See *Cleft lip.*
Lip anesthesia, from mental nerve injury, 313
Lip switch technique, for hydroxylapatite augmentation, 322, 322–323, 324
Load, redirection of, Hollow-Basket implant design and, 255
Lumbar spine, pain in, and edentulous bone loss, 14
Lymph nodes, activity in antibody production following bone graft, 27
Lymphatic system, penetration of, and cancer treatment, 348

Lymphatic system (*Continued*)
  restoration of continuity following skin grafts, 34
Lymphocyte culture (MLC) reactivity, mixed, definition of, 23

Major connectors, on subperiosteal implant framework, definition of, 271
Mallet, spring-driven, 293
Mandible
  allogeneic
    as crib, in mandibular reconstruction after injury, 439–440, 440
    availability of, 371
    for PBCM grafts within allogeneic cribs, 371–374
    rehydration of, 371
    tissue preparation for graft with crib, 371–372, 372
    use of, reserved for large defects, 374
  alveolar ridge reconstruction with hydroxylapatite, 318, 319–321, 322, 322–323, 324, 324
  anatomy and physiology of, and edentulous bone loss, 10
  anteroposterior deficiency of, surgical procedures for, 479–481
  anteroposterior excess of, surgical procedures for, 478–479, 478–479
  atrophic, interposed bone graft augmentation of, 145–147
    staple bone plate for, 187
    total onlay graft for, 143–145
    with lack of keratinized attached mucosa, 44
  augmentation of, choosing procedure for, 143
    goals of, 143
    surgical procedures for, 143–164
    with hydroxylapatite, 47
    with rib autograft, prior to staple bone plate insertion, 189, 190
  avulsion injuries of, 429, 429
  blood supply to, and edentulous bone loss, 11
  bone resorption in, 43
  Branemark implants on, success rate of, 221
  buccal surface of, concavity in, and graft adaptation, 89
  continuous, as goal of reconstruction, 361
  deficiency of, in case presentation, 495
  edentulous, patterns of, 9
    stages and treatment planning, 56t, 56–57
    surgical management of, 117
  epithelialization on lingual side of, 90
  fracture of, and graft resorption, 154
    as complication of modified visor osteotomy, 153
    during osteotomy, treatment for, 153–154
  freeze-dried, allogeneic, 371
  height of, and indications for vestibuloplasty, 93
  measurement of, prior to staple bone plate implant, 180
  inferior border of, at removal of staple bone plate, 197
  obtaining impression of, for subperiosteal implant, 273, 274
  prefabricated, Silastic, to maintain space and facial contour after injury, 432

Mandible (*Continued*)
  preparation of, prior to subperiosteal implant, 270, 271
  procedures for surgical management of soft tissue problems of, 69–98
  prognathic, appearance of, and edentulous bone loss, 127
    correction of, 505
    in case presentation, 499, 499
  prosthetic reconstruction of, case study of, 154–161, 154–161
    postoperative considerations, 152–154
    potential complications from, 153
  reconstruction of, after injury, methods of, 435
    difficulties with, 349, 349
    following tumor resection, staple bone plate use in, 189, 191
    graft systems for, 435–442
    rigid internal fixation for, 410
    with hydroxylapatite and staple bone plate, 337, 337–338 338, 339
  rehabilitation to retrain muscles controlling, after cancer treatment, 353
  resorption of, and vestibuloplasty with skin graft, 71
  restoring strength to stage IV, 57
  retrognathic, edentulous patient with, and esthetics, 46
  ridge model for, and shaping and sizing rib graft, 144
  ridge relation to maxilla, following tooth loss, 49
  skeletal fixation to maintain position of, after surgery, 497, 498
  surgical prosthetic reconstruction of, 142–161
    intra-oral examination prior to, 142–143
Mandibular continuity defects, reconstruction of, 355, 358–412
  after cancer treatment
    and prosthetic considerations, 351–355, 356–357
    classification of, 351–352, 352
    cosmetic deficiencies from, 353
    physiologic concerns with, 352–353
    prosthetic management for, 353–355
    psychological deficiencies from, 353
  allogeneic ilia technique for, 374–379
  allogeneic mandibles technique for, 371–374
    results of, 373, 374, 375
  allogeneic split-rib technique for, 380–386
  biologic basis of, 355, 358–361
  from resection of, 353
  goals of, 361–362
  surgical phase of treatment for, 353–354
  surgical techniques for, 362–365
  transcutaneous approach for, 362
Mandibular denture, improved retention of, with skin-lined pockets, 108
  stability of, and vestibule depth in mylohyoid origin area, 97, 97
  unstable, surgical solution for, 48
Mandibular guide flange prosthesis, 354, 354–355
Mandibular staple bone plate implants, 175, 179–197, 199
  and hydroxylapatite augmentation, 337–338, 337–338
  complications of, 169t
  configuration for, 179, 179

Mandibular staple bone plate implants (Continued)
  consent form for, 181
  drill holes for, 184, *184*
  for injury repair, 192–193, *192–196*, 196–197
  future of, 197
  indications and contraindications for, 180
  inferior border of mandible at removal of, 197
  insertion of, 185, *185*
  instruments for, 181, *182*
  materials for, 179
  mobility of, infection complicated by, 192
  patient selection for, 179–180
  postoperative management of, 186
  preoperative preparation for, 180–181
  problems with, 186
  prosthetic reconstruction with, 186–187
  study of, results of, 168
  success of, 168
  surgical and prosthetic summary for, 187
  surgical technique for placement of, *182*, 182–186, *184–186*
  versatility of, 187–197
Mandibular subperiosteal implant, *178*, 269–281, *270*. See also *Subperiosteal mandibular implants.*
Mandibular torus, removal of, 66–67, *67*
Marrow
  packing in onlay bone grafting, 122
  removal of, impact of, on antibody production, and bone graft, 26
  storage of, 121
  viable autogenous, coating of, on TCP (Ca$_3$(PO$_4$)$_2$ implants, and implant success, 311
Mastication, improvement of, with maxillary occlusal plane prosthesis, 355
  maximum force of, measured in molar area, 199
Maxilla
  advancement of, with unilateral alveolar cleft, 461, 464, *464–468*
  anatomy and physiology of, and edentulous bone loss, 10
  anterior, correction of atrophy in, with rib grafts, 122
  anterior atrophy of, 133t
    with adequate tuberosity, case study of, 138–141, *139–141*
  anteroposterior deficiency of, surgical procedures for, 476–477
  anteroposterior excess of, surgical procedures for, 477–478
  atrophic, autologous onlay bone grafts for, vs allogeneic onlay grafts, 119
    totally, with good palatal vault form, 123t
    with poor palatal vault form, 118t
    with adequate palatal vault form, case study of, 137–138, *137–139*
  augmentation of, with freeze-dried bone, 119
  avulsion injuries of, 429
  bone resorption in, 43
  Branemark implants on, success rate of, 221
  deficiency of, 117t
    in case presentation, 484
    surgical procedures for, 118t
  dental alveolar protrusion, correction for, in case presentation, 502, *503*

Maxilla (Continued)
  downfracturing of, 134, *135*
    mobilization and, 124, *125*
    segmentalization of, to correct transverse deficiency, 127, *127–128*
  edentulous, surgical management of, 117
    treatment plan for, factors affecting, 57–58
  edentulous bone loss in, *119*
    contributing reasons for, 118
    preoperative evaluation of, 118
    types of, 117
  excess, three-piece osteotomy to correct, in case presentation, 491
  growth of, after palatal surgery, 448
  impression of, made prior to buccal inlay vestibuloplasty, 110
  maintenance of posterior segments' positions with temporary prosthesis, 490
  prosthetic management of defects of, 417–420
    extirpative surgical phase, 417–418
    follow-up schedule for, 420
    interim phase of, 418–419
    reconstructive-rehabilitative phase of, 419–420
  reconstruction of, after cancer treatment, 412–423
    goals of, 413
    soft tissue assessment in, 414
    surgical approach to, 412–417
    surgical technique for, 414–416
  after injury, 442
    cosmetic reasons for, 420
    problem with transoral bone grafts for, 416, *416*
    with hydroxylapatite, 315, *317*, 318, *339*
  resection of, deficiencies from, 417
  ridge relation to mandible, following tooth loss, 49
  stabilized with allogeneic bone block, after correction of transverse deficiency, 128, *128*
  surgical management for soft tissue problems, 98–115
  surgical prosthetic reconstruction of, 117–142
    postoperative management for, 136
  total osteotomy with palatal vault extension, case study of, 141–142, *141–142*
Maxillary arch bar, in case presentation, 487–488
Maxillary canine, eruption of, alveolar cleft grafting prior to, 453, *454*
Maxillary cast, 417–418, *418*
Maxillary inclined plane prosthesis, 354, *354*
Maxillary lateral vestibule, scarring of, in cleft patients, 449
Maxillary occlusal plane prosthesis, 355, *355*
Maxillary occlusal table prosthesis, 355, *355*
Maxillary palatal splint, 67
Maxillary sinus, pneumatization of, radiograph to determine extent of, 62
Maxillary tuberosity reduction, 62–64, *63*
  with local vestibuloplasty, 64
Maxillary vestibuloplasties
  buccal inlay, 109–115
    constant use of splint or denture following, 114
    controversy over, 109
    indications for, 109, *110*
    with skin graft, 98–104

Maxillofacial injuries, 429–446
  early care of, 430, *431*, *432*, 432–433
  intermediate care of, 433
  priority of, vs other injuries, 430
  reconstructive care of, 433–445, *436–441*, *443*
    potential complications in, 442, 444
    timing of procedures for, 445
  summary of treatment for, 445–446
Maxillofacial prostheses. See *Prostheses, maxillofacial.*
Maxillomandibular fixation, in mandibular continuity defect treatment, 353
Maxillomandibular malrelations, as factor in denture success, 45
Maxillomandibular surgery, for cleft patients, 470
  simultaneous. See also *Jaw surgery, combined.*
Menopause, influence on bone loss, 4
Mental foramen, caudal margin, removing bony ridge from, 79, *79*
  exposure of, avoided in supraperiosteal dissection, 93, *94*
Mental nerve
  and edentulous bone loss, 9
  dissection of, vestibuloplasties involving, 92
  in mandibular augmentation with hydroxylapatite, 318, *319*
  paresthesia in, and mental N-V bundle dissection, 87
    decreased incidence of, after anterior osteotomy, 152
  position of, after mandibular resorption, and implant support for denture, 198
  potential injury to, 313
  relation of, to ridge, and periosteum elevation, 318
Mental neuropathy, modified mucosal dissection to reduce, 318, *319–321*
Mental neurovascular (N-V) bundle
  and supraperiosteal dissection in VSG, 78
  and three-piece augmentation osteotomy, 150
  avoiding trauma to, 79, 273, *273*, 284
  in TPS Screw implantation, 239
  dissection of, and paresthesia, 79, 87
  pain from prosthesis impinging on, 270, *270*
  potential for impression material below, 274–275
  skin graft sutures in relation to, 88
Mentalis muscle, dissection of, and chin droop, *78*, *79*, 92
  in mandibular augmentation with hydroxylapatite, 318
Metabolic disorders, as relative contraindication for tissue augmentation, 52
Metacarpophalangeal joint replacements, osseointegrated screws as anchor for, 223
Metallic contamination, avoidance of, for Branemark implants, 217
Metallic implant materials, mechanical properties of, 308, 308t
Metals
  biocompatibility of, as implant material, 201
  electrode potential of, 201t
  implants from, mechanical properties of, 200t
  oxide from, as corrosion protection, 201
  strength of, as implant material, 200
  types of, present in humans, 201

INDEX / **519**

Methotrexate (MTX), immunosuppression of bone graft recipient with, 29
Methylmethacrylate implants, disadvantages of, 306
Methylprednisolone, after mandibular prosthetic reconstruction, 152
  after maxillary prosthetic reconstruction, 136
MHC. See *Histocompatibility (HLA) complex, major.*
Mice, bone graft healing study in, 29
  major histocompatibility complex for, 21
  orthotopic cortical bone allografts in, alloantibody response to, 26–27
Microvascular grafts, anastomosis, for mandibular reconstruction after injury, 441–442
  iliac crest, 392–393, *393*, *394*
  rib periosteal, 391–392, *391*, *392*
Minor connectors, on subperiosteal implant framework, definition of, 271
Mixed lymphocyte culture (MLC) reactivity, definition of, 23
Modeling, definition of, 1
Monofilament material, for sutures, 82
  nylon, for circummandibular ligatures, 84
Moon face, and edentulous bone loss, 14
Mouth floor, lowering of, as only process, 90, 90–91, *91*
  as surgical option to improve denture function, 46
  in Stage I edentulous mandible, 56
  vestibuloplasties with, 69–90
  swelling of, and bleeding, 97
  with mylohyoid relaxed and contracted, *70*
Mucogingival junction, demarcation of, in onlay bone grafting, 121
Muco-osseous flap, use to create contoured ridge, 62
Mucoperiosteal flap procedure, for Branemark implants, 217, *218*
  in modified visor osteotomy, 147
Mucosa
  attached, importance of, to staple implant, *181*
  bearing-surface, resurfacing to improve denture function, 44
  beyond the mucogingival junction, poorly suited for stress from dentures, 44
  buccal, as support for maxillary bone graft, 414
    split-thickness, disadvantages as graft, 36
  denture-bearing surface, as factor in success of denture, 44
  keratinization of, 44
  keratinized attached, atrophic mandible with lack of, 44
  palatal, definition of, 36
  separating from submucosa, 105, *105*
  skin as substitute for, in oral cavity, 36
  split-thickness, use for oral cavity grafts, 36
  suturing techniques for, after maxillofacial injury, 430
  water-tight closure for, 444
Mucosal dissection, in mandibular augmentation, modification of, 318, *319–321*
  in maxillary augmentation with hydroxylapatite, *317*

Mucosal flap techniques, for hydroxylapatite mandibular augmentation, 322–323
Mucosal grafts
  after stent removal, 96
  buccal, inappropriateness for bearing surface for dentures, 44
  contraindications for, 50–52, 51t
  crestally pedicled, 91–92, *92*
    incision for, 92, *92*
    suture for, 92, *93*
  donor site, suture closing of, 94
  for mandibular anterior vestibuloplasty, 94, *95*
  for maxilla reconstruction, 58
  free, mandibular anterior vestibuloplasty with, 92–97
  meshed palatal, over interpositional bone allografts, 152
  palatal, 107–108, *107–109*. See also *Palatal mucosal grafts.*
  suturing of, 94, *95*, 96
  postoperative conditions of, 96
  thinning, 94
Mucosal vestibuloplasties, and hydroxylapatite augmentation, recommendations for, 344
Muscle attachments, dissection from periosteum, in vestibuloplasty with skin graft, 78
Muscles, alveolar bone loss and, 48
  attachments of, and edentulous bone loss, 9
  in mucosal graft, avoiding, 94
Musculoskeletal system, in patient evaluation for edentulous bone loss, 12, 14
Mylohyoid area vestibuloplasties, 97–98, *97–99*
Mylohyoid artery, and subperiosteal dissection, 98
Mylohyoid muscle
  and subperiosteal dissection, 98
  bleeding from, 97
  detachment of, and mouth floor lowering, 56
  dissection from mouth floor, 98
  exposed by retraction following mucosa incision, *80*
  prominence of, after three-piece augmentation osteotomy, 150
  sectioning, 80, *81*
Mylohyoid ridge
  as supporting part of dental prosthesis, 208
  exposed, *98*
  management in vestibuloplasty with skin graft, 72, *72*
  reduction of, 99
  resorption of sharp edge of, 80
Myocutaneous flaps, latissimus dorsi, problems with, *405*, 405–406
  to correct soft tissue defects, 404–406, *404–406*
  pectoralis major, ischemic necrosis of skin paddle of, *404*
  problems with, 403
  sutures for, 402, *403*
  to correct soft tissue defects, 402–403, *402*, *403*
  vs osteomyocutaneous flap, 403
  to improve recipient tissue bed, 350
  without bone, for improving soft-tissue recipient beds, 391
Myotomies, contraindications for, 50–52, 51t

Nasal defect, prosthesis placement for, *421*
Nasal floor, closure of, in maxillary advancement with unilateral cleft graft, 465
Nasal intubation, for vestibuloplasty with skin graft, 74
Nasal mucosa, repairs to, and allogeneic bone grafts, 124
Nasal prosthesis, with marginal separation, 422, *422*
Nasal septum, release of, and maxilla downfracturing, 134, *135*
  sectioning of, in palatal vault osteotomy, 129, *131*
Nasogastric tubes, for confinement of hydroxylapatite particles, 314, *315*
Nasopalatine neurovascular bundle, and edentulous bone loss, 9
Nausea, postoperative, prevention of, 86
Necrotic border zone, healing of, after implant insertion, 214
Nerve grafts
  and bone graft techniques, 408
  autogenous, 406–410
    timing of, 406
  bone sheath formed about distal end of, 408, *409*
  length of, 408
  results of, *410*
  selection of patients for, 408
Nerve(s)
  alveolar. See *Alveolar nerve.*
  lateral femoral cutaneous, 162
  lingual, avoiding during lingual dissection, 80
    immediate grafting for, 406
    paresthesia of, 87
  mental. See *Mental nerve.*
  sural, as donor nerve for grafting, 406
    harvesting of, 407, *407*
    vs greater auricular nerve, for graft, 408
  tagging during graft process, 408
Neurologic examination, for patient with edentulous bone loss, 14
Nutrition. See *Diet.*
Nutritional analysis, triphasic, 12, 13t
N-V bundle, mental. See *Mental neurovascular (N-V) bundle.*

Obesity, extreme, and edentulous bone loss, 13
Oblique ostectomy, for cancer treatment in tonsillar or retromolar areas, 348, 349
Obturator, soft tissue repair to eliminate need for, 442
  surgical, 418, *418*
Obturator prosthesis, definitive, 419, *419*
  interim, 418, *419*
Onlay bone grafts, 118–122, 118t. See also *Bone grafts, onlay.*
Opsite-type dressing, on skin graft donor site, 76
Optical chamber, 213
Oral cavity
  environment of, 199
  evaluation of, prior to implant decision, 170, 170–171
  precancerous lesions in, as contraindication for soft tissue procedures, 52
  skin as mucosal substitute in, 36

520 / INDEX

Oral cavity (Continued)
  transplantation problems unique to, 25
  transplanted tissue in, functional in nonviable state, 25
Oral contamination, minimizing in oral and maxillofacial bone grafts, 33
Oral hygiene
  after mandibular prosthetic reconstruction, 153
  after maxillary prosthetic reconstruction, 136
  after ramus frame implant insertion, 287
  after subperiosteal implant, 278
  and candidate selection for implant, 169–170
  and papillary hyperplasia of palatal vault, 68
Oral membranes, suturing techniques for, after maxillofacial injury, 430
Oral mucosa, perforation of, 444
  water-tight closure of, 444
Oral perforation, accidental, correcting for, in mandibular reconstruction, 365
Oral tissue transplantation, contraction in, 35–36
Oral-nasal communications, in soft tissue assessment in cancer patients, 414
Oral-nasal fistula. See Fistula, oral-nasal.
Orbital defect, prosthesis placement for, 421
Organ transplants, as contraindication for transmucosal implants, 54
  as relative contraindication for soft tissue procedures, 52
Orthognathic surgery, for cleft patient, 453, 459
Orthokeratosis, and skin grafts, 35
Orthotopic cortical bone allografts, alloantibody response to, in mice, 26–27
Osseointegrated implant system. See also Branemark implants.
  and elimination of connective tissue layer, 197
  anteriorly placed, for Stage IV mandible, 57
  as surgical option to improve denture function, 47
  extra-oral, 223
  future impact on denture use, 43
  in maxilla, restrictions on use of, 57
  in Stage I mandible, 56
  in Stage II mandible, 56
  utilization of, for prosthesis retention after injury, 442
Osseointegrated screws, as anchor for metacarpophalangeal joint replacements, 223
Osseointegration
  and bone condensation around implant, 216
  definition of, 211
  loading of implants and, 215
  necrotic border zone at implant insertion and, 214
  time limits for occurrence of, 221
Ostectomies, horizontal, for cancer treatment in tonsillar or retromolar areas, 348
  oblique, for cancer treatment in tonsillar or retromolar areas, 348, 349
  to improve denture function, 45
  vertical subcondylar, for cancer treatment in tonsillar or retromolar areas, 349, 349
Osteitis fibrosa cystica, in periodontal trauma, renal osteodystrophy and, 7

Osteoconduction, occurrence of, in graft healing, 31–32
Osteodystrophy, renal, in uremia, 7
Osteogenesis
  bone graft material induction of, 435
  mechanism of, enhanced with hyperbaric oxygen, 396
  occurrence of, in graft healing, 31
  phase one, enhancement of, with high cancellous-to-cortical ratio, 360
  phase two, recipient bed characteristics and, 360
  two-phase theory of, 358, 358, 359
Osteoinduction, occurrence of, in graft healing, 31
Osteomalacia, and edentulous bone loss, 4t, 6
  serum calcium levels in, 15
Osteomyelitis, as relative contraindication for soft tissue procedures, 52
Osteomyocutaneous flap, undergoing ischemic necrosis, 390, 391
  vs pectoralis major myocutaneous flap, 403
Osteomyocutaneous grafts, for irradiated cancer patients, 388–391, 389, 390
  for mandibular reconstruction after injury, 441
Osteopenia, definition of, 4
Osteoporosis
  and edentulous bone loss, 4t, 4–6
  as contraindication for transmucosal implants, 55
  bone mineral loss in, rate of, 5
  bone shape changes in, 3
  clinical signs and symptoms of, 5
  histologic appearance of, 4
  postmenopausal, 4
  radiographic appearance of, 5, 5–6
  senile, 4
  serum calcium levels in, 15
  serum phosphate levels in, 15
  treatment of, 6
Osteotomies
  anterior, with posterior onlay graft, 150–152
    long-term results of, 152
  anterior horizontal, with interposed allogeneic block graft, case study of, 158, 158–161
  anterior maxillary, 133t, 133–136
    indications and contraindications for, 133
    surgical technique for, 134–136, 135, 136
  anterior segmental, 150, 151
  bilateral intra-oral vertical ramus, for correcting prognathic mandible, 505
  bilateral posterior maxillary, model surgery of, 488
  combined with vestibuloplasty to correct anterior maxillary edentulous bone loss, 133, 134
  high to low, 127
  in maxillary advancement with bilateral cleft graft, 469
  interdental, in case presentation, 487
  interpositional, disadvantages of, 306
  intra-oral sagittal split ramus, for edentulous patients, 479–481
  mandibular fracture during, treatment for, 153–154
  maxillary, with simultaneous alveolar cleft grafts, 453
  modified, with allogeneic bone grafts, infection following, 153

Osteotomies (Continued)
  palatal vault, 128–129, 129–133, 129t, 142
    indications for, 129
    surgical technique for, 129
  problems of, on edentulous patients, 46
  sagittal split, for mandibular advancement and retrusions in cleft patients, 459
  in case presentation, 500
  sandwich, for interposed bone graft augmentation, 146, 146, 147
    patient activities during healing from, 154
  segmental maxillary, to reduce maxillary excess, 477–478
  three-piece, to correct maxillary excess, in case presentation, 491
  three-piece augmentation procedure, 149–150, 149, 150
    nerve sensibility testing after, 150t
  to improve denture function, 45
  total maxillary
    with advancement, 127–128
    with interpositional grafting, 122–126
      surgical procedure for, 124–126
    with palatal vault elevation, 128, 128
    with palatal vault extension, case study of, 141–142, 141–142
  transoral vertical ramus, for edentulous patients, 478
Overdenture support, titanium inserts for, 227, 227
Oxygen tensions, of irradiated tissue, vs nonirradiated tissue, 394

Palatal appliances, problems from wearing of, 448–449
Palatal closure, in maxillary advancement with unilateral cleft graft, 465
Palatal grafts, disadvantages of, 36
Palatal mucosa, definition of, 36
  protection of, during anterior maxillary osteotomy, 134
Palatal mucosal grafts, 107–108, 107–109
  advantages and disadvantages of, 108
  donor site for, 107–108, 107–108
  inadequate quantity of, and placement of, 108, 109
  long-term result of, 109
Palatal papillary hyperplasia removal, 68
Palatal screw fixation, stent outline for, 100
Palatal torus, definition of, 67
  removal, 67–68
Palatal vault, elevation of, total maxillary osteotomy with, 128, 128
  papillary hyperplasia removal from, 68
  poor form of, total maxillary atrophy with, 118t
Palatal vault osteotomies, 128–129, 129–133, 142. See also Osteotomies, palatal vault.
Palate
  avulsive injuries of, early care of, 432
  cleft, 447t, 447–448. See also Clefts, facial.
  hard, freeing of, 129, 131
  repair of, 443
  surgical elevation of, and maxilla reconstruction, 58

Palatine vessels, preservation of, in palatal vault osteotomy, 129, *130*
Papillary hyperplasia, in cleft patients, 448–449, *450*
 removal from palatal vault, 68
Papilledema, and edentulous bone loss, 14
Parallelism, of Core-Vent Implants, *229*
 surveyor for checking, *280*
Parathyroid hormone (PTH), serum levels of, in edentulous bone loss, 15
Paresthesia
 after mandibular prosthetic reconstruction, 153
 lingual nerve, 87
 of lower lip, probability in VSG, 71
 potential for, during direct bone impression phase of subperiosteal implant, 273
Particulate bone. See also *Bone chips.*
Particulate bone and cancellous marrow grafts
 for maxillary reconstruction, 414–415, *415*
 graft material, compression of, into crib, *384–385, 387*
 with allogeneic bone cribs, 368–397
  after injury, 439–441
  allogeneic ilia technique, 374–379
  allogeneic mandible technique, 371–374
  results of, *373, 374, 375*
 with allogeneic split rib segments for cribs, 380–386
  results of, 382
 with alloplastic cribs, 365, *366–368, 367–368, 370*
  after injury, 438–439, *439*
Particulate cancellous bone and marrow, packing of, at interface for iliac crest graft, 437
Patient assessment, after cancer treatment, for mandibular continuity defects, 351–355, *356–357*
 for reconstruction and rehabilitation, 347–355
 surgical concerns of, 347–351
Patient management, after alveolar ridge reconstruction, 325, 329
 prior to alveolar ridge reconstruction with hydroxylapatite, 312–314
 reconstructive edentulous, recommendations for, 341, 344
Patients
 cancer, 420–426. See also *Cancer patients.*
 denture, initial interview of, 42, *42, 43*
 discussion with, prior to vestibuloplasty with skin graft, 71–72
  prior to crestally pedicled mucosal graft, 91
  prior to submucous vestibuloplasty, 104
 edentulous. See *Edentulous patients.*
 education of, prior to implant, 181
 evaluation of, prior to vestibuloplasty with skin graft and mouth floor lowering, 72
 older, and recipient beds for skin grafts, 34
 partially dentate, with deformities, 482–483
  diagnosis and treatment planning for, 482
  postsurgical management of, 483

Patients (*Continued*)
 partially dentate, surgical considerations for, 482–483
 selection of, for mandibular staple bone plate, 179–180
 with clefts, special problems of, 448–449, *449–451*
PBCM grafts. See *Particulate bone and cancellous marrow grafts.*
PCI (polysulfone coping insert), 226–227, *227*
Pectoralis major myocutaneous flaps
 ischemic necrosis of skin paddle of, *404*
 to correct soft tissue defects, 402–403, *402, 403*
 problems with, 403
 sutures for, 402, *403*
 vs osteomyocutaneous flap, 403
Penicillin
 after alveolar ridge reconstruction, 313, 325
 after Branemark implants insertion, 218
 for use with bone grafting, 153
 prophylactic treatment with, after mandibular reconstruction, 364
Penrose drain, after maxillofacial injury, 433
Perialveolar method, of stent fixation, 103
Perialveolar wiring, stent for, 100
Periodontal lesions, and calcium phosphate implants vs cancellous bone autografts, 311
Periodontal ligament, tooth attachment with, 211
Perioral area, avulsive wounds in, 430
Periosteum
 and maxillary vestibuloplasty incision, 100
 bone remodeling in, 2
 host connective tissue bed functioning as, *359*
 in maxillary augmentation with hydroxylapatite, *317*
 mucosal flap grafted to, *104, 104–105*
 possibility of exposure following vestibuloplasty with skin graft, 87
 prevention of unnecessary loss of, 82
 skin grafted to, *70*
 soft tissue cleared from, for vestibuloplasty with skin graft, 78
 soft tissue on, problems with, 105
Peripheral struts, on subperiosteal implant framework, definition of, 271
Personal hygiene, quality of, and implant contraindications, 55
Personality disorders, as relative contraindication for soft tissue procedures, 52
Pharyngeal flaps, evaluation of, in cleft patients, 452, *452*
Pharyngeal pack, 77
 removal of, 86, 89
Phonation, improvement of, with maxillary occlusal plane prosthesis, 355
Phosphate, high intake of, and alveolar bone loss, 7
 serum levels of, in edentulous bone loss, 15
 urinary levels of, in edentulous bone loss, 15
Phosphate ions, from implants, studies of, 308–309
Photographs, as record prior to implant surgery, 175, *177*
Photon absorption densitometry, for bone mineral determination, 6

Photon absorption densitometry (*Continued*)
 for patient with edentulous bone loss, 14–15
Physical examination, for patients with edentulous bone loss, 13–14
Pin fixation, biphasic extraskeletal, to stabilize bone fragments, 432, *433*
 extraskeletal, for bone graft after maxillofacial injury, 435
Plaque, instructions for control of, for cancer patients, 425
 problems with, after Branemark implants, 222
Plasma cells, and immunity transfer, 27
Plasma spray surface, on Hollow-Basket implants, 254
Plasma spraying, process of, for TPS implant, 234, *234*
Plasmatic imbibition, following skin grafts, 34
Polycarbonate plug for interface analysis, *209*
Polyglycolic acid suture material, 82
Polymers, biocompatibility of, as implant material, 200–201
 strength of, as implant material, 200
Polymethylmethacrylate (PMMA), host rejection of, as implant material, 340
 limits to use of, as implant material, 200
Polysulfone coping insert (PCI), 226–227, *227*
Polytetrafluoroethylene (Teflon), limits to use of, as implant material, 200
Polyvinyl ether impression material, 274
Porosity, of implant surface, effect of, 234
Pregnancy, as contraindication for surgical procedures, 50, 52, 53
Preprosthetic procedures, 61–68
Pressure dressing, following vestibuloplasty with skin graft, 86
 following skin graft suturing technique, 89
 importance to success of crestally pedicled mucosal graft, 92, *93*
Primary contraction, of skin graft, definition of, 35
Primary (first-set) rejection, of graft, definition of, 23
Prognathism, mandibular, characteristics related to, 45
 due to ridge resorption, 45–46
 pseudo-, advanced resorption as cause of, 46
 treatment of, and esthetics, 46
Proplast implants, disadvantages of, 306
Prosthesis
 dental. See *Dentures.*
 detachable fixed, titanium screw for, 230, *231*
 extra-oral, materials for, 421, *422–423*
 fixed, titanium coping insert for, 226, *227*
 for Branemark implants, 218–219, *219*
 function of, in rehabilitation after cancer treatment, 353
 interim obturator, 418, *418*
 mandibular guide flange, 354, *354–355*
 maxillary inclined plane, 354, *354*
 maxillary occlusal plane, 355, *355*
 maxillary occlusal table, 355, *355*
 maxillofacial, effect of scar bands on use of, 413
  three-point stability required by, 413
  to restore deformities from cancer treatment, 413

Prosthesis (Continued)
  osseous bulk restoration to support, 361
  temporary
    after blade-vent implant insertion, 252
    after surgical deformity correction in partially edentulous patients, 483
    fabrication of, 280
    for subperiosteal implant, 276, 277
    timing of insertion of, for cleft patients, 452
    transitional, during control program, prior to implant surgery, 170
Prosthetic management, phases of, for mandibular continuity defect cancer patient, 353–355
Prosthetic materials, hard-tissue, 307. See also *Hydroxylapatite*.
Prosthetics, and alveolar bone loss, 8–9
Prosthodontic loading, and edentulous bone loss, 8–9
Prosthodontist, clinical evaluation by, prior to surgery for maxillary edentulous bone loss, 118
  roles in evaluation of totally edentulous patient with deformities, 476
Protaform
  characteristics of, 110
  on splint for palatal mucosal graft donor site, 108
  placement of, in vestibuloplasty with skin graft, 85–86, *86*
  stent modified with, *112*
  use next to skin graft, 85
Protrusion, bimaxillary, in case presentation, *492*
Proximal muscle weakness, and edentulous bone loss, 14
Pseudo-periodontium, 197
Pseudohypoparathyroidism, serum calcium levels in, 15
Pseudoprognathism, advanced resorption as cause of, 46
Psychiatric disorders, as relative contraindication for soft tissue procedures, 52
Psychological factors, and evaluation for vestibuloplasty with skin graft, 72
  and patient's reaction to dentures, 42
Psychologists, referral of denture patient to, 42
PTH (parathyroid hormone), serum levels of, in edentulous bone loss, 15

RA-2 Ramus frame implants, 288, 290–296, *291*, *292*
  advantages of, vs basic Ramus frame, 290
  disadvantages of, 290–291
  guidelines for insertion of, 291–292
  preliminary preparation for, 292
  surgical preparation for, 292
  surgical procedure for, 292–294, *293–295*
Radiation caries, fluoride to reduce, 425
Radiation treatment. See also *Irradiated tissue*.
  and soft tissue recipient bed quality, 350
  as contraindication for transmucosal implants, 53–54
  dysphagia from, 348
Radical neck dissection, ipsilateral, 347–348, *348*
  vs functional neck dissection, 348, *348*

Radiographs
  and implant template, to determine implant length, 237, *237*
  as aid for implant planning, 171, 173–175, *171–175*
  importance of, in mandible reconstruction, 143
  panoramic, evaluation prior to vestibuloplasty with skin graft, 72, *72*
  required for maxillary edentulous bone loss treatment planning, 118
Ramus, continuity defects including, split-rib cribs for, 380, *383*
Ramus frame implants, *281*, 281–296. See also *RA-2 Ramus frame implants*.
  advantages and disadvantages of, 281
  advantages of RA-2 Ramus frame over, 290
  and mandible strength, 57
  conclusions on, 296
  failures of, 294–295
  instruments for, *283*
  patient preparation for, 282
  patient selection for, 281
  permanent fixation of lower denture and, 288
  postoperative care and medication for, 287–288
  preliminary preparation for, 281–282
  removing, 295–296, *296*
  surgical preparation for, 282
  surgical procedure for, 282–284, 286, *283–289*
  sutures after insertion of, 286, *287*
Ratchet, for TPS screw implant insertion, *235*
Recipient tissue bed
  adapting skin graft to, 89
  assessment of, for maxillary reconstruction, 414
  characteristics of, and phase-two osteogenesis, 360
  complications of, 442, 444
  dissection of, in mandibular reconstruction after cancer surgery, 362, *362*
  for bone grafts, 434
    functioning as periosteum, *359*
    site variables in, 32–33
    vascular quality of, 32
  for skin grafts. See *Skin grafts, recipient beds for*.
  hyperbaric oxygen to enhance, for irradiated cancer patients, 394–397, *394–397*
  hypocellular, hypovascular, or hypoxic, and graft success potential, 387–388
  irradiated, exposure of, to hyperbaric oxygen, 388, *388*, *389*
Reconstructive surgery
  after cancer treatment, timing of, 350–351
  intra-oral, prior to transmandibular implant, 204
  of cancer patients, vs rehabilitation, 424–426
  preprosthetic
    anatomic factors and treatment planning, 56
    diseases and conditions affecting, 50
    goal with Stage I mandible, 56
    goals of, 49
    options, 46–47
    patient history and examination, 49–55

Reconstructive surgery (Continued)
  preprosthetic, possible procedures, 48t
  prosthodontic aspects of, 41–47
  surgical aspects of, 47–58
  treatment planning, prosthodontic and surgical aspects of, 41–60
Reconstructive-rehabilitative phase, of patient treatment for mandibular continuity defect, 354–355
  of prosthodontic treatment for maxillary defects, 419–420
Rehabilitation, of cancer patients, extra-oral, 420–423, *421*
  programs for, 423–424
  vs reconstruction, 424–426
Rejection
  accelerated, 27
  acute, of graft, definition of, 23
  chronic, of graft, definition of, 23–24
  definition of, 23
  first-set, of graft, definition of, 23
  of skin grafts, diagnosis and prevention of, 24
  stages in, *24*
  treatment of. See *Immunosuppression*.
  of transplant, mechanism of, 19
  other immunologic factors in, 28
  secondary, of graft, definition of, 23
Remodeling, steps in, 1
Renal failure, chronic, as contraindication for surgical procedures, 52, 54
Resorption
  after anterior maxillary osteotomy, 134
  after Branemark implants, 222
  after hemimaxilla reconstruction, 416
  after hydroxylapatite ridge augmentation, studies of, 332, 334, *334*, *335*
  after interposed bone graft to mandible, 146
  after modified visor osteotomy, 149
  and graft bone sequestered areas, 31
  and nonresorbable hydroxylapatite for Stage IV mandible reconstruction, 57
  as factor affecting denture success, 43
  avoidance of, peak loads on implants and, 231
  beneath implants in Stage I mandible, 56
  bone morphogenetic protein and, 360
  definition of, 1
  hydroxylapatite potential for reducing, 56
  hydroxylapatite-bone augmentation vs hydroxylapatite only augmentation, 334
  in alveolar ridge, 305
  in mandible and maxilla, 43
  in remodeling, 2, *2*, *3*
  inhibiting, 43
  mandibular prognathism due to, 45–46
  metallic cribs and, 360, *360*, *361*
  of allogeneic bone, 368, 370
  of allogeneic ilia cribs, 377, *380*
  of allogeneic mandible cribs, 371
  of bone grafts, 361
    rate of, 305–306
  of edentulous maxillary ridge, 119
  of graft after mandibular fracture, 154
  of maxilla, tense facial skin and, 414
  of maxillary alveolar process, prevention of, teeth arrangement on upper denture and, 208
  prevention of. See also *Alveolar ridge, preservation of*.
  rate of, for total onlay grafts, 145

INDEX / 523

Resorption (Continued)
  slower mandibular, as objective of vestibuloplasty with skin graft, 71
  soft tissue contractions as cause of, in maxilla, 416, *416*, *417*
Resorption remodeling, in osteogenesis, 358
Retina, hemorrhage of, and edentulous bone loss, 14
Retraction, for lingual dissection, 79, *80*
Retractors, Davis nested, 77, *77*
Retroauricular region, titanium implants in, 223
Retrognathic mandible, edentulous patient with, and esthetics, 46
Retromolar area, incision at, in buccolabial dissection, 78
  treatment for tumor in, 348–349
Revascularization process, and resorption rate in maxilla, 416
Rhesus monkeys, in utero allogeneic bone transplant studies in, 29
Rib grafts
  allogeneic, for maxillary reconstruction, 415, *415*
  alternate method for use in total onlay mandibular graft, 145, *145*
  autogenous, for mandibular reconstruction after injury, 437
  on bony-deficient maxilla, 118
  costochondral, for mandibular reconstruction after injury, 440, *441*
  donor site for, postoperative care of, 164
    surgery for, 162, 164, *164*
  fixation techniques for, *120*, *121*, 121
  harvest for, complications of, 442
  hydroxylapatite particles used with, 344
  microvascular periosteal, for irradiated cancer patients, 391–392, *391*, *392*
  onlay, case study of, 154–155, *154*, *155*
  placement of, in mandible reconstruction, 144
  preparation of rib for, 121
  for total onlay graft to mandible, 144
  stainless steel wire for fixation of, 121–122
  storage of, 121
  success of, *393*
  wiring of, to mandible, 144
Rib resection, for graft harvest, complications of, 442
Ridge. See also *Alveolar ridge*; *Edentulous ridge*.
  atrophic. See also *Mandible, atrophic*; *Maxilla, atrophic*.
  osseous reconstruction of, 117–165
Rigid internal fixation, in cancer patient reconstruction, 410
Running, long-distance, and sural nerve for grafting, 407

Sagittal split osteotomy for mandibular advancement and retrusions in cleft patients, 459
Saline injection, to ease cutting of mucosal graft, 94, *95*
Saline solution, for bone graft storage, 362
  for skin graft, 76
  to minimize heat damage, 284
Saliva. See also *Xerostomia*.
  pH of, 199

Sandwich osteotomies, for interposed bone graft augmentation, 146, *146*. See also *Visor osteotomy, modified*.
  problems with, 147
  patient activities during healing from, 154
Sapphire, single crystal
  as material for endosseous implant, 296–299, *297–299*
  forms of, 297
  failures of, 298
  indications for use of, 298
Scar tissue
  and sensation in grafted skin, 36
  during cleft repair procedures, *451*, 451–452
  effect of, on quality of recipient tissue bed, 434
    on use of maxillofacial prosthesis, 413
  elimination of, prior to bone graft, 32
  exophytic, removal of, and secondary epithelialization procedure, 106
  from mandibular anterior vestibuloplasty, 94, *95*
  hypertrophic, prevention of, 91
  in cancer patients, cribs unsuited for, 368
SCM (sternocleidomastoid muscle), 348, *398*
Scoliosis, and edentulous bone loss, 14
Screw form, for implant, research on, 212
Sebaceous glands, and skin grafts, 36
Secondary contraction, of skin grafts, definition of, 35–36
Secondary epithelialization, overexposed mature areas of hydroxylapatite augmentation, 107
Secondary rejection, of graft, 23
Secondary struts, on subperiosteal implant framework, definition of, 271
Second-set reaction, to osseous allograft, 27
Segmental replacements, and calcium phosphate implants vs cancellous bone autografts, 311
Semifunctional implants, definition of, 199
Semilunar tissue punch, 248, 252
Sensation, in skin grafts, 35, 36
Septal screw method, of stent fixation, 103
Sequestration of graft bone, and resorption, 31
Seroma, separating skin graft from bed, 34
Serum, accumulation under skin graft, preventing, 89, *90*
Silastic mandibles, prefabricated, to maintain space and facial contour after injury, 432
Silastic tubing, for suture ends in mouth floor lowering, 90, *91*
Silicone implants, disadvantages of, 306
Single crystal sapphire, 296–299, *297–299*. See also *Sapphire, single crystal*.
Sintering process, 307
Skeletal envelopes, 2, 2t
  normal progress of bone turnover in, *2*
Skeletal fixation, to maintain mandibular position, in case presentation, *497*, *498*
Skeletal pin fixation, external, for cancer patient reconstruction, 412, *412*, *413*
Skin, as load-bearing tissue for dentures, 70
  grafted, characteristics of, 35–36

Skin grafts, 33–36
  and accessory skin structures, 36
  autogenous, on bearing surface mucosa, 44
  characteristics required for success of, 33–34
  classification of, 33
  contraindications for, 50–52, 51t
  definition of, 33
  donor site, dressing of, 75–76
    postoperative discomfort at, after vestibuloplasty with skin graft, 71
    weeping of, 87
  for maxilla reconstruction, 58
  growth patterns of, 36
  history, 69
  identifying external and dermal surfaces, 85
  infection and contamination of, 35
  intra-oral placement of, with suturing technique, 88, *88*
  placement on stent, 85
  recipient beds for
    characteristics of, and sensation in grafted skin, 36
    comparative vascularity of, 33–34
    factors preventing proper contact with, 34–35
    postoperative discomfort of, following VSG, 71
  rejection of, and immunologic basis for delayed healing, 29
  stages in, 24
  removing bacteria prior to, 35
  split-thickness, definition of, 33
  storing, 76, *76*
  stretching with finger pressure, 88, *88*
  success of, and stent removal, 86
  suturing technique for, 90
  test cut examination for, 75
  thickness of, and interface contraction, 33
  trimming excess skin from, 89, *89*
  variables affecting cut depth, 75
  vascularization of, 34
  with vestibuloplasties
    after alveolar ridge reconstruction, 313
    and hydroxylapatite augmentation, recommendations for, 344
    fixation methods for, 72–73
    graft table setup for, 74t
    graft-taking setup, for, 74t
    permanence of fixation to mandible after, 71
    suture technique for, 87–90, *88*, *89*
    width determination in, 74
Skin-lined pockets, 108
Skin-mucosal junction, denture irritation of, following isolated vestibuloplasty, 91
Slide-tape programs, for cancer patients, 423
Sliding visor osteotomies. See *Visor osteotomies*.
Smell, loss of, iodophor solution and, 182
Social workers, referral of denture patient to, 42
Soft tissue
  and atrophic mandible ridge reconstruction, 152
  as factor affecting denture success, 43–44
  assessment of, in maxilla reconstruction after cancer treatment, 414

524 / INDEX

Soft tissue (*Continued*)
  attachment to bony fragments after injury, maintenance of, 430
  closure for total onlay graft, 145
  contraction of, as cause of resorption, 416, *416*, *417*
  dissection of, in mandibular reconstruction in cancer patient, 362
  evaluation of, in cleft patients, 452
  healing of, effect of bone fragment movement on, 433
  inflammation of, and hydroxylapatite particle shape, 336, *337*
  quantitative defects in cancer patients, 397–410
  recipient bed, determination of thickness of, 350
    factors affecting quality of, after cancer treatment, 350
  recommendations for correcting abnormalities of, 341
  reconstruction of, after injury, 444
    timing of, 444
  removing bulk after blade-vent implant insertion, 251–252
  repair of, in intra-oral areas, 442, *443*
  resorption and problems with, 48–49
  response of, to calcium phosphate implants, 310, *310*
  status of, after Branemark implants, 222
  surgical management of problems, 69–116
  surgical options, to improve denture function, 46
  surgical procedures, contraindications for, 50–52, 51t
  wound management of, in maxillofacial injury, 430
Soft-tissue procedures, and hydroxylapatite augmentation, recommendations for, 344
Softic, for definitive obturator prosthesis, 419
Sphincter, development of, following buccal inlay vestibuloplasty, 110
Spinal fusions, and calcium phosphate implants vs cancellous bone autografts, 311
Spleen cells, and immunity transfer, 27
Splints. See also *Gunning splints*.
  after surgical deformity correction in partially edentulous patients, 482–483
  constant use of, after buccal inlay vestibuloplasty, 114
  construction of, to control hydroxylapatite particles, 314
  definitive transitional, construction of, 110
  for hydroxylapatite augmentation with mucosal flap technique, 324
  for mandibular positioning, in case presentation, *496*, *498*
  for use after alveolar ridge reconstruction with hydroxylapatite, 313, *313*, *314*
  immediate transitional, construction of, 110
    placement of, 112
  insertion in maxillary augmentation with hydroxylapatite, 318
  maxillary palatal, use after palatal torus removal, 67
  removal after alveolar ridge reconstruction, 325

Splints (*Continued*)
  transitional, 113, *113*
    immediate insertion of, 113
    stent to construct surgical tray for, 114
Split-rib segments, allogeneic
  cost and availability of, 383
  for costochondral graft, 384, *385*, *386*
  for cribs, 380, 380–385, *381*
  in mandibular reconstruction after injury, 440
Split-thickness skin grafts. See *Skin grafts, split-thickness*.
Stability, importance of, in TPS implant, 234
Stabilization, after intra-oral sagittal split ramus osteotomy, for edentulous patients, 480–481
Stainless steel, as implant material, research on, 212
Staple bone plates, mandibular, 175, 179–197, 199. See also *Mandibular staple bone plate implants*.
Stent
  care during buccal inlay vestibuloplasty, 111–112, *112*
  construction of, for buccal inlay vestibuloplasty, 110
    for maxillary vestibuloplasty, 98, 100, *100*
    for vestibuloplasty with skin graft, 84–85
  fixation of, for maxillary vestibuloplasty, 98
    outline for, 100
    perialveolar method of, 103
    septal screw method of, 103
  for buccal inlay vestibuloplasty, *111*
  for mucosal graft, 94
  for skin graft fixation, in vestibuloplasty with skin graft, 73, *73*
  for submucous vestibuloplasty, 105, *105*
  placing and securing, 85–86
  placing skin graft on, 85
  removal of, after vestibuloplasties, 86
    after maxillary vestibuloplasty, 103–104
    after mylohyoid area vestibuloplasty, 98
  transpalatal fixation of, *103*, 103
    alternative to, 103
  use for construction of impression tray, 113, *114*
  use of, in procedure to correct anteroposterior deficiency of maxilla, 477
  with attached split-thickness skin graft, 113
Sternocleidomastoid muscle, retention of, in functional neck dissection, 348
  vascular anatomy of, *398*
Sternocleidomastoid muscular flap, to correct soft tissue defects in cancer patients, 397–402, *398*
  access to, *398*, *399*, *399*
  before and after, *400*
  closure of, 400, *400*
Sternocleidomastoid myocutaneous flaps, to correct soft tissue defects, 401–402, *401*, *402*
  for closure after mandibular reconstruction, 363, *364*, *364*
Steroids, after mandibular staple bone plate implant, 186
  after mandibular prosthetic reconstruction, 152–153

Steroids (*Continued*)
  after maxillary prosthetic reconstruction, 136
  prolonged use of, as relative contraindication for soft tissue procedures, 51
  treatment with, after alveolar ridge reconstruction, 314
Stone casts, for Branemark implant prosthesis, 218, *219*
Strength, of implant materials, 199–200
Stress, distribution of, with Core-Vent implant and Core-Vent attachment, 228
  minimization of, to healing tissue from interim obturator prosthesis, 418–419
Struts, on subperiosteal implant framework, definition of, 271
Study casts, for preoperative implant study, 175
  in case presentation, *488*
  mock surgery on, in case presentation, *496*, *496*, *498*
Submandibular sutures, 85
  removing, 90
Submucosal implants, disadvantages of, 306
Submucosal tissue, positioning of, in submucous vestibuloplasty, 105
Submucous vestibuloplasties, 104–106. See also *Vestibuloplasties, submucous*.
Subperiosteal implants, 175
  on Stage VI mandible, problems of, 57
  success of, 168
Subperiosteal mandibular implants, *178*, 269–281, *270*
  direct bone impression for (Stage I), 271–276
  early, 269
  framework for, 271, *272*
    examination after return from lab, 276
    insertion of (Stage II), 276–278
    laboratory fabrication of, 280
    radiograph of, *277*
    seating of, 277, *277*
  laboratory phase for, 278–281
  long-term results of, *278*
  natural opposing dentition as contraindication for, 270, *271*
  patient selection for, 270–271
  phases of, 271
  temporary prosthesis for, fabrication of, 280
Sulcus depth, for dissection during vestibuloplasty with skin graft, 87
Sulcus maintenance, after alveolar ridge reconstruction, 325
Sulcus obliteration, modified mucosal dissection to reduce, 318, *319*–*321*
Superior border rib grafting techniques, of bone augmentation, problems with, 47
Supramid, 82
  and suture abcess, 87
  for circummandibular ligatures, 84
Supraperiosteal dissection, for mandibular anterior vestibuloplasty, 93, *94*
  in vestibuloplasty with skin graft, 78
Sural nerve, as donor nerve for grafting, 406
  harvesting of, 407, *407*
  vs greater auricular nerve, for graft, 408
Surgical bite rim, laboratory fabrication of, 278, *279*
  placement of, 275
Surgical obturator, 418, *418*
Surveyor, for checking parallelism, *280*

INDEX / 525

Survival theory. See *Osteogenesis*.
Suture abcess, potential for, in vestibuloplasty with skin graft, 87
Suture material
  for alveoloplasties, 62
  for intra-oral wounds, 433
  for maxillary vestibuloplasty, 101
  for submandibular sutures, 82
  nonabsorbable, and graft fixation by sutures, 82
    length of, and later removal, 82
Sutures. See also *Closure*.
  after direct bone impression, 276, 276
  avoiding stress on, from chewing, 136
  for grafts
    onlay bone, 122, 123
    skin graft fixation with vestibuloplasty, 73
    skin graft placement, with vestibuloplasty, 87–90, 88, 89
    and crestal tissue, 81–82
    and lingual dissection, 80
  for implants
    blade-vent, 252, 252
    Branemark, et type "C," 257–258
    Hollow-Basket type "E," 259
    subperiosteal implant framework, 277, 278
    TPS screw, 241, 241
  for osteotomies, maxillary, with interpositional grafting, 126, 127
    palatal vault, 129, 133
  for unilateral cleft repair, 456, 456
  for vestibuloplasties
    buccal inlay, 110
    mandibular anterior, 94, 95
    removal of, 90
    submandibular, 82–84, 82–84
    submucous, 105
    nonresorbable submandibular, and stent removal, 86
    with mouth floor lowering process, 90
    position in lingual mucosa for vestibuloplasty with skin graft, 82
  to create self-retaining flaps for mandible bone impression, 273, 274
Swallowing, difficulty in, and sectioning of genioglossi, 81
Sweat glands, and skin grafts, 36
Symphysis
  reconstruction of, rigid internal fixation for, 410
  resected, reconstruction difficulties with, 349, 349
  resorption of, after transmandibular implant, 210
  vascularized soft-tissue bulk for, 402
Syringe, beveled, for delivery of hydroxylapatite particles, 314, 316
  for injection of hydroxylapatite in mandibular augmentation, 318, 319
Systemic bone disease. See *Bone disease, systemic*.

Tachycardia, and edentulous bone loss, 14
Tantalum, as implant material, problems with, 201
TCI (titanium coping insert), 226, 227
TCP [(Ca$_3$(PO$_4$)$_2$)], 307
  porous bioresorbable, studies of, 311–312
  porous ceramic, bioresorption of, 307

TCP [(Ca$_3$(PO$_4$)$_2$)] implants, and coating of calcitonin or marrow, 311
Technetium-99 (^{99}Tc) diphosphonate bone scan, 386
Teeth
  extraction of, and immediate hydroxylapatite implants, 340, 341
  in cleft region, problems with, 448
  natural, and deformity correction in partially edentulous patients, 482
    Core-Vent implant use with, 227
    maintenance of, in cancer patients, 425
    mandibular, included as fixed restorative component of prosthetic reconstruction, 186
    staple bone plate use with, 189, 192
  on interim obturator prosthesis, 419
  removal of
    considerations at time of, 56
    rest fracturing during, 61
    vs retention, in osteotomy, in case presentation, 491
    vs salvage of, after injury, 432
  single replacement of, Hollow-Basket "F" implant for, 267
  with Core-Vent implant, 224, 225
Teflon (polytetrafluoroethylene), limits to use of, as implant material, 200
Temporization, of blade-vent implant, 252
Tenting, and skin graft on periosteum, 89, 89
Tetany, and edentulous bone loss, 14
Thermoplastic materials, stent modification with, 110
Thiersch graft, history of, 69
Thinness, extreme, and edentulous bone loss, 13
Thoracic kyphosis, and edentulous bone loss, 14
Three-H phenomenon, 387
Thrombin dressing, on skin graft donor site, 75
Thymus-derived (T) lymphocytes, human D loci antigens recognized by, 21
Thyrotoxicosis, serum calcium levels in, 15
Tissue, irradiated, 387–397, 388. See also *Irradiated tissue*.
Tissue bars, cast, to splint together Core-Vent Implants, 229
  laboratory procedures for construction of, simplified with TSI, 230–231, 232
  resilient, evaluation of need for, 227
Tissue bed. See *Recipient tissue bed*.
Tissue punch, semilunar, 248, 252
Tissue typing, definition of, 23
  unnecessary for AAA bone recipients, 30
Titanium
  as implant material, research on, 211–212, 212
  corrosion of, 201
  for Hollow-Basket Systems, 255
  host rejection of, as implant material, 340
  properties of, 233
  toxicity of, 201
Titanium coping insert (TCI), for fixed prosthesis, 226, 227
Titanium implants, in retroauricular region, 223
Titanium Plasma Spray (TPS) Implant System, 231–245
  anesthesia for, 237

Titanium plasma spray (TPS) implant system (*Continued*)
  engineering considerations of, 231, 233
  implantation procedures for, 237, 238–245, 239–241, 243, 245
  insertion of, 235, 241–242, 241, 242
  physical characteristics of, 233, 233–236
  positioning of, 240
  preoperative procedure for, 237
  splinting of, 237
  summary of, 245
  treatment of complications from, 245
Titanium plasma-sprayed surface, for implant, 266
Titanium screw inserts (TSI), 227, 228–231, 228–230
  restoration options with, 230
Titanium washer, 229, 229
Tobacco use, effect on implants, 55
  in cancer patients, 425
Tongue
  abnormal positions of, classes of, 44–45, 45
  irritation of, minimizing, in maxillary vestibuloplasty, 103
  lacerations of, 432
  normal position, definition of, 44
  posture and function of, as predictor of denture success, 44–45
  swelling of, and mylohyoid muscle bleeding, 97
Tongue mass, surgical removal of tumor and, 355
Tongue tie, correction of, 65–66
Tonsillar areas, treatment for tumor in, 348–349
Tooth. See *Teeth*.
Toxicity, and calcium phosphate implants, 308–309
TPS implant system. See *Titanium Plasma Spray (TPS) Implant System*.
TPS screw implants, 174, 178
Trabecular system, bone loss in osteoporosis, 4–5
  bone remodeling in, 2
Transcutaneous oxygen measurements, vs number of hyperbaric oxygen sessions, graph of, 389
Transfer copings, in TPS screw implant system, 236, 236
Transiliac bone biopsy, for bone mineral determination, 6, 6
Transitional prosthesis, during control program, prior to implant surgery, 170
Transmandibular implants, 197–211, 197
  anatomic aspect of, 198
  and dental prosthesis function, research on, 210
  choice of material for, 202–203
  complications from, research on, 209–210
  copper allergy as contraindication for, 203
  design of, 198, 198–199, 200
  development of, 198
  embryologic aspects of, 198
  indications and contraindications for, 204
  instrumentation for, 203
  research on, 209–210
  summary of, 210–211
  surgical technique for, 204–206, 204–208, 208
  unfavorable side effect of, research on, 210

Transoral bone grafts, problem with, for maxillary reconstruction, 416, *416*
Transosteal implants. See *Mandibular staple bone plate implants.*
Transpalatal arch retainer, for cleft patients, 452
Transpalatal fixation, stent for, 103
Transplant material, bone, availability of, 25
Transplantation, factors eliminating potential donor for, 23
  general principles of, 19
  in oral cavity, problems unique to, 25
Transplantation antigens, 19, 20
  detection of, in bone cells, 26
  source of, in grafts, 24
Transposition flaps, for closure after mandibular reconstruction, 363–364, *364*
Transverse deficiency, correction of, by segmentalization of downfractured maxilla, *127*, 127–128
Trauma, and edentulous bone loss, 8
  minimizing, during preparation for Branemark implants, 218
Trephine
  use for Hollow-Basket "C" implant insertion, 257, *257*
  use for Hollow-Basket "E" implant insertion, 258–259, *259*
  use to prepare site for Core-Vent implant, 226
  vs solid drill, for Hollow-Basket "F" implant site, 268
Triphasic nutritional analysis, 12, 13t
TSI (titanium screw inserts), 227, 228–231, *228–230*
Tuberoplasties, 64–65, *65*
  closure following, 64–65
  success of, 58
Tuberosity, excess, removal of, 62–64, *63*
  with local vestibuloplasty, 64
Tubinger implant, 199
Tumors, removal of, and tongue mass reduction, 355
  recurrent, recognition of, and reconstruction timing, 351
Twist drill, for insertion of TPS screw implant, 235, *235*
  for site preparation for Hollow-Basket "H" implant, 260, 261, *261*
  for site preparation for Hollow-Basket "K" implant, 262–264, *264*

University of Miami/HBO protocol, *374*, 395–396. See also *Hyperbaric oxygen therapy.*
  results from, *388*
Urinary system, in patient evaluation for edentulous bone loss, 13

Vascular bed, for skin graft success, 33
Vascular system, within porous calcium phosphate implants, problems with, 311

Vascularization process, of skin graft, effect of hematoma on, 35
Vasoconstrictor, for hemostasis in vestibuloplasty with skin graft, 74
  for secondary epithelialization procedure, 106
  in submucous vestibuloplasty, 105
  prior to lingual dissection, 79
Vents, in implants, 255, *255*
Vertical reference lines, and total maxillary osteotomy, 124
Vertical subcondylar ostectomy, for cancer treatment in tonsillar or retromolar areas, 349, *349*
Vestibular depth, need for, in genioglossi areas, 87
Vestibular mucosa, ballooning of, 100
Vestibuloplasties
  after alveolar ridge reconstruction with hydroxylapatite, 329
  after anterior osteotomy with posterior onlay graft, 152
  after maxillary reconstruction in cancer patients, 414
  after modified visor osteotomy, 149
  after osteotomy with bone graft, 152
  alternate lateral procedure for tuberosity with, 64
  combined with osteotomy to correct anterior maxillary edentulous bone loss, *133*, *134*
  contraindications for, 50–52, 51t
    complete resorption as, 305
  displeasing effects of, 92–93
  for Stage III mandible, 57
  history of, 47–48
  indications for, 305
    and mandible height, 93
    prior to mandibular staple bone plate implant, 180
  instruments for, 75t
  localized, frenum correction with, 65–66
  mandibular anterior, with free mucosal graft, 92–97
  maxillary, 98–104. See also *Maxillary vestibuloplasties.*
  maxillary buccal inlay, 114
  maxillary tuberosity reduction with local, 64
  mucosal, and hydroxylapatite augmentation, 344
  mylohyoid area, 97–98, *97–99*
  recommendations for surgical management of reconstructive edentulous patient, 341
  required following total onlay mandibular graft, 145
  skin grafts over, complications from, 107
  submucous, 104–106
    for maxilla reconstruction, 58
    results of, 104
    stent for, 105, *105*
  suture technique for skin graft placement, 87–90, *88*, *89*
  with skin graft, as surgical option to improve denture function, 46

Vestibuloplasties (*Continued*)
  with skin grafting and mouth floor lowering, 69–90
    complications of, 87
    draping patient for, 77
    follow-up on, 86
    good results from, 87
    history of, 69–70
    long-term evaluation of, 71
    objectives of, 70–71
    oral cavity preparation for, 77
    postoperative care of, 86
    preliminary details of, 71–73
    stent removal after, 86
    surgical procedure for, 74–86
    technique alterations for suturing method in, 73
Visor osteotomies, disadvantages of, 306
  for interposed bone graft augmentation, 146, *146*
  modified, 146, *146*, 147–150
    major drawback of, 149
    mandibular fracture as complication of, 153
    patient activities during healing from, 154
Vitamin D overdose, serum calcium levels in, 15
Vitreous carbon, host rejection of, as implant material, 340
Vitreous carbon implants, success of, 168
VSG. See *Vestibuloplasties, with skin grafting.*

Walking, long-distance, and sural nerve for grafting, 407
Weber-Ferguson incision, modified, for maxillary reconstruction, 414, *414*
Wires, for circummandibular ligatures, 84
  exposed, treatment of, after osteotomy, 153
Wound management, in maxillofacial injuries, 430–433
  drain in, 433
  for bone, 430, 433
  for soft tissue, 430
  intra-oral, 432–433
Wounds, intermediate care of, after maxillofacial injury, 433
  open, healing process for, 36

Xenografts, as substitutes for autogenous bone grafts, 30–31
  definition of, 20
Xerostomia, in cancer patients, 425

Z-plasty, for frena removal, 65, *66*
Zirconium, as implant material, research on, 212